Examination Review for Ultrasound

Examination Review for Ultrasound

Abdomen & Obstetrics and Gynecology

Third Edition

Steven M. Penny, MA, RT(R), RDMS

Sonography Programs Director
Health, Wellness, and Human Services Department
Johnston Community College
Smithfield, North Carolina

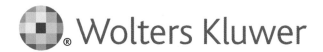 Wolters Kluwer

Philadelphia • Baltimore • New York • London
Buenos Aires • Hong Kong • Sydney • Tokyo

Acquisitions Editor: Nicole Dernoski
Development Editor: Eric McDermott
Editorial Coordinator: Remington Fernando
Marketing Manager: Kirstin Watrud
Production Project Manager: Barton Dudlick
Manager, Graphic Arts & Design: Stephen Druding
Manufacturing Coordinator: Beth Welsh
Prepress Vendor: S4Carlisle Publishing Services

Third edition

9 8 7 6 5 4 3 2

Printed in Mexico

Library of Congress Cataloging-in-Publication Data

ISBN-13: 978-1-9751-8548-0
ISBN-10: 1-975185-48-X

Cataloging in Publication data available on request from publisher.

shop.lww.com

Dedication

To the Architect—I know that I can do nothing without the strength and ability that You continue to provide. Thank you for sending your blameless Lamb to die on that old, rugged cross for me. Thank you for allowing me to share my knowledge with others and for guiding my career.

To Ted M. Penny—You lived your life to truly serve your family and gave so much of yourself to provide for us. I understand that suffering is a part of everyone's life. You suffered for many years, and we watched as you slowly left us in small, and sometimes, drastic ways. But I know in my heart, with certainty, that we will meet again someday.

To Linda Penny—Thank you for taking care of my father and for all of us. You will receive your reward someday for all the sacrifices that you made for him and for others. I love you and want you to know that I am grateful that you were chosen to be my mother.

To Lisa—I have been blessed beyond what I deserve to have you as part of my life. You take care of me and the kids and make sacrifices daily that you likely think go unnoticed. I want you to know that they are indeed noticed, and that I feel so fortunate to have you as my wife. I love you and I know that marrying you was one of the best decisions that I have ever made or will ever make.

To Devin and Reagan—I love you both and I want to thank you for turning out to be the best kids a father could ask for. Remember, "Enter by the narrow gate. For the gate is wide and the way is easy that leads to destruction." If you continue to seek God's will in your life, you will see that He will direct your path, and although you will have trials and tribulations, He will never fail you.

Preface

I am grateful to have the opportunity to report to you that the second edition of *Examination Review for Ultrasound: Abdomen & Obstetrics and Gynecology* proved to be yet another successful resource for study preparation for thousands of ambitious students of sonography across the globe. To this day, it remains one of the most well-known, highest-reviewed, and best-selling sonography textbooks available.

The concept and format of the first edition of the book was unique from the beginning. Before its inception, there was never really an easy-to-read narrative-style review book that could be used for examination preparation for the challenging sonography examinations offered by the American Registry for Diagnostic Medical Sonography (ARDMS) and the American Registry of Radiologic Technologists (ARRT).

It has been recognized that, for most people, the opportunity to have a succinctly written *physical* book as a resource is educationally priceless. Though this is anecdotal, through my own educational experience, most of my students greatly value the feeling of turning the tangible page as they read and study. Nonetheless, we have tried to provide a resource for the entire audience. Indeed, for those of you who have embraced electronic readers, an e-edition of this book has been created. This book has an online component as well, including a question/answer bank—with explanations—that can be accessed with the code provided on the back of the front cover.

Objective

The primary role of this book has never been altered. Clearly, it has been fashioned to serve as a registry review resource for learners who are preparing to take the national certification examinations offered by the ARDMS and ARRT. The sonographic specialties included in this book are, again, abdomen (which includes small parts), gynecology, and obstetrics. It does contain some limited sonographic physics principles in both major sections as well, specifically artifacts. For a more thorough review of sonographic physics, I would like to direct the reader to the physics companion to this text—*Examination Review for Ultrasound: Sonographic Principles & Instrumentation*.

The construction of this book is yet again partly based on the outlines provided by the ARDMS and ARRT certification organization. One may find these outlines at the corresponding websites. Accordingly, the foundation of the book remains the same, with new and updated information offered throughout. For instructors who have registry review classes, it may also be used in the classroom setting to reinforce the curriculum.

Lastly, it is interesting to note that a supplementary clinical reference book role for this book has manifested over the years. Thus, it may be noted that *Examination Review for Ultrasound: Abdomen & Obstetrics and Gynecology, Third Edition* is not just a book that can be used for registry review alone, but it is also a book that one can utilize in the classroom, or even place in a backpack and take to the clinical setting. When it arrives in the clinical setting, there it can certainly aid in the daily training of a sonography student. And as the preparation and successful completion of the examinations are achieved, the book can remain on the shelf in the ultrasound room, where it can continue to serve as a resource for the hard-working, frontline sonographer.

Organization

In general, the book is again divided into three sections: Section I, Abdominal Sonography Review; Section II, Gynecologic Sonography Review; and Section III, Obstetric Sonography Review. Each chapter follows a similar path that was established in the first and second editions. Key terms are provided in each chapter and are highlighted in the chapters as well. The key terms allow for a rapid assessment of one's familiarity with the subject and provide a quick reference for the reader. Each chapter begins with an introduction, and then a review of basic anatomy, function, and specific sonographically relevant information. The narrative aspect of this book is once more written in a clear-cut manner, offering the most essential facts about the topic, many times providing tables or boxes that include both clinical and sonographic findings. Thus, the pathology of each organ/system/section is included in each chapter as well.

"Sound Off" boxes can be found throughout each chapter, which is a tool that is valuable and effective for highlighting unique key points about specific topics. These boxes may also provide a specific way to recall vital information. Tables and many new, high-quality *color* diagrams, sonographic images, and anatomic drawings further enhance the straightforward narrative. New to this edition are 60 review questions per chapter, with some of the questions even including images. With a total of 1,920 review questions in this latest edition, one should certainly be capable of gaging comprehension of each chapter's content. The answers to these questions can be found in the back of the book. Also, each chapter now has a *Bonus Review* section. The *Bonus Review* may include images of procedures, other diagnostic tests, diagrams, or even unique sonographic case studies or helpful tips.

Section I—Abdominal Sonography Review—has many noteworthy changes in this latest edition. In Chapter 1, a brief section is included concerning the Focused Assessment with Sonography in Trauma (*FAST*) examination. It also contains a convenient summary table of some of the more popular sonographic signs for abdominal imaging. Doppler artifact color images and descriptions can be found in Chapter 1 too. The *Bonus Review* section for this chapter includes labeled images of normal computed tomography anatomy of the abdomen, which should prove useful. In Chapter 2, more color liver Doppler, TIPS evaluation, and liver transplant assessment diagrams and images can be found. In Chapter 4, a normal magnetic resonance cholangiopancreatography can be seen, as well as a routine endoscopic retrograde cholangiopancreatography. Chapter 5 includes more on pancreatic transplantation and Doppler assessment of such a transplant. Chapter 7 includes more images and diagrams concerning renal cystic disease. In Chapter 10—The Gastrointestinal Tract and Abdominal Wall— the reader will find more information about bowel disorders and abdominal hernias. Last, Chapter 14, which is the chapter concerning musculoskeletal and superficial structures, includes more information and scanning techniques for developmental dysplasia of the infant hip, as well as information concerning the knee, breast, and foreign objects.

In Section II—Gynecologic Sonography Review— there are some important additions as well. For example, in Chapter 16, enhanced information regarding the bony pelvis, female pelvic muscles, and pelvic vasculature can be found. In Chapter 17, the reader will find more three-dimensional images of uterine anomalies, as well as better images of uterine pathology. Also, distributed throughout the other gynecologic chapters, the user will find superior sonographic images, helpful drawings, and essential diagrams.

In Section III—Obstetric Sonography Review— several revisions include more information on fetal lie and presentation, and artifacts (Chapter 22), an expanded review of the fetal heart, fetal heart scan planes (including the 3-vessel and trachea view), and more color Doppler images of the heart (Chapter 27). More information concerning cloacal anomalies (Chapter 29), and fetal environment and maternal complications (Chapter 32) is offered as well.

Additional Resources

The certification review should not conclude without accessing the associated electronic resources. As mentioned earlier, we have provided several resources for this book, including a mock registry examination that can be attempted by accessing the VitalSource eBook by following the instructions and using the code provided at the beginning of the book. This exam simulator will provide the user with more intense "registry-like" questions, with topics that can be selected and answers that provide rationale. Instructors can use the faculty resources as well, which include an image bank and helpful PowerPoint presentations aimed at review.

Final Note

As with the previous two editions, my hope is that this book continues to effectively assist those who choose it as a resource. It is an honor for me to be able to continue updating this textbook, and to help my colleagues, or future colleagues, in this unique manner. My prayer is that this book will serve you, your students, and your patients well. I would like to state that though we may never meet, I am grateful to you for choosing to utilize this book. And whether you chose *Examination Review for Ultrasound: Abdomen & Obstetrics and Gynecology, Third Edition* as a certification review book, to help educate the next generation of sonographers, or perhaps simply as a clinical resource, I want to say thank you for doing so.

Steven M. Penny

Acknowledgments

I would like to thank my acquisitions editor, Nicole Dernoski, for encouraging me to write this third edition. Thanks to all the workers behind the scenes at Wolters Kluwer, especially Eric McDermott, whom I have teamed up with successfully over the years to produce several of my books.

To my brother, Jeff Penny, and his family, Tammy, Nick, and Mackenzie, thanks each of you for your continued support and encouragement.

Thanks to the leadership and my colleagues at Johnston Community College, including Ann Jackson, Catherine Rominski, and Ashley Mielcarek. To all of my students, thank you for challenging me to continually learn more about the profession that I have grown to truly love.

I would also like to thank Susan Raatz Stephenson for her contribution of several of the figures for the cover of this book.

Test-Taking Tips

"By failing to prepare, you are preparing to fail."
—Ben Franklin

The national certification examinations offered by the American Registry for Diagnostic Medical Sonography (ARDMS) and the American Registry of Radiologic Technologists (ARRT) are not easy. These exams should be difficult because they have been created to test your knowledge of a vital imaging modality that can save people's lives. Consequently, preparing for and challenging these exams should not be approached dispassionately. There are many resources on test taking that you can access at your local library and online. Below are three basic steps, which include tips for getting organized, studying, and preparing for these significant certification exams.

Step 1—Get Organized and Schedule the Exam

Both the ARDMS (ardms.org) and ARRT (arrt.org) provide content outlines for each of their certification examination. In fact, the content of this book is based on these content outlines, and accordingly this book includes pertinent information on each topic. However, you can use these content outlines as a guide for focused study as well. Keep your study materials—which should include all the resources you obtained throughout your sonography education—organized by these content outlines. School lecture notes, note cards, quizzes, and any other test-taking materials should be organized well before you begin to study.

Once you have organized your study materials, you should apply for the exam and then try to consider the best time to attempt it. When scheduling the examination, consider all of your other obligations (e.g., family responsibilities, vacations, job requirements) and allow for an ample amount of time to study so that you are thoroughly prepared on the examination day. Do not postpone scheduling the exam. Scheduling the examination will provide you with a firm date, and it will hopefully help those of you who suffer from procrastination to focus on test preparation.

Step 2—Establish a Study Routine and Study Schedule

Next, because you have your deadline, find a quiet place to study and develop a study routine and schedule. Your study space should be quiet and free from distractions, like television and your cell phone (stay off of social media). The study schedule that you create for yourself should be realistic. That is to say, do not schedule 2 hours each night to study if you know that you will not be dedicated to that schedule. Instead, it may be best to schedule one solid hour each night. Also, studying in 45-minute increments with 15 minute breaks may work best for some. You can create your own deadlines on your schedule and strive to meet them. Be sure to study at least for a few minutes every day to maintain momentum going into the exam.

The amount of time one requires to study will vary per individual. Only *you* know how much time *you* need to study, so if you struggle with certain topics, then allow for extra time to focus more attention on those topics. It may be best to review those topics you are most familiar with first, and as the exam approaches, review the topics that you struggle with just before your attempt, with the hopes of making the challenging information more readily accessible.

Most people know what manner they prepare for an exam best. Some test takers find flashcard useful, some create their own notes from reading, whereas others may simply read and choose to gradually answer registry review questions. A study group may be helpful for some as well. Nonetheless, the main concern of your studies should be *learning* the material and not just *memorizing* it to pass the exam. By learning the information, you will most likely be successful on the exam, with the added benefit of being able to apply your knowledge in your daily clinical practice as a registered sonographer.

Step 3—Confidently Attempt the Exam

Test anxiety is a challenge for many people. Some tips for reducing anxiety include eating well, getting plenty of rest and exercise, keeping a positive attitude, and taking practice tests. The ARDMS offers some tips for exam-day success, which include getting a good night's sleep before exam day, knowing how long it takes to get to the testing center (traffic included), being early to the testing center, and being familiar with all of the test center requirements, like testing day registrant identification specifications. Currently, the ARDMS specialty examinations consist of 170 questions. The questions are in multiple choice format. The specialty exams may also include advanced item type questions referred to as *hotspot* questions. These questions require that the test taker use the cursor to mark the correct answer directly on the image.

Multiple choice questions consist of the stem—which is the question—and four possible answers to choose from. The correct answer must be included along with three other options referred to as distractors. You should read the question cautiously first and try to answer the question before looking at the provided choices. If your given answer is provided, it will most likely be the correct choice to make. If you do not know the answer immediately, then try to eliminate the choices you know are incorrect. For these exams, you are allowed to mark questions and return to answer them later. You can also make changes before final submission. But be careful, it may be best to not change any of your answers. You should only make changes to questions that you feel confident you have answered incorrectly because for many of us our first impulse or guess is correct.

Bibliography

ARDMS.org. Review our tips for examination day success. Accessed February 27, 2022. https://www.ardms.org/get-certified/rdms/abdomen/

Fry R. *Surefire Study Success: Surefire Tips to Improve Your Test-Taking Skills.* Rosen Publishing Group; 2016.

Hill J. Test taking tips to give you an edge. *Biomed Instrum Technol.* 2009;43(3):223–224.

Mary KL. *Test-taking strategies for CNOR certification. AORN J.* 2007;85(2):315–332.

Medoff L. *Stressed Out Students' Guide to Dealing with Tests.* Kaplan Inc; 2008.

Contents

Abdominal Sonography Overview

Introduction

A summary of abdominal sonography practice is provided in this chapter. Accordingly, the subsequent chapters will build on the foundation established in this chapter. Indeed, many of the conditions listed in this chapter will be discussed in much greater detail in the later chapters. It is important for the sonographer to obtain and recognize vital clinical information from patients, including laboratory results and other data that are obtained through patient inquiry. This chapter offers a summary of relevant laboratory findings, imaging artifacts, a brief overview of physics and instrumentation, and infection control. Cross-referencing of potential information that may be encountered on the abdominal certification examination offered by the American Registry for Diagnostic Medical Sonography (www.ardms.org) and the abdominal portion of the examination offered by the American Registry of Radiologic Technologists (www.arrt.org) has been performed to establish this chapter. Finally, in the "Bonus Review" section, basic images of computed tomography of the abdomen, with labeled anatomy, are provided with a schematic indicating the possible surface projections of visceral pain.

Key Terms

anemia—a condition in which the red blood cell count or the hemoglobin is decreased

anticoagulation therapy—drug therapy in which anticoagulant medications are given to a patient to slow down the rate at which that patient's blood clots

ascites—a collection of abdominal fluid within the peritoneal cavity

chromaffin cells—the cells in the adrenal medulla that secrete epinephrine and norepinephrine

clinical findings—the information gathered by obtaining a clinical history

clinical history—a patient's signs and symptoms, pertinent illnesses, past surgeries, laboratory findings, and the results of other diagnostic testing

coagulopathies—disorders that result from the body's inability to coagulate or form blood clots; also referred to as bleeding disorders

compound imaging—ultrasound imaging tool that utilizes electronic beam steering of the transducer array in order to obtain many overlapping scans from varying angles, thus improving image resolution and reducing artifacts; also referred to as compound spatial imaging or SonoCT

computed tomography—an imaging modality that uses X-ray to obtain cross-sectional images of the body in multiple planes; also referred to as CT or computerized axial tomography (CAT scan)

elastography—a sonographic technique employed to evaluate tissue based on stiffness

endoscopy—a means of looking inside of the human body using an endoscope

exudate ascites—a collection of abdominal fluid within the peritoneal cavity that may be associated with cancer

fluid–fluid level—a distinctive line seen within a cyst representing the layering of two different fluid densities

gastrin—hormone produced by the stomach lining that is used to regulate the release of digestive acid

harmonics imaging—ultrasound imaging tool that utilizes nonlinear propagation of ultrasound as it travels through the body in order to improve axial and lateral resolution and reduce imaging artifacts; also referred to as tissue harmonic imaging

hematocrit—a laboratory value that indicates the amount of red blood cells in the blood

homeostasis—the body's ability or tendency to maintain internal equilibrium by adjusting its physiologic processes

hyperthyroidism—a condition that results from the overproduction of thyroid hormones

hypoglycemia—low blood sugar

hypothyroidism—a condition that results from the underproduction of thyroid hormones

intraluminal—located within the lumen or opening of an organ or structure

intraperitoneal—located within the parietal peritoneum

Kaposi sarcoma—cancer that causes lesions to develop on the skin and other places; often associated with AIDS

leukocytosis—an elevated white blood cell count

lymphadenopathy—disease or enlargement of the lymph nodes

lymphedema—buildup of lymph that is most likely caused by the obstruction of lymph drainage

magnetic resonance imaging—imaging modality that uses magnetic waves to obtain images of the human body in various planes

mass effect—the displacement or alteration of normal anatomy that is located adjacent to a tumor

Morison Pouch—the space between the liver and the right kidney; also referred to as the posterior right subhepatic space

multiloculated—having many cavities

mural nodules—small solid internal projections of tissue originating from the wall of a cyst

nosocomial infections—hospital-acquired infections

nuclear medicine—a diagnostic imaging modality that utilizes the administration of radionuclides into the human body for an analysis of the function of organs or for the treatment of various abnormalities

occult—hidden

oncocytes—large cells of glandular origin

paracentesis—a procedure that uses a needle to drain fluid from the abdominal cavity for diagnostic and/or therapeutic reasons

parietal peritoneum—the portion of the peritoneum that lines the abdominal and pelvic cavities

pineal gland—endocrine gland located in the brain that secretes melatonin

radiography—a diagnostic imaging modality that uses ionizing radiation for imaging bones, joints, organs, and some other soft tissue structures

retroperitoneal—posterior to the peritoneum

serosal fluid—fluid that is secreted by the serous membranes to reduce friction in the peritoneal and other cavities of the body

signs—objective proof of a disease such as abnormal laboratory findings and fever

sonographic findings—information gathered by performing a sonographic examination

space of Retzius—the space between the urinary bladder and the pubic bone; also referred to as the retropubic space

standoff pad—a gel pad that is used to provide some distance between the transducer face and the skin surface, allowing superficial structures to be imaged more clearly

symptoms—any subjective evidence of a disease such as nausea, weakness, or numbness

thoracentesis—a procedure that uses a needle to drain fluid from the pleural cavity for either diagnostic or therapeutic reasons

thymus gland—gland of the immune and lymphatic system located in the chest

transudate ascites—a collection of abdominal fluid within the peritoneal cavity often associated with cirrhosis

tumor markers—biomarkers found in blood, urine, or other body tissues that elevate in response to cancer

unilocular—having a single cavity

visceral peritoneum—the portion of the peritoneum that is closely applied to each organ

visceromegaly—enlargement of an organ

voiding cystourethrogram—a radiographic examination used to evaluate the lower urinary tract, where a contrast agent is instilled into the urinary bladder by means of urethral catheterization

Wilson disease—a congenital disorder that causes a person to retain excess copper

SONOGRAPHIC TERMINOLOGY, DIRECTIONAL TERMINOLOGY, AND PRACTICE GUIDELINES

Sonographers must have an understanding of common directional terms utilized in abdominal imaging and patient positions (Table 1-1; Figs. 1-1 and 1-2). Moreover, before beginning the examination, the sonographer must have a fundamental appreciation of the sonographic terminology, commonly used sonographic descriptive terms, and abdominal scanning planes and image orientation (Table 1-2; Fig. 1-3). Abdominal sonograms may be requested for various reasons. The American Institute of Ultrasound in Medicine (AIUM) publishes

TABLE 1-1 Common directional or relational terms	
Directional Term	**Definition**
Anterior (ventral)	Toward the front of the body or the front of a body part
Contralateral	On the opposite side of the body
Deep	Away from the surface of the body or structure
Distal	Farther away from the point of attachment or origin of an extremity to the trunk of the body
Inferior (caudal)	Toward the feet or away from the head; a structure that is lower than another part of the body; the lower part of an organ or structure
Ipsilateral	On the same side of the body
Lateral	Away from the midline of the body or pertaining to the side; situated at or on the side
Medial	Toward the middle (midline) of the body or organ
Posterior (dorsal)	Toward the back or behind another structure
Proximal	Toward the origin or attachment of a structure to the trunk
Superficial	Closer to the surface of the body or structure
Superior (cranial)	Toward the head or higher in the body

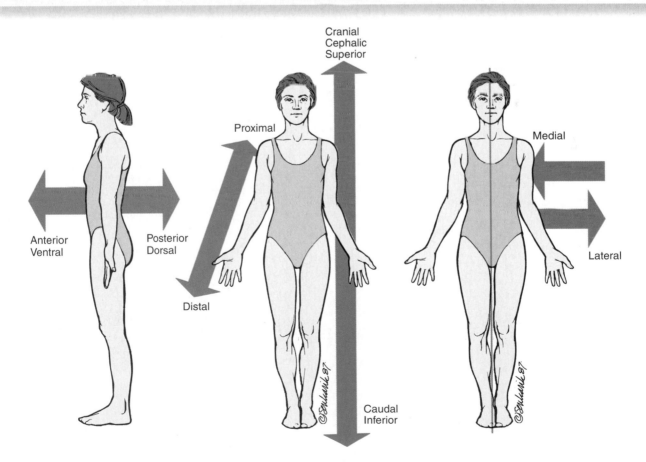

Figure 1-1 Commonly used directional terms.

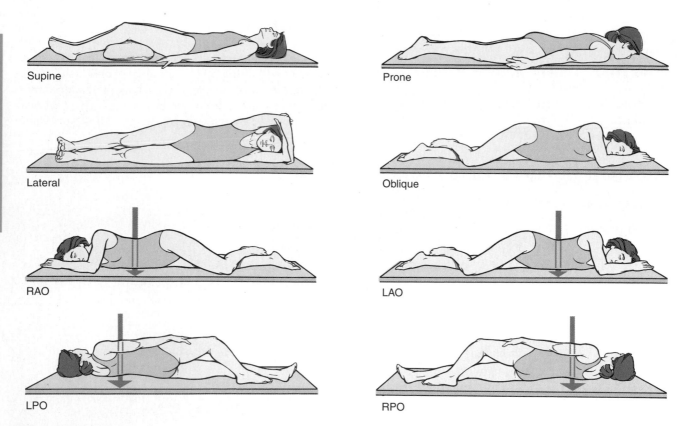

Figure 1-2 Common patient positions. RAO, right anterior oblique; LAO, left anterior oblique; LPO, left posterior oblique; RPO, right posterior oblique

TABLE 1-2 Sonographic descriptive terms

Sonographic Descriptive Term	Definition	Examples
Anechoic	Without echoes	Gallbladder Simple renal cyst
Complex	Having both cystic and solid components	Hemorrhagic cyst Hepatic abscess
Echogenic	Structure that produces echoes; comparative term	Fatty liver Chronic renal disease
Heterogeneous	Of differing composition	Graves disease Diffuse liver metastasis
Homogeneous	Of uniform composition	Normal liver Normal testicle
Hyperechoic	Having many echoes	Cavernous hemangioma Angiomyolipoma
Hypoechoic	Having few echoes	Hepatic adenoma Thyroid adenoma
Isoechoic	Having the same echogenicity	Focal nodular hyperplasia

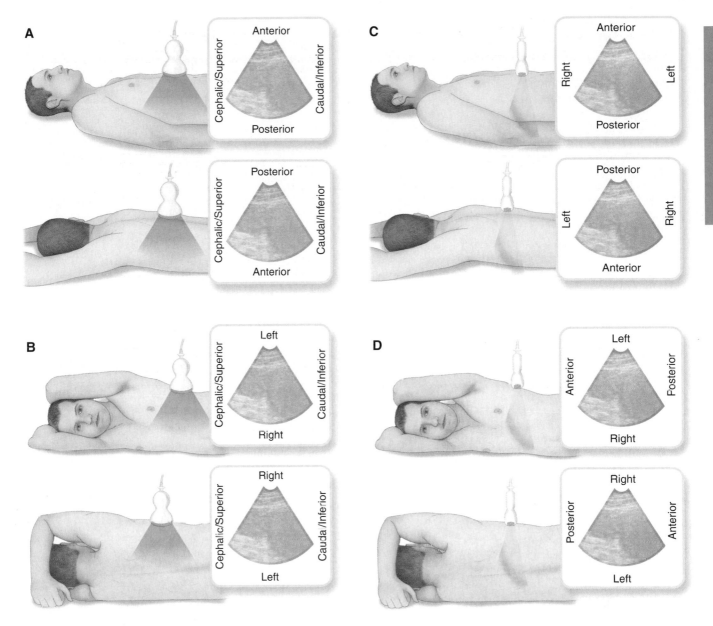

Figure 1-3 Image presentation. **A.** Longitudinal sagittal plane. **B.** Longitudinal coronal plane scanning on the lateral left or right surface. **C.** Transverse plane, anterior or posterior surface. **D.** Transverse plane, left or right lateral surface.

the practice guidelines for an abdominal sonogram on its website at www.aium.org (Table 1-3).

SONOGRAPHIC DESCRIPTION OF ABNORMAL FINDINGS

An appreciation and recognition of sonographic pathology is vital for every sonographer. They must not only be able to recognize the normal echogenicity of organs and structures but also be capable of identifying abnormalities. The normal echogenicity of the abdominal organs from greatest (brightest) to least

(darkest) is as follows: renal sinus → pancreas → spleen → liver → renal cortex → renal pyramids → gallbladder. Therefore, if the right kidney appears more echogenic than the liver, both the liver and the right kidney must be closely examined for a cause of this deviant sonographic finding.

SOUND OFF
The normal echogenicity of the abdominal organs from greatest (brightest) to least (darkest) is as follows: renal sinus → pancreas → spleen → liver → renal cortex → renal pyramids → gallbladder.

TABLE 1-3 AIUM indications for abdomen and/or retroperitoneum sonogram

AIUM Indications for an Ultrasound Examination of the Abdomen and/or Retroperitoneum[a]

- Abdominal, flank, and/or back pain
- Signs or symptoms that may be referred from the abdominal and/or retroperitoneal regions, such as jaundice or hematuria
- Palpable abnormalities such as an abdominal mass or organomegaly
- Abnormal laboratory values or abnormal findings on other imaging examinations suggestive of abdominal and/or retroperitoneal pathology
- Follow-up of known or suspected abnormalities in the abdomen and/or retroperitoneum
- Search for metastatic disease or an **occult** primary neoplasm
- Evaluation of cirrhosis, portal hypertension, and transjugular intrahepatic portosystemic shunt (TIPS) stents; screening for hepatoma; and evaluation of the liver in conjunction with liver elastography
- Abdominal trauma
- Evaluation of urinary tract infection and hydronephrosis
- Evaluation of uncontrolled hypertension and suspected renal artery stenosis
- Search for the presence of free or loculated peritoneal and/or retroperitoneal fluid
- Evaluation of suspected congenital abnormalities
- Evaluation of suspected hypertrophic pyloric stenosis, intussusception, necrotizing enterocolotis, or any other bowel abnormalities
- Pretransplantation and posttransplantation evaluation
- Planning for and guiding an invasive procedure

An abdominal and/or retroperitoneal ultrasound examination should be performed when there is a valid medical reason. There are no absolute contraindications.

[a]This is a limited list of indications. Other indications exist.
AIUM, American Institute of Ultrasound in Medicine.

Pathology is often described sonographically, relative to surrounding or adjacent tissue. For example, a hepatic mass may be described as hyperechoic compared to the surrounding echotexture of the normal liver. Solid tumors may be hyperechoic (occasionally described as echogenic), hypoechoic, homogeneous, heterogeneous, complex, isoechoic, cystic, or a combination of these. For example, a renal mass may be described as a hypoechoic mass with a central area of increased echogenicity.

A cyst must fit certain criteria to be referred to as a simple cyst sonographically. Simple cysts have smooth walls or borders, demonstrate *t*hrough transmission (acoustic enhancement), are *a*nechoic, and are *r*ound in shape (*STAR* criteria). Other features that are common to simple cysts include the presence of a clearly defined posterior wall, reverberation artifact, and edge shadowing. Occasionally, with higher frequency transducers that have superior resolution, a diminutive amount of internal debris may be noted within a simple cyst.

Cysts that have a large amount of internal debris, septations, **mural nodules**, contain a **fluid–fluid level**, or other components, may be described as complex. Cysts may also be referred to as **multiloculated** or **unilocular**. Although simple cysts may not be worrisome, complex or complicated cysts may be followed closely or further analyzed with another imaging modality. Figure 1-4 demonstrates the sonographic difference between a simple cyst, solid mass, and a complex cystic mass.

> 🔊 **SOUND OFF**
> A simple cyst should have *s*mooth walls, demonstrate *t*hrough transmission (acoustic enhancement), be completely *a*nechoic, and be *r*ound in shape (STAR criteria).

PATIENT PREPARATION FOR AN ABDOMINAL SONOGRAM

Patients who are required to undergo an abdominal sonogram, and particularly patients who still have a gallbladder, need to fast for 8 hours, although some authors suggest that only a 6-hour fast may be warranted. However, diagnostic studies can be obtained in the nonfasting patient, especially those patients who require an emergency sonogram. The purpose of fasting is to ensure that the gallbladder is fully distended and to potentially reduce the amount of upper abdominal gas that may inhibit diagnostic accuracy. For renal

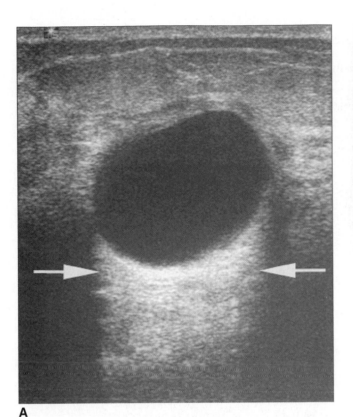

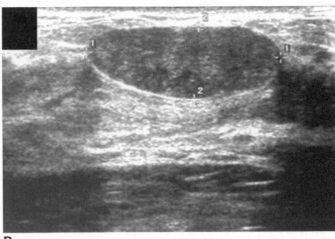

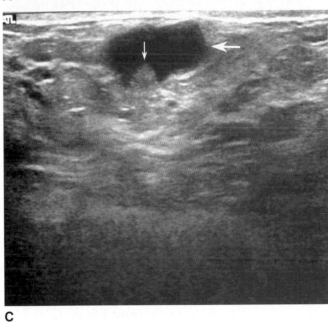

Figure 1-4 Simple cyst, solid mass, and complex cystic mass. **A.** A simple breast cyst demonstrating acoustic enhancement (*between arrows*), smooth borders, and anechoic appearance. **B.** Solid mass. A solid hypoechoic breast mass is imaged here in the transverse plane. **C.** Complex. Predominantly cystic mass (*large arrow*) with a solid mural nodule (*small arrow*) and posterior acoustic enhancement.

sonograms, the patient is not typically required to fast, although some facilities may recommend that the patient be well hydrated. This is true especially if the urinary bladder needs to be assessed sonographically for **intraluminal** masses, wall irregularities, or urinary stones. Small part sonography, such as scrotal and thyroid imaging, does not require patient preparation.

The timing and order of imaging studies is also important. Diabetic patients need to be scheduled early in the morning for studies that require fasting in order to prevent symptoms and complications related to **hypoglycemia**. Abdominal sonography should also be performed prior to radiographic examinations that utilize barium contrast agents. For pediatric patients who must undergo renal sonography and urologic radiographic examinations, such as a **voiding cystourethrogram**, the renal sonogram is typically performed first.

GATHERING A CLINICAL HISTORY AND LABORATORY FINDINGS

Although the patient–sonographer interaction is exceedingly important, a review of prior examinations and relevant documents should be performed by the sonographer before any contact with the patient. The sonographic imaging process should be clearly explained to the patient and a thorough **clinical history** obtained prior to performing each examination. Gathering a thorough clinical history includes a review of reports from previous sonograms, **computed tomography** (CT) scans, **magnetic resonance imaging** studies, **nuclear medicine** examinations, **radiography** procedures, **endoscopy** examinations, and any additional related laboratory and diagnostic report available. Moreover, sonographers must be capable of analyzing the clinical complaints of their patients. This practice will aid not only in clinical practice but also in answering complex certification examination questions. By correlating **clinical findings** with **sonographic findings**, the sonographer can directly impact the patient's outcome by providing the most targeted examination possible. Furthermore, when faced with a complicated, in-depth registry question, the test taker should be capable of eliminating information that is not applicable, to answer the question appropriately. Helpful information can be gathered from patient inquiry or from analyzing the registry review question at hand.

Although not all patients visit the sonography department with laboratory results (labs) in hand, sonographers must be capable of analyzing labs when they are available. For most inpatients and emergency room patients, lab results from blood work and/or a urinalysis will be electronically available. Although an increase in most labs reveals evidence of an abnormality, some lab levels decrease with certain abnormalities. For example, **leukocytosis**, or an elevation in white blood cell (WBC) count, in general, indicates the presence of an inflammatory response owing to infection. Patients who have some form of "itis" (such as cholecystitis or pancreatitis), or possibly even an abscess, will most likely have an abnormal WBC count with existing infection. Conversely, a decrease in **hematocrit** can indicate bleeding. Patients who have suffered recent trauma or have an active hemorrhage will most likely have a decreased hematocrit level. These two labs should be kept in mind during the study. Other labs and specific associated pathologies will be included in organ-specific chapters. A summary of labs can be found in Table 1-4 for quick broad reference (Table 1-4).

TABLE 1-4 Basic overview of commonly encountered and relevant laboratory findings for abdominal imaging

Lab	Results
Alanine aminotransferase	↑ Biliary tree disease ↑ Pancreatic disease ↑ Hepatic disease
Albumin	↓ Liver damage
Alkaline phosphatase	↑ Biliary obstruction ↑ Liver cancer ↑ Pancreatic disease ↑ Gallstones ↓ **Wilson disease**
Aspartate aminotransferase	↑ Liver damage ↑ Pancreatic disease
Bilirubin	↑ Liver disease ↑ Biliary obstruction ↑ Other systemic disorders and syndromes
Gamma-glutamyl transferase	↑ Liver disease ↑ Biliary obstruction
PTT	↑ Liver disease ↑ Hereditary **coagulopathies** ↓ Vitamin K (deficiency) ↑ **Anticoagulation therapy**
PT	↑ Liver disease ↑ Bleeding abnormalities ↑ Anticoagulation therapy
Urobilirubin (urine test)	↑ Liver disease ↑ Biliary obstruction
Calcitonin	↑ Thyroid cancer ↑ Lung cancer ↑ **Anemia**
Thyroid-stimulating hormone	↑ **Hypothyroidism** ↓ **Hyperthyroidism**
Thyroxine (T_4) or free thyroxine	↑ Hyperthyroidism ↓ Hypothyroidism
Triiodothyronine (T_3)	↑ Hyperthyroidism ↓ Hypothyroidism
BUN	↑ Renal disease ↑ Renal obstruction ↑ Dehydration ↑ Gastrointestinal bleeding ↑ Congestive heart failure
Creatinine	↑ Renal damage ↑ Renal infection ↑ Renal obstruction
Amylase	↑ Pancreatic disorders ↑ Gallbladder disease ↑ Biliary or pancreatic obstruction

TABLE 1-4 Basic overview of commonly encountered and relevant laboratory findings for abdominal imaging (*continued*)

Lab	Results
Lipase	↑ Pancreatic disorders ↑ Gallbladder disease ↑ Biliary or pancreatic obstruction
Serum calcium	↑ Parathyroid abnormalities
Prostatic-specific antigen	↑ Prostate abnormalities
Hematocrit	↓ Hemorrhage
WBC	↑ Inflammatory disease/infection

BUN, blood urea nitrogen; PT, prothrombin time; PTT, partial thromboplastin time; WBC, white blood cell.

🔊)) SOUND OFF
Patients who have some form of "itis" (such as cholecystitis or pancreatitis), or possibly even an abscess, will most likely have an abnormal WBC count with existing infection.

BASIC PATIENT CARE AND EMERGENCY SITUATIONS IN ABDOMINAL IMAGING

Sonographers must be capable of providing basic patient care for every patient equitably and in a timely manner. Although sonographers may spend a limited amount of time with each patient, they must also be prepared for emergency situations and know how to respond. Basic patient care includes the assessment of body temperature, pulse, respiration, and blood pressure if needed (Table 1-5). Sonographers should be competent at transferring patients safely from wheelchairs and stretchers to the examination stretcher, being mindful of intravenous

TABLE 1-5 Normal numbers or ranges for basic patient care assessment

Basic Patient Assessment	
Body temperature	98.6° F (oral)
Adult pulse	60–100 beats/min
Adult blood pressure	<120/80 mm Hg
Adult respiration	12–20 breaths/min

therapy, postsurgical, and urinary catheter needs. For patients with intravenous therapy, the intravenous fluid bag should be continually elevated to prevent retrograde flow. For urinary catheter care, the urinary bag should be placed below the level of the urinary bladder to prevent retrograde urine flow that could result in a urinary tract infection. One of the most common causes of **nosocomial infections**, or hospital-acquired infections, is the urinary tract infection.

INFECTION CONTROL AND TRANSDUCER CARE

The cycle of infection may be depicted as a succession of steps (Fig. 1-5). Sonographers should continually employ standard precautions and good hygiene to prevent the spread of infection. Standard precautions are put into place to reduce the risk of microorganism transmission in the clinical setting. Standard precautions, formerly referred to as universal precautions, include (1) hand hygiene, (2) the use of personal protective equipment, (3) safe injection practices, (4) sharps safety (5) respiratory hygiene and coughing etiquette (6) sterile instruments and devices and (7) clean and disinfected environmental surfaces. These precautions apply to blood, nonintact skin, mucous membranes, contaminated equipment, and all other body fluids, except for sweat. It is important to note that standard precautions are often supplemented with transmission-based precautions, including contact and droplet or airborne route precautions.

The use of proper hand-washing and hand-cleaning techniques is one of the most effective means of preventing the spread of infection. The Centers for Disease Control now recommends that healthcare workers employ an alcohol-based hand rub as the primary mode of hand hygiene in the clinical setting. Traditional hand-washing should be used as well when time permits, especially in situations when the hands are visibly soiled. Sonographers should also utilize personal protective equipment, such as gloves, gowns, face shields, and masks, when clinically applicable. Gloves, which are made of latex, nonlatex, or other synthetic material, should be worn during the sonographic examination and should be changed between patients. The sonographers should be mindful of the potential for patient latex allergies and adapt accordingly by using another form of synthetic gloves.

Medical asepsis refers to the practices used to render an object or area free of pathogenic microorganisms. Although medical asepsis includes hand-washing, it also includes the use of disinfectants in the clinical setting, as well as the use of transducer or probe covers. Probe covers should be used for endocavity examinations, such as endovaginal and endorectal imaging. The use of sterile or nonsterile probe covers for these examinations

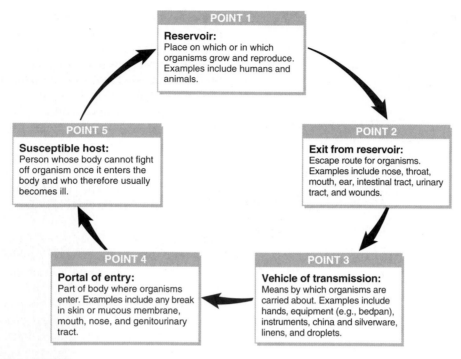

Figure 1-5 The cycle of infection.

is recommended by some institutions. Transducers used during invasive procedures should be covered with a sterile probe cover, and sterile ultrasound gel should be utilized.

Following each examination, the transducer, ultrasound machine, stretcher, and any other equipment used during the examination should be thoroughly disinfected. The transducer should be cleaned with a disinfectant spray or wipe as recommended by the institution and manufacturer. Endocavity transducers should undergo high-level disinfection in some manner after each examination. Lastly, to prevent the spread of infection, sonographers should maintain good personal hygiene and health.

INVASIVE AND STERILE PROCEDURES

Patient preparation for invasive procedures varies among clinical facilities. However, informed consent from the patient and laboratory results are universally obtained. Laboratory findings, including an analysis of prothrombin time (PT), partial thromboplastin time (PTT), international normalizing ratio, fibrinogen, and platelets, are used to evaluate the patient for coagulopathies. Sterile field preparation is performed prior to the procedure as well, and sterile asepsis, also referred to as surgical asepsis, must be maintained (Table 1-6). Of course, sterile asepsis is always practiced in the surgical suite. Some invasive procedures that are commonly performed in the sonography department include **thoracentesis**,

paracentesis, organ biopsies, mass biopsies, and abscess drainages. Biopsies can be performed using a freehand technique or under ultrasound guidance using a needle guide that attaches to the transducer. They may also be described as fine needle aspiration (FNA), which uses a thin needle and a syringe, or a core biopsy, which uses a much larger diameter needle to obtain a substantial tissue sample. An example of an FNA would be that of

TABLE 1-6 Ten vital rules of surgical asepsis to remember

1. Always know which area and items are sterile and which are not
2. If the sterility of an object is questionable, it is considered nonsterile.
3. If it has been recognized that an item has become nonsterile, immediate action is required.
4. A sterile field must never be left unmonitored. If a sterile field is left unattended, it is considered nonsterile.
5. A sterile person does not lean across a sterile field.
6. A sterile field ends at the level of the tabletop.
7. Cuffs of a sterile gown are not considered sterile.
8. The edges of a sterile wrapper are not considered sterile.
9. If one sterile person must pass another, they must pass back-to-back.
10. Coughing, sneezing, or excessive talking over a sterile field leads to contamination.

a thyroid biopsy, whereas an example of a core biopsy would be a liver biopsy.

INSTRUMENTATION

Although a thorough physics review is beyond the scope of this book, there are several topics that must be addressed in preparation for the abdominal examination. Sonographic images are typically recorded and stored in a picture-archiving and communication system (PACS). PACS allows for both easy storage and comparison between sonographic findings and straightforward correlation between other imaging modality findings. PACS systems vary per institution.

General abdominal imaging requires the use of a transducer that balances penetration with high-quality resolution. In general, the higher the frequency employed, the poorer the penetration ability, but the better the resolution. Conversely, the lower frequencies provide better penetration with a sacrifice in resolution. Transducers that may be used for abdominal and small part sonographic imaging include linear array, matrix array, curved or convex array, phased array, or vector or sector array. Higher frequency linear array transducers (7.5 to 18 MHz or higher when appropriate) should be used for superficial structures, such as thyroid, scrotum, breast, musculoskeletal (MSK) imaging, and some gastrointestinal examinations (e.g., appendix and pylorus). A **standoff pad** or a mound of gel may be used

for imaging some superficial structures, such as splinters, superficial mass, or foreign objects just below the skin surface. Lower frequency curved array transducers (2.0 to 5.0 MHz) are employed for general abdominal imaging for the assessment of deeper or larger structures such as the liver, abdominal aorta, or pancreas. When applicable, sonographers should utilize technology such as power Doppler, color Doppler, pulsed Doppler, **harmonics imaging**, **compound imaging**, extended-field of view, **elastography**, and three-dimensional (3D) sonography to reinforce diagnostic accuracy. Sonographic protocols must always be malleable and case specific.

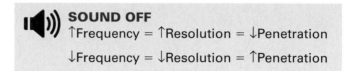

SOUND OFF

$\uparrow$Frequency = $\uparrow$Resolution = $\downarrow$Penetration

$\downarrow$Frequency = $\downarrow$Resolution = $\uparrow$Penetration

IMAGING AND DOPPLER ARTIFACTS

Gray-scale, or brightness mode (B-mode), provides a two-dimensional (2D) image of the human body in real time. Real-time imaging provides anatomy and motion, much like watching a live video of the internal structure being analyzed. Abdominal sonography involves careful analysis of vital structures. Often, artifacts will be observed during real-time imaging or during Doppler utilization (Tables 1-7 and 1-8). Sonographers may employ various technologies or techniques to reduce the presence of

TABLE 1-7 Two-dimensional real-time imaging artifacts

Artifact	Explanation	Example
Anisotropy	Occurs when the sound beam strikes a structure in a non-perpendicular manner, resulting in a loss of the true echogenicity of the structure	May occur when imaging tendons (Fig. 1-6)

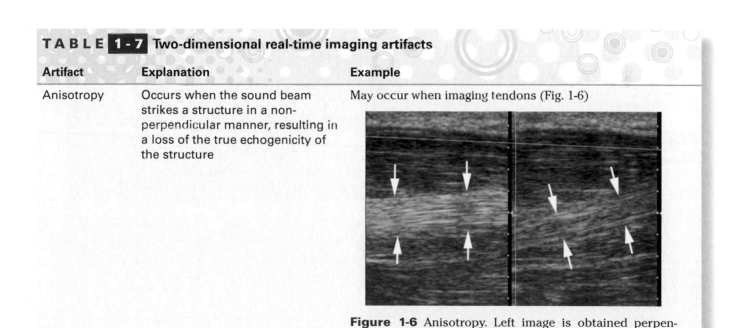

Figure 1-6 Anisotropy. Left image is obtained perpendicular to the tendon (*arrows*), whereas the right image has been obtained in an obliqued orientation to the tendon.

(*continued*)

T A B L E 1 - 7 Two-dimensional real-time imaging artifacts (*continued*)

Artifact	Explanation	Example
Comet-tail	Artifact caused by several small, highly reflective interfaces	Seen with adenomyomatosis of the gallbladder (Fig. 1-7)

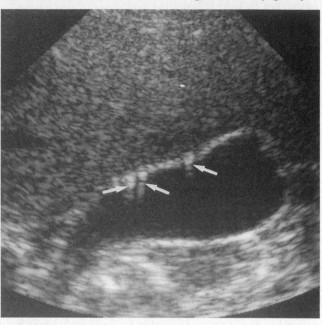

Figure 1-7 Comet-tail artifact (*arrows*).

| Dirty shadowing | Caused by air or bowel gas | Most often seen emanating from bowel; may be seen posterior to gas within an abscess (Fig. 1-8) |

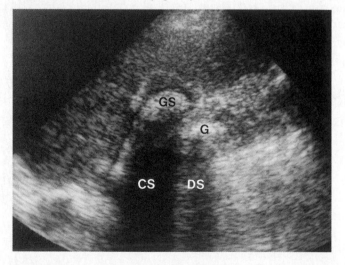

Figure 1-8 Dirty shadowing (*DS*) produced by gas (*G*). Clean shadow (*CS*) produced by gallstone (*GS*).

T A B L E 1 - 7 **Two-dimensional real-time imaging artifacts (*continued*)**

Artifact	Explanation	Example
Edge shadowing	Reflective or refractive effect seen deep to the margins of a round structure that has a significantly different speed of sound compared to surrounding tissue; may be termed refractive shadowing	Often seen arising from cystic structures and appears as narrow shadow lines originating at the edge of these structures (Fig. 1-9)

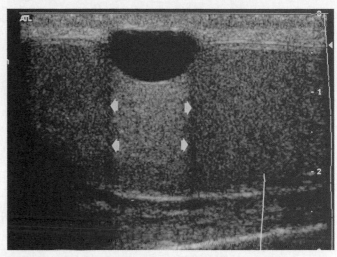

Figure 1-9 Edge artifact (*arrowheads*).

Mirror image	Produced by a strong specular reflector and results in a copy of the anatomy being placed deeper than the correct location	Seen posterior to the liver and diaphragm (Fig. 1-10); can also been seen in Doppler modes as well

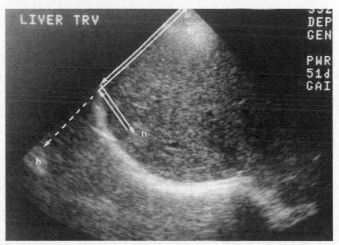

Figure 1-10 Mirror image artifact of a hemangioma (*h*) of the liver. The artifact is identified by the *broken arrow* outside of the liver.

(*continued*)

TABLE 1-7 Two-dimensional real-time imaging artifacts (*continued*)

Artifact	Explanation	Example
(Posterior) Acoustic enhancement	Produced when the sound beam is barely attenuated through a fluid or a fluid-filled structure; may occasionally be referred to as through transmission	Seen posterior to fluid-filled structures such as the gallbladder and renal cysts. Also, seen with pleural effusions and with ascites (Fig. 1-11) 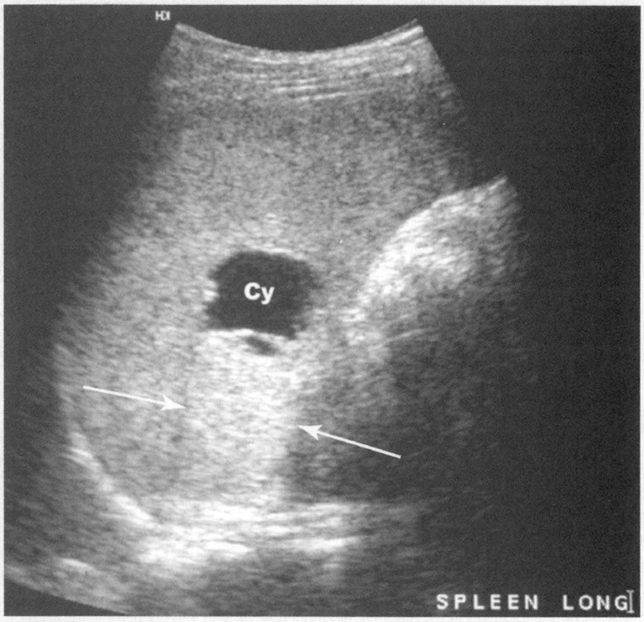
Refraction	Caused by the bending of the ultrasound beam when it passes through an interface between two tissues with vastly dissimilar speeds of sound and the angle of the approach is not perpendicular	Seen when imaging through the rectus muscles of the abdominal wall (Fig. 1-12)

Figure 1-11 Acoustic enhancement or through transmission (*arrows*) seen posterior to a liver cyst (*Cy*).

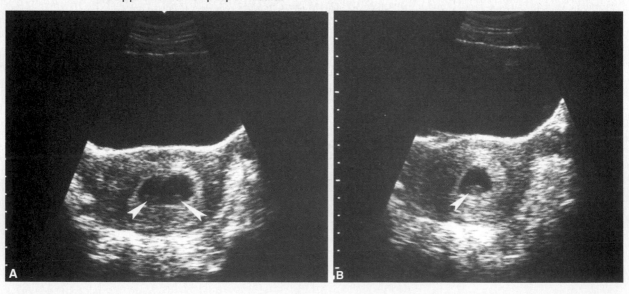

Figure 1-12 Refraction caused by the anterior abdominal muscles, producing the appearance of two gestational sacs (**A**, *arrowheads*) when there was truly only one (**B**, *arrowhead*). By changing the angle of insonation, the artifact is removed.

TABLE 1-7 Two-dimensional real-time imaging artifacts (*continued*)

Artifact	Explanation	Example
Reverberation artifact	Caused by a large acoustic interface and subsequent production of false echoes	Seen as an echogenic region in the anterior aspect of the gallbladder or other fluid-filled structures (Fig. 1-13)

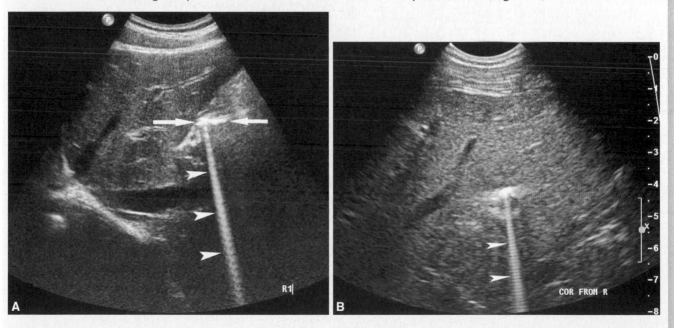

Figure 1-13 Reverberation. **A.** Reverberation in the anterior aspect of the urinary bladder (*arrows*). **B.** Changing the scanning angle minimizes the artifact.

Ring-down artifact	Artifact that appears as a solid streak or a chain of parallel bands radiating away from a structure	Seen emanating from gas bubbles within the abdomen; can help to identify the presence of air in a structure, such as in the case of pneumobilia (Fig. 1-14)

Figure 1-14 Ring-down artifact. **A** and **B.** Air (between *arrows* in **A**) producing ring-down artifact (*arrowheads* in **A** and **B**).

Shadowing	Caused by attenuation of the sound beam	Seen posterior to bone, and calculi like gallstones and renal stones (see label CS in Fig. 1-8)

(*continued*)

T A B L E 1 - 7 Two-dimensional real-time imaging artifacts (*continued*)

Artifact	Explanation	Example
Side lobes	Caused by sound beams that are peripheral to the main sound beam	Seen as low-level echoes within fluid, mimicking sludge, debris, or pus within a fluid-filled structure like the gallbladder (Fig. 1-15)

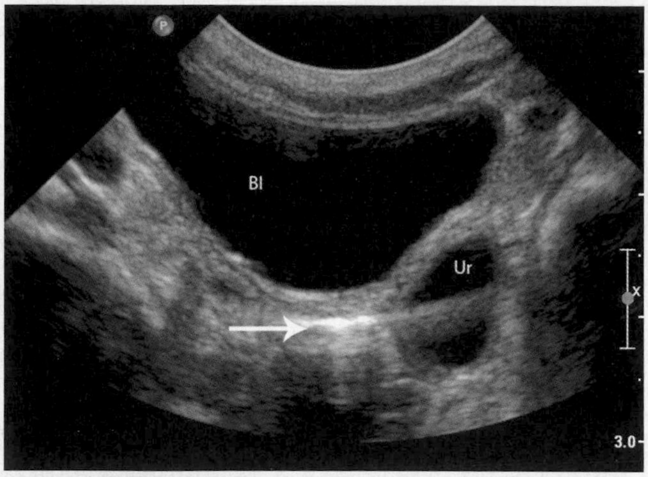

Figure 1-15 Side lobe artifact from air (*arrow*) within the rectum extending into the fluid-filled dilated ureter (*Ur*) that lies adjacent to the urinary bladder (*Bl*).

Artifact	Explanation	Example
Slice thickness	Caused by compression from 3D to 2D images	Simulates false echoes that could resemble sludge or debris in the urinary bladder or gallbladder (Fig. 1-16)

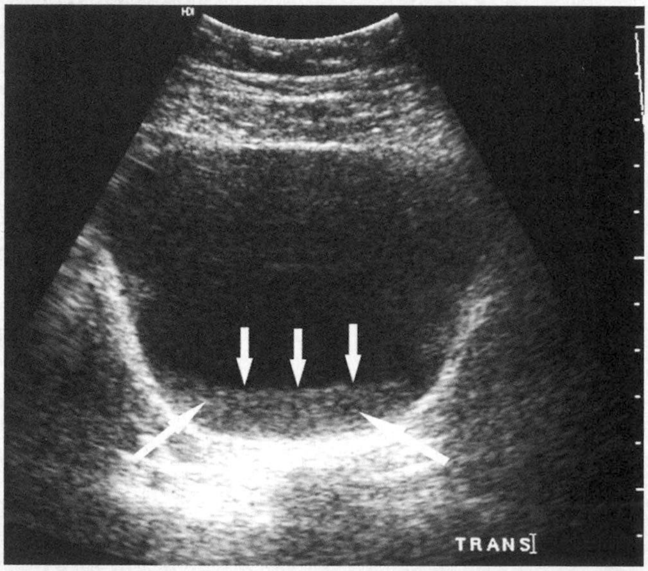

Figure 1-16 Slice thickness artifact produces false layering debris (*arrows*) within the urinary bladder.

TABLE 1-8 Doppler artifacts

Doppler Artifact	Explanation	Adjustment
Absent Doppler signal	Could be caused by low gain, low frequency, high wall filter, or too high velocity scale	• Decrease PRF • Turn up spectral gain • Decrease the wall filter • Open the sample gate
Aliasing	Occurs when the Doppler sampling rate (pulse-repetition frequency) is not high enough to accurately display the Doppler frequency shift	• Increase the pulse-repetition frequency. • Adjust the baseline. • Switch to a lower transmitted frequency. • Increase the angle of insonation to decrease Doppler shift (Figs. 1-17 and 1-18).

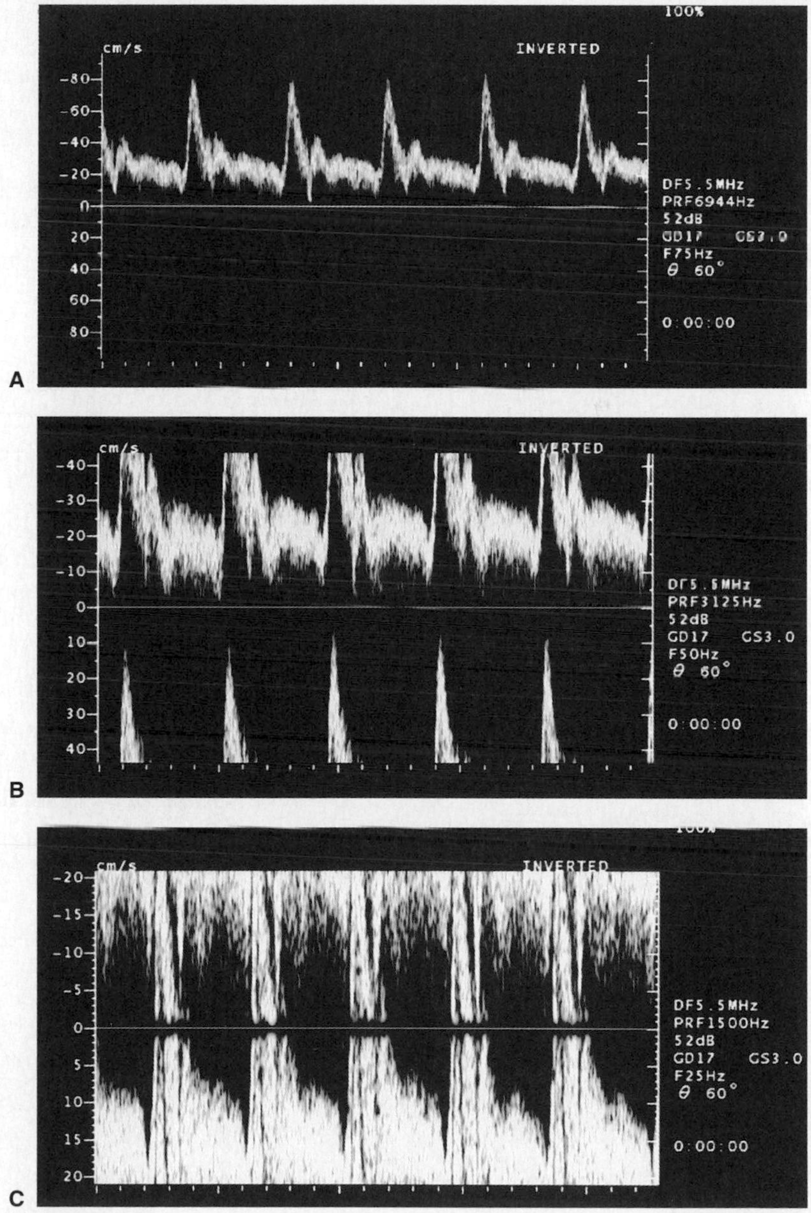

Figure 1-17 Pulsed Doppler aliasing. **A.** Pulsed waveform of internal carotid shows normal systolic peaks. **B.** Sampling rate set too low demonstrating aliasing. **C.** Further decrease in sampling rate produces more aliasing.

(*continued*)

TABLE 1-8 Doppler artifacts (*continued*)

Doppler Artifact	Explanation	Adjustment
		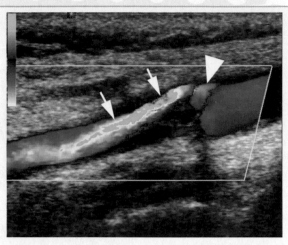

Figure 1-18 Color Doppler aliasing. The *arrows* demonstrate localized aliasing within a stenotic internal carotid artery. The *arrowhead* demonstrates a true reversal of flow.

| Doppler noise | Caused by inappropriately high Doppler settings | Reduce color gain setting or adjust wall filter (Fig. 1-19) |

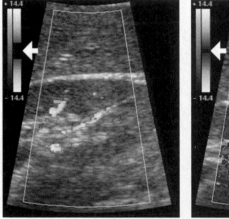 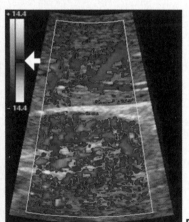

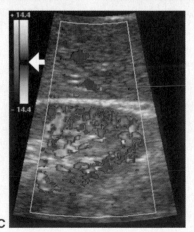

Figure 1-19 Doppler noise and the wall filter (*arrow*). **A.** High filter setting produces minimal flow detection. **B.** Low filter setting produces excessive noise. **C.** Medium filter setting eliminates noise and correctly depicts flow.

T A B L E 1 - 8 Doppler artifacts (*continued*)

Doppler Artifact	Explanation	Adjustment
Flow directional abnormalities	Caused by the sound beam striking a vessel at a 90-degree angle, producing an area void of color	Change the angle of insonation
Twinkle artifact	Occurs behind strong, granular, and irregular surfaces like crystals, calculi, or calcifications	Artifact that is actually useful at identifying small kidney or biliary stones (Fig. 1-20)

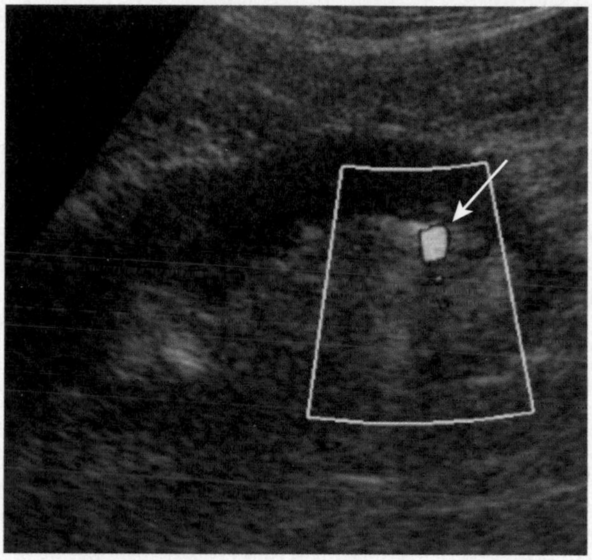

Figure 1-20 Twinkle artifact (*arrow*) seen posterior to a small kidney stone.

artifacts. For example, harmonic imaging can reduce reverberation and side lobe artifacts, whereas compound imaging may reduce speckle and clutter. Furthermore, simply manipulating the transducer slightly or altering the angle of insonation may eliminate some artifacts.

BODY SYSTEMS AND ABDOMINAL CAVITY

Overview of Body Systems

Throughout the following chapters, specific vital details will be provided for both normal and abnormal conditions that can be demonstrated with sonography. However, a fundamental understanding of several of the body systems is an important commission for the sonographer. The body consists of many mutually supporting body systems. These systems work together to preserve **homeostasis**, the body's tendency to maintain internal equilibrium by adjusting internal processes. These systems include the cardiovascular system, endocrine system, lymphatic system, MSK system, nervous system, and reproductive system. The excretory system includes the digestive system, urinary system, and respiratory system. Table 1-9 provides some insight into the basic functions of these systems and relevant topics to keep in mind as you study the various components that are applicable to abdominal sonographic imaging (Table 1-9).

Although a detailed comprehension of cardiac system function and circuitry may not be compulsory for the abdominal sonographer, you should have a fundamental understanding of blood circulation to enhance your grasp of some abdominal anatomy and pathologic processes. The cardiovascular system has both a pulmonary and systemic function. The pulmonary circulation provides blood to the lungs and drains the lungs as well, whereas the systemic circulation provides this same function for the rest of the body's organs and structures.

T A B L E **1 - 9** **Functions and structures of body systems**

Body System	Primary Function	Organs or Structures
Cardiovascular	Supplies the body with oxygen, nutrients, hormones, and WBCs and removes waste and toxins by pumping and transferring blood	Arteries and arterioles Capillaries Heart Veins and venules
Digestive	Provides metabolism, nutrient uptake, energy storage, and the excretion of waste	Liver Gallbladder Pancreas Esophagus Mouth Small and large bowel Stomach
Endocrine	It is involved in the secretion of hormones into the blood to control many different body functions. The hypothalamus in the brain controls the pituitary gland's secretion of various hormones, which in turn controls the secretion of hormones by endocrine organs or glands.	Adrenal glands Liver Ovaries Pancreas Parathyroid glands **Pineal gland** Pituitary gland (anterior and posterior) Testicles Thyroid gland
Exocrine	Secretes hormones or juices through ducts	Breast Pancreas Salivary glands (parotid glands, submandibular glands, and sublingual glands) Liver
Lymphatic	Collection and transportation of excess fluid, absorption of fats (which are eventually sent to the liver), and immune response	Adenoids Bone marrow Lymph nodes Spleen **Thymus gland** Tonsils
MSK	Provides the structural support system for the body	Cartilage Connective tissue Joints Ligaments Muscles Tendons
Nervous	Controls almost every organ system and structure in the body	Brain Spinal cord Nerves
Respiratory	Supplies the body with oxygen and removes carbon dioxide from the blood	Bronchus Larynx Lungs Nasal cavity Pharynx Trachea

TABLE 1-9 Functions and structures of body systems (*continued*)

Body System	Primary Function	Organs or Structures
Reproductive	Produces new life	Male: Epididymis Prostate gland Scrotum Testes Vas deferens Female: Fallopian tubes Ovaries Uterus Vagina
Urinary	Maintains chemical and water balance, regulates blood pressure, and filters waste products from the blood	Kidneys Ureters Urethra Urinary bladder

MSK, musculoskeletal; WBCs, white blood cells.

The heart consists of four chambers: two atria and two ventricles. Blood returning to the heart from the systemic circulation is via the superior vena cava and the inferior vena cava (IVC). The superior vena cava and the IVC empty into the right atrium of the heart. Thus, recognizing an enlargement of IVC during an abdominal sonogram can be indicative of right-sided heart failure. Although the heart is not specifically imaged by the abdominal sonographer, the fluid around the heart, termed a pericardial effusion, may be noted during an abdominal sonogram. Also, fluid within the chest cavity, termed a pleural effusion, may be noted. Vascularity of the abdomen can be evaluated with sonography with real-time, pulsed Doppler, and color or power Doppler. Although there are a few exclusions, the typical pattern of blood flow is as follows: arterioles → capillary → venule → vein.

The digestive system can be evaluated with sonography for various indications. The esophagus may be seen while imaging the liver, especially in the sagittal plane when analyzing the left lobe of the liver. Although gastritis may be demonstrated, the adult stomach is not often analyzed specifically with sonography. However, the distal portion of the pediatric stomach can be evaluated for pyloric stenosis. The intestines may be examined for disorders such as intussusception, volvulus, diverticulitis, and appendicitis. Tumors of the gastrointestinal tract may be seen with sonography as well. Of course, the accessory organs of the digestive system, such as the liver, gallbladder, and pancreas are readily imaged with sonography.

The glands of the endocrine system, specifically the thyroid gland, parathyroid glands, adrenal glands, and testicles, are imaged by abdominal sonographers (Fig. 1-21). Endocrine glands release their hormones directly into the bloodstream. Exocrine glands, such as the salivary glands, release their enzymes through ducts. Some organs, such as the pancreas and testicles, have both exocrine and endocrine functions. Whereas the pancreatic endocrine function is to produce the hormones, including insulin, glucagon, and somatostatin, the exocrine function is to produce digestive enzymes, including amylase, lipase, sodium bicarbonate, and others. The testicular endocrine function is to produce testosterone, whereas the testicular exocrine function is to produce and transport sperm.

◀))) SOUND OFF
Endocrine organs release hormones into the bloodstream, whereas exocrine organs use ducts. Remember, *exocrine exit* through ducts.

The lymphatic system plays a vital role in the immune response. Small structures known as lymph nodes are scattered throughout the body and serve the purpose of filtering lymphatic fluid of foreign material (Fig. 1-22). The lymphatic system also plays an important role in the transportation of lymphatic fluid or lymph, and thus fluid balance. This fluid makes its way through lymphatic channels to the thoracic duct, ultimately to be returned to the systemic circulation via the heart. A buildup of lymphatic fluid, most likely caused by obstruction of this drainage process with subsequent swelling, is referred to as **lymphedema**. Lymph nodes, which contain lymphocytes and macrophages, are commonly imaged by the sonographer in the neck, the groin, the armpit, and perhaps, when enlarged, they may be seen within the abdomen. Enlargement of a lymph node may

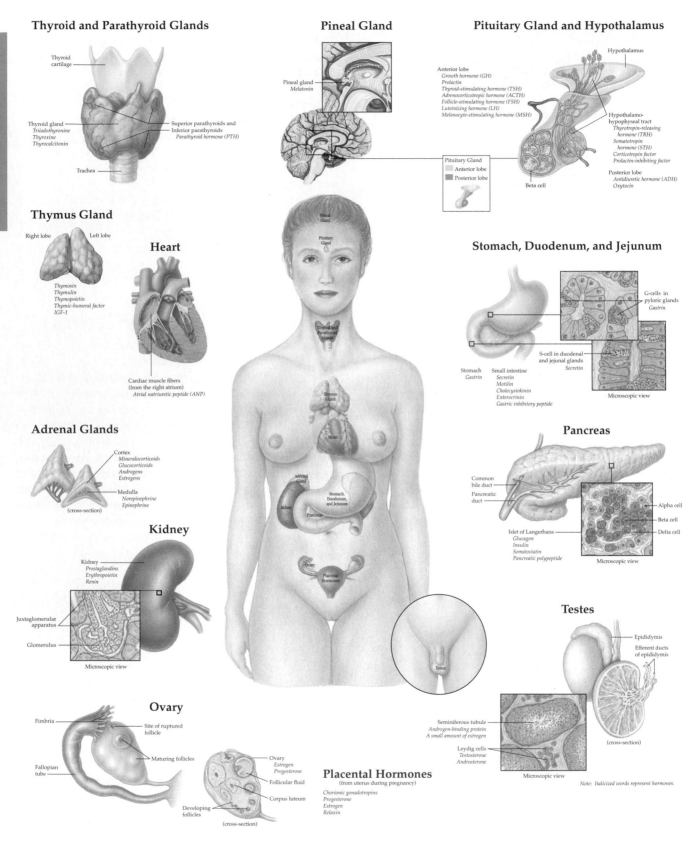

Thyroid and Parathyroid Glands

Thyroid cartilage

Thyroid gland
Triiodothyronine
Thyroxine
Thyrocalcitonin

Superior parathyroids and Inferior parathyroids
Parathyroid hormone (PTH)

Trachea

Pineal Gland

Pineal gland
Melatonin

Pituitary Gland and Hypothalamus

Hypothalamus

Anterior lobe
Growth hormone (GH)
Prolactin
Thyroid-stimulating hormone (TSH)
Adrenocorticotropic hormone (ACTH)
Follicle-stimulating hormone (FSH)
Luteinizing hormone (LH)
Melanocyte-stimulating hormone (MSH)

Hypothalamo-hypophyseal tract
Thyrotropin-releasing hormone (TRH)
Somatotropin hormone (STH)
Corticotropin factor
Prolactin-inhibiting factor

Posterior lobe
Antidiuretic hormone (ADH)
Oxytocin

Beta cell

Pituitary Gland
☐ Anterior lobe
☐ Posterior lobe

Thymus Gland

Right lobe   Left lobe

Thymosin
Thymulin
Thymopoietin
Thymic-humoral factor
IGF-1

Heart

Cardiac muscle fibers (from the right atrium)
Atrial natriuretic peptide (ANP)

Stomach, Duodenum, and Jejunum

G-cells in pyloric glands
Gastrin

S-cell in duodenal and jejunal glands
Secretin

Stomach
Gastrin

Small intestine
Secretin
Motilin
Cholecystokinin
Enterocrinin
Gastric inhibitory peptide

Microscopic view

Adrenal Glands

Cortex
Mineralocorticoids
Glucocorticoids
Androgens
Estrogens

Medulla
Norepinephrine
Epinephrine

(cross-section)

Pancreas

Common bile duct
Pancreatic duct

Alpha cell
Beta cell
Delta cell

Islet of Langerhans
Glucagon
Insulin
Somatostatin
Pancreatic polypeptide

Microscopic view

Kidney

Kidney
Prostaglandins
Erythropoietin
Renin

Juxtaglomerular apparatus

Glomerulus

Microscopic view

Testes

Epididymis
Efferent ducts of epididymis

Seminiferous tubule
Androgen-binding protein
A small amount of estrogen

Leydig cells
Testosterone
Androsterone

(cross-section)

Microscopic view

Note: Italicized words represent hormones.

Ovary

Fimbria

Site of ruptured follicle

Maturing follicles

Fallopian tube

Ovary
Estrogen
Progesterone

Follicular fluid

Corpus luteum

Developing follicles

(cross-section)

Placental Hormones
(from uterus during pregnancy)

Chorionic gonadotropins
Progesterone
Estrogen
Relaxin

Figure 1-21 Endocrine system.

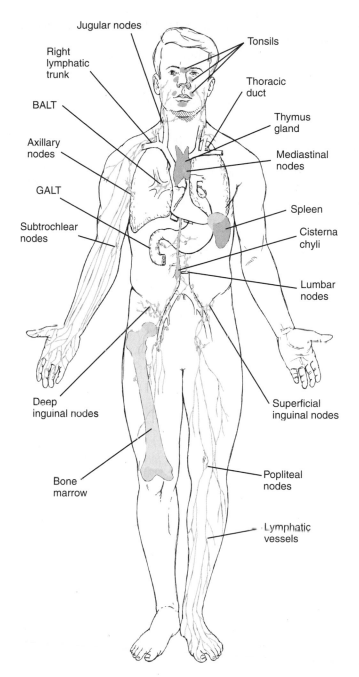

be useful at detecting many pathologic complications of the MSK system, including joint effusions and tendon tears or ruptures.

Both the male and the female reproductive systems can be readily imaged with sonography. For abdominal sonography, one must understand the function and anatomy of male reproductive organs and structures, including the penis, scrotum, testes, and prostate gland. Testicular torsion and infection of the testicles and epididymis are among the common indications for scrotal sonography.

The urinary tract consists of an upper and a lower part. The upper urinary tract includes the kidney and ureters, whereas the lower part includes the bladder and urethra. The kidneys function to regulate blood volume, filter the blood, and regulate blood pressure. The kidneys produce urine, which is comprised of waste products, such as urea. Urine flows from the paired kidneys down the paired ureters and is temporarily stored in the urinary bladder before exiting the body via the urethra. Sonography can be used to evaluate the urinary tract for obstruction, tumors, and renal calculi, as well as to perform an overall assessment of other disorders that can inhibit the system's functions.

Abdominal Cavity

The double lining of the abdominal cavity is the peritoneum. The peritoneum consists of a parietal and visceral layer. The **parietal peritoneum** forms a closed sac, except for two openings in the female pelvis, which permits passage of the fallopian tubes from the uterus to the ovaries. Furthermore, each organ is covered by a layer of **visceral peritoneum**, which is essentially the organ's serosal layer.

Some abdominal organs are considered **intra-peritoneal** and others **retroperitoneal** (Tables 1-10 and 1-11). The retroperitoneal structures are only covered anteriorly with peritoneum. The abdominal parietal peritoneum can be divided into two sections: the

Figure 1-22 Lymphatic system. *BALT*, bronchus-associated lymphoid tissue; *GALT*, gut-associated lymphoid tissue.

be referred to as **lymphadenopathy**. The largest mass of lymphatic tissue is the spleen. Other lymphatic system components include the thymus gland in the chest and the tonsils and adenoids in the neck.

The MSK system provides the framework for the human body. It comprises bones, muscles, tendons, ligaments, and joints. Although there is an additional certification covering MSK sonography offered by the American Registry for Diagnostic Medical Sonography (ARDMS), the abdominal sonographer may be called upon to analyze some MSK structures, including the pediatric hip and the Achilles tendon. Sonography can

TABLE 1-10 The list of intraperitoneal organs
Gallbladder
Liver (except for the bare area)
Ovaries
Spleen (except for splenic hilum)
Stomach
Appendix
Transverse colon
First part of the duodenum
Jejunum
Ileum
Sigmoid colon

TABLE 1-11 The list of retroperitoneal organs

Abdominal lymph nodes
Adrenal glands
Aorta
Ascending and descending colon
Most of the duodenum
IVC
Kidneys
Pancreas
Prostate gland
Ureters
Urinary bladder
Uterus

IVC, inferior vena cava.

greater sac and the lesser sac. The greater sac extends from the diaphragm to the pelvis, whereas the lesser sac is located posterior to the stomach. Potential spaces, which are essentially outpouching in the peritoneum, exist between the organs (Table 1-12).

These spaces provide an area for fluid to collect in the abdomen and pelvis. **Ascites** is an abnormal collection of abdominal fluid in these spaces. It can be found in association with several pathologies (Table 1-13). Ascites can be a single fluid, such as serosal fluid, pus, blood, or urine, or it may be a combination of fluids. **Exudate ascites** can be a malignant form of ascites. It may appear as complex fluid with loculations and produce matting of the bowel. Benign ascites, or **transudate ascites**, consists of **serosal fluid** and typically appears simple and anechoic.

TABLE 1-12 The location and significance of the peritoneal cavity spaces

Peritoneal Cavity Spaces	Location and Significant Points
Subphrenic spaces	• Inferior to the diaphragm • Divided into right and left
Subhepatic spaces	• Divided into right (anterior and posterior) and left • Right subhepatic space is located between the right lobe of the liver and right kidney. • Posterior right subhepatic space or hepatorenal recess is also referred to as **Morison Pouch.** • Left subhepatic space is located between the left lobe of liver and stomach.
Retropubic space	• Between the pubic bone and urinary bladder • Also referred to as the **space of Retzius**
Lesser sac	• Between the stomach and pancreas • Common location for pancreatic pseudocysts
Paracolic gutters (Fig. 1-23)	• Extend alongside the ascending and descending colon on both sides of the abdomen
Posterior cul-de-sac	• Male: between the urinary bladder and rectum; also referred to as the rectovesical pouch • Female: between the uterus and rectum; also referred to as pouch of Douglas and rectouterine pouch
Anterior cul-de-sac	• Between the urinary bladder and uterus • Also called the vesicouterine pouch in females

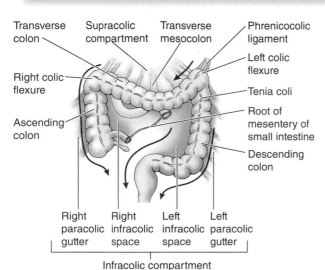

Transverse colon
Supracolic compartment
Transverse mesocolon
Phrenicocolic ligament
Right colic flexure
Left colic flexure
Tenia coli
Ascending colon
Root of mesentery of small intestine
Descending colon

Right paracolic gutter
Right infracolic space
Left infracolic space
Left paracolic gutter

Infracolic compartment

Figure 1-23 Paracolic gutters and ascites. This figure demonstrates the typical flow (*arrows*) of abdominal fluid (ascites) and other materials that may occur in the abdomen from the supracolic compartment to the infracolic compartment.

TABLE 1-13 Pathologies associated with ascites

Abdominal trauma
Acute cholecystitis
Cirrhosis
Congestive heart failure
Ectopic pregnancy
Malignancy
Portal hypertension
Ruptured abdominal aortic aneurysm

SONOGRAPHIC ABDOMINAL PATHOLOGY OVERVIEW

A mass, also referred to as a neoplasm or tumor, may be benign, potentially malignant (precancerous), or malignant. Whereas malignant, or cancerous, tumors both invade adjacent tissue and have the potential to metastasize to other parts of the body, a benign tumor, although certainly not normal, typically does not invade neighboring tissue and does not metastasize. Metastasis can occur via the blood stream or lymphatic system, and cancer can be staged according to its progression (Fig. 1-24). It is important to note that some benign tumors have the potential for progressing to cancer. Also, tumors, whether benign or malignant, may also displace adjacent anatomy, termed **mass effect**, causing secondary clinical complaints such as pain.

A synopsis of the most common benign and malignant adult abdominal solid masses encountered with sonography is provided in Tables 1-14 and 1-15, respectively. Though a description of each mass and the most common abdominal location is provided, each of these masses will be further discussed in the following chapters. A synopsis of the most common pediatric malignant abdominal masses encountered with sonography is provided in Table 1-16. A common theme that one can recognize is the presence of the word part "blast" in these childhood malignant tumors.

🔊 **SOUND OFF**
The word part "blast," as in hepato*blast*oma, often refers to a childhood malignancy.

As a screening modality, sonography has some challenges in regard to predicting whether a mass is benign or malignant. However, there are several clinical findings that can be indicators for the presence of malignancy. These indicators may present as **signs** or **symptoms**. A sign is something that can be observed by others and is therefore objective. An example of a sign is fever, vomiting, and elevated laboratory tests. A symptom is something felt by the person themselves, such as nausea, a headache, or abdominal pain, and is therefore subjective. In general, patients with cancer may present with vague signs and symptoms, such as unexplained weight loss, fever, fatigue, pain, and possible skin changes. Throughout this text, signs and symptoms will be placed together in tables and referred to as clinical findings. Clinical findings also include laboratory results. Some labs can be used as **tumor markers**. Tumor markers are substances produced by cancer cells or organs in response to cancer (Table 1-17).

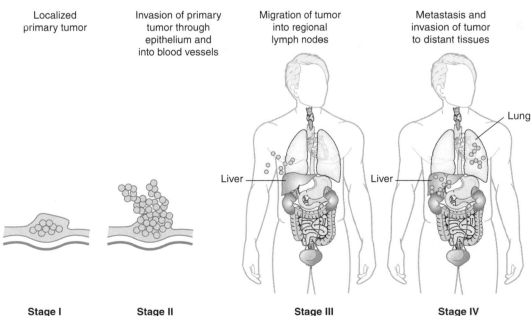

Cancer Staging and Progression

Localized primary tumor

Invasion of primary tumor through epithelium and into blood vessels

Migration of tumor into regional lymph nodes

Metastasis and invasion of tumor to distant tissues

Lung

Liver

Liver

Stage I   Stage II   Stage III   Stage IV

Figure 1-24 Generalized cancer staging and progression. This simplified diagram is an example of numerous factors are used in combination to define cancer stage; these include tumor size, extent of invasion, lymph node involvement, metastasis, and histologic assessments.

Abdominal Sonography Overview

TABLE 1-14 Common locations of benign abdominal/small part tumors

Benign Abdominal Tumor	Description	Common (Abdominal) Location
Adenoma	Tumor of glandular origin	Most organs
Adrenal rest tumor	Tumor containing adrenal tissue	Testicle
Angiomyolipoma	Tumor of blood vessels, muscle, and fat	Kidney
Focal nodular hyperplasia	Abnormal accumulation of cells within a focal region of an organ	Liver
Granuloma	Tumor consisting of a group of inflammatory cells	Liver and spleen
Gastrinoma	Tumor that secretes **gastrin**	Pancreas
Hamartoma	Tumor consisting of an overgrowth of normal cells of an organ	Kidney
Hemangioma	Tumor consisting of blood vessels	Liver, spleen, and kidney
Hematoma	Localized collection of blood	Anywhere an organ/tissue is affected by trauma
Insulinoma	Tumor that secretes insulin	Pancreas
Lipoma	Tumor that consists of fat	Liver, spleen, kidney, and superficial locations
Oncocytoma	Tumor consisting of **oncocytes**	Kidney
Pheochromocytoma	Tumor that consists of **chromaffin cells** of the adrenal gland	Adrenal gland
Teratoma	Tumor that consists of tissue from all three germ cell layers	Testicle/ovary
Urinoma	Localized collection of urine	Adjacent to a kidney transplant

TABLE 1-15 Common locations of malignant abdominal/small part tumors

Malignant Abdominal Tumor	Description	Common (Abdominal) Location
Adenocarcinoma	Cancer of glandular origin	Pancreas and gastrointestinal tract
Angiosarcoma	Cancer in the lining of vessels (lymphatic or vascular)	Spleen
Choriocarcinoma	Cancer that consists of trophoblastic cells	Testicle
Cholangiocarcinoma	Cancer of the bile ducts	Biliary tree
Cystadenocarcinoma	Cancer that is fundamentally adenocarcinoma with cystic components	Pancreas
Embryonal cell carcinoma	Cancer that is of germ cell origin	Testicle
Follicular carcinoma	Cancer of aggressive abnormal epithelial cells	Thyroid
Hepatocellular carcinoma (hepatoma)	Cancer that originates in the hepatocytes	Liver
Hypernephroma (renal cell carcinoma)	Cancer that originates in the tubules of the kidney	Kidney
Leukemia (focal)	Cancer of the blood cells	Spleen, kidney, liver, and testicle
Lymphoma	Cancer of the lymphatic system; classified as Hodgkin or non-Hodgkin lymphoma	Spleen, kidney, and testicle
Medullary carcinoma	Cancer originating from the parafollicular cells of the thyroid	Thyroid

TABLE 1-15 Common locations of malignant abdominal/small part tumors (*continued*)

Malignant Abdominal Tumor	Description	Common (Abdominal) Location
Papillary carcinoma	Cancer that has formation of many irregular, fingerlike projections	Thyroid
Seminoma	Cancer that originates in the seminiferous tubules	Testicle
Transitional cell carcinoma	Cancer that originates in the transitional epithelium of an organ or structure	Bladder, ureter, and kidney
Yolk sac tumor	Cancer that is of germ cell origin	Testicle

TABLE 1-16 Common locations of malignant pediatric abdominal masses

Solid Pediatric Malignant Abdominal Mass	Common Location
Hepatoblastoma	Liver
Nephroblastoma (Wilms tumor)	Kidney
Neuroblastoma	Adrenal gland

TABLE 1-17 Basic overview of tumor markers relevant to abdominal imaging that may be elevated with some cancers

Abdominal/Small Part Tumor Marker	Possible Cancer Present[a]
Alpha-fetoprotein	Liver, ovarian, or testicular cancers
Bladder tumor antigen (BTA)	Urinary tract
BRCA1 and BRCA2 gene mutations	Breast and ovarian cancers
CA-15-3	Breast cancers
CA-19-9	Pancreatic, biliary tract, stomach, and colon cancers
CA-125	Ovarian cancers
Calcitonin	Medullary thyroid cancer
Carcinoembryonic antigen	Colorectal cancer
Beta-hCG	Testicular cancers and malignant germ cell tumors
LDH	Testicular, ovarian, and other malignant germ cell tumors
PSA	Prostate cancer

[a]Some benign conditions may cause an increase in these labs. Beta-hCG, human chorionic gonadotropin; LDH, lactate dehydrogenase; PSA, prostate-specific antigen.

There are many syndromes, multisystem disorders, and diseases that will be encountered during the study of abdominal pathology. A summary of these is provided in Table 1-18. It should be kept in mind that a syndrome is a group of clinically observable findings that exist together and allow for classification, whereas a disease is the result of the incorrect functioning of an organ or body system that can result from many different issues, including genetic predisposition, infection, and environmental factors. Some diseases have associated syndromes. Lastly, for convenience, a table of common abdominal sonographic "signs" has been provided in Table 1-19. These will be noted throughout the subsequent chapters.

FOCUSED ASSESSMENT WITH SONOGRAPHY FOR TRAUMA AND EXTENDED FOCUSED ASSESSMENT WITH SONOGRAPHY FOR TRAUMA EXAM

Because sonography is safe, highly effective, and portable, some institutions may employ the focused assessment with sonography for trauma (FAST) examination to evaluate emergency patients. FAST examination is a form of point-of-care sonography that is utilized to assess the abdomen and pelvis for free fluid secondary to traumatic injury. This free fluid may be indicative of internal hemorrhage. An extended FAST (eFAST) exam may also include an evaluation of the lungs for the presence of pneumothorax and the heart for pericardial effusions. If appropriately trained, it may be performed by physicians, physician extenders, emergency medical personnel (e.g., in an ambulance), and sonographers.

Several views may be obtained of the abdomen and chest, including views of the right upper quadrant, left upper quadrant, pelvis, pericardium, anterior thorax, right and left pericolic gutters, pleural spaces, parasternal region, and apex of the heart. As with any assessment of the abdomen/chest, the examination should be performed in at least two orthogonal planes and representative images obtained. Guidelines for FAST examination have been established by the AIUM. More information is available at the AIUM website, https://www.aium.org/resources/guidelines/fast.pdf

TABLE 1-18 Summary of multisystem disorders, diseases, or syndromes

Multisystem Disorder, Disease, or Syndrome	Synopsis	Affected Structures or Organs
Addison disease	Primary adrenal gland insufficiency where the glands produce too little cortisol and aldosterone	Adrenal glands
Autosomal dominant polycystic kidney disease	Inherited condition that causes cysts in multiple organs; usually seen in adults later in life, but may be discovered earlier	Kidneys, liver, spleen, and pancreas
Autosomal recessive polycystic kidney disease	Inherited condition that causes cysts in the kidneys, renal failure, and hepatic fibrosis; usually discovered in utero or in newborns	Kidneys and liver
AIDS and HIV	Virus that attacks the immune system	Liver, spleen, lymph nodes, and skin tumors (**Kaposi sarcoma**)
Beckwith–Wiedemann syndrome	Growth disorder that causes enlargement of many organs and structures; increased risk for kidney and liver cancer in children	Skull, abdominal **visceromegaly**, and tongue (macroglossia)
Budd–Chiari syndrome	Narrowing or occlusion of the hepatic veins and possibly IVC	Liver and IVC
Caroli disease	Ectasia or narrowing of the bile ducts	Biliary tract
Conn syndrome	Results from high levels of aldosterone; can be caused by adrenal adenoma	Adrenal glands
Crohn disease	Autoimmune disease that causes chronic inflammation of the gastrointestinal tract	Gastrointestinal tract
Cruveilhier–Baumgarten syndrome	Cirrhosis, portal hypertension, and dilation of the umbilical and paraumbilical veins	Liver
Cushing syndrome	Results from high levels of cortisol; can be caused by adrenal adenoma	Adrenal glands
Cystic fibrosis	Inherited disorder in which mucus secreting glands produce thick and sticky secretions instead of normal secretions	Lungs, pancreas, and other digestive organs
Diabetes	Caused by hyposecretion or hypoactivity of insulin Type 1—Early onset (juvenile or young adult) Type 2—Adult onset	Multiple organs including eyes, extremities, kidneys, nerves, and vasculature
Fitz-Hugh–Curtis syndrome	Rare complication of pelvic inflammatory disease causing inflammation of the tissue around the liver	Liver
Graves disease	Associated with hyperthyroidism	Thyroid
Hashimoto disease	Associated with hypothyroidism	Thyroid
Hemochromatosis	Associated with iron overload	Liver
Henoch–Schonlein purpura	Autoimmune disorder and form of vasculitis associated with purple spots on the skin, gastrointestinal complications, joint pain, and possibly renal failure	Kidneys
Hepatorenal syndrome	Form of progressive renal failure associated with severe liver damage often secondary to cirrhosis	Liver and kidneys
Inflammatory bowel disease	Chronic inflammation of all or parts of the bowel	Small bowel and colon
Irritable bowel syndrome	Results from hypersensitivity of nerves in the wall of the gastrointestinal tract; results in abdominal discomfort and irregular bowel movements	Gastrointestinal tract
Ischemic bowel disease	Results from decreased blood flow to the intestines resulting in damaged bowel tissue owing to inadequate oxygenation	Small bowel and colon

TABLE 1-18 Summary of multisystem disorders, diseases, or syndromes (*continued*)

Multisystem Disorder, Disease, or Syndrome	Synopsis	Affected Structures or Organs
Klinefelter syndrome	Genetic condition in which a male has an extra X chromosome	Testicles and male breast
Marfan syndrome	Disorder of the connective tissue	Heart, vascular structures, and skeleton
Mirizzi syndrome	Jaundice, pain, and fever associated with a stone lodged in the cystic duct	Liver, gallbladder, and biliary tract
Nephrotic syndrome	Damaged filtration of the kidneys that causes excessive protein in the urine (proteinuria)	Kidneys, swelling of feet and ankles
Nutcracker syndrome	Syndrome often associated with complications that result from the compression of the left renal vein as it travels between the superior mesenteric artery and abdominal aorta	Testicles
Peyronie disease	Condition resulting from the buildup of fibrous tissue within the penis	Penis
Prune belly syndrome	Syndrome resulting from the maldevelopment of the fetal abdominal musculature secondary to an extremely enlarged fetal urinary bladder	Kidneys, abdominal musculature, bladder, urethra
Sarcoidosis	Inflammatory disease that results in granulomas and possibly scar tissue development in multiple organs	Liver, spleen, kidneys, testicles, lymphatics, and lungs
Sickle cell anemia (disease)	Form of hemolytic anemia in which the body produces abnormally shaped red blood cells	Liver, kidneys, spleen, eyes, bones, and gallbladder
Sjögren syndrome	Autoimmune disease that affects all glands that produce moisture	Salivary glands, eyes, nose, skin, and mouth
Tuberculosis	Infectious disease spread through the air	Lungs, lymphatics, and testicles
Tuberous sclerosis	Rare genetic disorder that leads to the development of tumors (hamartomas) within various organs	Brain, heart, and kidneys (hamartomas in the kidney may be called angiomyolipoma)
Von Gierke disease	Condition resulting from the body's inability to break down glycogen; also called Type 1 glycogen storage disease	Liver
von Hippel–Lindau disease	Rare genetic disorder characterized by cysts and tumors in various organs; results in von Hippel–Lindau syndrome	Pancreas, kidneys, and adrenal glands
Wilson disease	Congenital disorder that causes the body to accumulate excess copper	Liver
Zinner syndrome	Syndrome that consists of unilateral renal agenesis, ipsilateral seminal vesicle cyst, and ejaculatory duct obstruction	Seminal vesicles and kidneys
Zollinger–Ellison syndrome	Tumor (gastrinoma) in the pancreas or intestine that causes an increase in the production of gastrin	Pancreas and stomach (produces excessive stomach acid)

Many of these diseases, syndromes, or conditions affect other organs. This is a condensed list for the purpose of focused study. IVC, inferior vena cava.

TABLE 1-19 Abdominal signs, location, and a brief description

Abdominal Sign	Location	Description
Ball-on-the-wall sign	Gallbladder	Appearance of a gallbladder polyp
Barcode sign	Lungs	Abnormal M-mode appearance of lung sliding indicating pneumothorax
Blue dot sign	Scrotum	Torsed appendage of the testicle that can be seen superficially
Central dot sign	Intrahepatic biliary ducts	Echogenic dot in dilated intrahepatic ducts associated with Caroli disease
Cervix sign	Pyloric sphincter of stomach	Appearance of pyloric stenosis in the long axis
Champaign sign	Gallbladder	Air within the gallbladder wall associated with emphysematous cholecystitis
Cinnamon bun sign	Bowel	Short axis appearance of intussusception
Double-duct sign	Pancreatic duct and common bile duct	Dilatation of both the pancreatic and common bile duct
Doughnut sign (target sign)	Pyloric sphincter of stomach	Appearance of pyloric stenosis in the short axis
Keyboard sign	Small bowel	Seen in small bowel obstruction
McBurney sign	Appendix	Pain over McBurney point in the right lower quadrant
Mickey sign	Liver	Cross section appearance of the porta hepatis
Murphy sign	Right upper quadrant	Pain with probe pressure over the gallbladder
Olive sign	Pyloric sphincter of stomach	Palpable hypertrophic pyloric muscle associated with pyloric stenosis
Parallel tube sign (shotgun sign)	Liver hilum	Dilatation of both the common duct and portal vein
Pseudogallbladder sign	Liver	Cystic structure noted in the gallbladder fossa without evidence of an actual gallbladder; associated with biliary atresia in children
Pseudokidney sign	Bowel	Longitudinal appearance of intussusception (may be used for some bowel masses also)
Rovsing sign	Appendix	Right lower quadrant pain when the left lower quadrant is palpated
Sandwich sign	Abdominal aorta and IVC	Abnormal abdominal lymph node enlargement associated with retroperitoneal lymphadenopathy
Seashore sign	Lungs	Normal M-mode tracing of lung sliding
Starry sky sign	Liver	Bright portal triads seen with hepatitis
Thyroid in the belly sign	Appendix	Hyperechoic edematous tissue surrounding an inflamed appendix
Thyroid inferno (sign)	Thyroid	Hypervascular thyroid tissue noted with color Doppler
Triangle cord sign	Liver hilum	Avascular, triangular, or tubular structure representing fibrous replacement of duct associated with biliary atresia
Turtleback sign	Liver	Calcified septa and fibrosis associated with schistosomiasis
Wall-echo-shadow (WES) sign	Gallbladder	Appearance of a gallbladder completely filled with stones
Water lily sign	Liver	Pericyst surrounding a free floating endocyst; associated with a hydatid liver cyst
Whirlpool sign	Gallbladder	Cystic duct appearance with color Doppler associated with gallbladder torsion
Yin–yang sign	Pseudoaneurysm	Swirling blood flow within a pseudoaneurysm demonstrated with color Doppler

IVC, inferior vena cava.

REVIEW QUESTIONS

1. What artifact is demonstrated by the arrow in Figure 1-25?
   a. Doppler noise artifact
   b. Twinkle artifact
   c. Aliasing
   d. Slice thickness

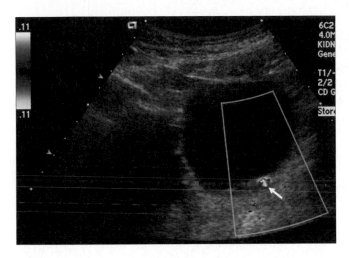

Figure 1-25

2. A patient with cholecystitis most likely has an elevation in which of the following labs?
   a. Alpha-fetoprotein
   b. WBC count
   c. Lactate dehydrogenase (LDH)
   d. Chromaffin

3. What is the cause of the artifact demonstrated in Figure 1-26?
   a. Attenuation of the sound beam resulting in false echoes
   b. Sound beams that strike a structure that is not perpendicular to the main sound beam
   c. Sound beam that is barely attenuated resulting in false echoes
   d. Large acoustic interface resulting in false echoes

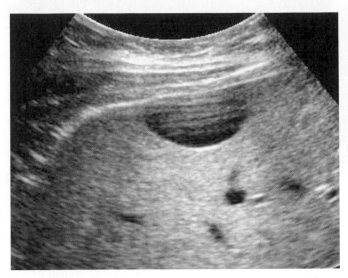

Figure 1-26

4. What is the name of the artifact demonstrated in Figure 1-26?
   a. Reverberation
   b. Noise
   c. Ring down
   d. Refraction

5. Transitional cell carcinoma is commonly found in all of the following locations except the:
   a. liver.
   b. renal pelvis.
   c. urinary bladder.
   d. ureter.

6. What is the artifact identified by the arrows in Figure 1-27?
   a. Side lobes
   b. Ring-down artifact
   c. Refraction
   d. Comet-tail

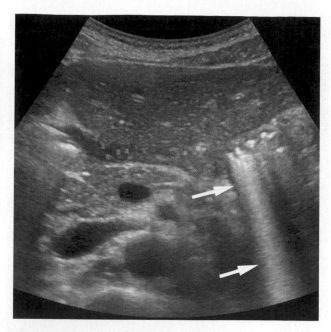

Figure 1-27

7. The neuroblastoma is a malignant pediatric mass commonly found in the:
   a. kidney.
   b. liver.
   c. adrenal gland.
   d. pancreas.

8. What is a biomarker produced by a cancerous tumor or an organ or structure in response to cancer?
   a. Oncocyte
   b. Tumor marker
   c. Lymphadenopathy
   d. Homeostatin

9. The pheochromocytoma is a benign mass commonly located in the:
   a. testicle.
   b. thyroid gland.
   c. adrenal gland.
   d. liver.

10. A tumor that is of similar echotexture to normal liver tissue is discovered in the liver of an asymptomatic patient. What is the echogenicity of the tumor?
    a. Echogenic
    b. Hypoechoic
    c. Isoechoic
    d. Hypodense

11. What is the artifact termed that is being identified by the arrow in Figure 1-28?
    a. Doppler aliasing
    b. Slice thickness
    c. Doppler noise
    d. Mirror image

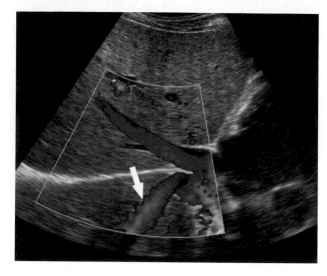

Figure 1-28

12. Which of the following is not considered to be an intraperitoneal organ?
    a. Liver
    b. Pancreas
    c. Gallbladder
    d. Spleen

13. In Figure 1-29, the sonographer has adjusted the pulse repetition frequency (PRF) to correct what sonographic artifact?
    a. Aliasing
    b. Doppler noise
    c. Refraction
    d. Overall gain

A

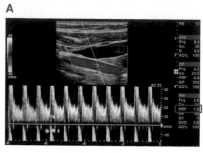

PRF = 1.6 kHz

B

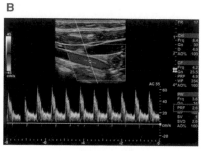

PRF = 2.6 kHz

Figure 1-29

14. Which of the following are not considered retroperitoneal organs?
    a. Abdominal lymph nodes
    b. Adrenal glands
    c. Kidneys
    d. Ovaries

15. What is another name for Morison Pouch?
    a. Posterior right subhepatic space
    b. Anterior subhepatic space
    c. Posterior cul-de-sac
    d. Anterior cul-de-sac

16. The hypernephroma may also be referred to as the:
    a. nephroblastoma.
    b. neuroblastoma.
    c. hepatocellular carcinoma.
    d. renal cell carcinoma.

17. An artifact caused by several small, highly reflective interfaces, such as gas bubbles, describes:
    a. mirror image artifact.
    b. posterior shadowing.
    c. comet-tail artifact.
    d. ring-down artifact.

18. The term cholangiocarcinoma denotes:
    a. bile duct carcinoma.
    b. hepatic carcinoma.
    c. pancreatic carcinoma.
    d. splenic carcinoma.

19. What artifact is identified by the white arrow in Figure 1-30?
    a. Grating lobe
    b. Reverberation
    c. Ring down
    d. Side lobe

20. Which of the following occurs when the Doppler sampling rate (pulse repetition frequency) is not high enough to display the Doppler frequency shift?
    a. Doppler noise
    b. Aliasing
    c. Mirror image
    d. Twinkle artifact

21. The hepatoma is a:
    a. benign tumor of the spleen.
    b. benign tumor of the liver.
    c. malignant tumor of the pancreas.
    d. malignant tumor of the liver.

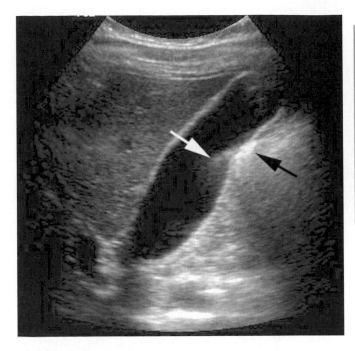

Figure 1-30

22. What artifact is identified by the white arrow in Figure 1-31?
    a. Anisotropy
    b. Dirty shadowing
    c. Comet-tail
    d. Reverberation

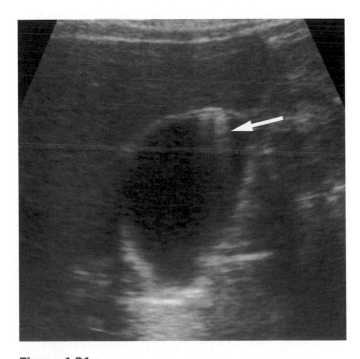

Figure 1-31

23. The hepatoblastoma is a:
    a. benign tumor of the pediatric liver.
    b. malignant tumor of the adult liver.
    c. malignant tumor of the pediatric liver.
    d. malignant tumor of the pediatric adrenal gland.

24. Which of the following is the space located between the pancreas and the stomach?
    a. Morison Pouch
    b. Lesser sac
    c. Space of Retzius
    d. Pouch of Douglas

25. Which of the following is another name for the Wilms tumor?
    a. Nephroblastoma
    b. Hepatoblastoma
    c. Neuroblastoma
    d. Hepatoma

26. An angiosarcoma would most likely be discovered in the:
    a. rectum.
    b. gallbladder.
    c. spleen.
    d. pancreas.

27. Image A in Figure 1-32 is a transverse view of the upper abdomen with the transducer positioned lateral to the midline. Image B is obtained with the transducer positioned directly over the rectus muscle in the midline. What is the artifact demonstrated in Image B?
    a. Side lobe
    b. Refraction
    c. Mirror image
    d. Slice thickness

28. Which of the following is not an endocrine organ or structure?
    a. Thymus
    b. Pancreas
    c. Thyroid
    d. Spleen

29. Which of the following is an artifact that alters the echogenicity of a tendon?
    a. Acoustic enhancement
    b. Anisotropy
    c. Ring-down artifact
    d. Mirror image artifact

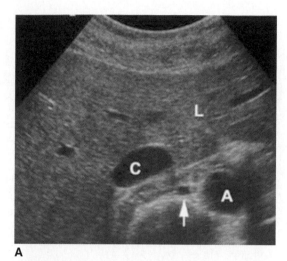

A

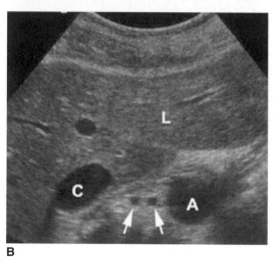

B

Figure 1-32

30. The gastrinoma would most likely be discovered in the:
    a. pancreas.
    b. adrenal gland.
    c. stomach.
    d. spleen.

31. What is the cause of the artifact identified by the white arrow in Figure 1-33?
    a. Extraneous sound beams
    b. Non-perpendicular sound beams that are peripheral to the main sound beam
    c. Perpendicular sound beams that interact negatively to the main sound beam
    d. Partial attenuation of the sound beam

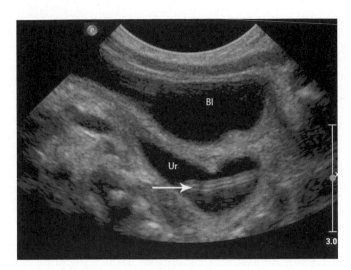

Figure 1-33

32. What artifact is demonstrated in Figure 1-34, image A?
    a. Aliasing
    b. Slice thickness
    c. Power enhancement
    d. Doppler noise

33. Of the list below, which is considered to be an intraperitoneal organ?
    a. Left kidney
    b. Aorta
    c. IVC
    d. Liver

34. Which of the following is considered to be a malignant testicular neoplasm?
    a. Neuroblastoma
    b. Hepatoma
    c. Yolk sac tumor
    d. Hamartoma

35. Which of the following is caused by the bending of the ultrasound beam when it passes through an interface between two tissues with vastly dissimilar speeds of sound and the angle of the approach is not perpendicular?
    a. Comet-tail
    b. Refraction
    c. Reverberation
    d. Acoustic enhancement

36. These potential spaces extend alongside the ascending and descending colon on both sides of the abdomen.
    a. Paracolic gutters
    b. Periumbilical gutters
    c. Greater gutters
    d. Pericentric gutters

37. This common tumor of the kidney consists of blood vessels, muscle, and fat.
    a. Hemangioma
    b. Angiomyolipoma
    c. Oncocytoma
    d. Lipoma

38. Which of the following is not a salivary gland?
    a. Thyroid gland
    b. Parotid gland
    c. Submandibular gland
    d. Sublingual gland

39. Which of the following is not a pediatric malignant tumor?
    a. Hepatoblastoma
    b. Neuroblastoma
    c. Pheochromocytoma
    d. Nephroblastoma

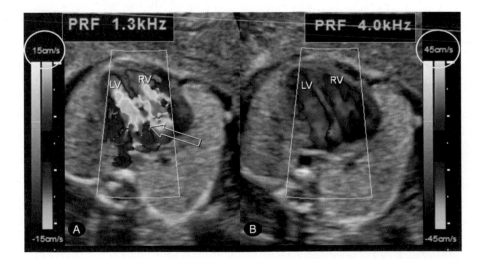

Figure 1-34

40. A tumor that consists of tissue from all three germ cell layers is the:
    a. pheochromocytoma.
    b. hamartoma.
    c. adrenal rest tumor.
    d. teratoma.

41. Which of the following would be considered a sign of disease?
    a. Nausea
    b. Elevated WBC
    c. Headache
    d. Abdominal pain

42. Which of the following laboratory values would be most helpful in evaluating a patient who has suffered from recent trauma?
    a. WBC count
    b. Alpha-fetoprotein
    c. Blood urea nitrogen (BUN)
    d. Hematocrit

43. The insulinoma is a:
    a. malignant pediatric adrenal tumor.
    b. benign pancreatic tumor.
    c. malignant pediatric tumor.
    d. benign liver tumor.

44. A tumor that consists of a group of inflammatory cells best describes the:
    a. hematoma.
    b. hepatoma.
    c. lymphoma.
    d. granuloma.

45. A tumor that consists of a focal collection of blood best describes the:
    a. hematoma.
    b. hamartoma.
    c. lipoma.
    d. angiomyolipoma.

46. Which of the following is a tumor marker that may be used in cases of suspected testicular malignancy?
    a. BUN
    b. Creatinine
    c. Human chorionic gonadotropin (beta-hCG)
    d. Calcitonin

47. The malignant testicular tumor that consists of trophoblastic cells is the:
    a. choriocarcinoma.
    b. yolk sac tumor.
    c. teratoma.
    d. insulinoma.

48. What is the artifact most likely encountered posterior to a gallstone?
    a. Acoustic enhancement
    b. Shadowing
    c. Ring down
    d. Reverberation

49. A collection of abdominal fluid within the peritoneal cavity often associated with cancer is termed:
    a. transudate ascites.
    b. chromaffin ascites.
    c. peritoneal ascites.
    d. exudate ascites.

50. Which of the following occurs behind strong, granular, and irregular surfaces like crystals, calculi, or calcifications such as a kidney stone?
    a. Twinkle artifact
    b. Refraction
    c. Anisotropy
    d. Side lobes

51. Which of the following has both an endocrine and an exocrine function?
    a. Adrenal glands
    b. Spleen
    c. Pancreas
    d. Duodenum

52. Which of the following would be most likely associated with ascites?
    a. Cirrhosis
    b. Gallstones
    c. Gastroesophageal reflux disease
    d. Cervical lymphadenopathy

53. What does elastography analyze?
    a. Cancer characteristics of a mass
    b. Tissue stiffness
    c. Blood flow
    d. Spatial imaging

54. Which of the following techniques utilizes nonlinear propagation of ultrasound as it travels through the body in order to improve axial and lateral resolution?
    a. Compound imaging
    b. Convex imaging
    c. Computerized tomographic imaging
    d. Harmonics imaging

55. Which of the following would disqualify a cyst from being a simple cyst?
    a. Anechoic echogenicity
    b. Mural nodule
    c. Edge artifact
    d. Acoustic enhancement

56. Which of the following would indicate renal disease if elevated?
    a. Calcitonin
    b. Bilirubin
    c. Creatinine
    d. Albumin

57. What is another name for the space of Retzius?
    a. Morison Pouch
    b. Posterior cul-de-sac
    c. Retropubic space
    d. Anterior cul-de-sac

58. Which of the following imaging modalities does not utilize X-ray or radionuclides to obtain diagnostic information?
    a. Radiography
    b. Computed tomography
    c. Nuclear medicine
    d. Magnetic resonance imaging

59. What is among the most common hospital-acquired infections?
    a. Urinary tract infection
    b. Tuberculosis
    c. Mononucleosis
    d. Strep infection

60. What is a rare genetic disorder characterized by cysts and tumors in various organs?
    a. Zinner disease
    b. von Hippel–Lindau disease
    c. Zollinger–Ellison disease
    d. Wilson disease

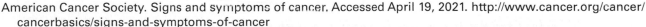

SUGGESTED READINGS

American Cancer Society. Signs and symptoms of cancer. Accessed April 19, 2021. http://www.cancer.org/cancer/cancerbasics/signs-and-symptoms-of-cancer

American Institute of Ultrasound in Medicine. AIUM practice parameter for the performance of an ultrasound of the abdomen and/or retroperitoneum. Accessed April 12, 2021. https://www.aium.org/accreditation/specialties/abdominal.aspx

American Institute of Ultrasound in Medicine. AIUM practice parameter for the performance of the focused assessment with sonography for trauma (FAST) examination. https://www.aium.org/resources/guidelines/fast.pdf

Curry RA, Tempkin BB. Sonography: Introduction to Normal Structure and Function. 5th ed. Elsevier; 2021:33–39, 55–88, & 113–128.

Hertzberg BS, Middleton WD. Ultrasound: The Requisites. 3rd ed. Elsevier; 2016:32.

Hopkins TB. Lab Notes: Guide to Lab and Diagnostic Tests. 2nd ed. F.A. Davis Company; 2009.

National Cancer Institute. Tumor markers in common use. Accessed April 18, 2021. https://www.cancer.gov/about-cancer/diagnosis-staging/diagnosis/tumor-markers-list

Penny SM. Introduction to Sonography and Patient Care. 2nd ed. Wolters Kluwer; 2021:70–76, 250–278, 307–420, & 462–464.

Sanders RC, Hall-Terracciano B. Clinical Sonography: A Practical Guide. 5th ed. Wolters Kluwer; 2016:61–93 & 399.

Siegel MJ. Pediatric Sonography. 5th ed. Wolters Kluwer; 2019:1–39.

BONUS REVIEW!

Surface Projections of Visceral Pain (Fig. 1-35)

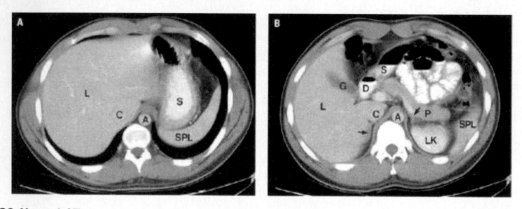

Liver, gallbladder, and duodenum (resulting from irritation of diaphragm)

Duodenum, head of pancreas
Gallbladder
Liver
Appendix
Cecum and ascending colon

Stomach
Spleen
Small intestine (*pink*)
Sigmoid colon
Kidney and ureter

Gallbladder
Liver

A. Anterior View

B. Posterior View

Figure 1-35 Surface projections of visceral pain. Colored regions indicate the possible visceral location of pathology that can cause associated pain.

Normal Computed Tomography Anatomy (Fig. 1-36)

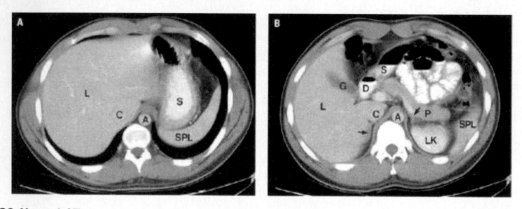

Figure 1-36 Normal CT anatomy. **A.** Diaphragmatic hiatus. Note the collapsed esophagus immediately anterior to the aorta. *L*, liver; *C*, inferior vena cava; *A*, aorta; *S*, stomach; *SPL*, spleen. **B.** The pancreatic body and tail are located immediately anterior to the splenic vein. Note the superior end of the gallbladder fossa, which is located immediately caudal to the interlobar fissure. An air–oral contrast material level is present in the second portion of the duodenum. Both adrenal glands are visible in this section (*arrows*). *L*, liver; *G*, gallbladder; *D*, duodenum; *C*, inferior vena cava; *S*, stomach; *A*, aorta; *P*, pancreatic tail; *LK*, left kidney; *SPL*, spleen.

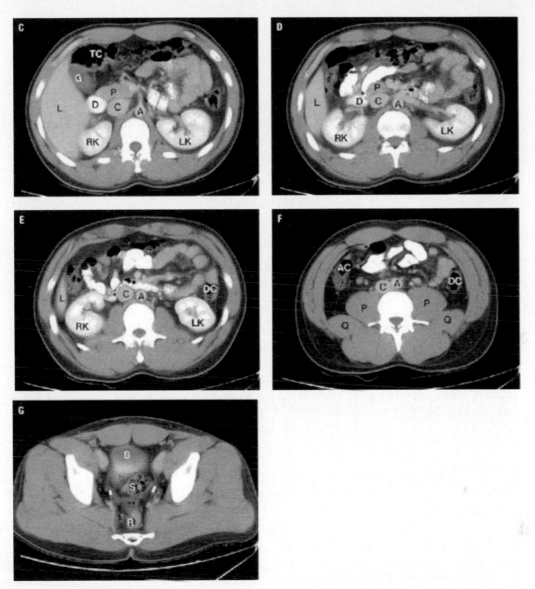

Figure 1-36 (*continued*) **C.** Pancreatic head. At the level of the superior mesenteric artery origin, an elongated but homogeneous pancreatic head has no contour abnormalities. The duodenum is filled with contrast material on this image. Note the close relationship between the hepatic flexure, the gallbladder, and the liver. *L*, liver; *G*, gallbladder; *TC*, transverse colon; *D*, duodenum; *RK*, right kidney; *P*, pancreatic head; *C*, inferior vena cava; *S*, stomach; *A*, aorta; *LK*, left kidney. **D.** The third portion of the duodenum. Note the contrast-filled duodenum crossing anterior to the inferior vena cava and the aorta immediately posterior to the superior mesenteric artery and vein at the upper end of the root of the small bowel mesentery. *L*, liver; *RK*, right kidney; *D*, duodenum; *P*, pancreatic head; *C*, inferior vena cava; *A*, aorta; *LK*, left kidney. **E.** Kidneys. Image at the level of the left splenic vein shows the inferior portion of the right lobe of the liver. The superior mesenteric vein and artery are visible in the root of the small bowel mesentery. *L*, liver; *RK*, right kidney; *C*, inferior vena cava; *A*, aorta; *DC*, descending colon; *LK*, left kidney. **F.** Paracolic gutters. In the normal individual, the paracolic gutter is a potential space between the parietal peritoneum of the body wall and the visceral peritoneum surrounding the ascending and descending colon. Note the multiple small arteries and veins coursing through the mesentery. *AC*, ascending colon; *P*, psoas muscle; *Q*, quadratus lumborum muscle; *C*, inferior vena cava; *A*, aorta; *DC*, descending colon. **G.** Peritoneal reflection. This image is below the anterior surface of the peritoneal reflection where the parietal peritoneum covers the dome of the bladder. *B*, bladder; *S*, sigmoid colon; *R*, rectum.

The Liver

Introduction

The liver is a vital organ. Therefore, much attention should be paid to the significance of comprehending its function and the various pathologic changes that can distort its sonographic appearance. This chapter provides an overview of the normal sonographic anatomy, as well as many pathologic processes of the liver. Because there are numerous conditions that can involve the liver, pathology has been categorized as either focal or diffuse diseases. The clinical findings and sonographic features of these pathologies are also provided. This chapter also includes a section on contrast-enhanced sonography of the liver. In the "Bonus Review" section, computed tomography and magnetic resonance imaging images of the liver with metastasis and cirrhosis are provided.

Key Terms

alcoholic liver disease—liver injury resulting from alcohol abuse

amebic hepatic abscess—an abscess that develops from a parasite that grows in the colon and invades the liver via the portal vein

anastomosis—the surgical connection between two structures

arteriovenous fistula—an abnormal passageway between an artery and a vein

autoimmune disorders—disorders in which the body's immune system attacks and destroys healthy tissues and/or organs

autosomal dominant polycystic kidney disease—an inherited disease that results in the development of renal, liver, and pancreatic cysts typically late in life; also referred to as adult polycystic kidney disease

bare area—the region of the liver not covered by peritoneum

Beckwith–Wiedemann syndrome—a growth disorder syndrome synonymous with enlargement of several organs, including the skull, tongue, and liver; children with this disorder are prone to several childhood cancers, including within the liver and kidney

biloma—a collection of bile within the abdomen; can be intrahepatic or extrahepatic in location

Budd–Chiari syndrome—a syndrome described as the occlusion of the hepatic veins, with possible coexisting occlusion of the inferior vena cava

caput medusae—recognizable dilation of the superficial veins of the abdomen

cavernous hemangioma—the most common benign liver tumor

cholangitis—inflammation of the bile ducts

cirrhosis—condition defined as hepatocyte death, fibrosis and necrosis of the liver, and the subsequent development of regenerating nodules

conjugated bilirubin—the water soluble form of bilirubin that is excreted into the intestines in bile and excreted in the stool; also referred to a direct bilirubin

The Liver

contrast-enhanced (liver) ultrasound—sonographic imaging that includes the injection of a contrast agent intravenously to better enhance the borders of liver lesions and to analyze those lesions for possible signs of malignancy

Couinaud classification—system used to separate the liver into eight surgical segments; used to describe functional liver anatomy

Cruveilhier–Baumgarten syndrome—syndrome characterized by cirrhosis, portal hypertension, and dilation of the umbilical and paraumbilical veins

cystic fibrosis—genetic disorder linked with the development of scar tissue accumulation within the lungs, liver, pancreas, kidneys, and/or intestines

diaphragmatic slip—a pseudomass of the liver seen on sonography resulting from hypertrophied diaphragmatic muscle bundles

dysentery—infection of the bowel which leads to diarrhea that may contain mucus and/or blood

echinococcal cyst—see hydatid liver cyst

Echinococcus granulosus—a parasite responsible for the development of hydatid liver cysts

Epstein–Barr virus—the virus responsible for mononucleosis and other potential complications

facial telangiectasia—dilated or broken vessels located near the surface of the skin on the face that appears as threadlike red lines; commonly referred to as spider veins

falciform ligament—ligament that attaches the liver to the anterior abdominal wall

fatty liver—a reversible disease characterized by deposits of fat within the hepatocytes; also referred to as hepatic steatosis

fetor hepaticus—bad breath secondary to end-stage liver disease and the liver's inability to filter toxins; often accompanies cirrhosis, portal hypertension, and hepatic encephalopathy

focal fatty infiltration—manifestation of fatty liver disease in which fat deposits are localized

focal fatty sparing—manifestation of fatty liver disease in which an area of the liver is spared from fatty infiltration

focal nodular hyperplasia—a benign liver mass composed of a combination of hepatocytes and fibrous tissue that typically contains a central scar

gastroesophageal junction—the junction between the stomach and the esophagus

Glisson capsule—the thin fibrous casing of the liver

gynecomastia—enlargement of the male breast

hematemesis—vomiting blood

hematoma—a localized collection of blood

hemochromatosis—an inherited disease characterized by disproportionate absorption of dietary iron

hemopoiesis—the formation and development of blood cells

hepatic candidiasis—a hepatic mass that results from the spread of fungus in the blood to the liver

hepatic encephalopathy—a condition in which a patient becomes confused or suffers from intermittent loss of consciousness secondary to the overexposure of the brain to toxic chemicals that the liver would normally remove from the body

hepatic jaundice—jaundice resulting from the liver's inability to conjugate bilirubin; may be caused by conditions such as viral hepatitis, toxins, drugs, cirrhosis, and liver cancer

hepatic steatosis—see fatty liver

hepatitis—inflammation of the liver

hepatocellular adenoma—a benign liver mass often associated with the use of oral contraceptives

hepatocellular carcinoma—the primary form of liver cancer

hepatofugal—blood flow away from the liver

hepatoma—the malignant tumor associated with hepatocellular carcinoma; primary liver cancer

hepatomegaly—enlargement of the liver

hepatopetal—blood flow toward the liver

hepatorenal syndrome—the development of renal impairment and possible renal failure because of chronic liver disease

hepatosplenomegaly—concurrent enlargement of the spleen and liver

hydatid liver cyst—a liver cyst that develops from a tapeworm that lives in dog feces; also referred to as an echinococcal cyst because it originates from the parasite *Echinococcus granulosus*

hyperbilirubinemia—elevated levels of serum bilirubin

hyperlipidemia—abnormally high levels of fats within the blood (i.e., high cholesterol and high triglycerides)

hypovolemia—decreased blood volume

idiopathic—no recognizable cause; from an unknown origin

immunocompromised—a patient who has a weakened immune system

inferior vena cava web—rare condition characterized by obstruction of the inferior vena cava by membranous or fibrous bands; can cause obstruction of the hepatic veins leading to Budd–Chiari syndrome

inflammatory bowel disease—chronic inflammation of all or parts of the bowel

ischemic bowel disease—condition that results from decreased blood flow to the intestines resulting in damaged bowel tissue owing to inadequate oxygenation; also referred to as intestinal ischemia

jaundice—broad clinical term referring to the yellowish discoloration of the skin, mucous membranes, and sclerae; found with liver disease and/or biliary obstruction

kernicterus—brain damage from bilirubin exposure in a newborn with jaundice

Kupffer cells—specialized macrophages within the liver that engulf pathogens and damaged cells

leukocytosis—an elevated white blood cell count

ligamentum teres—ligament that forms part of the edge of the falciform ligament of the liver, connecting the liver to the umbilicus; a remnant of the left umbilical vein; also referred to as the round ligament of the liver

ligamentum venosum—remnant of the fetal ductus venosus; appears as a hyperechoic linear ligament between the caudate lobe and left lobe of the liver

lipoma—a benign fatty tumor

liver fibrosis—the development of scar tissue within the liver as a result of the liver repeatedly trying to repair itself

liver hilum—the area of the liver where the common bile duct exits the liver and portal vein and hepatic artery enter the liver; also referred to as the porta hepatis

low-resistance flow—a flow pattern that characteristically has antegrade flow throughout the cardiac cycle

malaise—feeling of uneasiness

malignant degeneration—the deterioration of a benign mass into a malignancy

mass effect—the displacement or alteration of normal anatomy that is located adjacent to a tumor

metabolic syndrome—condition that includes hypertension, hyperglycemia, excessive body fat around the waist, elevated cholesterol, and nonalcoholic fatty liver disease

monophasic—vascular flow yielding a single phase

necrosis—death of tissue

palmar erythema—reddening of the palms

periportal cuffing—an increase in the echogenicity of the portal triads as seen in hepatitis and other conditions

pneumobilia—air within the biliary tree

porta hepatis—the area of the liver where the portal vein and hepatic artery enter and the hepatic duct exit; also referred to as the liver hilum

portal hypertension—the elevation of blood pressure within the portal venous system

portal triads—an assembly of a small branch of the portal vein, bile duct, and hepatic artery that surround each liver lobule

portal vein thrombosis—the development of clot within the portal vein

posthepatic jaundice—elevation in bilirubin caused by an obstruction of bile flow, typically by either a gallstone lodged in the biliary tract or pancreatic mass

prehepatic jaundice—when the liver cannot process the amount of hemolysis of the red blood cells, resulting in a buildup of circulating bilirubin in the bloodstream

pseudocirrhosis—nodular appearance of the liver caused by multiple metastatic tumors

pseudomass—false mass

purpura—blood spots under the skin that may appear purple

pyogenic liver abscess—a liver abscess that can result from the spread of infection from inflammatory conditions such as appendicitis, diverticulitis, cholecystitis, cholangitis, and endocarditis

quadrate lobe—the medial segment of the left lobe

recanalization—the reopening of canals or pathways

Riedel lobe—a tongue-like extension of the right hepatic lobe

sequela—an illness resulting from another disease, trauma, or injury

serpiginous—twisted or snake-like pattern

shear wave elastography—elastography technique that utilizes a standard ultrasound transducer with elastography technology to obtain information about the stiffness of tissue as in the case of liver fibrosis or cirrhosis

situs inversus—condition in which the organs of the abdomen and chest are on the opposite sides of the body (e.g., the liver is within the left upper quadrant instead of the right upper quadrant)

spider nevi—a cluster of vessels noted on the skin that have a web-like pattern; singular form is nevus

splanchnic circulation—blood flow to the major gastrointestinal organs including the stomach, liver, spleen, pancreas, and small and large intestines; consists of the celiac artery, superior mesenteric artery, and inferior mesenteric artery

splenomegaly—enlargement of the spleen

***starry sky* sign**—the sonographic sign associated with the appearance of periportal cuffing in which there is an increased echogenicity of the walls of the portal triads that may be associated with hepatitis

steatohepatitis—a type of fatty liver disease that causes inflammation of the liver

total bilirubin—obtained by adding unconjugated and conjugated bilirubin

total parental hyperalimentation—procedure in which an individual receives vitamin and nutrients through a vein, often the subclavian vein

transient elastography—imaging technique that utilizes a special transducer to assess the liver and other organs for signs of fibrosis and cirrhosis; used to measure the stiffness of tissue

transjugular intrahepatic portosystemic shunt (TIPS)—the therapy for portal hypertension that involves the placement of a stent between the portal veins and hepatic veins to reduce portal systemic pressure

triphasic—vascular flow yielding three phases

unconjugated bilirubin—the non–water soluble form of bilirubin that travels to the liver via the bloodstream;

eventually converted to conjugated bilirubin by the liver; also referred to as indirect bilirubin

von Gierke disease—condition in which the body does not have the ability to break down glycogen; also referred to as glycogen storage disease type 1

von Hippel–Lindau disease—an inherited disease that includes the development of cysts within the liver, pancreas, and other organs

Wilson disease—a congenital disorder that causes the body to accumulate excess copper

ANATOMY AND PHYSIOLOGY OF THE LIVER

The liver is an essential organ (Table 2-1). In early embryonic life, the liver is responsible for **hemopoiesis**. The function of the liver can be analyzed with certain laboratory tests (Table 2-2). It is the largest parenchymal organ in the body, with the majority of its bulk—the right lobe—located in the right upper quadrant, whereas the left lobe is positioned within the epigastrium and may traverse the midline and extend

T A B L E 2 - 1 Vital functions of the liver

1. Carbohydrate metabolism
2. Fat (lipid) metabolism
3. Amino acid metabolism
4. Removal of waste products
5. Vitamin and mineral storage
6. Drug inactivation
7. Synthesis and secretion of bile
8. Blood reservoir
9. Lymph production
10. Detoxification

T A B L E 2 - 2 Specific liver function test, results, and associated abnormalities

Liver Function Test	Result	Associated Abnormality
Albumin	Decrease	Chronic liver disease[a] **Cirrhosis**
ALP	Increase	Cirrhosis Extrahepatic biliary obstruction Gallstones **Hepatitis** Metastatic liver disease Pancreatic carcinoma
ALT	Increase	Biliary tract obstruction Hepatitis Hepatocellular disease Obstructive **jaundice**
AST	Increase	Cirrhosis **Fatty liver** Hepatitis Metastatic liver disease
Gamma-glutamyl transferase	Increase	Diffuse liver disease Posthepatic obstruction
LDH	Increase	Cirrhosis Hepatitis Obstructive jaundice
Serum bilirubin	Increase	Unconjugated (direct) bilirubin: acute hepatocellular disease Conjugated (indirect) bilirubin: biliary tract obstruction Total bilirubin: cirrhosis, hepatitis, and other liver cell diseases
PT		Prolonged PT: metastasis of the liver and hepatitis Shortened PT: extrahepatic duct obstruction
AFP	Increase	**Hepatocellular carcinoma (hepatoma)** Hepatoblastoma

[a]This is an abbreviated list of complications for review purposes, because other complications may exist.
AFP, alpha-fetoprotein; ALP, alkaline phosphatase; ALT, alanine aminotransferase; AST, aspartate aminotransferase; LDH, lactate dehydrogenase; PT, prothrombin.

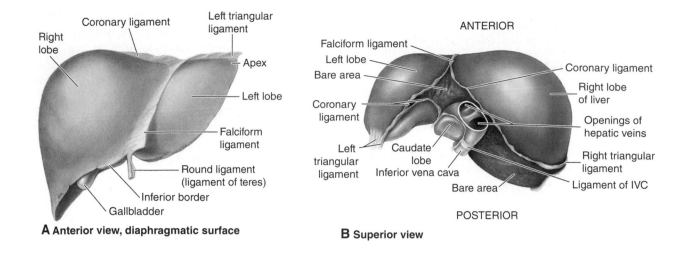

A Anterior view, diaphragmatic surface

B Superior view

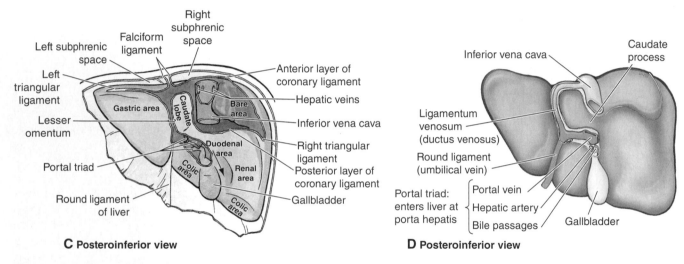

C Posteroinferior view

D Posteroinferior view

Figure 2-1 The surfaces of the liver.

into the left hypochondrium (Fig. 2-1). In some persons, the liver may actually come in contact with the spleen.

The liver is considered an intraperitoneal organ, with only a small portion left uncovered, including the **bare area**, the area of the **falciform ligament**, the gallbladder fossa, the **porta hepatis**, and an area adjacent to the inferior vena cava (IVC). The liver is also covered by **Glisson capsule**, a thin fibrous casing. It is composed of three main hepatic lobes—right, left, and caudate. Each hepatic lobe can be further divided into thousands of liver lobules. Lobules contain hepatocytes, biliary epithelial cells, and **Kupffer cells**. Each lobule is also surrounded by **portal triads**, which are composed of small branches of the portal vein, bile duct, and hepatic artery.

LOBES OF THE LIVER

The **Couinaud classification** is a system used to separate the liver into eight surgical segments and to describe functional liver anatomy (Fig. 2-2). However,

fundamentally, the liver can be divided into three primary hepatic lobes: right, left, and caudate (Table 2-3). An additional anatomic lobe, the **quadrate lobe**, is located between the gallbladder fossa and the

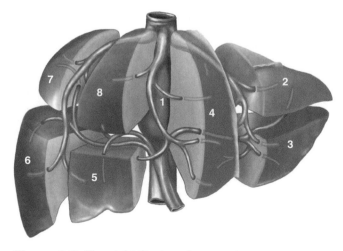

Figure 2-2 The eight Couinaud segments.

The Liver

TABLE 2-3 Useful landmarks for separating the hepatic segments and lobes

Right hepatic vein Right intersegmental fissure	Separates the anterior segment of the right lobe from the posterior segment of the right lobe
Middle hepatic vein Main lobar fissure Gallbladder fossa	Separates the right lobe from the left lobe (these are located between the anterior segment of the right lobe and the medial segment of the left lobe)
Left hepatic vein Left intersegmental fissure Ligamentum teres Falciform ligament	Separates the left lateral segment of the left lobe from the left medial segment of the left lobe

round ligament. However, sonographically this lobe is referred to as the medial segment of the left lobe, and thus it is usually not considered one of the main hepatic lobes.

SOUND OFF
The liver is composed of a right lobe, left lobe, and caudate lobe.

The right hepatic lobe is the largest lobe. It takes up most of the right upper quadrant. The right lobe can be divided into an anterior and posterior segment by the right hepatic vein, which lies within the right intersegmental fissure. The right lobe can be separated from the left lobe by the middle hepatic vein, which lies within the main lobar fissure. The right and left lobes are also separated by the gallbladder fossa.

The left lobe is much smaller than the right lobe. It is located within the epigastrium and may extend to the left hypochondrium. The left lobe may be divided into a medial and lateral segment by the left hepatic vein, which lies within the left intersegmental fissure. These segments can also be separated by the **ligamentum teres** and **falciform ligament**.

The caudate lobe, which has its own separate blood supply and venous drainage, is the smallest hepatic lobe. It is also located within the epigastrium and is bounded anteriorly by the **ligamentum venosum** and posteriorly by the IVC. Thus, the caudate lobe can be separated from the left lobe by the ligamentum venosum.

SOUND OFF
The medial segment of the left lobe may also be referred to as the quadrate lobe.

LIVER VASCULATURE OVERVIEW

It is important to note that the liver has a dual blood supply. The main portal vein provides the majority of hepatic perfusion (Table 2-4). Although this may seem perplexing, given that in many situations the purpose of a vein is to drain an organ, one must remember that one of the primary functions of the liver is to essentially be the major blood filter for the body, including detoxification and blood storage. Much of the blood within the main portal vein originates from the intestines and, consequently, the blood contains intestinally absorbed beneficial nutrients and toxins that must undergo refining in the liver.

The liver also receives some of its blood supply via **splanchnic circulation**, which describes blood flow to

TABLE 2-4 Differentiating features of the portal and hepatic veins

Feature	Portal Veins	Hepatic Vein
Doppler characteristics	Hepatopetal and monophasic with some variation with breathing	Hepatofugal and triphasic
Function	Transports blood to the liver from the intestines and other organs	Drain blood from the liver and deposits it into the IVC
Location	Main portal vein enters the liver at the porta hepatis *Intra*segmental (within segments)	Upper aspect of the liver *Inter*segmental (between segments) *Inter*lobar (between lobes)
Number and Pattern	Main portal vein branches into left and right Decrease in size as they approach the diaphragm	Three (right, middle, left), but some persons may have extra Increase in size as they approach the diaphragm
Sonographic appearance	Hyperechoic walls	Thin walls (perpendicular incidence may cause a brighter appearing wall)

the major gastrointestinal organs, including the liver, spleen, pancreas, small intestines, and large intestines. The primary vessels of splanchnic circulation are the celiac artery, superior mesenteric artery, and inferior mesenteric artery. One of the main branches of the celiac artery (also referred to as the celiac trunk or celiac axis) is the common hepatic artery. The common hepatic artery thus transports highly oxygenated blood directly to the liver from the abdominal aorta. The following sections will provide more details about liver vasculature.

Portal Veins

The main portal vein enters the liver at the porta hepatis, also referred to as the **liver hilum**. The main portal vein is created by the union of the superior mesenteric vein and splenic vein (Fig. 2-3). The merger of these two vessels and occasionally the inferior mesenteric vein, which typically takes place posterior to the neck of the pancreas and anterior to the IVC, is an area referred to as the portal confluence, portal

splenic confluence, or portovenous confluence. The portal vein provides the liver with approximately 75% of its total blood supply. The blood within the portal vein is partially oxygenated because it is derived from the intestines.

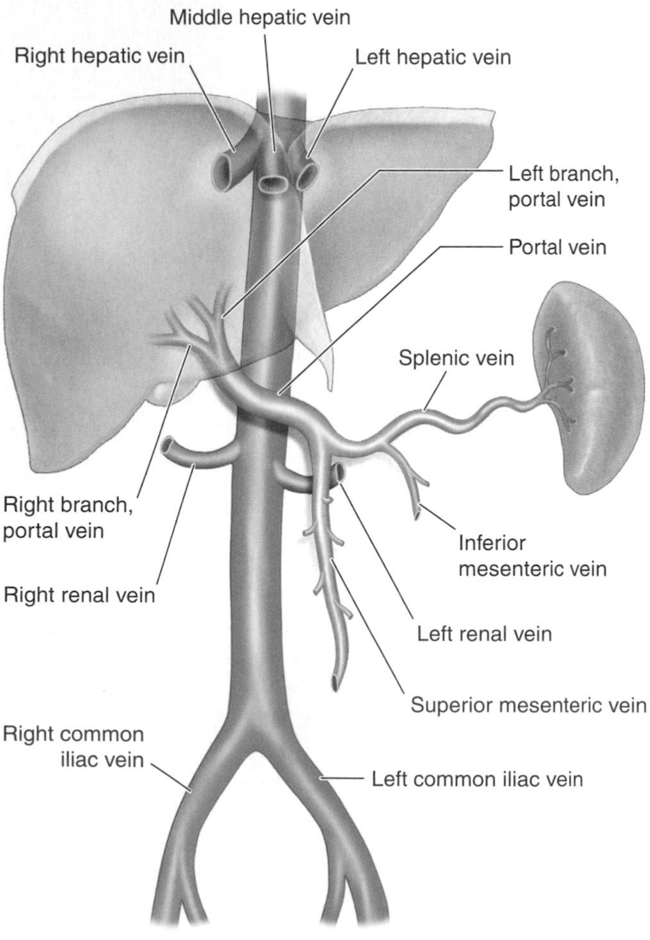

> 🔊 **SOUND OFF**
> Both the main portal vein and the hepatic artery transport oxygenated blood to the liver.

As the main portal vein enters the liver, it splits into the right and left portal veins (Fig. 2-4). The right portal vein, like the right hepatic lobe, is separated into an anterior and posterior division. The left portal vein, like the left hepatic lobe, is separated into a medial and lateral division. These vessels supply blood to their related segments. The diameter of the main portal vein can vary with respiration, although typically it measures less than 13 mm in the anteroposterior dimension (Fig. 2-5). Enlargement of the portal vein is often indicative of **portal hypertension**. Normal portal veins decrease in size as they approach the diaphragm. They are also considered intrasegmental because they course within the segments of the liver. On a sonogram, their walls appear much brighter than those of the hepatic veins. This may be because of an increase in the amount of collagen within their walls. Normal flow within the portal veins should be **hepatopetal** and **monophasic**, with some variation noted with respiratory changes (Fig. 2-6). In addition, scanning after a meal will often demonstrate an increase in portal vein flow.

Figure 2-3 The construction of the portal venous system.

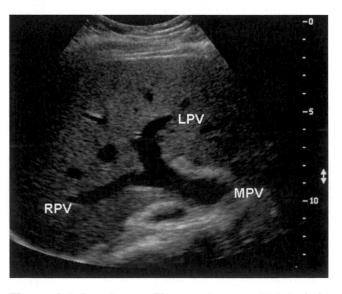

Figure 2-4 Portal veins. The portal veins, which include the main portal vein (*MPV*) that gives rise to the right portal vein (*RPV*) and left portal vein (*LPV*), are easily identified by their echogenic wall.

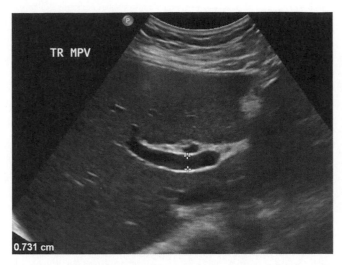

Figure 2-5 Measurement of the main portal vein. The main portal vein (*MPV*) should not exceed 1.3 cm. TR, transverse

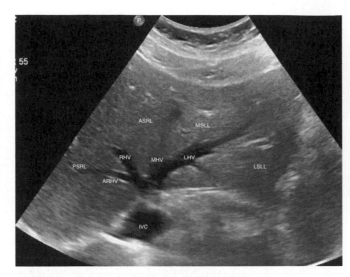

Figure 2-7 Hepatic veins. The left hepatic vein (*LHV*), middle hepatic vein (*MHV*), and right hepatic vein (*RHV*) are noted in this image. The *LHV* can be used to separate the left lateral segment (*LLS*) from the left medial segment (*LMS*). The *RHV* can be used to separate the right anterior segment (*RAS*) from the right posterior segment (*RPS*). The *MHV* can be used to separate the left lobe from the right lobe.

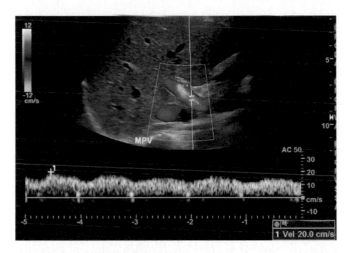

Figure 2-6 Normal hepatopetal flow (*red*) within the main portal vein (*MPV*) depicts monophasic flow with some respiratory variation.

> ◀)) **SOUND OFF**
> The portal veins branch into corresponding branches that match the segments of the liver (right portal = anterior and posterior branches; left portal = medial and lateral branches). The portal veins also typically have brighter walls compared with the hepatic veins.

Hepatic Veins

Most persons have three hepatic veins: right, middle, and left. These veins drain into the IVC. They are considered both intersegmental and interlobar because they are located between the segments and the lobes (Fig. 2-7). As mentioned earlier, they are readily used to

distinguish the hepatic segments. Unlike the portal veins, the hepatic veins increase in size as they approach the diaphragm. Hepatic veins have a **triphasic** blood flow pattern secondary to their association with the right atrium and atrial contraction (Fig. 2-8). Enlargement of the hepatic veins and IVC is seen with right-sided heart failure, and occlusion or narrowing of the hepatic veins is seen with **Budd–Chiari syndrome**.

The Porta Hepatis and the Hepatic Artery

The porta hepatis may also be referred to as the liver hilum. The three structures located within the porta hepatis are the main portal vein, common bile duct, and hepatic artery. The common hepatic artery carries oxygenated blood to the liver from the abdominal aorta. It is a branch of the celiac artery, the first main branch of the abdominal aorta as it passes below the diaphragm. The normal, **low-resistance flow** pattern of the hepatic artery can be noted with Doppler imaging (Fig. 2-9). Typically, the hepatic artery takes a course anterior to the main portal vein in the porta hepatis. When a longitudinally oriented image is obtained of this area, the artery can be noted anterior to the main portal vein and posterior to the common bile duct (Fig. 2-10). The *Mickey* sign describes the transverse image taken of the porta hepatis (Fig. 2-11). In some persons, the relationship between the artery and common bile duct is reversed.

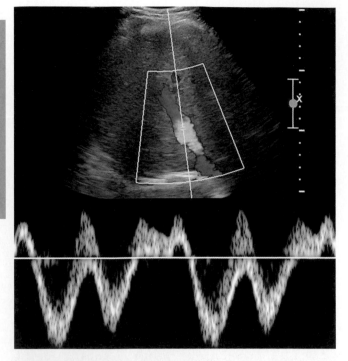

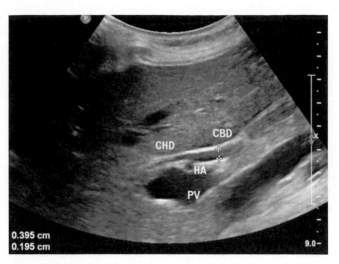

Figure 2-10 Porta hepatis. The portal vein (*PV*), common bile duct (*CBD*), and hepatic artery (*HA*) comprise the porta hepatis. Common hepatic duct (*CHD*).

Figure 2-8 Doppler signal of the normal right hepatic vein.

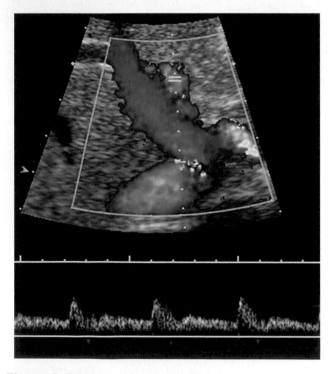

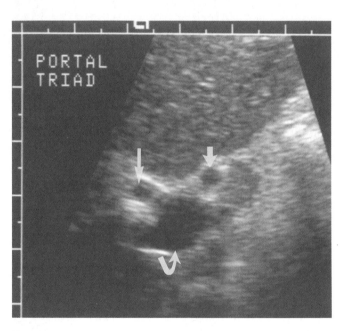

Figure 2-11 Mickey mouse sign. Transverse image of the porta hepatis. The face of Mickey is the portal vein (*curved arrow*), the hepatic artery is the left ear (*short arrow*), and the common bile duct is the right ear (*long arrow*).

Figure 2-9 Doppler signal of the hepatic artery.

LIGAMENTS AND FISSURES OF THE LIVER

Two readily identifiable ligaments may be noted within the normal liver during a sonogram: the ligamentum venosum and the falciform ligament. In utero, the umbilical vein supplies the fetus with oxygenated blood. The umbilical vein travels to the liver and bifurcates into a left and a right branch. The right branch, also referred to as the ductus venosus, shunts blood directly into the fetal IVC. Shortly after birth, the ductus venosus collapses and becomes the ligamentum venosum. The left umbilical vein connects directly to the left portal vein. After birth, it becomes a fibrous cord referred to as the ligamentum teres or round ligament. The ligamentum teres ascends along the falciform ligament. **Recanalization** of the paraumbilical vein in the ligamentum teres can occur in the presence of portal hypertension.

Sonographically, ligaments appear hyperechoic because of the fat located within and around them. The ligamentum venosum, which appears as a hyperechoic linear structure, can be noted anterior to the caudate lobe, between the caudate lobe and left hepatic lobe (Fig. 2-12). The falciform ligament can be appreciated near the left portal vein in most persons. In the transverse scan plane, it often appears as a

hyperechoic, triangle-shaped structure between the left and right hepatic lobes (Fig. 2-13). It is important to note that some texts may refer to the area of the falciform ligament as the ligamentum teres. Thus, it is vital to understand that the ligamentum teres is potentially identifiable with sonography within the lower margins of the falciform ligament. The main lobar fissure, which houses the middle hepatic vein, may also be identifiable in many persons. It is seen in the sagittal oblique plane as a hyperechoic line, which seems to connect the neck of the gallbladder to the right portal vein (Fig. 2-14). The main lobar fissure may be used to separate the right and left hepatic lobes. Finally, although not a true fissure, occasionally, a **diaphragmatic slip**

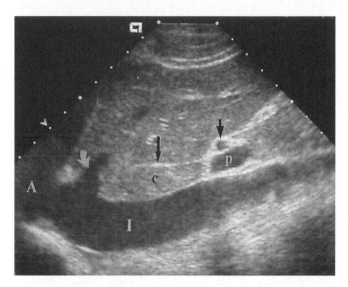

Figure 2-12 Caudate lobe. The caudate lobe (*c*) is located between the ligamentum venosum (*long arrow*) and the inferior vena cava (*I*). The inferior vena cava terminates at the heart's right atrium (*A*). The *curved arrow* indicates the right hepatic vein. Also seen are the portal vein (*p*) and hepatic artery (*short arrow*).

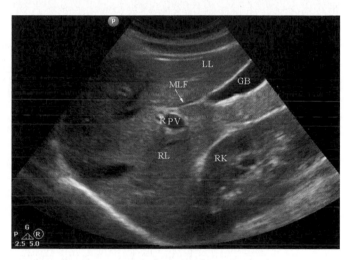

Figure 2-14 Sagittal oblique image of the liver demonstrating the right lobe (*RL*), left lobe (*LL*), and right kidney (*RK*). The main lobar fissure (*MLF*), the right portal vein (*RPV*), and gallbladder (*GB*) can be visualized well.

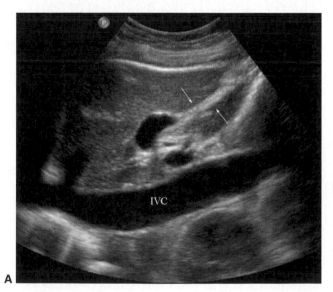

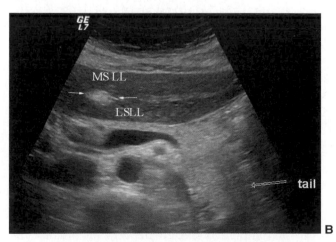

Figure 2-13 The falciform ligament is seen in sagittal (**A**) between the *arrows* and transverse (**B**) between the *arrows*. *IVC*, inferior vena cava; *MSLL*, medial segment left lobe; *LSLL*, lateral segment left lobe.

The Liver

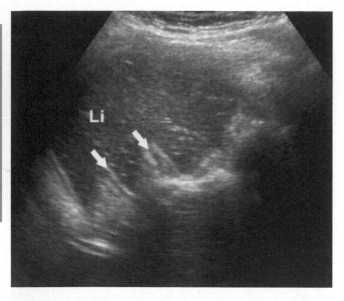

Figure 2-15 Diaphragmatic slip. There are two diaphragmatic slips (*arrows*) noted in this transverse image of the liver (*Li*).

or diaphragmatic muscular bundles may present as a **pseudomass** on sonography (Fig 2-15). Diaphragmatic slip, which typically occurs in older patients, is caused by hypertrophied diaphragmatic muscle bundles. It appears as hyperechoic strands extending from the diaphragm in the sagittal plane and may be confused for a hyperechoic mass in the transverse plane.

ANATOMIC VARIANTS OF THE LIVER

A **Riedel lobe** can be described as a tongue-like extension of the right hepatic lobe. This anatomic variant is more often seen in women. Riedel lobe may extend inferiorly as far as the iliac crest. To differentiate Riedel lobe from **hepatomegaly**, one could examine the left lobe for coexisting enlargement. An additional variant of the liver is the papillary process of the caudate lobe. This inferior extension of the caudate lobe can resemble a mass. If a papillary process is suspected, it may be prudent to evaluate the caudate lobe in both transverse and sagittal scan planes. Other anomalies of the liver include **situs inversus**, agenesis of a lobe, and there are many vascular variations, including missing or extra vessels.

SONOGRAPHY OF THE LIVER

A sonogram of the liver can be ordered for many reasons. The patient should fast for a period of 8 hours if the entire right upper quadrant is to be evaluated. Whereas some facilities may only require 4 hours of fasting, some

may not require any special patient preparation if only the liver is being examined with sonography, as in the situation where a brief follow-up for findings identified with other imaging modalities such as computed tomography (CT) or magnetic resonance imaging (MRI).

The normal liver is homogeneous. Its echogenicity is either equal to or slightly greater than the parenchyma of the normal right kidney, and it is slightly less echogenic than that of the normal spleen. In addition, when compared with the pancreas, the liver is slightly less echogenic in an adult. The liver measures approximately 13 to 15 cm in length in an adult. Although many studies differ, hepatomegaly is often suspected if the liver measures greater than 15.5 cm in the midhepatic or midclavicular line. One study suggested that the most accurate measurement of the right lobe can be obtained from the uppermost right hemidiaphragm to the inferior tip of the right lobe using a horizontal plane parallel to the anterior liver wall through the midaxillary line. Conversely, indirect sonographic signs have been suggested (Table 2-5; Fig. 2-16). And as mentioned earlier, in some individuals, particularly females, Riedel lobe can mistakenly suggest

TABLE 2-5 Indirect signs of hepatomegaly
• Extension of right lobe beyond the lower pole of the right kidney (without evidence of Riedel lobe)
• Rounding of the inferior tip of the right lobe
• Extension of left lobe well into the left upper quadrant

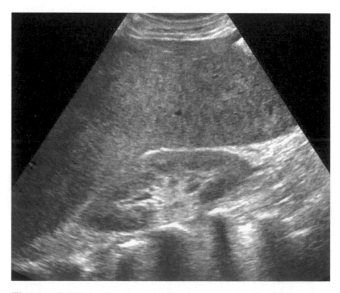

Figure 2-16 Indirect sign of hepatomegaly. In this patient with AIDS, the liver is enlarged and clearly extends beyond the lower pole of the right kidney.

hepatomegaly; so careful correlation with clinical history is strongly warranted when hepatomegaly is suspected sonographically.

> **SOUND OFF**
> Careful correlation with clinical history—especially an analysis of current laboratory findings—is strongly warranted when hepatomegaly is suspected sonographically.

LIVER PATHOLOGY

Overview of Jaundice and Bilirubin

In the upcoming section covering pathology of the liver, there will be several conditions that can result in **jaundice**. In general, jaundice is defined as the yellowish discoloration of the skin, mucous membranes, and sclerae of the eyes because of **hyperbilirubinemia**. Thus, one vital laboratory finding to assess before conducting a right upper quadrant sonogram is the serum bilirubin test. Bilirubin is the yellowish compound that results from the breakdown of hemoglobin that is found in red blood cells. Therefore, when the body has a buildup of bilirubin, this is what results in the yellowing of the skin and sclera of the eyes with jaundice.

Bilirubin may be described as either unconjugated (indirect), conjugated (direct), or total bilirubin. **Unconjugated bilirubin** is the non–water soluble form of bilirubin that travels to the liver via the bloodstream. It is eventually converted to conjugated bilirubin by the liver. **Conjugated bilirubin** is the water soluble form of bilirubin that is excreted into the intestines in bile and passed in the stool. **Total bilirubin** is calculated by adding the direct and indirect bilirubin levels. Excessive bilirubin may also be found in the urine.

In adults, jaundice can be described as prehepatic, hepatic, and posthepatic. **Prehepatic jaundice** occurs when the liver cannot process the amount of hemolysis of the red blood cells, resulting in a buildup of circulating (unconjugated) bilirubin in the bloodstream. One cause of prehepatic jaundice is a hemolytic disorder referred to as sickle cell disease. **Hepatic jaundice** results from the liver's inability to conjugate bilirubin and thus may be caused by conditions such as viral hepatitis, toxins, drugs, cirrhosis, and liver cancer. Hepatic jaundice may lead to an elevation in either unconjugated bilirubin or conjugated bilirubin because the liver either lacks the ability to conjugate the bilirubin or secrete it. **Posthepatic jaundice** will lead to an elevation in conjugated bilirubin and is caused by an obstruction of bile flow, typically by either a gallstone lodged in the biliary tract or a pancreatic mass. Posthepatic jaundice may also be referred to as obstructive jaundice.

> **SOUND OFF**
> An increase in conjugated (direct) bilirubin tends to be associated with gallstones or a pancreatic mass, whereas unconjugated (indirect) bilirubin tends to increase in the presence of hepatocellular disease, such as hepatitis and cirrhosis.

Diffuse Liver Disease
Fatty Liver Disease (Hepatic Steatosis)

Fatty liver disease, also referred to as **hepatic steatosis**, is a disorder characterized by fatty deposits (triglycerides) within the hepatocytes. It can be classified as alcoholic fatty liver disease or nonalcoholic fatty liver disease. Alcoholic fatty liver disease results from the chronic abuse of alcohol. The causes of nonalcoholic fatty liver disease include starvation, obesity, chemotherapy, diabetes mellitus, **hyperlipidemia**, pregnancy, glycogen storage disease or **von Gierke disease** (glycogen storage disease type 1), **total parental hyperalimentation**, severe hepatitis, **cystic fibrosis**, intestinal bypass surgery for obesity, and the use of some drugs such as corticosteroids. Nonalcoholic fatty liver disease has been cited as the most common liver disorder in the Western world and, subsequently, it is the most common cause of chronic liver disease, hepatic failure, and liver cancer. In many instances, nonalcoholic fatty liver disease is both acquired and reversible.

Fatty liver disease is said to be the hepatic manifestation of a disorder known as **metabolic syndrome** and it can lead to **steatohepatitis**. Steatohepatitis, which is inflammation of the liver secondary to fatty liver disease, can be caused by alcohol or the previously mentioned nonalcoholic conditions (nonalcoholic steatohepatitis or NASH). Steatohepatitis has been shown to be a precursor for chronic liver disease, leading to **liver fibrosis**, cirrhosis, and hepatocellular carcinoma (HCC) in some individuals. In many situations, a biopsy is warranted to accurately diagnose steatohepatitis.

Although fatty liver is often asymptomatic, patients may present clinically with elevated liver function tests. Fatty liver can be described as mild, moderate, or severe based on the sonographic visualization of both the hepatic vasculature and diaphragm. Fatty changes within the liver can also be diffuse or focal. Diffuse infiltration will cause the liver to appear diffusely echogenic, and it will be more difficult to penetrate. Frequently, in the presence of diffuse fatty infiltration, the walls of the hepatic vasculature and diaphragm will not be easily imaged, secondary to the attenuation of the sound beam (Fig. 2-17).

Sonographically, the liver segment affected by **focal fatty infiltration** will appear as an area of increased echogenicity and can thus appear much like a solid,

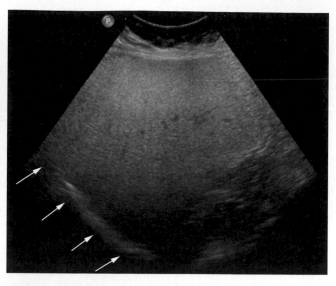

Figure 2-17 Sagittal image of a diffusely fatty liver that demonstrates the inability to clearly visualize the diaphragm (*arrows*).

hyperechoic mass (Fig. 2-18). Alternatively, **focal fatty sparing** of the liver can occur. In this circumstance, the liver is involved with diffuse fatty infiltration, with certain areas spared. This area of sparing can appear much like a solid, hypoechoic mass or possibly even fluid (Fig. 2-19).

Both focal fatty infiltration and focal fatty sparing occur in essentially the same places. It is much more likely that the signs of sparing and infiltration be identified adjacent to the gallbladder, near the porta hepatis, and the left medial segment. Although both of these abnormalities may mimic solid masses, they will not produce **mass effect** and therefore should not distort adjacent anatomy.

CLINICAL FINDINGS OF FATTY LIVER DISEASE

1. Asymptomatic
2. Alcohol abuse
3. Chemotherapy
4. Diabetes mellitus
5. Elevated liver function test (specifically AST and ALT)
6. Hyperlipidemia
7. Obesity
8. Pregnancy

SONOGRAPHIC FINDINGS OF DIFFUSE FATTY LIVER DISEASE

1. Diffusely echogenic liver
2. Increased attenuation of the sound beam
3. Wall of the hepatic vasculature and diaphragm will not be easily imaged

SONOGRAPHIC FINDINGS OF FOCAL FATTY INFILTRATION

1. Hyperechoic area adjacent to the gallbladder, near the porta hepatis, or part of a lobe may appear echogenic

SONOGRAPHIC FINDINGS OF FOCAL FATTY SPARING

1. Hypoechoic area adjacent to the gallbladder, near the porta hepatis, or part of a lobe or an entire lobe may be spared
2. Can appear much like pericholecystic fluid when identified adjacent to the gallbladder

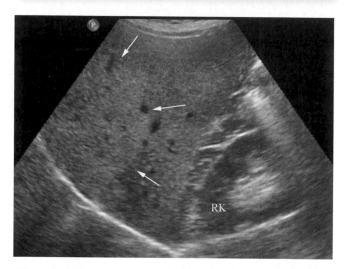

Figure 2-18 Sagittal image of the liver demonstrating an area of focal fatty infiltration (*arrows*) *RK*, right kidney.

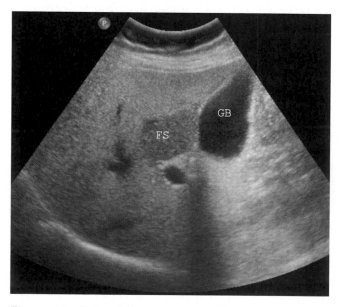

Figure 2-19 Focal fatty sparing (*FS*) is noted in this sagittal image of the liver adjacent to the gallbladder (*GB*).

Hepatitis

Hepatitis is inflammation of the liver, which can ultimately lead to cirrhosis, portal hypertension, and HCC. Hepatitis can be acute or chronic. Acute hepatitis is said to resolve within 4 months, whereas chronic hepatitis persists beyond 6 months. Hepatitis comes in many forms, including hepatitis A, B, C, D, E, and G. The two most common forms are hepatitis A and B.

Hepatitis A is spread by fecal–oral route in contaminated water or food. Hepatitis B is spread by contact with contaminated body fluids, mother-to-infant transmission, or inadvertent blood contact, as seen in the case of intravenous drug abuse or occupational exposure. An additional concern for healthcare workers is work-related exposure to hepatitis C. This form of hepatitis is also spread by means of contact with blood and body fluids, including needlesticks, tattoos or body piercings, and high-risk sexual contact. Currently, hepatitis C is the leading indication for liver transplantation in the United States. Fortunately, newer drug regimens exist that have a high success rate for removing hepatitis C from the body.

Hepatitis may also be triggered by reactions to systemic viruses such as herpes simplex virus and **Epstein–Barr virus**. Chronic hepatitis can be caused by **Wilson disease**, **hemochromatosis**, and **autoimmune disorders**, or it can be drug induced. Both Wilson disease and hemochromatosis are inherited conditions. Wilson disease is an autosomal-recessive disorder that results in the excessive accumulation of copper in the liver, brain, and other tissues. Eventually, the accumulation of copper in the hepatocytes results in their dysfunction, initially manifesting as fatty liver disease, and ultimately progressing to liver failure, hepatitis, and liver fibrosis. Hemochromatosis is characterized by disproportionate absorption of dietary iron. Patients with hemochromatosis also typically have a history of diabetes, hypogonadism, skin pigmentation, heart disease, and arthritis.

> **))) SOUND OFF**
> Wilson disease results from excessive copper accumulation, whereas hemochromatosis results from excessive iron. If a patient has either of these diseases, sonographers should evaluate the liver for signs of chronic hepatitis.

Hepatitis is often a clinical diagnosis. Patients with any form of hepatitis can experience a wide range of clinical troubles, including fever, chills, nausea, vomiting, fatigue, **hepatosplenomegaly**, dark urine, and jaundice. However, the jaundice related to hepatitis is on a cellular level and is not associated with biliary obstruction. As mentioned earlier, this is referred to as hepatic jaundice and is, thus, considered nonobstructive. Elevation in liver chemistries or liver function—specifically prothrombin time (PT), alkaline phosphatase (ALP), aspartate aminotransferase (AST), alanine aminotransferase (ALT), lactate dehydrogenase (LDH), and serum bilirubin levels—is often apparent as well. ALT is a more specific indicator of hepatic injury. Impaired liver function, as a result of hepatitis and other hepatic diseases, may lead to **hepatic encephalopathy**, a condition in which a patient becomes confused or suffers from intermittent loss of consciousness secondary to the overexposure of the brain to toxic chemicals that the liver would normally remove from the body. In newborns, brain damage can occur with severe jaundice as a result of bilirubin exposure, a condition referred to as **kernicterus**.

Sonographically, a patient with hepatitis may initially have a completely normal-appearing liver. With time, hepatomegaly and **splenomegaly**, termed hepatosplenomegaly, can be observed with sonography. As the liver enlarges, it tends to become more hypoechoic. **Periportal cuffing** may be seen in some patients with hepatitis, although this is not always a specific finding. Periportal cuffing is described as an increase in the echogenicity of the walls of the portal triads. The sonographic manifestation of this phenomenon is referred to as the ***starry sky*** sign (Fig. 2-20). The gallbladder wall may also be thickened in the presence of hepatitis.

> **))) SOUND OFF**
> Sonographically, the liver may appear normal with hepatitis or demonstrate evidence of periportal cuffing and gallbladder wall thickening.

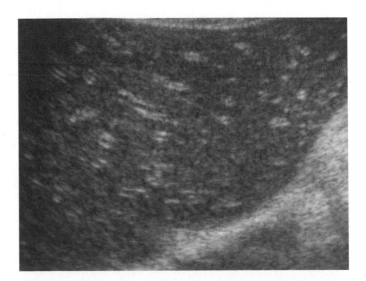

Figure 2-20 Transverse image of the liver demonstrates the *starry sky* appearance frequently associated with hepatitis.

CLINICAL FINDINGS OF HEPATITIS

1. Chills
2. Dark urine
3. Elevated liver function tests (specifically ALP, ALT, AST, LDH, PT, and total bilirubin)
4. Fatigue
5. Fever
6. Hepatosplenomegaly
7. Jaundice
8. Nausea
9. Vomiting

SONOGRAPHIC FINDINGS OF HEPATITIS

1. Normal liver
2. Enlarged, hypoechoic liver
3. Periportal cuffing with *starry sky*
4. Gallbladder wall thickening

Cirrhosis

Cirrhosis, also known specifically as liver or hepatic cirrhosis, is a devastating liver disorder that is defined as hepatocyte death, liver fibrosis and **necrosis** of the liver, and the subsequent development of regenerating nodules. Common **sequela** of cirrhosis includes portal hypertension, the development of varicosities within the abdomen, **portal vein thrombosis**, splenomegaly, HCC, and **hepatorenal syndrome**. The most common cause of cirrhosis is alcoholism. In fact, (alcoholic) cirrhosis is actually a type of **alcoholic liver disease**. The definition of significant alcohol consumption has been suggested to be more than 210 g of alcohol per week in men and more than 140 g per week for women. Cirrhosis can also be caused by Wilson disease, primary biliary cirrhosis, hepatitis, **cholangitis**, and hemochromatosis.

Patients may have normal laboratory findings until cirrhosis advances into end-stage liver disease. However, when laboratory abnormalities are evident, they include elevation in AST, LDH, ALT, and bilirubin. Patients may present with jaundice, fatigue, weight loss, diarrhea, initial hepatomegaly, ascites, **spider nevi**, **purpura**, **palmar erythema**, **gynecomastia**, **fetor hepaticus**, **facial telangiectasia**, hepatic encephalopathy, **caput medusae**, muscle wasting, testicular atrophy, and hemorrhoids (Fig. 2-21).

> 🔊 **SOUND OFF**
> Remember this possibly pathway of disease:
> Alcoholism → hepatic steatosis (fatty liver) → steatohepatitis → cirrhosis → portal hypertension → portal vein thrombosis → hepatocellular carcinoma

Sonographic findings of cirrhosis include an echogenic, small right lobe, an enlarged caudate and left

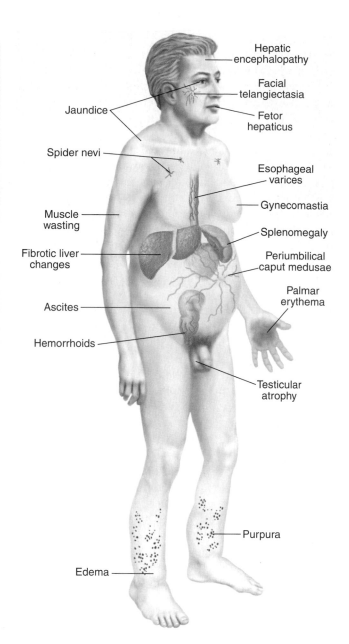

Figure 2-21 Clinical findings of cirrhosis.

lobe, nodular surface irregularity, coarse echotexture, ascites, and splenomegaly (Figs. 2-22 to 2-24). Cirrhosis caused by alcoholism will lead to the development of nodules that typically measure less than 1 cm (termed micronodular), whereas cirrhosis caused by hepatitis will lead to the development of larger nodules that measure between 1 and 5 cm (termed macronodular). Larger nodules may be readily seen when ascites surrounds the liver. If ascites is not present, a high-frequency linear transducer can be used to analyze the liver surface for evidence of surface nodularity or lumps (See Fig. 2-23 B).

Possible Doppler findings in patients with cirrhosis include monophasic flow within the hepatic veins and **hepatofugal** flow within the portal veins. Recall, normal

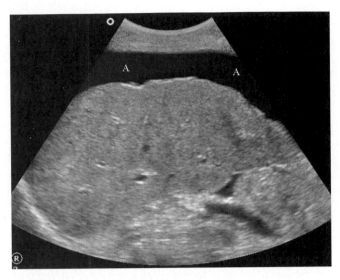

Figure 2-22 Ascites (*A*) is noted surrounding this liver that is affected by cirrhosis. Note the irregular, nodular contour of the liver.

flow within the main portal vein should be hepatopetal. These vascular complications are both findings consistent with advanced cirrhosis and portal hypertension. With these findings, the sonographer is encouraged to further investigate the liver and abdomen for further signs of portal hypertension, portal vein thrombosis, and HCC.

SOUND OFF
When you suspect cirrhosis, always look for signs of portal hypertension, portal vein thrombosis, and hepatocellular carcinoma.

CLINICAL FINDINGS OF CIRRHOSIS

1. Ascites
2. Diarrhea
3. Abnormal liver function tests (specifically elevated ALP, ALT, AST, bilirubin, PT, partial prothrombin time [PTT], total protein, and decreased albumin)
4. Fatigue
5. Hepatomegaly (initial)
6. Jaundice
7. Splenomegaly
8. Weight loss with muscle wasting
9. Caput medusae
10. Spider nevi
11. Palmar erythema
12. Gynecomastia
13. Fetor hepaticus
14. Facial telangiectasia
15. Hepatic encephalopathy
16. Testicular atrophy
17. Hemorrhoids

SONOGRAPHIC FINDINGS OF CIRRHOSIS

1. Hepatosplenomegaly (initial)
2. Shrunken, echogenic right lobe of the liver
3. Enlarged caudate and left lobes
4. Nodular surface irregularity
5. Coarse echotexture
6. Splenomegaly
7. Ascites
8. Monophasic flow within the hepatic veins
9. Hepatofugal flow within the portal veins

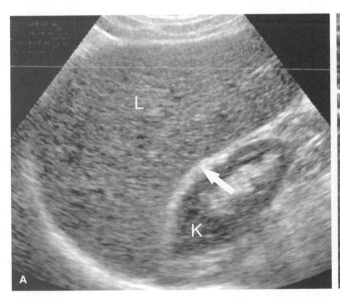
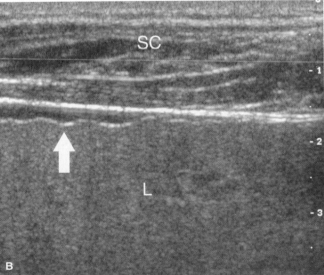

Figure 2-23 A. Note the course echotexture of the liver (*L*) damaged by cirrhosis and the irregular echogenicity of the liver compared to the kidney (*K*). **B.** A linear transducer is employed to analyze the surface (*arrow*) of the liver (*L*). *SC,* subcutaneous tissue.

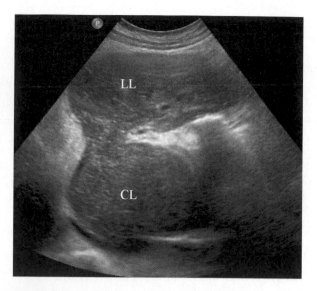

Figure 2-24 Enlargement of the caudate lobe (*CL*) compared to the left lobe (*LL*) is noted in this patient with cirrhosis.

Liver Fibrosis and Liver Elastography

Liver fibrosis, also referred to as hepatic fibrosis, results in the development of scar tissue within the liver as it attempts to repair itself. It has been demonstrated that liver stiffness (i.e., the stiffer the liver tissue the more fibrosis present) correlates with cirrhosis complication, including variceal hemorrhage, ascites, and HCC, all of which are signs of advanced cirrhosis and portal hypertension. Elastography of the liver has become a valuable imaging tool for the analysis of the degree of liver fibrosis in those with predisposing conditions, such as NASH or alcoholic liver disease. Essentially, as the amount of fibrosis of the liver increases, the stiffness of the liver increases as well. Consequently, the stiffer the liver tissue, the higher the level of tissue stiffness indicated on an elastogram (Fig. 2-25). There are two fundamental forms of elastography—**transient elastography** and **shear wave elastography**. With transient elastography, there is no imaging guidance

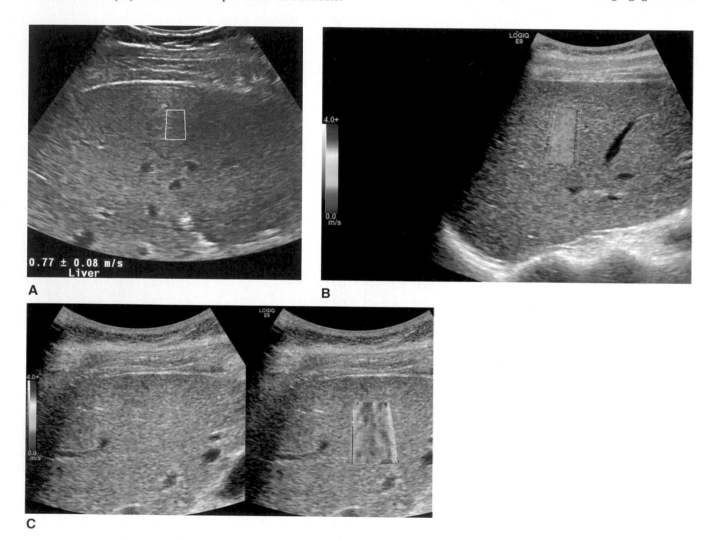

Figure 2-25 Elastography of the liver. **A.** Point shear wave elastogram of a normal liver with proper placement of the region of interest (*ROI*). **B.** The 2D shear wave elastogram uses a larger box and a color map to show areas of normal or abnormal tissue. This is a normal patient because the only color seen is blue. **C.** This patient has areas of red in the ROI, which is compatible with stiff tissue. The red and yellow areas represent areas of stiff tissue. This patient had a cirrhotic liver.

and there are dedicated point-of-care ultrasound devices, such as the FDA-approved FibroScan, that may be utilized as well. Most often, an elastogram of the liver is obtained by a sonographer during a sonogram of the liver utilizing the shear wave elastography application included as part of the ultrasound unit.

> **◀))) SOUND OFF**
> Elastography is used to evaluate the stiffness of the liver. Essentially, the stiffer the liver tissue, the more fibrosis present.

Portal Hypertension

Portal hypertension is the elevation of blood pressure within the portal venous system. The pressure within the portal vein can be altered by several abnormalities. The most common cause of portal hypertension is cirrhosis. However, portal hypertension can also result from portal vein thrombosis, hepatic vein thrombosis, IVC thrombosis, or compression of the portal veins by a tumor in the liver or an adjacent organ.

Recall that normal flow toward the liver within the portal vein is termed hepatopetal. With cirrhosis, the liver becomes fibrotic or scarred and more difficult to perfuse. Consequently, the blood traveling into the liver via the main portal vein meets greater vascular resistance. Therefore, the pressure within the portal veins increases, resulting in portal hypertension. The hepatic artery, which also brings blood into the liver, has to increase its supply as well, and will consequently enlarge. The flow within the portal vein can eventually become reversed—termed hepatofugal (Fig. 2-26). Portosystemic collaterals and varicosities can consequently develop within the abdomen as a result of the body's attempt to repair itself by channeling blood away from the damaged liver (Table 2-6).

> **◀))) SOUND OFF**
> Because the liver becomes so scarred with cirrhosis, the blood flowing to the liver meets greater vascular resistance, resulting in portal hypertension or high blood pressure within the portal veins.

One of the most common sonographically identifiable collaterals in portal hypertension is the recanalization of the paraumbilical vein, also termed a patent paraumbilical vein (Figs. 2-27 and 2-28). The umbilical vein, which is associated with the left portal vein, ligamentum teres, and falciform ligament, becomes open again (as it once was in utero) and shunts blood away from the liver and into the inferior epigastric veins or superior epigastric vein—termed **Cruveilhier–Baumgarten syndrome**.

Abdominal varicosities may be noted near the splenic hilum, renal hilum, and **gastroesophageal**

junction (Fig. 2-29). Furthermore, sonographic evidence of enlargement and reversed flow within the coronary

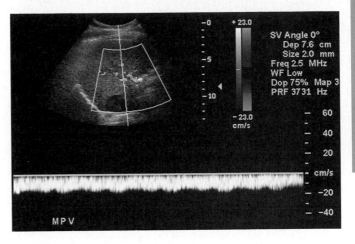

Figure 2-26 Hepatofugal flow. Blood flow is demonstrated away from the liver in the main portal vein with spectral Doppler and color Doppler in the presence of portal hypertension.

TABLE 2-6 Examples of portosystemic collaterals that may result from portal hypertension

1. Coronary vein
2. Short gastric vein
3. Gastrorenal pathway
4. Splenorenal pathway
5. Umbilical vein
6. Anterior abdominal wall vein
7. Superior mesenteric vein

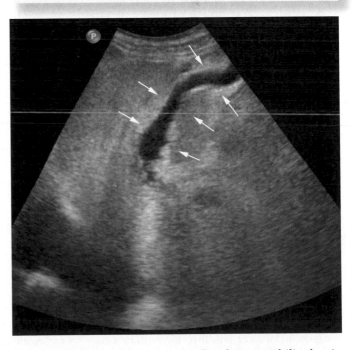

Figure 2-27 A patent or recanalized paraumbilical vein (*arrows*) is noted extended from the left lobe of this patient who is suffering from cirrhosis and portal hypertension.

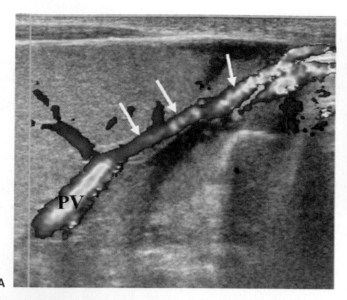
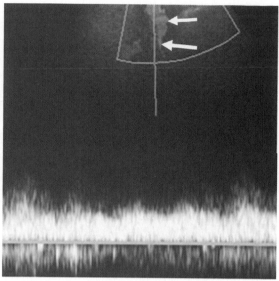

Figure 2-28 A. Recanalized paraumbilical vein (*arrows*) is demonstrated extended from the left portal vein (*PV*) toward the anterior abdominal wall in a patient with portal hypertension. **B.** Pulsed Doppler scan shows hepatofugal flow (away from the liver) in the paraumbilical vein (*arrows*).

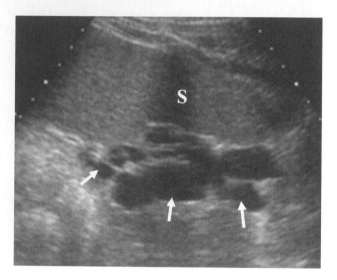

Figure 2-29 In a patient with portal hypertension, splenic varices (*arrows*) are noted adjacent to the spleen (*S*) in the area of the splenic hilum.

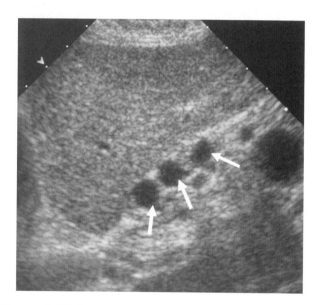

Figure 2-30 Enlarged coronary vein (*arrows*) can be seen posterior to the left lobe in a patient with portal hypertension.

vein, also referred to as the left gastric vein, may be seen with portal hypertension (Fig. 2-30). In some individuals, the normal coronary vein can be seen arising from the splenic vein and extending superiorly toward the left. With portal hypertension, the coronary vein will demonstrate abnormal flow toward the esophagus and will measure greater than 6 mm. Unfortunately, shunting of blood toward the esophagus increases the risk for esophageal hemorrhage and death.

Enlargement of the portal vein with portal hypertension is often apparent, especially prior to collateral development. Along with hepatofugal flow, the portal vein diameter will exceed 13 mm in the anteroposterior dimension, and the superior mesenteric vein will exceed

10 mm. This irregular, and often stagnant flow, increases the patient's likelihood of developing portal vein thrombosis. Essentially, patients with portal hypertension will have many of the same sonographic findings of cirrhosis, including ascites and splenomegaly, with the addition of portal vascular and shunting abnormalities and the development of collateral channels.

◀))) SOUND OFF
With portal hypertension, the portal vein diameter will exceed 13 mm in the anteroposterior dimension, and flow may reverse within the portal vein, which is termed hepatofugal flow.

Clinical features of portal hypertension often mimic cirrhosis. **Hematemesis**, if present, is an ominous sign of ruptured esophageal varices because it markedly increases mortality and morbidity. Other clinical findings of portal hypertension include hepatic encephalopathy, recognizable dilation of the superficial veins of the abdomen (termed caput medusae), and tremors.

Surgical shunts may be placed to reduce the likelihood of complications resulting from portal hypertension. Surgically placed shunts include the portocaval shunt, splenorenal shunt, and mesocaval shunt. A common, minimally invasive interventional treatment for portal hypertension is by means of a **transjugular intrahepatic portosystemic shunt** (TIPS). Although it is only a temporary treatment for portal hypertension, this therapy involves the placement of a stent between the portal veins and hepatic veins to shunt blood and reduce portal systemic pressure. The TIPS is often evaluated for patency with Doppler sonography (see "Liver Doppler, Transjugular Intrahepatic Portosystemic Shunt Evaluation, and Liver Transplant Assessment" section in this chapter).

> **◀))) SOUND OFF**
> If cirrhosis is suspected the sonographer should closely analyze the *left portal vein* for evidence of recanalization of the paraumbilical vein. The recanalized paraumbilical vein will extend from the left portal vein, continue through the left lobe, and may travel inferiorly toward the umbilicus.

CLINICAL FINDINGS OF PORTAL HYPERTENSION

1. Abnormal liver function tests
2. Ascites
3. Diarrhea
4. Fatigue
5. Palpated hepatomegaly (initially)
6. Hepatic encephalopathy
7. Caput medusae
8. Tremors
9. Gastrointestinal bleeding
10. Jaundice

SONOGRAPHIC FINDINGS OF PORTAL HYPERTENSION

1. Hepatomegaly (initially)
2. Shrunken right lobe of the liver
3. Enlarged caudate lobe of the liver
4. Nodular surface irregularity
5. Coarse echotexture
6. Splenomegaly
7. Ascites

8. Monophasic flow within the hepatic veins
9. Hepatofugal flow within the portal veins
10. Enlargement of the portal vein (diameter will exceed 13 mm in the anteroposterior dimension)
11. Enlargement of the superior mesenteric vein
12. Enlargement and reversed flow within the coronary vein
13. Enlarged hepatic arteries
14. Abdominal varicosities at the splenic hilum, renal hilum, and gastroesophageal junction
15. Patent paraumbilical vein (also called a recanalized paraumbilical vein)

Portal Vein Compression and Portal Vein Thrombosis

Portal vein compression, which subsequently leads to portal vein obstruction, is most commonly caused by tumors from adjacent organs or lymphadenopathy. Portal vein thrombosis is the development of clot within the portal vein. Portal vein thrombosis is seen in conditions such as hepatocellular carcinoma, portal hypertension, pancreatitis, cholecystitis, pregnancy, oral contraceptive use, and surgery. Thrombus can completely occlude the portal vein. In this case, the development of collaterals within the portal vein region will occur. These small vessels try to shunt blood around the clot. This results in a mesh of tiny blood vessels in the area of the portal vein, termed cavernous transformation of the portal vein. In addition, as the disease progresses, larger collaterals can develop.

Patients may complain of abdominal pain, low-grade fever, **leukocytosis**, **hypovolemia**, elevated liver function tests, and nausea and vomiting. Initial sonographic evaluation of portal vein thrombus may be difficult because clot can be isoechoic to the surrounding circulating blood. With time, thrombus will become more echogenic and may be more noticeable within the portal vein (Fig. 2-31). The cavernous transformation of the portal veins will appear as wormlike or **serpiginous** vessels within the region of the portal vein (Fig. 2-32). Portal occlusion can also be the result of tumor invasion within the portal vein. Because of the compromise to hepatic blood flow, color Doppler should be used to evaluate the vascularity of liver.

> **◀))) SOUND OFF**
> Cavernous transformation of the portal vein is a sequela of portal vein thrombosis. With cavernous transformation of the portal vein, there will be evidence of multiple serpiginous or tortuous vessels in the region of the porta hepatis.

CLINICAL FINDINGS OF PORTAL VEIN THROMBOSIS

1. Abdominal pain
2. Elevated liver function tests
3. Hypovolemia
4. Leukocytosis
5. Low-grade fever
6. Nausea
7. Vomiting

SONOGRAPHIC FINDINGS OF PORTAL VEIN THROMBOSIS

1. Echogenic thrombus within the portal vein
2. Cavernous transformation of the portal veins will appear as wormlike or serpiginous vessels within the region of the portal vein

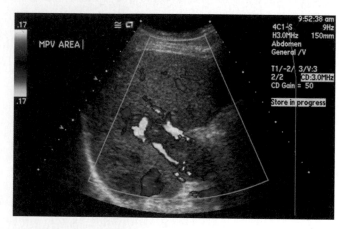

Figure 2-31 Color Doppler image of the main portal vein reveals portal vein thrombosis that is isoechoic to the liver parenchyma.

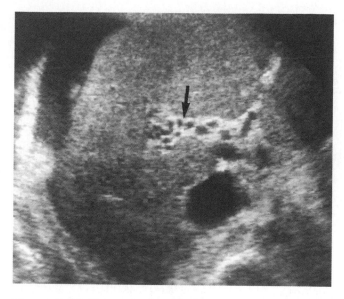

Figure 2-32 Cavernous transformation of the portal vein. Transverse image through the porta hepatis demonstrates multiple, small collateral vessels (*arrow*) in the area of the portal vein.

CLINICAL FINDINGS OF PORTAL VENOUS GAS

1. Recent bout of diverticulitis, appendicitis, inflammatory bowel disease, bowel obstruction, ulcers within the bowel, gastrointestinal cancer, or invasive procedures that involve stent placement (TIPS) or endoscopic analysis of the bowel

SONOGRAPHIC FINDINGS OF PORTAL VENOUS GAS

1. Small, bright reflectors are noted within the circulating blood inside the portal vein.
2. Larger air collections may produce ring-down artifact.

Portal Venous Gas

Gas within the portal veins or mesenteric veins that results from **ischemic bowel disease** is typically fatal. However, portal venous gas may also be associated with diverticulitis, appendicitis, **inflammatory bowel disease**, bowel obstructions, ulcers within the bowel, gastrointestinal cancer, and invasive procedures that involve stent placement or endoscopic analysis of the bowel. The sonographic findings of portal venous gas are consistent with evidence of small, bright reflectors noted within the circulating blood inside the portal vein. Larger air collections may produce ring-down artifact. Care should be taken to not confuse portal venous gas with **pneumobilia**, which is air located within the biliary ducts.

Budd–Chiari Syndrome

Budd–Chiari syndrome is described as the occlusion of the hepatic veins, with possible coexisting occlusion of the IVC (Fig. 2-33). Budd–Chiari syndrome can be seen secondary to a congenital webbing disorder (**inferior vena cava web**), coagulation abnormalities, tumor invasion from HCC, thrombosis, oral contraceptive use, pregnancy, and trauma. Clinical symptoms of this abnormality, when found in female patients on oral contraception, include ascites, right upper quadrant pain, hepatomegaly, and possibly splenomegaly. Other patients may suffer from extensive upper abdominal pain and elevated liver function test. Sonographic findings include the nonvisualization or reduced visualization of

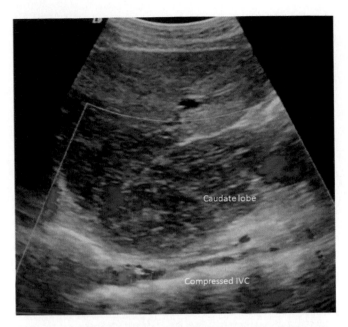

Figure 2-33 Budd–Chiari syndrome. Compression of the inferior vena cava (*IVC*) is noted in this patient with an enlarged heterogenous caudate lobe.

the hepatic veins. Thrombus may be noted within the hepatic veins, the caudate lobe may be enlarged, and color Doppler will often yield evidence of absent flow within the hepatic veins. The IVC may also be narrowed.

CLINICAL FINDINGS OF BUDD–CHIARI SYNDROME

1. Ascites
2. Elevated liver function test
3. Hepatomegaly
4. Splenomegaly
5. Upper abdominal pain

SONOGRAPHIC FINDINGS OF BUDD–CHIARI SYNDROME

1. Nonvisualization or reduced visualization of the hepatic veins
2. Thrombus within the hepatic veins
3. Enlarged caudate lobe
4. Lack of flow within the hepatic veins with color Doppler
5. Narrowing of the IVC

◀)) SOUND OFF
Budd–Chiari syndrome is characterized by occlusion of the hepatic veins and possibly the IVC.

Hepatorenal Syndrome and Liver Failure

Hepatorenal syndrome is the development of renal impairment and possible renal failure as a result of chronic liver disease and liver failure. Consequently, cirrhosis is a common cause of hepatorenal syndrome. In fact, as many as half of patients admitted to the hospital with complications of cirrhosis may be suffering from acute kidney injury because of coexisting hepatorenal syndrome. With hepatorenal syndrome, there is reduced glomerular filtration rate and increased creatinine, though the kidneys may appear normal sonographically. Patients also suffer from nervous system changes and decreased cardiovascular function. Key clinical findings include reduced glomerular filtration rate and an increase in serum creatinine in the presence of cirrhosis or other causes of liver failure. Sonographic findings will be consistent with cirrhosis. The prognosis for individuals with hepatorenal syndrome is poor, with many requiring liver transplantation.

CLINICAL FINDINGS OF HEPATORENAL SYNDROME

1. History of cirrhosis or other cause of liver failure
2. Reduced glomerular filtration rate
3. Increased serum creatinine
4. Decreased urine output

SONOGRAPHIC FINDINGS OF HEPATORENAL SYNDROME

1. Sonographic findings consistent with cirrhosis
2. Kidneys may appear normal.

Focal Liver Disease

Hepatic Cysts

True hepatic cysts are usually not encountered until middle age, and they may be solitary and **idiopathic**. (Fig. 2-34). Hepatic cysts may also be associated with **autosomal dominant polycystic kidney disease** (ADPKD). Clinically, hepatic cysts associated with ADPKD may be asymptomatic and they may not always alter liver function tests. They tend to be multiple, and they may not always conform to the sonographic appearance of a simple cyst because their shape can be somewhat irregular. Clusters of cysts with jagged walls may be noted, which may produce a complex appearance (Fig. 2-35). However, all other simple cyst criteria should be present, including a smooth wall and the presence of posterior acoustic enhancement, and they should be entirely anechoic. Complex hepatic cysts are often caused by hemorrhage and may have internal echoes, thick walls, calcification, or solid components.

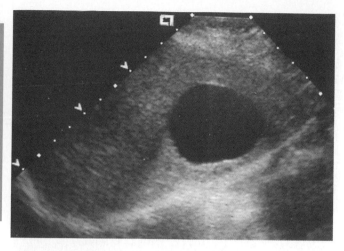

Figure 2-34 Benign hepatic cyst. This liver mass has well-defined borders, is completely anechoic, has thin walls, and demonstrates posterior enhancement.

When pain occurs because of hepatic cysts, it may be caused by hemorrhage, infection, or be secondary to mass effect. Hepatic cysts may also be noted in patients with **von Hippel–Lindau disease**.

CLINICAL FINDINGS OF HEPATIC CYSTS

1. Asymptomatic
2. Possible normal liver function tests
3. ADPKD
4. Hemorrhagic or large cysts may cause right upper quadrant pain.

SONOGRAPHIC FINDINGS OF HEPATIC CYSTS

1. Anechoic mass or masses with posterior enhancement
2. May have irregular shapes
3. Clusters of cysts may be noted

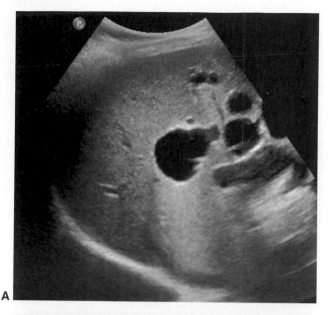

A

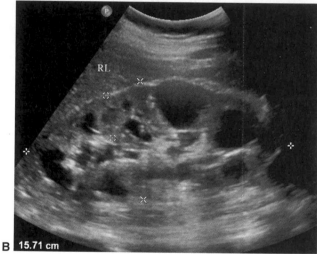

B | 15.71 cm

Figure 2-35 ADPKD cysts. This appearance of hepatic cysts (**A**) is commonly associated with cysts of the kidney affected by ADPKD (**B**). *ADPKD*, autosomal dominant polycystic kidney disease; *RL*, right lobe.

Hydatid Liver Cyst

A **hydatid liver cyst** may also be referred to as an **echinococcal cyst**. These cysts develop most commonly from a parasite referred to as *Echinococcus granulosus*. This parasite is a tapeworm that lives in dog feces. Food, such as vegetables, contaminated by the infected feces is consumed indirectly by sheep, cattle, goat, and possibly humans (Fig. 2-36). Therefore, there is a higher prevalence of hydatid disease in sheep- and cattle-raising countries such as the Middle East, Australia, and the Mediterranean. The parasite moves from the bowel through the portal vein to enter the liver.

Clinically, patients present with a low-grade fever and right upper quadrant tenderness. Other signs and symptoms include nausea, obstructive jaundice, leukocytosis, and a slight raise in alkaline phosphatase. The sonographic appearance is variable. A hydatid cyst may appear as an anechoic mass containing some debris. This debris is referred to as hydatid sand. The cyst is composed of an endocyst, and a pericyst or ectocyst. The endocyst, contained within the pericyst, may disconnect from the pericyst, and its wall may be clearly identified floating within the larger cyst. This has been referred to as the *water lily* sign.

A hydatid cyst may also appear as cyst within a cyst. This has been described as a *mother* cyst containing a *daugther cyst*. This sonographic description is highly specific for hydatid disease (Fig. 2-37). The mass may also contain some elements of dense calcification. Surgical

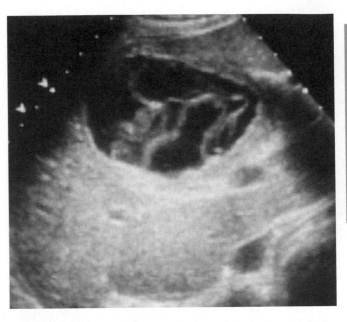

Figure 2-37 Hydatid disease. Transverse image of the liver demonstrates a complex mass containing a detached membrane, which is the typical appearance of a hydatid cyst.

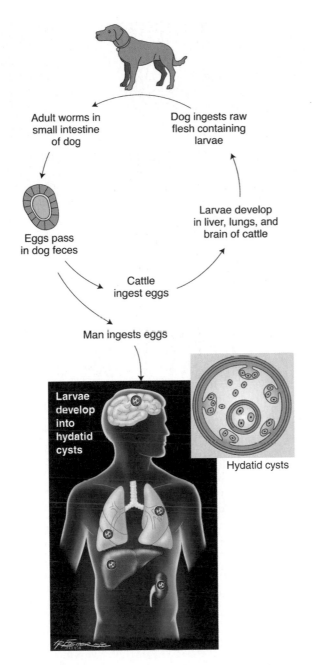

Hydatid cysts

Figure 2-36 Life cycle of an *Echinococcus granulosus*.

resection, catheter drainage, or medical treatment may be used to manage a hydatid liver cyst. Unfortunately, cyst ruptures could lead to anaphylactic shock.

CLINICAL FINDINGS OF A HYDATID LIVER CYST

1. Leukocytosis
2. Low-grade fever
3. Nausea
4. Obstructive jaundice
5. Right upper quadrant tenderness
6. Possible recent travel abroad

SONOGRAPHIC FINDINGS OF A HYDATID LIVER CYST

1. Anechoic mass containing some debris (hydatid sand)
2. *Water lily* sign appears as an endocyst floating within the pericyst
3. *Mother* cyst containing one or more smaller *daughter* cysts
4. Mass may contain some elements of dense calcification

Amebic Hepatic Abscess

An **amebic hepatic abscess** comes from the parasite *Entamoeba histolytica* that grows in the colon and invades the liver via the portal vein. It is typically transmitted through contaminated water found in places such as Mexico, Central America, South America, Asia, India, and Africa. Therefore, patients who present with amebic abscesses may have traveled out of the country recently. Clinical features may be hepatomegaly, right upper quadrant pain, general **malaise**, or signs of **dysentery**, which include bloody diarrhea, abdominal pain, and fever.

Laboratory findings may include leukocytosis, elevated liver function tests, and mild anemia. Like other abscesses, amebic abscesses have variable sonographic appearances. They are typically round, hypoechoic or anechoic, contain debris, and have some acoustic enhancement. Amebic abscesses are most often noted within the right lobe of the liver near the capsule.

They may also be multiple and appear hypoechoic or contain a fluid-debris level (Fig. 2-38). Often, they are indistinguishable sonographically from a **pyogenic liver abscess** and therefore require a serologic confirmation. These masses are typically treated medically, although aspiration may be performed. Complications include rupture or extension into the chest or peritoneal cavity, resulting in a high mortality rate if not treated efficiently.

CLINICAL FINDINGS OF AN AMEBIC HEPATIC ABSCESS

1. Hepatomegaly
2. Right upper quadrant or general abdominal pain
3. General malaise
4. Diarrhea (possibly bloody)
5. Fever
6. Leukocytosis
7. Elevated liver function tests
8. Mild anemia
9. Possible recent travel abroad

SONOGRAPHIC FINDINGS OF AN AMEBIC HEPATIC ABSCESS

1. Round, hypoechoic or anechoic mass or masses
2. May contain debris (with fluid-debris layering)
3. Acoustic enhancement

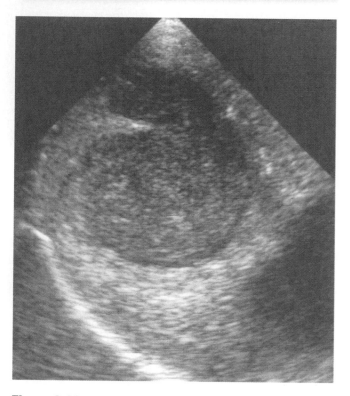

Figure 2-38 Amebic abscess. This amebic abscess appears as a hypoechoic mass surrounded by a hypoechoic wall.

Schistosomiasis

Schistosomiasis is the hepatic infestation of the parasite *schistosoma*. Schistosomiasis is fundamentally a flatworm parasite. It may also be referred to as snail fever or bilharzia. Schistosomiasis is rare in the United States. Though found in many countries, there are varying forms in Africa, the Mediterranean, China, and South America. Schistosomiasis is said to be one of the most common causes of hepatic fibrosis in the world. The disease is transmitted in contaminated water that contains certain types of snails that release the parasites. The parasites can then penetrate the skin of individuals as they bathe or utilize the water for other purposes. The eggs of the worms can travel to the liver, intestines, lungs, and bladder. Clinical findings include fever, hepatomegaly, abdominal pain, and diarrhea that may contain blood. Sonographic findings include evidence of periportal thickening and possibly bull's-eye lesions that have an anechoic center surrounded by a hyperechoic rim. In the case of chronic schistosomiasis, there may be evidence of the *turtleback* sign, which is calcified septa and fibrosis resembling the rounded part of a turtle's shell.

CLINICAL FINDINGS OF SCHISTOSOMIASIS

1. Fever
2. Hepatomegaly
3. Abdominal pain
4. Diarrhea (may contain blood)

SONOGRAPHIC FINDINGS OF SCHISTOSOMIASIS

1. *Bull's-eye* lesion
2. Anechoic center surrounded by hyperechoic ring
3. Periportal thickening
4. *Turtleback* sign (chronic appearance)

Pyogenic Hepatic Abscess

A pyogenic hepatic abscess can result from the spread of infection from inflammatory conditions such as appendicitis, diverticulitis, cholecystitis, cholangitis, or endocarditis. The bacteria enter the liver through the portal vein, hepatic artery, or biliary tree or from an operative procedure. Clinical symptoms of a pyogenic abscess include fever, leukocytosis, possible abnormal liver function tests, right upper quadrant pain, and hepatomegaly. The sonographic findings of a hepatic abscess are variable (Fig. 2-39). It may appear as a complex cyst with thick walls. It may also contain debris, septations, and/or gas. The gas (air) within the abscess may produce dirty shadowing or ring-down artifact.

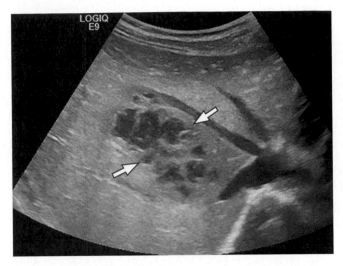

Figure 2-39 Pyogenic abscess. Transverse image of the liver containing a complex mass with indistinct borders (between *arrows*).

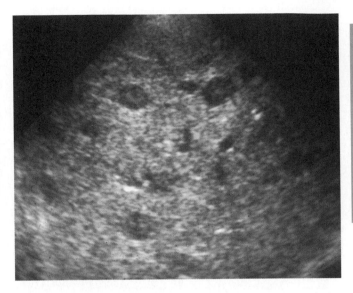

Figure 2-40 Candidiasis. This transverse image of the liver demonstrates multiple hypoechoic lesions that appear as small bull's-eyes scattered throughout the organ.

CLINICAL FINDINGS OF A PYOGENIC HEPATIC ABSCESS

1. Fever
2. Hepatomegaly
3. Leukocytosis
4. Possible abnormal liver function tests
5. Right upper quadrant pain

CLINICAL FINDINGS OF HEPATIC CANDIDIASIS

1. Immunocompromised patients including cancer patients, recent organ transplant patients, and patients with human immunodeficiency virus
2. Right upper quadrant pain
3. Fever
4. Hepatomegaly

SONOGRAPHIC FINDINGS OF A PYOGENIC HEPATIC ABSCESS

1. Complex cyst with thick walls
2. Mass may contain debris, septations, and/or gas.
3. The air within the abscess may produce dirty shadowing or ring-down artifact.

SONOGRAPHIC FINDINGS OF HEPATIC CANDIDIASIS

1. Multiple masses with hyperechoic central portions and hypoechoic borders (may be described as *target, halo,* or *bull's-eye* lesions)
2. These masses are typically 1 cm or smaller in size.
3. Older lesions may calcify.

Hepatic Candidiasis

Hepatic candidiasis results from the spread of fungus, namely *Candida albicans,* in the blood to the liver. Those who are prone to developing hepatic candidiasis are typically **immunocompromised** in some way. For example, cancer patients, recent organ transplant patients, and those with human immunodeficiency virus are more prone to develop this type of fungal abscess within their liver. Besides being immunocompromised, patients may have right upper quadrant pain, fever, and hepatomegaly. Sonographic findings include multiple hyperechoic (central portion) masses with hypoechoic borders. These masses may be described as *target, halo,* or *bull's-eye* lesions and are typically 1 cm or smaller in size (Fig. 2-40). Older lesions may calcify.

Cavernous Hemangioma

The most common benign liver tumor is the **cavernous hemangioma**. Although they can be found in men, they are more commonly discovered in women. Hepatic hemangiomas are usually incidentally detected and asymptomatic. The most common location of the cavernous hemangioma is within the right lobe of the liver. They characteristically appear as a small, hyperechoic mass measuring less than 3 cm, although some may be quite large and are referred to as giant hemangiomas (Fig. 2-41). Occasionally, posterior enhancement may be seen. Although hemangiomas are comprised of blood vessels, detectable flow may not be seen with color Doppler because the flow within the

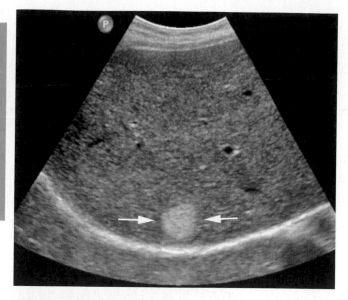

Figure 2-41 Cavernous hemangioma. A hyperechoic mass (*arrows*) is noted within the right lobe of the liver.

vessels tends to be exceedingly slow. Unfortunately, hemangiomas may occasionally appear hypoechoic or complex, and therefore they can be sonographically indistinguishable from metastatic liver disease. There may also be multiple hemangiomas present, further complicating the sonographic diagnosis and consequently leading to other imaging or biopsy.

> 🔊 **SOUND OFF**
> The cavernous hemangioma is the most common benign liver mass. It is most often found in women in the right hepatic lobe.

CLINICAL FINDINGS OF A CAVERNOUS HEMANGIOMA

1. Asymptomatic

SONOGRAPHIC FINDINGS OF A CAVERNOUS HEMANGIOMA

1. Small, hyperechoic mass
2. Most often found in the right lobe

Focal Nodular Hyperplasia

Focal nodular hyperplasia (FNH) has been cited as the second most common benign liver tumor and more commonly incidentally discovered in women. The mass is composed of a combination of hepatocytes

and fibrous tissue. Patients who have FNH are most often asymptomatic, but if the mass impinges upon surrounding anatomy or if hemorrhage occurs, pain will most likely ensue. Although the mass is not caused by oral contraceptive use, it may enlarge because of oral contraceptive use as a result of estrogen exposure.

> 🔊 **SOUND OFF**
> Although FNH is not caused by oral contraceptive use, the mass tends to be estrogen-dependent and, thus, can grow as a result of oral contraceptive use.

Sonographically, FNH may have varying sonographic appearances, including isoechoic, echogenic, and hypoechoic (Fig. 2-42). It typically contains a central stellate (star-like) scar that is not always detected with sonography but is readily identified with CT and MRI. The central scar, when seen, will appear as a hypoechoic or hyperechoic, linear structure within the mass. Hypervascularity within the scar can be identified by using color Doppler. FNH has been referred to as a *stealth lesion* because it may be difficult to identify secondary to its slight sonographic disparity from normal liver parenchyma.

CLINICAL FINDINGS OF FOCAL NODULAR HYPERPLASIA

1. Asymptomatic

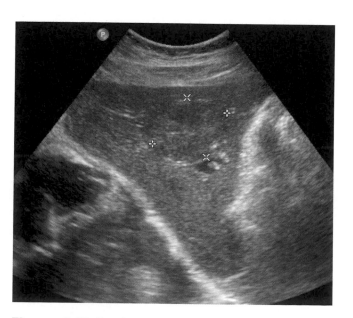

Figure 2-42 Focal nodular hyperplasia. An isoechoic mass (between *calipers*) is noted within the left lobe of the liver.

SONOGRAPHIC FINDINGS OF FOCAL NODULAR HYPERPLASIA

1. Isoechoic, hyperechoic, or hypoechoic mass
2. Central scar may appear as hyperechoic or hypoechoic linear structure within the mass and will often reveal hypervascularity with color Doppler.

SOUND OFF
FNH often contains a central stellate scar and may be referred to as a *stealth lesion* because it may not be readily identifiable sonographically.

Hepatocellular Adenoma

The **hepatocellular adenoma**, which may also be referred to as a hepatic adenoma or liver cell adenoma, is a rare benign liver tumor. It is often associated with the use of oral contraceptives. Patients are typically asymptomatic though hemorrhage of the tumor will often to abdominal pain. Because of hemorrhage, and a small propensity to become malignant (termed **malignant degeneration**), hepatic adenomas are often surgically removed. There may be multiple adenomas present at the time of discovery. The sonographic appearance of a hepatic adenoma is variable, and although a solid, hypoechoic echogenicity is common, they may be hyperechoic, isoechoic, or have mixed echogenicities (Fig. 2-43).

SOUND OFF
Hepatic adenomas can be caused by oral contraceptive use.

CLINICAL FINDINGS OF A HEPATOCELLULAR ADENOMA

1. Asymptomatic
2. Oral contraceptive use
3. Pain occurs with hemorrhage

SONOGRAPHIC FINDINGS OF A HEPATOCELLULAR ADENOMA

1. Mostly hypoechoic
2. May be hyperechoic, isoechoic, or be comprised of mixed echogenicities

Hepatic Lipoma

The hepatic **lipoma** is rarely encountered. Patients are asymptomatic, and its sonographic appearance is that of a hyperechoic mass.

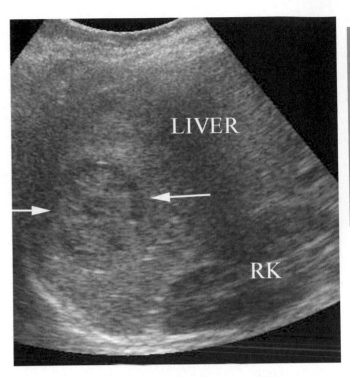

Figure 2-43 Hepatic adenoma. This well-circumscribed mass (between *arrows*) is a hepatic adenoma located within the right lobe of the liver, superior to the right kidney (*RK*).

CLINICAL FINDINGS OF HEPATIC LIPOMA

1. Asymptomatic

SONOGRAPHIC FINDINGS OF HEPATIC LIPOMA

1. Hyperechoic mass

Hepatic Hematoma

A hepatic **hematoma** can be a consequence of trauma or surgery. Patients will have pain and a decreased hematocrit. Hematomas can be located within the liver parenchyma, termed intrahepatic, or around the liver, which is termed subcapsular (under Glisson capsule). Hematomas can appear solid or complex depending on their age. Initial hemorrhage appears echogenic with the development of clot, and over time as it resolves, it may appear more cystic or complex. Focal hematomas have been known to calcify as well. Therefore, in the acute stage, an intrahepatic hematoma adjacent to the liver may be difficult to visualize with sonography because it may be isoechoic to the normal hepatic tissue. When the subcapsular hematoma is anechoic, it may appear similar to ascites surrounding the liver (Fig. 2-44).

Following trauma to the liver, an abnormal passageway between an artery and vein—termed **arteriovenous fistula**—can result. Arteriovenous fistulas may also be

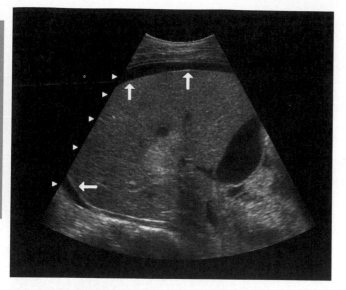

Figure 2-44 This older hematoma (*arrows*) has become anechoic. Fresh hematomas may appear isoechoic to normal liver tissue.

discovered following a liver biopsy, cholangiography, or hepatic surgery. Multiple anechoic spaces will be noted in the area of the fistula, and color Doppler can be used to prove that the mass is vascular in origin. Flow is typically from the higher-pressure arterial system to the venous system. Color Doppler will yield turbulent high-velocity flow within the connection.

CLINICAL FINDINGS OF HEPATIC HEMATOMA

1. Trauma
2. Recent surgery
3. Pain
4. Decreased hematocrit

SONOGRAPHIC FINDINGS OF HEPATIC HEMATOMA

1. Fresh clot may appear hyperechoic.
2. Older hemorrhage can appear anechoic or complex.
3. May be intrahepatic or subcapsular
4. Assess for signs of an arteriovenous fistula

Liver Cancer

Hepatocellular Carcinoma

HCC is the most common primary form of liver cancer. It is important to note that HCC it is not encountered as often as metastatic liver disease. HCC is most often seen in men and frequently accompanied by cirrhosis or chronic hepatitis. The malignant mass associated with HCC is referred to as a hepatoma. Other causes

include hemochromatosis, von Gierke disease, and Wilson disease. Hepatomas can invade the portal veins or hepatic veins. Occlusion of the hepatic veins, with possible tumor invasion into the IVC, is termed Budd–Chiari syndrome, and thus the sonographic evaluation of pertinent vasculature is warranted for evidence of tumor thrombus. Color Doppler may yield evidence of hypervascularity within the mass, although this is not a specific indicator for malignancy.

Clinically, patients with HCC will have possible abnormal liver function tests, signs of cirrhosis, history of chronic hepatitis, unexplained weight loss, hepatomegaly, fever, abdominal swelling with ascites, and perhaps a palpable mass. A tumor marker for HCC is serum alpha-fetoprotein (AFP). In the fetus, AFP is produced in large amounts by the liver, whereas in the adult, low levels of AFP exist. Most patients with HCC will have an elevated AFP. This occurs because AFP is produced in excess by the malignant hepatocytes that make up the tumor.

The sonographic findings of HCC are unpredictable. There may be an individual mass or multiple masses present at the time of diagnosis. HCC may appear as a solitary, small, hypoechoic mass, or as heterogeneous masses scattered throughout the liver (Fig. 2-45). A hypoechoic halo may be noted around the hepatoma as well, yielding the *target* or *bull's-eye* pattern. The target lesion will yield a hypoechoic rim, with the center of the mass often isoechoic to normal liver tissue.

🔊 SOUND OFF
The tumor marker for hepatocellular carcinoma is AFP.

CLINICAL FINDINGS OF HEPATOCELLULAR CARCINOMA

1. Elevated AFP
2. Abnormal liver function tests (possibly)
3. Cirrhosis
4. Chronic hepatitis
5. Unexplained weight loss
6. Hepatomegaly
7. Fever
8. Palpable mass
9. Abdominal swelling with ascites

SONOGRAPHIC FINDINGS OF HEPATOCELLULAR CARCINOMA

1. Solitary, hypoechoic mass
2. Heterogeneous masses scattered throughout the liver
3. Mass with a hypoechoic halo and central echogenic portion (*target* or *bull's-eye* lesion)
4. Possible ascites

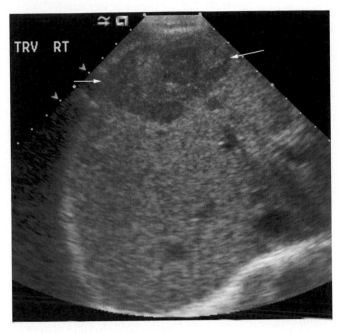

Figure 2-45 Hepatoma. This solid, hypoechoic mass (between *arrows*) was found to be hepatocellular carcinoma.

Hepatic Metastasis

The liver is a common location for metastatic disease to manifest in the abdomen. Metastatic liver disease is the most common form of liver cancer. Because it is much more common than primary liver cancer (cancer that starts in the liver). The malignant cells from other sites enter the liver through the portal veins or lymphatic channels. Primary cancers that metastasize to the liver include the gallbladder, colon, stomach, pancreas, breast, and lung, with the latter being the most common primary source. Patients with hepatic metastasis may present with weight loss, jaundice, right upper quadrant pain, hepatomegaly, and ascites. However, in about half of patients, there are no clinical signs or symptoms, including the possibility of normal liver function tests initially.

The sonographic findings of metastatic liver disease are variable, often depending on the location of the primary cancer. Metastatic cancer from the gastrointestinal tract and pancreas tends to be calcified tumors. Hyperechoic masses tend to arise from the gastrointestinal tract as well, most commonly the colon, but they may also be from the kidney, pancreas, or biliary tree. Hypoechoic masses may be from the breast, lung, or lymphoma. Cystic metastatic masses within the liver have also been seen with ovarian cancers. Metastatic disease in the liver can appear as an individual mass, several large masses, or diffuse involvement (Figs. 2-46 and 2-47). Target lesions are also common with metastasis and may be the expression of lung or colon metastasis within the liver, although they may be the manifestation of many forms of cancer. Diffuse metastasis can produce an appearance of

a nodular liver—termed **pseudocirrhosis**. Thus, a high-frequency linear transducer can be employed when surface irregularity is suspected to identify smaller lesions.

> 🔊 **SOUND OFF**
> Although HCC is the most common *primary* form of liver cancer—meaning that it develops in the liver—the *most common* cancer discovered in the liver is metastasis from some other primary location.

CLINICAL FINDINGS OF HEPATIC METASTASIS

1. Abnormal liver function test (possibly)
2. Weight loss
3. Jaundice
4. Right upper quadrant pain
5. Hepatomegaly
6. Abdominal swelling with ascites

SONOGRAPHIC FINDINGS OF HEPATIC METASTASIS

1. Hyperechoic, hypoechoic, calcified, cystic, or heterogeneous masses
2. Mass or masses demonstrating a hypoechoic rim and central echogenic region
3. Diffusely heterogeneous liver
4. Possible ascites

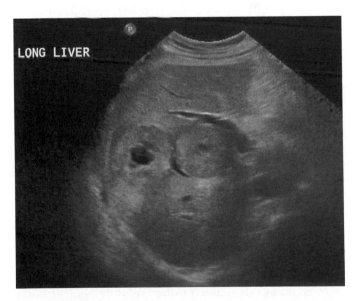

Figure 2-46 Metastatic liver disease. These masses were found in a patient with metastatic liver disease originating in the rectum.

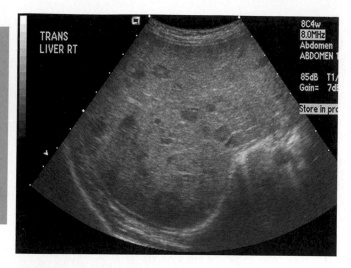

Figure 2-47 Pediatric metastatic liver disease. This image is of a 1-year-old patient with metastatic liver disease originating in the adrenal gland as a neuroblastoma.

LIVER DOPPLER, TRANSJUGULAR INTRAHEPATIC PORTOSYSTEMIC SHUNT EVALUATION, AND LIVER TRANSPLANT ASSESSMENT

Doppler assessment of the liver can be performed using both color Doppler and spectral Doppler. Normal flow within the portal veins should be hepatopetal, continuous, monophasic, and have low velocity—typically between 20 and 40 cm per second (see Fig. 2-6). Some variation of flow may be seen with variations in breathing. Because of their close association with left atrium, the hepatic veins typically demonstrate a triphasic flow pattern (see Fig. 2-8). Flow assessment should be obtained at the end of respiration if possible because deep inspiration may result in blunting or complete loss of hepatic vein pulsatility. The hepatic artery should demonstrate a continuous, low-resistance waveform pattern, with a quick upstroke, and gradual deceleration with diastole (see Fig. 2-9). The normal resistive index of the hepatic artery is said to be between 0.5 and 0.8.

◀))) SOUND OFF
Normal flow within the portal veins should be hepatopetal, continuous, monophasic, and have low velocity, whereas the hepatic veins are triphasic.

In patients with advanced cirrhosis and portal hypertension, a TIPS stent may be inserted via the jugular vein and ultimately placed between a hepatic vein and intrahepatic portion of the portal vein (Fig. 2-48). Most often, the shunt is created between the right portal vein and the right hepatic vein and a bridging stent is left in place. This procedure reduces the amount of blood flow to the liver by rerouting the blood coming from the portal vein to the hepatic vein, ultimately sending the blood back to the heart. The primary goal of TIPS is to prevent the rupture and hemorrhage of gastroesophageal and other varices, an occurrence that is often fatal.

Sonographically, TIPS appears as a highly echogenic tube within the liver (Fig. 2-49). The sonographer may be asked to perform both preoperative and postoperative imaging, including a liver Doppler evaluation. For pre-TIPS assessment, care should be taken to analyze each vascular structure for evidence of abnormal flow patterns and thrombosis. Postoperative imaging of TIPS should include an evaluation of the shunt for patency throughout (Fig. 2-50). A baseline study, including Doppler interrogation, is vital to establish the patient's individualized standard. It may be noted that flow within the right and left portal veins typically reverses after stent placement. The normal flow velocity within the shunt ranges between 90 and 190 cm per second. The signs of TIPS failure include signs of thrombus within the shunt, stenosis of the shunt, stenosis of the hepatic vein, reversal of intrahepatic flow, flow void next to the shunt, reversal of hepatic venous flow, drop in shunt velocity between examinations, and abnormally high or low shunt velocity (Fig. 2-51).

◀))) SOUND OFF
TIPS is typically located between the right portal vein and the right hepatic vein.

The sonographer may be called upon to analyze a liver transplant. Recall that hepatitis C is the most common disease requiring a liver transplant, closely followed by alcoholic liver disease and cirrhosis. Although techniques may vary, typically the transplanted liver is attached end to end to the native portal vein and hepatic artery—termed **anastomosis**—and a *piggy back* attachment is made between the donor and recipient IVC (Fig. 2-52). With sonography, a liver transplant should appear similar to a normal native liver. All vasculature, including the portal veins, hepatic veins, hepatic artery, and IVC, should be evaluated with color and spectral Doppler, should appear patent and have normal waveforms.

Although often with acute rejection the liver appears normal, suspicion should arise when the liver appears diffusely heterogeneous. Hepatic artery thrombosis is the most common vascular complication of a liver transplant (Fig. 2-53). When hepatic artery thrombosis is suspected, the sonographer should closely evaluate the liver for signs of infarction, which appears as hypoechoic wedge-shaped area scattered throughout the periphery of the liver. Other complications include biliary strictures, cholangitis, biliary sludge and stones, hepatic artery stenosis, a hepatic artery

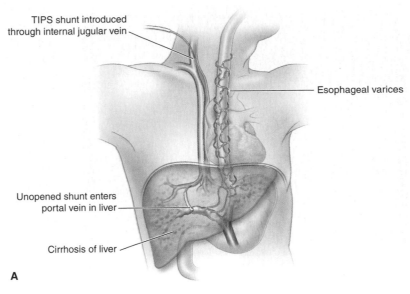

TIPS shunt introduced through internal jugular vein

Esophageal varices

Unopened shunt enters portal vein in liver

Cirrhosis of liver

A

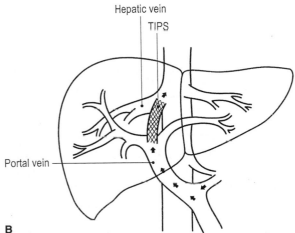

Hepatic vein
TIPS
Portal vein

B

Figure 2-48 Transjugular intrahepatic portosystemic shunt (*TIPS*) placement. **A.** The TIPS is placed between the hepatic vein and portal vein. **B.** Normal flow through the shunt allows blood to be directed from the portal vein into the hepatic vein.

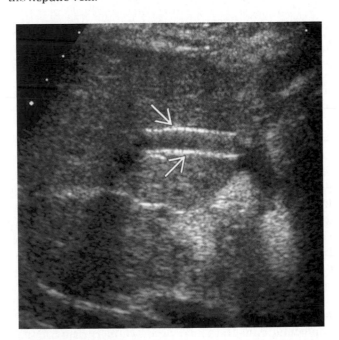

Figure 2-49 *TIPS* sonographic appearance. The wall of the TIPS appears highly echogenic. *TIPS*, transjugular intrahepatic portosystemic shunt.

pseudoaneurysm, celiac artery stenosis, portal vein stenosis and thrombosis, and fluid collections, including ascites, a hematoma, **biloma**, and abscess. If present, stenoses, strictures, and pseudoaneurysms are often discovered at the anastomotic site.

PEDIATRIC LIVER PATHOLOGY

Infantile Hemangioendothelioma

Infantile hemangioendothelioma is the most common benign liver childhood tumor. These masses are typically identified in the first few weeks or months of life, because they may cause hepatomegaly or be accompanied by hemangiomas of the skin. The sonographic findings of these masses are variable.

CLINICAL FINDINGS OF INFANTILE HEMANGIOENDOTHELIOMA

1. Pediatric patient
2. May cause hepatomegaly
3. May be accompanied by hemangiomas of the skin

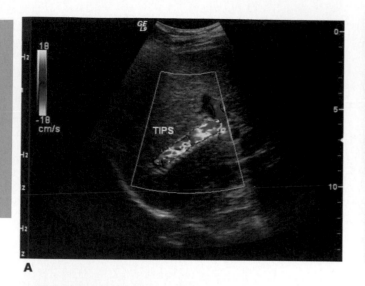
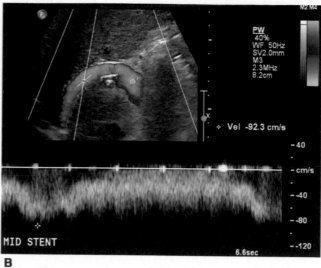

Figure 2-50 *TIPS* with color. **A.** Color image of a normal TIPS. **B.** Spectral waveform of a normal TIPS. *TIPS*, transjugular intrahepatic portosystemic shunt.

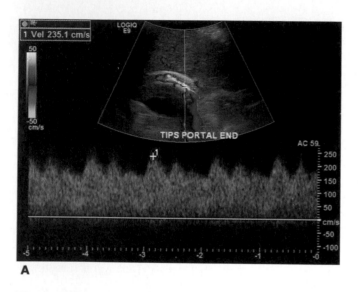
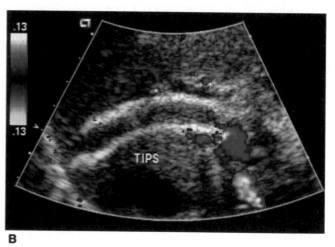

Figure 2-51 *TIPS* failure. **A.** This stenotic TIPS is yielding an elevated velocity of 235 cm/s. **B.** This shunt lacks color-flow filling, and echogenic material (thrombus) can be noted within the shunt. *TIPS*, transjugular intrahepatic portosystemic shunt.

SONOGRAPHIC FINDINGS OF INFANTILE HEMANGIOENDOTHELIOMA

1. Homogeneous or complex hepatic mass
2. May contain calcification or cystic spaces

Hepatoblastoma

Hepatoblastoma is a malignant pediatric liver tumor. It has been cited as the most common malignant tumor of childhood. These aggressive tumors are most often discovered before the age of 5 years, with half of the cases identified in children less than 2 years old. There is a high incidence of hepatoblastoma in children who have **Beckwith–Wiedemann syndrome**. Like liver carcinoma in adults, hepatoblastomas will often cause an elevation in AFP. These tumors can invade surrounding vasculature and may also obstruct the biliary tree. Clinically, these young patients may be asymptomatic or present with hepatomegaly and/or a palpable abdominal mass. They may also suffer from jaundice, abdominal pain, weight loss, and anorexia. The sonographic findings of a hepatoblastoma are that of a solid, hyperechoic, or heterogeneous mass. This mass may also contain calcifications.

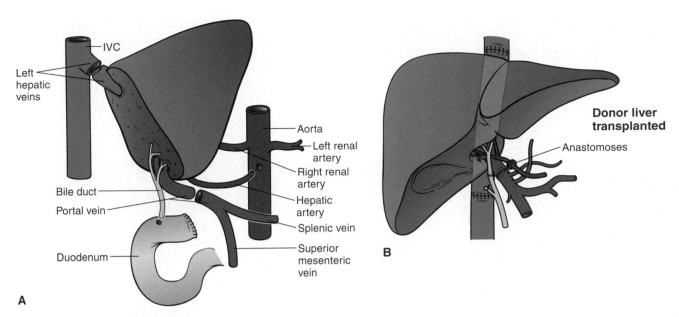

Figure 2-52 Partial and complete liver transplant. **A.** Living-donor left lateral liver transplant anastomoses: end-to-end anastomosis of the portal veins and hepatic arteries, end-to-side anastomosis between the donor inferior vena cava and common stump of the recipient hepatic veins, and biliary duct to small bowel (hepaticojejunostomy). **B.** Whole-liver transplant anastomoses: end-to-end anastomosis of hepatic arteries and portal veins, piggy back anastomosis between the donor and recipient inferior vena cava, and end-to-end biliary duct anastomosis. *IVC*, inferior vena cava.

CLINICAL FINDINGS OF HEPATOBLASTOMA

1. Pediatric patient
2. May be asymptomatic
3. Palpable abdominal mass
4. Hepatomegaly
5. Abdominal pain
6. Weight loss
7. Anorexia
8. Elevated AFP
9. Jaundice

SONOGRAPHIC FINDINGS OF HEPATOBLASTOMA

1. Solid, hyperechoic, or heterogeneous mass
2. Mass may contain some calcifications

🔊 SOUND OFF
Children with Beckwith–Wiedemann syndrome are often screened with sonography for the early detection of hepatoblastomas.

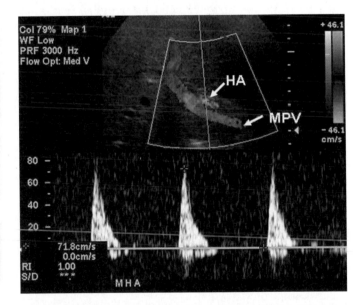

Figure 2-53 Hepatic artery thrombosis. Duplex Doppler image of the main hepatic artery (*HA*) immediately posttransplantation procedure demonstrating complete absence of diastolic flow and with a RI = 1.0. MPV, main portal vein

CONTRAST-ENHANCED ULTRASOUND OF THE LIVER

There are limitations of gray-scale sonography for the identification of masses within a fatty or cirrhotic liver. Some hepatic masses may not be seen without the use of **contrast-enhanced (liver) ultrasound** (CEUS). CEUS utilizes a contrast agent that is injected into the patient intravenously in order to aid in the identification of liver lesions and to assess those lesions for signs of malignancy. The contrast agent contains microbubbles of gas that have a lipid or protein shell. The microbubbles are smaller than red blood cells and are thus allowed to move into the capillaries. The contrast agent travels to the liver and aids in the delineation of masses.

The liver is assessed during phases, including the initial arterial and early portal venous phases and the later phase of contrast *washout*. Contrast can also predict whether a mass is likely malignant, with some researchers finding that contrast-enhanced ultrasound can have a 95% specificity for determining whether a mass is benign (Fig. 2-54). Within a matter of minutes, scanning is complete, and the gas is released through the respiratory tract of the patient, with little to no side effects. Contrast agents can be used for pediatric imaging of the liver as well.

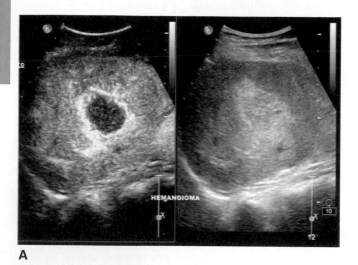

A

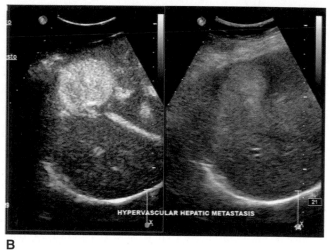

B

Figure 2-54 Contrast-enhanced sonography. **A.** Contrast-enhanced ultrasound of the liver demonstrates a benign cavernous hemangioma. **B.** Contrast-enhanced ultrasound of the liver in another patient reveals a hypervascular metastatic liver lesion.

REVIEW QUESTIONS

1. The patient in Figure 2-55 presented with right upper quadrant pain and elevated AFP. What is the most likely diagnosis?
   a. Hepatic hematoma
   b. Hemangioma
   c. Hepatoma
   d. Focal nodular hyperplasia

2. Which of the following benign liver masses is typically isoechoic and contains a central scar?
   a. Hepatoblastoma
   b. Cavernous hemangioma
   c. Hamartoma
   d. Focal nodular hyperplasia

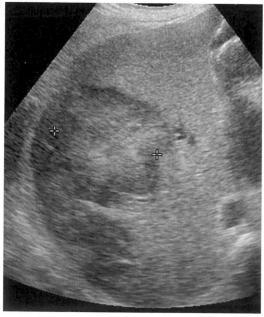

Figure 2-55

3. The covering of the liver is referred to as:
   a. Glisson capsule.
   b. Gerota fascia.
   c. Morison pouch.
   d. hepatic fascia.

4. The left lobe of the liver can be separated from the right lobe by the:
   a. right hepatic vein.
   b. middle hepatic vein.
   c. left hepatic vein.
   d. falciform ligament.

5. The TIPS shunt is placed:
   a. between the main hepatic artery and main portal vein.
   b. between a portal vein and hepatic vein.
   c. between the common hepatic duct and common bile duct.
   d. between a portal vein and hepatic artery.

6. Which of the following is the likely diagnosis for the patient in Figure 2-56?
   a. Hepatitis
   b. Hepatic steatosis
   c. Cirrhosis
   d. Steatohepatitis

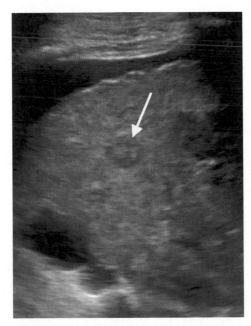

Figure 2-56

7. What is the arrow in Figure 2-56 most likely indicating?
   a. Metastatic liver disease
   b. Hemangioma
   c. Amebic hepatic abscess
   d. Hepatoma

8. The right lobe of the liver is divided into segments by the:
   a. middle lobar fissure.
   b. middle hepatic vein.
   c. right hepatic vein.
   d. left hepatic vein.

9. The right intersegmental fissure contains the:
   a. right hepatic vein.
   b. middle hepatic vein.
   c. left portal vein.
   d. right portal vein.

10. The main portal vein divides into:
    a. middle, left, and right branches.
    b. left and right branches.
    c. anterior and posterior branches.
    d. medial and lateral branches.

11. Which of the following is the patient suffering from in Figure 2-57?
    a. Hepatopetal flow with hepatitis
    b. Hepatofugal flow with hepatitis
    c. Hepatopetal flow with portal hypertension
    d. Hepatofugal flow with portal hypertension

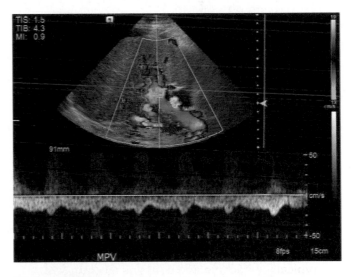

Figure 2-57

12. What is the normal velocity range of the structure being analyzed with the sample gate in Figure 2-57?
    a. 20 to 40 cm per second
    b. 90 to 100 cm per second
    c. 0.5 to 0.8 cm per second
    d. 1.2 to 1.3 cm per second

13. The ligamentum teres can be used to separate the:
    a. medial and lateral segments of the left lobe.
    b. medial and posterior segments of the right lobe.
    c. anterior and medial segments of the left lobe.
    d. anterior and posterior segments of the right lobe.

14. The main lobar fissure contains the:
    a. right hepatic vein.
    b. middle hepatic vein.
    c. main portal vein.
    d. right portal vein.

15. All of the following are located within the porta hepatis except:
    a. main portal vein.
    b. common bile duct.
    c. hepatic artery.
    d. middle hepatic vein.

16. Right-sided heart failure often leads to enlargement of the:
    a. abdominal aorta.
    b. IVC and hepatic veins.
    c. IVC and portal veins.
    d. portal veins and spleen.

17. The mass noted by the arrow in Figure 2-58 was discovered in an asymptomatic 22-year-old female patient. What is the most likely diagnosis?
    a. Focal nodular hyperplasia
    b. Fibroma
    c. Cavernous hemangioma
    d. Lipoma

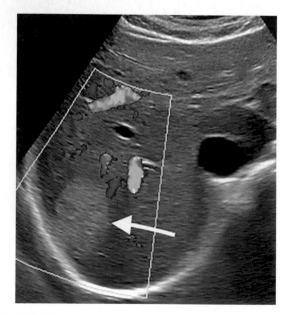

Figure 2-58

18. Which of the following is typically transmitted through contaminated water found in places such as Mexico, Central America, South America, Asia, India, and Africa?
    a. Amebic liver abscess
    b. Hydatid liver cyst
    c. Candidiasis
    d. Hepatoma

19. The right portal vein divides into:
    a. middle, left, and right branches.
    b. left and right branches.
    c. anterior and posterior branches.
    d. medial and lateral branches.

20. The diameter of the portal vein should not exceed:
    a. 4 mm.
    b. 8 mm.
    c. 10 mm.
    d. 13 mm.

21. The right lobe of the liver can be divided into:
    a. medial and lateral segments.
    b. medial and posterior segments.
    c. anterior and medial segments.
    d. anterior and posterior segments.

22. Which of the following is true about the portal veins?
    a. Portal veins carry deoxygenated blood away from the liver.
    b. Portal veins have brighter walls than the hepatic veins.
    c. Portal veins should demonstrate hepatofugal flow.
    d. Portal veins increase in diameter as they approach the diaphragm.

23. The left lobe of the liver can be divided into:
    a. medial and lateral segments.
    b. medial and posterior segments.
    c. anterior and medial segments.
    d. anterior and posterior segments.

24. Normal flow within the hepatic artery should demonstrate a:
    a. high-resistance waveform pattern, with a slow upstroke, and gradual deceleration with diastole.
    b. low-resistance waveform pattern, with a quick upstroke, and gradual deceleration with diastole.
    c. low-resistance waveform pattern, with a slow upstroke, and gradual acceleration with diastole.
    d. high-resistance waveform patter, with a quick upstroke, and gradual deceleration with diastole.

25. The patient in Figure 2-59 would be most likely suffering from:
    a. cirrhosis.
    b. portal hypertension.
    c. autosomal dominant polycystic kidney disease.
    d. *Echinococcus granulosis.*

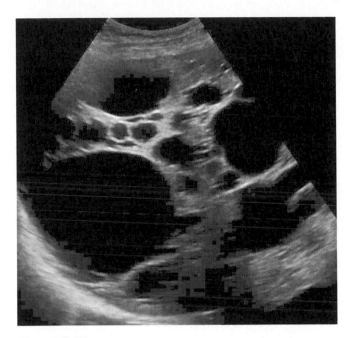

Figure 2-59

26. Budd–Chiari syndrome leads to a reduction in the size of the:
    a. hepatic arteries.
    b. portal veins.
    c. hepatic veins.
    d. common bile duct.

27. A tongue-like extension of the right lobe of the liver is termed:
    a. papillary lobe.
    b. focal hepatomegaly.
    c. Riedel lobe.
    d. Morison lobe.

28. The left portal vein divides into:
    a. middle, left, and right branches.
    b. left and right branches.
    c. anterior and posterior branches.
    d. medial and lateral branches.

29. The left umbilical vein after birth becomes the:
    a. falciform ligament.
    b. main lobar fissure.
    c. ligamentum teres.
    d. ligamentum venosum.

30. Normal flow within the hepatic veins is said to be:
    a. biphasic.
    b. irregular.
    c. high resistant.
    d. triphasic.

31. The inferior extension of the caudate lobe is referred to as:
    a. papillary process.
    b. focal hepatomegaly.
    c. Riedel process.
    d. Morison lobe.

32. The patient in Figure 2-60 has other sonographic findings including splenomegaly and hepatofugal flow within the main portal vein. What are the three unlabeled arrows in this image identifying?
    a. Irregular superior mesenteric artery
    b. Esophageal varices
    c. Splenic varices
    d. Atrophic coronary artery

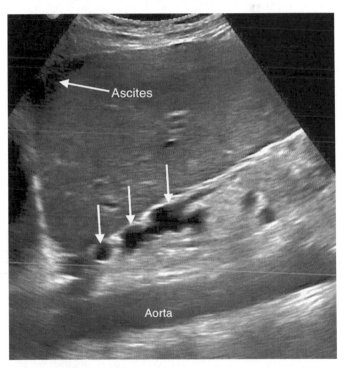

Figure 2-60

33. What other sonographic findings would also most likely be evident in the patient with Figure 2-60?
    a. Periportal cuffing
    b. *Water lily* sign
    c. Subcapsular hematoma
    d. Shrunken right lobe

34. The patient in Figure 2-60 would least likely be suffering from which of the following clinical findings?
    a. Hepatic encephalopathy
    b. Narrowing of the hepatic veins
    c. Caput medusa
    d. Tremors

35. Which of the following is the most common reason for a liver transplant?
    a. Hepatocellular carcinoma
    b. Hepatitis C
    c. Hepatitis B
    d. Hepatic metastasis

36. Clinical findings of fatty infiltration of the liver include:
    a. elevated liver function labs.
    b. fever.
    c. fatigue.
    d. weight loss.

37. Shortly after birth, the ductus venosus collapses and becomes the:
    a. falciform ligament.
    b. main lobar fissure.
    c. ligamentum teres.
    d. ligamentum venosum.

38. Sonographically, when the liver is difficult to penetrate and diffusely echogenic, this is indicative of:
    a. portal vein thrombosis.
    b. metastatic liver disease.
    c. primary liver carcinoma.
    d. fatty liver disease.

39. The most common cause of cirrhosis is:
    a. portal hypertension.
    b. hepatitis.
    c. alcoholism.
    d. cholangitis.

40. Clinical findings of hepatitis include all of the following except:
    a. jaundice.
    b. fever.
    c. chills.
    d. pericholecystic fluid.

41. What form of hepatic abnormality are immunocompromised patients more prone to develop?
    a. Hepatic adenoma
    b. Amebic abscess
    c. Hydatid liver abscess
    d. Candidiasis

42. All of the following are sequela of cirrhosis except:
    a. portal vein thrombosis.
    b. hepatic artery contraction.
    c. portal hypertension.
    d. splenomegaly.

43. Normal flow toward the liver in the portal veins is termed:
    a. hepatopetal.
    b. hepatofugal.

44. Which of the following masses would be most worrisome for malignancy?
    a. Echogenic mass
    b. Cystic mass with posterior enhancement
    c. Isoechoic mass with a central scar
    d. Hyperechoic mass with a hypoechoic halo

45. Which of the following statements is true of hepatic adenomas?
    a. Hepatic adenomas are more common in males.
    b. Hepatic adenomas are also referred to as a *stealth lesion*.
    c. Hepatic adenomas typically contain air owing to bacterial formation.
    d. Hepatic adenomas can undergo malignant degeneration.

46. Which of the following is the most common cancer found in the liver?
    a. Hepatocellular carcinoma
    b. Adenocarcinoma
    c. Metastatic liver disease
    d. Hepatoblastoma

47. Which hepatic mass is closely associated with oral contraceptive use?
    a. Hepatic adenoma
    b. Hepatic hypernephroma
    c. Hepatic hamartoma
    d. Hepatic hemangioma

48. Which of the following is considered the most common benign childhood hepatic mass?
    a. Hepatoblastoma
    b. Hepatoma
    c. Hematoma
    d. Hemangioendothelioma

49. All of the following are clinical findings of hepatocellular carcinoma except:
    a. reduction in AFP.
    b. unexplained weight loss.
    c. fever.
    d. cirrhosis.

50. The childhood syndrome Beckwith–Wiedemann is associated with an increased risk for developing:
    a. hepatoblastoma.
    b. cirrhosis.
    c. portal hypertension.
    d. hepatitis.

51. Which of the following is associated with *E. granulosus*?
    a. Candidiasis
    b. Amebic liver abscess
    c. Hydatid liver cyst
    d. Hepatocellular carcinoma

52. Which of the following laboratory findings would be most likely associated with a decrease in albumin?
    a. Hepatic steatosis
    b. Hepatic steatohepatitis
    c. Cirrhosis
    d. Hepatitis

53. Which of the following are the cells of the liver responsible for engulfing pathogens and damaged cells?
    a. Kupffer
    b. Morrison
    c. Hepatocytes
    d. Epstein

54. What liver pathology is associated with periportal cuffing?
    a. Candidiasis
    b. Amebic hepatic abscess
    c. Steatosis
    d. Hepatitis

55. Which of the following is an inherited disease characterized by disproportionate absorption of dietary iron?
    a. Wilson disease
    b. Hemochromatosis
    c. von Gierke syndrome
    d. von Hippel–Lindau disease

56. What inherited disease is linked with the development of cysts in the liver and other organs?
    a. von Gierke disease
    b. Wilson disease
    c. Epstein–Barr disease
    d. von Hippel–Lindau disease

57. Wilson disease will present sonographic similar to what disorder?
    a. Hepatitis
    b. Portal hypertension
    c. Budd–Chiari syndrome
    d. Focal fatty infiltration

58. Cavernous transformation of the portal vein is found in the presence of:
    a. portal venous gas.
    b. portal vein thrombosis.
    c. autosomal dominant polycystic liver disease.
    d. multiple hydatid liver cysts.

59. Which of the following hepatic lesions may occur following a recent bout of appendicitis, diverticulitis, or cholecystitis?
    a. Focal nodular hyperplasia
    b. Pyogenic hepatic abscess
    c. Echinococcal abscess
    d. Amebic liver abscess

60. The patient in Figure 2-61 is a 5-year-old female patient who presented with increased abdominal girth. What is the most likely etiology of this mass?
    a. Hematoma
    b. Pyogenic liver abscess
    c. Hepatoblastoma
    d. Hepatoma

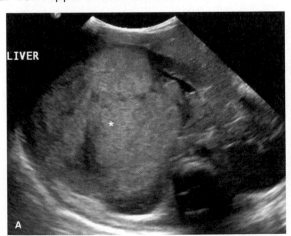
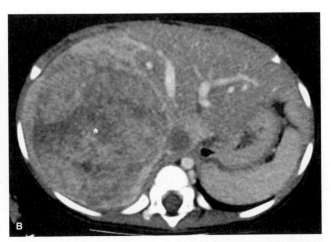

Figure 2-61

The Liver

SUGGESTED READINGS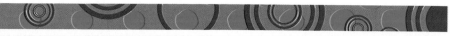

Curry RA, Prince M. *Sonography: Introduction to Normal Structure and Function*. 5th ed. Elsevier; 2021:113–128 & 167–186.

El-Ali A, Davis JC, Cickelli JM, Squires JH. Contrast-enhanced ultrasound of liver lesions in children. *Pediatr Radiol*. 2019;49(11):1422–1432.

Fargo MV, Grogan SP, Saguil A. Evaluation of jaundice in adults. *Am Fam Physician*. 2017;95(3):164–168.

Federle MP, Jeffrey RB, Woodward PJ, et al. *Diagnostic Imaging: Abdomen*. 2nd ed. Amirsys; 2010:III-1-2–III-1-168.

Ginès P, Solà E, Angeli P, Wong F, Nadim MK, Kamath PS. Hepatorenal syndrome. *Nat Rev Dis Primers*. 2018;4(1):23.

Henningsen C, Kuntz K, Youngs D. *Clinical Guide to Sonography: Exercises for Critical Thinking*. 2nd ed. Elsevier; 2014:8–39.

Hertzberg BS, Middleton WD. *Ultrasound: The Requisites*. 3rd ed. Elsevier; 2016:51–88.

Kawamura DM, Nolan TD. *Diagnostic Medical Sonography: Abdomen and Superficial Structures*. 4th ed. Wolters Kluwer; 2018:101–170 & 739–756.

Krawczyk M, Bonfrate L, Portincasa P. Nonalcoholic fatty liver disease. *Best Pract Res*. 2010;24(5):695–708.

Kupinski AM. *Diagnostic Medical Sonography: The Vascular System*. Lippincott Williams & Wilkins; 2013:333–373.

Kwo PY, Cohen SM, Lim JK. ACG clinical guideline: evaluation of abnormal liver chemistries. *Am J Gastroenterol*. 2017;112(1):18–35.

Liao Y, Yeh C, Huang K, Tsui P, Yang K. Metabolic characteristics of a novel ultrasound quantitative diagnostic index for nonalcoholic fatty liver disease. *Sci Rep*. 2019;9:7922.

McCann C, Penny SM. Focal nodular hyperplasia: case study, imaging, and treatment. *J Diagn Med Sonogr*. 2013;29(1):17–23.

Pang JXQ, Zimmer S, Niu S, et al. Liver stiffness by transient elastography predicts liver-related complications and mortality in patients with chronic liver disease. *PLoS One*. 2014;9(4):e95776.

Penny SM. Alcoholic liver disease. *Radiol Technol*. 2013;84(6):577–592.

Riestra-Candelaria BL, Rodríguez-Mojica W, Vázquez-Quiñones LE, et al. Ultrasound accu-racy of liver length measurement with cadaveric specimens. *J Diagn Med Sonogr*. 2016;32(1):12–19.

Rumack CM, Wilson SR, Charboneau JW, et al. *Diagnostic Ultrasound*. 4th ed. Elsevier; 2011:78–145, 639–707, 1800–1843.

Sanders RC, Hall-Terracciano B. *Clinical Sonography: A Practical Guide*. 5th ed. Wolters Kluwer; 2016:436–451, 525–545.

Scheiber IF, Brůha R, Dušek P. Pathogenesis of Wilson disease. In: Członkowska A, Schilsky ML, eds. *Handbook of Clinical Neurology*. Vol 142. 3rd series. Elsevier; 2017:43–55. doi:10.1016/B978-0-444-63625-6.00005-7

Siegel MJ. *Pediatric Sonography*. 5th ed. Wolters Kluwer; 2019:211–272.

Tan EC, Tai MS, Chan W, Mahadeva S. Association between non-alcoholic fatty liver disease evaluated by transient elastography with extracranial carotid atherosclerosis in a multiethnic Asian community. *JGH Open*. 2019;3:117–125.

Utako P, Emyoo T, Anothaisintawee T, Yamashiki N, Thakkinstian A, Sobhonslidsuk A. Clinical outcomes after liver transplantation for hepatorenal syndrome: a systematic review and meta-analysis. *BioMed Res Int*. 2018;2018:5362810.

Metastasis on Computed Tomography (Fig. 2-62)

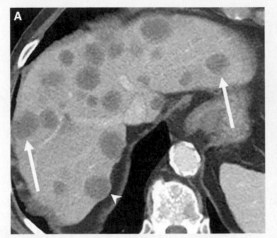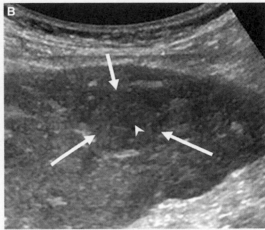

Figure 2-62 **A.** Computed tomography (*CT*) with IV contrast enhancement in the portal venous phase demonstrates the typical appearance of metastases with multiple low-attenuation masses scattered throughout the liver (*arrows*), some of which distort the normal parenchymal architecture (*arrowhead*). **B.** Sonogram of the same patient demonstrating a solid hypoechoic mass (*arrow*) with a central region of lower echogenicity (*arrowhead*) offering a somewhat target appearance.

Cirrhosis on Computed Tomography and MRI (Fig. 2-63)

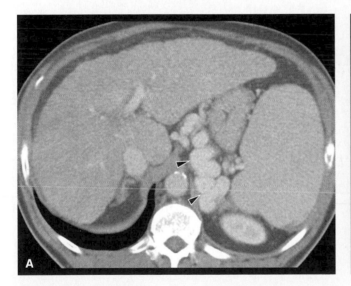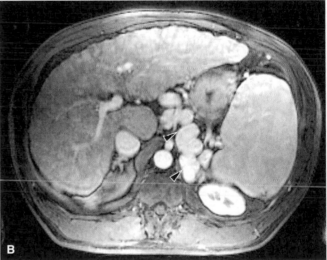

Figure 2-63 Cirrhosis with portosystemic collateral veins. Axial enhanced soft tissue window setting CT **(A)** and axial enhanced T1-weighted fat-suppressed MR **(B)** images show nodularity of the hepatic contour with hypertrophy of the caudate and left hepatic lobes. Splenomegaly and portosystemic collateral veins (*arrowheads*) are indicative of portal venous hypertension.

3

The Gallbladder

Introduction

Sonography is often the initial imaging modality of choice for the identification of biliary disease. Therefore, patients who present with clinical signs and symptoms suggesting biliary disease must be systematically examined by the sonographer. This chapter reviews anatomy, physiology, and pathology of the gallbladder. In the "Bonus Review" section, images of a hepatobiliary iminodiacetic acid scan (HIDA), cholecystostomy procedure, and computed tomography of cholecystitis are provided.

Key Terms

acalculous cholecystitis—the inflammation of the gallbladder without associated gallstones

acute cholecystitis—the sudden onset of gallbladder inflammation

adenomyomatosis—benign hyperplasia of the gallbladder wall

"ball-on-the-wall" sign—when a polyp appears to be a round object, like a ball, that is stuck to the gallbladder wall

biliary colic—pain located in the right upper quadrant in the area of the gallbladder

champagne sign—the effect of dirty shadowing, reverberation, or ring-down artifact caused by gas or gas bubbles produced by bacteria within the nondependent (typically anterior) gallbladder wall

cholecystectomy—the surgical removal of the gallbladder

cholecystokinin—the hormone produced by the duodenum that causes the gallbladder to contract

choledocholithiasis—the presence of a gallstone or gallstones within the biliary tree

cholelithiasis—gallstone(s)

cholesterolosis—a condition that results from the disturbance in cholesterol metabolism and accumulation of

cholesterol typically within a focal region of the gallbladder wall; may be diffuse and referred to as a strawberry gallbladder

chronic cholecystitis—cholecystitis that results from the intermittent obstruction of the cystic duct by gallstones

chyme—partially digested food from the stomach

comet-tail artifact—artifact caused by several small, highly reflective interfaces

Courvoisier gallbladder—the clinical detection of an enlarged, palpable gallbladder caused by a biliary obstruction in the area of the pancreatic head; typically caused by a pancreatic head mass

Crohn disease—chronic inflammatory bowel disease that leads to thickening and scarring of the bowel walls, leading to chronic pain and recurrent bowel obstructions

cystic duct—the duct that connects the gallbladder to the common hepatic duct

duplication of the gallbladder—having two gallbladders that are often, but not always, paired with their own cystic ducts

emphysematous—abnormal distention of an organ with air or gas

empyema—the presence or collection of pus

floating gallbladder—a gallbladder that is highly mobile and thus prone to torsion

gallbladder torsion—the twisting of the vascular supply to the gallbladder

Hartmann pouch—an outpouching of the gallbladder neck

hemolytic anemia—a condition that results in the destruction of red blood cells

hepatization of the gallbladder—situation in which the gallbladder is completely filled with tumefactive sludge, causing the gallbladder to appear isoechoic to the liver tissue

hydropic gallbladder—an enlarged gallbladder; also referred to as mucocele of the gallbladder

hyperalimentation—the intravenous administration of nutrients and vitamins

hyperplastic cholecystosis—a group of proliferative and degenerative gallbladder disorders, which includes both adenomyomatosis and cholesterolosis

hypoalbuminemia—abnormal low level of albumin in the blood; albumin is a protein produced in the liver

intercostal sonographic imaging—performing sonographic imaging between the ribs

interposition of the gallbladder—rare anomaly of the biliary tree where the main hepatic ducts drain directly into the gallbladder and the gallbladder drains directly into the common bile duct; may lead to childhood jaundice, enlarged gallbladder, and intermittent abdominal pain

intrahepatic gallbladder—a gallbladder that is completely surrounded by the hepatic parenchyma

junctional fold—a fold in the neck of the gallbladder

Kawasaki disease—a condition associated with vasculitis and can affect the lymph node, skin, and mucous membranes; also referred to as mucocutaneous lymph node syndrome

leukocytosis—an elevated white blood cell count

Murphy sign—pain directly over the gallbladder with applied probe pressure

parity—the total number of completed pregnancies that have reached the age of viability

pericholecystic fluid—fluid around the gallbladder

peritonitis—inflammation of the peritoneal lining

Phrygian cap—gallbladder variant when the gallbladder fundus is folded onto itself

porcelain gallbladder—the calcification of all or part of the gallbladder wall

postprandial—after a meal

Rokitansky–Aschoff sinuses—tiny pockets within the gallbladder wall

sepsis—a life-threatening condition caused by the body's response to a systemic infection; also referred to as blood poisoning; results in a number of issues including low blood pressure, rapid heart beat, and fever

septate gallbladder—a gallbladder that has one or more septa within its lumen; a gallbladder with several septa; may be referred to as a multiseptate gallbladder

sequela—an illness resulting from another disease, trauma, or injury

sickle cell disease—form of hemolytic anemia typically found in Africans or people of African descent; characterized by dysfunctional sickle-shaped red blood cells

spiral valves of Heister—folds located within the cystic duct that prevent it from collapsing and distending

suppurative cholecystitis—complication of acute cholecystitis characterized by pus accumulation within the gallbladder

total parenteral nutrition—the feeding of a person intravenously

tumefactive sludge—thick sludge

wall–echo–shadow sign—shadowing from the gallbladder fossa produced by a gallbladder that is completely filled with gallstones

whirlpool sign—the sonographic sign of gallbladder torsion when color Doppler is applied to the spiraled, twisted cystic artery

xanthogranulomatous cholecystitis—rare chronic gallbladder infection characterized by intramural accumulation of inflammatory cells; noted sonographically as asymmetrical thickening of the gallbladder wall and intraluminal echogenic debris

ANATOMY AND PHYSIOLOGY OF THE GALLBLADDER

The gallbladder, which is located posterior to the right lobe of the liver within the gallbladder fossa, is considered an intraperitoneal organ. Although the location of the gallbladder relies on the position of the patient, a useful landmark to locate the gallbladder fossa is the main lobar fissure (see Fig. 2-14). This pear-shaped sac is used to store and concentrate bile that is produced by the liver. It has three distinct layers within its walls. The mucosal layer is the innermost layer. It consists of multiple folds and rugae. The middle layer of the wall is the fibromuscular layer, whereas the outer is the serosal layer.

The gallbladder has a neck, body, and fundus. The neck is contiguous with the **cystic duct**, which connects the gallbladder to the rest of the biliary system at the level of the common hepatic duct. The portion of the biliary tree that lies distal to the union of the cystic duct with the hepatic duct is the common bile duct. The fundus is the most dependent portion of the gallbladder and, therefore, is a common location for gallstones, also referred to as **cholelithiasis**, to collect.

> **◀)) SOUND OFF**
> The most common location of gallstones is in the fundus because it is the most dependent part of the gallbladder.

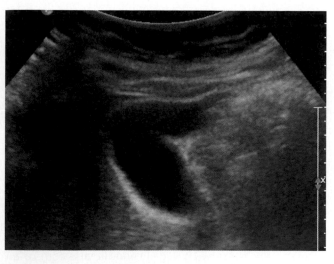

Figure 3-1 Longitudinal image of the gallbladder yielding evidence of a Phrygian cap.

Blood supply to the gallbladder is via the cystic artery, typically a small branch of the right hepatic artery. As **chyme** leaves the stomach, the hormone **cholecystokinin** is released by the enteroendocrine cells of the duodenum, causing the gallbladder to contract. Bile consequently flows from the gallbladder through the cystic duct and into the common bile duct. Although the most common variant in gallbladder shape is the **Phrygian cap** (Fig. 3-1), other variants may be noted (Table 3-1). Other positional and developmental anomalies of the gallbladder include **interposition of the gallbladder**, **duplication of the gallbladder**, **floating gallbladder**, septate gallbladder, agenesis of the gallbladder, and hypoplasia. Although the occurrence is rare, the floating variant does have potential for twisting of the blood supply, resulting in a condition termed **gallbladder torsion** or gallbladder volvulus, in which the patient will present with right upper quadrant pain and a sonographic finding referred to as the **"whirlpool" sign**, which is the spiral appearance of the cystic artery when color Doppler is applied. The gallbladder can also be located on the left side, midline, or right lower quadrant. A gallbladder that is totally surrounded by the hepatic parenchyma is termed an **intrahepatic gallbladder**.

SONOGRAPHY OF THE GALLBLADDER

A gallbladder sonogram should be performed after the patient has had nothing to eat for at least 4 hours, although a period of 8 hours is optimal. The normal gallbladder appears sonographically as an anechoic, pear-shaped structure in the sagittal plane (Fig. 3-2). A true transverse image of the gallbladder will typically yield an anechoic circle. It is helpful in most situations to scan at the level of the main lobar fissure and right portal vein to find the gallbladder. The size of gallbladder is variable, although the normal ranges are said to be 8 to 10 cm in length and no more than 4 to 5 cm in diameter. Most authors agree that a gallbladder that measures over 4 cm in transverse should evoke special scrutiny of the biliary tract for signs of obstruction. A gallbladder volume can be obtained by using the formula: $V = 0.523$ $(L \times W \times H)$. It normally holds around 40 ml of bile, but varies slightly per individual.

The gallbladder should be evaluated in the supine, left lateral decubitus, prone, upright, and any other position needed to demonstrate the mobility—or lack of mobility—of any apparent intraluminal objects like gallstones or polyps (Fig. 3-3). **Intercostal sonographic imaging** should be employed, especially if midline visualization is obstructed by overlying bowel gas.

The gallbladder neck and fundus should be examined closely because these locations are common sites for gallstones to become lodged or to accumulate. The gallbladder wall, which can be focally or diffusely thickened, should measure no more than 3 mm (Tables 3-2 and 3-3). There are several causes of nonvisualization of the gallbladder, with the most obvious being a previous **cholecystectomy** (Table 3-4). Occasionally, patients are poor historians and are unclear if they have had a laparoscopic cholecystectomy. Clarification may

TABLE 3-1 Normal variants of the gallbladder	
Normal Variants in Gallbladder Shape	**Sonographic Description**
Bilobed gallbladder	Hourglass appearance
Septate gallbladder	Appears as thin separations within the gallbladder
Phrygian cap (most common variant)	Gallbladder fundus is folded onto itself (Fig. 3-1)
Hartmann pouch	Outpouching of gallbladder neck
Junctional fold	Prominent fold located at the junction of the gallbladder neck

The Gallbladder

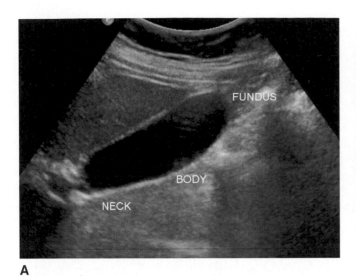

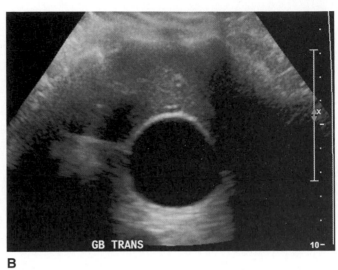

Figure 3-2 Sonographic images of the normal gallbladder. **A.** Longitudinal gallbladder. The distal fundus is more bulbous, whereas the neck is the narrowest portion. **B.** Transverse mid-gallbladder at the body with a normal-appearing wall.

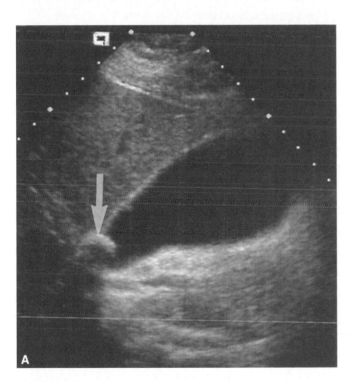

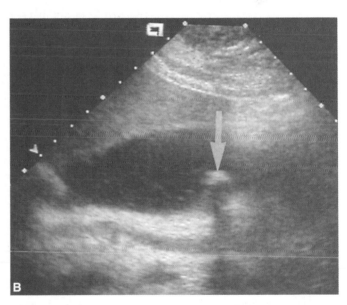

Figure 3-3 Rolling gallstone. **A.** The patient is in the supine position, and the gallstone (*arrow*) is located within the neck of the gallbladder. **B.** The patient has been rolled into the left lateral decubitus position, and the gallstone (*arrow*) moves into the fundus of the gallbladder.

be obtained by simply noting evidence of superficial abdominal scars (Fig. 3-4). It is important to note that patients who have had a recent cholecystectomy may have some residual fluid located within the gallbladder fossa. Right upper quadrant sonography may also be needed to further assess these patients for residual **choledocholithiasis** or postoperative complications, such as those associated with a laparoscopically injured hepatic artery or common bile duct.

When clinical findings and sonographic findings found in this chapter are consistent with gallbladder disease, the sonographer should closely evaluate the liver, other parts of the biliary tree, and pancreas for additional complications such as intrahepatic and extrahepatic biliary tree obstruction and pancreatitis. Helpful labs to evaluate in the presence of suspected gallbladder disease include alkaline phosphatase (ALP), alanine aminotransferase (ALT),

TABLE 3-2 Sources of diffuse gallbladder wall thickening

Postprandial
Acute cholecystitis
Chronic cholecystitis
Adenomyomatosis
Hepatic dysfunction (e.g., hepatitis, cirrhosis)
Benign ascites
Hypoalbuminemia
AIDS cholangiopathy
Congestive heart failure
Gallbladder carcinoma

TABLE 3-3 Sources of focal gallbladder wall thickening

Gallbladder polyp
Adenomyomatosis
Gallbladder carcinoma
Adhered gallstone

TABLE 3-4 Causes of nonvisualization of the gallbladder

Cholecystectomy
Gallbladder completely filled with stones (**wall–echo–shadow sign** or WES sign)
Postprandial
Chronic cholecystitis (collapse and fibrosis of the gallbladder)
Ectopic location
Agenesis
Hepatization of the gallbladder (caused by **tumefactive sludge**)
Air-filled gallbladder or **emphysematous** cholecystitis

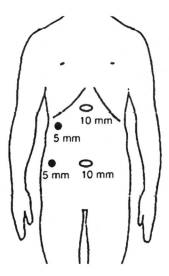

Figure 3-4 Typical location of abdominal scars following a laparoscopic cholecystectomy. If the patient is unclear about past cholecystectomy and a gallbladder is not visualized, assess the patient for signs of abdominal scars in these locations.

GALLBLADDER PATHOLOGY

Cholelithiasis

Biliary stones that form within the gallbladder are called gallstones, or cholelithiasis. Gallstones typically consist of a mixture of cholesterol, calcium bilirubinate, and calcium carbonate. Cholelithiasis formation has been associated with many risk factors and predisposing conditions (Table 3-5). Gallstones are more commonly seen in female patients. Moreover, patients who are fat, female, fertile, flatulent, fair, and forty—the six F's—have been shown to have higher incidence of gallstones. Gallstones have been found in children, newborns, and the fetus. Pediatric patients who have **hemolytic anemia**, such as **sickle cell disease**, and patients with **Crohn disease** have an increased risk for developing gallstones.

Clinically, patients who have gallstones may be asymptomatic. But because gallstones are mobile, **biliary colic** can occur, as well as other biliary tree complications. Chapter 3 will provide more details concerning biliary tree

TABLE 3-5 Risk factors and predisposing conditions for cholelithiasis

Obesity
Pregnancy
Increased **parity**
Gestational diabetes
Estrogen therapy
Oral contraceptive use
Rapid weight loss programs
Hemolytic disorder
Crohn disease
Total parenteral nutrition

bilirubin, gamma-glutamyltransferase (GGT), lactate dehydrogenase (LDH), and white blood cell count (WBC). Among this list, ALT, ALP, and bilirubin may be most beneficial for determining evidence of gallbladder and bile duct disease.

◀))) SOUND OFF
ALT, ALP, and bilirubin may be most beneficial for determining evidence of gallbladder and bile duct disease.

pathology. (Fig. 3-5). Other clinical findings of gallstones include abdominal pain after fatty meals, epigastric pain, nausea and vomiting, and pain that radiates to the shoulders. Sonographically, a cholelithiasis appears as a mobile, echogenic structure within the gallbladder lumen that produces an acoustic shadow (Fig. 3-6). A gallbladder that is completely filled with gallstones may exhibit the wall–echo–shadow (WES) sign. In this situation, only the gallbladder wall and shadowing from the gallbladder fossa are observable (Fig. 3-7). It is important to note that tiny folds within the cystic duct, the **spiral valves of Heister**, can also produce a posterior shadow, and therefore, small gallstones may be suspected. Changing the patient position and altering scanning planes can often resolve this dilemma. Small gallstones may become adhered to the gallbladder wall and may also not produce a well-defined acoustic shadow. The twinkle artifact—which occurs posterior to a strong, granular, and irregular surface like crystals, calculi, or calcifications—may be used to identify a small gallstone in the neck of the gallbladder or perhaps to differentiate an adhered, small gallstone from a gallbladder polyp (Fig. 3-8).

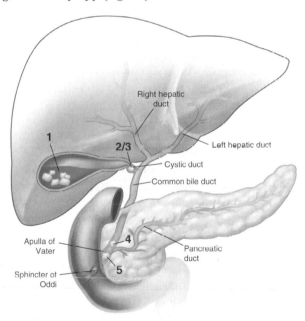

Figure 3-5 Biliary tree complications as a result of cholelithiasis. A patient may have simple cholelithiasis (1), with gallstones located in the gallbladder, but not causing obstruction. Biliary colic (2) is pain in the area of the gallbladder. It may occur after a fatty meal when the gallbladder contracts and pushes bile and stones into the cystic duct. Bile duct spasm and swelling causes irritation and waves of pain. The stone may return to the gallbladder lumen and pain may subside. Cholecystitis (3) occurs when the stone causes sustained obstruction of the cystic duct, resulting in acute inflammation of the gallbladder wall. Choledocholithiasis (4) are gallstones located in the bile ducts. Cholangitis (5) is inflammation of the bile ducts that can occur when gallstones become lodged in the ampulla of Vater.

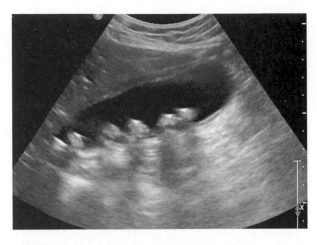

Figure 3-6 Cholelithiasis. Multiple shadowing, echogenic gallstones are noted within this gallbladder.

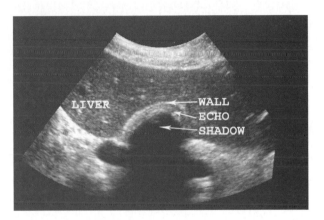

Figure 3-7 *WES* sign. Sonogram of the liver and gallbladder fossa reveals the WES sign which denotes a gallbladder that is completely filled with gallstones. *WES*, wall–echo–shadow.

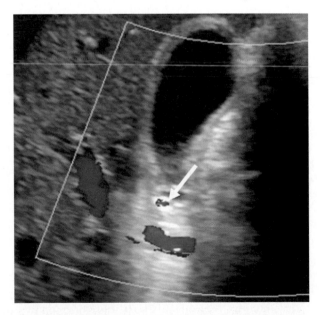

Figure 3-8 Twinkle sign. Color Doppler demonstrates a small gallstone producing the twinkle artifact (*arrow*).

CLINICAL FINDINGS OF CHOLELITHIASIS

1. Asymptomatic
2. Biliary colic
3. Abdominal pain after fatty meals
4. Epigastric pain
5. Nausea and vomiting
6. Pain that radiates to the shoulders

SONOGRAPHIC FINDINGS OF CHOLELITHIASIS

1. Echogenic, mobile, shadowing structure(s) within the lumen of the gallbladder
2. Stones that lodge within the cystic duct or neck of the gallbladder may not move
3. WES sign may be present (gallbladder completely filled with stones)

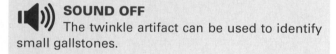

SOUND OFF

The twinkle artifact can be used to identify small gallstones.

Gallbladder Sludge

Sludge, or viscid bile, within the gallbladder is most often associated with biliary stasis. Sludge may be found in patients who have coexisting gallstones or gallbladder carcinoma and in those suffering from jaundice, liver disease, **hyperalimentation**, or **sepsis**. In addition, patients who have undergone an extended period of fasting or are on **total parenteral nutrition** may have gallbladder sludge. Sludge is typically asymptomatic.

Sonographically, sludge appears as a collection of low-level, nonshadowing, dependent echoes within the gallbladder lumen (Fig. 3-9). When sludge is visualized, the sonographer should closely evaluate the gallbladder for signs of small gallstones and other possible sonographic markers of cholecystitis (Fig. 3-10). Occasionally, sludge can be thick and mimic an intraluminal gallbladder mass. This is referred to as tumefactive sludge. The mobility of this type of sludge should be observed vigilantly. If sludge does not move with patient positioning, suspicion of a solid gallbladder mass may arise, and thus, color Doppler should be used to evaluate for signs of vascularity. Tumefactive sludge may also form into sludge balls, which are typically mobile and will not produce an acoustic shadow. The gallbladder can also completely fill with tumefactive sludge, causing the gallbladder to appear isoechoic to the liver tissue, a condition referred to as hepatization of the gallbladder (Fig. 3-11).

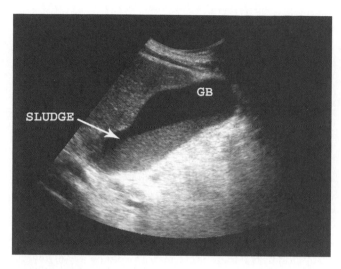

Figure 3-9 Sludge. Sagittal image of the gallbladder (*GB*) demonstrates layering sludge.

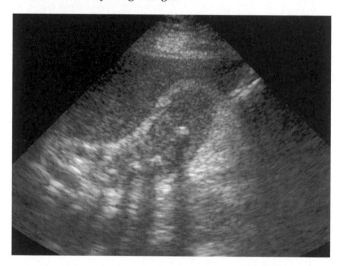

Figure 3-10 Sludge and stones. Sagittal image of the gallbladder that contains both sludge, and small, shadowing stones. The gallbladder wall is also prominent.

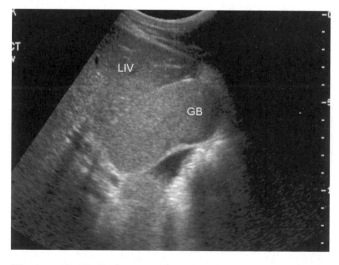

Figure 3-11 Sagittal image of a gallbladder (*GB*) demonstrating hepatization, in which the GB is filled with sludge and is consequently isoechoic to the liver (*LIV*).

CLINICAL FINDINGS OF GALLBLADDER SLUDGE

1. Asymptomatic
2. Any reason for biliary stasis (e.g., total parenteral nutrition, extended period of fasting)

SONOGRAPHIC FINDINGS OF GALLBLADDER SLUDGE

1. A collection of low-level, nonshadowing, dependent echoes within the gallbladder lumen

Gallbladder Polyps

A gallbladder polyp is a projection of tissue from the gallbladder wall that protrudes into the lumen of the gallbladder. Cholesterol polyps are the most common type of gallbladder polyps. They tend to be small, measure less than 10 mm, and are the result of an accumulation of cholesterol and triglycerides within the gallbladder wall, thus causing an elevation in the gallbladder mucosal layer. Polyps may be solitary or multiple and will appear sonographically as hyperechoic, nonshadowing, and nonmobile projections of tissue. Although most polyps have a stalk, the stalk may not always be seen, and thus, they typically yield the **"ball-on-the-wall" sign** because the polyp appears to be a round object, like a ball, that is stuck to the gallbladder wall. When a sonographer varies the patient's position, polyps will neither shadow nor move (Fig. 3-12). Most polyps are benign and incidentally discovered. However, a rapidly growing polyp or large polyp is worrisome for gallbladder carcinoma (see "Gallbladder Carcinoma" section in this chapter).

Gallbladder polyps are often seen with **cholesterolosis** that results from the disturbance in cholesterol

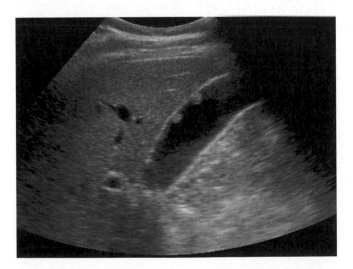

Figure 3-12 Gallbladder polyps. Two polyps are noted attached to the anterior wall of this gallbladder.

metabolism and accumulation of cholesterol typically within a focal region of gallbladder wall. Cholesterolosis is considered a subset of **hyperplastic cholecystosis**, and it may also cause a diffuse polypoid appearance of the gallbladder referred to as a strawberry gallbladder, although this is not distinct on imaging but rather noted upon pathological investigation. Hyperplastic cholecystosis also includes adenomyomatosis.

CLINICAL FINDINGS OF POLYPS

1. Asymptomatic

SONOGRAPHIC FINDINGS OF POLYPS

1. Hyperechoic, nonshadowing, and nonmobile mass that projects from the gallbladder wall into the gallbladder lumen

🔊))) **SOUND OFF**
Hyperplastic cholecystosis, which is a group of proliferative and degenerative gallbladder disorders, includes both adenomyomatosis and cholesterolosis.

Adenomyomatosis

Adenomyomatosis is literally interpreted as "the dissemination of glands within the muscle" of the gallbladder. Like cholesterolosis, it is a form of hyperplastic cholecystosis of the gallbladder. With adenomyomatosis, the luminal epithelium is hyperplastic, and the muscular layer becomes thickened, producing diverticuli or tiny pockets called **Rokitansky–Aschoff sinuses**. These sinuses may contain cholesterol crystals that produce **comet-tail artifact** that is most often seen protruding into the gallbladder lumen from the anterior wall (Fig. 3-13). Adenomyomatosis can be focal or diffuse and is clinically silent and most often insignificant.

CLINICAL FINDINGS OF ADENOMYOMATOSIS

1. Asymptomatic

SONOGRAPHIC FINDINGS OF ADENOMYOMATOSIS

1. Focal or diffuse thickening of the gallbladder wall
2. Comet-tail artifact that projects from the gallbladder wall into the lumen of the gallbladder

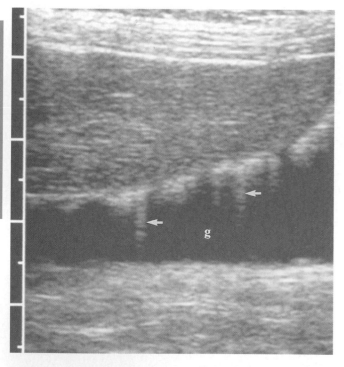

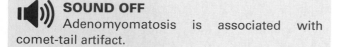

Figure 3-13 Adenomyomatosis of the gallbladder. Characteristic comet-tail artifact (*arrows*) is produced by cholesterol crystals located in the Rokitansky–Aschoff sinuses of the anterior gallbladder (*g*) wall.

> **SOUND OFF**
> Adenomyomatosis is associated with comet-tail artifact.

Acute Cholecystitis

The sudden onset of gallbladder inflammation is referred to as acute cholecystitis. The most common cause of acute cholecystitis is a gallstone that has become lodged in the cystic duct or neck of the gallbladder. **Leukocytosis** is often associated with acute cholecystitis. Other laboratory findings may include an elevation in ALP and ALT. Bilirubin may also be elevated if obstruction to the ducts occurs. Recall, if the bile ducts are obstructed, the patient will also likely be suffering from posthepatic jaundice. Besides right upper quadrant or epigastric pain, patients often complain of focal tenderness over the gallbladder with transducer pressure when the gallbladder is inflamed. This is termed a positive sonographic **Murphy sign** (Fig. 3-14). Other sonographic findings include gallstones, **pericholecystic fluid**, sludge, and thickening of the gallbladder wall, which may contain pockets of edematous fluid creating a striated appearance (Fig. 3-15). When acute cholecystitis is suspected, the sonographer should closely evaluate

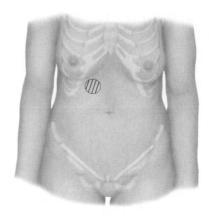

Figure 3-14 Murphy sign. Location of Murphy sign. This location will be tender with transducer pressure in the presence of cholecystitis and possibly other right upper quadrant maladies.

the gallbladder for the progression of the disease to gangrenous cholecystitis, gallbladder perforation, and other **sequela** mentioned in this chapter.

> **SOUND OFF**
> The presence of gallstones and a positive sonographic Murphy sign is a strong indicator of acute cholecystitis.

CLINICAL FINDINGS OF ACUTE CHOLECYSTITIS

1. Right upper quadrant tenderness
2. Epigastric or abdominal pain
3. Leukocytosis
4. Possible elevation in ALP, ALT, GGT, and bilirubin (with obstruction)
5. Fever
6. Pain that radiates to the shoulders
7. Nausea and vomiting
8. Jaundice may be present if there is an obstruction of the bile ducts

SONOGRAPHIC FINDINGS OF ACUTE CHOLECYSTITIS

1. Gallstones (evaluate the neck and cystic duct for a possible lodged stone)
2. Positive sonographic Murphy sign
3. Gallbladder wall thickening
4. Gallbladder enlargement
5. Pericholecystic fluid
6. Sludge

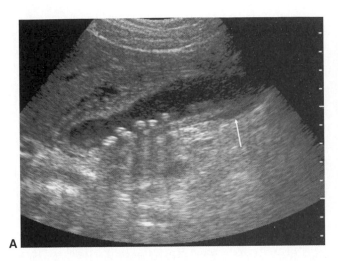
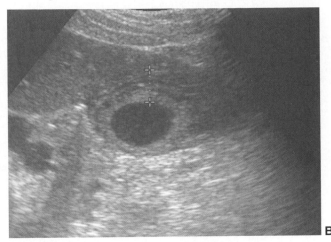

Figure 3-15 Acute cholecystitis. Sagittal **(A)** and transverse **(B)** images of a patient with a positive Murphy sign reveal an inflamed gallbladder containing gallstones and sludge, a thickened gallbladder wall (*calipers*), and pericholecystic fluid (*arrow*). Note that the wall appears striated.

Gangrenous Cholecystitis and Gallbladder Perforation

Gangrenous cholecystitis can be a direct evolution of acute cholecystitis. In addition to the sonographic findings of acute cholecystitis, gangrenous cholecystitis includes focal wall necrosis, bulges of the gallbladder wall, sloughed membranes, and ulcerative craters. Perforation, or rupture, of the gallbladder has a high mortality and morbidity rate secondary to **peritonitis**. A distinct gallbladder wall tear may be noted with sonography, and the gallbladder may appear irregular in shape (Fig. 3-16). Clinically, the patient does not always demonstrate the sonographic Murphy sign.

CLINICAL FINDINGS OF GANGRENOUS CHOLECYSTITIS AND GALLBLADDER PERFORATION

1. Right upper quadrant pain
2. Epigastric or abdominal pain
3. Leukocytosis
4. Possible elevation in ALP, ALT, GGT, and bilirubin (with obstruction)
5. Fever
6. Pain that radiates to the shoulders
7. Nausea and vomiting

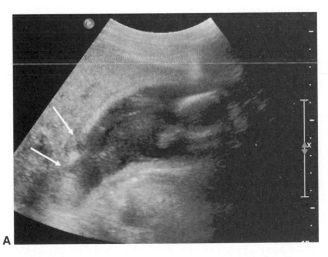
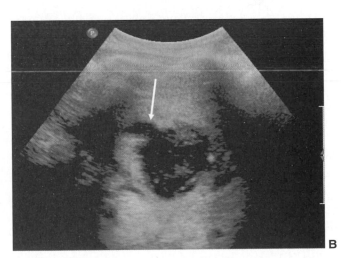

Figure 3-16 Gallbladder perforation. Longitudinal **(A)** and transverse **(B)** images in a patient with gallbladder perforation. The defect seen on the anterior wall (*arrows*) is better demonstrated in the transverse section. Debris is also located within the gallbladder lumen.

SONOGRAPHIC FINDINGS OF GANGRENOUS CHOLECYSTITIS AND GALLBLADDER PERFORATION

1. Gallstones (evaluate the neck and cystic duct for a possible lodged stone)
2. Loss of the sonographic Murphy sign
3. Gallbladder wall thickening with a possible perceptible wall tear
4. Focal wall necrosis, bulges of the gallbladder wall, sloughed membranes, and ulcerative craters
5. Gallbladder loses typically its shape
6. Pericholecystic fluid
7. Sludge

Emphysematous Cholecystitis

Emphysematous cholecystitis, most often discovered in diabetic patients, is a form of acute cholecystitis that is caused by gas-forming infection invading the gallbladder lumen, wall, or both. The gas or gas bubbles produced by the bacteria within the gallbladder wall will lead to the manifestation of dirty shadowing, reverberation, or ring-down artifact, and these gas bubbles may rise to the nondependent wall of the gallbladder (most likely the anterior wall), producing a sonographic sign referred to as the **"champagne" sign** (Fig. 3-17). Although patients with emphysematous cholecystitis may not have a positive Murphy sign and other clinical symptoms associated with acute cholecystitis, this form of the disease can lead to gallbladder perforation or sepsis and become fatal quickly.

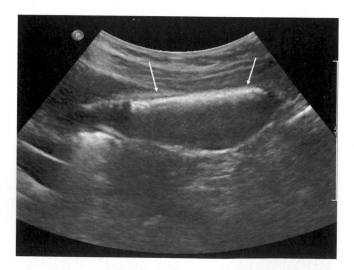

Figure 3-17 Emphysematous cholecystitis. Longitudinal sonogram of a gallbladder that contains air (*arrows*) within its anterior wall secondary to emphysematous cholecystitis. This may be referred to as the "champagne" sign.

CLINICAL FINDINGS OF EMPHYSEMATOUS CHOLECYSTITIS

1. Diabetic patient
2. Right upper quadrant pain, possibly without Murphy sign
3. Fever
4. Can progress to **sepsis**

SONOGRAPHIC FINDINGS OF EMPHYSEMATOUS CHOLECYSTITIS

1. Dirty shadowing reverberation, or ring-down artifact emanating from the gallbladder wall or gallbladder lumen consistent with air
2. Champagne sign (gas bubbles within the gallbladder wall—like the bubbles in champagne—may rise to the nondependent wall of the gallbladder)

🔊 **SOUND OFF**
Emphysematous cholecystitis is most often discovered in diabetic patients.

Chronic Cholecystitis

Chronic cholecystitis results from the intermittent obstruction of the cystic duct by gallstones, resulting in multiple bouts of acute cholecystitis. Clinical findings for chronic cholecystitis include intolerance to fatty foods and a nontender gallbladder. Sonographically, the gallbladder wall will appear thickened, and there may be evidence of WES sign. There may be an elevation in ALP, AST, and ALT.

CLINICAL FINDINGS OF CHRONIC CHOLECYSTITIS

1. Intolerance to fatty foods because of subsequent abdominal pain
2. Nontender gallbladder

SONOGRAPHIC FINDINGS OF CHRONIC CHOLECYSTITIS

1. Contracted gallbladder
2. WES sign
3. Gallstones
4. Wall thickening

Acalculous Cholecystitis

Acalculous cholecystitis presents with all of the symptoms and sonographic findings of cholecystitis, except no gallstones are present (Fig. 3-18). This form of acute cholecystitis is more commonly found in children, recently hospitalized patients, or those who are immunocompromised.

CLINICAL FINDINGS OF ACALCULOUS CHOLECYSTITIS

1. Right upper quadrant tenderness
2. Epigastric or abdominal pain
3. Leukocytosis

SONOGRAPHIC FINDINGS OF ACALCULOUS CHOLECYSTITIS

1. Positive sonographic Murphy sign
2. Gallbladder wall thickening
3. Pericholecystic fluid
4. Sludge

Other Forms of Cholecystitis

One differential diagnosis of gangrenous cholecystitis is **empyema** of the gallbladder, also referred to as **suppurative cholecystitis**, in which the gallbladder is filled with purulent material, commonly referred to as pus. Pus will appear as echogenic material within the lumen of the gallbladder and possible within the ducts as well. Biliary obstruction may also be present.

Although it may be difficult to diagnose sonographically, chronic infection of the gallbladder may also result in **xanthogranulomatous cholecystitis**. This disorder is rare, and it is characterized by the intramural accumulation of inflammatory cells. Sonographically, xanthogranulomatous cholecystitis will demonstrate asymmetrical thickening of the gallbladder wall and intraluminal echogenic debris. Echogenic pericholecystic fat may be visualized as well.

Gallbladder Enlargement

The gallbladder should not exceed 4 to 5 cm in width and 8 to 10 cm in length. The transverse measurement is more indicative of gallbladder enlargement. And again, if the gallbladder transverse measurement exceeds 4 cm, especially in those with clinical indicators of obstruction, then careful analysis of the biliary tract should ensue. An enlarged gallbladder can be caused by a blockage of the cystic duct or other parts of the biliary tree. This may be referred to as a **hydropic gallbladder**, also referred to as a mucocele of the gallbladder (Fig. 3-19). Patients with a hydropic gallbladder may be asymptomatic or may complain of epigastric pain, nausea, and/or vomiting. An enlarged gallbladder is often palpable on physical examination. **Courvoisier gallbladder** describes the clinical detection of an enlarged, palpable gallbladder caused by a pancreatic head mass. Patients with Courvoisier gallbladder also typically have painless jaundice. Gallbladder hydrops in older infants and children may be associated with **Kawasaki disease**, which is a condition associated with vasculitis and can affect the lymph node, skin, and mucous membranes.

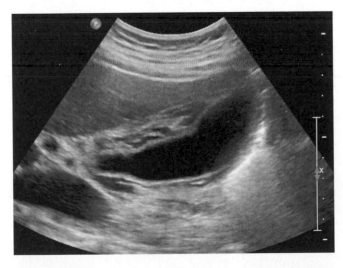

Figure 3-18 Acalculous cholecystitis. Longitudinal image of a gallbladder demonstrating a striated, thickened wall. Although the patient complained of a positive Murphy sign and fever, no gallstones were identified within the gallbladder.

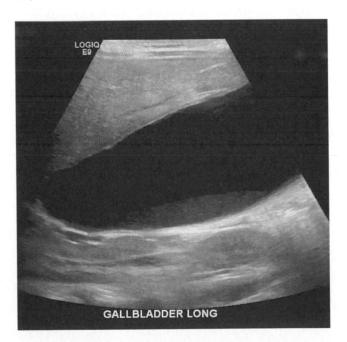

Figure 3-19 Hydropic gallbladder. The longitudinal scan of the gallbladder demonstrates a drastically enlarged gallbladder with thin walls. Some echogenic foci are demonstrated within the lumen of the gallbladder, adjacent to the posterior gallbladder wall, likely indicative of sludge.

CLINICAL FINDINGS OF GALLBLADDER ENLARGEMENT

1. Palpable gallbladder
2. Could suffer from painless jaundice (Courvoisier gallbladder)
3. Possible elevation in ALP, ALT, GGT, and bilirubin (with obstruction)

SONOGRAPHIC FINDINGS OF GALLBLADDER ENLARGEMENT

1. Gallbladder measures greater than 4 to 5 cm in diameter or greater than 8 to 10 cm in length
2. Search for obstructive entities such as choledocholithiasis or pancreatic mass

CLINICAL FINDINGS OF PORCELAIN GALLBLADDER

1. Asymptomatic

SONOGRAPHIC FINDINGS OF PORCELAIN GALLBLADDER

1. Calcification of the gallbladder wall recognized by a echogenic curvilinear structure within the gallbladder fossa with shadowing
2. The identification of the calcified posterior wall of the gallbladder is helpful to differentiate porcelain gallbladder from WES sign
3. Signs of chronic cholecystitis and gallstones may be present

Porcelain Gallbladder

A **porcelain gallbladder**, which is classically clinically silent, results from the calcification of the gallbladder wall. It is sonographically recognized by the presence of an echogenic curvilinear structure within the gallbladder fossa with shadowing. Dense calcification of the gallbladder wall may appear sonographically similar to WES sign or the air seen with emphysematous cholecystitis. Thus, clinical findings should be closely evaluated. With WES sign, the posterior wall of the gallbladder is typically obscured by extensive shadowing. Therefore, the identification of the calcified posterior wall of the gallbladder is helpful to differentiate porcelain gallbladder from WES sign, although radiography or computed tomography is often utilized to confirm the diagnosis (Fig. 3-20). Gallstones and chronic inflammation are linked with porcelain gallbladder, and although current research studies reject the connection, there was once a suspected increased risk for those with a porcelain gallbladder to development gallbladder carcinoma.

SOUND OFF

The identification of the calcified posterior wall of the gallbladder is helpful to differentiate porcelain gallbladder from WES sign. With WES sign, the posterior wall is typically obscured by the shadowing gallstones within the gallbladder, while the posterior wall will often be seen with porcelain gallbladder.

Gallbladder Carcinoma

Although it is the most common cancer of the biliary tract, gallbladder carcinoma is rare. It is thought to be caused by chronic irritation of the gallbladder wall by gallstones. Therefore, gallbladder carcinoma is almost always associated with gallstones, and the mass may actually contain gallstones. Furthermore, there appears to be an increased risk for developing gallbladder carcinoma in patients who suffer from chronic cholecystitis. Patients may

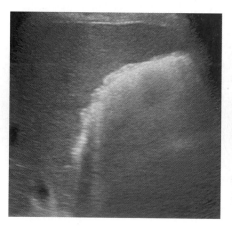 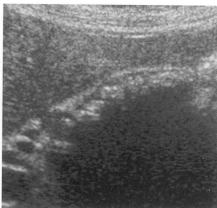 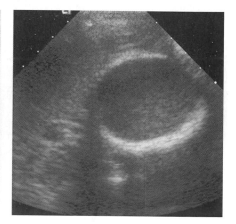

Figure 3-20 Differing sonographic appearances of emphysematous cholecystitis (*left image*), wall–echo–shadow sign (*middle image*), and porcelain gallbladder (*right image*).

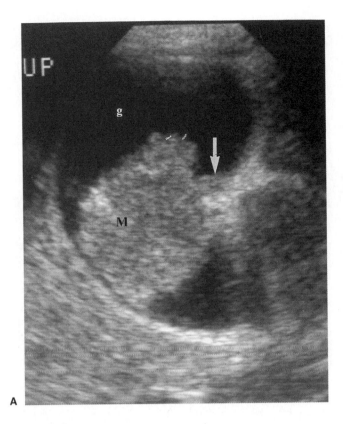

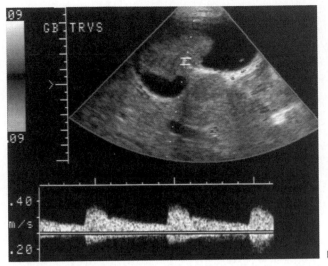

Figure 3-21 Gallbladder carcinoma. **A.** An irregular mass (*M*) projects into the gallbladder (*g*) lumen from a stalk (*arrow*). **B.** Spectral Doppler shows arterial flow within the mass.

be asymptomatic at the time of detection, or they may suffer from nausea, vomiting, unexplained weight loss, right upper quadrant pain, jaundice, or hepatomegaly.

Gallbladder carcinoma may appear sonographically as a distinct, nonmobile, hypoechoic mass within the lumen of gallbladder or as diffuse gallbladder wall thickening. It may also appear as an irregular polypoid mass that completely fills the gallbladder fossa, and it may have invaded the adjacent liver tissue at the time of diagnosis. Whenever a mass is visualized within the gallbladder lumen, it should be measured. Gallbladder carcinoma is suspected if a polyp or mass within the gallbladder measures greater than 1 cm. When confused with tumefactive sludge, color Doppler can reveal vessels within the malignancy (Fig. 3-21). The most common metastatic disease of the gallbladder is malignant melanoma. It is difficult to sonographically differentiate metastasis from primary gallbladder cancer.

CLINICAL FINDINGS OF GALLBLADDER CARCINOMA

1. Weight loss
2. Right upper quadrant pain
3. Jaundice
4. Nausea and vomiting
5. Hepatomegaly
6. Possible elevation in ALP, ALT, GGT, and bilirubin (with obstruction)

SONOGRAPHIC FINDINGS OF GALLBLADDER CARCINOMA

1. Nonmobile mass within the gallbladder lumen that measures greater than 1 cm
2. Diffuse or focal gallbladder wall thickening
3. Irregular mass that may completely fill the gallbladder fossa
4. Invasion of the mass into surrounding liver tissue

REVIEW QUESTIONS

1. Hepatization of the gallbladder occurs when the gallbladder:
   a. perforates.
   b. becomes hydropic.
   c. fills with sludge.
   d. undergoes torsion.

2. What is the most likely diagnosis for Figure 3-22?
   a. Acute cholecystitis
   b. Adenomyomatosis
   c. Emphysematous cholecystitis
   d. Gallbladder polyps

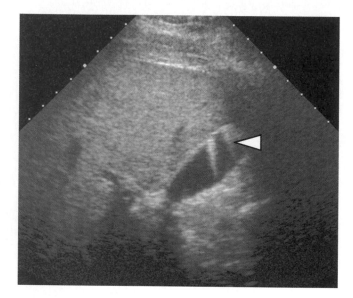

Figure 3-22

3. A 71-year-old patient presents to the emergency department with painless jaundice and an enlarged, palpable gallbladder. These findings are highly suspicious for:
   a. acute cholecystitis.
   b. chronic cholecystitis.
   c. Courvoisier gallbladder.
   d. porcelain gallbladder.

4. The innermost layer of the gallbladder wall is the:
   a. fibromuscular layer.
   b. mucosal layer.
   c. serosal layer.
   d. muscularis layer.

5. Which of the following would not be a laboratory finding typically analyzed with suspected gallbladder disease?
   a. ALP
   b. ALT
   c. Bilirubin
   d. Alpha-fetoprotein

6. A 34-year-old patient in Figure 3-23 presented with a positive Murphy sign and elevated WBC. What is the most likely diagnosis?
   a. Acalculous cholecystitis
   b. Chronic cholecystitis
   c. Acute cholecystitis
   d. Emphysematous cholecystitis

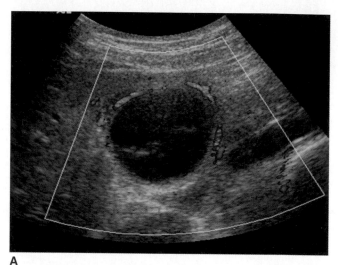

A

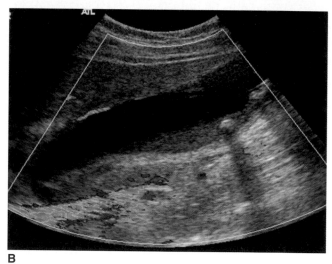

B

Figure 3-23

7. The cystic artery is most often a direct branch of the:
   a. main pancreatic artery.
   b. celiac artery.
   c. right hepatic artery.
   d. left hepatic artery.

8. The middle layer of the gallbladder wall is the:
   a. fibromuscular layer.
   b. mucosal layer.
   c. serosal layer.
   d. muscularis layer.

9. Which structure is a useful landmark for identifying the gallbladder?
   a. Main lobar fissure
   b. Hepatoduodenal ligament
   c. Falciform ligament
   d. Ligamentum venosum

10. Which of the following would be least likely to cause focal gallbladder wall thickening?
    a. Gallbladder polyp
    b. Adenomyomatosis
    c. Ascites
    d. Adhered gallstone

11. What hormone causes the gallbladder to contract?
    a. Estrogen
    b. Cholecystokinin
    c. Bilirubin
    d. Biliverdin

12. The gallbladder wall should measure not more than:
    a. 5 mm.
    b. 6 mm.
    c. 4 mm.
    d. 3 mm.

13. Which of the following is associated with cholelithiasis and is characteristically found in Africans or people of African descent?
    a. Sickle cell disease
    b. Gallbladder torsion
    c. Cholesterolosis
    d. Arland–Berlin syndrome

14. The direct blood supply to the gallbladder is the:
    a. cholecystic artery.
    b. common hepatic artery.
    c. main portal vein.
    d. cystic artery.

15. The outermost layer of the gallbladder wall is the:
    a. fibromuscular layer.
    b. mucosal layer.
    c. serosal layer.
    d. muscularis layer.

16. Which part of the gallbladder is involved in Hartmann pouch?
    a. Neck
    b. Fundus
    c. Body
    d. Phrygian cap

17. The gallbladder is connected to the biliary tree by the:
    a. common hepatic duct.
    b. common bile duct.
    c. cystic duct.
    d. right hepatic duct.

18. At which level of the gallbladder is the junctional fold found?
    a. Neck
    b. Fundus
    c. Body
    d. Phrygian cap

19. Empyema of the gallbladder denotes:
    a. gallbladder hydrops.
    b. gallbladder filled with pus.
    c. gallbladder completely filled with air.
    d. gallbladder completely filled with polyps.

20. What is/are cholelithiasis?
    a. Inflammation of the gallbladder
    b. Gallstones
    c. Hyperplasia of the gallbladder wall
    d. Polyps within the biliary tree

21. The diffuse polypoid appearance of the gallbladder referred to as strawberry gallbladder is seen with:
    a. cholesterolosis.
    b. adenomyomatosis.
    c. cholangitis.
    d. Kawasaki disease.

22. The most common variant of gallbladder shape is the:
    a. Phrygian cap.
    b. Hartmann pouch.
    c. septated gallbladder.
    d. junctional fold.

23. The diameter of the gallbladder should not exceed:
    a. 8 cm.
    b. 5 cm.
    c. 7 mm.
    d. 3 cm.

24. Patients who suffer from acute cholecystitis that leads to perforation and rupture have a high mortality and morbidity rate secondary to:
    a. exudate.
    b. peritonitis.
    c. cholesterolosis.
    d. pancreatic carcinoma.

25. All of the following are sources of diffuse gallbladder wall thickening except:
    a. acute cholecystitis.
    b. AIDS.
    c. hepatitis.
    d. gallbladder polyp.

26. Which statement is not true of cholelithiasis?
    a. Men have an increased likelihood of developing cholelithiasis compared to women.
    b. Patients who have been or are pregnant have an increased occurrence of cholelithiasis.

c. A rapid weight loss may increase the likelihood of developing cholelithiasis.

d. Patients who have hemolytic disorders have an increased occurrence of cholelithiasis.

27. WES sign denotes:
a. the presence of a gallstone lodged in the cystic duct.
b. multiple biliary stones and biliary dilatation.
c. a gallbladder filled with cholelithiasis.
d. the sonographic sign of a porcelain gallbladder.

28. Which of the following is the most likely clinical finding of adenomyomatosis?
a. Murphy sign
b. Hepatitis
c. Congestive heart failure
d. Asymptomatic

29. Tumefactive sludge can resemble the sonographic appearance of:
a. cholelithiasis.
b. gallbladder carcinoma.
c. cholecystitis.
d. adenomyomatosis.

30. The champagne sign is associated with:
a. adenomyomatosis.
b. cholangiocarcinoma.
c. emphysematous cholecystitis.
d. acalculous cholecystitis.

31. The sequela of acute cholecystitis that is associated with a tear in the gallbladder wall is:
a. emphysematous cholecystitis.
b. membranous cholecystitis.
c. chronic cholecystitis.
d. gallbladder perforation.

32. A 32-year-old female patient presents to the sonography department with vague abdominal pain. The sonographic investigation of the gallbladder reveals a focal area of gallbladder wall thickening that produces comet-tail artifact. These findings are consistent with:
a. gangrenous cholecystitis.
b. gallbladder perforation.
c. acalculous cholecystitis.
d. adenomyomatosis.

33. Which of the following would not be a finding of acalculous cholecystitis?
a. Gallbladder wall thickening
b. Pericholecystic fluid
c. Cholelithiasis
d. Positive Murphy sign

34. Intermittent obstruction of the cystic duct by a gallstone results in:
a. emphysematous cholecystitis.
b. gangrenous cholecystitis.
c. chronic cholecystitis.
d. acute cholecystitis.

35. Which of the following is not a risk factor for the development of gallstones?
a. Phrygian cap
b. Pregnancy
c. Total parenteral nutrition
d. Oral contraceptive use

36. A nonmobile, nonshadowing focus is seen within the gallbladder lumen. This most likely represents a:
a. gallstone.
b. gallbladder carcinoma.
c. gallbladder polyp.
d. sludge ball.

37. Focal tenderness over the gallbladder with probe pressure describes:
a. Murphy sign.
b. strawberry sign.
c. Courvoisier sign.
d. hydrops sign.

38. Diabetic patients suffering from acute cholecystitis have an increased risk for developing:
a. emphysematous cholecystitis.
b. gangrenous cholecystitis.
c. chronic cholecystitis.
d. gallbladder torsion.

39. Cholesterol crystals within the Rokitansky–Aschoff sinuses are found with:
a. acute cholecystitis.
b. acalculous cholecystitis.
c. adenomyomatosis.
d. gallbladder perforation.

40. The spiral valves of Heister are found within the:
a. gallbladder neck.
b. cystic duct.
c. gallbladder fundus.
d. gallbladder wall.

41. Which of the following would yield a gallbladder with an hourglass appearance?
a. Hartmann pouch
b. Phrygian cap
c. Junctional fold
d. Bilobed

42. With which of the following is Courvoisier gallbladder associated?
    a. A pancreatic head mass
    b. A stone in the cystic duct
    c. Cholecystitis
    d. Chronic diverticulitis

43. Calcification of the gallbladder wall is termed:
    a. concrete gallbladder.
    b. Heister syndrome.
    c. porcelain gallbladder.
    d. hyperplastic cholecystosis.

44. What produces the hormone cholecystokinin?
    a. Gallbladder
    b. Anterior pituitary gland
    c. Duodenum
    d. Pancreas

45. What is the artifact associated with adenomyomatosis?
    a. Comet tail
    b. Reverberation
    c. Acoustic shadowing
    d. Twinkle

46. Which of the following is a condition associated with vasculitis and gallbladder hydrops?
    a. Kawasaki disease
    b. Beckwith–Wiedemann syndrome
    c. Sickle cell disease
    d. Multiple hepatic hemangioma

47. Unconjugated bilirubin may also be referred to as:
    a. conjugated bilirubin.
    b. total bilirubin.
    c. direct bilirubin.
    d. indirect bilirubin.

48. Which of the following may not be a clinical or sonographic finding in patients with emphysematous cholecystitis?
    a. Diabetes
    b. Gas formation in the wall of the gallbladder
    c. Fever
    d. Murphy sign

49. Which of the following is a rare chronic gallbladder infection characterized by intramural accumulation of inflammatory cells?
    a. Gallbladder perforation
    b. Adenomyomatosis
    c. Xanthogranulomatous cholecystitis
    d. Emphysematous cholecystitis

50. Which of the following would most likely be associated with gallstones or biliary tree obstruction?
    a. Elevated direct bilirubin
    b. Elevated indirect bilirubin
    c. Decreased conjugated bilirubin
    d. Decreased unconjugated bilirubin

51. What is the most likely diagnosis for this asymptomatic patient in Figure 3-24?
    a. Chronic cholecystitis
    b. Emphysematous cholecystitis
    c. Porcelain gallbladder
    d. Champaign sign

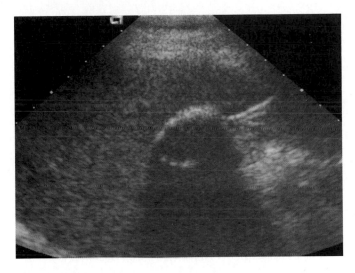

Figure 3-24

52. Which of the following is associated focal wall necrosis, bulges in the gallbladder wall, sloughing membranes, and ulcerative craters?
    a. Porcelain gallbladder
    b. Adenomyomatosis
    c. Gangrenous cholecystitis
    d. Emphysematous cholecystitis

53. What condition may increase the likelihood of developing gallbladder carcinoma?
    a. Porcelain gallbladder
    b. Chronic cholecystitis
    c. Hydropic gallbladder
    d. Gallbladder perforation

54. Gallbladder carcinoma may be suspected when a gallbladder polyp exceeds:
    a. 1 cm.
    b. 2 mm.
    c. 5 mm.
    d. 8 mm.

The Gallbladder

55. Which of the following would increase the likelihood of suffering from gallbladder torsion?
    a. Floating gallbladder
    b. Gallstones
    c. Acalculous cholecystitis
    d. AIDS cholangiopathy

56. Which of the following is a result of an accumulation of cholesterol and triglycerides within the gallbladder wall?
    a. Gallstone
    b. Gallbladder carcinoma
    c. Gallbladder polyp
    d. Xanthogranulomatous cholecystitis

57. Which of the following is not a section of the gallbladder?
    a. Neck
    b. Body
    c. Fundus
    d. Head

58. What is another name for empyema of the gallbladder?
    a. Caroli disease
    b. Emphysematous cholecystitis
    c. Suppurative cholecystitis
    d. Gallbladder hydrops

59. Which of the following could be a likely cause of a hydropic gallbladder?
    a. Multiple gallbladder polyps
    b. Gallstone in the cystic duct
    c. Phrygian cap
    d. Hartman pouch

60. What clinical finding is not typically associated with gallbladder carcinoma?
    a. Weight gain
    b. Hepatomegaly
    c. Jaundice
    d. Elevation in ALP

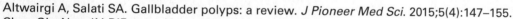

SUGGESTED READINGS

Altwairgi A, Salati SA. Gallbladder polyps: a review. *J Pioneer Med Sci.* 2015;5(4):147–155.

Chen GL, Akmal Y, DiFronzo AL, et al. Porcelain gallbladder: no longer an indication for prophylactic cholecystectomy. *Am Surg.* 2015;81(10):936–940.

Colecchia A, Larocca A, Scaioli E, et al. Natural history of small gallbladder polyps is benign: evidence from a clinical and pathogenetic study. *Am J Gastroenterol.* 2009;104(3):624–629.

Curry RA, Tempkin BB. *Sonography: Introduction to Normal Structure and Function.* 5th ed. Elsevier; 2021:189–208.

Federle MP, Jeffrey RB, Woodward PJ, et al. *Diagnostic Imaging: Abdomen.* 2nd ed. Amirsys; 2010:III-2-2–III-2-82.

French DG, Allen PD, Ellsmere JC. The diagnostic accuracy of trans-abdominal ultrasonography needs to be considered when managing gallbladder polyps. *Surg Endosc.* 2013;27(11):4021–4025.

Henningsen C, Kuntz K, Youngs D. *Clinical Guide to Sonography: Exercises for Critical Thinking.* 2nd ed. Elsevier; 2014:2–8 & 100–102.

Hertzberg BS, Middleton WD. *Ultrasound: The Requisites.* 3rd ed. Elsevier; 2016:32–50 & 89–102.

Kawamura DM, Nolan TD. *Diagnostic Medical Sonography: Abdomen and Superficial Structures.* 4th ed. Wolters Kluwer; 2018:171–211.

Rumack CM, Wilson SR, Charboneau JW, et al. *Diagnostic Ultrasound.* 4th ed. Elsevier; 2011:172–215 & 1800–1844.

Safwan M, Penny SM. Emphysematous cholecystitis: a deadly twist to a common disease. *J Diagn Med Sonogr.* 2016;32(3):131–137.

Sanders RC, Hall-Terracciano B. *Clinical Sonography: A Practical Guide.* 5th ed. Wolters Kluwer; 2016:421–435.

Siegel MJ. *Pediatric Sonography.* 5th ed. Wolters Kluwer; 2019:273–304.

BONUS REVIEW!

Hepatobiliary Iminodiacetic Acid Scan (Fig. 3-25)

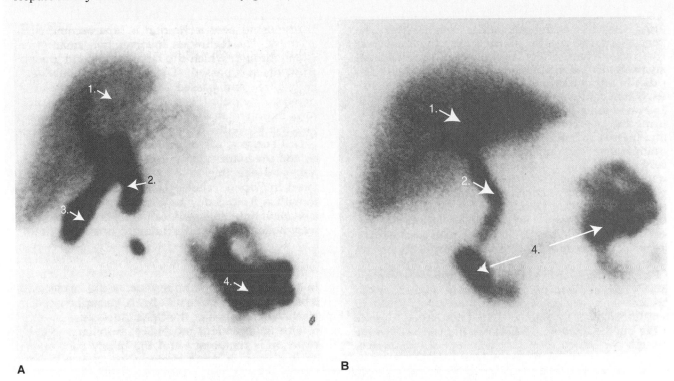

A

B

Figure 3-25 Image of the nuclear medicine examination referred to as a hepatobiliary iminodiacetic acid (HIDA) scan. This examination is used to evaluate the function of liver, gallbladder, and bile ducts. **A,** With and **B,** without visualization of the gallbladder. 1. Liver; 2. Common bile duct; 3. Gallbladder; 4. Activity in intestine.

Cholecystostomy Procedure (Fig. 3-26)

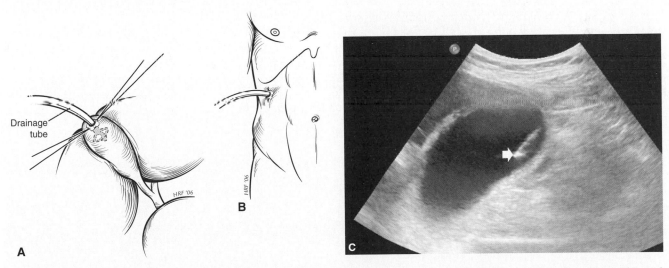

Drainage tube

HRF '06

HRF '06

A

B

C

Figure 3-26 Cholecystostomy procedure. A drainage tube is secured to the gallbladder wall by a suture **(A)** and to the abdominal wall by a skin suture **(B)** to allow percutaneous drainage of the gallbladder. **C.** A sonogram of the gallbladder demonstrating needle placement into the distended gallbladder (*arrowhead*) during ultrasound-guided cholecystostomy tube placement.

(continued)

BONUS REVIEW! (*continued*)

Cholecystitis on Computed Tomography (Fig. 3-27)

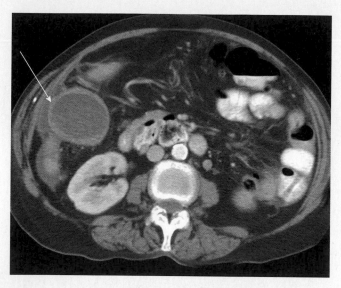

Figure 3-27 Axial-enhanced computed tomography image through the upper abdomen shows a dilated thick-walled gallbladder with pericholecystic fluid (*arrow*) secondary to acute cholecystitis.

The Bile Ducts

Introduction

Sonography has become the modality of choice in the evaluation of the bile ducts for suspected disease. This chapter provides normal anatomy and pathology of the biliary tree. In the "Bonus Review" section, diagram and radiographic images of an endoscopic retrograde cholangiopancreatography (ERCP), anatomy that can be noted on a magnetic resonance cholangiopancreatography (MRCP), and a sonographic image of a biliary stent are provided.

Key Terms

acute pancreatitis—inflammation of the pancreas secondary to the leakage of pancreatic enzymes from the acinar cells into the parenchyma of the organ

ampulla of Vater—the merging point of the pancreatic duct and common bile duct just before the sphincter of Oddi; also referred to as the hepatopancreatic ampulla

ascariasis—an infection of the small intestine that is caused by *Ascaris lumbricoides*, a parasitic roundworm

biliary atresia—a congenital disease described as the narrowing or obliteration of all or a portion of the biliary tree

biliary colic—pain secondary to a blockage of the biliary tree

biliary stasis—a condition in which bile is stagnant and allowed to develop into sludge or stones

bilirubin—a yellowish pigment found in bile that is produced by the breakdown of old red blood cells by the liver

biliverdin—a green pigment found in the bile

Caroli disease—a congenital disorder characterized by segmental dilatation of the intrahepatic ducts

central dot sign—the presence of echogenic dots in the nondependent part of the dilated duct representing small fibrovascular bundles; seen with Caroli disease

Charcot triad—fever, right upper quadrant pain, and jaundice associated with cholangitis

cholangiocarcinoma—primary bile duct cancer

cholangiography—a radiographic procedure in which contrast is injected into the bile ducts to assess for the presence of disease

cholangitis—inflammation of the bile ducts

chronic pancreatitis—the recurring destruction of the pancreatic tissue that results in atrophy, fibrosis, scarring, and the development of calcifications within the gland

double-duct sign—coexisting dilation of the common bile duct and pancreatic duct

endoscopic retrograde cholangiopancreatography—endoscopic procedure that utilizes fluoroscopy to evaluate the biliary tree and pancreas

hepatopancreatic ampulla—the level of the biliary tree where the common bile duct and the main pancreatic duct meet; may also be referred to as the ampulla of Vater

hepatopancreatic sphincter—the muscle that controls the emptying of bile and pancreatic juices into the duodenum; may also be referred to as the sphincter of Oddi

inflammatory bowel disease—chronic inflammation of all or part of the bowel

Klatskin tumor—a malignant biliary tumor located at the junction of the right and left hepatic ducts

Mirizzi syndrome—a clinical condition when the patient presents with jaundice, pain, and fever secondary to a lodged stone in the cystic duct causing compression of the common duct

parallel tube sign—the enlargement of the common duct to the size of the adjacent portal vein within the porta hepatis

pneumobilia—air within the biliary tree

pruritus—severe itchiness of the skin

pseudogallbladder sign—a sign associated with biliary atresia in children where there is evidence of a cystic structure in the gallbladder fossa without the presence of an actual gallbladder

shotgun sign—the enlargement of the common duct to the size of the adjacent portal vein within the porta hepatis; also referred to as the parallel tube sign

sphincter of Oddi—the muscle that controls the emptying of bile and pancreatic juices into the duodenum; also referred to as the hepatopancreatic sphincter

triangular cord sign—a sign associated with biliary atresia in children that is described as an avascular, echogenic, triangular, or tubular structure anterior to the portal vein, representing the replacement of the extrahepatic duct with fibrous tissue in the porta hepatis

ulcerative colitis—an inflammatory bowel disease that leads to the development of ulcers within the bowel

ANATOMY AND PHYSIOLOGY OF THE BILE DUCTS

Bile, a vital digestive fluid, is produced by the liver. Cholesterol is a major component of bile, although it includes other key elements that aid in digestion such as **bilirubin**, **biliverdin**, and bile acids. The function of the biliary tree is to provide a conduit for bile to drain from the liver into the small intestine (Fig. 4-1). Bile first accumulates in the small intrahepatic biliary radicles that are located throughout the liver. These tiny ducts are scattered throughout the liver parenchyma and are part of the portal triads. Each portal triad contains a small branch of the hepatic artery, portal vein, and intrahepatic ducts (biliary radicles). From these small biliary radicles, bile flows into either the right or left hepatic duct. The right and left hepatic ducts eventually unite to form the common hepatic duct. Bile then travels only a short distance to the gallbladder, where it is concentrated and stored.

The gallbladder is attached to the biliary tree by the cystic duct. The point of attachment of the cystic duct to the gallbladder marks the proximal margin of the common bile duct. The cystic duct contains tiny structures called the spiral valves of Heister. These small projections of tissue prevent the cystic duct from collapsing or distending. When stimulated by cholecystokinin—produced by the duodenum—the gallbladder contracts and empties bile into the biliary tree at the level of the proximal common bile duct. Bile travels from the common bile duct toward the duodenum, where it meets the main pancreatic duct at the **ampulla of Vater** or **hepatopancreatic ampulla**. There, pancreatic juices and bile are mixed. The **sphincter of Oddi**, also referred to as the **hepatopancreatic sphincter**, is the opening that allows bile and pancreatic juices to flow into the duodenum. The fluid is mixed with chyme in the duodenum, and appropriate chemical reactions ensue.

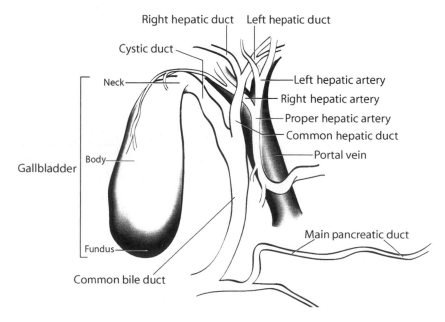

Figure 4-1 Normal anatomy of the biliary tree, gallbladder, and adjacent vasculature.

> **SOUND OFF**
> Bile flow = liver → biliary radicles → right or left hepatic duct → common hepatic duct → cystic duct → gallbladder → common bile duct → ampulla of Vater → sphincter of Oddi → duodenum

SONOGRAPHY OF THE BILE DUCTS

Although a period of 8 hours is optimal, patients should have nothing to eat or drink for at least 4 hours before a sonogram of the biliary tree is performed. The entire biliary tree should be examined. Although the common bile duct can often be differentiated from the common hepatic duct if it recognized posterior to the head of the pancreas or inferior to the gallbladder neck, delineation may be difficult at times. For this reason, many sonographers and interpreting physicians may describe the portion of the biliary tree that is located at the porta hepatis as the common duct.

In general, a common bile duct diameter that exceeds 6 mm is typically considered abnormal, and thus, the cause of dilatation should systematically be investigated through diligent scanning of the entire right upper quadrant, including the complete biliary tree, liver, gallbladder, and pancreas (Fig. 4-2). For the sonographer, when an enlarged portion of the biliary tree is identified, a more thorough inquiry of the patient's clinical history should also ensue, for the obtained measurement of the biliary tree is only part of the overall patient assessment, and thus, the

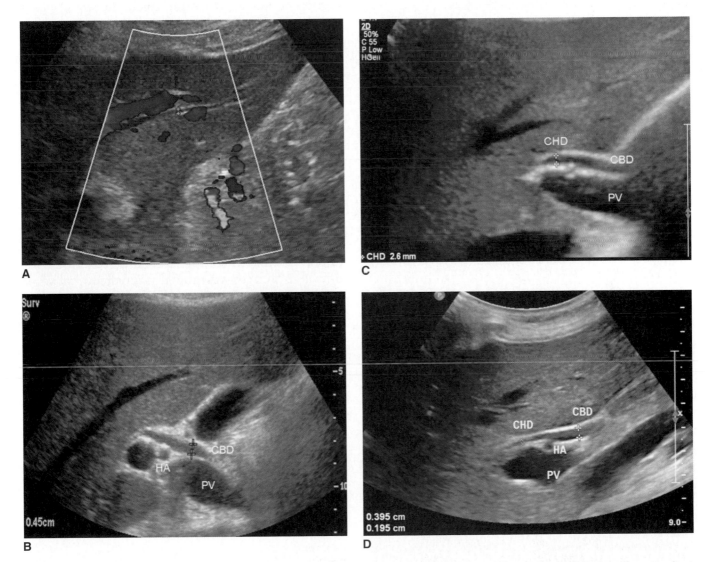

Figure 4-2 Normal measurements of the bile ducts. The ducts are measured inner wall to inner wall. **A.** Intrahepatic duct (*between calipers*). **B.** Common bile duct (*CBD*), less than 8 mm (*between calipers*), and **C.** common hepatic duct (*CHD*), less than 6 mm at the porta hepatis. Normal duct measurements at the porta hepatis. **D.** Both the common hepatic duct (CHD) and common bile duct (CBD) are noted in this image. *HA*, hepatic artery; *PV*, portal vein.

entire clinical picture must be appreciated in order to assist the interpreting physician in making the correct diagnosis. For example, some authors claim that the normal anteroposterior diameter of the common duct in adults at the level of the porta hepatis is between 1 and 7 mm. For patients older than 60 years or who have had a cholecystectomy, a maximum diameter of 10 mm may be considered normal if the patient is asymptomatic. Thus, clinical history is vital. Laboratory results, such alanine aminotransferase (ALT), alkaline phosphatase (ALP), serum bilirubin, gamma-glutamyltransferase (GGT), and urobilirubin, are often elevated in the presence of biliary obstruction or disease. Also, liver function and pancreatic laboratory results—specifically amylase and lipase—should be closely evaluated when biliary abnormalities are suspected. The intrahepatic ducts are considered dilated if they exceed 2 mm (see Fig. 4-2).

Caliper placement when measuring the duct should be from inner-to-inner wall. The double-barrel "**shotgun sign**" or "**parallel tube sign**" describes the enlargement of the common duct to the size of the adjacent portal vein within the porta hepatis (Fig. 4-3). Also, coexisting dilation of the common bile duct and pancreatic duct has been referred to as the "**double-duct sign.**" When these finding are present, color Doppler is helpful for delineating the vasculature from bile ducts.

> **🔊)) SOUND OFF**
> When biliary tree obstruction or disease is suspected, look for an elevation in ALP, ALT, serum bilirubin, GGT, and urobilirubin.

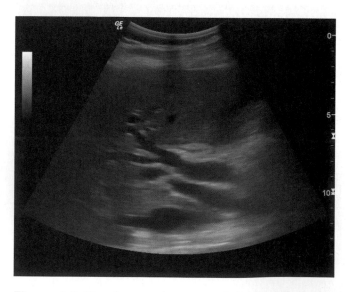

Figure 4-3 The shotgun sign or parallel tube sign. In this image, the common duct is as large, if not slightly larger, than the main portal vein at the level of the porta hepatis.

PATHOLOGY OF THE BILE DUCTS

Biliary Obstruction and Jaundice

Understanding the origin and flow of bile from the liver to the duodenum is imperative to determine the level of biliary obstruction. The origin of bile is within the liver, which is considered the proximal portion of the biliary tree. Conversely, the common bile duct segment closest to the pancreatic head is considered the most distal segment of the biliary tree. As a rule, biliary dilatation will occur proximal to the level of obstruction. The common bile duct, the cystic duct, and part of the common hepatic duct are considered extrahepatic in location. All other portions of the biliary tree are considered intrahepatic. The most common level for an obstruction to occur is the distal common bile duct. In most instances, the extrahepatic ducts will dilate first. Therefore, with obstruction of the distal common bile duct, there will be eventual dilatation of the common bile duct, gallbladder, common hepatic duct, and intrahepatic ducts. The most common causes of common bile duct obstruction are choledocholithiasis, **chronic pancreatitis**, **acute pancreatitis**, and pancreatic carcinoma.

As a result of an obstruction within the biliary tree, the patient will eventually suffer from posthepatic (obstructive) jaundice. Recall, jaundice occurs as a consequence of bilirubin accumulation within the tissues of the body. Bilirubin, which is a yellowish pigment found in bile, can turn the skin and the whites of the eyes—the sclerae—yellow if allowed to accumulate. Accordingly, excessive bilirubin in the body leads to elevated serum bilirubin. And although biliary obstruction is a common cause of jaundice, remember that it can also occur with other conditions, including hepatitis, cirrhosis, liver carcinoma, pancreatic carcinoma, and hemolytic disorders. Consequently, an important assignment for the sonographer is to perform a thorough investigation of the jaundiced patient's clinical history. Lastly, infant jaundice is typically caused by the inability of the newborn liver to eliminate bilirubin from the bloodstream. It is often treated successfully with phototherapy.

> **🔊)) SOUND OFF**
> The most common level for an obstruction to occur is the distal common bile duct.

Choledocholithiasis

Whenever **biliary stasis** occurs, gallstone formation is probable. Choledocholithiasis describes the presence of gallstones within the bile ducts (Fig. 4-4).

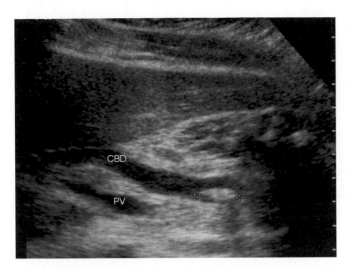

Figure 4-4 Choledocholithiasis. Sonographic image of choledocholithiasis (between calipers). *CBD*, common bile duct; *PV*, portal vein.

However, if biliary obstruction has occurred because of choledocholithiasis, the patient will have jaundice, elevated bilirubin, ALP, and ALT and likely right upper quadrant pain. Stones located within the duct will typically appear as echogenic, shadowing foci; however, about 20% of the time these stones may not shadow.

An uncommon manifestation of choledocholithiasis is **Mirizzi syndrome**. It is a clinical condition in which the patient presents with jaundice, pain, and fever secondary to a lodged stone in the cystic duct with subsequent compression of the common duct (Fig. 4-5). The sonographic findings and symptoms may appear much like those found with cholecystitis. Mirizzi syndrome may be suspected with sonography, but typically, it is diagnosed by **cholangiography** or **endoscopic retrograde cholangiopancreatography (ERCP)**.

Stones typically form in the gallbladder and pass into the biliary tree. Rarely, they can form in the ducts themselves, although some conditions increase the incidence of primary biliary tree stones. Gallstones located within the common bile duct are considered the most common cause of obstructive jaundice. Most stones will be located near the ampulla of Vater and can be difficult to image secondary to neighboring bowel gas shadows. It is important to note that patients presenting with biliary symptoms who have recently undergone a cholecystectomy should be closely evaluated for retained gallstones located within the biliary tree.

Patients with choledocholithiasis may be asymptomatic, and the biliary ducts may be normal in caliber.

CLINICAL FINDINGS OF CHOLEDOCHOLITHIASIS

1. Jaundice
2. Elevated ALP, ALT, and GGT, and bilirubin (with obstruction)
3. Right upper quadrant pain

SONOGRAPHIC FINDINGS OF CHOLEDOCHOLITHIASIS

1. Echogenic foci within the bile duct that may or may not shadow
2. May have biliary dilatation but not always

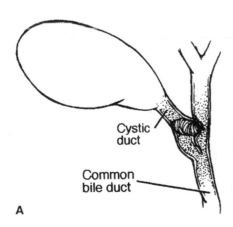

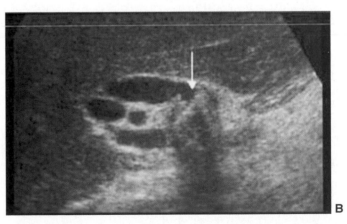

Figure 4-5 Mirizzi syndrome. **A.** Mirizzi syndrome is the clinical condition when a patient presents with jaundice, pain, and fever because of a stone that is lodged in the cystic duct with compression of the common duct. **B.** A stone (*arrow*) is noted to be lodged in the cystic duct, compressing the common bile duct and leading to obstruction and dilation of the extrahepatic biliary tree.

> **◀))) SOUND OFF**
> Mirizzi syndrome is a clinical condition caused by compression of the common duct secondary to a stone that is lodged in the cystic duct.

Cholangitis

Inflammation of the biliary ducts is termed **cholangitis**. When the bile duct walls thicken greater than 5 mm, one should suspect some form of cholangitis. Indeed, if the biliary duct wall appears visible thickened at any time, cholangitis should be suspected (Fig. 4-6).

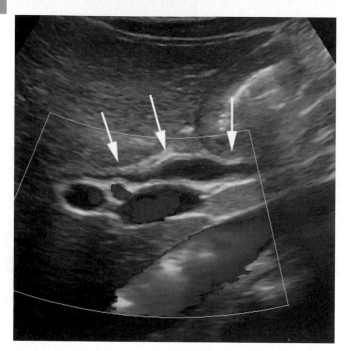

Figure 4-6 Cholangitis. Color Doppler image of the common bile duct (*arrows*) indicates thickening of the bile duct walls, which is sonographic evidence of cholangitis. This patient had sclerosing cholangitis.

The most common cause of cholangitis is often some type of obstructive disease, as in the case of choledocholithiasis. This may be referred to as acute bacterial or ascending cholangitis. There are several other types of cholangitis, including AIDS, Oriental (recurrent pyogenic cholangitis), and sclerosing (Table 4-1). Patients with acute bacterial cholangitis are often present with fever, right upper quadrant pain, and jaundice, a condition referred to a **Charcot triad**. They may also suffer from leukocytosis and elevated ALP and bilirubin. All of the variants of cholangitis have similar sonographic findings that include some degree of biliary dilatation, biliary sludge, and bile duct wall thickening. Cholangitis can lead to cirrhosis and portal hypertension.

CLINICAL FINDINGS OF CHOLANGITIS

1. Charcot triad: fever, right upper quadrant pain, and jaundice
2. Leukocytosis
3. Elevated ALP, ALT, GGT, and bilirubin (with obstruction)

SONOGRAPHIC FINDINGS OF CHOLANGITIS

1. Biliary dilatation
2. Biliary sludge or pus
3. Choledocholithiasis
4. Bile duct wall thickening

> **◀))) SOUND OFF**
> Charcot triad is fever, right upper quadrant pain, and jaundice.

TABLE 4-1 Types of cholangitis	
Type of Cholangitis	**Important Points**
Acute bacterial cholangitis	• Caused by bacterial accumulation secondary to obstruction • Bacteria can be introduced during an ERCP for choledocholithiasis • Pus may be noted within the bile ducts as low-level echoes
AIDS cholangitis	• Associated with advance HIV and AIDS • Most often results from infection with *Cryptosporidium* or cytomegalovirus
Oriental cholangitis	• Endemic to Asia • Seen in America because of immigration
Sclerosing cholangitis	• Characterized by fibrotic thickening of the bile ducts • Most often affects young men • Associated with **inflammatory bowel disease** or **ulcerative colitis** • Increased risk for cholangiocarcinoma

ERCP, endoscopic retrograde cholangiopancreatography.

Pneumobilia

Pneumobilia is defined as air within the biliary tree. Pneumobilia may be associated with recent biliary or gastric surgery, emphysematous or prolonged acute cholecystitis, or fistula formation. Pneumobilia is diagnosed sonographically when echogenic linear structures are seen within the ducts (Fig. 4-7). It may be difficult to differentiate pneumobilia from intrahepatic stones. However, air within the bile ducts may be linear in appearance and will most often produce ring-down artifact and have dirty shadowing, whereas intrahepatic stones will produce an acoustic shadow if large enough.

CLINICAL FINDINGS OF PNEUMOBILIA

1. Recent biliary or gastric surgery, emphysematous or acute cholecystitis, or fistula formation
2. Symptoms of acute cholecystitis

SONOGRAPHIC FINDINGS OF PNEUMOBILIA

1. Echogenic linear structures within the ducts that produce ring-down artifacts and dirty shadowing

Ascariasis

Ascariasis is an infection of the small intestine that is caused by *Ascaris lumbricoides*, a parasitic roundworm. The roundworm, which is transmitted the fecal–oral route, develops in the small intestine and makes its way to the biliary tree via the ampulla of Vater. Some patients may be asymptomatic, whereas others may complain of **biliary colic**, or have symptoms of inflammation of the biliary tree, gallbladder, or pancreas. Sonographically, the worm will be noted within the biliary duct as an echogenic linear structure, and its movement with real-time imaging confirms diagnosis.

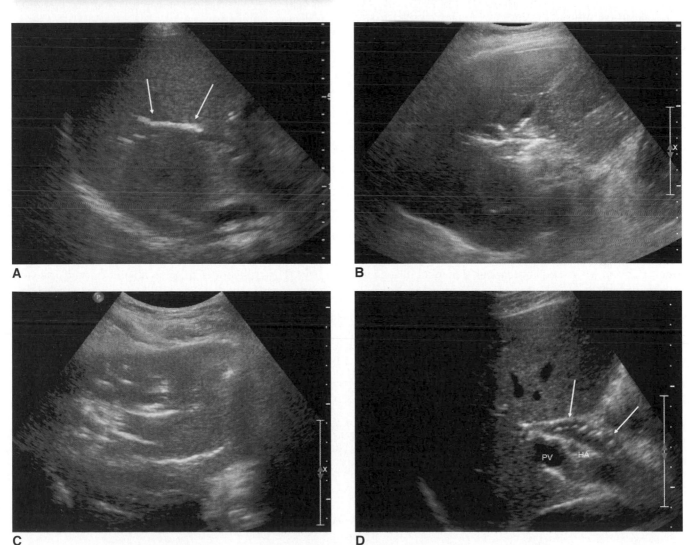

Figure 4-7 Pneumobilia. **A & B.** The echogenic air (*arrows*) and posterior dirty shadowing are seen in the right hepatic lobe. **C.** Diffuse, extensive air within the intrahepatic ducts follows the branching pattern of the ducts and portal venous tree. The air moved under real-time observation. **D.** Air (*arrows*) was seen within the common bile duct after a liver transplant. *HA*, hepatic artery; *PV*, portal vein.

CLINICAL FINDINGS OF ASCARIASIS

1. Asymptomatic
2. May have symptoms of inflammation of the biliary tree, gallbladder, or pancreas

SONOGRAPHIC FINDINGS OF ASCARIASIS

1. The worm will be noted within the biliary duct as an echogenic linear structure in the sagittal plane
2. Movement of the worm within the duct confirms diagnosis

Cholangiocarcinoma and Klatskin Tumors

Primary biliary tree cancer is referred to as **cholangiocarcinoma**. Primary sclerosing cholangitis is the most common risk factor for cholangiocarcinoma, whereas recurrent biliary infections and stone disease also increase the risk. It can have an intrahepatic or extrahepatic location, both of which carry a poor prognosis. **Klatskin tumors** are the most common manifestation of cholangiocarcinoma. These tumors are located at the junction of the right and left hepatic ducts and cause dilatation of the intrahepatic ducts. Patients will present with jaundice, **pruritus**, unexplained weight loss, and abdominal pain. Laboratory findings include an elevated serum bilirubin and ALP. Sonographically, dilated intrahepatic ducts that abruptly terminate at the level of the tumor are suggestive of cholangiocarcinoma (Fig. 4-8). Occasionally, a solid mass may be noted within the liver or ducts. Cholangiocarcinoma is most often adenocarcinoma, but other forms of biliary cancer can occur, such as squamous cell carcinoma and cystadenocarcinoma.

CLINICAL FINDINGS OF CHOLANGIOCARCINOMA

1. Jaundice
2. Pruritus
3. Unexplained weight loss
4. Abdominal pain
5. Elevated bilirubin
6. Elevated ALP

SONOGRAPHIC FINDINGS OF CHOLANGIOCARCINOMA

1. Dilated intrahepatic ducts that abruptly terminate at the level of the tumor
2. A solid mass may be noted within the liver or ducts

🔊 SOUND OFF
Klatskin tumors are located at the junction of the right and left hepatic ducts and cause dilatation of the intrahepatic ducts.

PEDIATRIC PATHOLOGY OF THE BILE DUCTS

Biliary Atresia

Biliary atresia is a congenital disease that is thought to be caused by a viral infection at birth, although some think it may be an inherited disorder. It is a disease with a poor prognosis that is described as the narrowing or obliteration of all or a portion of the biliary tree. Eventually, infants suffer from cirrhosis and portal hypertension. Sonographically, biliary atresia will appear as absent ducts. The gallbladder may be absent or small as well. There may be evidence of the **"triangular cord sign,"**

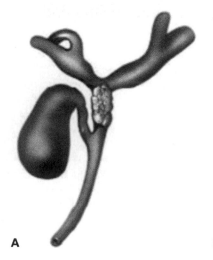
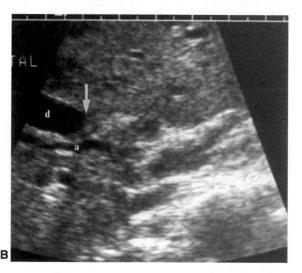

Figure 4-8 Klatskin tumor and cholangiocarcinoma. **A.** A Klatskin tumor is the most common form of cholangiocarcinoma. It is located at the junction of the right and left hepatic ducts, leading to dilation of the intrahepatic ducts. **B.** The dilated common bile duct (*d*) abruptly ends at a small cholangiocarcinoma (*arrow*) that fills the duct. The hepatic artery (*a*) is also noted in this image.

which is an avascular, echogenic, triangular, or tubular structure anterior to the portal vein, representing the replacement of the extrahepatic duct with fibrous tissue in the porta hepatis (Fig. 4-9). Also, the "**pseudogallbladder sign**" may be demonstrated, which appears as a cystic structure in the area of the gallbladder fossa without evidence of an actual gallbladder. Eventually, sonographic features of cirrhosis and portal hypertension will be seen if the disorder is not treated. Clinical findings can be confused with neonatal hepatitis. Both atresia and hepatitis include elevated AST, ALT, and bilirubin. However, unlike neonatal hepatitis, which can be treated medically, biliary atresia is often fatal without surgical intervention.

CLINICAL FINDINGS OF BILIARY ATRESIA

1. Neonatal jaundice
2. Elevated AST, ALT, and bilirubin

SONOGRAPHIC FINDINGS OF BILIARY ATRESIA

1. Absent biliary ducts
2. Triangular cord sign (avascular, echogenic, triangular, or tubular structure anterior to the portal vein)
3. Pseudogallbladder sign (cystic structure in the area of the gallbladder fossa without evidence of a true gallbladder)
4. Sonographic signs of cirrhosis and portal hypertension (see Chapter 2)

Choledochal Cyst

There are four different types of choledochal cysts, with the most common being described as the cystic dilatation of the common bile duct. They are usually discovered in infancy or in the first decade of life. Patients with a choledochal cyst present with an abdominal mass, jaundice, pain, and fever. Choledochal cysts can lead

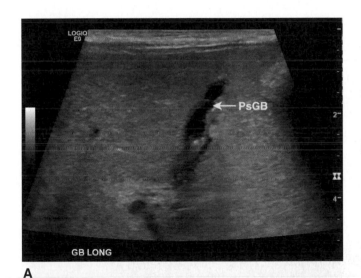

A

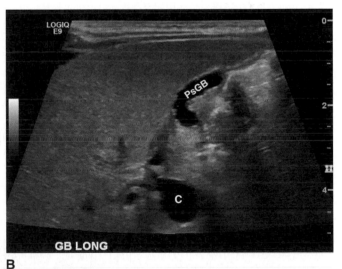

B

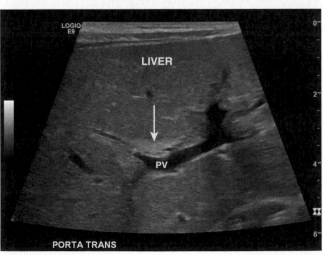

C

Figure 4-9 Biliary atresia. **A.** Longitudinal scan of an atretic gallbladder in a patient with biliary atresia. A pseudogallbladder sign (*PsGB*) is defined as a fluid-filled structure in the gallbladder fossa measuring less than 15 mm in length without a defined gallbladder wall. **B.** A choledochal cyst (*C*) noted within the area of the porta hepatis in the same patient. **C.** The triangular cord sign (*arrow*) refers to a triangular echogenic anterior wall of the right portal vein (*PV*) that measures more than 4 mm in thickness on a longitudinal scan. This sign is specific for diagnosis of biliary atresia.

to cholangitis, portal hypertension, pancreatitis, and liver failure. Sonographic findings of a choledochal cyst include a fusiform cystic mass in the area of the porta hepatis and biliary dilatation (Fig. 4-10).

CLINICAL FINDINGS OF A CHOLEDOCHAL CYST

1. Jaundice
2. Pain
3. Fever

SONOGRAPHIC FINDINGS OF A CHOLEDOCHAL CYST

1. Cystic mass in the area of the porta hepatis (separate from the gallbladder)
2. Biliary dilatation

Caroli Disease

Caroli disease, or Caroli syndrome, is a congenital disorder characterized by segmental dilatation of the intrahepatic ducts. It is often seen in association with cystic renal disease

and may precede the development of cholangiocarcinoma, a hepatic abscess, cholangitis, and sepsis. Patients may present with pain, fever, jaundice, or signs of portal hypertension. Sonographic findings include segmental dilatation of the intrahepatic ducts. The **"central dot sign"** may also be noted, which is described as the presence of echogenic dots in the nondependent part of the dilated duct representing small fibrovascular bundles (Fig. 4-11).

CLINICAL FINDINGS OF CAROLI DISEASE

1. Pain
2. Fever
3. Jaundice
4. Signs of portal hypertension (see Chapter 2)

SONOGRAPHIC FINDINGS OF CAROLI DISEASE

1. Segmental dilatation of the intrahepatic ducts
2. The patient may also have cystic renal disease
3. Central dot sign (echogenic dots in the nondependent part of the dilated duct)

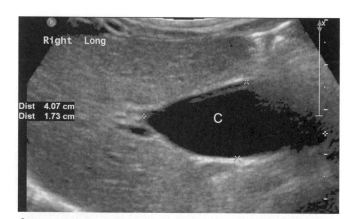

A

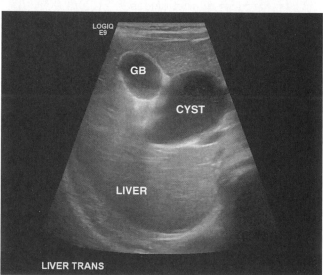

C

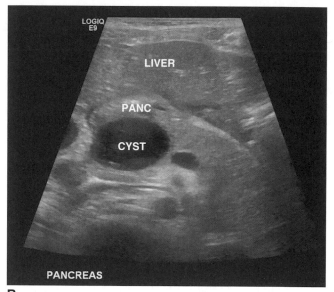

B

Figure 4-10 Choledochal cyst. **A.** A longitudinal image of the right upper quadrant shows fusiform dilation of the common bile duct (*between calipers*). **B.** A choledochal cyst is noted posterior to the head of the pancreas. **C.** A transvers image of the liver reveals a choledochal cyst imaged posterior to the gallbladder (*GB*).

The Bile Ducts

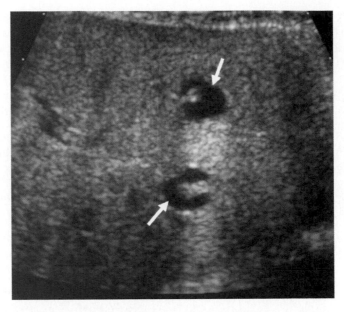

Figure 4-11 Central dot sign and Caroli disease. Image of the liver with dilated ducts (*arrows*) demonstrating the "central dot" sign associated with Caroli disease that are representing small fibromuscular bundles.

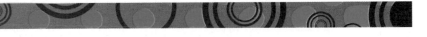

REVIEW QUESTIONS

1. A congenital disease that is described as narrowing or obliteration of the bile ducts is referred to as:
   a. Caroli disease.
   b. Mirizzi disease.
   c. choledochal cysts.
   d. biliary atresia.

2. Ascariasis is:
   a. a form of biliary tree carcinoma.
   b. a congenital disorder characterized by segmental dilatation of the intrahepatic ducts.
   c. caused by a parasitic roundworm.
   d. a type of ringworm that invades the liver.

3. Primary biliary tree cancer is referred to as:
   a. gallbladder carcinoma.
   b. biloma.
   c. cholangiocarcinoma.
   d. lymphangioma.

4. Which of the following is associated with Charcot triad?
   a. Cholangitis
   b. Cholesterolosis
   c. Klatskin tumor
   d. Choledochal cyst

5. The merging point of the pancreatic duct and common bile duct at the level of duodenum is referred to as the:
   a. sphincter of Oddi.
   b. ampulla of Vater.
   c. common bile duct.
   d. cystic duct.

6. Which of the following would be the least helpful laboratory value to analyze in patients with suspected biliary tract disease?
   a. ALT
   b. ALP
   c. GGT
   d. Creatinine

7. A gallstone located within the biliary tree is referred to as:
   a. cholecystitis.
   b. choledocholithiasis.
   c. cholangitis.
   d. cholangiocarcinoma.

8. Which of the following disorders is associated with the sonographic triangular cord sign?
   a. Cholangitis
   b. Choledocholithiasis
   c. Biliary atresia
   d. Ascariasis

9. The yellowish staining of the whites of the eyes and the skin secondary to a liver disorder or biliary obstruction is referred to as:
   a. AIDS cholangitis.
   b. pruritus.
   c. jaundice.
   d. bilirubinemia.

10. The Klatskin tumor is located:
    a. at the junction of the right and left hepatic ducts.
    b. at the junction of the cystic and common bile duct.
    c. at the junction of the common bile duct and common hepatic duct.
    d. between the pancreatic head and the duodenum.

11. Inflammation of the bile ducts is referred to as:
    a. pneumobilia.
    b. choledocholithiasis.
    c. cholelithiasis.
    d. cholangitis.

12. A patient presents with jaundice, pain, and fever secondary to an impacted stone in the cystic duct. This is referred to as:
    a. Caroli syndrome.
    b. Mirizzi syndrome.
    c. choledochal cysts.
    d. biliary atresia.

13. Air within the biliary tree is referred to as:
    a. pneumobilia.
    b. cholangitis.
    c. choledocholithiasis.
    d. cholesterolosis.

14. The presence of an echogenic dot in the nondependent part of a dilated duct representing small fibrovascular bundles is seen with:
    a. Caroli disease.
    b. choledochal cysts.
    c. biliary atresia.
    d. Mirizzi syndrome.

15. The spiral valves of Heister are located within the:
    a. common bile duct.
    b. pancreatic duct.
    c. common hepatic duct.
    d. cystic duct.

16. Which of the following is characterized by fibrotic thickening of the bile ducts, found most often in young males, and is associated with inflammatory bowel disease or ulcerative colitis?
    a. Ulcerative biliary atresia
    b. Oriental cholangitis
    c. Sclerosing cholangitis
    d. AIDS biliary atresia

17. If a gallstone, causing obstruction, is located within the distal common hepatic duct, which of the following would become dilated?
    a. Main pancreatic duct
    b. Gallbladder only
    c. Intrahepatic ducts
    d. Distal common bile duct

18. Which of the following is considered the most proximal portion of the biliary tree?
    a. Intrahepatic radicles
    b. Cystic duct
    c. Common hepatic duct
    d. Common bile duct

19. Pneumobilia will produce:
    a. through transmission.
    b. ring-down artifact.
    c. acoustic shadowing.
    d. edge artifact.

20. Which of the following would be the most distal portion of the biliary tree?
    a. Common bile duct
    b. Common hepatic duct
    c. Gallbladder
    d. Intrahepatic radicles

21. Which of the following could accidentally introduce bacteria into the biliary tree and thus cause cholangitis?
    a. Computed tomography
    b. ERCP
    c. Magnetic resonance imaging
    d. Radiography

22. If an obstructive biliary calculus is located within the distal common duct, which of the following could ultimately dilate?
    a. Common bile duct only
    b. Gallbladder and cystic duct
    c. Common hepatic duct and intrahepatic ducts
    d. Common bile duct, gallbladder, common hepatic duct, and intrahepatic ducts

23. The muscle that controls the emptying of bile and pancreatic juices into the duodenum is the:
    a. cystic duct.
    b. ampulla of Vater.
    c. sphincter of Oddi.
    d. common bile duct.

24. The most common level for biliary obstruction to occur is the:
    a. junction of the right and left hepatic ducts.
    b. proximal common hepatic duct.
    c. distal common bile duct.
    d. cystic duct.

25. A 32-year-old female patient presents to the sonography department with a history of fever, leukocytosis, and right upper quadrant pain. Sonographically, you visualize dilated bile ducts that have thickened walls and contain sludge. What is the most likely diagnosis?
    a. Choledocholithiasis
    b. Cholangitis
    c. Mirizzi syndrome
    d. Biliary atresia

26. Sonographically, you visualize scattered echogenic linear structures within the liver parenchyma that produce ring-down artifact. What is the most likely diagnosis?
    a. Pneumobilia
    b. Choledocholithiasis
    c. Sludge balls
    d. Cholesterolosis

27. A 64-year-old man presents to the sonography department for a right upper quadrant sonogram. He is complaining of abdominal pain, weight loss, and pruritus. Sonographically, you visualize an area of dilated ducts that abruptly end. What is the most likely diagnosis?
    a. Biliary atresia
    b. Choledocholithiasis
    c. Caroli syndrome
    d. Cholangiocarcinoma

28. An abdominal sonogram is ordered for an infant in the intensive care unit who is suffering from jaundice and fever. Sonographically, you visualize an anechoic mass within the common bile duct that is causing a focal enlargement. This is most suggestive of:
    a. cholangiocarcinoma.
    b. Mirizzi syndrome.
    c. choledochal cyst.
    d. biliary atresia.

29. All of the following are clinical findings consistent with cholangiocarcinoma except:
    a. pruritus.
    b. weight loss.
    c. elevated bilirubin.
    d. dilation of the intrahepatic ducts.

30. Which of the following is not associated with the development of pneumobilia?
    a. Cholangiopneumonia
    b. Gastric surgery
    c. Acute cholecystitis
    d. Fistula formation

31. A Klatskin tumor is a manifestation of:
    a. lymphocytic carcinoma.
    b. cholangiocarcinoma.
    c. pancreatic carcinoma.
    d. gallbladder carcinoma.

32. The biliary duct wall should never measure more than:
    a. 2 mm.
    b. 9 mm.
    c. 4 mm.
    d. 5 mm.

33. Clinical findings of choledocholithiasis include all of the following except:
    a. jaundice.
    b. elevated bilirubin.
    c. elevated blood urea nitrogen.
    d. elevated ALP.

34. Which segment of the biliary tree tends to dilate first with obstruction?
    a. Intrahepatic
    b. Extrahepatic

35. Which of the following is not a plausible cause of common bile duct obstruction in adults?
    a. Choledocholithiasis
    b. Chronic pancreatitis
    c. Choledochal cyst
    d. Pancreatic carcinoma

36. All of the following are forms of cholangitis except:
    a. acute bacterial.
    b. AIDS.
    c. oriental.
    d. parabolic.

37. The yellowish pigment found in bile that is produced by the breakdown of old red blood cells by the liver is:
    a. biliverdin.
    b. bilirubin.
    c. cholesterol.
    d. chyme.

38. Which of the following is typically found in pediatric patients and is described as the cystic dilation of the common bile duct?
    a. Biliary atresia
    b. Mirizzi syndrome
    c. Caroli disease
    d. Choledochal cyst

39. For patients older than 60 years, or those who have had a cholecystectomy, a maximum diameter of _____ may be considered normal.
    a. 1 cm
    b. 12 mm
    c. 14 mm
    d. 1.5 cm

40. Which of the following would be the most common cause of obstructive jaundice?
    a. Klatskin tumor
    b. Cholangiocarcinoma
    c. Biliary atresia
    d. Choledocholithiasis

41. The patient in Figure 4-12 recently underwent surgery following a bout of emphysematous cholecystitis. Which of the following is the most likely etiology of the pathology noted by the arrows?
    a. Biliary atresia
    b. Cholangitis
    c. Pneumobilia
    d. Choledochal cysts

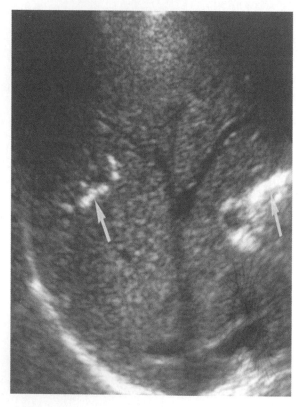

Figure 4-12

42. Which of the following is associated with the "pseudogallbladder" sign?
    a. Biliary strictures
    b. Charcot triad
    c. Pruritus
    d. Biliary atresia

43. Which of the following clinical findings would be least likely noted concerning the patient in Figure 4-13?
    a. Triangular cord sign
    b. Jaundice
    c. Elevated bilirubin
    d. Elevated ALP

44. What does the arrow in Figure 4-14 indicate?
    a. Cystic artery
    b. Cystic duct
    c. Hepatic artery
    d. Common hepatic duct

45. What pathology can be noted in Figure 4-14?
    a. Choledocholithiasis
    b. Cholecystitis
    c. Pneumobilia
    d. Cholangitis

46. Which of the following is a fluoroscopic procedure typically performed in the radiology department that involves an analysis of the biliary tree and pancreas?
    a. MRCP
    b. ERCP
    c. Nuclear medicine cholangiography
    d. Cholangiofluoroscopy

47. Which of the following is associated with a biliary obstruction?
    a. Posthepatic jaundice
    b. Prehepatic jaundice
    c. Hepatic jaundice
    d. Biliary jaundice

48. What is another name for the sphincter of Oddi?
    a. Vatorial sphincter
    b. Proximal duodenal sphincter
    c. Common biliary sphincter
    d. Hepatopancreatic sphincter

49. Among the following list, which of the following is located just distal to the cystic duct?
    a. Right hepatic duct
    b. Common hepatic duct
    c. Duct of Wirsung
    d. Common bile duct

50. Sever itchiness of the skin is referred to as:
    a. pruritus.
    b. kernicterus.
    c. cellulitis.
    d. subcutaneous edemitis.

51. Enlargement of the common bile duct and pancreatic duct is referred to as the:
    a. double-barrel shotgun sign.
    b. parallel tube sign.
    c. Mirizzi sign.
    d. double-duct sign.

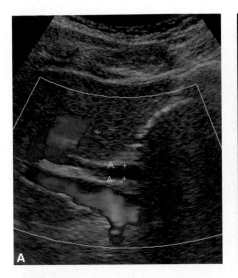
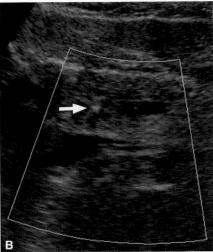
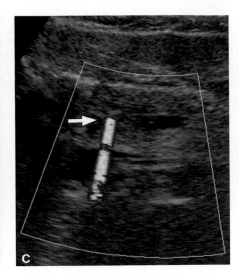

Figure 4-13

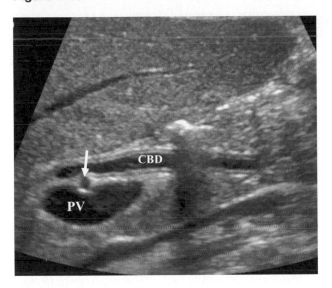

Figure 4-14

52. Which of the following is not a sonographic finding of cholangitis?
    a. Biliary dilatation
    b. Biliary sludge
    c. Choledocholithiasis
    d. Triangular cord sign

53. Which of the following is the most common risk factor for cholangiocarcinoma?
    a. Pruritus
    b. Biliary atresia
    c. Sclerosing cholangitis
    d. Choledocholithiasis

54. What is the most common location of choledocholithiasis?
    a. Near the ampulla of Vater
    b. Near the pancreatic neck
    c. Within the common hepatic duct
    d. Within the proximal common bile duct

55. Which type of cholangitis is found in severely immunocompromised patients and results from infections caused by *Cryptosporidium* or cytomegalovirus?
    a. Sclerosing cholangitis
    b. AIDS cholangitis
    c. Oriental cholangitis
    d. Acute bacterial cholangitis

56. What is the most common form of cholangiocarcinoma?
    a. Adenocarcinoma
    b. Squamous cell carcinoma
    c. Melanoma
    d. Serous cystadenocarcinoma

57. How is ascariasis transmitted?
    a. Blood transfusion
    b. Contaminated water
    c. Fecal–oral route
    d. Inhalation of spores

58. Infants with biliary atresia often ultimately suffer from:
    a. choledocholithiasis.
    b. cirrhosis.
    c. cholecystitis.
    d. pneumobilia.

59. The pathology in Figure 4-15 was identified in a patient complaining of right upper quadrant pain and fever. What do the arrows most likely represent?
    a. Bile duct sludge
    b. Cholangitis
    c. Choledocholithiasis
    d. Intrahepatic thrombus

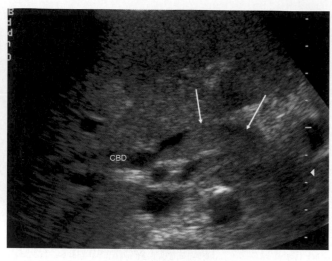

Figure 4-15

60. Which of the following is the major component of bile?
    a. Salt
    b. Spent hepatocytes
    c. Cholesterol
    d. Amylase

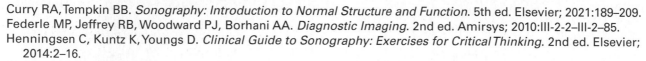

SUGGESTED READINGS

Curry RA, Tempkin BB. *Sonography: Introduction to Normal Structure and Function*. 5th ed. Elsevier; 2021:189–209.

Federle MP, Jeffrey RB, Woodward PJ, Borhani AA. *Diagnostic Imaging*. 2nd ed. Amirsys; 2010:III-2-2–III-2–85.

Henningsen C, Kuntz K, Youngs D. *Clinical Guide to Sonography: Exercises for Critical Thinking*. 2nd ed. Elsevier; 2014:2–16.

Hertzberg BS, Middleton WD. *Ultrasound: The Requisites*. 3rd ed. Elsevier; 2016:89–102.

Kawamura DM, Nolan TD. *Diagnostic Medical Sonography: Abdomen and Superficial Structures*. 4th ed. Wolters Kluwer; 2018:171–212 & 611–654.

Lee JG. Diagnosis and management of acute cholangitis. *Nat Clin Pract Gastroenterol Hepatol*. 2009;6(9):533–541.

Rumack CM, Wilson SR, Charboneau JW, et al. *Diagnostic Ultrasound*. 4th ed. Elsevier; 2011:172–215 & 1800–1844.

Sanders RC, Hall-Terracciano B. *Clinical Sonography: A Practical Guide*. 5th ed. Wolters Kluwer; 2016:421–451.

Siegel MJ. *Pediatric Sonography*. 5th ed. Wolters Kluwer; 2019:273–303.

BONUS REVIEW!

Biliary Stent (Fig. 4-16)

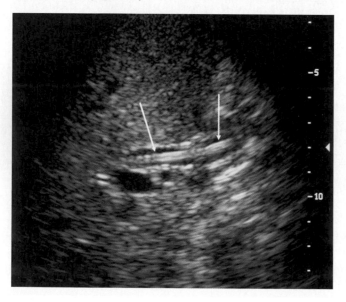

Figure 4-16 Biliary stent. Echogenic parallel lines (*arrows*) within the common bile duct represent a biliary stent. Stents are placed in the biliary tree to act as a conduit for bile.

The Bile Ducts

Endoscopic Retrograde Cholangiopancreatography (Fig. 4-17)

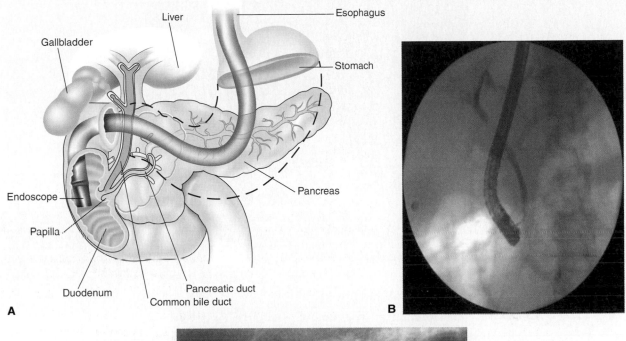

A

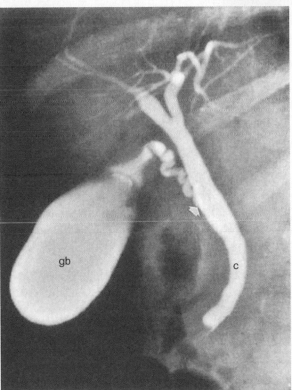

C

Figure 4-17 Endoscopic retrograde cholangiopancreatography (*ERCP*). **A.** During an ERCP, an endoscope is inserted into the mouth, down the esophagus, through the stomach, and into the proximal duodenum. A contrast medium is injected into the pancreatic and bile ducts in preparation for radiography. **B.** Completed ERCP showing a patent common bile duct and absence of filling defects. **C.** Different radiographic view (contrast appears white in this image) demonstrating filling of the gallbladder (*gb*) and common bile duct (*c*). The tortuous cystic duct (*arrow*) is also noted.

(*continued*)

Magnetic Resonance Cholangiopancreatography (Fig. 4-18)

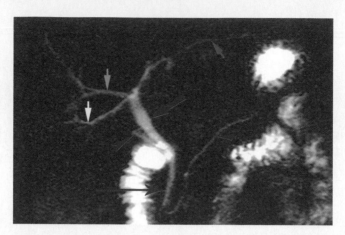

Figure 4-18 Normal magnetic resonance cholangiopancreatography (*MRCP*). Image from an MRCP in a patient who has had a cholecystectomy shows the cystic duct remnant (*red arrowhead*), common bile duct (*long red arrow*), common hepatic duct (*fat red arrow*), pancreatic duct (*small red arrow*), left hepatic duct (*small blue arrow*), anterior branch of the right hepatic duct (*small yellow arrow*), and posterior branch of the right hepatic (*small green arrow*). An MRCP is utilized to evaluate the biliary tree for masses, postsurgical complications, and many other issues with the use of contrast.

The Pancreas

Introduction

This chapter contains information about normal pancreatic anatomy and pancreatic abnormalities that may be noted during a sonographic examination. The reviewer should be attentive to detailed clinical findings because many of the abnormalities mentioned in this chapter can appear sonographically similar. The "Bonus Review" section includes several computed tomography (CT) images of pancreatitis.

Key Terms

acinar cells—the cells of the pancreas that carry out the exocrine function and, therefore, produce amylase, lipase, sodium bicarbonate, and other digestive enzymes

annular pancreas—congenital anomaly of the pancreas that results in the maldevelopment of the pancreas in which the most ventral part of the pancreas encases the duodenum and may consequently lead to duodenal obstruction

chronic pancreatitis—the recurring destruction of the pancreatic tissue that results in atrophy, fibrosis with scarring, and the development of calcification within the gland

cystic fibrosis—inherited disorder that can affect the lungs, liver, pancreas, and other organs; this disorder changes how the body creates mucus and sweat

double-duct sign—coexisting enlargement of the common bile duct and pancreatic duct

duct of Santorini—the accessory duct of the pancreas

duct of Wirsung—the main pancreatic duct

duodenum—the first segment of the small intestine

endoscopic retrograde cholangiopancreatography—endoscopic procedure that utilizes fluoroscopy (radiographic imaging) to evaluate the biliary tree and pancreas

gallstone pancreatitis—form of pancreatitis associated with gallstones and pancreatic duct obstruction

gastrinoma—an islet cell tumor found within the cells of the pancreas that may produce an abundance of gastrin

hemorrhagic pancreatitis—form of pancreatitis associated with bleeding within or around the pancreas

hyperamylasemia—elevated amylase

hyperparathyroidism—the presence of elevated parathyroid hormone

ileus—bowel obstruction caused by the lack of normal peristalsis

insulinoma—an islet cell tumor found within the beta cells of the pancreas that may produce an abundance of insulin

interstitial edematous pancreatitis—most common form of pancreatitis; associated with inflammation of the pancreas and peripancreatic tissue without necrosis

islet cell tumors—tumor found within the islets of Langerhans of the pancreas

islets of Langerhans—small islands of tissue found within the pancreas that produce insulin and glucagon

lesser sac—a peritoneal cavity located between the stomach and the pancreas where fluid can accumulate

necrosis—death of tissue

necrotizing pancreatitis—severe form of acute pancreatitis in which there is death of the pancreatic tissue

pancreatic adenocarcinoma—the most common form of pancreatic malignancy, typically found within the head of the pancreas

pancreatic divisum—congenital anomaly of the pancreas that results in a shortened main pancreatic duct that only works to drain the pancreatic head and not the entire pancreas

pancreaticoduodenectomy—the surgical procedure in which the head of the pancreas, the gallbladder, some of the bile ducts, and the proximal duodenum are removed because of a malignant pancreatic neoplasm; also referred to as the Whipple procedure

pancreatic pseudocyst—a cyst surrounded by fibrous tissue that consists of pancreatic enzymes that have leaked from the pancreas

pancreatic steatosis—fatty infiltration of the pancreas; may be classified as alcoholic or nonalcoholic; may also be referred to as a fatty pancreas

phlegmon—the peripancreatic fluid collection that results from the inflammation of the pancreas

uncinate process—a posteromedial extension of the pancreatic head

von Hippel–Lindau disease—a hereditary disease that includes the development of cysts within the pancreas and other organs

Whipple procedure—see pancreaticoduodenectomy

Whipple triad—a group of clinical indicators of a functional insulinoma; includes hypoglycemia, low fasting glucose, and relief with intravenous glucose administration

Zollinger–Ellison syndrome—the syndrome that includes an excessive secretion of acid by the stomach caused by the presence of a functional gastrinoma within the pancreas

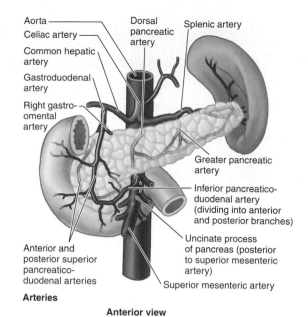

Figure 5-1 Diagrams of the surrounding anatomy and vasculature of the pancreas.

ANATOMY AND PHYSIOLOGY OF THE PANCREAS

The pancreas develops initially in the embryo from two separate parts that eventually fuse together to constitute its typical comma-shaped appearance. It is located within the epigastrium between the C-loop of the **duodenum** and the splenic hilum (Fig. 5-1). It consists of four main parts: head, neck, body, and tail. In some individuals, there exists a posteromedial extension of the pancreatic head, referred to as the **uncinate process**. Although some of the pancreatic head may be covered by peritoneum, the pancreas is a retroperitoneal organ. The organ functions as both an exocrine and an endocrine gland.

> **◀))) SOUND OFF**
> The pancreas is both an exocrine gland (uses ducts to transport digestive juices) and an endocrine gland (releases hormone directly into the bloodstream).

Primarily, the pancreas is an exocrine gland that aids in digestion (Table 5-1). The **acinar cells** of the pancreas carry out the exocrine function because they produce vital digestive enzymes, such as amylase and lipase, and sodium bicarbonate. The pancreas also produces trypsin, chymotrypsin, and carboxypolypeptidase as

TABLE 5-1 Exocrine function of the pancreas

1. Amylase: digests carbohydrates and converts starch to sugar
2. Lipase: digests fats and converts fats to fatty acids and glycerol
3. Sodium bicarbonate: neutralizes stomach acid
4. Trypsin, chymotrypsin, and carboxypolypeptidase: breaks down proteins

part of its exocrine function. These pancreatic enzymes drain from the pancreas into the main pancreatic duct, or **duct of Wirsung**, which travels the length of the pancreas (Fig. 5-2). An accessory duct, the **duct of Santorini**, which is typically a branch of the main pancreatic duct, has a separate minor sphincter into the duodenum. The slightly raised area into the lumen of duodenum, upon which the sphincter is located, is referred to as the minor duodenal papilla or accessory papilla. From the main pancreatic duct, the enzymes collect in the ampulla of Vater, also referred to as the hepatopancreatic ampulla. At the ampulla of Vater,

the pancreatic digestive enzymes are mixed with bile from the liver and released into the duodenum through the major sphincter, or sphincter of Oddi. The sphincter of Oddi rests upon another raised area within the duodenal lumen, referred to as the major duodenal papilla (papilla of Vater). Relaxation and the consequent opening of the sphincter of Oddi is triggered by cholecystokinin released by the duodenum because of the presence of chyme. Therefore, cholecystokinin causes the simultaneous contraction of the gallbladder and relaxation of the sphincter of Oddi. The breakdown of the various food products into useful derivatives for the body ensues once the pancreatic enzymes and bile mix with chyme in the proximal portion of the duodenum.

The endocrine function of the pancreas is performed by the **islets of Langerhans**. These clusters of tissue, which are dispersed like islands throughout the pancreas, are composed of alpha, beta, and delta cells (Table 5-2). The islets of Langerhans produce vital hormones, including insulin and glucagon, which are released directly into the bloodstream. Glucagon promotes the release of glucose by the liver, which, in turn, increases blood sugar levels. Insulin stimulates the body to use up glucagon to produce energy.

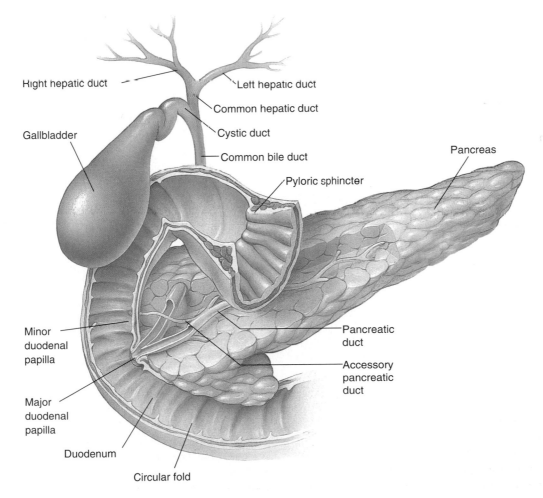

Figure 5-2 Diagram of the biliary tree and the pancreas.

TABLE 5-2 Endocrine function of the pancreas

Alpha cells	Glucagon	Promotes the release of glucose by the liver (increases blood sugar level)
Beta cells	Insulin	Stimulates the body's use of glucagon
Delta cells	Somatostatin	Restrains insulin and glucose level

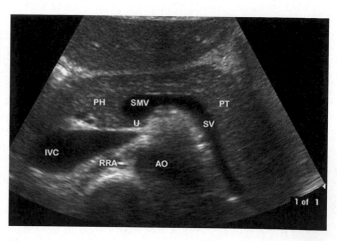

Figure 5-3 Transverse sonogram of the pancreas demonstrating adjacent vasculature. The pancreatic head (*PH*) is noted right lateral to the superior mesenteric vein (*SMV*). The splenic vein (*SV*) can be seen outlining the posterior aspect of the pancreatic tail (*PT*). *AO*, aorta; *IVC*, inferior vena cava; *RRA*, right renal artery; *U*, uncinate process.

VASCULAR ANATOMY OF THE PANCREAS

The arterial blood supply to the head of the pancreas is via the gastroduodenal artery. The body and tail of the pancreas receive their blood supply from the splenic and superior mesenteric arteries. Venous drainage is achieved by means of the splenic vein, superior mesenteric vein, inferior mesenteric vein, and portal vein (see Fig. 5-1).

SONOGRAPHY OF THE PANCREAS

Rarely, the pancreas is imaged without including the complete right upper quadrant. A thorough evaluation of the bile ducts and gallbladder for associated abnormalities is generally required. The pancreas can frequently be a neglected abdominal organ because of the challenge that it presents for the sonographer. Adjacent bowel gas and body habitus are two obstacles that the sonographer encounters when attempting to assess the pancreas using sound. To improve visualization of the pancreatic head, the sonographer can ask the patient to drink a small cup of water (should protocols allow). The water, once in the stomach and C-loop of the duodenum, may provide an enhanced view of the pancreatic head in most individuals. In addition, left lateral decubitus position may help improve visualization of the pancreatic head. To better visualize the pancreatic tail area, the sonographer can scan through the left kidney and spleen while the patient is in the right lateral decubitus position. Upright scanning can furthermore be exceedingly helpful.

The pancreas is identified sonographically by its neighboring vasculature (Fig. 5-3, Table 5-3). The normal echogenicity of the pancreas is greater than that of the liver, and equal to, or greater than, that of the spleen in the adult. In some adults, the pancreas may appear peculiarly diffusely hyperechoic, representing **pancreatic steatosis**. The pediatric

TABLE 5-3 Adjacent vasculature associated with the pancreas

Part of the Pancreas	Adjacent Vasculature
Pancreatic head	Right lateral to superior mesenteric vein Anterior to inferior vena cava and inferior to portal vein
Uncinate process	Posterior to superior mesenteric vein; may completely surround superior mesenteric vein Anterior to aorta
Pancreatic neck	Anterior to portal confluence
Pancreatic body	Anterior to superior mesenteric vein, splenic vein, and superior mesenteric artery
Pancreatic tail	Splenic vein marks posterior border of pancreatic tail

pancreas may appear more hypoechoic because of the lack of fat surrounding the pancreas in younger patients. In the transverse plane, two round anechoic structures may be noted within the pancreatic head. The anterior structure is the gastroduodenal artery, and the more posterior structure is the common bile duct (Fig. 5-4).

Depending upon the resolution of the ultrasound system and size of the patient, the normal main pancreatic duct may be noted during a routine sonographic examination. It will appear as an anechoic tube, consisting of two parallel lines, with an anechoic

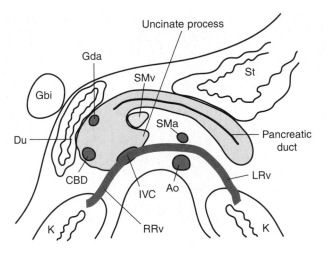

Figure 5-4 Transverse pancreas. Transverse drawing of pancreatic anatomy demonstrating the gallbladder (*Gbi*), duodenum (*Du*), stomach (*St*), kidneys (*K*), inferior vena cava (*IVC*), aorta (*Ao*), superior mesenteric artery (*SMa*), superior mesenteric vein (*SMv*), right renal vein (*RRv*), left renal vein (*LRv*), common bile duct (*CBD*), gastroduodenal artery (*Gda*), uncinate process of the pancreas, and the pancreatic duct.

lumen. The anteroposterior diameter of the main pancreatic duct should not exceed 2 mm. Color-flow Doppler imaging is helpful to differentiate the splenic artery from the main pancreatic duct because these two structures can have parallel paths within the body. The

sonographic analysis of the pancreas may include measurements of the various parts of the organ. The pancreas is typically measured in the anteroposterior dimension in the transverse scan plane. The normal measurement of the pancreatic head and body is between 2 and 3 cm, whereas the tail should measure between 1 and 2 cm. Clinical history should always be considered when pancreatic enlargement is suspected.

> ### SOUND OFF
> The splenic artery, which takes a similar path within the abdomen, may be confused for a dilated main pancreatic duct, and thus, color Doppler should be utilized to differentiate the two structures.

CONGENITAL ANOMALIES OF THE PANCREAS

The two most common congenital anomalies of the pancreas are **pancreatic divisum** and **annular pancreas** (Fig. 5-5). Pancreatic divisum, which is the most common congenital variant of pancreatic anatomy, results from abnormal fusion of the pancreatic ducts during embryologic development. Pancreatic divisum results in a shortened main pancreatic duct (duct of Wirsung)

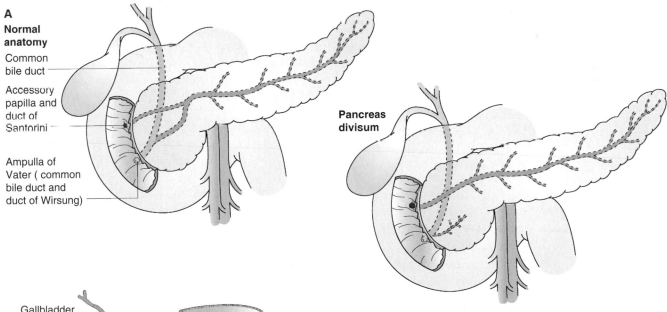

A
Normal anatomy
Common bile duct
Accessory papilla and duct of Santorini
Ampulla of Vater (common bile duct and duct of Wirsung)

Pancreas divisum

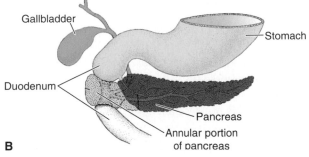

Gallbladder
Stomach
Duodenum
Pancreas
Annular portion of pancreas
B

Figure 5-5 Pancreatic variants. **A.** Pancreatic divisum results in no communication between the main pancreatic duct and the accessory duct. The main pancreatic duct is short or may be completely absent, whereas most of the pancreas is drained by the accessory duct into the much smaller accessory papilla. For quick comparison, normal ductal anatomy is provided as well. **B.** Annular pancreas is the variant in which the head of the pancreas wraps around the duodenum, effectively causing a bowel obstruction.

that works to drain only the pancreatic head and not the entire pancreas. The accessory duct (duct of Santorini), which is much smaller than the main pancreatic duct, is, therefore, forced to drain the rest of the pancreas and empty a larger-than-normal amount of pancreatic juices through the minor sphincter. This abnormal duct arrangement causes a functional obstruction, disallowing proper pancreatic drainage and increasing the risk for pancreatic inflammation secondary to the obstruction. Therefore, although these individuals may be asymptomatic, some may be prone to suffer from both chronic and acute pancreatitis. The annular pancreas results from the maldevelopment of the two embryologic elements of the pancreas. With an annular pancreas, the most ventral part of the pancreas encases the duodenum and may consequently lead to duodenal obstruction. Neither variant is definitively diagnosed sonographically, but rather with other imaging modalities, including CT, magnetic resonance imaging (MRI), and, possibly, radiography.

> ◀))) **SOUND OFF**
> Pancreatic divisum, which is the most common congenital variant of the pancreas, can lead to both acute and chronic pancreatitis.

PATHOLOGY OF THE PANCREAS

Distinctive Forms of Pancreatitis

Though this chapter focuses primarily on the broader definitions and clinical presentations of acute and chronic pancreatitis, it may be beneficial to have a basic understanding concerning the differentiation between the various descriptive forms of pancreatitis. Table 5-4

provides a summary of several of the more distinct forms of pancreatitis.

Acute Pancreatitis

Acute pancreatitis is the inflammation of the pancreas secondary to the leakage of pancreatic enzymes from the acinar cells into the parenchyma of the organ. These enzymes can destroy the pancreatic tissue and the tissues surrounding the pancreas. The most common causes of acute pancreatitis are alcohol abuse and biliary tract disease, such as choledocholithiasis. Other causes of acute pancreatitis include post **endoscopic retrograde cholangiopancreatography** and trauma.

Though acute pancreatitis can be specifically denoted as in Table 5-4, often, acute pancreatitis is divided into either interstitial edematous pancreatitis or necrotizing pancreatitis. Interstitial edematous pancreatitis is more common and better manageable, whereas necrotizing pancreatitis may be fatal. There are several specific clinical findings that suggest acute pancreatitis. The patient will complain of abdominal pain and back pain and have an elevation in blood glucose (hyperglycemia), leukocytosis, serum amylase, and lipase. Amylase levels will rise first, and within 72 hours, an accompanying rise in lipase should occur. Lipase appears to be more specific for diagnosing pancreatitis because **hyperamylasemia** can be associated with other abnormalities. Alanine aminotransferase (ALT) is typically elevated with gallstone pancreatitis. Patients suffering from acute pancreatitis may find reprieve from symptoms in certain positions. For example, the supine position is often most painful, whereas sitting or leaning forward may temporarily relieve pain.

TABLE 5-4 Specific forms or categories of pancreatitis	
Specific Form or Category of Pancreatitis	**Explanation and Unique Feature**
Gallstone pancreatitis	Pancreatitis associated with gallstones and concurrent obstruction of the pancreatic duct
Hemorrhagic pancreatitis	Pancreatitis associated with bleeding within or around the pancreas; high rate of morbidity and mortality
Autoimmune pancreatitis	Form of chronic pancreatitis that results from the body's immune system attacking the pancreas
Groove pancreatitis	Uncommon form of chronic pancreatitis found in the head of the pancreas with associated inflammation of the common bile duct and second portion of the duodenum
Necrotizing pancreatitis	Form of acute pancreatitis resulting in the **necrosis** of the pancreatic parenchyma and the tissue surrounding the pancreas; high rate of morbidity and mortality
Interstitial edematous pancreatitis	Most common form of acute pancreatitis; associated with inflammation of the pancreatic parenchyma and peripancreatic tissues; necrosis is not present

Milder cases of pancreatitis can resolve spontaneously. Higher mortality rates are associated with acute pancreatitis when the disease progresses and leads to severe necrosis and hemorrhage of the organ, termed *necrotizing pancreatitis* and *hemorrhagic pancreatitis*, respectively. In these situations, patients may suffer from shock, **ileus**, and have a decreased hematocrit secondary to hemorrhage.

Unfortunately, sonography is not always successful at diagnosing cases of acute pancreatitis because the pancreas may appear completely normal with mild disease. But it can provide useful information as to the size and echogenicity of the gland and determine whether any peripancreatic fluid collections exist. This peripancreatic fluid collection may be referred to as **phlegmon**. The involvement of the gland can be focal or diffuse. Focal pancreatitis will lead to an enlargement of the gland in a particular segment, most often in the head, appearing as a hypoechoic region. This manifestation of pancreatitis can resemble a neoplasm, and a close investigation of laboratory findings and other imaging is often required in such cases (Fig. 5-6).

Diffuse enlargement of the gland can also occur with pancreatitis, and with this manifestation, the entire pancreas will most likely become enlarged and hypoechoic (Fig. 5-7). The pancreatic margins may appear ill-defined with areas of fluid collections noted within and around the pancreas. Both focal and diffuse acute pancreatitis can lead to hemorrhage, peripancreatic fluid collections, and a **pancreatic pseudocyst**. With moderate and severe pancreatitis,

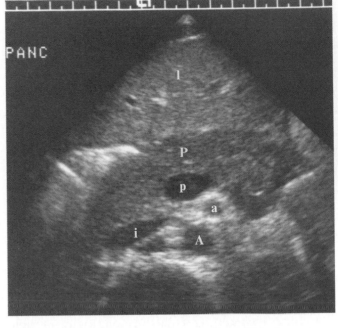

Figure 5-7 Diffuse acute pancreatitis. This transverse image of a diffusely enlarged and hypoechoic pancreas (*P*) demonstrates diffuse acute pancreatitis. Also seen in this image are the portal confluence (*p*), superior mesenteric artery (*a*), aorta (*A*), inferior vena cava (*i*), and liver (*l*).

the body will attempt to encapsulate the damaging digestive enzymes that leak from the pancreas and form a pseudocyst. One of the more common sites for a pancreatic pseudocyst is the **lesser sac**, which is located between the pancreas and the stomach, although pseudocysts may be found as far away as the groin. A pancreatic pseudocyst will appear as an anechoic mass with posterior enhancement, although it may contain some internal echoes (Fig. 5-8). Vascular complications can also arise secondary to the destructive influence of the pancreatic enzymes on adjacent vascular structures.

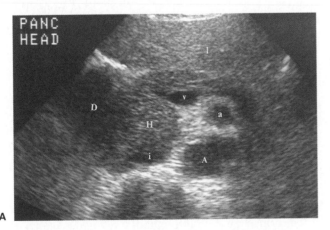
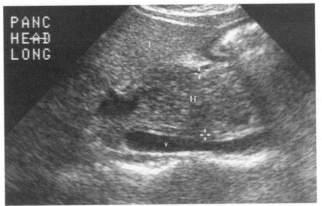

Figure 5-6 Focal acute pancreatitis. **A.** Transverse image of the pancreas reveals the duodenum (*D*), liver (*l*), inferior vena cava (*i*), aorta (*A*), superior mesenteric artery (*a*), superior mesenteric vein (*v*), and an enlarged pancreatic head (*H*). **B.** Longitudinal image of the pancreatic head (*H*) between *calipers*.

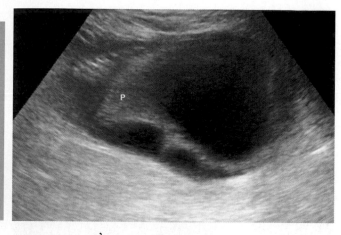

Figure 5-8 Pancreatic pseudocyst. Pancreatic pseudocyst. Longitudinal image showing pancreatic pseudocysts arising from the tail of the pancreas (*P*) in a patient with acute pancreatitis.

The more common vascular complications include thrombosis of the splenic vein and pseudoaneurysm of the splenic artery.

> ◄))) **SOUND OFF**
> Diffuse acute pancreatitis will result in a diffusely enlarged, hypoechoic gland.

CLINICAL FINDINGS OF ACUTE PANCREATITIS

1. Elevated amylase (within 24 hours)
2. Elevated lipase (within 72 hours)
3. Leukocytosis
4. Elevated ALT and other liver function labs when biliary obstruction is present
5. Abdominal pain (especially in the supine position)
6. Back pain
7. Fever
8. Nausea and vomiting
9. Severe acute pancreatitis may lead to hemorrhage and a decreased hematocrit

SONOGRAPHIC FINDINGS OF ACUTE PANCREATITIS

1. The pancreas may appear normal
2. Diffusely enlarged, hypoechoic pancreas (diffuse manifestation)
3. Focal hypoechoic area within the pancreas (focal manifestation)
4. Unencapsulated anechoic fluid collection surrounding all or part of the pancreas (peripancreatic fluid)
5. Pancreatic pseudocyst

6. Abscess formation can occur and is seen as echogenic fluid containing gas bubbles
7. Biliary obstruction may be present (possibly choledocholithiasis)
8. Vascular complications such as splenic vein thrombosis and pseudoaneurysm of the splenic artery

Chronic Pancreatitis

Repeated bouts of pancreatic inflammation can lead to **chronic pancreatitis**, but not all patients who have a history of acute pancreatitis will develop chronic pancreatitis. Like acute pancreatitis, chronic pancreatitis is often caused by chronic alcohol abuse. But other causes exist, including **hyperparathyroidism**, congenital anomalies (pancreatic divisum), genetic disorders, pancreatic duct obstruction, and trauma. When destruction of the pancreatic tissue recurs, it can result in atrophy, fibrosis (scarring), and the development of calcifications within the gland.

Although patients may be completely asymptomatic, they may present with a possible elevation in alkaline phosphatase (ALP), amylase and lipase, persistent epigastric and back pain, and jaundice. Patients may also suffer from weight loss, anorexia, vomiting, and constipation.

Sonographically, the pancreas will appear small, heterogeneous, or hyperechoic and have poor margins. Calcifications are often noted throughout the parenchyma of the organ, although they may be confined to the pancreatic ducts (Fig. 5-9). This, in turn, can lead to pancreatic duct

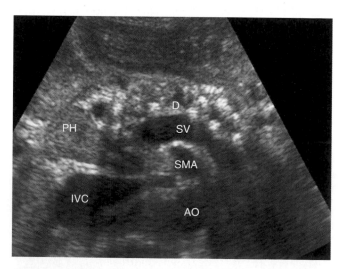

Figure 5-9 Chronic pancreatitis. Transverse image of the pancreas in a patient with chronic pancreatitis. Calcifications are seen throughout the body and tail of the pancreas. Aorta (*AO*), pancreatic duct (*D*), inferior vena cava (*IVC*), pancreatic head (*PH*), superior mesenteric artery (*SMA*), splenic vein (*SV*).

and biliary dilatation. Like acute pancreatitis, chronic pancreatitis can affect only a segment of the pancreas. In addition, up to 40% of the time, there will be pseudocyst formation in association with chronic pancreatitis, and there is the possibility of portosplenic vein thrombosis.

> ### 🔊 SOUND OFF
> Chronic pancreatitis can result in an atrophic, hyperechoic pancreas with calcifications and a prominent pancreatic duct.

CLINICAL FINDINGS OF CHRONIC PANCREATITIS

1. Asymptomatic
2. Persistent epigastric pain
3. Jaundice
4. Back pain
5. Possible elevation in amylase or lipase (but they may remain normal)
6. Possible elevation in ALP
7. Anorexia
8. Vomiting
9. Weight loss
10. Constipation

SONOGRAPHIC FINDINGS OF CHRONIC PANCREATITIS

1. Heterogeneous, or hyperechoic, atrophic gland with poor margins
2. Calcifications within the gland
3. Pancreatic pseudocyst
4. Dilated pancreatic duct
5. Stone(s) within the pancreatic duct that may lead to biliary obstruction
6. Possible portosplenic vein thrombosis

Pancreatic Adenocarcinoma

Pancreatic adenocarcinoma, also referred to as pancreatic ductal adenocarcinoma or simply pancreatic ductal carcinoma, is the most common primary pancreatic malignancy, and it is most commonly discovered in men. This disease often presents late clinically, resulting in a delay in detection and treatment. Risk factors for pancreatic adenocarcinoma include a history of cigarette smoking, diabetes mellitus, chronic pancreatitis, and high-fat diet. There are also some genetic predispositions in some individuals.

Pancreatic cancer is the fourth most common cause of cancer-related deaths in men. The most common location of a pancreatic adenocarcinoma is within the pancreatic head, although it may be seen in other parts of the pancreas. If located within the head of the pancreas, this mass will often lead to obstruction of the

common bile duct and Courvoisier gallbladder. Recall that Courvoisier gallbladder describes the clinical detection of an enlarged, palpable gallbladder that may be caused by a (potentially malignant) pancreatic head mass (Fig. 5-10). The patient frequently has jaundice secondary to the obstruction of the common bile duct by the mass (Fig. 5-11). Other clinical features include elevated amylase and/or lipase, nausea, persistent back or epigastric pain, weight loss, and loss of appetite.

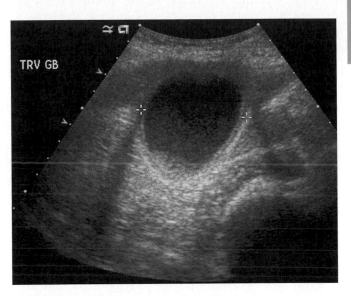

Figure 5-10 Courvoisier gallbladder. This gallbladder (*between calipers*) was enlarged, measuring greater than 5 cm in width, contained sludge, and was associated with a malignant pancreatic head mass. TRV, transverse; GB, gallbladder

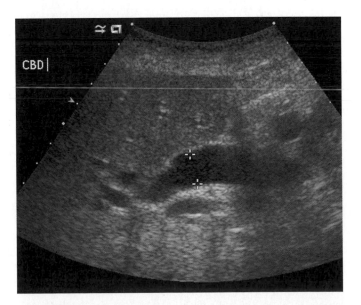

Figure 5-11 Dilated common bile duct. This dilated common bile duct (*between calipers*) measured more than 2 cm in diameter. It was associated with a malignant pancreatic head mass. CBD, common bile duct

🔊 **SOUND OFF**
Pancreatic adenocarcinoma is most commonly found in the head of the pancreas.

Sonographically, the most common appearance of pancreatic adenocarcinoma is a hypoechoic mass in the head of the pancreas (Fig. 5-12). Obstruction of both the common bile duct and the pancreatic duct may be present, a condition known as the **double-duct sign**. Pancreatic adenocarcinoma can be staged. With stage I, the mass is confined to the pancreas. Stage II involves local lymph node involvement, whereas with stage III, there is evidence of distant metastasis.

Consequently, the liver and other abdominal organs should be evaluated carefully for possible metastasis when a pancreatic mass is discovered sonographically. The surgical procedure that is performed on patients with pancreatic adenocarcinoma is referred to as the **Whipple procedure**. The Whipple procedure may also be called a **pancreaticoduodenectomy**. This procedure is the removal of the head of the pancreas, the gallbladder, some of the bile ducts, and the proximal duodenum.

CLINICAL FINDINGS OF PANCREATIC ADENOCARCINOMA

1. Elevated amylase and/or lipase
2. Loss of appetite
3. Weight loss
4. Jaundice
5. Courvoisier gallbladder (enlarged palpable gallbladder)
6. Epigastric pain
7. Elevated ALP and, possibly, other liver function labs associated with biliary obstruction
8. History of cigarette smoking, diabetes mellitus, or chronic pancreatitis

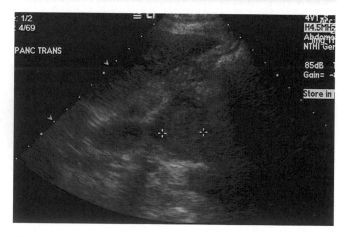

Figure 5-12 Pancreatic carcinoma. A solid hypoechoic mass (*between calipers*) representing pancreatic carcinoma is noted in the head of the pancreas.

SONOGRAPHIC FINDINGS OF PANCREATIC ADENOCARCINOMA

1. Hypoechoic mass in the head of the pancreas
2. Dilated common bile duct and pancreatic duct (double-duct sign)
3. Liver and other abdominal organs should be evaluated for possible metastasis
4. Enlarged (hydropic) gallbladder

🔊 **SOUND OFF**
Courvoisier gallbladder occurs when the gallbladder is palpable because it is enlarged. This is due to the presence of a (potentially malignant) pancreatic head mass that leads to biliary obstruction and the backup of a large amount of bile in the gallbladder.

Pancreatic Cystadenomas and Cystadenocarcinoma

A cystadenoma within the pancreas may be referred to as either a (microcystic) serous cystadenoma or (macrocystic) mucinous cystadenoma. Serous tumors are small and always benign, whereas mucinous tumors are larger and have malignant potential. When malignant, the mucinous tumors are referred to as mucinous cystadenocarcinomas. They are most often found within the body and tail of the pancreas. Patients with these masses present later than those with pancreatic head masses and may be asymptomatic initially. When symptomatic, patients often complain of epigastric pain, weight loss, palpable mass, and jaundice. The sonographic appearance of a benign serous cystadenoma is that of a small cystic mass, in that sonographically may actually appear solid and echogenic secondary to the small size of the cysts. A mucinous cystadenoma or cystadenocarcinoma most often appears as a multilocular cystic mass that may contain mural nodules and calcifications. There may be associated dilation of the pancreatic duct as well.

🔊 **SOUND OFF**
Pancreatic cystadenocarcinoma is most often found in the body or tail of the pancreas.

CLINICAL FINDINGS OF CYSTADENOMAS AND CYSTADENOCARCINOMAS

1. May be asymptomatic initially
2. Epigastric pain
3. Weight loss
4. Palpable mass
5. Jaundice

SONOGRAPHIC FINDINGS OF SEROUS CYSTADENOMA

1. Cystic mass
2. May actually appear solid and echogenic secondary to the small size of the cysts

SONOGRAPHIC FINDINGS OF MUCINOUS CYSTADENOMA AND CYSTADENOCARCINOMA

1. Multilocular cystic masses that may contain mural nodules and calcifications
2. There may be associated dilation of the pancreatic duct

Islet Cell Tumors

Recall, it is the islet of Langerhans that house the endocrine tissue of the pancreas. Consequently, endocrine tumors can be found within the islets of Langerhans. These are referred to as **islet cell tumors** or pancreatic neuroendocrine tumors. There are two common types of islet cell tumors: the **insulinoma** and the **gastrinoma**. These slow-growing tumors can be either functional or nonfunctional. Among the two, insulinomas are more common. Insulinomas are usually solitary, whereas gastrinomas are often multiple and difficult to image (Fig. 5-13). The functional gastrinomas can produce **Zollinger–Ellison syndrome**, which is described as the excessive secretion of acid by the stomach that leads to peptic ulcers. Functional insulinomas can cause hypoglycemia. The **Whipple triad**

is a group of clinical indicators of a functional insulinoma, which includes hypoglycemia, low fasting glucose, and relief with intravenous glucose administration. Patients with insulinomas may also present with palpitations, sweating, tremors, and headaches, and they may even eventually suffer from diabetic coma.

When seen, the most common sonographic appearance of an islet cell tumor is that of a small, hypoechoic mass that may contain calcifications. Islet cell tumors can be malignant or benign, with the functioning tumors most often appearing hypervascular with color Doppler interrogation. Endoscopic and intraoperative sonography have been utilized to detect small islet cell tumors. Several additional islet cell tumors exist, including the somatostatinoma, the glucagonoma, and the vasoactive intestinal peptide tumor or VIPoma.

CLINICAL FINDINGS OF ISLET CELL TUMORS

1. Insulinoma: hypoglycemia, low fasting glucose, and relief with intravenous glucose administration (Whipple triad)
2. Gastrinoma: Zollinger–Ellison syndrome

SONOGRAPHIC FINDINGS OF ISLET CELL TUMORS

1. Hypoechoic mass that may contain calcifications
2. Hypervascularity may be present with color Doppler
3. Visualization is challenging because of their small size

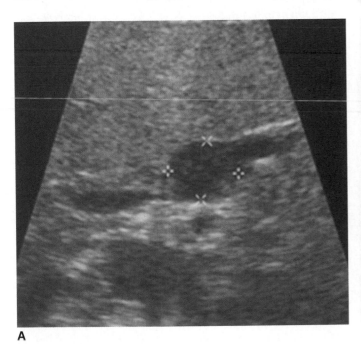
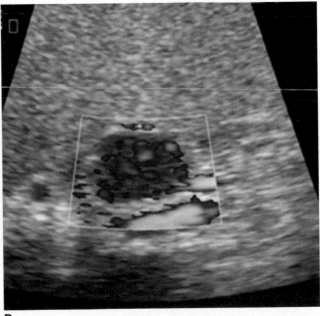

A   **B**

Figure 5-13 Insulinoma. Insulinoma. **A.** A hypoechoic mass is noted within the pancreas (*between calipers*). **B.** The mass appears to be highly vascular.

🔊))) SOUND OFF
Functional gastrinomas can produce Zollinger–Ellison syndrome, which is described as the excessive secretion of acid by the stomach that leads to peptic ulcers.

True Pancreatic Cysts

Cysts noted within the pancreas may be seen with **von Hippel–Lindau disease**, **cystic fibrosis**, or autosomal dominant polycystic kidney disease (ADPKD), the latter of which is associated with the development of cysts in many organs (Fig. 5-14). Caution should be taken to ensure that the patient does not have a pancreatic pseudocyst, which is most often associated with a history of acute or chronic pancreatitis.

CLINICAL FINDINGS OF TRUE PANCREATIC CYSTS

1. Possible history of von Hippel–Lindau disease or cystic fibrosis
2. Possible history of ADPKD

SONOGRAPHIC FINDINGS OF TRUE PANCREATIC CYSTS

1. Well-defined, anechoic mass with posterior enhancement

🔊))) SOUND OFF
von Hippel–Lindau disease is associated with cysts in the pancreas.

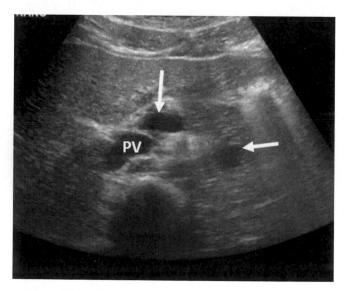

Figure 5-14 Pancreatic cysts and von Hippel–Lindau disease. Transverse sonogram of the pancreas shows cysts (*arrows*) in the pancreatic body and tail. *PV*, portal vein.

Pancreatic Transplant Assessment

Transplantation of the pancreas can occur for several reasons, including treating severe type 1 diabetes. Transplantation techniques can vary, however; and in up to 80% of the time, patients undergo a renal transplant at the same time. If this occurs, the pancreas is placed within the right side of the abdomen and the renal transplant is placed on the left. There are two common types of transplantation techniques—exocrine bladder drainage and exocrine enteric drainage.

With exocrine bladder drainage, the vasculature of the donor pancreas is anastomosed to the recipient's common iliac vessels and the donor duodenum is anastomosed to the urinary bladder. Thus, the recipient's urinary bladder is used to expel the pancreatic secretions. This procedure has been associated with many drawbacks, including dehydration and bladder irritation.

The other type of pancreatic transplantation, which is more common, is referred to as exocrine enteric drainage, in which case the donor's duodenum is anastomosed to a loop of jejunum (Fig. 5-15). With this technique, the splenic and superior mesenteric arteries are connected with the donor iliac arteries in what is referred to as a "Y" graft. The donor common iliac portion is anastomosed to the recipient's common iliac artery and external iliac artery. These transplants may be located in the right upper quadrant or on the right side and have a vertical orientation within the body.

The sonographic assessment of a pancreatic transplant includes a general evaluation of vascularity, the pancreatic parenchyma, and a search for fluid collections (Table 5-5). The pancreatic parenchyma should be homogeneous and may be hypoechoic just after transplantation, but a hypoechoic transplant may also be a sign of pancreatitis or acute rejection, so close clinical evaluation is warranted (Fig. 5-16). With rejection, the pancreas may also appear heterogeneous. Elevated resistive indices are often indicative of acute rejection as well. With chronic rejection, the pancreas can appear more hyperechoic, atrophic, and contain calcifications.

An appreciation of the surgical transplant technique will help guide the sonographer in the analysis of the various vascular anastomoses because there can be several vascular complications (Table 5-6). Color Doppler, pulsed Doppler, and power Doppler can all be used to evaluate the vasculature of the transplant. Thrombosis of the graft, whether arterial or venous, is a common complication, and it typically occurs shortly after surgery (Fig. 5-17). Graft thrombosis must be suspected if no flow can be detected within the gland. Other complications include pancreatitis, arterial stenosis, pseudoaneurysms, and fluid collections, such as hematomas and urinomas (with exocrine bladder drainage). An ultrasound-guided transplant biopsy may be performed to differentiate rejection from other complications if needed.

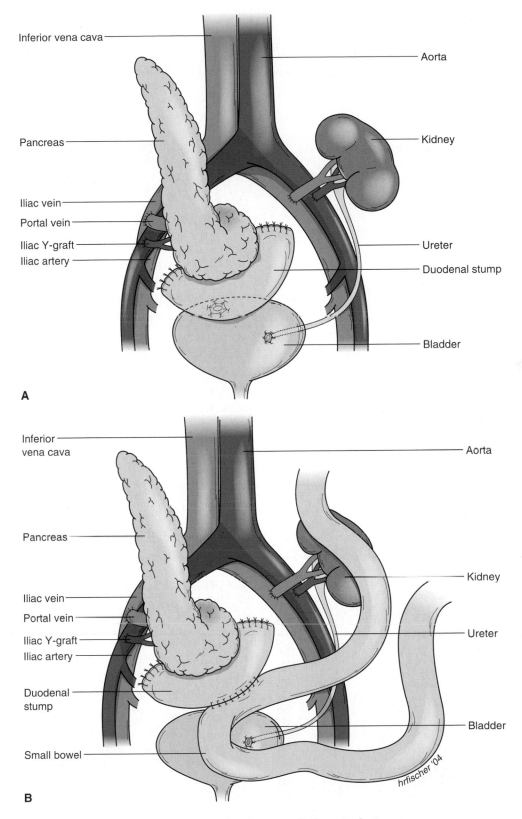

Figure 5-15 Pancreatic transplant. **A.** Exocrine bladder drainage. **B.** Enteric drainage.

SONOGRAPHIC FINDINGS OF CHRONIC PANCREATIC TRANSPLANT REJECTION

1. Hyperechoic echotexture
2. Atrophy
3. Pancreas may contain calcifications

SONOGRAPHIC FINDINGS OF ACUTE PANCREATIC TRANSPLANT REJECTION

1. Hypoechoic or heterogeneous gland
2. Elevated resistive indices

TABLE 5-5 Pancreatic transplant fluid collections

- Abscess
- Ascites
- Hematoma
- Urinoma (secondary to anastomosis problems at urinary bladder)
- Pseudocysts

TABLE 5-6 Pancreatic transplant vascular complications

- Arterial stenosis: focal areas of increased velocities
- Arterial thrombosis
- Graft thrombosis
- Pseudoaneurysms
- Splenic vein thrombosis: elevated pulsed-wave Doppler resistive index in the arterial inflow Doppler waveform, often >1.0; absent splenic inflow
- Strictures: evident with turbulent flow

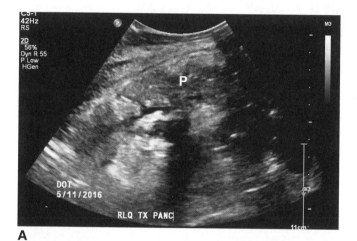

A

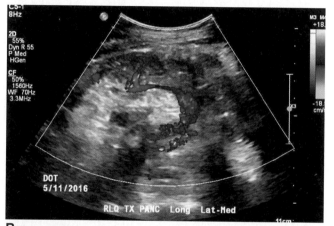

B

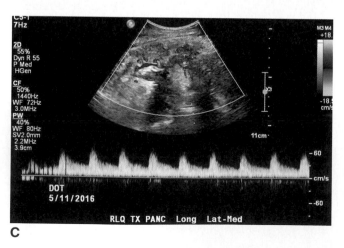

C

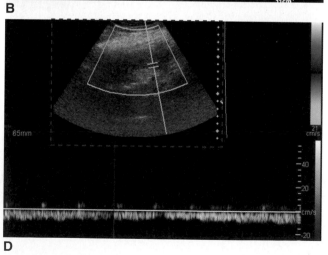

D

Figure 5-16 Pancreatic transplant sonogram. **A.** Grayscale evaluation. The longitudinal image of the normal pancreas (*P*) transplant located in the pelvis shows normal echogenicity similar to a native pancreas. **B.** Color Doppler evaluation. The longitudinal section of the pancreas demonstrates vascular patency and perfusion of the allograft. **C** and **D.** Spectral Doppler evaluation. The images of the transplanted pancreas sonograms document the presence of both (**C**) arterial flow and (**D**) venous patency.

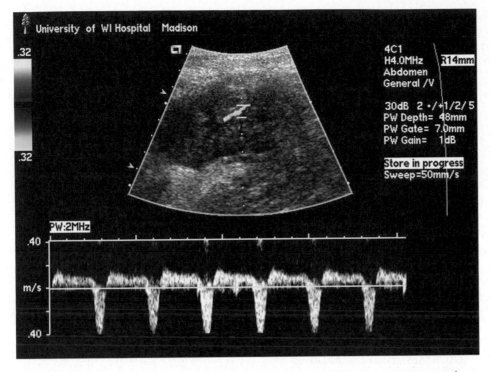

Figure 5-17 Reversed diastolic flow in a patient with venous thrombosis of his pancreatic transplant.

REVIEW QUESTIONS

1. What results in a shortened main pancreatic duct that works to drain only the pancreatic head and not the entire pancreas?
   a. Pancreatic divisum
   b. Annular pancreas
   c. Acute pancreatitis
   d. Zollinger–Ellison syndrome

2. All of the following are part of the exocrine function of the pancreas except for the:
   a. production of lipase.
   b. production of glucagon.
   c. production of amylase.
   d. production of sodium bicarbonate.

3. What is another name for the accessory duct of the pancreas?
   a. Duct of Santorini
   b. Duct of Langerhans
   c. Duct of Oddi
   d. Duct of Wirsung

4. Which of the following results from the maldevelopment of the two embryologic elements of the pancreas and consequent obstruction of the duodenum?
   a. Pancreatic divisum
   b. Annular pancreas
   c. Whipple syndrome
   d. Zollinger–Ellison syndrome

5. Which of the following is associated with development of cysts within the pancreas?
   a. Autosomal recessive polycystic kidney disease
   b. von Hippel–Lindau disease
   c. Zollinger–Ellison syndrome
   d. Endoscopic retrograde cholangiopancreatography

6. The most common form of malignancy of the pancreas is:
   a. cystadenocarcinoma.
   b. islet cell tumors.
   c. cystadenoma.
   d. adenocarcinoma.

7. The Whipple procedure is performed on patients who have:
   a. chronic pancreatitis.
   b. acute pancreatitis.
   c. pancreatic carcinoma.
   d. pancreatic transplants.

8. Which of the following is the enzyme released by the pancreas that neutralizes stomach acid?
   a. Insulin
   b. Somatostatin
   c. Glycogen
   d. Sodium bicarbonate

9. The most common location of adenocarcinoma of the pancreas is within the:
   a. head of the pancreas.
   b. neck of the pancreas.
   c. body of the pancreas.
   d. tail of the pancreas.

10. Which of the following is a peripancreatic fluid collection that results from the inflammation of the pancreas?
    a. Pus
    b. Trypsin
    c. Phlegmon
    d. Chyme

11. The most common location of focal pancreatitis is within the:
    a. head of the pancreas.
    b. neck of the pancreas.
    c. body of the pancreas.
    d. tail of the pancreas.

12. All of the following are sonographic features of chronic pancreatitis except:
    a. dilated pancreatic duct.
    b. calcifications within the pancreas.
    c. pancreatic pseudocyst.
    d. diffusely hypoechoic pancreas.

13. Which of the following would be the least likely complication of a pancreatic transplant?
    a. Hematoma
    b. Biloma
    c. Ascites
    d. Urinoma

14. All of the following are classic clinical features of acute pancreatitis except:
    a. leukocytosis.
    b. back pain.
    c. weight gain.
    d. fever.

15. Which of the following laboratory values appears to be more specific for acute pancreatitis?
    a. Amylase
    b. Lipase
    c. Aspartate aminotransferase
    d. Serum glutamic oxaloacetic transaminase

16. Which type of pancreatic transplantation is more common?
    a. Exocrine enteric drainage
    b. Exocrine bladder drainage
    c. Endocrine bladder drainage
    d. Endocrine enteric drainage

17. One of the most common locations for a pancreatic pseudocyst is within the:
    a. paracolic gutters.
    b. groin.
    c. spleen.
    d. lesser sac.

18. Which of the following would be the least likely cause of acute pancreatitis?
    a. Alcohol abuse
    b. Hepatitis
    c. Trauma
    d. Gallstones

19. Which of the following is the most common islet cell tumor?
    a. Granuloma
    b. Gastrinoma
    c. Insulinoma
    d. Cystadenoma

20. Which of the following laboratory findings elevates first in the presence of acute pancreatitis?
    a. Amylase
    b. ALP
    c. ALT
    d. Lipase

21. Courvoisier gallbladder is found in the presence of:
    a. hepatitis.
    b. cholecystitis and chronic pancreatitis.
    c. adenocarcinoma in the head of the pancreas.
    d. islet cell tumor in the tail of the pancreas.

22. A gastrinoma of the pancreas can produce:
    a. autosomal recessive polycystic kidney disease.
    b. von Hippel–Lindau disease.
    c. Zollinger–Ellison syndrome.
    d. hyperinsulinemia.

23. The muscle that controls the emptying of bile and pancreatic juices into the duodenum is the:
    a. sphincter of Vater.
    b. sphincter of Oddi.
    c. ampulla of Vater.
    d. ampulla of Oddi.

24. What is another name of the main pancreatic duct?
    a. Duct of Santorini
    b. Duct of Langerhans
    c. Duct of Oddi
    d. Duct of Wirsung

25. All of the following are clinical findings associated with pancreatic adenocarcinoma except:
    a. epigastric pain.
    b. weight loss.
    c. jaundice.
    d. decreased amylase and lipase.

26. The portion of the bowel that encompasses the head of the pancreas is the:
    a. duodenum.
    b. jejunum.
    c. ileum.
    d. cecum.

27. Which cells perform the exocrine function of the pancreas?
    a. Whipple cells
    b. Islets of Langerhans
    c. Delta cells
    d. Acinar cells

28. The most common echogenicity of an acutely inflamed pancreas is:
    a. anechoic.
    b. hyperechoic.
    c. hypoechoic.
    d. calcified.

29. Which of the following would be the most likely vascular complication of acute pancreatitis?
    a. Thrombosis in the splenic vein
    b. Pseudoaneurysm of the superior mesenteric artery
    c. Thrombosis of the main portal vein
    d. Stenosis of the superior mesenteric artery

30. The arterial blood supply to the head of the pancreas is via the:
    a. superior mesenteric artery.
    b. splenic artery.
    c. gastroduodenal artery.
    d. hepatic artery.

31. One clinical sign of an insulinoma is the presence of:
    a. hypoglycemia.
    b. elevated alpha-fetoprotein.
    c. hepatitis.
    d. Zollinger–Ellison syndrome.

32. What is the early sonographic appearance of acute pancreatitis?
    a. Calcifications within the gland
    b. Pancreatic pseudocyst
    c. Normal
    d. Hyperechoic glandular echotexture

33. Within which parts of the pancreas are mucinous cystadenocarcinomas most often located?
    a. Uncinate process and neck
    b. Head and neck
    c. Body and tail
    d. Fundus and neck

34. Coexisting obstruction of the common bile duct and pancreatic duct may be referred to as the:
    a. double-barrel shotgun sign.
    b. Courvoisier sign.
    c. Mirizzi sign.
    d. double-duct sign.

35. Courvoisier gallbladder is the:
    a. enlargement of the pancreatic duct secondary to coexisting masses within the pancreatic body and gallbladder.
    b. palpable gallbladder caused by a biliary obstruction in the area of the pancreatic head.
    c. gallbladder disorder associated with the buildup of cholesterol crystals within the gallbladder wall.
    d. type of gallbladder carcinoma that is the result of chronic cholecystitis.

36. The pancreas is an:
    a. intraperitoneal organ.
    b. retroperitoneal organ.

37. Which part of the pancreas is located right lateral to superior mesenteric vein, anterior to inferior vena cava, and inferior to portal vein?
    a. Head
    b. Neck
    c. Body
    d. Tail

38. What vascular structure outlines the pancreatic tail posteriorly?
    a. Superior mesenteric artery
    b. Inferior mesenteric vein
    c. Portal confluence
    d. Splenic vein

39. Which part of the pancreas is located anterior to portal confluence?
    a. Uncinate process
    b. Pancreatic body
    c. Pancreatic neck
    d. Pancreatic tail

40. Which of the following is the hormone released by the pancreas that encourages the body's use of glucagon?
    a. Insulin
    b. Somatostatin
    c. Glycogen
    d. Sodium bicarbonate

41. What are the cells of the pancreas that produce amylase and lipase?
    a. Acinar
    b. Beta
    c. Delta
    d. Alpha

42. The pancreatic tail is located medial to the:
    a. duodenum.
    b. jejunum.
    c. splenic hilum.
    d. liver hilum.

43. Which of the following would be most likely to increase an individual's likelihood of developing chronic pancreatitis?
    a. Hashimoto thyroiditis
    b. Splenic varices
    c. Hepatitis
    d. Hyperparathyroidism

44. A 52-year-old female patient in Figure 5-18 has weight loss, a palpable gallbladder, and elevated ALP. What does the arrow in this image indicate?
    a. Splenic vein
    b. Superior mesenteric vein
    c. Common bile duct
    d. Main pancreatic duct

45. Given the patient's history in Figure 5-18, what are calipers in the image most likely measuring?
    a. Pancreatic adenocarcinoma
    b. Insulinoma
    c. Pancreatic adenoma
    d. Pancreatic cystadenocarcinoma

46. The patient in Figure 5-19 presented with back pain and elevated amylase. What is the most likely diagnosis?
    a. Gastrinoma
    b. Acute pancreatitis
    c. Chronic pancreatitis
    d. Pancreatic adenocarcinoma

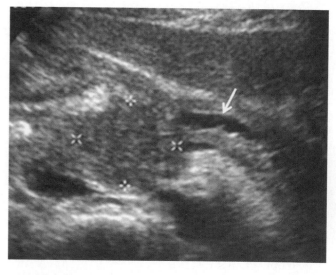

Figure 5-18

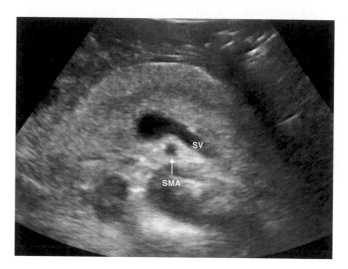

Figure 5-19

47. What is the most common form of pancreatitis?
    a. Hemorrhagic pancreatitis
    b. Necrotizing pancreatitis
    c. Interstitial edematous pancreatitis
    d. Hereditary pancreatitis

48. Which of the following is not included in the Whipple triad?
    a. Hypertension
    b. Hypoglycemia
    c. Low fasting glucose
    d. Relief with intravenous glucose administration

49. What does the Whipple triad indicate?
    a. Gastrinoma
    b. Insulinoma
    c. Somatostinoma
    d. Pancreatic adenocarcinoma

50. What performs the endocrine function of the pancreas?
    a. Islets of Langerhans
    b. Acinar cells
    c. Main pancreatic duct
    d. Pancreatocytes

51. What other structure is also typically transplanted simultaneously with the pancreas?
    a. Spleen
    b. Bladder
    c. Kidney
    d. Left lobe of the liver

52. Cystic fibrosis is associated with an increased risk of:
    a. pancreatic cysts.
    b. pancreatic calcifications.
    c. pancreatic duct stones.
    d. pancreatic cystadenocarcinoma.

53. Amylase converts:
    a. sugar to starch.
    b. starch to sugar.
    c. sugar to fat.
    d. fat to starch.

54. Which of the following would best describe the sonographic appearance of acute pancreatitis?
    a. Hyperechoic and atrophic
    b. Calcifications throughout an enlarged gland with an enlarged main pancreatic duct
    c. Hypoechoic and atrophic
    d. Hypoechoic and enlarged

55. Which of the following would best describe the sonographic appearance of chronic pancreatitis?
    a. Atrophic, hyperechoic gland with parenchymal calcifications and enlarged main pancreatic duct
    b. Enlarged gland with parenchymal calcifications and diffuse edema
    c. Shrunken, hypoechoic gland with intraparenchymal irregularities
    d. Enlarged gland, peripancreatic fluid, intraparenchymal hypoechoic foci, and intraductal sludge

56. Which of the following vascular complication would be most likely associated with acute pancreatitis?
    a. Renal vein thrombosis
    b. Inferior mesenteric vein aneurysm
    c. Abdominal aortic aneurysm
    d. Splenic vein thrombosis

57. What is the most common sonographic appearance of pancreatic adenocarcinoma?
    a. Hyperechoic mass
    b. Hypoechoic mass
    c. Anechoic mass
    d. Calcified mass

58. What is another name for the Whipple procedure?
    a. Hepato-pancreatectomy
    b. Duodenectomy
    c. Pancreaticoduodenectomy
    d. Renopancreaticoduodenectomy

59. Which of the following would be the least likely sonographic finding in a patient with acute pancreatitis?
    a. Pancreatic pseudocyst
    b. Phlegmon
    c. Choledocholithiasis
    d. Periportal cuffing

60. What part of the pancreas is located posterior to the superior mesenteric vein?
    a. Uncinate process
    b. Pancreatic tail
    c. Pancreatic neck
    d. Pancreatic head

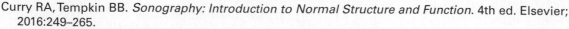

SUGGESTED READINGS

Curry RA, Tempkin BB. *Sonography: Introduction to Normal Structure and Function.* 4th ed. Elsevier; 2016:249–265.

Federle MP, Jeffrey RB, Woodward PJ. *Diagnostic Imaging: Abdomen.* 2nd ed. Amirsys; 2010:III-3-3–III-3-71.

Henningsen C, Kuntz K, Youngs D. *Clinical Guide to Sonography: Exercises for Critical Thinking.* 2nd ed. Elsevier; 2014:40–49.

Hertzberg BS, Middleton WD. *Ultrasound: The Requisites.* 3rd ed. Elsevier; 2016:179–191.

Jani B, Rzouq F, Saligram S, et al. Groove pancreatitis: a rare form of chronic pancreatitis. *N Am J Med Sci.* 2015;7(11):529–532.

Kawamura DM, Nolan TD. *Diagnostic Medical Sonography: Abdomen and Superficial Structures.* 3rd ed. Wolters Kluwer; 2018:213–228 & 739–756.

Penny SM. Clinical signs of pancreatitis. *Radiol Technol.* 2012:83(6):561–577.

Rumack CM, Wilson SR, Charboneau W, et al. *Diagnostic Ultrasound.* 4th ed. Elsevier; 2011:392–428, 639–707, & 1918–1921.

Sanders RC, Hall-Terracciano B. *Clinical Sonography: A Practical Guide.* 5th ed. Wolters Kluwer; 2016:396–407 & 525–545.

Shya JY, Sainani NI, Anik Sahni V, et al. Necrotizing pancreatitis: diagnosis, imaging, and intervention. *Radiographics.* 2014;34:1218–1239.

Siegel MJ. *Pediatric Sonography.* 4th ed. Wolters Kluwer; 2011:478–491.

Smits MM, van Geenen EJM. The clinical significance of pancreatic steatosis. *Nat Rev Gastroenterol Hepatol.* 2011;8(3):169–177.

BONUS REVIEW!

Acute Pancreatitis on Computed Tomography (Fig. 5-20)

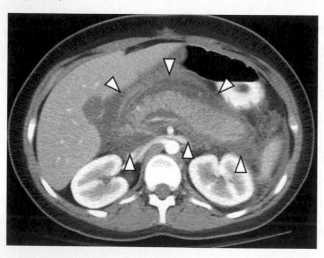

Figure 5-20 Acute pancreatitis on computed tomography. This image demonstrates the diffuse enlargement of the pancreas in a young patient with notable peripancreatic fluid and inflammatory tissue (*arrowheads*).

BONUS REVIEW! (*continued*)

Pancreatic Pseudocyst on Computed Tomography (Fig. 5-21)

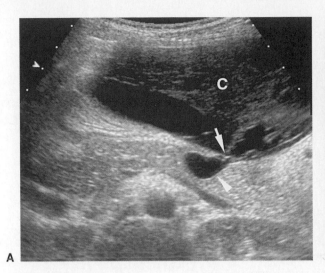
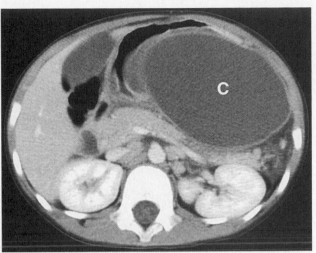

Figure 5-21 Pancreatic pseudocyst. **A.** Transverse image of a well-defined pseudocyst (*C*) with internal septations anterior to the pancreatic body. There is communication with a small cyst (*arrowhead*) in the body of the pancreas (*arrow*). **B.** Computed tomography image also demonstrates the pseudocyst (*C*) in the pancreatic body and tail with associated inflammatory changes in the peripancreatic fat.

Chronic Pancreatitis on Computed Tomography (Fig. 5-22)

Pancreatic Carcinoma on Computed Tomography (Fig. 5-23)

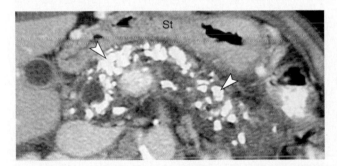

Figure 5-22 Chronic pancreatitis on computed tomography. Multiple calcifications (*arrowheads*) are noted within this pancreas affected by chronic pancreatitis resulting from alcoholism. *St*, stomach.

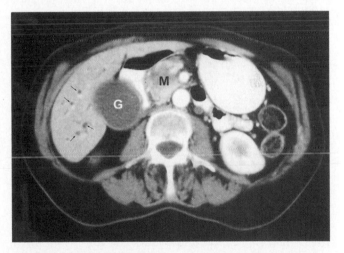

Figure 5-23 Computed tomography image of a malignant pancreatic mass (*M*). This image also depicts a massively dilated gallbladder (*G*) and dilated intrahepatic ducts (*arrows*).

The Spleen

Introduction

Sonography is often used in conjunction with other imaging modalities in the follow-up of pathologic processes affecting the spleen. This chapter will provide an overview of splenic anatomy, function, and pathology. The "Bonus Review" section contains images of splenomegaly and splenic rupture on computed tomography.

Key Terms

accessory spleen—a small, round island of splenic tissue often located near the splenic hilum or near the tail of the pancreas; also referred to as a splenule, a splenunculus, or a supernumerary spleen

angiosarcoma—a rare malignant tumor of the spleen that is derived from blood vessels

asplenia—congenital absence of the spleen

autosplenectomy—the gradual fibrosis and dysfunction of the spleen secondary to a disease

bacteremia—presence of bacteria in the blood

bacterial endocarditis—an infection of the surface of the heart that can spread to other organs

Beckwith–Wiedemann syndrome—a growth disorder syndrome synonymous with enlargement of several organs including the skull, tongue, and liver

blunt trauma—non-penetrating injury to the body

concave—having a rounded inward surface

convex—having a rounded exterior surface

culling—the splenic process of removing irregular red blood cells from the bloodstream

Epstein–Barr infection—a herpesvirus that can lead to infectious mononucleosis

erythropoiesis—the process of making red blood cells

extramedullary hematopoiesis—the spleen's hematopoietic function which can return in cases of severe anemia

granulomas—small echogenic calcifications that result from inflammation of the tissue in that area

granulomatous disease—an inherited disease that disrupts the normal immune system and causes it to malfunction, resulting in immunodeficiency; chronic inflammation can lead to the development of granulomas in several organs

hemangioma—a benign tumor composed of blood vessels

heterotaxia syndromes—a group of inherited syndromes in which the organs of the chest and abdomen are abnormally arranged; often includes either asplenia or polysplenia and many other anomalies

histoplasmosis—a disease that results from the inhalation of an airborne fungus that can affect the lungs and may spread to other organs

Hodgkin lymphoma—carcinoma of the lymphocytes that has a relatively high recovery rate; cancer of the lymphatic system

hydatid cyst—a cyst that results from the parasitic infestation of an organ by a tapeworm

hypersplenism—an overactive spleen; cytopenia caused by splenomegaly

leukopenia—a reduction in the number of leukocytes in the blood

lysis—breaking down of a cellular membrane

mononucleosis—an infectious disease caused by the Epstein–Barr virus

non-Hodgkin lymphoma—carcinoma of the lymphocytes; cancer of the lymphatic system

osteomyelitis—bone infection caused by fungus or bacteria

pitting—the splenic process of cleaning red blood cells of unwanted material

polysplenia—having many small islands of splenic tissue

portal hypertension—the elevation of blood pressure within the portal venous system

red pulp—specialized tissue within the spleen that performs its phagocytic function

Reed–Sternberg cells—the cells that indicate the presence of Hodgkin lymphoma

reticuloendothelial system—phagocytic system of the body that helps remove dead and toxic particles from the blood

sarcoidosis—a systemic disease that results in the development of granulomas throughout the body

sickle cell anemia—an inherited disease in which the body produces abnormally shaped red blood cells

splenectomy—surgical removal of the spleen

splenic cleft—a congenital anomaly in which the spleen is divided into two portions by a band of tissue

splenic hamartoma—benign splenic mass that has been associated with Beckwith–Wiedemann syndrome and tuberous sclerosis

splenic infarct—an area within the spleen that has become necrotic owing to a lack of oxygen

splenic lymphangioma—benign tumor composed of lymph spaces

splenic torsion—the twisting of the splenic vasculature causing a disruption in blood supply to the spleen and subsequent ischemia

splenomegaly—enlargement of the spleen

splenosis—the implantation of ectopic splenic tissue possibly secondary to splenic rupture

splenule—an accessory spleen

tuberous sclerosis—a systemic disorder that leads to the development of tumors (hamartomas) within various organs

wandering spleen—a highly mobile spleen

white pulp—specialized lymphatic tissue within the spleen

ANATOMY AND PHYSIOLOGY OF THE SPLEEN

The spleen, which is the largest structure of the **reticuloendothelial system**, is an intraperitoneal organ located within the left upper quadrant of the abdomen whose primary function is to filter the peripheral blood (Tables 6-1 and 6-2; Fig. 6-1). The gastrosplenic ligament attaches the spleen to the stomach, placing the spleen inferior to the diaphragm and posterolateral to the stomach. The spleen, which has a **concave** inferior surface and a **convex** superior surface, is also considered the largest lymphatic organ of the body. It begins to develop around the 5th week of gestation. In the fetus, it is responsible for **erythropoiesis**. In children, it plays an important role in defense against infection, whereas in adults, it produces lymphocytes and monocytes. Although red blood cell production in the adult is primarily performed by the bone marrow, the spleen's hematopoietic function can return in cases of severe anemia. This is referred to as **extramedullary hematopoiesis**.

The spleen is composed of specialized tissues called **white pulp** and **red pulp**. Leukocytes, or white blood cells (WBCs), play a vital role in the body's ability to fight infections and many diseases. There are several different types of WBCs, including lymphocytes. The white pulp of the spleen produces and houses lymphocytes, thus this tissue carries out the spleen's lymphatic function.

The red pulp, which contains red blood cells and macrophages, performs the phagocytic function of the spleen. Phagocytes engulf and destroy pathogens. The spleen also removes irregular red blood cells from the bloodstream through a process called **culling**. It can also clean red blood cells of unwanted material, a process called **pitting**.

TABLE 6-1 Anatomy bordering the spleen

Inferior to the diaphragm
Posterolateral to the stomach
Superior to the left kidney
Lateral to the adrenal gland and pancreatic tail

TABLE 6-2 Functions of the spleen

1. Defense against disease
2. Hematopoiesis/erythropoiesis
3. Destruction and removal of flawed red blood cells and platelets
4. Blood reservoir
5. Storage of iron

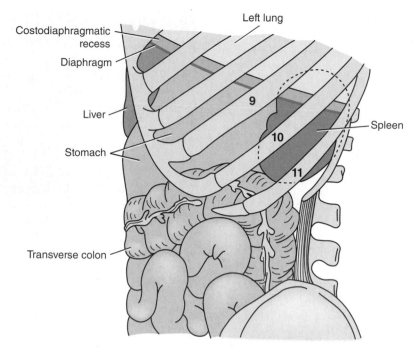

Figure 6-1 Location of the spleen and the adjacent anatomy 9,9th rib; 10,10th rib; 11,11th rib.

> ### ◀)) SOUND OFF
> Culling removes irregular red blood cells, whereas pitting cleans the cells of unwanted material.

VASCULAR ANATOMY OF THE SPLEEN

The splenic artery is a branch of the celiac trunk, which may also be referred to as the celiac artery or celiac axis. From the trunk, the splenic artery courses laterally toward the spleen (Fig. 6-2). It marks the superior border of the pancreatic body and tail. Therefore, the splenic artery can be confused sonographically for the main

pancreatic duct in some patients. The splenic artery enters the spleen at the splenic hilum superior and anterior to the splenic vein. A Doppler evaluation of the splenic artery normally demonstrates a low-resistance flow pattern (Fig. 6-3).

The splenic vein exits the spleen and travels along the posterior border of the pancreatic tail and body. It joins with the superior mesenteric vein posterior to the pancreatic neck to form the portal vein. Flow within the splenic vein will be toward the liver. In the setting of some pathologic conditions, the splenic vein should certainly be carefully evaluated. For example, the sonographic investigation of the splenic

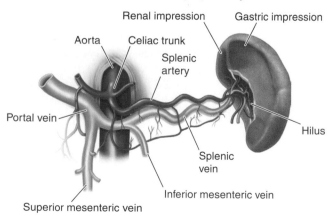

Figure 6-2 The circulation of the spleen, including the splenic vein and splenic artery.

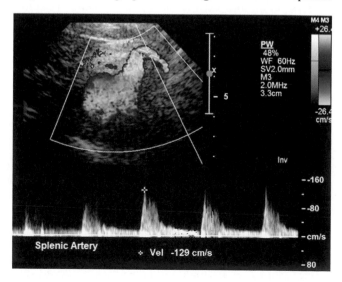

Figure 6-3 The normal splenic artery waveform demonstrates a low-pulsatility Doppler signal.

vein in the presence of pancreatitis may reveal splenic vein thrombosis. Occasionally, the splenic vein may be invaded by a malignant tumor as well, a condition referred to as tumor thrombus.

> ### 🔊 SOUND OFF
> The splenic artery can be confused for the main pancreatic duct in some patients because it takes a similar course in the body.

SONOGRAPHY OF THE SPLEEN

Most often, the spleen is best visualized with deep inspiration, with the patient lying on his or her right side. The sonographic appearance of a normal spleen is frequently isoechoic to the liver, although it may be slightly more echogenic. As stated earlier, the adult spleen has a concave, pointed inferior margin and a convex superior border, revealing a typical crescent moon shape on sonography. The size of the spleen in the adult varies with age and sex. The spleen decreases in size with advancing age and may enlarge—which is termed **splenomegaly**—when pathology is present. The splenic hilum, located along the medial surface of the spleen, is the location of the splenic vessels.

> ### 🔊 SOUND OFF
> The spleen is typically either isoechoic or more hypoechoic to the liver.

CONGENITAL ANOMALIES AND VARIANTS

Some persons may have an **accessory spleen**, also referred to as a **splenule**, a splenunculus, or a supernumerary spleen. This small, round island of splenic tissue is typically located near the splenic hilum or possibly near the tail of the pancreas. An accessory spleen will appear isoechoic to the spleen (Fig. 6-4). It is important to note that an accessory spleen is often located in a region in which other pathology may be present, and thus it may be mistaken for more worrisome conditions. For example, it may be confused not only for a splenic mass but also a pancreatic tail mass, a left adrenal mass, or possibly a mass located in the upper pole of the left kidney. Consequently, the sonographer should measure the tissue and try to determine if that tissue is truly an accessory spleen or rather a mass located on or within other organs that are located in the left upper quadrant.

The spleen may also appear to be divided by a hyperechoic line in some individuals, which is a

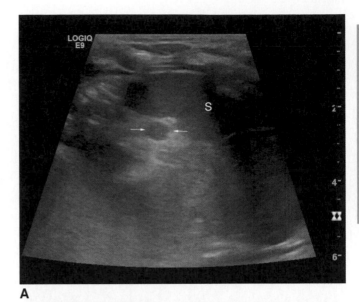

A

B

Figure 6-4 Accessory spleen. Transverse (**A**) and longitudinal (**B**) images of the spleen (*S*) with an adjacent accessory spleen (*arrows*) noted in the area of the splenic hilum.

common anomaly termed **splenic cleft**. Conversely, two uncommon congenital anomalies are **asplenia** and **polysplenia**. Whereas asplenia is the congenital absence of the spleen, polysplenia leads to the development of multiple small masses of splenic tissue. Both asplenia and polysplenia have been associated with some complex cardiac malformations and the abnormal location of other organs—termed **heterotaxia syndromes**.

> ### 🔊 SOUND OFF
> An accessory spleen may also be referred to as a splenule, splenunculus, or supernumerary spleen.

Though exceedingly rare, the spleen may also be identified as a **wandering spleen**, in which case the splenic ligaments are absent or underdeveloped, thus allowing the opportunity for the spleen to be highly mobile and often positioned well into the lower abdomen. Unfortunately, an individual with a wandering spleen could suffer from **splenic torsion** because the vessels of the spleen may twist secondary to the hypermobility of the organ. The resulting vascular torsion can lead to a splenic infarction (see section "Splenic Infarct" in this chapter).

 SOUND OFF
A wandering spleen may undergo splenic torsion.

PATHOLOGY OF THE SPLEEN

Clinical Importance of White Blood Cell Count Assessment

Recall, lymphocytes are a type of leukocyte found in the spleen, and thus it would be prudent to evaluate each patient's WBC before performing an abdominal sonogram. Leukocytosis is an increase in the number of WBCs in the blood. Typically, leukocytosis is the body's normal response to infection or inflammation. However, leukocytosis may also be a sign of more worrisome conditions such as cancer, including acute leukemia.

Leukopenia is a reduction in the number of leukocytes in the blood. Leukopenia may be caused by many conditions such as leukemia, **Hodgkin lymphoma**, **hypersplenism**, viral infections, and diabetes mellitus. Leukopenia can also be the result of radiation and chemotherapy treatments.

Splenomegaly

The most common abnormality of the spleen is splenomegaly. Enlargement of the spleen can be manually suspected on physical examination and subsequently confirmed using sonography. Although the splenic size varies with age, gender, and body sizes, the spleen should never measure more than 12 to 13 cm in length and 6 cm in thickness in adults. Suspicion of splenomegaly should arise however when the spleen extends beyond the inferior pole of the left kidney. As the spleen enlarges, it tends to become more hypoechoic.

The most common cause of splenomegaly is **portal hypertension**. And when portal hypertension is suspected as the cause of splenomegaly, the sonographer should closely evaluate the splenic hilum for evidence of abdominal varices seen in this condition (Fig. 6-5). Other causes of splenomegaly include trauma,

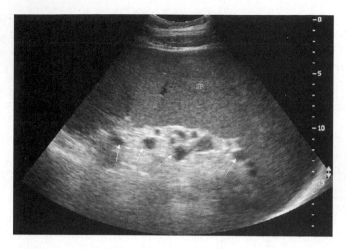

Figure 6-5 Splenomegaly. Transverse image of an enlarged spleen (*SP*) in a patient with cirrhosis and portal hypertension. Note that there are multiple prominent blood vessels adjacent to the splenic hilum (*arrows*).

leukemia, lymphoma, a pediatric **sickle cell anemia** crisis, **granulomatous disease**, and infections, such as endocarditis, acquired immunodeficiency syndrome (AIDS), and hepatitis. **Epstein–Barr infection**, which is associated with infectious **mononucleosis**, will typically result in splenomegaly in both adults and children. It is important to note that massive splenomegaly can lead to spontaneous splenic rupture. The implantation of ectopic splenic tissue, also referred to as **splenosis**, can occur following splenic rupture. In this situation, the ectopic tissue can resemble a mass.

SOUND OFF
The most common cause of splenomegaly is portal hypertension.

CLINICAL FINDINGS OF SPLENOMEGALY

1. Palpable, enlarged spleen
2. Hemolytic abnormalities (sickle cell anemia)
3. Trauma
4. Infection
5. History of cirrhosis, trauma, leukemia, or lymphoma
6. Leukocytosis and/or elevated red blood cell count
7. Possible left upper quadrant pain or discomfort

SONOGRAPHIC FINDINGS OF SPLENOMEGALY

1. Enlargement of the spleen to greater than 12 to 13 cm in length or 6 cm in thickness
2. Spleen extends beyond the inferior pole of the left kidney

Splenic Cysts

Most often, true splenic cysts, also referred to as an epithelial cyst, will have thin walls, an anechoic center, and posterior enhancement (Fig. 6-6). However, cysts found in the spleen can appear complex, particularly those associated with trauma (see section "Splenic Trauma" in this chapter). Other complex-appearing cysts could be displaced pancreatic pseudocysts, an abscess, congenital cysts, **hydatid cysts**, cystic metastasis, or even cystic manifestation of primary cancers. The hydatid cyst, which is most often the result of the tapeworm *Echinococcus granulosus*, will have a similar sonographic appearance and clinical findings to those found in the liver (see section "Hydatid Liver Cyst" in Chapter 2). Cysts found in the spleen may also be associated with autosomal dominant polycystic kidney disease.

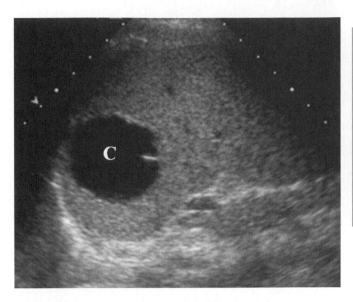

Figure 6-6 Splenic cyst. A simple splenic cyst (*C*) is noted in this patient.

CLINICAL FINDINGS OF SIMPLE SPLENIC CYSTS
1. Asymptomatic
2. Pain can occur with hemorrhage

SONOGRAPHIC FINDINGS OF SIMPLE SPLENIC CYSTS
1. Round
2. Smooth-walled mass
3. Anechoic mass
4. Posterior enhancement

Splenic Abscesses

Though uncommon, a pyogenic abscess can develop in the spleen. This may be caused by *Staphylococcus aureus*, *Streptococcus*, or even *Salmonella*. Clinical findings of a splenic abscess may include fever, leukocytosis, left upper quadrant tenderness, left flank or shoulder pain, and splenomegaly. A splenic abscess will most likely have a complex appearance, but it can also be completely hypoechoic, and possibly contain debris or gas (Fig. 6-7). As with any pyogenic abscess, the air and gas produced by the bacteria within a splenic abscess

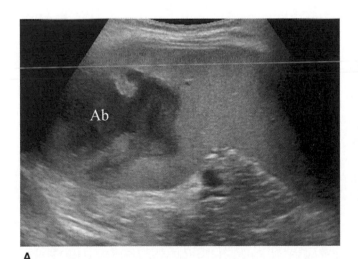

A

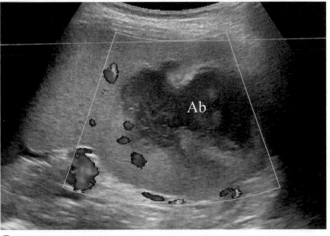

B

Figure 6-7 Pyogenic splenic abscess. **A.** Longitudinal sonogram reveals an irregular, heterogeneous mass, representing a pyogenic abscess (*Ab*) in the spleen. **B.** Color Doppler image shows flow in the adjacent parenchyma, but absence of vascularity within the abscess (*Ab*) confirming its complex cystic nature. Staphylococcus aureus grew on blood culture.

can produce dirty shadowing or ring-down artifact. Color Doppler interrogation will often yield increased vascularity around an abscess but not within it.

A history of **bacteremia** increases the patient's likelihood of developing a pyogenic abscess. Thus, disease processes that may lead to abscess development within the spleen include **bacterial endocarditis**, diverticulitis, **osteomyelitis**, and possibly pelvic infections.

CLINICAL FINDINGS OF SPLENIC ABSCESSES

1. Fever
2. Leukocytosis
3. Left upper quadrant tenderness
4. Left flank or shoulder pain
5. Splenomegaly

SONOGRAPHIC FINDINGS OF SPLENIC ABSCESSES

1. Complex appearance
2. May contain debris or gas (that produces dirty shadowing or ring down)
3. Can be completely hypoechoic
4. Fungal abscess may appear as small solid masses or have a target or *bull's-eye* appearance
5. Color Doppler will demonstrate increased flow around the mass but not within it

The spleen can also be affected by a fungal abscess, most often resulting from *Candida*. Fungal abscesses may be small and have a target or *bull's-eye* appearance (Fig. 6-8). These patients are often immuno compromised.

Splenic Infarct

Tissue that has been deprived of oxygen will eventually die. This is referred to as an infarct. Clinically, patients often suffer from the sudden onset of left upper quadrant pain. A **splenic infarct** may be caused by sickle cell disease, bacterial endocarditis, tumor embolization, vasculitis, and lymphoma. It will appear as a hypoechoic, wedge-shaped mass within the spleen in the acute stage (Fig. 6-9). In the chronic stage, splenic infarcts tend to appear more echogenic compared with adjacent normal splenic tissue.

🔊 SOUND OFF
The splenic infarct is typically seen sonographically as a hypoechoic, wedge-shaped mass.

CLINICAL FINDINGS OF A SPLENIC INFARCT

1. Sudden onset of left upper quadrant pain

SONOGRAPHIC FINDINGS OF A SPLENIC INFARCT

1. Acute infarct—hypoechoic, wedge-shaped mass within the spleen
2. Chronic infarct—hyperechoic, wedge-shaped mass within the spleen

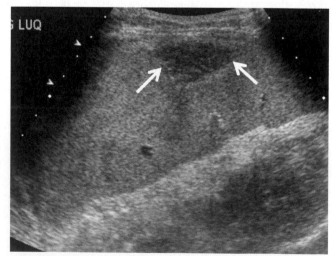

Figure 6-9 Splenic infarct. Infarcts often appear as wedge-shaped hypoechoic areas (*arrows*) within the spleen.

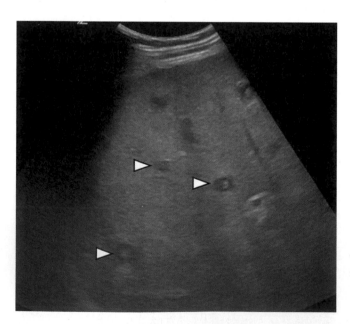

Figure 6-8 Splenic fungal abscesses in a patient with leukemia. Longitudinal sonographic image of the spleen demonstrates multiple small hypoechoic abscesses (*arrowheads*) within the spleen, some of which have a target or *bull's-eye* appearance.

Splenic Trauma

The spleen is often injured in cases of **blunt trauma**. Although sonography may not be the initial modality of choice immediately following trauma, it is often utilized to evaluate the spleen once the initial diagnosis of splenic trauma is established. Patients who suffer from splenic trauma complain of left upper quadrant pain and may have decreased hematocrit. A hematoma within the spleen can be difficult to identify with sonography, because it may appear isoechoic to the splenic tissue and can be located either subcapsular or within the splenic parenchyma. The evolution of a splenic hematoma as it undergoes **lysis** may range from complex or hypoechoic (early in the event) to echogenic or isoechoic and then back to hypoechoic or anechoic as the hematoma resolves (Fig. 6-10). Occasionally, a laceration may be noted as an echogenic line within the spleen immediately following trauma. In time, hemorrhagic cysts that result from trauma may eventually have calcified walls. Also, as mentioned earlier in this chapter, splenic rupture can lead to implants of ectopic splenic tissue referred to as splenosis. These masses of splenic tissue have a similar sonographic appearance to normal splenic tissue and, when found in unusual locations, can be mistaken for more worrisome neoplasms. Patients who suffer from trauma resulting in severe damage to the spleen may have to undergo a surgical **splenectomy**. The spleen may also be removed secondary to cancer, severe splenomegaly, or other pathology that inhibits normal function.

CLINICAL FINDINGS OF SPLENIC TRAUMA

1. Blunt trauma to the left upper quadrant
2. Severe left upper quadrant pain
3. Decreased hematocrit level indicating active bleeding

SONOGRAPHIC FINDINGS OF SPLENIC TRAUMA

1. Acute hemorrhage—complex or hypoechoic
2. Middle stage—echogenic (with clot formation) or isoechoic
3. Later stages of hemorrhage—anechoic or hypoechoic
4. Chronic hematomas may have a complex appearance or calcified walls

Splenic Hemangioma

The **hemangioma** is the most common benign tumor of the spleen. A splenic hemangioma will most often appear as a well-defined, hyperechoic mass (Fig. 6-11). The patient with a hemangioma will be asymptomatic, although pain may occur with hemorrhage.

◀)) SOUND OFF
The most common mass of the spleen is the benign hemangioma.

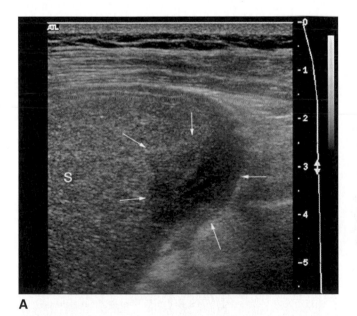
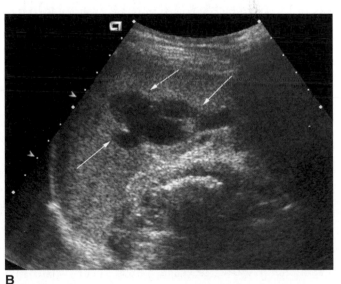

A   **B**

Figure 6-10 Splenic hematoma. **A.** Longitudinal scan of the spleen (*S*) demonstrating a resolving splenic hematoma (*arrows*). **B.** Longitudinal image of the spleen in a patient 6 months post-blunt abdominal trauma demonstrating a resolving hematoma (*arrows*).

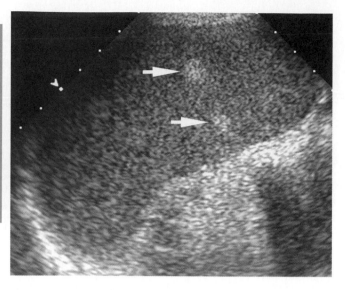

Figure 6-11 Splenic hemangiomas. Two hyperechoic masses (*arrows*) are noted within this spleen.

CLINICAL FINDINGS OF A SPLENIC HEMANGIOMA

1. Asymptomatic
2. Pain occurs with hemorrhage

SONOGRAPHIC FINDINGS OF A SPLENIC HEMANGIOMA

1. Well-defined, hyperechoic mass

Granulomatous Disease in the Spleen

Occasionally, small echogenic foci may be seen throughout the spleen. These small foci most often represent **granulomas**. They can be individual or multiple and may produce an acoustic shadow. Granulomas can be found in patients who have a history of **histoplasmosis**, tuberculosis, or **sarcoidosis**. Whereas granulomas tend to be small, larger calcifications may result from the resolution of splenic hematomas, infarctions, abscesses, neoplasms, or infection.

CLINICAL FINDINGS OF GRANULOMATOUS DISEASE IN THE SPLEEN

1. Asymptomatic
2. May have a history of histoplasmosis, tuberculosis, or sarcoidosis

SONOGRAPHIC FINDINGS OF GRANULOMATOUS DISEASE IN THE SPLEEN

1. Small, echogenic foci that may shadow

Splenic Hamartoma

The **splenic hamartoma** is benign and typically appears as a hypoechoic mass, though the sonographic appearance can be variable. These tumors have been associated with **Beckwith–Wiedemann syndrome** and **tuberous sclerosis**. They are typically asymptomatic. Color Doppler may yield hypervascularity.

CLINICAL FINDINGS OF SPLENIC HAMARTOMA

1. Asymptomatic
2. Pain can occur with rupture
3. Patient may have a history of Beckwith–Wiedemann syndrome or tuberous sclerosis

SONOGRAPHIC FINDINGS OF SPLENIC HAMARTOMA

1. Hypoechoic mass or masses (echotexture can vary however)
2. Color Doppler may reveal hypervascularity

Malignant Diseases of the Spleen

Patients with splenic malignancy may suffer from left upper quadrant pain, fever, weight loss, and malaise. Although exceedingly rare, the primary malignant tumor of the spleen is an **angiosarcoma**. Angiosarcomas will appear sonographically as a complex or solid mass. More often, lymphoma and leukemia rather than angiosarcoma will involve the spleen, with lymphoma being cited as the most common malignancy of the spleen. Diffuse involvement of lymphoma or leukemia will often produce splenomegaly. These malignant processes can also manifest as a focal disease and be recognized as a hypoechoic mass or masses scattered throughout spleen (Fig. 6-12). However, focal masses are less commonly seen with leukemia.

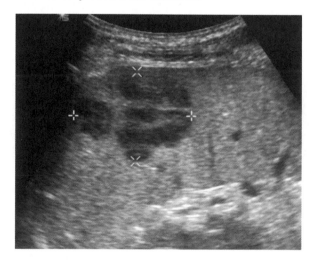

Figure 6-12 Lymphoma. Transverse image of the spleen in a patient with Hodgkin lymphoma reveals a hypoechoic mass (*between calipers*).

Lymphoma can be classified as Hodgkin lymphoma or **non-Hodgkin lymphoma**. Both are malignant disorders affecting the lymphocytes, with subsequent immune system compromise. The differentiation between these two types of cancers is performed microscopically. The presence of **Reed–Sternberg cells** indicates Hodgkin lymphoma. Hodgkin lymphoma can be treated and carries a high recovery rate. The other form of lymphoma, non-Hodgkin lymphoma, is not as easily managed but more common. Metastatic disease to the spleen is rare and occurs late in the disease process. The most common primary locations are the breast, lung, skin (melanoma), and ovary.

CLINICAL FINDINGS OF SPLENIC MALIGNANCY

1. LUQ pain
2. Fever
3. Weight loss
4. Malaise

SONOGRAPHIC FINDINGS OF SPLENIC MALIGNANCY

1. Diffuse—splenomegaly
2. Focal—hypoechoic masses

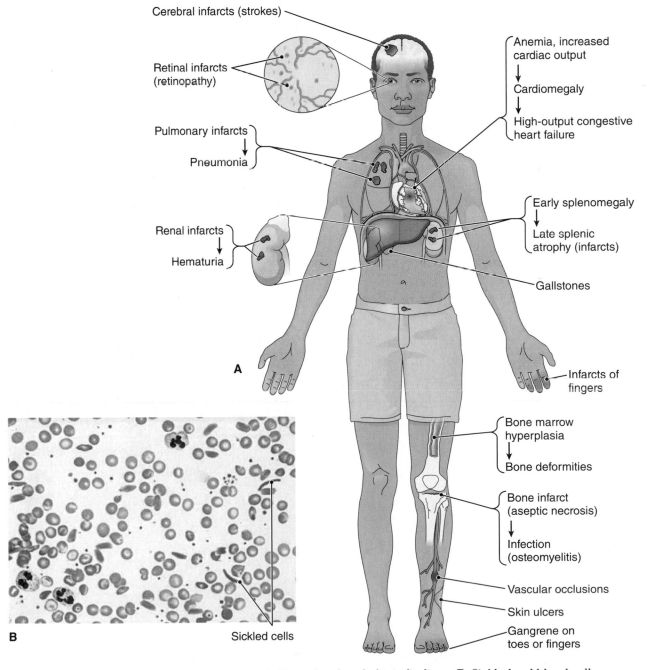

Figure 6-13 Complication of sickle cell disease. **A.** Clinical and pathologic findings. **B.** Sickled red blood cells.

🔊)) SOUND OFF
Hodgkin lymphoma has a better chance of recovery compared to non-Hodgkin lymphoma.

PEDIATRIC PATHOLOGY OF THE SPLEEN

Splenic Lymphangioma

The **splenic lymphangioma** is a benign lesion that is a congenital malformation of the lymphatic system. It is comprised of both lymphatic and blood vessels. Sonographically, lymphangiomas appear as multicystic masses that contain hypoechoic or anechoic locules and hyperechoic septations. Patients often suffer from splenomegaly as well. Lymphangiomas are most identified in children. Clinically, a child with a splenic lymphangioma would most likely complain of nausea, LUQ pain, and abdominal distention.

Sickle Cell Anemia

Sickle cell disease is a group of inherited blood disorders that affects hemoglobin and includes a disorder referred to as sickle cell anemia. Those with sickle cell anemia have abnormal, crescent-shaped red blood cells that tend to attach to each other and obstruct normal vascular channels, causing many clinical complications (Fig. 6-13). Sickle cell anemia is found more frequently in African-American, Middle East, Mediterranean, and Hispanic children of Caribbean descent in the United States.

CLINICAL FINDINGS OF SPLENIC LYMPHANGIOMA

1. Nausea
2. LUQ pain
3. Abdominal distention

SONOGRAPHIC FINDINGS OF SPLENIC LYMPHANGIOMA

1. Multicystic masses
2. Masses may contain hypoechoic or anechoic locules and hyperechoic septations

As mentioned earlier, a child suffering from sickle cell anemia often has an enlarged spleen during a sickle cell crisis. Occasionally, focal masses of normal splenic tissue may be noted (Fig. 6-14). However, with time and with recurrent sickle cell crises, the spleen will eventually become fibrotic and atrophy. The wasting-away of the spleen in this manner is caused by multiple infarctions and is termed **autosplenectomy**. Patients undergoing a sickle cell crisis may have decreased hematocrit and complain of bone pain. These patients are at increased risk for gallstones, multiple organ damage, blindness, and stroke.

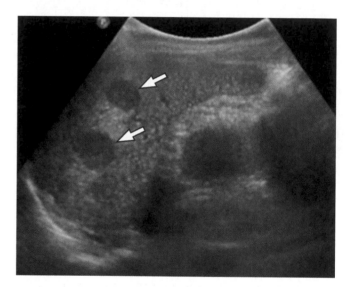

Figure 6-14 Sickle cell disease. Longitudinal sonographic image demonstrating rounded, hypoechoic lesions (*arrows*) within the spleen, which were later determined to be islands of normal splenic tissue in this spleen damaged by sickle cell disease.

REVIEW QUESTIONS

1. A 15-year-old male patient presents to the sonography department with a history of left-sided trauma 5 years earlier. He currently has no LUQ discomfort. The sonographic findings of the spleen include a mass that contains a calcification producing distinct posterior shadowing. What is the most likely diagnosis?
   a. Splenic hemangioma
   b. Splenic hamartoma
   c. Splenic lymphangioma
   d. Splenic hematoma

2. A 25-year-old female patient presents to the sonography department for a complete abdominal sonogram. She complains of right lower quadrant pain and nausea. The right upper abdomen appears normal. A small mass is noted in the area of the splenic hilum. This mass appears isoechoic to the spleen. What does this most likely represent?
   a. Pancreatic cystadenocarcinoma
   b. Splenic hemangioma
   c. Splenunculus
   d. Neuroblastoma

3. A rare malignant tumor of the spleen that consists of blood vessels is a/an:
   a. lymphoma.
   b. angiosarcoma.
   c. hemangioma.
   d. granuloma.

4. A 48-year-old male patient with a history of severe, sudden onset of left upper quadrant pain without trauma presents to the sonography department for a sonogram of the spleen. You visualize a wedge-shaped, hypoechoic area within the spleen. This most likely represents a:
   a. splenic infarct.
   b. splenic hematoma.
   c. splenic hemangioma.
   d. splenic metastasis.

5. A patient with a wandering spleen would have an increased risk for:
   a. splenic infection.
   b. splenosis.
   c. splenic carcinoma.
   d. splenic torsion.

6. What is the most common sonographic appearance of a splenic hemangioma?
   a. Hyperechoic
   b. Hypoechoic
   c. Anechoic
   d. Complex

7. The process of making red blood cells is termed:
   a. erythropoiesis.
   b. leukopoiesis.
   c. histopoiesis.
   d. anemia.

8. Multiple, small echogenic foci scattered throughout the spleen in a patient with a history of toxoplasmosis most likely represent:
   a. sarcoidosis.
   b. granulomas.
   c. lymphangiomas.
   d. hemangiomas.

9. The splenic artery marks the:
   a. posterior aspect of the pancreatic body and tail.
   b. superior aspect of the pancreatic body and tail.
   c. medial surface of the pancreatic body and tail.
   d. lateral aspect of the pancreatic body and tail.

10. The most common cause of splenomegaly is:
    a. hepatitis.
    b. portal hypertension.
    c. lymphoma.
    d. trauma.

11. The splenic hamartoma may be discovered more often in individuals with a history of:
    a. HIV.
    b. splenic carcinoma.
    c. tuberous sclerosis.
    d. Meckel–Gruber syndrome.

12. The type of tissue within the spleen that is responsible for its phagocytic function is the:
    a. red pulp.
    b. white pulp.
    c. culling pulp.
    d. pitting pulp.

13. A 32-year-old female patient presents to the sonography department for an abdominal sonogram. An evaluation of the spleen reveals a 1-cm, rounded, echogenic mass within the spleen that does not produce acoustic shadowing. What is the most likely diagnosis?
    a. Pheochromocytoma
    b. Lipoma
    c. Splenic metastasis
    d. Hemangioma

14. Which of the following is a benign lesion that is a congenital malformation of the lymphatic system?
    a. Lymphangioma
    b. Hemangioma
    c. Angiosarcoma
    d. Myeloma

15. The spleen is a/an:
    a. intraperitoneal organ.
    b. retroperitoneal organ.

16. The type of tissue within the spleen that is responsible for its lymphatic function is the:
    a. red pulp.
    b. white pulp.
    c. culling segment.
    d. pitting segment.

17. Which of the following children would least likely suffer from sickle cell anemia?
    a. African-American
    b. Caucasian
    c. Middle Eastern
    d. Mediterranean

18. The splenic vein marks the:
    a. posterior aspect of the pancreatic body and tail.
    b. anterior aspect of the pancreatic body and tail.
    c. medial surface of the pancreatic body and tail.
    d. lateral aspect of the pancreatic body and tail.

19. All of the following are functions of the spleen except:
    a. storage of iron.
    b. defense against disease.
    c. blood reservoir.
    d. destruction of phagocytic cells.

20. A 26-year-old patient with a long-standing history of multiple sickle cell crises and subsequent splenic infarctions presents to the sonography department for an abdominal sonogram. After thoroughly evaluating the left upper quadrant, only a fraction of splenic tissue can be identified. This describes the process of:
    a. splenomicroly.
    b. asplenia.
    c. autosplenectomy.
    d. splenosis.

21. Where is the most common location of an accessory spleen?
    a. Superior to the spleen
    b. Medial to the diaphragm and left kidney
    c. Splenic hilum
    d. Anterior to the pancreatic body

22. All of the following can be associated with splenomegaly except:
    a. trauma.
    b. hemolytic abnormalities.
    c. mononucleosis.
    d. pancreatitis.

23. What is the splenic process of cleaning red blood cells of unwanted material?
    a. Pitting
    b. Plucking
    c. Culling
    d. Coring

24. Diffuse involvement of lymphoma or leukemia of the spleen will often lead to:
    a. splenomegaly.
    b. splenic atrophy.
    c. Epstein–Barr infection.
    d. splenic torsion.

25. The splenic artery originates at the:
    a. superior mesenteric artery.
    b. inferior phrenic artery.
    c. celiac trunk.
    d. gastroduodenal artery.

26. Which of the following is a congenital anomaly in which the spleen is divided into two portions by a band of tissue?
    a. Splenic infarct
    b. Splenic cleft
    c. Splenosis
    d. Splenic imperfecta

27. A 35-year-old male patient presents to the sonography department for an abdominal sonogram with a history of abdominal pain and histoplasmosis. What are you more likely to identify within the spleen?
    a. Multiple histomas
    b. Multiple hemangiomas
    c. Multiple metastatic lesions
    d. Multiple granulomas

28. A 14-year-old male patient presents to the sonography department after falling from his bicycle. An abdominal sonogram reveals a complex-appearing mass within the spleen. This most likely represents a:
    a. splenic hemangioma.
    b. splenic granuloma.
    c. splenic hematoma.
    d. splenic infarct.

29. A sickle cell crisis will often lead to:
    a. splenic metastasis.
    b. sarcoidosis.
    c. splenomegaly.
    d. wandering spleen.

30. Epstein–Barr infection is best described as:
    a. a herpesvirus that can lead to infectious mononucleosis.
    b. a herpesvirus that is often associated with splenic granulomatous disease.
    c. an infection that results in sickle cell anemia in children.
    d. an infection within a splenic hematoma following blunt trauma.

31. The spleen removes irregular cells from the bloodstream through a process called:
    a. pitting.
    b. culling.
    c. crimping.
    d. amassing.

32. An area within the spleen that has become necrotic because of a lack of oxygen is referred to as a:
    a. splenic hemangioma.
    b. splenic hematoma.
    c. splenic infarct.
    d. granuloma.

33. What systemic disease results in the development of granulomas within the spleen and throughout the body?
    a. Granulomatosis
    b. Sarcoidosis
    c. Sickle cell anemia
    d. Beckwith–Wiedemann syndrome

34. A complex cyst that results from the parasitic infestation of the spleen by a tapeworm is the:
    a. bacterial endocarditic cyst.
    b. choledochal cyst.
    c. hydatid cyst.
    d. candidiasis.

35. From the list below, what is the most likely clinical finding of a patient who has a splenic hemangioma?
    a. Fever
    b. Decreased hematocrit
    c. Elevated white blood cell count
    d. Asymptomatic

36. In a patient with suspected lymphoma, the presence of Reed–Sternberg cells indicates:
    a. Hodgkin lymphoma.
    b. non-Hodgkin lymphoma.
    c. metastatic liver disease.
    d. splenic infarction.

37. Which of the following describes the implantation of ectopic splenic tissue possibly secondary to splenic rupture?
    a. Splenosis
    b. Polysplenia
    c. Asplenia
    d. Wandering spleen

38. All of the following are true of the spleen except:
    a. it is the largest structure of the reticuloendothelial system.
    b. the primary objective of the spleen is to filter the peripheral blood.
    c. the spleen has a convex inferior margin and a concave superior border.
    d. the spleen is considered the largest lymphatic organ.

39. The splenic vein joins with what structure posterior to the pancreatic neck to form the portal vein?
    a. Inferior mesenteric artery
    b. Superior mesenteric vein
    c. Inferior mesenteric artery
    d. Main hepatic vein

40. Small echogenic foci scattered throughout the spleen most likely represent:
    a. multiple benign hemangioma.
    b. multiple benign hematomas.
    c. multiple benign granulomas.
    d. malignant lymphoma.

41. Which of the following would be least likely associated with splenomegaly?
    a. Beckwith–Wiedemann syndrome
    b. Cirrhosis
    c. Blunt trauma
    d. Extramedullary erythropoiesis

42. What is the primary malignant tumor of the spleen?
    a. Leukemia
    b. Hemangioma
    c. Angiosarcoma
    d. Granuloma

43. Which of the following would most likely appear as a target lesion in the spleen?
    a. Fungal abscess
    b. Pyogenic abscess
    c. Hydatid disease
    d. Angiomyosarcoma

44. The abnormality noted in Figure 6-15, most likely represents a:
    a. splenic infarct.
    b. splenic cyst.
    c. splenic abscess.
    d. splenic hamartoma.

45. Which of the following would be least likely associated with the sonographic appearance of the abnormality noted in Figure 6-15?
    a. Trauma
    b. *Echinococcus granulosus*
    c. Autosomal dominant polycystic kidney disease
    d. Splenic hamartoma

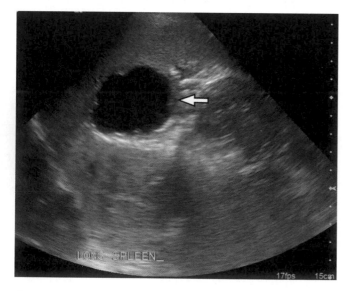

Figure 6-15

46. What would be the most likely sonographic appearance of a chronic infarct in the spleen?
    a. Hyperechoic, wedge-shaped mass
    b. Hypoechoic, irregular-shaped mass with posterior shadowing
    c. Anechoic mass
    d. Splenomegaly with multiple hypoechoic masses throughout

47. A patient with a history of bacteremia would have an increased risk at developing a:
    a. splenic hemangioma.
    b. splenic infarct.
    c. splenic abscess.
    d. splenic granuloma.

48. What is the most common benign mass of the spleen?
    a. Lymphangioma
    b. Hemangioma
    c. Hamartoma
    d. Splenic infarct

49. Which of the following would be least likely associated with the development of granulomas within the spleen?
    a. Bacterial endocarditis
    b. Tuberculosis
    c. Histoplasmosis
    d. Sarcoidosis

50. A 51-year-old patient presents to the sonography department with a history of fever, left flank pain, and splenomegaly. Sonographically, you identify a complex mass with internal components. Which of the following findings would be the most likely indicator that the mass is likely a pyogenic splenic abscess?
    a. A fluid-fluid level
    b. Hyperechogenicity of the borders
    c. Dirty shadowing emanating from the mass
    d. Posterior enhancement emanating from the mass

51. Which type of splenic cancer has a relatively high recovery rate?
    a. Hodgkin lymphoma
    b. non-Hodgkin lymphoma
    c. Adenocarcinoma
    d. Cystadenocarcinoma

52. Patients who suffer from sickle cell anemia have an increased risk for:
    a. hemangiomas.
    b. hamartomas.
    c. hydatid cysts.
    d. gallstones.

53. The spleen is located:
    a. medial to the pancreatic tail.
    b. superior and medial to the hepatic flexure.
    c. posterolateral to the stomach.
    d. medial to the caudate lobe.

54. The abnormality identified by the arrows in Figure 6-16 was discovered in a patient suffering from acute left upper quadrant pain and a history of sickle cell disease. What is the most likely diagnosis?
    a. Splenic hemangioma
    b. Splenic hematoma
    c. Splenic infarct
    d. Splenic pyogenic abscess

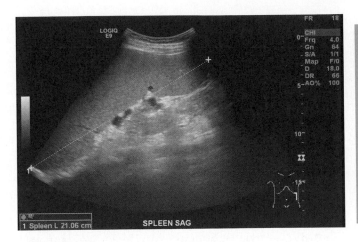

Figure 6-17

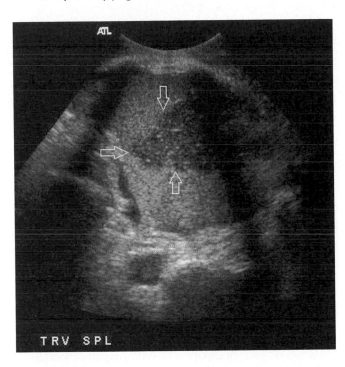

Figure 6-16

55. The patient in Figure 6-17 is a 43-year-old male patient who was also suffering from jaundice, weight loss, and ascites. What other sonographic finding would be most likely discovered in this patient?
    a. Hepatofugal flow within the portal veins
    b. Hypoechoic pancreatic echotexture
    c. Webbing of the hepatic veins
    d. Periportal cuffing

56. Heterotaxia syndromes may be associated with both cardiac malformation and:
    a. splenic infarcts.
    b. polysplenia.
    c. splenosis.
    d. splenic carcinoma.

57. Which of the following best describes histoplasmosis?
    a. Inherited disease that disrupts the normal immune system
    b. Disease that results from inhaling airborne fungus
    c. Abnormal arrangement of the abdominal organs
    d. System disease that affects the shape of red blood cells

58. What attaches the spleen to the stomach?
    a. Gastrostomach fissure
    b. Splenorenal tendon
    c. Renogastric tendon
    d. Gastrosplenic ligament

59. The normal spleen is:
    a. more anechoic than the gallbladder.
    b. more echogenic than the liver.
    c. more hyperechoic than left renal sinus.
    d. more heterogenous than the pancreas.

60. Which of the following best describes leukopenia?
    a. Decreased level of splenic cells
    b. Decreased level of red blood cells
    c. Decreased level of white blood cells
    d. Decreased level of hemoglobin

SUGGESTED READINGS

Curry RA, Tempkin BB. *Sonography: Introduction to Normal Structure and Function.* 5th ed. Elsevier; 2021:271–281.

Federle MP, Jeffrey RB, Woodward PJ, et al. *Diagnostic Imaging: Abdomen.* 2nd ed. Amirsys; 2010:II-7-2–II-7-39.

Hagen-Ansert SL. *Textbook of Diagnostic Sonography.* 7th ed. Elsevier; 2012:422–439.

Henningsen C, Kuntz K, Youngs D. *Clinical Guide to Sonography: Exercises for Critical Thinking.* 2nd ed. Elsevier; 2014:88–99.

Hertzberg BS, Middleton WD. *Ultrasound: The Requisites.* 3rd ed. Elsevier; 2016:192–203.

Kawamura DM, Nolan TD. *Diagnostic Medical Sonography: Abdomen and Superficial Structures.* 4th ed. Wolters Kluwer; 2018:229–246 & 611–654.

Rumack CM, Wilson SR, Charboneau JW, et al. *Diagnostic Ultrasound.* 4th ed. Elsevier; 2011:146–171 & 1800–1844.

Sanders RC, Hall-Terracciano B. *Clinical Sonography: A Practical Guide.* 5th ed. Wolters Kluwer; 2016:466–478.

Siegel MJ. *Pediatric Sonography.* 5th ed. Wolters Kluwer; 2019:304–345.

BONUS REVIEW!

Splenomegaly on Computed Tomography (CT) (Fig. 6-18)

Splenic Rupture on CT (Fig. 6-19)

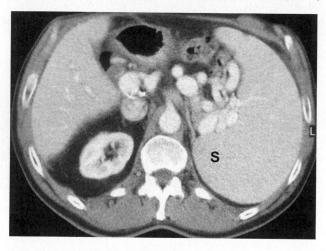

Figure 6-18 Splenomegaly (*S*) on CT.

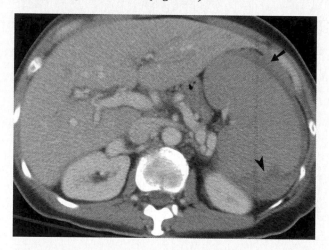

Figure 6-19 Splenic rupture on CT. Spontaneous splenic rupture. Contrast-enhanced CT of the upper abdomen demonstrates splenomegaly and posteriorly located splenic laceration (*arrowhead*). There is small amount of perisplenic hematoma (*arrow*) identified in this patient with leukemia.

The Urinary Tract

Introduction

This chapter provides an overview of the anatomy of the kidneys, ureters, and bladder. In addition, pathology of the urinary tract is explained. This chapter provides important vascular anatomy of the urinary tract, as well as renal vascular complications and basic transplant assessment. In the "Bonus Review" section, images of radiography, computed tomography (CT), and magnetic resonance imaging (MRI) are provided.

Key Terms

acquired renal cystic disease—a cystic disease of the kidney that is often the result of chronic hemodialysis

acute pyelonephritis—an inflammation of the kidney or kidneys secondary to infection

acute renal failure—a sudden decrease in renal function

acute tubular necrosis—damage to the tubule cells within the kidneys that results in renal failure

amyloidosis—the accumulation of the abnormal protein amyloid in the kidneys and other organs that can lead to organ damage, as well as renal failure

angiomyolipoma—a common benign renal tumor that consists of a network of blood vessels, muscle, and fat

autosomal dominant polycystic kidney disease—an inherited renal disease that results in the development of renal, liver, and pancreatic cysts late in life; also referred to as adult polycystic kidney disease

autosomal recessive polycystic kidney disease—an inherited renal disease that results in bilateral enlargement of the fetal kidneys and microscopic renal cysts; also referred to as infantile polycystic kidney disease

azotemia—an excess of urea or other nitrogenous compounds in the blood

bacteriuria—the presence of bacteria in the urine

benign prostatic hypertrophy—benign enlargement of the prostate gland

bladder diverticulum—an outpouching of the urinary bladder wall

blood urea nitrogen—a measure of the amount of nitrogen in the blood in the form of urea

chronic pyelonephritis—chronic inflammation of the kidney or kidneys

chronic renal failure—the gradual decrease in renal function over time

columns of Bertin—an extension of the renal cortex located between the renal pyramids

congenital hydronephrosis—the dilation of the renal collecting system at birth

cortical nephrocalcinosis—the accumulation of calcium within the cortex of the kidney

cortical thinning—the thinning of the (renal) cortex

corticomedullary differentiation—the ability to sonographically distinguish between the normal cortex and medullary portions of the kidney

creatinine—a chemical waste molecule that is generated from muscle metabolism and excreted in the urine

cystitis—inflammation of the urinary bladder

detrusor muscle—the muscle that controls the appropriate emptying of the urinary bladder

dirty shadowing—shadowing seen posterior to gas or air

dysuria—painful or difficult urination

emphysematous pyelonephritis—the formation of air within the kidney parenchyma secondary to bacterial infiltration

end-stage renal disease—medical condition in which the kidneys fail to function adequately, thus requiring the use of dialysis

exophytic—growing outward

flank pain—pain in one side of the body between the upper abdomen and the back

Gerota fascia—the fibrous envelope of tissue that surrounds the kidney and adrenal gland

glomerular filtration rate—blood test that is used to evaluate the overall function of glomeruli, which are the small blood filters located within the kidney

glomeruli—small blood filters located at the beginning of the nephron

glomerulonephritis—an infection of the kidney glomeruli

gross hematuria—blood within the urine that is visible to the naked eye

hematoma—a localized collection of blood

hematuria—blood within the urine; can be described as microscopic or gross

hemodialysis—form of dialysis that utilizes a machine that essentially acts as a kidney whereby it extracts the patient's blood, filters it, and returns the filtered blood to the patient

Henoch–Schönlein purpura—an autoimmune disorder and form of vasculitis associated with purple spots on the skin, gastrointestinal complications, joint pain, and possibly kidney failure; mostly occurs in childhood

homeostasis—maintenance of normal body physiology

hydronephrosis—the dilation of the renal collecting system resulting from the obstruction of the flow of urine from the kidney(s) to the bladder; also referred to as pelvocaliectasis or pelvicaliectasis

hydroureter—distention of the ureter with fluid because of obstruction

hyperkalemia—abnormally high levels of potassium in the blood

hypernephroma—carcinoma of the kidney; also referred to as renal cell carcinoma

hypovolemia—decreased blood volume

immunocompromised—the state of having an immune system that is impaired for some reason

infantile polycystic kidney disease—an inherited renal disease that results in bilateral enlargement of the fetal kidneys and microscopic renal cysts; also referred to as autosomal recessive polycystic kidney disease

lactate dehydrogenase—an enzyme found within the blood that may be used to monitor renal function; may also be used as a tumor marker

lymphocele—a collection of lymphatic fluid

malaise—the feeling of uneasiness

medullary nephrocalcinosis—the accumulation of calcium within the medulla of the renal parenchyma

medullary sponge kidney—a congenital disorder characterized by the accumulation of calcium within abnormally dilated collecting ducts located within the medulla

megacystis—an abnormally enlarged urinary bladder

megaureter—an enlarged ureter; can be congenital or acquired

moiety—division of the duplex collecting system, as in the upper pole moiety and the lower pole moiety

multicystic dysplastic kidney disease—a renal disease thought to be caused by an early renal obstruction; leads to the development of multiple noncommunicating cysts of varying sizes in the renal fossa

mural nodules—a small mass located on the wall of a structure

nephroblastoma—the most common solid malignant pediatric abdominal mass; may also be referred to as Wilms tumor

nephrocalcinosis—an accumulation of calcium within the renal parenchyma

nephrolithiasis—the urinary stones located within the kidney; kidney stones

nephron—the functional unit of the kidney

nephrotic syndrome—a kidney disorder caused by damage to the glomeruli that results in excess amounts of protein in the urine and the swelling of the ankles, face, and feet because of accumulation of excess water

neurogenic bladder—a bladder that is poorly functioning secondary to any type of neurologic disorder

nocturia—frequent urination at night

nuclear cystogram—a nuclear medicine examination of the urinary bladder and ureters

nutcracker syndrome—syndrome associated with clinical complications as a result of compression or entrapment of the left renal vein as it passes between the superior mesenteric artery and abdominal aorta

oliguria—scant or decreased urine output

oncocytoma—a benign renal tumor that is often found in men in their 60s

papillary projection—a small protrusion of tissue

pelvic congestion syndrome—syndrome that results from the compression of the left renal vein at the origin of the superior mesenteric artery; leads to lower abdominal and back pain after standing for long periods of time, dyspareunia, dysmenorrhea, abnormal uterine bleeding, chronic fatigue, and bowel issues

pelvic kidney—a kidney located within the pelvis

perinephric abscess—an abscess that surrounds the kidney

peritoneal dialysis—a form of dialysis that uses a solution that is instilled into the abdomen; uses diffusion and osmosis to filter waste products from the blood

pheochromocytoma—a benign, solid adrenal tumor associated with uncontrollable hypertension

posterior urethral valves—irregular thin membranes of tissue located within the male posterior urethra that do not allow urine to exit the urethra

proteinuria—protein within the urine

prune belly syndrome—a syndrome that is a consequence of the abdominal wall musculature being stretched by an extremely enlarged urinary bladder

pyonephrosis—the condition of having pus within the collecting system of the kidney

pyuria—pus within the urine

renal adenoma—a benign renal mass

renal artery stenosis—the narrowing of the renal artery

renal cell carcinoma—the carcinoma of the kidney; also referred to as hypernephroma

renal colic—a sharp pain in the lower back that radiates into the groin and is typically associated with the passage of a urinary stone through the ureter

renal cortex—the outer part of the renal parenchyma that is responsible for filtration

renal hamartoma—see angiomyolipoma

renal hemangioma—a benign renal mass that consists of blood vessels

renal hematoma—a collection of blood on or around the kidney that is typically associated with some form of trauma or perhaps an invasive kidney procedure

renal infarction—an area in the kidney that becomes necrotic because of a lack of oxygen; color Doppler most useful at demonstrating a focal or global absence of blood flow

renal lipoma—a fatty tumor on the kidney

renal medulla—the inner part of the renal parenchyma that is responsible for absorption

renal pyramids—cone-shaped structures located within the renal medulla that contain part of the nephron

renal sinus—the portion of the kidney containing the minor calices, major calices, renal pelvis, and infundibula

renal vein thrombosis—a blood clot located within the renal vein

renal:aorta ratio—a ratio calculated by dividing the highest renal artery velocity by the highest aortic velocity obtained at the level of the renal arteries

renin—enzyme produced by the kidneys that helps regulate blood pressure

renunculi—the two embryonic parenchymal tissue masses that combine to create the kidney; singular form is renunculus

retroperitoneal fibrosis—a disease characterized by the buildup of fibrous tissue within the retroperitoneum; this mass may involve the abdominal aorta, inferior vena cava, ureters, and sacrum

reverberation artifact—an artifact that results from a sound wave interacting with a large acoustic interface that repeatedly bounces back and forth from the interface to the transducer

schistosomiasis—a flatworm that enters humans by penetrating the skin

septation—a partition separating two or more cavities

Skene duct cyst—benign cyst that may be noted within the female urethra; may manifest as a Skene gland cyst

staghorn calculus—a large urinary stone that completely fills and takes the shape of the renal pelvis

subureteric Teflon injection—a treatment method for vesicoureteral reflux disease that uses a bulking agent to elevate the ureteral orifice and distal ureter, allowing for the normal flow of urine from the ureter into the bladder

tardus–parvus—the combination of a slow systolic upstroke and a decreased systolic velocity

trabeculae—muscular bundles

transitional cell carcinoma—a malignant tumor of the urinary tract that is often found within the urinary bladder or within the renal pelvis

trigone of the urinary bladder—the area within the urinary bladder where the two ureteral orifices and urethral orifice are located

tuberous sclerosis—a systemic disorder that leads to the development of tumors within various organs

tubo-ovarian abscess—a pelvic abscess involving the uterine tubes and ovaries that is often caused by pelvic inflammatory disease

twinkle sign—an artifact noted as an increased color Doppler signal posterior to a kidney stone or biliary stone

urachus—a tubular structure that is a remnant of embryonic development, which extends from the umbilicus to the apex of the bladder

ureteral jets—jets of urine that are the result of urine being forced into the urinary bladder from the ureters; can be demonstrated with color Doppler imaging

ureterocele—an abnormality in which the distal ureter projects into the urinary bladder

ureteropelvic junction—the junction of the ureter and renal pelvis

ureterovesicle junction—the junction of the ureter and urinary bladder

urethral caruncle—small benign lesions of the female urethra

urethritis—inflammation of the urethra

urinoma—a localized collection of urine; may appear complex or simple

urolithiasis—a urinary stone

uterine leiomyoma—a benign, smooth muscle tumor of the uterus; may also be referred to as a fibroid or uterine myoma

vesicoureteral reflux—the abnormal retrograde flow of urine from the urinary bladder into the ureter and possibly into the kidney(s)

voiding cystourethrogram—a radiographic examination that involves the assessment of the urinary bladder and distal ureter for urinary reflux and other abnormalities

von Hippel–Lindau syndrome—an inherited disorder characterized by tumors of the central nervous system and the development of cysts within the kidneys, renal cell carcinoma, and pheochromocytomas

Wilms tumor—the most common solid malignant pediatric abdominal mass; a malignant renal mass that may also be referred to as nephroblastoma

xanthogranulomatous pyelonephritis—a rare chronic form of pyelonephritis that is typically the result of a chronic obstructive process

ANATOMY AND PHYSIOLOGY OF THE KIDNEY

The urinary system consists of the upper urinary tract (kidneys and ureters) and the lower urinary tract (bladder and urethra). The functional unit of the kidney is the **nephron**. The nephron begins to function by the ninth week of gestation, although urine production begins between 11 and 13 weeks. A functional urinary tract is vital for the fetus because urine—produced by the fetal kidneys—comprises the majority of amniotic fluid.

Fundamentally, the kidneys are organs that are crucial for **homeostasis**. The kidneys detoxify and filter the blood; excrete metabolic waste; dynamically reabsorb amino acids, ions, glucose, and water. They also maintain normal pH, iron, and salt levels in the blood. The kidneys also work to regulate blood pressure by producing the enzyme **renin**, which is released by specialized cells adjacent to each **glomeruli**.

Each kidney is formed when two embryonic parenchymal masses combine. These kidney tissue masses are referred to as the **renunculi** or ranunculi. The kidneys initially develop within the pelvis and ascend into the fetal abdomen by 12 weeks gestation. This explains the occurrence of ectopic kidney locations, such as a **pelvic kidney**, which is the most common location of an ectopic kidney. However, this ascension can be arrested anywhere along the typical migratory path.

> 🔊 **SOUND OFF**
> The most common location of an ectopic kidney is within the pelvis.

Adult kidneys are bean-shaped organs that are retroperitoneal in location. The left kidney is located higher than the right because of the size of the liver, which occupies most of the right upper quadrant of the abdomen. The left kidney is also on average a little longer than the right kidney, although there is typically no more than a 2 cm difference between kidney lengths. However, suspicion of functional renal abnormalities may abound if there is a significant difference between kidney length, and certainly in these situations, clinical history should be correlated closely. Although the coverings of the kidney are indistinguishable on a sonogram, there are four that are present. The pararenal fat layer covers **Gerota fascia** and an additional fat layer known as the perirenal fat layer. The innermost covering of the kidney is the renal capsule. These layers protect the kidney and act as shock absorbers.

The kidneys are made up of two parts: the renal parenchyma and the renal sinus (Fig. 7-1). The parenchyma of the kidney consists of the **renal medulla** and **renal cortex**. The renal medulla, the inner part of the parenchyma, is responsible for absorption. It includes the **renal pyramids**. The renal cortex, which is responsible for filtration of the blood, is the outer part of the renal parenchyma. The **renal sinus** contains the renal collecting system that is composed of the minor calices, major calices, renal pelvis, and infundibula. The renal pelvis is a funnel-shaped structure that collects the urine before it moves into the ureter.

VASCULAR ANATOMY OF THE KIDNEYS

The renal arteries are branches of the abdominal aorta that are located just below the level of the superior mesenteric artery. Oxygenated blood travels through the renal arteries, which enter the renal hilum, and then into the segmental branches and subsequently into the interlobar arteries, which can be noted traveling between the renal pyramids (see Fig. 7-1). The interlobar arteries branch into the much smaller arcuate arteries at the base of the pyramids. The arcuate arteries then branch into the interlobular arteries, and into the afferent arterioles, which carry blood into the glomerulus for filtration. The right renal artery travels posterior to the

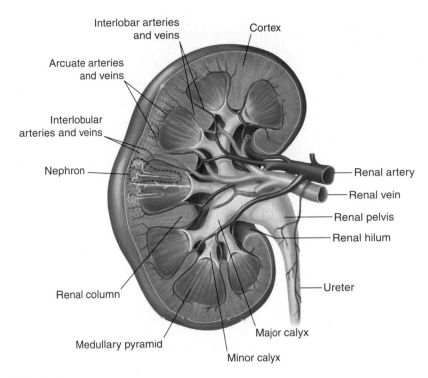

Figure 7-1 Anatomy of the kidney.

inferior vena cava (IVC), and is therefore longer than the left renal artery.

The renal veins exit the kidneys at their respective renal hilums and connect to the lateral aspects of the IVC. The left renal vein has to travel across the abdomen, between the superior mesenteric artery and abdominal aorta, and is therefore longer than the right renal vein. It is normal for the left renal vein to be smaller in diameter as it travels between the superior mesenteric artery and abdominal aorta, and then to appear more prominent beyond that point as it travels to the left kidney.

LABORATORY TESTS

Both urine and blood tests are used to evaluate renal function. A urinalysis for renal function includes, but is not limited to, an evaluation of the urine for bacteria (**bacteriuria**), pus (**pyuria**), blood (**hematuria**), and protein (**proteinuria**) (Table 7-1). Blood tests may be used to analyze levels of **blood urea nitrogen** (BUN), **creatinine**, **glomerular filtration rate** (GFR), and **lactate dehydrogenase** (LDH) (Table 7-2). BUN measures the amount of urea nitrogen, a byproduct of protein metabolism that occurs within the liver and is excreted by the kidneys. Creatinine, also excreted by the kidneys, measures the amount of creatinine phosphate found in the skeletal muscles. An elevation in either BUN or creatinine indicates some form of renal disease. The GFR—which utilizes creatinine, age, body size, and gender—can be used to evaluate the overall function of the kidneys.

LDH is an additional enzyme found within the blood that may be used to monitor renal function and other abnormalities, including some forms of cancer. LDH is found in nearly all tissues of the body. LDH elevates as a result of cell death. Therefore, an elevation in LDH is not a specific indicator for renal disease.

SONOGRAPHY OF THE KIDNEYS

The sonographic appearance of the kidneys differs with age, and multiple variants may be noted with sonography (Table 7-3). The most common congenital anomaly of the urinary tract is the duplex or duplicated collecting system (Fig. 7-2). Neonatal and pediatric kidneys may appear lobulated, have prominent renal pyramids, and/or have subtle sonographic distinctions between the renal cortex and renal sinus. Normal adult kidneys are elliptical in shape in the longitudinal plane and rounded in the transverse plane. Though renal size varies with age, gender, and other factors, in the adult, they typically measure approximately 8 to 13 cm in length, 2 to 3 cm in the anteroposterior dimension, and 4 to 5 cm in width.

> **SOUND OFF**
> The most common congenital anomaly of the urinary tract is the duplex or duplicated collecting system.

TABLE 7-1 Urinalysis and associated abnormalities

Urinalysis Results	Associated Abnormality
Bacteriuria	**Acute pyelonephritis**
	Urinary tract infections
Pyuria	Urinary tract infections
	Usually accompanied by bacteria
Hematuria	Acute and **chronic pyelonephritis**
	Hypernephroma (renal cell carcinoma)
	Renal infarction
	Trauma
	Urinary calculi
Proteinuria	Benign and malignant masses
	Glomerulonephritis
	Infection
	Nephrotic syndrome
	Acute or chronic pyelonephritis
	Urinary calculi
Urine pH (abnormal)	Urinary calculi (used to determine composition of stones)
Specific gravity	Low: renal failure and pyelonephritis
	High: dehydration
Elevated white blood cells (in urine)	Urinary tract infection

TABLE 7-2 Blood tests and associated abnormalities

Blood Test (Serum)	Elevation	Reduction
Blood urea nitrogen	Renal failure	Liver disease and failure
	Parenchymal disease	Malnutrition
	Renal obstruction	Overhydration
	Dehydration	Smoking
	Diabetes mellitus	Pregnancy
	Hemorrhage	
Creatinine	Renal failure	N/A
	Chronic nephritis	
	Renal obstruction	
	Diabetes mellitus	
	Reduced renal blood flow	
Glomerular filtration rate	N/A	Renal insufficiency or chronic renal disease
Lactate dehydrogenase	Renal infarction	N/A
	Chronic renal disease	
Total white blood cell	Infection or inflammation	Chemotherapy
		Radiation therapy
		Toxic reaction
Hematocrit	N/A	Acute hemorrhage

TABLE 7-3 Renal variants in appearance and location

Renal Variant	Description
Compensatory hypertrophy	Enlargement of the unaffected contralateral kidney with unilateral renal agenesis or compromised renal function
Dromedary hump (Fig. 7-3)	Bulge on the lateral border of the kidney (often on the left kidney) Will have the same echogenicity as the adjacent renal cortex
Duplex (duplicated) collecting system (the most common congenital anomaly of the urinary tract)	Division of the renal sinus. In this variant, there are two separate renal sinuses; they are referred to as an upper pole **moiety** and lower pole moiety. Obstruction to one or both of these collecting systems can occur. Two ureters drain separate portions of the kidney. A kidney with a duplex collecting system will typically measure longer than a normal size kidney.
Ectopic kidney	Pelvic kidney: one or both kidneys may be located within the pelvis; the pelvis is the most common location of an ectopic kidney. Crossed fused ectopia: both kidneys are fused and on the same side of the body. Thoracic kidney: kidney sits partially or completely in the chest.
Extrarenal pelvis	The renal pelvis is located outside of the renal hilum.
Fetal lobulation	Lobulated or bumpy outline to the kidney(s); can be seen in adults
Horseshoe kidneys	Two kidneys that cross the midline and connect at their lower poles by an isthmus The isthmus of the horseshoe kidneys travels anterior to the abdominal aorta and inferior vena cava
Hypertrophic column of Bertin	Enlargement of a renal column seen as an indentation of the renal sinus Actually are double layers of renal cortex
Junctional parenchymal defect (junctional line) (Fig. 7-4)	Results from the incomplete fusion of the two embryologic components (renunculi) of the kidney Appears as a hyperechoic, wedge-shaped structure on the anterior portion of the kidney; located between the upper and middle sections of the kidney
Malrotated kidney	The kidney sits in the renal fossa but is positioned off of the normal axis.
Renal agenesis	Congenital absence of the kidney Bilateral renal agenesis is typically not consistent with life.
Renal hypoplasia	The underdevelopment of the kidney in which there are too few nephrons Kidney will be smaller than normal.
Renal sinus lipomatosis (fibrolipomatosis)	Excessive fat within the renal pelvis Renal sinus will be large and echogenic.
Supernumerary kidney	A third, smaller kidney

The renal sinus is central in the kidney and has an echogenic appearance. The renal cortex appears as medium- to low-level echoes surrounding the central sinus. The normal cortex should be more hypoechoic than, or isoechoic to, the normal liver or the spleen. It should measure more than 1 cm in thickness. The term for this reduction in the thickness of the renal cortex is **cortical thinning**. Monitoring cortical thickness may especially be helpful for patients with chronic renal disease as well. Increased echogenicity of the renal cortex suggests intrinsic renal disease. Within the cortex, the triangular-shaped medullary pyramids may be noted separated by the **columns of Bertin**. Occasionally, the renal capsule may be observed in some cases. It appears as a highly reflective hyperechoic line surrounding the kidney.

SOUND OFF
Echogenicities of the kidney and adjacent structures are as follows: renal medulla < renal cortex ≤ liver < spleen < pancreas < diaphragm > renal sinus.

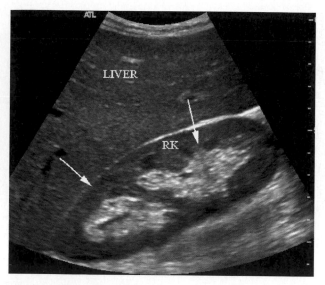

Figure 7-2 Duplex collecting system. Sagittal image of the right kidney (*RK*) revealing two distinct renal sinuses (*arrows*), separated by a band of parenchyma, denoting a duplicated collecting system.

KIDNEY PATHOLOGY

Renal Failure

Acute Renal Failure

A sudden decrease in renal function, typically over the course of days or weeks, is termed **acute renal failure** (ARF). The most common cause of ARF is **acute tubular necrosis**. With acute tubular necrosis, the kidney suffers from ischemic damage and subsequent cell destruction. Acute tubular necrosis may appear sonographically as a normal kidney initially, though it may also lead

to variable cortical changes and an elevated resistive index (RI) of greater than 0.7.

Other causes of ARF include **renal artery stenosis**, renal infection, urinary tract obstruction, polycystic kidney disease, metabolic disorders such as **amyloidosis**, and inflammatory conditions like **Henoch–Schönlein purpura**. Henoch–Schönlein purpura is an autoimmune, inflammatory vascular disease that mostly affects children and can permanently damage the kidneys. Clinical findings of ARF include elevated BUN, elevated creatinine, **oliguria**, hypertension, leukocytosis, hematuria, edema, and **hypovolemia**. Sonographically, the kidneys may appear normal or the cortex may appear hyperechoic. Once ARF is established, sonography is valuable at evaluating the overall appearance of the kidneys and determining if hydronephrosis is present in cases caused by urinary tract obstruction.

CLINICAL FINDINGS OF ACUTE RENAL FAILURE

1. Elevated BUN and creatinine
2. Oliguria
3. Hypertension
4. Leukocytosis
5. Hematuria
6. Edema
7. Hypovolemia

SONOGRAPHIC FINDINGS OF ACUTE RENAL FAILURE

1. Normal kidneys
2. May appear more echogenic
3. Hydronephrosis may be present.

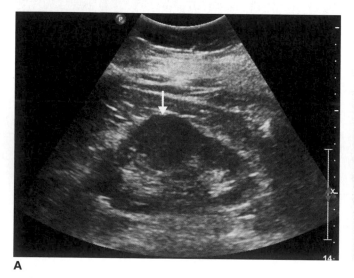

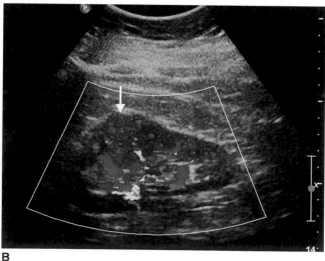

Figure 7-3 Dromedary hump (*arrows*). **A.** Gray-scale sonogram shows a focal bulge on the lateral border of the left kidney, consistent with a dromedary hump. **B.** Color Doppler image shows normal branching of the renal vasculature through the dromedary hump.

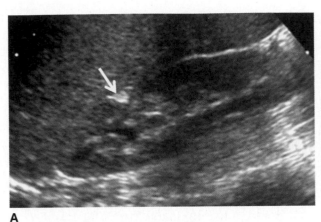
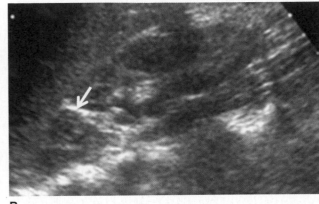

Figure 7-4 Junctional parenchymal defect or junctional line. The *arrows* in these images (**A** and **B**) denote the sonographic appearance of a junctional parenchymal defect.

> **◀)) SOUND OFF**
> The most common cause of ARF is acute tubular necrosis.

Chronic Renal Failure

The gradual decrease in renal function over time, typically months or years, is referred to as **chronic renal failure** (CRF). Kidneys that fail to function normally will lead to **end-stage renal disease**. The most common cause of CRF is diabetes mellitus. Other causes of CRF include, but are not limited to, glomerulonephritis, chronic pyelonephritis, metabolic disorders, chronic urinary tract obstruction, tuberculosis, renal vascular disease, and infection. Clinical findings include diabetes, **malaise**, elevated BUN, elevated creatinine, fatigue, hypertension, and **hyperkalemia**. Patients are typically placed on dialysis or a donor kidney may be needed. Sonographically, the kidneys will have cortical thinning, appear small and echogenic, and may contain cysts (Fig. 7-5). There is also typically loss of normal **corticomedullary differentiation**.

CLINICAL FINDINGS OF CHRONIC RENAL FAILURE
1. Diabetes mellitus
2. Malaise
3. Elevated BUN and creatinine
4. Fatigue
5. Hypertension
6. Hyperkalemia

SONOGRAPHIC FINDINGS OF CHRONIC RENAL FAILURE
1. Small, echogenic kidneys
2. Cortical thinning
3. Loss of normal corticomedullary differentiation
4. Renal cysts may be seen as well.

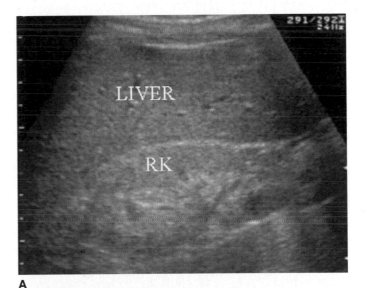
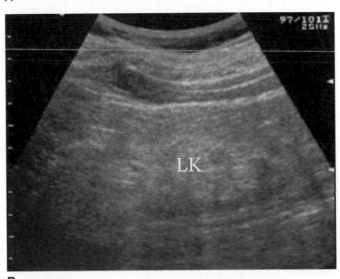

Figure 7-5 Chronic renal failure. The right kidney (*RK*) (**A**) and the left kidney (*LK*) (**B**) are notably more echogenic than normal, indicating chronic renal failure.

> 🔊 **SOUND OFF**
> The most common cause of CRF is diabetes mellitus.

Renal Failure and Dialysis

Patients suffering from renal failure may be forced to undergo dialysis treatment. This form of treatment is used to remove the accumulated urea, other waste materials, and excess water from patients whose kidney function is inadequate. Oftentimes, these patients are awaiting renal transplantation. Dialysis may be in the form of **hemodialysis**, hemofiltration, or **peritoneal dialysis**.

Both hemodialysis and hemofiltration utilize a machine that essentially acts as a kidney whereby it extracts the patient's blood, filters it, and returns the filtered blood to the patient. Peritoneal dialysis uses a solution that is instilled into the abdomen via a catheter. Through diffusion and osmosis, the solution allows for the filtration of waste. Because of the solution utilized in peritoneal dialysis, patients will often have a minimal amount of ascites noted during a sonographic examination of the abdomen and pelvis.

Renal Cystic Disease

Simple Renal Cyst

The simple cyst is the most common renal mass. A simple renal cyst should appear sonographically as an anechoic mass that is spherical, has smooth walls, posterior acoustic enhancement, and no internal echoes (Fig. 7-6). An anechoic mass that does not specifically meet all of these criteria is not considered a simple renal cyst. Although larger cysts may cause some pain as they compress adjacent renal tissue, they are typically asymptomatic and clinically insignificant. However, once one renal cyst is identified, the sonographer should more closely examine the kidneys for further cyst involvement.

Renal cysts can be peripelvic, parapelvic, cortical, or **exophytic** in location. A parapelvic cyst is one that originates in the renal parenchyma and protrudes into the renal sinus. They may be difficult to differentiate from a dilated renal pelvis. Peripelvic cysts are renal cysts that originate in the renal sinus. They may be difficult to differentiate from hydronephrosis. Small cortical cysts are located within the cortex and may be difficult to differentiate from prominent renal pyramids, especially if they are solitary. Renal cysts that appear to be projecting out away from the kidney may be termed "exophytic."

CLINICAL FINDINGS OF A SIMPLE RENAL CYST
1. Asymptomatic

SONOGRAPHIC FINDINGS OF A SIMPLE RENAL CYST
1. Spherical
2. Anechoic mass
3. Smooth walls (including a well-defined posterior wall)
4. Posterior acoustic enhancement
5. No internal echoes

Complex Renal Cysts

A cyst that does not meet all of the characteristics of a simple cyst will fall into the complex cyst category. It is important to note that renal cell carcinoma (RCC) may manifest as a multicystic mass. Therefore, when a cyst has characteristics that include a **septation**, internal debris, **mural nodules**, a **papillary projection**, or irregular borders, it becomes more worrisome for malignancy and is often followed up with further imaging or surgical intervention (Fig. 7-7). A wide range of sonographic findings may be noted with complex renal cysts (Table 7-4).

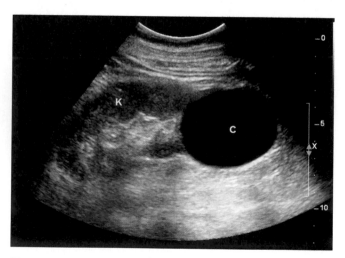

Figure 7-6 Simple renal cyst. A simple renal cyst (*C*) is noted on the lower pole of this kidney (*K*).

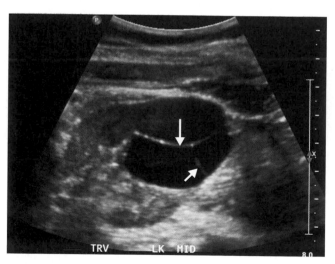

Figure 7-7 Complex renal cyst. This renal cyst has several septations (*arrows*).

Autosomal Dominant Polycystic Kidney Disease

Autosomal dominant polycystic kidney disease (ADPKD) is a hereditary disorder that may also be referred to as adult polycystic kidney disease. ADPKD can lie dormant for many years, often not manifesting in clinical symptoms until the person is in the third to fourth decade of life. Clinical symptoms include hypertension and decreasing renal function. In addition, the patient may suffer from a urinary tract infection, renal calculi, **flank pain**, hematuria, and have a palpable mass in the abdomen.

With ADPKD, the patient will develop numerous cortical renal cysts of varying sizes (Fig. 7-8). Cysts may also be found in other organs, including the pancreas, liver, testis, seminal vesicles, and spleen. In fact, ADPKD has a 40% association with polycystic liver disease. Many times, these patients ultimately suffer from end-stage renal disease and must be placed on dialysis, placing ADPKD among the top causes of CRF worldwide. Sonographically, the kidneys will appear enlarged and contain numerous renal cysts, with possible cysts identified in the pancreas, liver, and/or spleen.

CLINICAL FINDINGS OF AUTOSOMAL DOMINANT POLYCYSTIC KIDNEY DISEASE

1. Asymptomatic until third or fourth decade of life
2. Decreased renal function
3. Urinary tract infections
4. Renal calculi
5. Flank pain
6. Hematuria
7. Palpable abdominal mass

SONOGRAPHIC FINDINGS OF AUTOSOMAL DOMINANT POLYCYSTIC KIDNEY DISEASE

1. Bilateral enlarged kidneys that contain numerous cortical renal cysts
2. Possible cysts identified in the pancreas, liver, spleen, testis, and seminal vesicles

SOUND OFF
ADPKD is most often seen in adults. Just remember, adults are *dominant*.

Autosomal Recessive Polycystic Kidney Disease

Autosomal recessive polycystic kidney disease (ARPKD) is a hereditary disorder that may also be referred to as autosomal recessive polycystic renal disease or **infantile polycystic kidney disease**. ARPKD is characterized by dilation of the renal collecting tubules (Fig. 7-9). This disorder is often recognized in the fetus and can be confirmed with a postnatal sonographic examination. If perinatal death does not occur, patients often die secondary to complication of renal failure and portal hypertension from hepatic fibrosis. The typical sonographic findings of a newborn affected by ARPKD are bilateral, enlarged, echogenic kidneys, with a loss of corticomedullary differentiation (Fig. 7-10). A high-frequency transducer may be useful to demonstrate the abnormal renal architecture and small renal cysts.

TABLE 7-4 Clinical and sonographic findings of complex renal cyst

Complex Renal Cyst	Clinical Findings	Sonographic Findings
Renal cyst with internal calcifications	Previous history of a hemorrhagic or infected cyst Asymptomatic	Posterior shadowing from the calcification within the cyst
Hemorrhagic renal cyst	Simple cysts may bleed into themselves. Possible history of trauma Flank pain Hematuria	Anechoic, hypoechoic, hyperechoic, or complex mass, depending on the stage of hemolysis; chronic hemorrhagic cysts may also contain calcifications.
Infected renal cyst	Urinary tract infection Fever Flank pain Hematuria Leukocytosis	Internal debris Thick walls
Milk of calcium cyst	Asymptomatic	Fluid–fluid level within the cyst Milk of calcium will shadow and layer within the cyst.
Multilocular renal cyst	Previous history of a hemorrhagic or infected cyst Asymptomatic	Thin septations separating the locules of fluid No blood flow within the septations

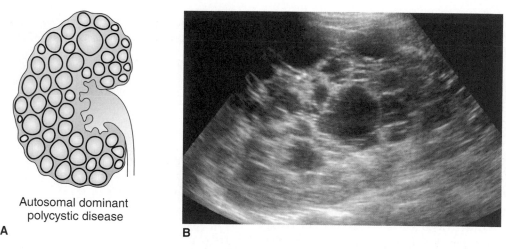

Figure 7-8 Autosomal dominant polycystic kidney disease (*ADPKD*). **A.** Drawing of autosomal dominant polycystic kidney disease. **B.** Advanced ADPKD results in the parenchyma being replaced by numerous noncommunicating cysts of varying sizes.

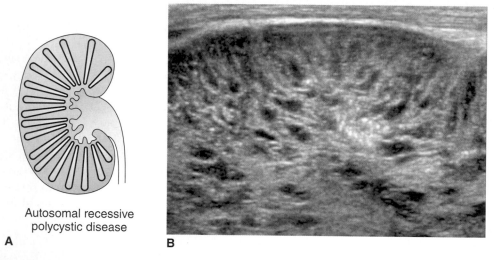

Figure 7-9 Autosomal recessive polycystic kidney disease (*ARPKD*). **A.** Drawing of ARPKD. **B.** High-frequency (12 MHz) image of the parenchyma of the kidney in a newborn demonstrates dilation of the collecting tubules that characterize ARPKD.

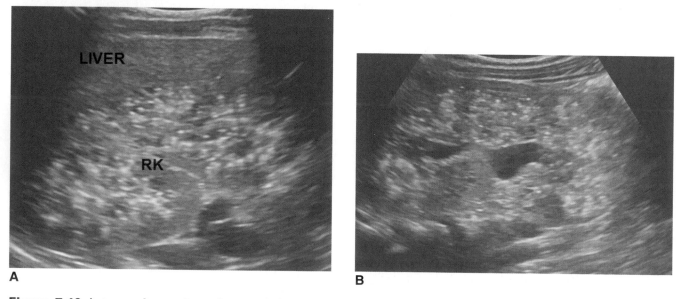

Figure 7-10 Autosomal recessive polycystic kidney disease. Longitudinal images of the right (**A**) and left (**B**) kidneys in a newborn patient with echogenic kidneys seen on a prenatal sonogram (*RK*, right kidney). Both kidneys are enlarged and normal renal pyramids are not seen.

CLINICAL FINDINGS OF AUTOSOMAL RECESSIVE POLYCYSTIC KIDNEY DISEASE

1. Clinical findings of renal failure
2. Abnormal liver function tests because of hepatic disease
3. Portal hypertension and hepatic fibrosis often ensue.

SONOGRAPHIC FINDINGS OF AUTOSOMAL RECESSIVE POLYCYSTIC KIDNEY DISEASE

1. Bilateral, enlarged echogenic kidneys
2. Loss of corticomedullary differentiation
3. High-frequency transducer may be useful to demonstrate the abnormal renal architecture and small renal cysts.

🔊 SOUND OFF
ARPKD is seen in children. Just remember, children are offered *recess* at school.

Multicystic Dysplastic Kidney Disease

Multicystic dysplastic kidney (MCDK) disease may also be referred to as multicystic dysplastic renal disease or multicystic renal dysplasia. MCDK is thought to be caused by an early, first-trimester obstruction of the ureter. There is typically no normal functioning renal tissue present in the kidney affected by MCDK. Therefore, if this condition is bilateral, it is fatal.

Clinically, MCDK may be asymptomatic and incidentally identified in the adult patient. The sonographic finding of MCDK is the identification of several, smooth-walled, noncommunicating cysts of varying sizes in the area of the renal fossa, which completely replaces all renal parenchyma (Fig. 7-11). In addition, as a result of the nonfunctioning kidney, the contralateral kidney will take over the function of the abnormal kidney and undergo compensatory hypertrophy.

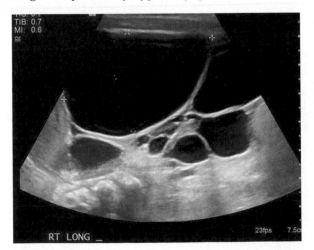

Figure 7-11 Multicystic dysplastic kidney (*MCDK*) disease of the right kidney at the age of 3 months showing multiple large cysts with minimal solid renal parenchyma noted.

CLINICAL FINDINGS OF MULTICYSTIC DYSPLASTIC KIDNEY DISEASE

1. Asymptomatic
2. Normal renal function

SONOGRAPHIC FINDINGS OF MULTICYSTIC DYSPLASTIC KIDNEY DISEASE

1. Unilateral, smooth-walled, noncommunicating cysts of varying sizes located within the renal fossa
2. Compensatory hypertrophy of the contralateral kidney

🔊 SOUND OFF
MCDK is thought to be caused by an early urinary tract obstruction. The MCDK kidney is nonfunctional. Bilateral MCDK is fatal.

Acquired Renal Cystic Disease

Acquired renal cystic disease is often the result of chronic hemodialysis. Patients with a history of dialysis and who have acquired renal cystic disease are at an increased risk for developing RCC. Sonographically, the kidneys will appear small initially during end-stage renal disease, with the development of some small cysts (Fig. 7-12). However, with time, the kidneys will enlarge and have numerous small cysts noted throughout the renal parenchyma. These cysts may also appear complex, and a thorough analysis for signs of RCC is warranted in these patients.

CLINICAL FINDINGS OF ACQUIRED RENAL CYSTIC DISEASE

1. Clinical findings of CRF
2. History of hemodialysis

SONOGRAPHIC FINDINGS OF ACQUIRED RENAL CYSTIC DISEASE

1. The kidneys will appear small initially during end-stage renal disease with some small cysts.
2. With time, the kidneys may enlarge and have numerous small cysts noted throughout the renal parenchyma.

🔊 SOUND OFF
Acquired renal cystic disease can result from hemodialysis.

von Hippel–Lindau Syndrome

von Hippel–Lindau syndrome, also referred to as von Hippel–Lindau disease, is an inherited disorder characterized by tumors of the central nervous system and orbits. Patients with this syndrome also have the

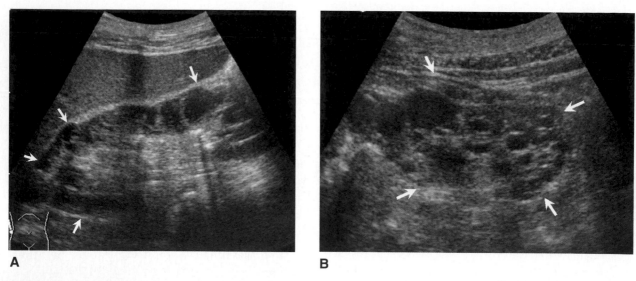

A

B

Figure 7-12 Dialysis related acquired renal cystic disease. Longitudinal images of the (**A**) right and (**B**) left kidneys reveal shrunken, echogenic, bilateral kidneys (*arrows*) consistent with chronic renal failure. Multiple small bilateral cysts are seen in this hemodialysis patient.

propensity to develop cysts within the kidneys, RCC, and **pheochromocytomas**, which are adrenal gland tumors, and have other complications (Fig. 7-13). Clinical symptoms are most often associated with the tumors in the central nervous system or eyes and not with the coexisting renal cystic disease. Sonographically, the kidneys affected by von Hippel–Lindau syndrome will have multiple renal cysts. These cysts have the potential to progress to RCC, so an evaluation for solid components within the cysts is exceedingly important.

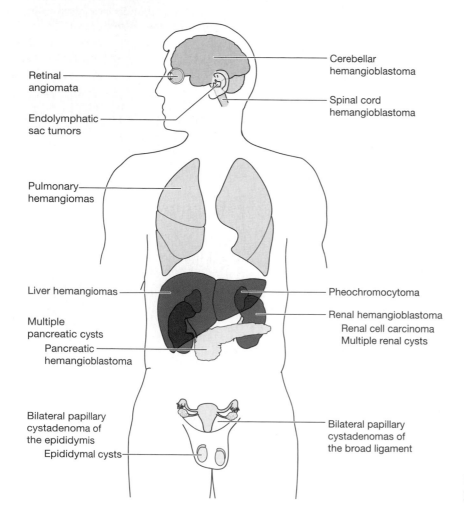

Figure 7-13 Features of von Hippel–Lindau syndrome.

CLINICAL FINDINGS OF VON HIPPEL–LINDAU SYNDROME

1. Symptoms of brain and/or an eye tumor(s)

SONOGRAPHIC FINDINGS OF VON HIPPEL–LINDAU SYNDROME

1. Multiple renal cysts
2. Cysts may be complex and have mural nodules (possible signs of RCC).
3. Cysts within the pancreas
4. Pheochromocytoma may be present.

■))) SOUND OFF
von Hippel–Lindau syndrome is characterized by possible tumors of the central nervous system, cysts within the kidneys, RCC, and pheochromocytomas.

Tuberous Sclerosis

Tuberous sclerosis is a systemic disorder that leads to the development of tumors within various organs. It is also seen in association with renal cystic disease and the accumulation of **angiomyolipomas** in the kidneys. Clinical findings of tuberous sclerosis include epilepsy and skin lesions of the face. Sonographically, a person suffering from tuberous sclerosis may have signs of bilateral, multiple renal cysts and evidence of bilateral angiomyolipomas (Fig. 7-14).

CLINICAL FINDINGS OF TUBEROUS SCLEROSIS

1. Epilepsy
2. Skin lesions of the face

SONOGRAPHIC FINDINGS OF TUBEROUS SCLEROSIS

1. Bilateral renal cysts
2. Bilateral angiomyolipomas

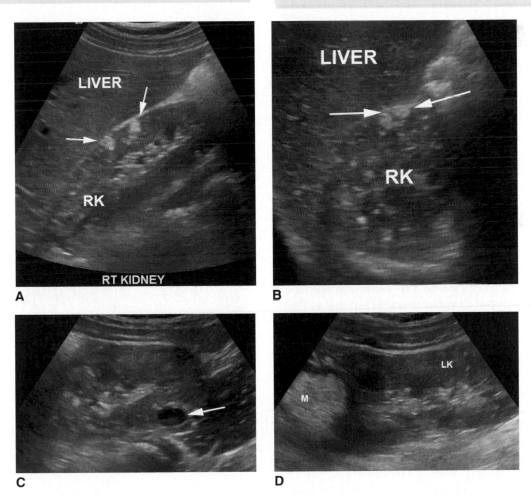

Figure 7-14 Tuberous sclerosis. **A.** Longitudinal image of the right kidney (*RK*) in a pediatric patient diagnosed with tuberous sclerosis. Two hyperechoic, homogeneous, solid masses (*arrows*) are seen in the renal cortex consistent with angiomyolipomas. **B.** Transverse image of the right kidney in a different patient demonstrates multiple echogenic foci seen throughout the renal cortex. The echogenic foci are angiomyolipomas. A larger angiomyolipoma (between *arrows*) is seen at the periphery of the cortex. **C.** Longitudinal image of the left kidney (*LK*) from the same patient as **B** again shows multiple echogenic foci throughout the cortex as well as a simple cyst (*arrow*) in the lower pole. **D.** Longitudinal image of the LK in a pediatric patient with tuberous sclerosis demonstrates an echogenic mass (*M*) arising from the upper pole.

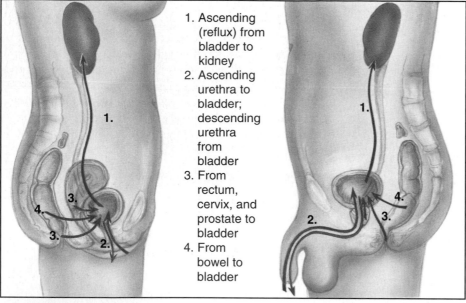

1. Ascending (reflux) from bladder to kidney
2. Ascending urethra to bladder; descending urethra from bladder
3. From rectum, cervix, and prostate to bladder
4. From bowel to bladder

Routes of Infection in the Urinary Tract

Figure 7-15 Urinary tract infections can result from various causes.

> **SOUND OFF**
> Tuberous sclerosis is associated with renal cysts and multiple, bilateral renal angiomyolipomas.

Renal Infection

A kidney infection, or pyelonephritis, is a serious medical condition that must be treated quickly and accurately to prevent permanent kidney damage. It can result from various causes, including the invasion of external bacteria from the genitalia into the bladder via the urethra, obstruction secondary to stones or masses, as well as distant infections that reach the kidney via the bloodstream (Fig. 7-15). One primary goal is to prevent permanent renal atrophy and scarring that results from pyelonephritis, as this can significantly diminish the function of the organ (Fig. 7-16). Sonographers should especially be aware of the clinical findings that are specific to urinary tract infections, as the sonographic findings may be allusive.

Acute Pyelonephritis

Acute pyelonephritis is an inflammation of the kidney or kidneys secondary to infection. Bacteria can spread to the kidney through the bloodstream or, more commonly, from the lower urinary tract (see Fig. 7-15). This type of infection is referred to as an ascending infection. The infection begins in the bladder and refluxes up through the ureters and into the kidney. It is most commonly encountered in women and is treated by antibiotics. Retrograde urine flow is also common in young children secondary to some structural defects. This will be discussed later in this chapter.

Clinically, patients present with flank pain, bacteriuria, pyuria, **dysuria**, urinary frequency, and leukocytosis. A patient with acute pyelonephritis may not have any sonographically identifiable abnormalities.

However, some findings consistent with acute pyelonephritis include renal enlargement, focal areas of altered echotexture, and compression of the renal sinus. Color Doppler may be helpful at identifying the susceptible area (Fig. 7-17). Complications of acute pyelonephritis include the development of a renal abscess, **pyonephrosis**, **xanthogranulomatous pyelonephritis**, **emphysematous pyelonephritis**, and chronic pyelonephritis.

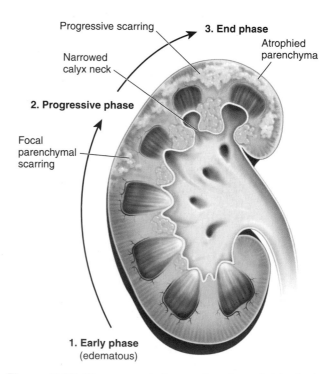

Progressive scarring

3. End phase

Atrophied parenchyma

Narrowed calyx neck

2. Progressive phase

Focal parenchymal scarring

1. Early phase (edematous)

Figure 7-16 Changes and phases of pyelonephritis. In the early phase, the kidney becomes enlarged, in the progressive phase scarring begins, whereas in the end phase, there is diffuse atrophy of the parenchyma.

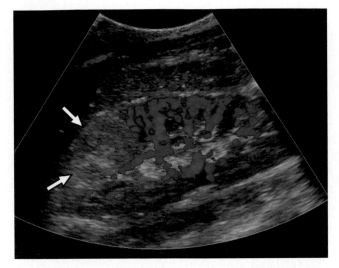

Figure 7-17 Acute pyelonephritis. Longitudinal color Doppler image of the right kidney shows a mass-like area of increased echogenicity (*arrows*) in the upper pole that has decreased blood flow compared to adjacent parenchyma.

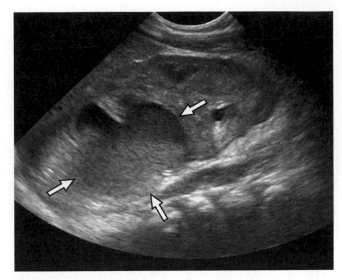

Figure 7-18 Pyonephrosis in a 3-month-old female with fever and pyuria. Longitudinal gray-scale image demonstrates echogenic fluid representing pus (*arrows*) filling the upper moiety collecting system of a duplex right kidney.

CLINICAL FINDINGS OF ACUTE PYELONEPHRITIS

1. Flank pain
2. Bacteriuria
3. Pyuria
4. Leukocytosis
5. Dysuria
6. Urinary frequency

CLINICAL FINDINGS OF PYONEPHROSIS

1. Pyuria
2. Bacteriuria
3. Fever
4. Flank pain
5. Leukocytosis

SONOGRAPHIC FINDINGS OF ACUTE PYELONEPHRITIS

1. May appear normal
2. Renal enlargement
3. Focal areas of altered echotexture
4. Compression of the renal sinus
5. Color Doppler may be useful in differentiating the infected renal parenchyma.

SONOGRAPHIC FINDINGS OF PYONEPHROSIS

1. Hydronephrosis
2. Pus and debris appear as internal, layering, low-level echoes within the dilated collecting system.

Pyonephrosis

Pyonephrosis describes the condition of having pus, also referred to as purulent material, within the collecting system of the kidney. The accumulation of pus is most likely caused by some obstructive process or infection that leads to urinary stasis, as seen in many cases of pyelonephritis. The patient will likely present with pyuria, bacteriuria, fever, flank pain, and leukocytosis. Sonographically, **hydronephrosis** will be evident. Within the dilated collecting system, thick pus or debris will appear as dependent layering, low-level echoes (Fig. 7-18).

Chronic Pyelonephritis

Recurrent kidney infections or chronic obstruction may lead to scarring of the calices and renal pelvis. This is referred to as chronic pyelonephritis. Chronic pyelonephritis can lead to xanthogranulomatous pyelonephritis and end-stage renal disease. Children with a history of **vesicoureteral reflux** (VUR) are at increased risk for developing chronic pyelonephritis (Fig. 7-19). Patients present clinically much like the patients with acute pyelonephritis in that they suffer from flank pain, fever, and evidence of a urinary tract infection. Sonographically, the kidneys will appear small, echogenic, and have lobulated borders. This lobulation is secondary to parenchymal scarring. A scar will appear as an echogenic area that extends from the renal sinus through the renal parenchyma.

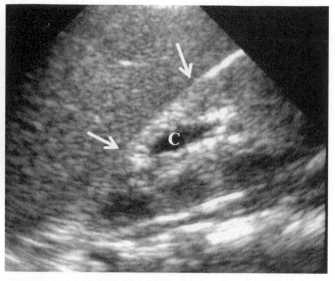

Figure 7-19 Chronic pyelonephritis. Longitudinal image of a 10-year-old boy showing a small echogenic left kidney with a dilated calyx (*C*) and overlying parenchymal atrophy (*arrows*).

CLINICAL FINDINGS OF CHRONIC PYELONEPHRITIS

1. Flank pain
2. Bacteriuria
3. Pyuria
4. Leukocytosis
5. Dysuria
6. Urinary frequency
7. History of VUR

SONOGRAPHIC FINDINGS OF CHRONIC PYELONEPHRITIS

1. Small, echogenic kidneys that have lobulated borders
2. Renal scar appears as an echogenic area within the kidney that extends from the renal sinus through the renal parenchyma.

🔊 SOUND OFF
A renal scar will appear as an echogenic area that extends from the renal sinus through the renal parenchyma.

Renal or Perinephric Abscess

A renal abscess can occur in regions of the kidney affected by pyelonephritis or be located adjacent to the kidney. A **perinephric abscess** is a collection of purulent material that has leaked through the capsule into the tissue surrounding the kidney. Patients with a renal abscess present with signs of a urinary tract infection, including high fever, flank pain, and leukocytosis. An abscess on sonography may appear anechoic, hypoechoic, or complex, depending on its contents. Gas development within the abscess produces **dirty shadowing** or **reverberation artifact**.

CLINICAL FINDINGS OF A RENAL OR PERINEPHRIC ABSCESS

1. Symptoms of pyelonephritis (pyuria, hematuria, and flank pain)
2. High fever
3. Flank pain
4. Leukocytosis

SONOGRAPHIC FINDINGS OF A RENAL OR PERINEPHRIC ABSCESS

1. Can appear anechoic, hypoechoic, or complex
2. Gas shadows or dirty shadowing may be present within the mass.

Emphysematous Pyelonephritis

A rare, and yet life-threatening, complication of pyelonephritis is emphysematous pyelonephritis. Although emphysematous pyelonephritis may be the result of a long-standing urinary tract obstruction, it is found more often in patients who have diabetes mellitus or who are **immunocompromised**. The term "emphysematous" denotes the formation of air within an organ. Consequently, with emphysematous pyelonephritis, bacterial formation allows gas to accumulate within the renal parenchyma. *Escherichia coli* infection is the most common culprit. These patients will be extremely ill and will present with a fever and flank pain. Sonographically, a highly echogenic area within the parenchyma containing air that produces reverberation artifact or dirty shadowing will be noted.

CLINICAL FINDINGS OF EMPHYSEMATOUS PYELONEPHRITIS

1. Diabetes mellitus
2. Immunocompromised patient
3. Fever
4. Flank pain
5. Leukocytosis

SONOGRAPHIC FINDINGS OF EMPHYSEMATOUS PYELONEPHRITIS

1. Gas or air within the renal parenchyma
2. Dirty shadowing or reverberation artifact coming from the renal parenchyma

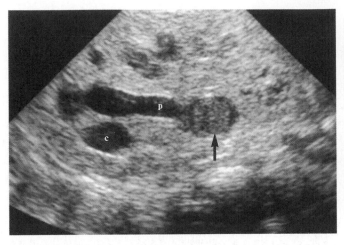

Figure 7-20 Fungus ball. Transverse image of the kidney in a 2-month-old infant with *Candida albicans* showing a dilated renal pelvis (*p*) and calices (*c*) that contain echogenic urine and a mobile fungal ball (*arrow*).

🔊 **SOUND OFF**
Emphysematous pyelonephritis is found more often in patients who have diabetes mellitus or who are immunocompromised. Dirty shadowing is often noted emanating from the renal parenchyma.

Xanthogranulomatous Pyelonephritis

Xanthogranulomatous pyelonephritis is uncommon and is typically caused by a chronic urinary tract obstruction and subsequent infection. The renal parenchyma is also replaced with granulomatous tissue. Clinical findings are consistent with urinary tract infection symptoms with dull or persistent flank pain, fever, and weight loss. With xanthogranulomatous pyelonephritis, a **staghorn calculus**, hydronephrosis, and perinephric fluid are often present. If antibiotic therapy is not effective, a nephrectomy is typically required.

CLINICAL FINDINGS OF XANTHOGRANULOMATOUS PYELONEPHRITIS

1. Dull or persistent flank pain
2. Pyuria
3. Hematuria
4. Fever
5. Leukocytosis

SONOGRAPHIC FINDINGS OF XANTHOGRANULOMATOUS PYELONEPHRITIS

1. Hydronephrosis
2. Staghorn calculus
3. Perinephric fluid collection

🔊 **SOUND OFF**
With xanthogranulomatous pyelonephritis, a staghorn calculus, hydronephrosis, and perinephric fluid are often present.

Renal Fungal Disease

The most common cause of fungal urinary tract infections is *Candida albicans*. Immunocompromised patients are at increased risk for developing a fungal infection within their kidneys. In addition, patients with a history of diabetes mellitus, intravenous drug abuse, and infants who have long-standing, indwelling catheters are more likely to suffer from renal fungal disease. Clinical symptoms include flank pain, fever, and chills. The sonographic findings may mimic several other abnormalities. However, when fungal balls are noted within the collecting system, the diagnosis of a renal fungal disease can be made (Fig. 7-20). Sonographically, fungal balls appear as echogenic, mobile, nonshadowing structures within the renal collecting system.

CLINICAL FINDINGS OF RENAL FUNGAL DISEASE

1. Immunocompromised person
2. Diabetes mellitus, intravenous drug abuse, or long-standing indwelling catheter
3. Infant with an indwelling catheter
4. Flank pain
5. Fever
6. Chills

SONOGRAPHIC FINDINGS OF RENAL FUNGAL DISEASE

1. Fungal balls appear as hyperechoic, non-shadowing, mobile structures within the renal collecting system.

Glomerulonephritis

Glomerulonephritis can be caused by a distant infection, such as strep throat, or an autoimmune reaction. Some conditions, such as lupus, have glomerulonephritis as a characteristic feature. The infection can lead to significant glomerular damage, and the kidneys can slowly shut down secondary to diminished filtration capabilities. Patients typically present with smoky urine, fever, proteinuria, hematuria, hypertension, and **azotemia**.

Glomerulonephritis can be acute or chronic. In the acute stage, the kidney may appear normal, enlarged, and have an overall increase in echogenicity. The renal pyramids may appear more prominent with acute glomerulonephritis. Chronic glomerulonephritis, the result of a long-standing infection, can lead to end-stage renal disease. Sonographically, chronic glomerulonephritis appears as an increase in the cortical echogenicity.

CLINICAL FINDINGS OF GLOMERULONEPHRITIS

1. Recent throat infection (acute)
2. Smoky urine
3. Hematuria
4. Proteinuria
5. Fever
6. Hypertension
7. Azotemia

SONOGRAPHIC FINDINGS OF ACUTE GLOMERULONEPHRITIS

1. Enlarged kidney(s) with increased echogenicity
2. Prominent renal pyramids

SONOGRAPHIC FINDINGS OF CHRONIC GLOMERULONEPHRITIS

1. Small, echogenic kidney(s)

■))) SOUND OFF
Glomerulonephritis can be caused by a distant throat infection like strep throat.

Parasitic Urinary Tract Infections

The most common renal parasitic infection is from **schistosomiasis**, which is a worm that enters humans by penetrating the skin. Although rare in the United States, clinically these patients present with hematuria, and may also have persistent fever. Sonographically, schistosomiasis is most often seen in the bladder, causing thickening of the bladder wall. Like the liver, the kidney can also succumb to *Echinococcus granulosus*, with the development of a hydatid cyst. Sonographically, the renal hydatid cyst depends on the stage of its maturation, as it may appear completely anechoic, contain a daughter cyst with internal debris, or appear as a complex mass with calcifications. Hydatid disease is most often found in sheep- and cattle-raising countries such as the Middle East, Australia, and the Mediterranean.

CLINICAL FINDINGS OF PARASITIC URINARY TRACT INFECTION

1. Hematuria
2. Flank pain
3. Pyuria
4. Dysuria
5. Possible recent travel out of the country (hydatid cyst: Middle East, Australia, and Mediterranean)

SONOGRAPHIC FINDINGS OF PARASITIC URINARY TRACT INFECTION

1. Schistosomiasis: bladder wall thickening
2. Hydatid cyst: depends on the stage of its maturation, as it may appear completely anechoic, contain a daughter cyst with internal debris, or appear as a complex mass with calcifications.

Urinary Tract Obstruction and Stones

Determining the Level of Urinary Tract Obstruction

To determine the level of urinary tract obstruction, one must have a fundamental understanding of the normal flow of urine from the kidneys to the external orifice of the urethra. Essentially, urine is created within the kidneys, travels down the ureters, collects in the bladder, and exits the urethra. Dilation of the urinary tract occurs proximal to the level of obstruction. Therefore, if there is distention of the ureter and dilation of the renal collecting system with a normal urinary bladder, the level of obstruction must be proximal to the urinary bladder, either within the ureter or at the level of the **ureterovesicle junction**.

Hydronephrosis and Renal Obstruction

Hydronephrosis is a broad term that is defined as the dilation of the renal collecting system secondary to the obstruction of normal urine flow. Accordingly, hydronephrosis is dilation of the calices, infundibula, and renal pelvis. Hydronephrosis may also be referred to as pyelocaliectasis and described more specifically according to which part of the kidney is dilated (Table 7-5). It may also be classified as mild, moderate, and severe or marked. Mild hydronephrosis is noted as distention of the renal pelvis, whereas moderate hydronephrosis is described as further progression of distention into the calices and medullary pyramids. Marked hydronephrosis extends into the cortex and causes severe thinning of the parenchyma.

TABLE 7-5 Terminology associated with hydronephrosis

Terminology for Hydronephrosis	Description
Caliectasis	Dilation of the calices
Pelviectasis (pyelectasis)	Dilation of the renal pelvis
Pelvicaliectasis (pelvocaliectasis)	Dilation of the calices and renal pelvis

There are many possible causes of a urinary tract obstruction (Fig. 7-21). Irregularities that lead to renal obstruction that are located inside the urinary tract are called intrinsic causes of hydronephrosis, and abnormalities that are located outside the urinary tract that lead to renal obstruction are referred to as extrinsic causes of hydronephrosis (Tables 7-6 and 7-7). Sonographically, hydronephrosis will appear as anechoic fluid filling all or part of the renal collecting system (Fig. 7-22). Hydronephrosis can also alter the renal artery RI within the arcuate or interlobar vessels, often leading to an RI that will be greater than 0.7.

False-Positive Hydronephrosis

The diagnosis of false-positive hydronephrosis can occur. For example, overdistention of the urinary bladder, parapelvic cysts, a prominent renal vein, and an extrarenal pelvis may all be a source of false-positive hydronephrosis. The use of color Doppler imaging and emptying the patient's bladder (postvoid imaging) are two methods that may be used to alleviate the uncertainty in these cases.

Urolithiasis

Urolithiasis is the presence of kidney stones anywhere within the urinary tract. More specifically, stones within the kidney may be referred to as renal calculi, kidney stones, renal stones, or **nephrolithiasis**. They are most often made of calcium oxalate and more frequently found in males. Stones can form in the kidney or in the bladder. A stone that completely fills

TABLE 7-6	Intrinsic causes of hydronephrosis

Urolithiasis
Congenital abnormality (vesicoureteral reflux, **posterior urethral valves**, and **ureterovesicle junction** obstruction)
Hematoma (blood clot)
Neoplasm
Ureteropelvic junction obstruction or ureteral stricture/scarring
Ureterocele

TABLE 7-7	Extrinsic causes of hydronephrosis

Benign prostatic hypertrophy
Neurogenic bladder
Pelvic masses (**uterine leiomyoma**, ovarian masses, **tubo-ovarian abscess**, and bowel masses)
Pregnancy
Retroperitoneal fibrosis
Surgery
Trauma
Urethritis

and takes on the shape of the renal pelvis is called a staghorn calculus.

If created in the kidney, urolithiasis can pass into the collecting system or ureter and cause obstruction. The most common location for a stone to become lodged in the urinary tract is the ureterovesicle junction, near the urinary bladder. Other frequently encountered places for stones to get trapped are just past the ureteropelvic junction, and at the pelvic brim where the ureter crosses the iliac vessels.

> **◀))) SOUND OFF**
> The most common location for a stone to become lodged in the urinary tract is the ureterovesicle junction, near the urinary bladder.

Kidney stones that are nonobstructing may not cause pain. Alternatively, obstructive stones can cause hematuria, **renal colic**, oliguria, and may lead to considerable urinary tract infections. Renal colic in men can cause testicular pain on the affected side. Renal stones less than 5 mm may be difficult to visualize sonographically. When seen, a kidney stone will appear as an echogenic focus that produces posterior acoustic shadowing (Fig. 7-23). The sonographic "**twinkle sign**"

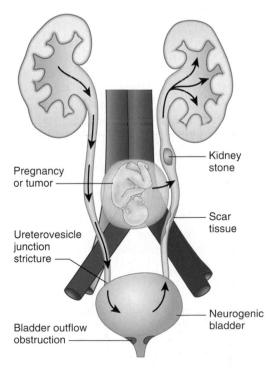

Figure 7-21 Several locations and causes of urinary tract obstruction.

Kidney stone

Scar tissue

Neurogenic bladder

Pregnancy or tumor

Ureterovesicle junction stricture

Bladder outflow obstruction

The Urinary Tract

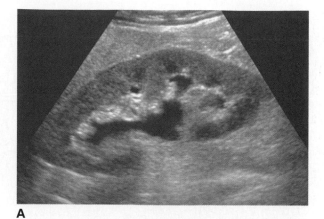

A

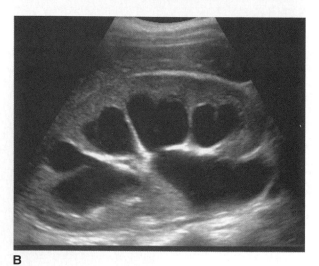

B

Figure 7-22 Hydronephrosis. Two longitudinal images of hydronephrotic kidneys. **A.** Mild hydronephrosis. **B.** Moderate hydronephrosis.

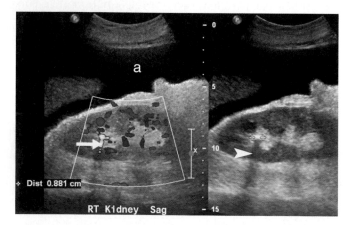

Figure 7-23 Twinkle artifact. The gray-scale image of the right kidney on the right shows a kidney stone (*between cursors*, +) casting an acoustic shadow (*arrowhead*). On the left the same image utilizing color Doppler shows blood flow in the kidney in red and blue colors and the amorphous color signal of the twinkle artifact (*arrow*) emanating from the stone. This patient also has ascites (*a*).

or "twinkle artifact" will be noted as an increased color Doppler signal posterior to a kidney stone. A urolithiasis that becomes lodged within the distal ureter may be better imaged with transvaginal scanning or by using a transperineal approach.

CLINICAL FINDINGS OF UROLITHIASIS
1. Hematuria
2. Renal colic
3. Oliguria
4. Urinary tract infection
5. Males may suffer from testicular pain.

SONOGRAPHIC FINDINGS OF UROLITHIASIS
1. Echogenic focus that produces acoustic shadowing
2. "Twinkle sign" seen posterior to the stone with the use of color Doppler
3. Hydronephrosis and dilation of ureter may be present.

Nephrocalcinosis and Medullary Sponge Kidney
Nephrocalcinosis is an accumulation of calcium within the renal parenchyma. There are two forms of nephrocalcinosis defined by their location: **medullary nephrocalcinosis** and **cortical nephrocalcinosis**. Although medullary nephrocalcinosis is commonly caused by hyperparathyroidism and associated with hypercalcemia, it may also be caused by a congenital defect known as **medullary sponge kidney**. Medullary sponge kidney is the accumulation of calcium within abnormally dilated collecting ducts located within the medulla. Clinically, patients with medullary sponge kidney may be asymptomatic or can have signs of infection and a history of urinary calculi. Medullary sponge kidney appears sonographically as highly echogenic renal pyramids that may shadow (Fig. 7-24). Nephrocalcinosis that occurs within the cortex is termed cortical nephrocalcinosis. It may be caused by hyperparathyroidism, AIDS, or found in association with some malignancies. Sonographically, cortical nephrocalcinosis appears as small calculi within the cortex.

CLINICAL FINDINGS OF NEPHROCALCINOSIS
1. Hypercalcemia
2. Hyperparathyroidism
3. Urinary tract infection
4. History of urinary calculi

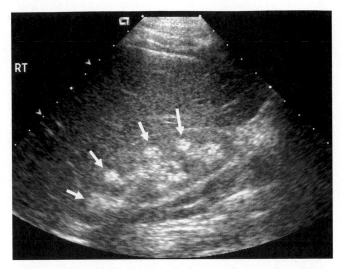

Figure 7-24 Medullary nephrocalcinosis. With nephrocalcinosis, the pyramids (*arrows*) are filled with small stones that may or may not produce acoustic shadowing.

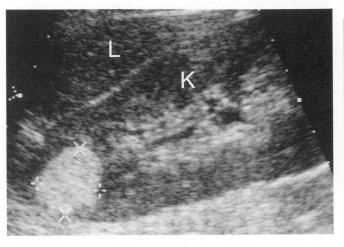

Figure 7-25 Angiomyolipoma. An image through the long axis of the right kidney (*K*) demonstrates a well-defined, uniformly hyperechoic tumor (*between calipers*) in the upper pole. This appearance is strongly suggestive of angiomyolipoma. *L*, liver.

SONOGRAPHIC FINDINGS OF NEPHROCALCINOSIS

1. Medullary nephrocalcinosis—echogenic renal pyramids—medullary sponge kidney
2. Cortical nephrocalcinosis—echogenic foci within the cortex

((•)) SOUND OFF
Medullary nephrocalcinosis is commonly caused by hyperparathyroidism and associated with hypercalcemia; it may also be caused by a congenital defect known as medullary sponge kidney.

Benign Masses of the Kidney

Angiomyolipoma

Angiomyolipoma is the most common benign renal tumor. It consists of a network of blood vessels, muscle, and fat. It may also be referred to as a **renal hamartoma**. These masses are frequently incidentally encountered and are unilateral and asymptomatic in the general population. However, patients with tuberous sclerosis have a tendency to have multiple and bilateral angiomyolipomas (see Fig. 7-14). If symptoms do occur, they will be secondary to hemorrhage within the mass. These symptoms include hematuria, pain, and/or hypertension.

Classically, the sonographic appearance of an angiomyolipoma is a solid, echogenic mass (Fig. 7-25). However, depending on the composition of the mass, the sonographic appearance may vary. Angiomyolipomas, in 20% to 30% of the cases, will shadow secondary to

its high-fat component. Because RCC rarely shadows, the acoustic shadowing seen posterior to a hyperechoic mass is helpful, but not always indicative of an angiomyolipoma.

CLINICAL FINDINGS OF ANGIOMYOLIPOMA

1. Asymptomatic in most individuals
2. Patients may have a history of tuberous sclerosis.
3. Pain, hematuria, and hypertension can occur with hemorrhage of the mass.

SONOGRAPHIC FINDINGS OF ANGIOMYOLIPOMA

1. Solid, hyperechoic mass
2. May produce acoustic shadowing
3. Tends to be multiple and bilateral with tuberous sclerosis

((•)) SOUND OFF
Angiomyolipoma is the most common benign renal tumor. Patients with tuberous sclerosis have a tendency to have multiple and bilateral angiomyolipomas.

Oncocytoma

Oncocytoma is a benign renal tumor that is often found in men in their 60s and is the second most common renal mass after angiomyolipoma. An oncocytoma is often asymptomatic but may produce pain or hematuria. A stellate (star-shaped) central scar may be noted within an oncocytoma. This scar results from a previous infarction within an oncocytoma. Sonographically, the mass is often difficult to differentiate from an RCC. It may appear as an isoechoic, hyperechoic, or hypoechoic mass. It may also contain the sonographically identifiable aforementioned hypoechoic central scar, although this finding is appreciated most often on a CT study. Nonetheless, a central scar within a renal mass does not necessarily indicate that the mass is an oncocytoma because RCC may also have a central scar. For this reason, surgical excision or biopsy is often warranted to differentiate the oncocytoma from RCC.

CLINICAL FINDINGS OF AN ONCOCYTOMA

1. Asymptomatic
2. May produce pain or hematuria

SONOGRAPHIC FINDINGS OF AN ONCOCYTOMA

1. Isoechoic, hyperechoic, or hypoechoic mass
2. May also contain a hypoechoic central scar

 SOUND OFF
Oncocytomas often contain a central scar.

Renal Hemangioma

Like benign hemangiomas found elsewhere in the body, **renal hemangioma** consists of a mass of blood vessels. They are most often asymptomatic and are encountered during the third or fourth decade of life. Again, pain and hematuria may result from hemorrhage within the mass. A hemangioma most often appears as a small hyperechoic mass on the kidney. Like other solid tumors of the kidney, a hemangioma may mimic RCC, and therefore further imaging, surgical intervention, or a biopsy may be performed.

CLINICAL FINDINGS OF A RENAL HEMANGIOMA

1. Asymptomatic
2. Hemorrhage of the mass can lead to pain and hematuria.

SONOGRAPHIC FINDINGS OF A RENAL HEMANGIOMA

1. Small, hyperechoic mass

Renal Lipoma

A lipoma is a benign fatty tumor. The **renal lipoma** is most often found in women, and they are typically asymptomatic. Sonographically, a renal lipoma will appear as well-circumscribed hyperechoic mass that typically measures less than 5 mm in diameter.

CLINICAL FINDINGS OF A RENAL LIPOMA

1. Asymptomatic

SONOGRAPHIC FINDINGS OF A RENAL LIPOMA

1. Well-circumscribed, hyperechoic mass

Renal Adenoma

A **renal adenoma** is a benign mass that appears sonographically similar to its malignant counterpart, RCC. Clinically, patients are most often asymptomatic, although larger tumors may lead to hematuria. Sonographically, a renal adenoma appears as a vascular hyperechoic mass with areas of internal calcifications that may produce acoustic shadowing. They typically measure less than 1 cm. Surgical excision or biopsy is often warranted to differentiate the renal adenoma from the RCC.

CLINICAL FINDINGS OF RENAL ADENOMA

1. Asymptomatic
2. May complain of hematuria

SONOGRAPHIC FINDINGS OF RENAL ADENOMA

1. Hyperechoic, vascular mass with internal calcifications
2. May produce acoustic shadowing

Trauma and Renal Hematoma

Hematomas are localized collections of blood. A **renal hematoma** may be the result of blunt trauma to the kidney region, surgical intervention or biopsy, and lithotripsy. Rarely, spontaneous hematomas can occur and can be the result of preexisting pathologic conditions or may be entirely idiopathic. Patients who have suffered trauma to the kidney(s) may complain of flank pain and/or general abdominal pain. They will also have evidence of decreased hematocrit and may have hematuria.

A renal fracture may be observed sonographically. The fracture appears as the linear absence of echoes, or a linear anechoic or hypoechoic region in the renal parenchyma. Blood may accumulate under the capsule (subcapsular), in the perinephric area (in Gerota fascia), in the pararenal area (anterior or posterior), or intramuscularly (in the psoas muscle) (Fig. 7-26).

Sonographically, the appearance of a hematoma is directly related to its location and the amount of time that has elapsed since the traumatic event. An acute

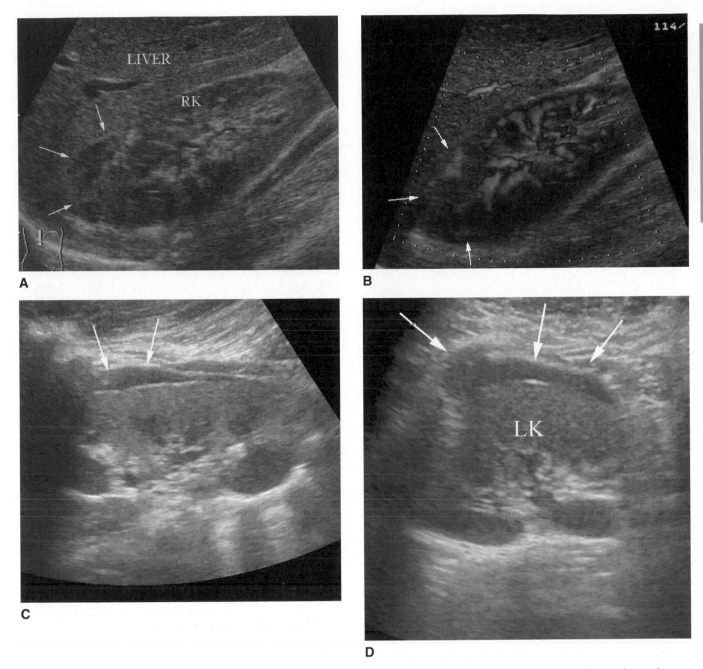

Figure 7-26 Renal trauma. **A.** Hematoma. Longitudinal image reveals irregular hypoechoic region (*arrows*) on the superior pole of this kidney in a patient who experienced blunt trauma. **B.** Power Doppler indicates no flow in the hypoechoic area (*arrows*). Based on the clinical and sonographic information, the diagnosis of hematoma was made. **C.** Longitudinal image of the left kidney demonstrates a hypoechoic collection anterior to the kidney (*arrows*). The collection lies between the echogenic renal capsule and the renal cortex. The hematoma follows the contour of the kidney as well. **D.** Transverse image demonstrates the fluid collection anterior to the kidney. *LK*, left kidney; *RK*, right kidney.

hemorrhage may appear anechoic initially, and then hyperechoic as clot collects in the area. With time, the blood can form into a focal tumor—a hematoma—which may appear complex, with varying degrees of anechoic, hypoechoic, and hyperechoic components. Eventually, the fluid will become anechoic again, as liquefaction takes place. Chronic hematomas may calcify and produce acoustic shadowing.

CLINICAL FINDINGS OF A RENAL HEMATOMA

1. History of some form of trauma to the kidney(s) (blunt trauma, stab wound, biopsy, or lithotripsy)
2. Flank pain
3. Abdominal pain
4. Hematuria
5. Decreased hematocrit

SONOGRAPHIC FINDINGS OF A RENAL HEMATOMA

1. Variable appearance depending on the stage of the blood and location
2. Blood may accumulate under the capsule (subcapsular), in the perinephric area (in Gerota fascia), in the pararenal area (anterior or posterior), or intramuscularly (in the psoas muscle).
3. Chronic hematomas may calcify and produce acoustic shadowing.

Malignant Renal Masses

Renal Cell Carcinoma

RCC may also be referred to as a hypernephroma or adenocarcinoma of the kidney. It is a primary form of renal cancer, meaning this form of cancer begins in the kidney, specifically originating from the renal tubular epithelium. Smoking, hypertension, obesity, and tuberous sclerosis increase the risk for developing RCC. In addition, there seems to be a strong association between RCC and von Hippel–Lindau disease. Patients who have acquired renal cystic disease from long-term dialysis are especially susceptible to develop RCC as well.

Unfortunately, frequently symptoms manifest late in the disease even though the tumor is moderately large. Patients may present with flank pain, a palpable mass, and **gross hematuria**. They may also suffer from unexplained weight loss and anorexia. The tumor can spread beyond the borders of the kidney and even into the renal vein and IVC, which is termed "tumor thrombus" (Fig. 7-27). The sonographic findings of RCC vary (Fig. 7-28). Often, the tumor is either hypoechoic or isoechoic to normal renal tissue, but can be hyperechoic as well. RCC can even have a complex cystic appearance. The ipsilateral renal vein and IVC should be analyzed closely for tumor invasion. Furthermore, the patient should be closely evaluated for evidence of distant metastasis, including scrutiny of the contralateral kidney, liver, and other major organs.

🔊)) SOUND OFF
RCC may be referred to as a hypernephroma. It has a strong link with smoking.

CLINICAL FINDINGS OF RENAL CELL CARCINOMA

1. Anorexia
2. Flank pain
3. Gross hematuria
4. Hypertension
5. Palpable mass
6. Smoker
7. Weight loss

SONOGRAPHIC FINDINGS OF RENAL CELL CARCINOMA

1. Hypoechoic, isoechoic, or hyperechoic solid mass on the kidney
2. Can have a complex cystic appearance as well
3. Check the renal vein and IVC for tumor invasion
4. Check for distant metastasis, including contralateral kidney and liver

Renal Transitional Cell Carcinoma

Transitional cell carcinoma (TCC) of the kidney is a malignant tumor that is most often found in the area of the renal pelvis. TCC may also be found within the ureter and urinary bladder (see section "Transitional Cell Carcinoma of the Bladder" in this chapter). Like RCC, patients who smoke are also at an increased risk for TCC.

TCC can cause focal dilation of the calices, and small lesions can be difficult to identify with sonography. Larger masses most often appear as hypoechoic or isoechoic masses within the renal sinus. Patients may present with gross hematuria and pain secondary to renal obstruction.

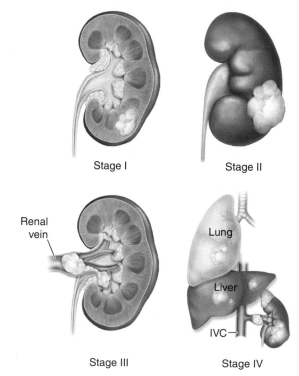

Stage I   Stage II

Renal vein

Lung

Liver

IVC

Stage III   Stage IV

Figure 7-27 Staging of renal cell carcinoma. In Stage I, the tumor is confined to the kidney and is small, whereas in Stage II, the tumor is larger, distorting the normal architecture of the kidney. In Stage III, the tumor often invades the adjacent vasculature, whereas Stage IV typically involves distant metastasis.

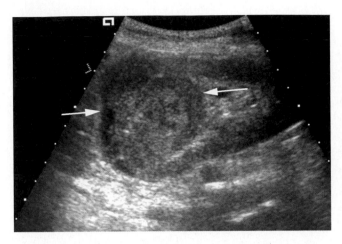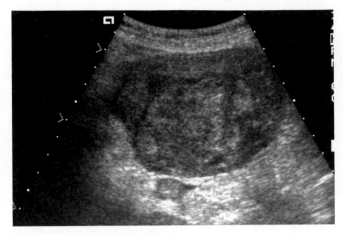

Figure 7-28 Renal cell carcinoma. Longitudinal (**left**) and transverse images (**right**) of the left kidney showing a heterogeneous solid lesion (*arrows*) in the superior pole.

CLINICAL FINDINGS OF RENAL TRANSITIONAL CELL CARCINOMA

1. Gross hematuria
2. Pain secondary to renal obstruction
3. History of smoking

SONOGRAPHIC FINDINGS OF RENAL TRANSITIONAL CELL CARCINOMA

1. Hypoechoic or isoechoic mass within the renal sinus
2. Varying degrees of hydronephrosis may be present.

🔊 SOUND OFF
TCC found in the kidney is most often located within the renal pelvis.

CLINICAL FINDINGS OF OTHER RENAL MALIGNANCIES

1. History of primary cancer (often lung or breast)
2. Hematuria
3. Fever
4. Weight loss

SONOGRAPHIC FINDINGS OF OTHER RENAL MALIGNANCIES

1. Bilateral, hypoechoic masses with lymphoma
2. Lymphoma or leukemia can manifest as an enlarged kidney.
3. Metastases have varying sonographic findings but are most often solid tumors that are hypoechoic or hyperechoic.

Metastases to the Kidney and Other Malignancies

Metastases to the kidneys are most often from the lungs or breast, with prostate, pancreas, and melanoma occurring less frequently. RCC can also metastasize from the contralateral kidney. These tumors appear as solid masses that are often hypoechoic or hyperechoic. Lymphoma and leukemia of the kidney will appear sonographically similar. Both can either result in a multiple, hypoechoic masses or be seen as bilateral, renal enlargement with a decrease in overall renal echogenicity. Lymphoma, which is most likely in the form of non-Hodgkin lymphoma, typically affects both kidneys. Patients who have a history of primary malignancy should be thoroughly evaluated for renal metastasis. Clinical findings may include hematuria, flank pain, fever, and weight loss.

RENAL VASCULAR ABNORMALITIES AND TRANSPLANT ASSESSMENT

Nutcracker Syndrome

Compression or entrapment of the left renal vein as it passes between the superior mesenteric artery and abdominal aorta is termed nutcracker syndrome or renal vein entrapment. Sonographically, the left renal vein will reveal elevated pressure with Doppler evaluation (see Chapter 9). In general, patients with nutcracker syndrome can present with proteinuria, hematuria, left-sided abdominal or flank pain, and pelvic pain. Male patients may complain of left testicular pain as well and may have a left-sided varicocele. Females with **nutcracker syndrome** may suffer from **pelvic congestion syndrome**, which includes lower abdominal and back pain after standing for long periods of time, dyspareunia, dysmenorrhea, abnormal uterine bleeding, chronic fatigue, and bowel issues. Sonographically, dilated veins may be noted within the female pelvis.

CLINICAL FINDINGS IN NUTCRACKER SYNDROME

1. Hematuria
2. Proteinuria
3. Possible left-sided abdominal or flank pain
4. Pelvic pain
5. Left-sided testicular pain
6. Left-sided varicocele
7. Females—pelvic congestion syndrome

SONOGRAPHIC FINDINGS OF NUTCRACKER SYNDROME

1. Compression of the left renal vein between the superior mesenteric artery and abdominal aorta
2. Elevated pressure within the left renal vein

Renal Artery Stenosis

Renal artery stenosis is a decrease in the diameter of the renal arteries. A common cause of renal artery stenosis is atherosclerosis (Fig. 7-29). Patients who have a history of smoking, diabetes, high cholesterol, and high blood pressure are inclined to develop renal artery stenosis. Patients who have existing renal artery stenosis often suffer from hypertension that does not respond to treatment. In younger female patients, fibromuscular disease may be the cause of renal artery stenosis.

The narrowing of the renal artery may be hemodynamically significant. The diagnosis of renal artery stenosis can be made sonographically, but it is often a challenging endeavor secondary to the patient's body habitus, the inability of the patient to suspend respiration, and overlying bowel gas. Renal artery stenosis can lead to renal infarction and irreparable renal compromise. Sonographic findings of renal artery stenosis include thickening and calcification of the renal artery, along with a **renal:aorta ratio** that is greater than 3.5, and possibly a **tardus–parvus** spectral waveform downstream from the stenosis, although this may not always be present (Fig. 7-30).

CLINICAL FINDINGS OF RENAL ARTERY STENOSIS

1. Smoker
2. High blood pressure
3. High cholesterol
4. Diabetes
5. Hypertension that does not respond to treatment

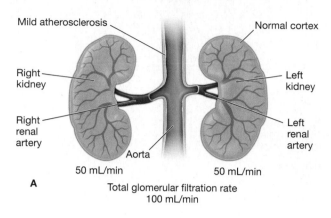

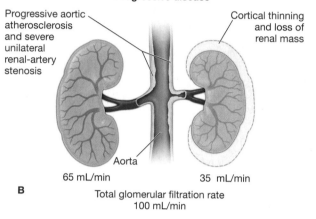

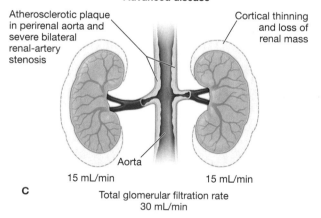

Figure 7-29 Renal artery stenosis. Progressive atherosclerosis, renal artery stenosis, and ischemic nephropathy. In the early phase (**A**), there is mild atherosclerosis of the perirenal abdominal aorta and normal renal function. As the disease progresses (**B**), there is progressive aortic atherosclerosis and severe unilateral renal artery stenosis. The left kidney is smaller than the right kidney, and there may be cortical thinning and decrease in renal blood flow. In advanced disease (**C**), there is bulky atherosclerotic plaque in the perirenal aorta and severe bilateral renal artery stenosis. Both kidneys are small, and there is marked cortical thinning and irregularity.

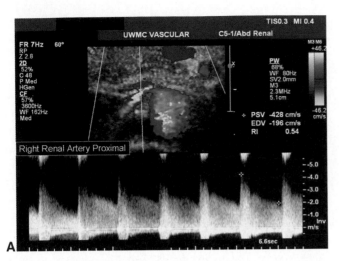
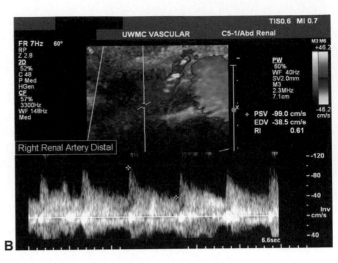

Figure 7-30 Renal artery stenosis. **A.** Abnormal spectral waveform from the proximal right renal artery. The PSV is 428 cm per second, and there is a visible Doppler bruit indicative of a hemodynamically significant stenosis. **B.** Spectral waveform from the distal right renal artery. Poststenotic turbulence is present with a PSV of 99 cm per second. PSV, peak systolic velocity

---

SONOGRAPHIC FINDINGS OF RENAL ARTERY STENOSIS

1. Thickening and calcification of the renal artery may be noted.
2. Renal to aorta ratio that is greater than 3.5
3. Possibly a tardus–parvus spectral waveform downstream from the stenosis

Renal Vein Thrombosis

Blood clot within the renal vein is termed **renal vein thrombosis**. It may be caused by renal tumors, trauma, renal infections, or be seen following a renal transplant. Patients typically present with flank pain and hematuria. The kidney that is completely blocked will increase in size and have a heterogeneous sonographic appearance. The renal vein itself will also enlarge, and Doppler signals will be absent. Sonographic identification of the clot is vital, although this can often be difficult.

CLINICAL FINDINGS OF RENAL VEIN THROMBOSIS

1. Pain
2. Hematuria

SONOGRAPHIC FINDINGS OF RENAL VEIN THROMBOSIS

1. Heterogeneous renal echotexture
2. Enlarged renal vein
3. Absent renal vein Doppler signals
4. Thrombus may not be seen.

Renal Transplant and Postsurgical Complications

Renal biopsy is often the best indicator of renal transplant rejection. However, although sonography is not the typical means for the diagnosis of renal transplant rejection, it is often utilized to provide an overall assessment for complications following transplantation. There are various conditions that lead to renal failure and the need for a renal transplant. The transplanted kidney, also referred to as the allograft, is placed within the right or left lower quadrant. The donor artery and vein is typically anastomosed (connected) to the external iliac artery and external iliac vein of the recipient. The donor ureter is attached to the recipient urinary bladder. The donor kidney should appear sonographically similar to a normal kidney. Mild pelviectasis is considered normal in the transplanted kidney. The native kidneys should be examined as well.

Doppler and spectral imaging is warranted to fully assess the functional state of the transplanted kidney. Spectral analysis of the interlobar arteries should be obtained in the upper, mid-, and lower regions of the kidney. The main renal artery should be analyzed with color and spectral Doppler at the anastomosis, proximal, and distal segments. The normal waveform should yield low resistance with continuous diastolic flow. The RIs should be 0.6 to 0.8, with anything over 0.9 considered abnormal. The renal vein should demonstrate normal continuous flow away from the kidney and may be examined at the anastomosis site with the iliac vein as well.

Postrenal transplant fluid collections are common and could be a **lymphocele**, **urinoma**, hematoma, or abscess. These fluid collections may appear similar with sonography, with most appearing echogenic, complex, or anechoic. Clinical signs of transplant rejection include anuria, oliguria, elevated creatinine and BUN, proteinuria, hypertension, and enlargement of the transplant.

Complications of a renal transplant include rejection, infection, obstruction, vascular stenosis, renal artery stenosis, renal artery thrombosis, renal vein thrombosis, pseudoaneurysm, and fistulas (Fig. 7-31). Renal artery stenosis is the most common vascular complication following renal transplantation. The sonographic indication of renal artery stenosis includes color aliasing and turbulent flow at the level of the anastomosis site. The diagnosis of renal artery stenosis in a renal transplant includes an elevated peak systolic velocity greater than 200 to 250 cm per second, renal artery to external iliac ratio greater than 2.0 to 3.0, and poststenotic turbulence.

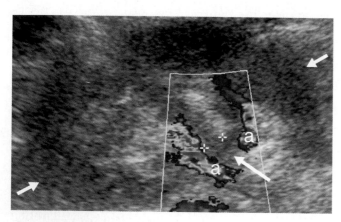

Figure 7-31 Renal vein thrombosis in a transplant kidney. Color Doppler ultrasound of a transplant kidney (*between small arrows*) on the second postoperative day shows blood flow in the renal arteries (*a*) but thrombus (*large arrow*) and no flow in the renal vein (*between cursors,* +). Acute thrombosis of the renal vein in a transplant kidney is a surgical emergency requiring immediate correction to save the kidney.

PEDIATRIC KIDNEY PATHOLOGY

Congenital Hydronephrosis

Congenital hydronephrosis can occur as a result of several conditions, which are mentioned in Table 7-8. The most common cause of congenital hydronephrosis in infants and children is a ureteropelvic junction obstruction. VUR may also be the cause of congenital hydronephrosis. VUR is the backward flow of urine from the urinary bladder into the ureter, and possibly all the way back into the kidney (discussed later in this chapter). It is graded based on its severity (Table 7-9).

Other causes of congenital hydronephrosis include posterior urethral valves and **prune belly syndrome**. Posterior urethral valves are folds of excessive urethral tissue found exclusively in males. Posterior urethral valves cause dilation of the bladder, both ureters, and both renal collecting systems. Prune belly syndrome is typically caused by **megacystis**, a massively dilated urinary bladder. This syndrome is mostly seen in male

TABLE 7-9 Grades of vesicoureteral reflux

Grade of Vesicoureteral Reflux	Description
I	Urine refluxes into the ureter only.
II	Urine refluxes into the ureter and the renal pelvis without hydronephrosis.
III	Urine refluxes into the ureter and the renal pelvis with hydronephrosis.
IV	Moderate hydronephrosis
V	Severe hydronephrosis

TABLE 7-8 Clinical and sonographic findings for causes of congenital hydronephrosis

Cause of Congenital Hydronephrosis	Clinical Findings	Sonographic Findings
Ureteropelvic junction obstruction	Palpable abdominal mass Abdominal distention Hematuria	Dilated renal collecting system Distal ureter not seen
Vesicoureteral reflux	Urinary tract infection Proteinuria	Kidneys may appear normal. Hydronephrosis may be present and may reduce after micturition. Possible scar formation in the kidneys
Posterior urethral valves	Male patient Urinary tract infection Voiding abnormalities	Large urinary bladder Dilated ureters Dilated bilateral renal collecting systems
Prune belly syndrome	Often discovered in utero Urinary tract infection Failure to thrive	Large urinary bladder Varying degrees of hydronephrosis Varying degrees of ureteral dilation

fetuses and is the result of a urethral abnormality, which in turn leads to a bladder outlet obstruction. Prune belly describes the result of the abdominal wall musculature being stretched by the extremely enlarged urinary bladder. Enlargement of the bladder, ureter, and the renal collecting system will occur. The triad of absent abdominal musculature, undescended testis, and urinary tract abnormalities is consistent with the diagnosis of prune belly syndrome.

Pediatric Vesicoureteral Reflux

VUR, which is the retrograde flow of urine from the bladder to the ureter, is a widespread malady in the pediatric population. Urine-containing bacterium that travels from the bladder, up the ureter, and into the kidney can result in a kidney infection with subsequent scarring and permanent damage to the renal parenchyma. VUR is most commonly caused by an abnormal angle of insertion of the distal ureter into the bladder at the ureterovesicle junction, resulting in a faulty valve. Patients with duplicated pelvicaliceal systems and complete ureteral duplication may suffer from VUR. With these individuals, the upper pole moiety in the duplex kidney is often prone to obstruction because of an irregular insertion of the ureter into the urinary bladder. This leads to the development of an obstructing ureterocele. The lower pole moiety in these individuals is prone to reflux. This assumption about the obstruction and refluxing components of the duplicated system is referred to as the Weigert–Meyer rule (Fig. 7-32).

> **◀)) SOUND OFF**
> The upper pole moiety in the duplex kidney is often prone to obstruction because of an irregular insertion of the ureter into the urinary bladder. This leads to the development of an obstructing ureterocele. The lower pole moiety in these individuals is prone to reflux.

Clinically, patients with VUR present with signs and symptoms of a urinary tract infection, such as an unexplained fever, irritability, flank pain, leukocytosis, bacteriuria, hematuria, urgency to void, and dysuria. Sonography is not highly sensitive for detecting VUR, though it is often utilized in conjunction with other tests if VUR is suspected. For example, patients with minimal reflux often have normal sonographic findings because reflux can be transient. However, long-standing and severe reflux can cause obvious enlargement of the ureter and dilation of the renal collecting system. A **voiding cystourethrogram** or a **nuclear cystogram** can be performed to provide a more definitive diagnosis of this condition. In patients with VUR and a duplicated system, the upper pole tends to demonstrate hydronephrosis secondary to the obstructing ureterocele, whereas the lower pole can also demonstrate hydronephrosis secondary to reflux. Bladder debris may be seen as well.

Treatment is focused on preventing renal scarring, which increases the risk of complications from permanent renal damage and even end-stage renal disease later in life. Mild VUR is typically treated with antibiotics, whereas severe forms may require surgical intervention or the use of a synthetic bulking agent that is injected endoscopically. The administration of this bulking agent may be referred to as a **subureteric Teflon injection** (STING). These STING agents elevate the ureteral orifice and distal ureter, allowing for the normal flow of urine from the ureter into the bladder. Although often effective, the STING procedure may not be as successful as other surgical means of treatment. Sonographically, the bulking agent appears as a hyperechoic structure in the area of the vesicoureteral junction that may produce acoustic shadowing.

> **CLINICAL FINDINGS OF VESICOURETERAL REFLUX**
>
> 1. May be asymptomatic
> 2. Unexplained fever
> 3. Irritability
> 4. Flank pain
> 5. Leukocytosis
> 6. Bacteriuria
> 7. Hematuria
> 8. Dysuria
> 9. Urgency to void

> **SONOGRAPHIC FINDINGS OF VESICOURETERAL REFLUX**
>
> 1. Patients with minimal reflux may have normal-appearing kidneys.
> 2. Hydronephrosis and/or hydroureter may be present.
> 3. Ureterocele may be seen in the bladder.
> 4. Bladder debris may be seen.

Pediatric Wilms Tumor

A **Wilms tumor** may also be referred to as a **nephroblastoma**. Wilms tumor is the most common solid malignant pediatric abdominal mass. It is typically discovered before the age of 5, with a mean age of 3. These tumors can grow reasonably large before discovery and can invade the renal vein and IVC. Nephroblastomas tend to metastasize to the liver and lungs. Clinically, these patients present with a palpable abdominal mass, abdominal pain, hematuria, fever, and hypertension. In addition, pediatric patients with Beckwith–Wiedemann syndrome have a tendency to

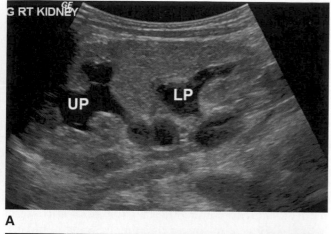

A

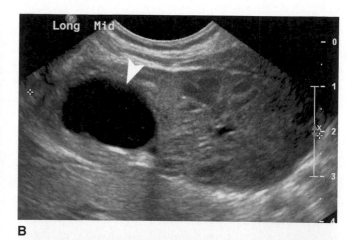

B

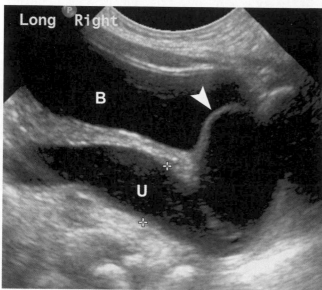

C

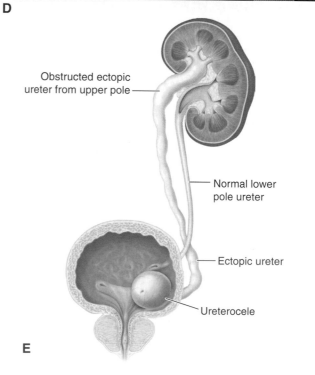

D

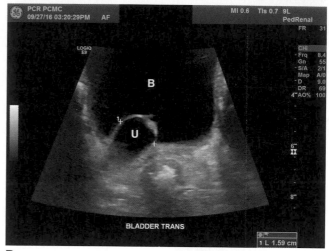

Obstructed ectopic ureter from upper pole

Normal lower pole ureter

Ectopic ureter

Ureterocele

E

Figure 7-32 Duplicating collecting systems. **A.** Longitudinal sonogram of the right kidney (*RK*) demonstrates a duplicated collecting system with a dilated upper (*UP*) and lower (*LP*) pole. **B.** Sonogram of another RK shows a duplex kidney with a dilated upper pole collecting system (*arrowhead*) and normal lower pole parenchyma. **C.** Longitudinal scan through the bladder (*B*) shows a dilated right ureter (*U*) emptying into an ectopic ureterocele (*arrowhead*). **D.** Transverse image of a pediatric bladder demonstrates a ureterocele that presents as a cyst with an echogenic wall (*U*) entering the base of the bladder (*B*). **E.** Weigert–Meyer rule describes the situation when an ectopic ureter from the upper pole moiety ends in a ureterocele in the bladder causing obstruction, whereas the lower pole moiety is prone to reflux.

develop Wilms tumors. Sonographically, a Wilms tumor appears as a large, solid, mostly echogenic mass that may contain anechoic or hypoechoic region (Fig. 7-33). Tumor invasion of the renal vein and IVC should be evaluated. In addition, a thorough evaluation of the abdominal organs for metastasis is necessary.

CLINICAL FINDINGS OF WILMS TUMOR

1. Palpable abdominal mass
2. Abdominal pain
3. Hematuria
4. Fever
5. Hypertension

SONOGRAPHIC FINDINGS OF WILMS TUMOR

1. Large, solid, mostly echogenic masses that may contain anechoic or hypoechoic areas
2. May also be isoechoic

SOUND OFF
Wilms tumor (nephroblastoma) is the most common solid malignant pediatric abdominal mass. It may be found in children with Beckwith–Wiedemann syndrome.

Urachal Anomalies

The **urachus** is a remnant of embryonic development. It is a tubular structure that extends from the umbilicus to the apex of the bladder (Fig. 7-34). During fetal life, the urachus normally closes. Failure of the urachus to close can result in a urachal anomaly. These include patent urachus (urachal fistula), urachal cyst, urachal sinus, or urachal diverticulum. A patent urachus will appear as an anechoic tube that extends from the umbilicus to the apex of the urinary bladder. Urachal cysts or a urachal sinus may also be encountered if closure is not complete. Urachal cyst and urachal diverticulum will appear as a cystic structure between the bladder and the umbilicus. A urachal sinus will appear as a linear, fluid-filled structure that is continuous with the umbilicus. Patients may be asymptomatic or can have signs of infection or a palpable anterior abdominal mass between the umbilicus and the urinary bladder.

CLINICAL FINDINGS OF URACHAL ANOMALIES

1. Possible signs of urinary tract infection
2. Palpable abdominal mass between the umbilicus and the urinary bladder

SONOGRAPHIC FINDINGS OF URACHAL ANOMALIES

1. Patent urachus will appear as an anechoic tube that extends from the umbilicus to the apex of the urinary bladder.
2. Urachal cyst and urachal diverticulum will appear as a cystic structure between the bladder and the umbilicus.
3. Urachal sinus will appear as a linear, fluid-filled structure that is continuous with the umbilicus.

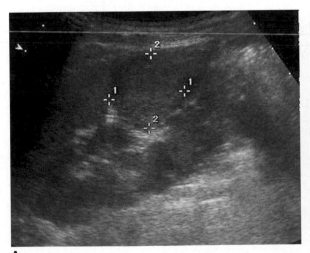 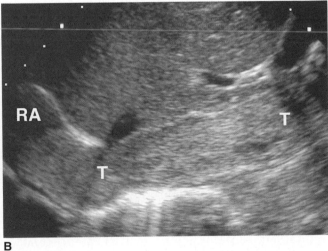

Figure 7-33 Wilms tumor. **A.** Longitudinal image of the kidney revealing an isoechoic mass (*between calipers*). It was proven to be a nephroblastoma (Wilms tumor). **B.** Longitudinal sonogram shows tumor thrombus (*T*) from a Wilms tumor in the inferior vena cava. The thrombus extends into the right atrium (*RA*).

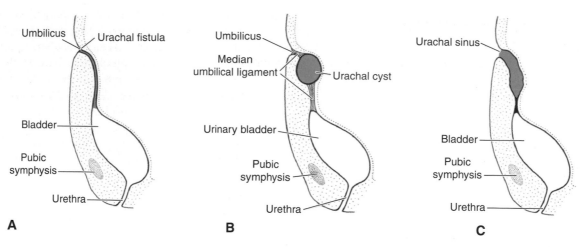

A   B   C

Figure 7-34 Urachal fistula (patent urachus). The withered allantois does not always resorb itself into a fibrous cord (the urachus, or median umbilical ligament) between the bladder and umbilicus. If the urachus remains patent, fluid can weep out of the umbilicus through a fistula (**A**) or can be trapped as a cyst (**B**). The urachus also may form a sinus connection to the outside, but not to the bladder (**C**).

ANATOMY AND PHYSIOLOGY OF THE URETERS

The ureters are bilateral muscular tubes that extend from the renal pelvis to the urinary bladder. The most proximal portion of the ureter is the point at which the ureter is attached to the renal pelvis. This is referred to as the ureteropelvic junction. The point at which the ureter meets the urinary bladder is referred to as the ureterovesicle junction. The ureters enter the bladder posteriorly at the superolateral margin of the trigone of the bladder. The purpose of the ureters is to propel urine from the kidneys to the urinary bladder. The ureters achieve this by means of peristalsis and gravity.

SONOGRAPHY OF THE URETERS

Normal ureters are not routinely imaged with sonography secondary to their small size. However, when enlarged and distended with urine, the ureters will appear as anechoic, tubular structures. Whenever identified with sonography, the ureters should be thoroughly evaluated for obstructive processes.

Ureteral jets can be demonstrated as well (Fig. 7-35). These jets result from urine being forced into the urinary bladder from the ureters. Color Doppler is employed over the inferoposterior aspect of the urinary bladder in the area of the ureteral orifices and trigone. Imaging of ureteral jets is performed to demonstrate ureteral patency in suspected cases of urinary obstruction. Urinary jets typically occur at least once every minute, though this is variable depending upon the hydration of the patient.

URETERAL PATHOLOGY

Ureteral Stones

The most common place for a urinary stone to become lodged is within the ureterovesicle junction, near the urinary bladder. A patient with a stone passing through the ureter may present with renal colic; pain in the groin, labia, or testicle on the side of stone; and possibly hematuria. A ureteral stone will appear as an echogenic focus within the ureter that produces an acoustic shadow. The twinkle sign can be used to prove the presence of a ureteral stone. Typically, the ureter is dilated proximal to the level of the stone.

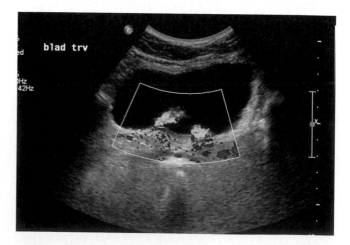

Figure 7-35 Bilateral ureteral jets. Transverse sonogram of the urinary bladder demonstrates ureteral jets. The size and frequency of the ureteral jets are variable depending on the hydration of the patient at the time of examination.

CLINICAL FINDINGS OF A URETERAL STONE

1. Renal colic
2. Pain in the groin, labia, or testicle on the side of the stone
3. Possible hematuria

SONOGRAPHIC FINDINGS OF A URETERAL STONE

1. Echogenic focus within the ureter that produces acoustic shadowing
2. Dilation of the ureter proximal to the stone

Ureterocele

A ureterocele is the cystic dilation of the ureter as it enters the bladder. Although ureteroceles are often asymptomatic, urinary stasis may result in the dilated area, and therefore infection and stone formation can occur. Ureteroceles are often associated with duplicated collecting systems, specifically the ureter that originates from the upper moiety. They may also be ectopic in location, causing obstruction of the contralateral ureter. Sonographically, a ureterocele appears as an anechoic, balloon-like structure within the lumen of the urinary bladder near the ureterovesicle junction (Fig. 7-36).

CLINICAL FINDINGS OF A URETEROCELE

1. Asymptomatic
2. Signs of a urinary tract infection

SONOGRAPHIC FINDINGS OF A URETEROCELE

1. Anechoic, balloon-like structure within the lumen of the urinary bladder near the ureterovesicle junction
2. Can be ectopic in location

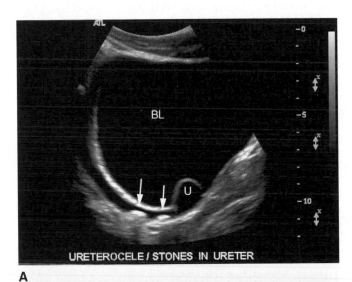

A

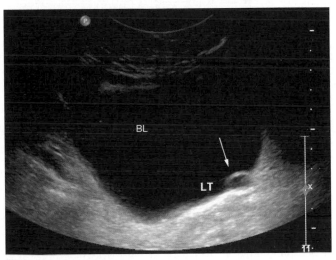

B

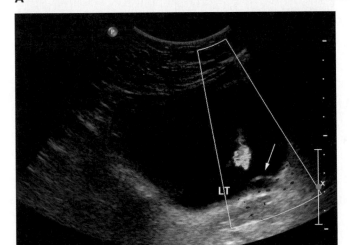

C

Figure 7-36 Ureterocele. **A.** Longitudinal image of the pelvis demonstrates a dilated ureter containing two echogenic calculi (*arrows*) and a thin-walled ureterocele (*U*) in the bladder lumen (*BL*). **B** and **C.** Transverse image of the urinary bladder shows a small thin-walled mass (*arrows*) projecting into the lumen of the bladder; color Doppler demonstrates the presence of a ureteral jet confirming the diagnosis of a small left ureterocele.

Megaureter and Hydroureter

A large ureter may be termed **megaureter** or **hydroureter** based on the cause of the enlargement. The ureter may be congenitally enlarged—megaureter—or associated with reflux or obstruction—hydroureter. Patients may be asymptomatic or have signs of a urinary tract infection. Sonographically, a dilated ureter will appear as an anechoic tube.

CLINICAL FINDINGS OF MEGAURETER AND HYDROURETER

1. Asymptomatic
2. Urinary tract infection

SONOGRAPHIC FINDINGS OF MEGAURETER AND HYDROURETER

1. Large, anechoic tubular structure that extends from the kidney to the urinary bladder; only a section may be enlarged, however.

ANATOMY AND PHYSIOLOGY OF THE URINARY BLADDER

The urinary bladder is a retroperitoneal organ that functions as a reservoir for urine. It is located in the pelvis, posterior to the symphysis pubis. In males, the urinary bladder is also positioned superior to the prostate gland and anterior to the seminal vesicles. In females, the urinary bladder is located anterior to the vagina, uterus, and rectum.

The bladder wall consists of four layers. From inner to outer, the layers of the bladder wall are the mucosa, submucosa, muscularis, and serosa. The **detrusor muscle** is located within the muscularis portion of the wall. This muscle controls the appropriate emptying of the urinary bladder. The trigone of the bladder is located inferiorly, at the base of the urinary bladder. Its location marks the single urethral opening and bilateral ureteral openings.

SONOGRAPHY OF THE URINARY BLADDER

Sonographically, the normal distended bladder appears as a smooth-walled, anechoic structure within the pelvis. In the transverse plane, it appears as a square-shaped organ; whereas in sagittal, the urinary bladder appears more elliptical. Much like a balloon, the normal empty urinary bladder will have a more evident or thicker appearing wall, whereas the bladder that is fully distended will have a thin wall. When the bladder wall is thickened, its diameter will exceed 4 mm in a distended state. The wall should be analyzed closely for irregularities. The volume of the bladder can be evaluated sonographically. A bladder volume can be obtained using the following formula: $L \times W \times H \times 0.56$. In As previously mentioned, patency of the ureters can be proven sonographically by demonstrating ureteral jets with color Doppler in the area of the trigone.

URINARY BLADDER PATHOLOGY

Neurogenic Bladder

A neurogenic bladder is one that is poorly functioning secondary to any type of neurologic disorder. Thus, a neurogenic bladder may be caused by brain or spinal trauma, congenital spinal abnormalities (e.g., spina bifida), diabetes, and several other conditions. In effect, what is really not working properly is the detrusor muscle surrounding the bladder. Clinical symptoms of a neurogenic bladder vary, as do sonographic findings. Patients may suffer from an unnecessary urgency to void or may rarely feel the need to urinate. Sonographic findings may include a normal bladder wall or a thickened bladder wall with identifiable **trabeculae**—termed trabeculated bladder (Fig. 7-37). A trabeculated bladder can also result from chronic bladder infections; therefore, a thorough clinical history is warranted. The patient may have an extremely distended urinary bladder, although they may lack the urgency to void. Postvoid images may demonstrate excessive urinary retention, thus bladder volume pre- and postvoid can be useful.

CLINICAL FINDINGS OF A NEUROGENIC BLADDER

1. Past history of brain or spinal trauma, congenital spinal abnormalities, or diabetes
2. Unnecessary urgency to void
3. Rarely feel the need to urinate

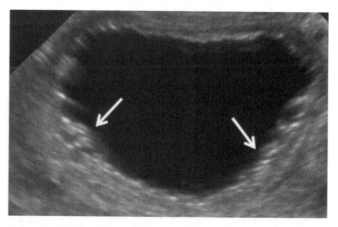

Figure 7-37 Trabeculated bladder. Longitudinal sonogram through the lower pelvis demonstrates a thickened and trabeculated bladder wall (*arrows*) resulting from posterior urethral valves in a neonate.

SONOGRAPHIC FINDINGS OF A NEUROGENIC BLADDER

1. Urinary bladder wall thickening
2. Trabeculae of the bladder wall
3. Postvoid images will show excessive urinary retention.
4. The patient may have a distended bladder but does not feel the need to urinate.
5. Bladder stones may be present.

SONOGRAPHIC FINDINGS OF A BLADDER DIVERTICULUM

1. Anechoic outpouching of the bladder wall
2. A visible neck connecting the diverticulum to the bladder

🔊 **SOUND OFF**
When a bladder diverticulum is suspected, the sonographer should try to visualize and demonstrate the neck of the diverticulum.

Bladder Diverticulum

A **bladder diverticulum** is an outpouching in the bladder wall. A diverticulum of the bladder may be associated with a urethral obstruction, or it may be congenital. Complications of a bladder diverticulum include bladder infection, ureteral obstruction, tumor development, and the spread of infection to the upper urinary tract. Patients can be asymptomatic. However, those who present with a urinary tract infection do so as a result of urinary stasis within the diverticulum. Sonographically, a bladder diverticulum will be noted as an outpouching of the bladder wall (Fig. 7-38). The sonographer should try to visualize and demonstrate the neck of the diverticulum. A color Doppler jet may be noted at the level of the neck of the diverticulum.

Cystitis

Inflammation of the urinary bladder is referred to as **cystitis**. Most likely, cystitis will appear sonographically as bladder wall thickening. When the bladder wall is thickened, its diameter will exceed 4 mm in a distended state. Cystitis is more common in women secondary to the short length of the urethra. The infection continues as an ascending infection, moving from the urethra into the bladder. Cystitis can present clinically with dysuria, urinary frequency, lower abdominal pain, **nocturia**, and even hematuria. Sonographically, the bladder wall may appear focally or diffusely thickened with decreased echogenity and measure greater than 4 mm in thickness. Chronic cystitis can lead to scarring and trabeculation of the bladder wall. Within the lumen, echogenic, layering material may be noted. Decubitus positioning can be helpful to differentiate bladder debris from focal wall thickening and bladder tumors.

CLINICAL FINDINGS OF A BLADDER DIVERTICULUM

1. Can be asymptomatic
2. Urinary tract infection

CLINICAL FINDINGS OF CYSTITIS

1. Dysuria
2. Urinary frequency
3. Lower abdominal pain
4. Nocturia
5. Hematuria

SONOGRAPHIC FINDINGS OF CYSTITIS

1. Hypoechoic bladder wall that may appear focally or diffusely thickened, measuring greater than 4 mm in thickness
2. Bladder may contain echogenic, layering material within its lumen.

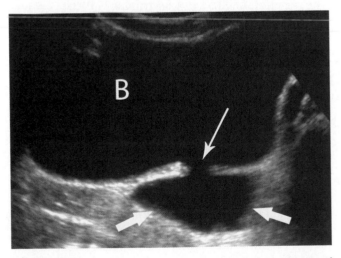

Figure 7-38 Bladder diverticulum. Transverse image of the bladder (*B*) shows a urine-filled diverticulum (*arrows*) with a narrow neck (*long arrow*) connecting it to the bladder.

🔊 **SOUND OFF**
The urinary bladder wall does not typically exceed 4 mm in a distended state.

Bladder Stones and Other Intraluminal Objects

Urolithiasis may be created or become trapped within the urinary bladder. They appear as echogenic, mobile structures that produce posterior acoustic shadowing. Blood clots may also be noted within the urinary bladder. A blood clot within the bladder will appear as an echogenic, nonshadowing mass that may be mobile or adhered to the bladder wall. Decubitus positioning can be helpful to differentiate mobile intraluminal bladder objects from focal wall thickening and bladder tumors.

SONOGRAPHIC APPEARANCE OF BLADDER STONES

1. Echogenic, mobile, shadowing foci within the lumen of the urinary bladder

SONOGRAPHIC APPEARANCE OF BLOOD CLOTS IN THE BLADDER

1. Echogenic, nonshadowing mass that may be mobile or adhered to the wall of the bladder

🔊 SOUND OFF
When an intraluminal bladder object or bladder wall mass is suspected, the sonographer should ask the patient to move into a decubitus position to determine the mobility of the object or mass.

Transitional Cell Carcinoma of the Bladder

The most common malignant tumor of the bladder is TCC. Patients typically present with gross hematuria and may pass some blood clots. The sonographic appearance of TCC within the urinary bladder is a smooth or papillary hypoechoic or hyperechoic mass that projects into the lumen of the bladder (Fig. 7-39). These masses must be differentiated from other intraluminal bladder abnormalities such as blood clots because blood clots may accompany a TCC. This can often be achieved by utilizing color Doppler. Color Doppler will often reveal vascularity within a solid tumor, whereas a blood clot will not yield any Doppler signals. In addition, a blood clot may be mobile, whereas a tumor will maintain its location as the patient changes position.

CLINICAL FINDINGS OF TRANSITIONAL CELL CARCINOMA OF THE BLADDER

1. Gross hematuria
2. May urinate blood clots

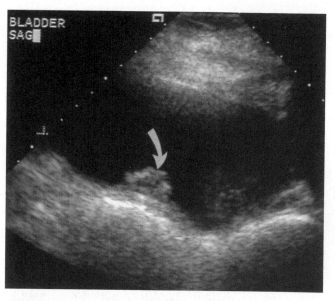

Figure 7-39 Transitional cell carcinoma. A solid mass (curved arrow) is noted within the urinary bladder.

SONOGRAPHIC FINDINGS OF TRANSITIONAL CELL CARCINOMA OF THE BLADDER

1. Smooth or papillary hypoechoic or hyperechoic mass that projects into the lumen of the bladder
2. A solid tumor will not be mobile and will often demonstrate vascularity.

🔊 SOUND OFF
The most common malignancy of the urinary bladder is TCC.

THE URETHRA

The urethra begins at the **trigone of the urinary bladder** and ends at the urethral orifice. Its purpose is to transport urine from the urinary bladder out of the body. The male urethra is longer than the female urethra. The urethra may be noted during sonographic examination of the female and male genital tracts. A portion of the male urethra is surrounded by the prostate gland. Therefore, enlargement of the gland, often occurring with benign prostatic hypertrophy, can lead to compression of the urethra, causing urinary obstruction. The female urethra can be better visualized with endovaginal, transperineal, or translabial sonographic imaging compared with the traditional transabdominal approach. Among the abnormalities that could possibly be noted sonographically within the female urethra include a urethral diverticulum or possibly a **Skene duct cyst**, also referred to as a Skene gland cyst. Though not typically noted with sonography, a **urethral caruncle** may be noted during a physical examination. Malignancies of the urethra may be noted with sonography as well.

REVIEW QUESTIONS

1. The sonographic finding in Figure 7-40 is most consistent with what diagnosis?
   a. ARF
   b. CRF
   c. MCDK
   d. ADPKD

2. What is the most common cause of the disorder noted in Figure 7-40?
   a. Diabetes mellitus
   b. Acute tubular necrosis
   c. Smoking
   d. Chronic pyonephrosis

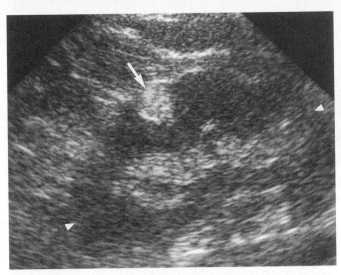

Figure 7-41

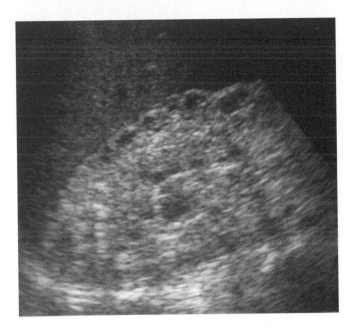

Figure 7-40

3. Which of the following is a cyst located within the female urethra?
   a. Nabothian cyst
   b. Gartner duct cyst
   c. Skene gland cyst
   d. Bulbourethral gland cyst

4. What is the arrow in Figure 7-41 most likely identifying in this asymptomatic patient?
   a. Hypernephroma
   b. Nephroblastoma
   c. Renal hemangioma
   d. Angiomyolipoma

5. The 41-year-old patient in Figure 7-42 had a clinical history that included decreased renal function, urinary tract infections, and a palpable abdominal mass. What is the most likely diagnosis?
   a. Acquired renal cystic disease
   b. ARPKD
   c. MCDK
   d. ADPKD

6. Which of the following would be most likely associated with the findings in Figure 7-42?
   a. Urinary tract infection
   b. Testicular torsion
   c. Hemihypertrophy
   d. Urachal anomaly

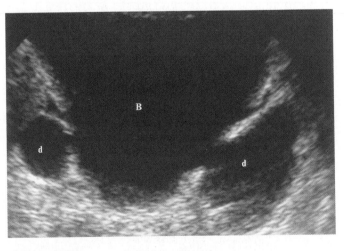

Figure 7-42

7. The 64-year-old patient in Figure 7-43 was suffering from anorexia, gross hematuria, flank pain, and had a history of smoking. Which of the following would be the most likely diagnosis for the mass (M) noted in this image?
   a. Hypernephroma
   b. Angiomyolipoma
   c. TCC
   d. Renal hematoma

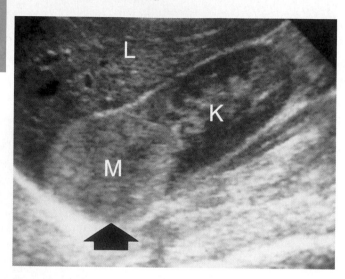

Figure 7-43

8. Which laboratory finding would be the most helpful for predicting evidence of a renal infarction?
   a. GFR
   b. Hematocrit
   c. Total white blood cell count
   d. LDH

9. Which of the following is described as a disorder caused by damage to the glomeruli, resulting in proteinuria and swelling of the ankles, face, and feet because of excess water retention?
   a. Diabetes mellitus
   b. Prune belly syndrome
   c. Nephrotic syndrome
   d. von Hippel–Lindau syndrome

10. What is a hallmark sonographic feature of a patient suffering from xanthogranulomatous pyelonephritis?
    a. Perinephric abscess
    b. Pheochromocytoma
    c. Renal infarction
    d. Staghorn calculous

11. What are the sonographic findings in Figure 7-44 consistent with?
    a. Multiple renal hemangiomas
    b. Medullary nephrocalcinosis
    c. Renal lipomatosis
    d. Schistosomiasis

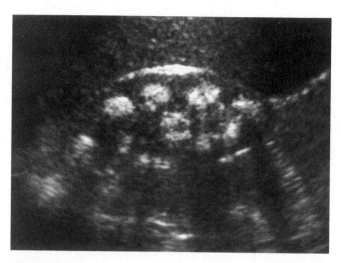

Figure 7-44

12. Which of the following would be least likely associated with Figure 7-44?
    a. Pyonephritis
    b. Hypercalcemia
    c. Urinary tract infection
    d. Hyperparathyroidism

13. What is the most common vascular complication following renal transplantation?
    a. Renal vein thrombosis
    b. Renal vein aneurysm
    c. Renal artery thrombosis
    d. Renal artery stenosis

14. What is the most common cause of prune belly syndrome?
    a. Urinoma
    b. Megacystis
    c. Nutcracker syndrome
    d. Azotemia

15. Which of the following is another name for Wilms tumor?
    a. Neuroblastoma
    b. Pheochromocytoma
    c. Renal hamartoma
    d. Nephroblastoma

16. Which of the following pediatric patients would be at an increased risk for developing a Wilms tumor?
    a. 4-year-old with Beckwith–Wiedemann syndrome
    b. 10-year-old with three renal infections
    c. 6-year-old with a duplicated collecting system
    d. 18-year-old with Marfan syndrome

17. Renal vein entrapment occurs:
    a. between the abdominal aorta and IVC.
    b. between the superior mesenteric vein and abdominal aorta.
    c. between the abdominal aorta and superior mesenteric artery.
    d. between the abdominal aorta and celiac artery.

18. Nutcracker syndrome affects the:
    a. left renal vein.
    b. left renal artery.
    c. right renal vein.
    d. right renal artery.

19. Figure 7-45 is an image of a 61-year-old male with gross hematuria. Which of the following would be the most likely diagnosis for the mass (M) noted in this transverse image?
    a. Renal adenoma
    b. TCC
    c. Renal hamartoma
    d. Renal hyponephroma

20. What enzyme is produced by the kidneys to assist in blood pressure regulation?
    a. BUN
    b. Creatinine
    c. Renin
    d. Trypsin

21. Which of the following is a childhood, autoimmune disease that results in the development of purple spots on the skin and possible renal failure?
    a. Henoch–Schönlein purpura
    b. Azotemia
    c. von Hippel–Lindau syndrome
    d. Xanthogranulomatous pyelonephritis

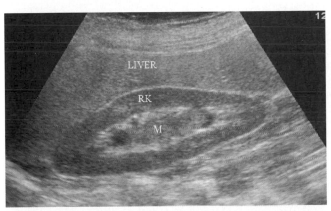

A

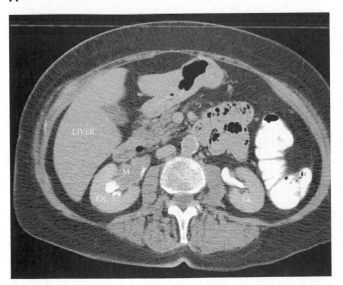

C

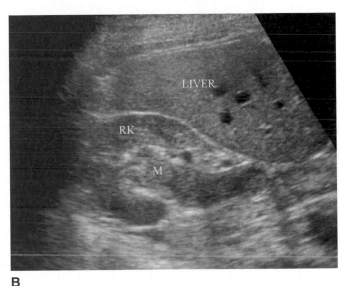

B

Figure 7-45

22. What is the functional unit of the kidney?
    a. Nephron
    b. Medulla
    c. Cortex
    d. Bowman capsule

23. Which of the following would be most indicative of renal artery stenosis?
    a. Decreased cortical echogenicity
    b. A renal to aorta ratio that is greater than 3.5
    c. Enlarged kidney
    d. Tardus–parvus waveform upstream to the stenosis

24. The kidneys are:
    a. intraperitoneal organs.
    b. retroperitoneal organs.
    c. both intraperitoneal and retroperitoneal organs.
    d. neither intraperitoneal nor retroperitoneal organs.

25. The protective capsule of the kidney is referred to as:
    a. Glisson capsule.
    b. perirenal capsule.
    c. renal capsule.
    d. renal cortex.

26. The vessel located anterior to the abdominal aorta and posterior to the superior mesenteric artery is the:
    a. celiac artery.
    b. left renal artery.
    c. right renal vein.
    d. left renal vein.

27. Which of the following would not be a typical clinical feature of renal transplant failure?
    a. Oliguria
    b. Proteinuria
    c. Hypotension
    d. Elevated creatinine

28. Enlargement of the unaffected contralateral kidney with unilateral renal agenesis or compromised renal function is referred to as:
    a. dromedary hypertrophy.
    b. renal hypoplasia.
    c. supernumerary kidney.
    d. compensatory hypertrophy.

29. A bulge on the lateral border of the kidney is referred to as:
    a. duplicated kidney.
    b. renal hypoplasia.
    c. dromedary hump.
    d. supernumerary kidney.

30. The most common congenital anomaly of the urinary tract is:
    a. horseshoe kidney.
    b. duplicated collecting system.
    c. renal agenesis.
    d. renal hypoplasia.

31. A renal scar most likely appears as:
    a. a hypoechoic mass in the renal parenchyma.
    b. a linear anechoic space in the renal cortex.
    c. a hyperechoic, rounded structure within the renal pyramid that shadows.
    d. an echogenic area that extends from the renal sinus through the renal parenchyma.

32. What is the most common location of an ectopic kidney?
    a. Thoracic cavity
    b. Pelvis
    c. Contralateral fossa
    d. Left upper quadrant

33. All of the following are clinical findings of ARF except:
    a. hematuria.
    b. hypertension.
    c. oliguria.
    d. decreased BUN and creatinine.

34. Which of the following is true regarding a duplex collecting system with complete ureteral duplication?
    a. The upper pole of the kidney suffers from reflux.
    b. The lower pole suffers from obstruction because of a varicocele.
    c. The upper pole suffers from obstruction because of a ureterocele.
    d. The lower pole suffers from deflux and hypertrophy.

35. Which of the following is the most common cause of CRF?
    a. Hypertension
    b. Diabetes mellitus
    c. ARPKD
    d. Acute tubular necrosis

36. What renal cystic disease would be most likely caused by and thus associated with hemodialysis?
    a. MCDK
    b. ADPKD
    c. Acquired renal cystic disease
    d. ARPKD

37. Sonographically, compared to normal kidneys, those affected by CRF will appear:
    a. normal in size with a decreased echogenicity.
    b. smaller in size and hypoechoic.
    c. larger in size and more echogenic.
    d. smaller in size and more echogenic.

38. Renal cysts that project out away from the kidney are termed:
    a. exophytic.
    b. perapelvic.
    c. cortical.
    d. peripelvic.

39. A female patient presents with a history of leukocytosis, dysuria, lower abdominal pain, and hematuria. Sonographically, the kidneys appear normal, although the bladder wall measures 6 mm in the distended state. What is the most likely diagnosis?
    a. Glomerulonephritis
    b. Xanthogranulomatous pyelonephritis
    c. Cystitis
    d. TCC of the bladder

40. The inherited disorder associated with the development of tumors of the central nervous system and orbits, renal cysts, and adrenal tumors is:
    a. tuberous sclerosis.
    b. tuberculosis.
    c. von Hippel–Lindau syndrome.
    d. MCDK.

41. What is the most likely location of TCC in the kidney?
    a. Cortex
    b. Medulla
    c. Minor calyx
    d. Renal pelvis

42. Which of the following is the most common cause of ARF?
    a. Hypertension
    b. Diabetes mellitus
    c. ARPKD
    d. Acute tubular necrosis

43. All of the following are characteristics of a complex cyst except:
    a. internal echoes.
    b. smooth walls.
    c. mural nodules.
    d. septations.

44. Which of the following renal findings would most likely present with a clinical finding of hematuria?
    a. Hemorrhagic renal cyst
    b. Milk of calcium renal cyst
    c. Simple renal cyst
    d. Angiomyolipoma

45. Which of the following would be considered the most common solid renal mass?
    a. Renal hematoma
    b. Angiomyolipoma
    c. Oncocytoma
    d. Hypernephroma

46. Infantile polycystic kidney disease may also be referred to as:
    a. ARPKD.
    b. ADPKD.
    c. MCDK.
    d. acquired renal cystic disease.

47. Which of the following best describes the sonographic appearance of a kidney affected by ARPKD?
    a. Bilateral enlarged, echogenic kidneys
    b. Unilateral, smooth-walled, noncommunicating cysts of varying sizes located within the renal fossa
    c. Small, echogenic kidneys
    d. Numerous, large, complex renal cysts

48. The systemic disorder associated with epilepsy that leads to the development of solid tumors in various organs, including angiomyolipomas of the kidneys, is:
    a. tuberous sclerosis.
    b. tuberculosis.
    c. von Hippel–Lindau syndrome.
    d. MCDK.

49. What is the most common clinical finding of a simple renal cyst?
    a. Hematuria
    b. Quadrant pain
    c. Elevated BUN
    d. Asymptomatic

50. Suspicion of cortical thinning should occur when the renal cortex measures:
    a. greater than 2 mm.
    b. less than 1 cm.
    c. greater than 5 mm.
    d. less than 3 cm.

51. Which of the following is not considered an extrinsic cause of hydronephrosis?
    a. Ureteral stricture
    b. Pregnancy
    c. Neurogenic bladder
    d. Uterine leiomyoma

52. Which of the following would be a common finding in a patient undergoing peritoneal dialysis?
    a. Hemorrhage
    b. Ascites
    c. Renal artery stenosis
    d. Renal vein thrombosis

53. The presence of purulent material within the renal collecting system is termed:
    a. pylotosis.
    b. pyelonephritis.
    c. pyonephrosis.
    d. emphysematous pyelonephritis.

54. The most common cause of fungal urinary tract infections is:
    a. *Candida albicans.*
    b. RCC.
    c. renal tract obstruction.
    d. urolithiasis.

55. Clinical findings of glomerulonephritis include all of the following except:
    a. proteinuria.
    b. throat infection.
    c. azotemia.
    d. hypercalcemia.

56. Which of the following is not considered an intrinsic cause of hydronephrosis?
    a. Ureterocele
    b. Urethritis
    c. Urolithiasis
    d. Ureteropelvic junction obstruction

57. Clinical findings of nephrocalcinosis include all of the following except:
    a. urinary tract infections.
    b. urinary calculi.
    c. hyperparathyroidism.
    d. weight loss.

58. Which of the following renal conditions is associated with the development of cysts within the pancreas and liver?
    a. ARPKD
    b. ADPKD
    c. MCDK
    d. Acquired renal cystic disease

59. A stone that completely fills the renal pelvis is referred to as a:
    a. calculus granulosis.
    b. staghorn calculus.
    c. twinkle stone.
    d. nephrocalcinotic calculus.

60. What is the most common location for a urolithiasis to become lodged?
    a. Ureteropelvic junction
    b. Midureter
    c. Urethra
    d. Ureterovesicle junction

SUGGESTED READINGS

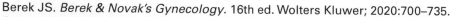

Berek JS. *Berek & Novak's Gynecology.* 16th ed. Wolters Kluwer; 2020:700–735.

Centers for Disease Control and Prevention. Parasites-Schistosomiasis. Accessed October 18, 2021. https://www.cdc.gov/parasites/schistosomiasis/disease.html

Curry RA, Prince M. *Sonography: Introduction to Normal Structure and Function.* 5th ed. Elsevier; 2020:227–252.

Federle MP, Jeffrey RB, Woodward PJ, et al. *Diagnostic Imaging: Abdomen.* 2nd ed. Amirsys; 2010:IV-3-2–IV-6-9.

Henningsen C, Kuntz K, Youngs D. *Clinical Guide to Sonography: Exercises for Critical Thinking.* 2nd ed. Elsevier; 2014:50–88 & 104–112.

Hertzberg BS, Middleton WD. *Ultrasound: The Requisites.* 3rd ed. Elsevier; 2016:103–178.

Kawamura DM, Nolan TD. *Diagnostic Medical Sonography: Abdomen and Superficial Structures.* 4th ed. Wolters Kluwer; 2018:271–356 & 739–756.

Kupinski AM. *Diagnostic Medical Sonography: The Vascular System.* Lippincott Williams & Wilkins; 2013: 305–322 & 349–361.

Penny SM. The pediatric urinary tract and medical imaging. *Radiol Technol.* 2016;87(4):425–442.

Rumack CM, Wilson SR, Charboneau JW, et al. *Diagnostic Ultrasound.* 4th ed. Elsevier; 2011:317–391, 639–707, & 1845–1890.

Sanders RC, Hall-Terracciano B. *Clinical Sonography: A Practical Guide.* 5th ed. Wolters Kluwer; 2016:525–625.

Siegel MJ. *Pediatric Sonography.* 5th ed. Wolters Kluwer; 2019:396–466.

Takeyama PH, Bhatt S, Dogra VS. Nutcracker syndrome. *Appl Radiol.* 2012. *Accessed* October 18, 2021. https://appliedradiology.com/articles/nutcracker-syndrome

The Urinary Tract

IVU and CT of Kidney Stone (Fig. 7-46)

A

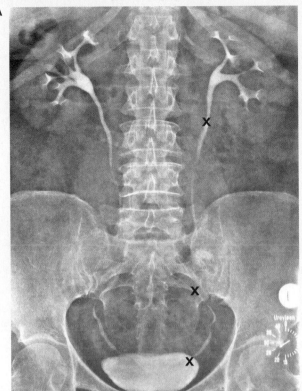

B

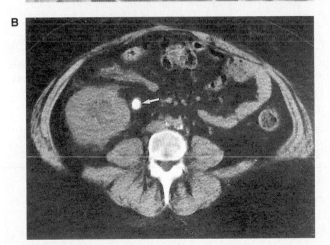

Figure 7-46 Intravenous urogram (*IVU*) of normal kidney and computed tomography (*CT*) of renal calculi. **A.** The IVU shows the normal collecting system of the kidney and the ureter. The ureters are normally constricted at three sites (*X*) where kidney stones most commonly cause obstruction. **B.** The CT scan shows a large, obstructing urolithiasis in the ureter (*arrow*).

ADPKD on CT (Fig. 7-47)

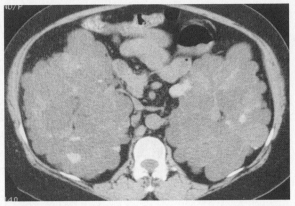

Figure 7-47 Autosomal dominant polycystic kidney disease (*ADPKD*) bilateral renal enlargement because of numerous cysts is demonstrated on this enhanced computed tomography (*CT*) examination.

RCC on MRI (Fig. 7-48)

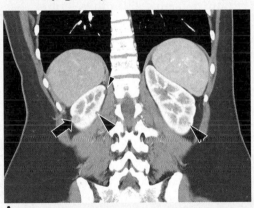

A

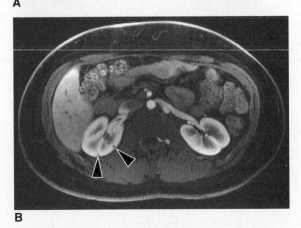

B

Figure 7-48 Renal cell carcinoma on magnetic resonance imaging (*MRI*). von Hippel–Lindau syndrome, bilateral renal cysts, and right kidney renal cell carcinoma in an 18-year-old woman. **A.** Coronal computed tomography (*CT*) image shows a small enhancing right lower zone renal mass (*arrow*), consistent with a renal cell carcinoma. Tiny additional cortical cysts (*arrowheads*) are also seen. **B.** Axial enhanced MRI shows numerous small renal cysts (*arrowheads*).

The Adrenal Glands

Introduction

The normal structure and function of the adrenal glands are presented in this chapter. Additionally, both adult and pediatric abnormalities are discussed. It is important to have a thorough appreciation of the clinical history of patients who are found to have solid adrenal tumors because many of their sonographic findings overlap. The "Bonus Review" section contains computed tomography (CT) and magnetic resonance imaging (MRI) images of an adrenal adenoma and neuroblastoma.

Key Terms

Addison disease—an endocrine disorder that results from hypofunction of the adrenal cortex

adipose—fat

adrenal adenoma—benign solid mass located within the adrenal glands

adrenal cysts—benign simple cysts located within the adrenal glands

adrenal rests—accessory adrenal gland tissue

adrenocorticotropic hormone (ACTH)—hormone secreted by the anterior pituitary gland, which controls the release of hormones by the adrenal glands

androgens—steroid hormones that regulate the development and circulation of secondary male characteristics

anoxia—lack of oxygen supply to the body, organ, or tissue

buffalo hump—excessive amount of fat on the back between the shoulders

congenital adrenal hyperplasia—a group of disorders in which there is a deficiency of cortisol production by the adrenal glands, although other hormones produced by the adrenal gland may be deficient as well

Conn syndrome—a syndrome caused by a functioning tumor within the adrenal cortex that produces excessive amounts of aldosterone

crus of the diaphragm—a tendinous structure that extends from the diaphragm to the vertebral column; there are two crura (plural for crus), a right crus and a left crus

Cushing disease—the presence of a brain tumor in the pituitary gland that increases the release of ACTH, resulting in Cushing syndrome

Cushing syndrome—a syndrome that results from an anterior pituitary gland or adrenal tumor that causes overproduction of cortisol by the adrenal glands

endocrine glands—glands that release their hormones directly into the bloodstream

Gerota fascia—the fibrous envelope of tissue that surrounds the kidney and adrenal gland

glucocorticoids—adrenal steroid hormones that include cortisol (hydrocortisone)

hirsutism—excessive hair growth in women in areas where hair growth is normally negligible

hypercortisolism—high levels of cortisol in the blood

hyperkalemia—high levels of potassium in the blood

hypernatremia—high levels of sodium in the blood

hyperpigmentation—the darkening of the skin

hypertension—high blood pressure

hypokalemia—low levels of potassium in the blood

hyponatremia—low levels of sodium in the blood

incidentaloma—an adrenal mass discovered incidentally during an imaging examination; the term may also be used for incidentally discovered masses in other organs or structures

male secondary sex characteristics—sexual characteristics typically attributed to males, such as the growth of body hair on the chest, underarms, abdomen, and face

mineralocorticoids—adrenal steroid hormones that include aldosterone

neuroblastoma—malignant tumor that can occur within the adrenal gland and anywhere within the sympathetic nervous system

pheochromocytoma—a hyperfunctioning, benign adrenal mass that causes the adrenal gland to release excessive amounts of epinephrine and norepinephrine into the bloodstream, leading to uncontrollable hypertension

striae—stretch marks

suprarenal glands—another name for the adrenal glands

tachycardia—abnormally rapid heart rate

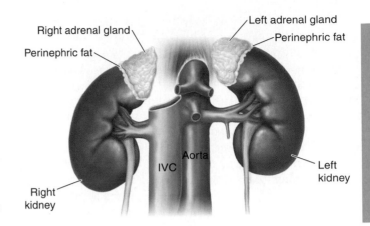

Figure 8-1 Position of the adrenal glands.

ANATOMY AND PHYSIOLOGY OF THE ADRENAL GLANDS

The paired adrenal glands, which are controlled by hormones produced by the hypothalamus, and subsequently the anterior pituitary gland, are retroperitoneal **endocrine glands** (Table 8-1; Fig. 8-1). This complex feedback system is referred to as the hypothalamic–pituitary–adrenal axis (Fig. 8-2). The hypothalamus controls the release of **adrenocorticotropic hormone** (ACTH) by the anterior pituitary gland, which in turn controls the release of hormones by the adrenal glands.

Each gland is composed of a medulla and a cortex. The cortex is the outer part of the adrenal gland. It is composed of three zones: zona glomerulosa, zona fasciculata, and zona reticularis. The adrenal cortex produces **glucocorticoids**, **mineralocorticoids**, and **androgens**. Among the hormones produced by the cortex is aldosterone, which is a mineralocorticoid

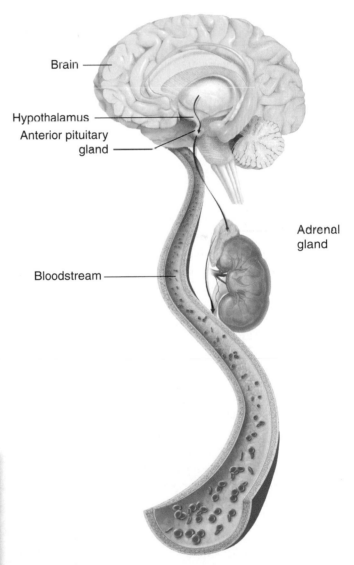

Figure 8-2 Hypothalamic–pituitary–adrenal axis. The hypothalamus controls the release of hormones by the anterior pituitary gland, which in turn controls the release of hormones by the adrenal gland.

TABLE 8-1 Location of the adrenal glands	
Location of Right Adrenal Gland	**Location of Left Adrenal Gland**
1. Posterior and right lateral to the inferior vena cava	1. Medial to the upper pole of the left kidney
2. Medial to the right lobe of the liver	2. Superior segment is located posterior to the lesser sac
3. Lateral to the **crus of the diaphragm**	3. Inferior segment is located posterior and lateral to the pancreas

(Tables 8-2 and 8-3). Aldosterone is responsible for regulating blood pressure by controlling the amounts of sodium and water in the body. The cortex furthermore produces androgenic hormones, which play a part in the development of **male secondary sex characteristics**, estrogens, and cortisol, which control the body's use of fat, carbohydrates, and protein. Last, the precursor hormone dehydroepiandrosterone, which the body uses to convert into other hormones, is also produced by the adrenal cortex.

The inner part of the adrenal glands, the medulla, produces epinephrine and norepinephrine. Epinephrine may also be referred to as adrenaline, and it is the primary hormone produced by the medulla. Both epinephrine and norepinephrine are responsible for the *flight-or-fight* response. Like the kidneys, the adrenal glands are enclosed in the **Gerota fascia**. It is important to note that individuals suffering adrenal complications may have variations in these hormones, consequently resulting in specific clinical findings.

> ◀))) **SOUND OFF**
> The adrenal glands are endocrine glands that are controlled by the release of ACTH by the anterior pituitary gland.

Vascular Anatomy of the Adrenal Glands

The adrenal glands may also be referred to as the **suprarenal glands**. They receive their blood supply by means of three arteries: the suprarenal branches of the inferior phrenic arteries, the suprarenal branches of the aorta, and the suprarenal branches of the renal arteries. Venous drainage is performed by means of the suprarenal veins. The right suprarenal vein drains directly into the inferior vena cava (IVC), whereas the left suprarenal vein drains into the left renal vein (Fig. 8-3).

TABLE 8-2 Hormones of the adrenal cortex
Aldosterone: responsible for regulating blood pressure by controlling the amounts of sodium and water in the body
Androgens: minimal impact on the development of male characteristics; supplementary and precursor hormones that contribute to testosterone production by the testicles
Cortisol (hydrocortisone): glucose metabolism, blood pressure regulation, immune function, inflammatory response
Estrogens: minimal impact on the development of female characteristics; supplementary and precursor hormones that contribute to estrogen production by the ovaries

TABLE 8-3 Hormones of the adrenal medulla
Epinephrine (adrenaline): accelerates heart rate, increasing blood pressure, opens airways in the lungs, narrows blood vessels in the skin and intestine to increase blood flow to major muscle groups
Norepinephrine: accelerates heart rate, increases blood pressure, contracts blood vessels

> ◀))) **SOUND OFF**
> The right suprarenal vein drains directly into the IVC, whereas the left suprarenal vein drains into the left renal vein.

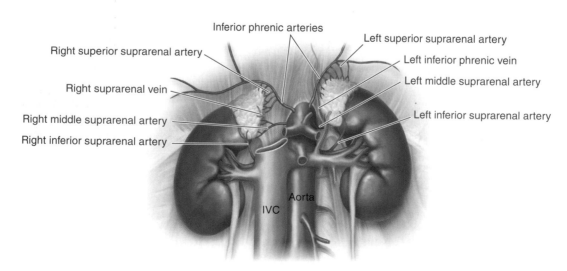

Figure 8-3 Vasculature of the adrenal glands.

SONOGRAPHY OF THE ADRENAL GLANDS

Although not routinely identified in the adult patient secondary to surrounding **adipose** tissue, the normal adrenal glands are often easily visualized in the fetus and in the pediatric patient as hypoechoic structures anterior, medial, and superior to the upper pole of each kidney (Fig. 8-4). Many of the pathologies discussed in this chapter may be incidentally discovered during an abdominal sonogram. Consequently, a mass discovered in this manner may be referred to as an **incidentaloma** because the patient is not presenting with clinical findings suggesting adrenal disease. With further follow-up, including a biochemical analysis and other imaging techniques, the mass may be determined to have little to no clinical significance. Nonetheless, if a mass is identified in the area of the adrenal gland, the sonographer should perform a thorough analysis of the mass, including providing measurements and color Doppler interrogation.

ADRENAL PATHOLOGY

Addison Disease

Addison disease, also referred to as primary adrenocortical insufficiency or chronic primary hypoadrenalism, is an endocrine disorder that results from the hypofunction of the adrenal cortex. Addison disease can be idiopathic, but it can also be caused by an autoimmune disorder, infection, or tuberculosis. With Addison disease, the cortex inadequately secretes corticosteroids as a result of partial or complete destruction of the adrenal glands. Some common clinical findings include an increase in the production of ACTH by the pituitary gland, hypotension, weakness and fatigue, loss of appetite and weight loss, and bronzing of the skin—termed **hyperpigmentation** (Fig. 8-5). Addison disease can also cause elevated liver enzymes, **hyperkalemia**, and **hyponatremia**. Although computed tomography (CT) is the imaging modality of choice to aid

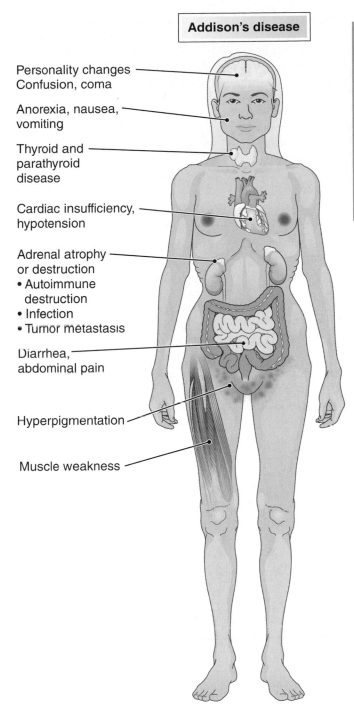

Addison's disease

Personality changes Confusion, coma

Anorexia, nausea, vomiting

Thyroid and parathyroid disease

Cardiac insufficiency, hypotension

Adrenal atrophy or destruction
• Autoimmune destruction
• Infection
• Tumor metastasis

Diarrhea, abdominal pain

Hyperpigmentation

Muscle weakness

Figure 8-5 Clinical signs of Addison disease.

in the diagnosis of Addison disease, the hemorrhagic, enlarged appearance of the adrenal glands in the acute stages of the disease could possibly be noted with sonography. The chronic form of the disease typically leads to atrophy and calcifications of the glands.

> 🔊 **SOUND OFF**
> Addison disease can be caused by an autoimmune disorder, infection, or tuberculosis and is associated with hyperkalemia, hyponatremia, and bronzing of the skin (hyperpigmentation).

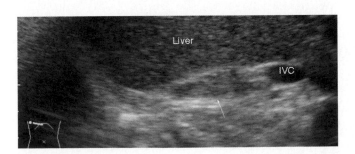

Figure 8-4 Sonographic appearance of the normal adrenal gland. The normal right adrenal gland (*arrow*) is noted in this patient in the transverse plane adjacent to the liver and inferior vena cava (*IVC*).

CLINICAL FINDINGS OF ADDISON DISEASE

1. Hypotension and cardiac insufficiency
2. Muscle weakness and fatigue
3. Loss of appetite and weight loss
4. Bronzing of the skin (hyperpigmentation)
5. Elevated liver enzymes
6. Hyperkalemia (high levels of potassium)
7. Hyponatremia (low levels of sodium)
8. Increased ACTH
9. Personality changes or confusion

SONOGRAPHIC FINDINGS OF ADDISON DISEASE

1. Enlarged appearance of the adrenal glands in the acute stages of the disease
2. Atrophic or calcified gland in the chronic stage (may be difficult to identify sonographically)

🔊 SOUND OFF
To recall the difference between the word parts *na*tremia and *ka*lemia, it should be remembered that the atomic symbol for sodium is *Na* whereas the atomic symbol for potassium is *K*.

Cushing Syndrome

Cushing syndrome can result from a tumor in the anterior pituitary gland (**Cushing disease**) or an adrenal tumor causing an increased cortisol secretion by the adrenal cortex—termed **hypercortisolism**. Cortisol plays an important role in glucose metabolism, blood pressure regulation, immune function, and inflammatory response. The tumor located within the adrenal gland is most likely and **adrenal adenoma** (see heading Adrenal Adenoma in this chapter). Patients can present with several ailments, including a **buffalo hump**, obesity, moon-shaped face, thinning arms and legs, poor wound healing, hypertension, red or purple **striae** over the abdomen and thighs, **hirsutism**, hyperglycemia, and severe fatigue (Fig. 8-6).

🔊 SOUND OFF
Cushing syndrome is the result of the overproduction of cortisol by the adrenal cortex and is associated with moon-shaped face, buffalo hump, and hypertension.

CLINICAL FINDINGS OF CUSHING SYNDROME

1. Obesity
2. Thinning arms and legs
3. Hypertension
4. Hirsutism

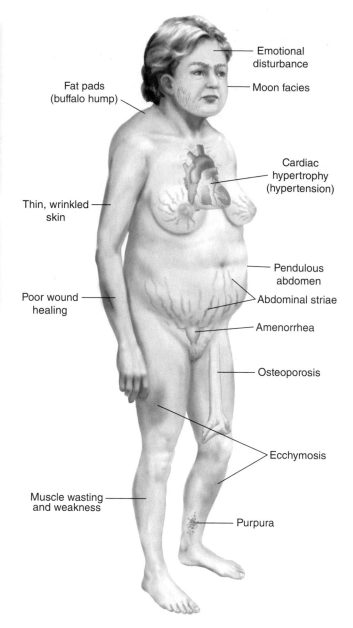

Figure 8-6 Clinical findings of Cushing syndrome.

5. Hyperglycemia
6. Severe fatigue
7. Poor wound healing
8. Buffalo hump
9. Moon-shaped face
10. Red or purple striae over the abdomen and thighs

SONOGRAPHIC FINDINGS OF CUSHING SYNDROME

1. Possible identification of an adrenal mass (most likely an adrenal adenoma)

Conn Syndrome

Conn syndrome, also referred to as primary hyperaldosteronism, results from high levels of aldosterone secretion by the adrenal cortex. Aldosterone is responsible for regulating blood pressure by controlling the amount of sodium and water in the body. Conn syndrome, like Cushing syndrome, can be caused by a functioning tumor within the adrenal cortex—most likely a benign, aldosterone-producing adrenal adenoma—that causes the adrenal gland to produce excessive amounts of aldosterone. Patients typically present with hypertension, excessive thirst, excessive urination, high levels of sodium in the blood (**hypernatremia**), and low levels of potassium in the blood (**hypokalemia**). As a result of low-potassium level, patients often complain of muscle cramps and weakness.

SOUND OFF
To recall the difference between the word parts *na*tremia and *k*alemia, it should be remembered that the atomic symbol for sodium is *Na* whereas the atomic symbol for potassium is *K*.

CLINICAL FINDINGS OF CONN SYNDROME

1. Hypertension
2. Excessive thirst
3. Excessive urination
4. High levels of sodium in the blood (hypernatremia)
5. Low levels of potassium in the blood (hypokalemia)
6. Muscle cramps and weakness

SONOGRAPHIC FINDINGS OF CONN SYNDROME

1. Possible identification of an adrenal mass (most likely an adrenal adenoma)

SOUND OFF
Conn syndrome results from high levels of aldosterone secretion by the adrenal cortex.

Adrenal Adenoma

The adrenal adenoma is the most common benign solid mass of the adrenal gland. It can be either hyperfunctioning or non-hyperfunctioning. As already established, hyperfunctioning adenomas are often seen in patients suffering from Cushing syndrome or Conn syndrome. Sonographically, an adrenal adenoma will most often appear as a solid, hypoechoic mass in the area of the adrenal gland (Fig. 8-7). Computed tomography or magnetic resonance imaging (MRI) may be needed to differentiate this mass from masses arising from adjacent organs, including the liver, spleen, or kidneys.

CLINICAL FINDINGS OF ADRENAL ADENOMAS

1. Signs and symptoms of Cushing syndrome
2. Signs and symptoms of Conn syndrome
3. May be asymptomatic

SONOGRAPHIC FINDINGS OF ADRENAL ADENOMAS

1. Solid, hypoechoic mass in the area of the adrenal gland

SOUND OFF
Adrenal adenomas can be found in patients suffering from Cushing syndrome or Conn syndrome.

Pheochromocytoma

As stated earlier, the adrenal glands play an important role in blood pressure regulation by secreting various

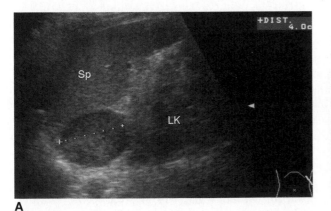
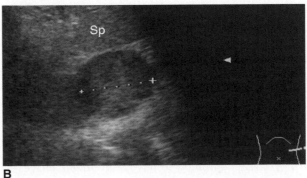

Figure 8-7 Adrenal adenoma. **A.** Sagittal image of a solid hypoechoic mass (between calipers) between the upper pole of the left kidney (*LK*) and spleen (*Sp*). **B.** The same mass (between *calipers*) was identified in the transverse plane. It was diagnosed as an adrenal adenoma.

hormones. The **pheochromocytoma**, which arises from the adrenal medulla, is typically a hyperfunctioning, benign adrenal mass that causes the adrenal gland to release excessive amounts of epinephrine and norepinephrine into the blood stream, thus leading to uncontrollable **hypertension**. However, pheochromocytomas can be malignant. Other clinical complaints of patients who have a pheochromocytoma include headaches, **tachycardia**, tremors, anxiety, and excessive sweating. A pheochromocytoma may appear as a large, hyperechoic mass in the area of the adrenal gland, but it can have various sonographic appearances (Fig. 8-8).

CLINICAL FINDINGS OF PHEOCHROMOCYTOMAS

1. Uncontrollable hypertension
2. Headaches
3. Tachycardia
4. Tremors
5. Anxiety
6. Excessive sweating

SONOGRAPHIC FINDINGS OF PHEOCHROMOCYTOMAS

1. Large, hyperechoic mass in the area of the adrenal gland
2. Can have various sonographic appearances including hypoechoic or diffusely heterogeneous

🔊 **SOUND OFF**
The pheochromocytoma is associated with uncontrollable hypertension.

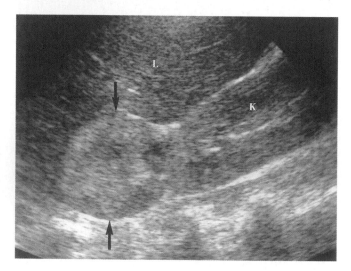

Figure 8-8 Pheochromocytoma. Longitudinal image of the liver (*L*) and right kidney (*K*) of a patient with severe hypertension revealing a heterogeneous, hyperechoic, solid right adrenal mass (*arrows*).

Adrenal Cysts

Adrenal cysts may be noted in the area of the adrenal gland and can often be difficult to separate from the liver, spleen, or upper pole of the kidneys. Simple cysts may be incidental findings with no clinical complaints provided. However, adrenal cysts that have a rim of calcification around them are much more worrisome for malignancy. Hemorrhage within an adrenal cyst, an infected cyst, and larger cysts may cause pain or other clinical symptoms. Sonographically, a simple adrenal cyst will typically be anechoic, round, and produce acoustic enhancement (Fig. 8-9).

CLINICAL FINDINGS OF ADRENAL CYSTS

1. Asymptomatic
2. Large, infected, or hemorrhagic cysts can cause pain

SONOGRAPHIC FINDINGS OF ADRENAL CYSTS

1. Anechoic
2. Round
3. Acoustic enhancement

Adrenal Rests

Accessory adrenal gland tissue, commonly referred to as **adrenal rests**, can be found within the testes, epididymis, ovaries, and inguinal canal. Adrenal rests disseminate during embryologic development and can form mass-like structures within the affected organs or structures. The cells are responsive to the secretion of ACTH by the pituitary gland. They are often associated with **congenital adrenal hyperplasia** and Cushing syndrome. More information about these masses can be found in Chapter 13.

🔊 **SOUND OFF**
In the male, adrenal rest tumors may be found in the testicles.

Adrenal Carcinoma and Metastasis

Primary adrenal carcinoma, such as adenocarcinoma, is rare. Malignant adrenal tumors will often produce the symptoms associated with Cushing syndrome because they may be functional tumors that impact hormone production. The adrenal glands are the fourth most common site of metastasis. Metastasis to the adrenal glands can originate in the lungs, breast, gastrointestinal tract, thyroid, pancreas, kidneys, or from lymphoma, leukemia, or melanoma. Specifically, there is a high probability that the primary sites are the lung, breast, or lymphoma in many patients. Cancer

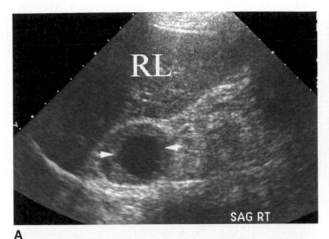

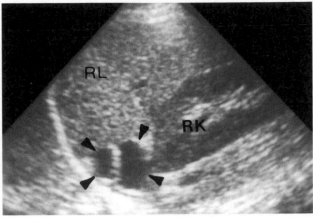

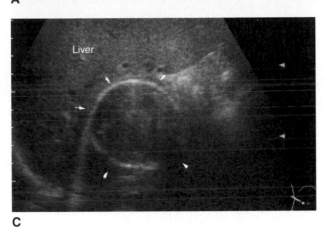

Figure 8-9 Adrenal cysts. **A.** Unilocular right adrenal gland cyst (*arrowheads*) posterior to the right liver lobe (*RL*) can be identified in this longitudinal image. **B.** Complex appearing cyst (*arrowheads*) was discovered in a symptomatic patient with right upper quadrant pain. **C.** Calcified cyst (*arrowheads*) is demonstrated in this transverse image posterior to the right liver lobe (*RL*) and superior to the right kidney (not seen). RK, right kidney.

of the adrenal gland can have various sonographic appearances, including that of a solid, hypoechoic mass, thus mimicking sonographic appearance of the benign adrenal adenoma. Cortical cancers tend to be large and have the tendency to invade the adrenal vein and IVC (Fig. 8-10).

CLINICAL FINDINGS OF ADRENAL CARCINOMA

1. May mimic symptoms of Cushing syndrome

SONOGRAPHIC FINDINGS OF ADRENAL CARCINOMA

1. Solid, hypoechoic mass
2. Large, heterogeneous mass

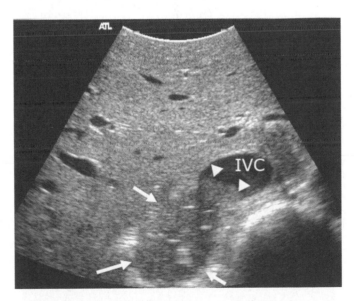

Figure 8-10 A solid, irregular-appearing mass is noted within the right adrenal gland (*arrows*) and extending into the inferior vena cava (*IVC*) (*arrowheads*).

PEDIATRIC ADRENAL PATHOLOGY

Neuroblastoma

The most common extracranial solid, malignant tumor in children is the **neuroblastoma**. It arises from the immature neural crest cells (neuroblasts) along the

sympathetic nervous system. Most patients will present with a palpable abdominal mass, abdominal pain, and bone pain, and metastasis is often present at the time of discovery. The child may also have blue or purple spots on the skin. Neuroblastomas, which arise from the adrenal medulla, typically present before 5 years of age, with the median age of diagnosis being 19 months. A neuroblastoma will appear as a solid, large (average size is 8 cm), heterogeneous mass that typically contains calcifications and can spread around the IVC and aorta (Fig. 8-11). In cases of a suspected neuroblastoma, the liver and other abdominal organs should be closely examined for metastatic involvement.

CLINICAL FINDINGS OF NEUROBLASTOMA

1. Palpable abdominal mass
2. Abdominal pain
3. Bone pain
4. Blue or purple skin lesions

SONOGRAPHIC FINDINGS OF NEUROBLASTOMA

1. Large, heterogeneous mass containing areas of calcification and hemorrhage located in the area of the adrenal gland
2. Metastasis often present at the time of discovery

SOUND OFF
The neuroblastoma is the most common extracranial solid, malignant tumor in children. Notable clinical features of the neuroblastoma are bone pain and skin lesions.

Adrenal Hemorrhage

The adrenal glands, particularly in stressed neonates following a traumatic birth or perinatal **anoxia**, can spontaneously hemorrhage. This often results in a heterogeneous-appearing mass in the area of the adrenal gland (Fig. 8-12). The resulting hematoma will be a rounded or triangle-shaped mass that appears echogenic during the acute stage, and with time it will become heterogeneous, hypoechoic, and cystic, and eventually completely resolve, although some residual calcifications may remain. This calcification may be prominent and produce an acoustic shadow. Patients with adrenal hemorrhage will present with an abdominal mass, jaundice, anemia, and an acute drop in hematocrit and blood pressure.

CLINICAL FINDINGS OF ADRENAL HEMORRHAGE

1. Abdominal mass
2. Jaundice
3. Anemia
4. Acute drop in hematocrit and blood pressure

SONOGRAPHIC FINDINGS OF ADRENAL HEMORRHAGE

1. Round or triangle-shaped mass in the area of the adrenal gland
2. Various sonographic appearances based on the age of hemorrhage
3. Echogenic during the acute stage
4. With time, it will become heterogeneous, hypoechoic, and possibly cystic.
5. Residual, shadowing calcifications may remain following resolution of the hemorrhage

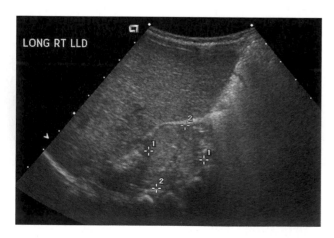

Figure 8-11 Neuroblastoma. This solid mass was proven to be a pediatric neuroblastoma. Coexisting liver metastasis was also present.

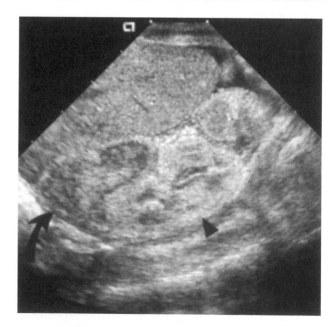

Figure 8-12 Adrenal hemorrhage. Longitudinal image in a premature 30-week-gestation infant showing acute hemorrhage in the right adrenal gland (*curved arrow*). The right kidney (*arrowhead*) is compressed by the hemorrhage.

REVIEW QUESTIONS

1. An abdominal sonogram is requested for a newborn in the intensive care unit. The newborn suffered from brief anoxia at birth and is now experiencing jaundice. Superior to the right kidney, a triangle-shaped, heterogeneous mass is visualized. What is the most likely diagnosis?
   a. Adrenal hemorrhage
   b. Adrenal adenoma
   c. Pheochromocytoma
   d. Cushing syndrome

2. All of the following are associated with Conn syndrome except:
   a. adrenal adenoma.
   b. hypertension.
   c. excessive thirst.
   d. thinning arms and legs.

3. When internal bleeding is suspected, what laboratory value is most useful for a sonographer to evaluate?
   a. Hematocrit
   b. Blood urea nitrogen
   c. Androgenic hormone
   d. Alkaline phosphatase

4. Which of the following mass-like lesions may be associated with congenital adrenal hyperplasia and found within the testes?
   a. Adrenal adenomas
   b. Adrenal rests
   c. Pheochromocytomas
   d. Neuroblastomas

5. The syndrome associated with hypertension, hyperglycemia, obesity, and an adrenal mass is:
   a. Edwards syndrome.
   b. Cushing syndrome.
   c. Juliet syndrome.
   d. Hirschsprung syndrome.

6. All of the following are true statements about the adrenal glands except:
   a. the adrenal glands are easily identified in the fetus.
   b. the adrenal glands are exocrine glands.
   c. the adrenal glands are composed of a medulla and cortex.
   d. the adrenal glands may also be referred to as the suprarenal glands.

7. The adrenal glands are surrounded by a connective tissue capsule called:
   a. Glisson capsule.
   b. adrenocortical fascia.
   c. Gerota fascia.
   d. Glisson fascia.

8. The left suprarenal vein drains directly into the:
   a. IVC.
   b. abdominal aorta.
   c. celiac trunk.
   d. left renal vein.

9. Conn syndrome results from:
   a. low levels of cortisol.
   b. high levels of cortisol.
   c. high levels of aldosterone.
   d. low levels of epinephrine.

10. With active internal hemorrhage, the patient's hematocrit will:
    a. increase.
    b. decrease.
    c. become stable.
    d. not change.

11. Which of the following would result in a buffalo hump and moon-shaped face?
    a. Conn syndrome
    b. Addison disease
    c. Androgenism
    d. Hypercortisolism

12. Which types of glands release their hormones directly into the bloodstream?
    a. Endocrine glands
    b. Exocrine glands

13. A localized collection of blood describes a:
    a. hemangioma.
    b. hematoma.
    c. hypertoma.
    d. hydrocele.

14. What is the cause of Cushing disease?
    a. Anterior pituitary gland tumor
    b. Adrenal hemorrhage
    c. Neuroblastoma
    d. Hyperaldosteronism

15. The arterial blood supply to the adrenal glands is accomplished by means of the:
    a. celiac trunk.
    b. subphrenic arteries.
    c. suprarenal arteries.
    d. superior mesenteric artery.

16. Bronzing of the skin is a clinical finding associated with:
    a. Addison disease.
    b. Cushing disease.
    c. Cushing syndrome.
    d. Conn syndrome.

17. Hyperfunctioning adrenal adenomas are associated with all of the following except:
    a. Cushing syndrome.
    b. Conn syndrome.
    c. hypoechoic mass in the area of the adrenal gland.
    d. acute drop in hematocrit.

18. Which of the following is also referred to as primary adrenocortical insufficiency?
    a. Conn syndrome
    b. Addison disease
    c. Cushing disease
    d. Congenital adrenal hyperplasia

19. The adrenal cortex produces all of the following except:
    a. cortisol.
    b. androgens.
    c. aldosterone.
    d. adrenaline.

20. Which of the following is produced by the adrenal medulla?
    a. Cortisol
    b. Aldosterone
    c. Norepinephrine
    d. Androgens

21. What is the term for low levels of sodium in the blood?
    a. Hypokalemia
    b. Hypopigmentation
    c. Hyponatremia
    d. Hypodisuria

22. Which of the following hormones are responsible for the *flight-or-fight* response?
    a. Epinephrine and norepinephrine
    b. Cortisol and androgens
    c. Cortisol and aldosterone
    d. ACTH and aldosterone

23. Which of the following is associated with hyponatremia?
    a. Cushing syndrome
    b. Conn syndrome
    c. Pheochromocytoma
    d. Addison disease

24. Which of the following best describes the location of the right adrenal gland?
    a. Posterior and lateral to the pancreas
    b. Medial to the lower pole of the right kidney
    c. Posterior and lateral to the IVC
    d. Medial to the crus of the diaphragm

25. Upon sonographic examination of the right upper quadrant in a 32-year-old female patient complaining of generalized abdominal pain, an anechoic mass with posterior enhancement superior and medial to the upper pole of the right kidney is visualized. This most likely represents a(n):
    a. adrenal metastatic lesion.
    b. pheochromocytoma.
    c. neuroblastoma.
    d. adrenal cyst.

26. The right suprarenal vein drains directly into the:
    a. IVC.
    b. abdominal aorta.
    c. celiac trunk.
    d. left renal vein.

27. The adrenal mass often associated with uncontrollable hypertension, tachycardia, and tremors is the:
    a. neuroblastoma.
    b. adrenal hematoma.
    c. oncocytoma.
    d. pheochromocytoma.

28. A 45-year-old obese woman with thin arms and legs, hypertension, and severe fatigue presents to the ultrasound department for an abdominal sonogram. Based on these clinical findings, the sonographer should evaluate the adrenal glands closely for signs of:
    a. Addison cyst.
    b. adrenal hemorrhage.
    c. adrenal adenoma.
    d. neuroblastoma.

29. The most common sonographic appearance of a pheochromocytoma is a(n):
    a. hyperechoic mass.
    b. hypoechoic mass.
    c. anechoic mass.
    d. complex mass.

30. The most common, extracranial, malignant mass in children is the:
    a. hepatoblastoma.
    b. hypernephroma.
    c. pheochromocytoma.
    d. neuroblastoma.

31. Which of the following is associated with hypernatremia?
    a. Cushing syndrome
    b. Conn syndrome
    c. Pheochromocytoma
    d. Addison disease

32. The most common sonographic appearance of a neuroblastoma is:
    a. hyperechoic mass.
    b. heterogeneous mass with calcifications.
    c. anechoic mass.
    d. hypoechoic mass.

33. The neuroblastoma typically presents before the age of:
    a. 1 year.
    b. 2 years.
    c. 4 years.
    d. 5 years.

34. Which hormone is responsible for regulating blood pressure by controlling the amounts of sodium and water in the body?
    a. Epinephrine
    b. Cortisol
    c. Aldosterone
    d. ACTH

35. Which hormone, secreted by the anterior pituitary gland, controls the release of hormones by the adrenal glands?
    a. Epinephrine
    b. Cortisol
    c. Aldosterone
    d. ACTH

36. All of the following are most likely a benign adrenal mass except:
    a. adrenal adenoma.
    b. neuroblastoma.
    c. pheochromocytoma.
    d. adrenal hematoma.

37. All of the following are clinical findings of a pheochromocytoma except:
    a. bradycardia.
    b. uncontrollable hypertension.
    c. excessive sweating.
    d. tremors.

38. Which plays a part in the development of male characteristics?
    a. Androgens
    b. Cortisol
    c. Aldosterone
    d. Hematocrit

39. The adrenal glands receive a portion of their blood supply from all of the following except the:
    a. suprarenal branches of the inferior phrenic arteries.
    b. suprarenal branches of the aorta.
    c. suprarenal branches of the renal arteries.
    d. suprarenal branches of the celiac trunk.

40. All of the following are true statements about the adrenal glands except:
    a. the adrenal glands play an important role in blood pressure regulation.
    b. the adrenal glands are easily identified in the fetus.
    c. the left adrenal gland is located lateral to the upper pole of the left kidney.
    d. the right adrenal gland is located medial to the right lobe of the liver.

41. Which of the following is associated with a deficiency of cortisol production by the adrenal gland?
    a. Conn syndrome
    b. Congenital adrenal hyperplasia
    c. Adrenocorticotropic deficiency syndrome
    d. Glucocortical deficiency syndrome

42. Which of the following would be least likely associated with an overproduction of the hormones released by the adrenal cortex?
    a. Cushing syndrome
    b. Adrenal adenoma
    c. Pheochromocytoma
    d. Conn syndrome

43. What is the term that may be used for an adrenal mass noted during an abdominal sonogram for unrelated clinical findings?
    a. Adrenaloma
    b. Fauxoma
    c. Corticoma
    d. Incidentaloma

44. Which of the following is a glucocorticoid?
    a. Cortisol
    b. Aldosterone
    c. Epinephrine
    d. Norepinephrine

45. Bone pain and purple skin lesions are clinical findings associated with what adrenal tumor?
    a. Pheochromocytoma
    b. Incidentaloma
    c. Neuroblastoma
    d. Adrenal adenoma

46. The patient in Figure 8-13 presented to the sonography department with a history of elevated liver function tests. What is the most likely pathology being identified by the curved arrow?
    a. Adrenal cyst
    b. Neuroblastoma
    c. Adrenal adenoma
    d. Pheochromocytoma

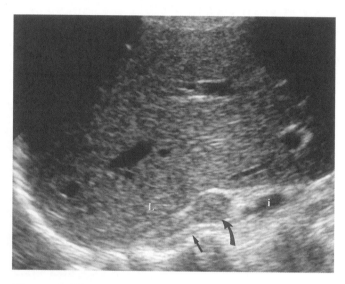

Figure 8-13

47. The patient in Figure 8-14 is a 36-year-old who presented with a history of anxiety, headaches, and excessive sweating. Based on the clinical history, what is the most likely etiology of the structure identified by the arrowheads in these images?
    a. Adrenal cyst
    b. Adrenal rest tumor
    c. Adrenal hemorrhage
    d. Pheochromocytoma

48. Which of the following is associated with excessive urination and hyperkalemia?
    a. Conn syndrome
    b. Cushing disease
    c. Cushing syndrome
    d. Addison disease

49. Which of the following is defined as excessive hair growth in women in areas where hair growth is normally negligible?
    a. Hypernatremia
    b. Hypercortisolism
    c. Hirsutism
    d. Addison syndrome

50. Hypernatremia is defined as:
    a. high levels of sodium in the blood.
    b. high levels of potassium in the blood.
    c. high levels of cortisol in the blood.
    d. high levels of nitrogen in the blood.

51. What adrenal disorder is associated with striae of the abdomen?
    a. Conn syndrome
    b. Addison disease
    c. Cushing syndrome
    d. Adrenocortical syndrome

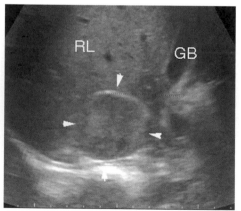

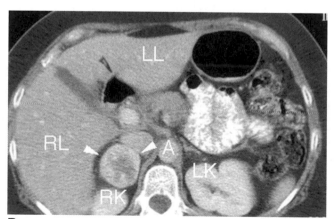

A

B

Figure 8-14

52. Hyperkalemia is defined as:
    a. high levels of potassium in the blood.
    b. high levels of sodium in the blood.
    c. high levels of nitrogen in the blood.
    d. high levels of aldosterone in the blood.

53. A 27-year-old patient presents to the sonography department with the sudden onset of hypotension, muscle weakness, and elevated liver enzymes. Evidence of hyperpigmentation is also noted. What sonographic finding would be most likely associated with this apparent clinical condition?
    a. Multiple masses within the adrenal glands
    b. Atrophy of the adrenal glands
    c. Bilateral adrenal hemorrhage
    d. Enlargement of the adrenal glands

54. The patient in Figure 8-15 was a 3-year-old girl who complained of abdominal pain and who had recent weight loss. What is the most likely diagnosis for the structure identified by the arrowheads?
    a. Adrenal adenoma
    b. Neuroblastoma
    c. Nephroblastoma
    d. Primary adrenal adenocarcinoma

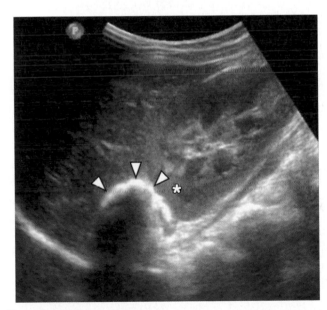

FIGURE 8-15

55. Figure 8-16 is a longitudinal right upper quadrant image of a newborn who was suffering from anemia, jaundice, and an acute drop in blood pressure. What is the most likely etiology of the structure identified by the red arrows?
    a. Adrenal hematoma
    b. Adrenal adenoma
    c. Neuroblastoma
    d. Adrenal metastasis

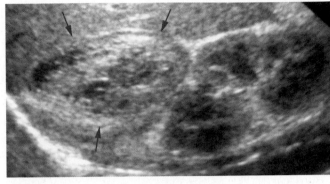

Figure 8-16

56. What are the tendinous structures that extend from the diaphragm to the vertebral column?
    a. Stria of the diaphragm
    b. Tendonae diaphramae
    c. Ligamentum diaphragmatum
    d. Crura of the diaphragm

57. Which of the following is not a zone of the adrenal cortex?
    a. Zona pellucida
    b. Zona glomerulosa
    c. Zona fasciculata
    d. Zona reticularis

58. Which of the following may also be referred to as chronic primary hypoadrenalism?
    a. Conn syndrome
    b. Addison disease
    c. Cushing disease
    d. Pheochromocytoma syndrome

59. What is another term for stretch marks?
    a. Crura
    b. Striae
    c. Plicae
    d. Cilia

60. What is the most likely sonographic appearance of a chronic adrenal hematoma?
    a. Solid, hypoechoic mass that produces acoustic enhancement
    b. Anechoic, triangular mass that produces shadowing
    c. Atrophic adrenal gland surrounded by an anechoic fluid collection
    d. Calcified mass that produces acoustic shadowing

The Adrenal Glands

SUGGESTED READINGS

Curry RA, Prince M. *Sonography: Introduction to Normal Structure and Function*. 5th ed. Elsevier; 2021:227–253.

Farrell TA. *Radiology 101*. 5th ed. Wolters Kluwer; 2020:168.

Federle MP, Jeffrey RB, Woodward PJ, et al. *Diagnostic Imaging: Abdomen*. 2nd ed. Amirsys; 2010:IV-2-2–IV-2-39.

Hagen-Ansert SL. *Textbook of Diagnostic Sonography*. 7th ed. Elsevier; 2012:448–457.

Henningsen C, Kuntz K, Youngs D. *Clinical Guide to Sonography: Exercises for Critical Thinking*. 2nd ed. Elsevier; 2014:102–104.

Hertzberg BS, Middleton WD. *Ultrasound: The Requisites*. 3rd ed. Elsevier; 2016:221–226.

Kawamura DM, Nolan TD. *Diagnostic Medical Sonography: Abdomen and Superficial Structures*. 4th ed. Wolters Kluwer; 2018:377–404.

Rumack CM, Wilson SR, Charboneau JW, et al. *Diagnostic Ultrasound*. 4th ed. Elsevier; 2011:429–446 & 1885–1888.

Siegel MJ. *Pediatric Sonography*. 5th ed. Wolters Kluwer; 2019:467–482.

BONUS REVIEW!

CT of an Adrenal Adenoma (Fig. 8-17)

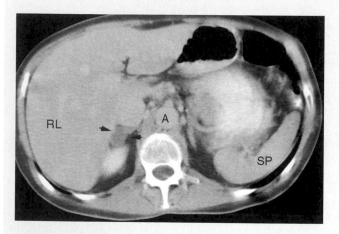

Figure 8-17 Computed tomography of an adrenal adenoma (between *arrowheads*). *RL*, right lobe of liver; *A*, aorta; *SP*, spleen

MRI of an Adrenal Adenoma (Fig. 8-18)

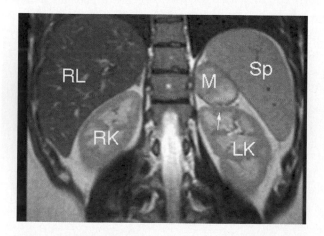

Figure 8-18 Magnetic resonance imaging coronal image of an adrenal adenoma (*M, arrow*). *RL*, right lobe of the liver; *RK*, right kidney; *LK*, left kidney; *Sp*, spleen

CT of a Neuroblastoma with Liver Metastasis (Fig. 8-19)

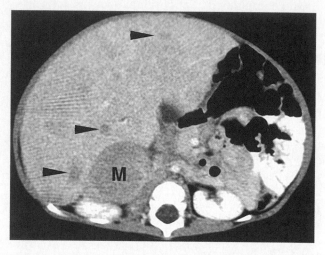

Figure 8-19 Neuroblastoma (*M*) on computed tomography with liver metastasis (*arrowheads*).

Abdominal Vasculature

Introduction

Although abdominal sonographers may not be required to have vascular credentials, they must have a fundamental understanding of the key vascular structures found in the abdomen, and indeed some may be required to perform many vascular sonograms. This chapter offers an explicit structural anatomy review of the vascular components that are associated with the abdominal aorta, inferior vena cava (IVC), and portal venous system. Pathology of the abdominal aorta and IVC is also presented. Vascular abnormalities of abdominal organs can be found in the specific organ chapters in this text. The "Bonus Review" section includes several magnetic resonance imaging and computed tomography images of vascular pathology.

Key Terms

abdominal aortic aneurysm (AAA)—enlargement of the diameter of the abdominal aorta to greater than 3 cm

aneurysm—any dilation of a blood vessel, whether focal or diffuse

atherosclerosis—a disease characterized by the accumulation of plaque within the walls of arteries

Budd–Chiari syndrome—a syndrome described as the occlusion of the hepatic veins, with possible coexisting occlusion of the inferior vena cava (IVC)

embolism—a blockage caused by an abnormal mass (embolus) within the bloodstream that hinders circulation downstream, leading to tissue damage

endovascular aortic stent graft repair—nonsurgical method for treating AAAs

false aneurysm—a contained rupture of a blood vessel that is most likely secondary to the disruption of one or more layers of that vessel's wall

false lumen—the residual channel of a vessel created by the accumulation of a clot within that vessel

fusiform—shaped like a spindle; wider in the middle and tapering toward the ends

hepatopetal—blood flow toward the liver

high-resistance flow—the flow pattern that results from small arteries or arterioles that are contracted, which produces an increase in the resistance to blood flow to the structure that is being supplied

intimal flap—observation of the intimal layer of a vessel as a result of a dissection

IVC filter—vascular filter placed in the IVC to prevent pulmonary emboli

low-resistance flow—the flow pattern characterized by persistent forward flow throughout the cardiac cycle

Marfan syndrome—a disorder of the connective tissue characterized by tall stature and aortic and mitral valve insufficiency

mycotic aneurysm—an aneurysm caused by infection

postprandial—after a meal

pseudoaneurysm—see key term false aneurysm

pulmonary embolus—blood clot that has traveled to the lungs and is obstructing the pulmonary arterial circulation; most often, the result of a deep venous thrombosis

saccular aneurysm—saclike dilation of a blood vessel

small bowel ischemia—a condition resulting in interruption or reduction of the blood supply to the small intestines

thrombus—blood clot

transitional cell carcinoma—a malignant tumor of the urinary tract that is often found within the urinary bladder or within the renal pelvis

true aneurysm—the enlargement of a vessel that involves all three layers of the wall

true lumen—the true or original channel within a vessel

tunica adventitia—the outer wall layer of a vessel

tunica intima—the inner wall layer of a vessel

tunica media—the middle, muscular layer of a vessel

Wilms tumor—the most common solid malignant pediatric abdominal mass; a malignant pediatric renal mass that may also be referred to as nephroblastoma

ANATOMY AND PHYSIOLOGY OF THE ABDOMINAL AORTA

The aorta, the largest artery in the body, originates at the left ventricle of the heart. The subdivision of the aorta within the chest is referred to as the thoracic aorta. Once the aorta passes through the aortic hiatus of the diaphragm, it is referred to as the abdominal aorta. It is retroperitoneal in location and positioned anterior to the spine, just left of the midline.

The walls of the aorta, and indeed all arteries and veins, consist of three layers. The innermost layer, closest to the flowing blood, is the **tunica intima**. The middle layer, or muscular layer, is referred to as the **tunica media**. The outermost layer is the **tunica adventitia** and may also be referred to as the tunica externa (Fig. 9-1). One important note is that arteries have a thicker tunica media.

The function of the abdominal aorta is to supply blood to the abdominal organs, pelvis, and lower extremities. The abdominal aorta has several important branches that are discussed in the following sections (Figs. 9-2 and 9-3). Most abdominal arteries are considered to have **low-resistance flow**, although some may have **high-resistance flow** at times (Figs. 9-4). The normal flow patterns of other pertinent abdominal arterial vessels are provided in Table 9-1.

Celiac Trunk

The celiac trunk may also be referred to as the celiac artery or celiac axis. It is the first main visceral branch

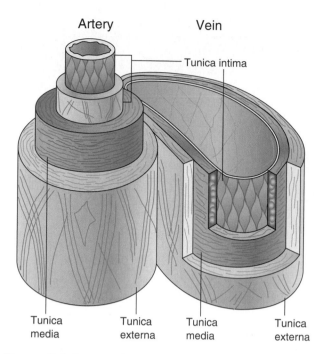

Figure 9-1 Layers of arteries and veins. Note: The tunica externa is also referred to as the tunica adventitia and the tunica media is thicker in an artery compared to a vein.

of the abdominal aorta, and its branches supply blood to several vital abdominal organs. The celiac trunk arises from the anterior aspect of the abdominal aorta, between the crura of the diaphragm. It branches into three arteries: the splenic artery, the common hepatic artery, and the left gastric artery. The common hepatic artery and splenic artery are readily seen in the transverse scan plane. Combined with the celiac trunk, these vessels have a *seagull* or *T*-shaped appearance (Fig. 9-5). Because of its small size, the left gastric artery is not typically seen with sonography. Flow within the celiac artery should be continuous and forward, whereas abnormal flow will have elevated velocities (Fig. 9-6).

The splenic artery travels in the direction of the left side of the patient, toward the spleen. Its route is tortuous. It can often be noted along the superior margin of the pancreas and may be confused for the main pancreatic duct. To differentiate the two vessels, color Doppler will confirm the artery. The splenic artery enters the splenic hilum and branches further into smaller arteries. Low-resistance flow should be noted within the normal splenic artery.

The common hepatic artery travels in the direction of the right side of the patient, toward the liver. It branches into the gastroduodenal artery at the level of the pancreatic head. After this point, the common hepatic artery becomes the proper hepatic artery. The proper hepatic artery enters the liver at the porta hepatis and branches further into the right and left

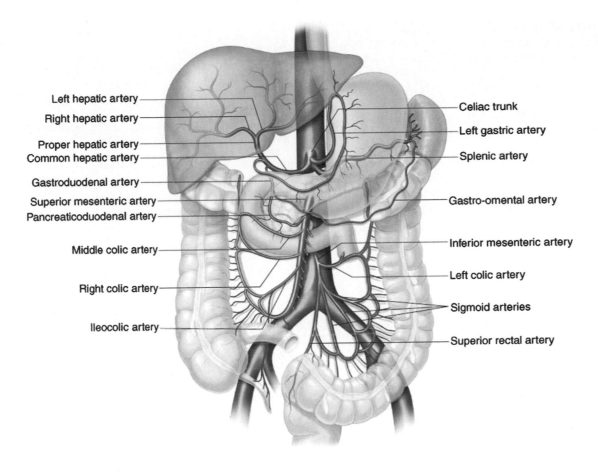

Left hepatic artery

Right hepatic artery

Proper hepatic artery

Common hepatic artery

Gastroduodenal artery

Superior mesenteric artery

Pancreaticoduodenal artery

Middle colic artery

Right colic artery

Ileocolic artery

Celiac trunk

Left gastric artery

Splenic artery

Gastro-omental artery

Inferior mesenteric artery

Left colic artery

Sigmoid arteries

Superior rectal artery

Figure 9-2 The abdominal aorta.

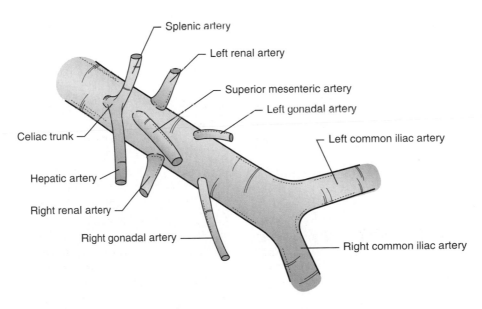

Splenic artery

Left renal artery

Superior mesenteric artery

Left gonadal artery

Left common iliac artery

Celiac trunk

Hepatic artery

Right renal artery

Right gonadal artery

Right common iliac artery

Figure 9-3 The main branches of the abdominal aorta.

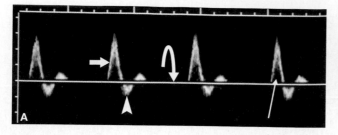
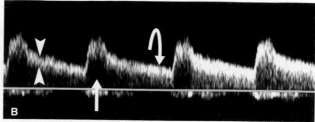

Figure 9-4 High-resistance and low-resistance Doppler spectrum. **A.** A high-resistance waveform is characterized by rapid systolic upstroke (*fat arrow*); low flow velocities or no flow during diastole (*curved arrow*); and, commonly, reversal of flow direction (*arrowhead*) in early diastole. A narrow Doppler spectrum and the *systolic window* (*skinny arrow*) are seen. **B.** A low-resistance waveform is characterized by relatively high flow velocities throughout all of diastole (*curved arrow*). The narrow spectrum (between *arrowheads*) and clean systolic window (*straight arrow*) are characteristic of laminar blood flow. Arteries that supply organs typically show low-resistance waveforms that represent continuous blood flow throughout the cardiac cycle.

TABLE 9-1 Abdominal arteries and normal flow patterns	
Abdominal Artery	**Normal Flow Pattern**
Abdominal aorta (PSV range 70–100 cm/s)	Suprarenal aorta = low-resistance flow Infrarenal aorta = high-resistance flow
Celiac artery (PSV range 98–105 cm/s)	Low-resistance flow
Common hepatic artery	Low-resistance flow
Common iliac artery	High-resistance flow
Splenic artery	Low-resistance flow
Superior mesenteric artery (PSV range 97–142 cm/s)	Fasting patient = high-resistance flow postprandial (30–90 min) = low-resistance flow
Renal arteries	Low-resistance flow

PSV, peak systolic velocity.

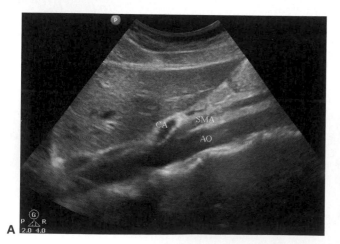
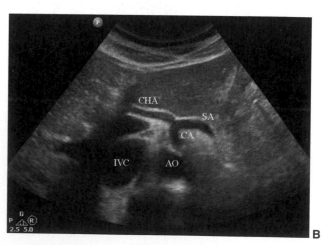

Figure 9-5 Celiac axis. **A.** In the longitudinal plane, the celiac artery (*CA*) can be seen branching from the anterior aorta (*AO*) proximal to the superior mesenteric artery (*SMA*). **B.** In the transverse plane, the CA can be seen branching from the abdominal aorta (*AO*) into the common hepatic artery (*CHA*) and splenic artery (*SA*). The inferior vena cava (*IVC*) can be noted right lateral to the aorta.

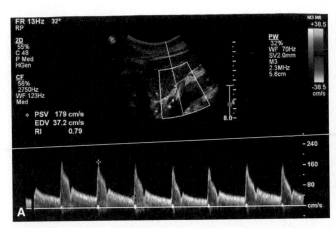
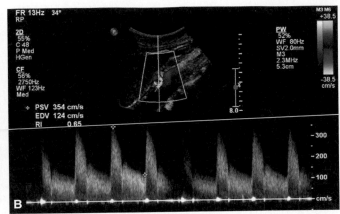

Figure 9-6 Normal and abnormal celiac artery. **A.** Normal flow within the celiac artery. **B.** Abnormal flow within the celiac artery reveals high velocities and abnormal waveforms.

hepatic arteries. One significant branch of the right hepatic artery is the cystic artery, which supplies blood to the gallbladder. The hepatic artery should yield low resistance and **hepatopetal** flow.

Superior Mesenteric Artery

The second main branch of the abdominal aorta is the superior mesenteric artery (SMA). The SMA typically originates along the anterior aspect of the abdominal aorta, just distal to the origin of the celiac trunk, although in some individuals, the SMA and celiac trunk originate at the same position. The SMA supplies blood to parts of the small intestines, some of the colon, and the pancreas. Sonographically, the SMA is readily identified by the echogenic fat layer surrounding it (Fig. 9-7). It is located posterior to the splenic vein and pancreas and left lateral to the superior mesenteric vein. The left renal

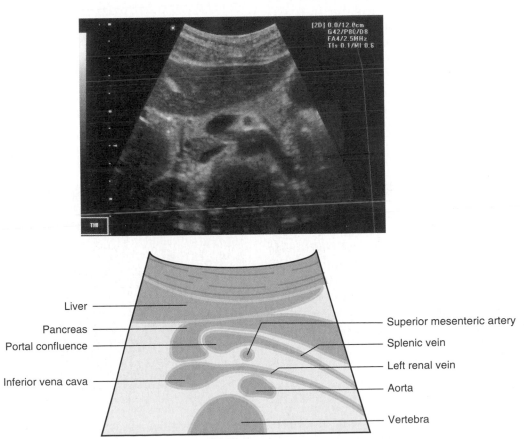

Figure 9-7 Superior mesenteric artery. Transverse view of the abdominal aorta at the level of the superior mesenteric artery. A sagittal sonographic image is noted in Figure 9-5.

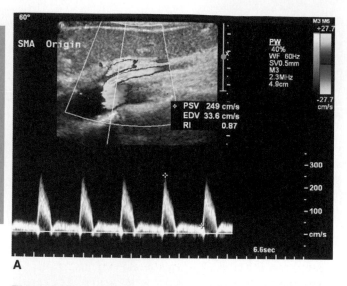

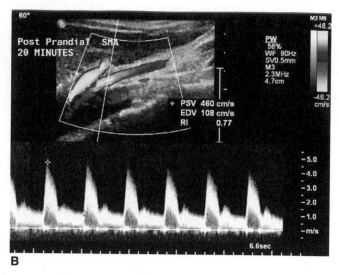

Figure 9-8 Fasting and postprandial flow velocities in a normal superior mesenteric artery (*SMA*). **A.** Color-flow image and Doppler spectral waveform in the fasting state with peak systolic velocity (*PSV*) of 249 cm per second and end-diastolic velocity (*EDV*) of 34 cm per second. **B.** Repeat evaluation 20 minutes after eating shows PSV of 460 cm per second and EDV of 108 cm per second.

vein should be noted posterior to the SMA and anterior to the abdominal aorta.

The SMA will exhibit high-resistance flow in fasting patients. However, 30 to 90 minutes **postprandial**, the SMA will yield a low-resistance waveform (Fig. 9-8). Sonography can aid in the diagnosis of **small bowel ischemia**. Patients with unexplained abdominal pain could be suffering from small bowel ischemia when this characteristic trend is not perceptible.

> 🔊 **SOUND OFF**
> The SMA will exhibit high-resistance flow in the fasting patient. However, 30 to 90 minutes postprandial, the SMA will yield a low-resistance waveform.

Renal Arteries

The third main visceral branches of the abdominal aorta are the paired renal arteries. They arise just below the level of the SMA (Fig. 9-9). The right renal artery originates from the right anterolateral aspect of the aorta and travels posterior to the IVC on its way to the right renal hilum (Fig. 9-10). The left renal artery originates from the left anterolateral aspect of the aorta and travels posterior to the left renal vein as it progresses to the left renal hilum.

Because the aorta is located on the left side of the abdomen, the right renal artery is much longer than the left renal artery. Duplication of the renal arteries is common. Normal renal arteries typically demonstrate low-resistance flow. Pathology of the renal arteries is discussed in Chapter 7.

> 🔊 **SOUND OFF**
> In the sagittal plane, the right renal artery may be identified as an anechoic circle posterior to the IVC.

Gonadal Arteries

The fourth branches, the gonadal arteries, arise from the anterior surface of the abdominal aorta, just below the renal artery level. Depending on the gender of the patient, they should be explicitly referred to as

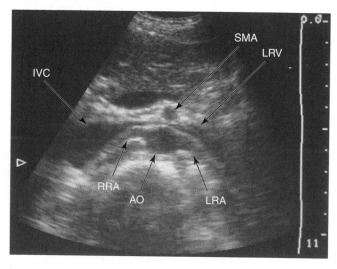

Figure 9-9 Renal arteries. Transverse image of the renal arteries revealing the inferior vena cava (*IVC*), superior mesenteric artery (*SMA*), abdominal aorta (*AO*), right renal artery (*RRA*), left renal artery (*LRA*), and the left renal vein (*LRV*).

The IMA may be difficult to image with sonography, but it may be seen in some slender patients.

Iliac Arteries

The aorta bifurcates at or near the level of the umbilicus. This point marks the origin of the right and left common iliac arteries. Color-flow Doppler may be used to identify this bifurcation.

SONOGRAPHY OF THE ABDOMINAL AORTA

The sonographic assessment of the abdominal aorta may be inhibited by gas or patient body habitus. Patient fasting can aid in evaluating the abdominal aorta with sonography. Applying transducer pressure or scanning from the left side could possibly improve visualization of the abdominal aorta in some patients as well. The normal aorta will be larger in diameter just below the diaphragm and progressively taper as it approaches the umbilicus. The aorta will also gradually be located more anteriorly in the abdomen as it travels away from the diaphragm as well.

The upper normal limit of the abdominal aorta just below the diaphragm is 2.5 cm in diameter. In the midabdomen, it will measure 2.0 cm or less, and the distal aorta should not exceed 1.8 cm. The common iliac arteries, which typically measure between 8 mm and 10 mm, are considered aneurysmal if their diameter exceeds 2.0 cm (Fig. 9-11). Normally, the

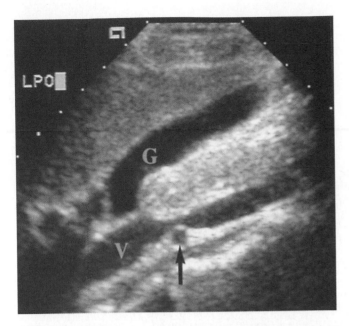

Figure 9-10 Right renal artery. Longitudinal image of the inferior vena cava (*V*) showing the right renal artery (*arrow*) crossing behind the cava. *G*, gallbladder.

the testicular or ovarian arteries. They are not generally imaged with sonography.

Inferior Mesenteric Artery

The inferior mesenteric artery (IMA) arises from the anterior surface of the abdominal aorta. It supplies blood to the transverse colon, descending colon, and rectum.

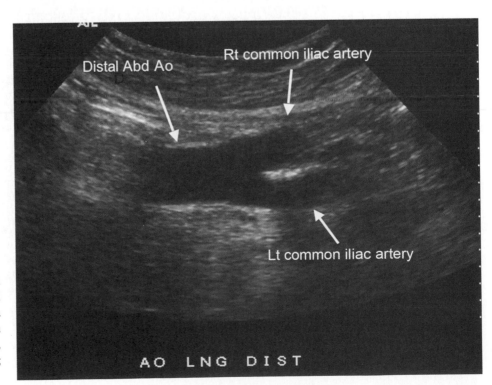

Figure 9-11 Aortic bifurcation. An image demonstrating the normal bifurcation of the abdominal aorta with both the right and left common iliac arteries visualized. Abd Ao, abdominal aorta; Rt, right; Lt, left; LNG, long; Dist, distal

spectral waveform of the proximal aorta superior to the abdominal visceral branches is considered low resistance, whereas the mid-to-distal abdominal aorta is typically high resistance. In fact, the normal spectral Doppler findings of the infrarenal aorta should show a triphasic, high-resistant flow pattern with reversal of flow in early diastole (Fig. 9-12).

> **SOUND OFF**
> Normally, the spectral waveform of the proximal aorta superior to the abdominal visceral branches is considered low resistance, whereas the distal abdominal aorta is typically high resistance.

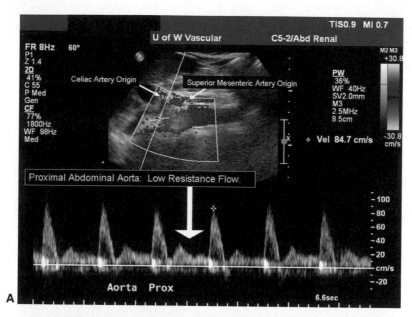

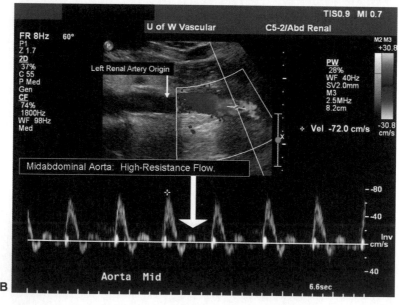

Figure 9-12 Normal abdominal aorta waveform. **A.** Duplex image demonstrates low-resistance spectral waveform in the abdominal aorta proximal to the renal artery origins. The Doppler sample volume is located at the level of the celiac and superior mesenteric artery origins. Forward flow is present throughout the cardiac cycle (*arrow*). **B.** High-resistance spectral waveform in the abdominal aorta distal to the renal artery origins. The Doppler sample volume is in the midabdominal aorta, distal to the level of the left renal artery origin. The flow pattern is triphasic with a reverse-flow component and a final brief forward-flow phase (*arrow*).

PATHOLOGY OF THE ABDOMINAL AORTA AND PSEUDOANEURYSMS

Abdominal Aortic Aneurysm

Any dilation of a blood vessel, whether focal or diffuse, is referred to as an **aneurysm** (Fig. 9-13). An aneurysm results from the weakening of the vessel wall. It can be described by the wall layers of the vessel that are affected. A **true aneurysm** involves all three layers of the vessel wall. Most **abdominal aortic aneurysms** (AAAs) are true aneurysms.

An AAA is present when the diameter of the abdominal aorta exceeds 3 cm. The most common shape of an AAA is **fusiform**. A fusiform aneurysm is one that has a gradual enlargement (Fig. 9-14). Aneurysms may also be saccular, which is described as the sudden dilation of a vessel. A **saccular aneurysm** is often spherical and can be large. Other aneurysmal shapes include berry, bulbous, eccentric, and dumbbell.

> 🔊 **SOUND OFF**
> An AAA is present when the diameter of the abdominal aorta exceeds 3 cm.

The most common location of an AAA is infrarenal. Determination of whether the renal arteries are involved in the aneurysm is vital because perfusion of the kidneys may be compromised. Distal aneurysm may also include the iliac arteries. Although the source of many AAAs is unknown, **atherosclerosis** has been cited as the most common cause of aneurysms in the United States. Aneurysms of the abdominal aorta have also been associated with **Marfan syndrome**, syphilis, familial inheritance, and infection (Fig. 9-15). An aneurysm caused by infection is referred to as a **mycotic aneurysm**. Although many patients who have an AAA have no symptoms, clinical findings may include evidence of a pulsatile abdominal mass, abdominal bruit, back pain, abdominal pain, or lower extremity pain.

Sonographically, an AAA is present when the abdominal aorta measures greater than 3 cm in diameter. The lumen may contain mural thrombus and varying amounts of calcification at the time of detection. The **true lumen** can be evaluated in contrast to the **false lumen**. The true lumen denotes the actual lumen of the aorta, including the **thrombus**, whereas the false lumen is the opening available after the narrowing from the thrombus has occurred (Fig. 9-16). Complications of an AAA include distal **embolism**, infection, dissection,

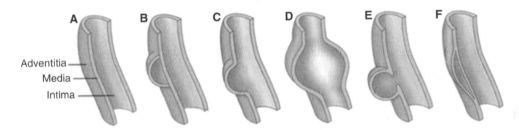

Figure 9-13 Types of abdominal aortic aneurysms. **A.** Normal artery. **B.** False aneurysm or pseudoaneurysm. **C.** True aneurysm. **D.** Fusiform aneurysm. **E.** Saccular aneurysm. **F.** Dissecting aneurysm.

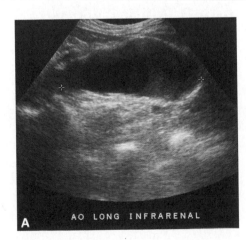
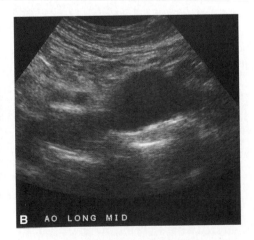

Figure 9-14 Fusiform and saccular abdominal aortic aneurysms (*AAAs*). **A.** A fusiform AAA. Notice the gradual dilation of the aorta. **B.** A saccular AAA. Notice the abrupt change in diameter from normal to enlarged.

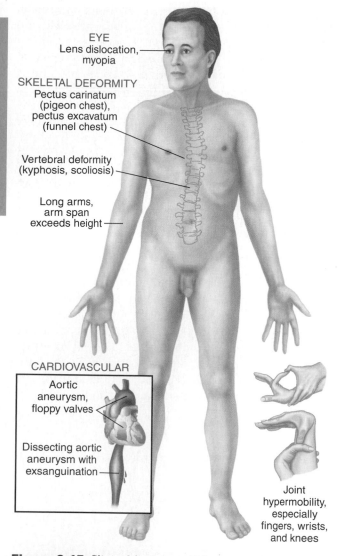

EYE
Lens dislocation, myopia

SKELETAL DEFORMITY
Pectus carinatum (pigeon chest), pectus excavatum (funnel chest)

Vertebral deformity (kyphosis, scoliosis)

Long arms, arm span exceeds height

CARDIOVASCULAR
Aortic aneurysm, floppy valves

Dissecting aortic aneurysm with exsanguination

Joint hypermobility, especially fingers, wrists, and knees

Figure 9-15 Clinical features of Marfan syndrome.

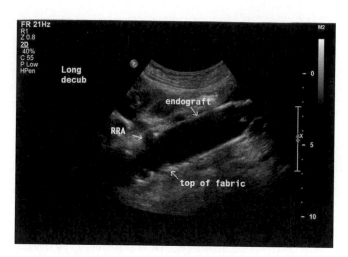

Figure 9-17 Aortic graft. The hyperechoic walls of the endograft can be seen in this image adjacent to the right renal artery (*RRA*). decub, decubitus

and rupture. The AAA may include dilation of the iliac vessels as well.

Treatment for an AAA includes open surgery and **endovascular aortic stent graft repair** (EVAR). Sonographically, an aortic graft will appear to have hyperechoic walls that are much brighter than the normal aortic walls (Fig. 9-17). The EVAR is delivered to the aorta by means of accessing the common femoral artery under angiographic guidance. The sonographic evaluation of the EVAR is for signs of patency or possibly an endoleak (Fig. 9-18). An endoleak results from the failure of the graft to isolate the aneurysm from circulation, resulting in flow disturbances and a propensity for aortic rupture. There are several types of EVAR, including a straight tube graft, bifurcated tube graft, and uni-iliac graft. Normal spectral Doppler characteristics within the graft are considered triphasic.

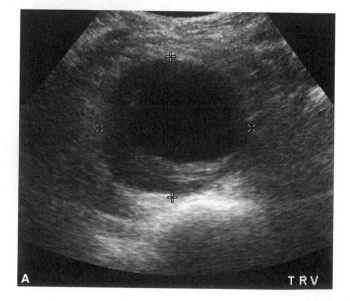

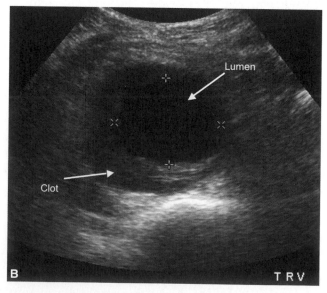

Figure 9-16 True lumen verses false lumen. **A.** Transverse abdominal aneurysm demonstrates the measurement of the entire abdominal aorta that contains notable clot within its borders (true lumen). **B.** The false lumen (between *calipers*) excludes the clot and is therefore the residual lumen.

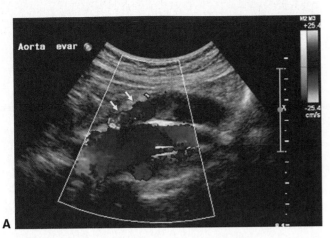
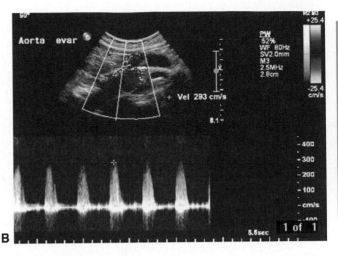

Figure 9-18 Type I endoleak at the proximal (aortic) attachment site of an endograft. **A.** Longitudinal color-flow Doppler image shows flow between the native arterial wall and endograft device into the aortic aneurysm sac (*arrows*). **B.** Doppler spectral waveform at the site of this endoleak shows a pulsatile arterial flow pattern.

CLINICAL FINDINGS OF AN ABDOMINAL AORTIC ANEURYSM

1. Pulsatile abdominal mass
2. Abdominal bruit
3. Back pain
4. Abdominal pain
5. Lower extremity pain

SONOGRAPHIC FINDINGS OF AN ABDOMINAL AORTIC ANEURYSM

1. Diameter of the abdominal aorta measures greater than 3 cm
2. Thrombus within the lumen of the aorta
3. Calcifications, along with the thrombus, may produce acoustic shadowing

Aortic Dissection

Dissection of the abdominal aorta occurs when there is a separation of the layers of the arterial wall, predominantly disturbing the intima. Clinical findings of aortic dissection include intense chest pain, hypertension, abdominal pain, lower back pain, and some neurologic symptoms. Those who have Marfan syndrome are at an increased risk for dissection. Sonographically, a linear echo flap, termed an **intimal flap**, may be noted within the aortic lumen. This flap may be visualized swaying in the current of the passing blood (Fig. 9-19). Color Doppler can be used to demonstrate flow within the layers of the dissection.

🔊 **SOUND OFF**
The sonographic visualization of an intimal flap is indicative of aortic dissection.

CLINICAL FINDINGS OF AN AORTIC DISSECTION

1. Intense chest pain
2. Hypertension
3. Abdominal pain
4. Lower back pain
5. Neurologic symptoms
6. Marfan syndrome

SONOGRAPHIC FINDINGS OF AN AORTIC DISSECTION

1. Possible AAA
2. Intimal flap may be noted within the aortic lumen

Abdominal Aortic Rupture

Rupture of the abdominal aorta has a high mortality and high morbidity rate. Specifically, aneurysms that measure greater than 7 cm in diameter are more prone to rupture. Clinical symptoms of aortic rupture include symptoms consistent with aortic aneurysms, with the addition of decreased hematocrit and hypotension. The patient may also complain of back pain, abdominal pain, lower extremity pain, and have a pulsatile abdominal mass. Sonographically, an abdominal aneurysm with an adjacent hematoma is diagnostic for aortic rupture.

CLINICAL FINDINGS OF AN AORTIC RUPTURE

1. Decreased hematocrit
2. Hypotension
3. Pulsatile abdominal mass
4. Abdominal bruit
5. Back pain
6. Abdominal pain
7. Lower extremity pain

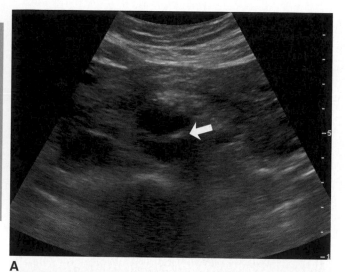

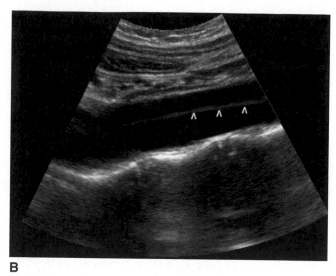

A

B

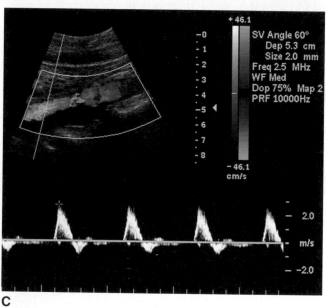

C

Figure 9-19 Dissecting aneurysm. **A.** Transverse of a dissecting aneurysm demonstrating a linear echo intimal flap (*arrow*) within the arterial lumen. **B.** On the longitudinal sonogram through the abdominal aorta, a thin linear echo flap (*carets*) is noted paralleling the anterior wall. **C.** The Doppler interrogation shows narrowing of an aorta flow with increased speed.

SONOGRAPHIC FINDINGS OF AN AORTIC RUPTURE

1. Abdominal aneurysm with an adjacent hematoma

Pseudoaneurysms

A **false aneurysm** may also be called a **pseudoaneurysm**. A pseudoaneurysm is a contained rupture of a blood vessel that is most likely secondary to the disruption of one or more layers of that vessel's wall. False aneurysms typically result from some type of injury to an artery, as seen with interventional procedures, surgery, or trauma. Pseudoaneurysms may also be associated with infection.

A common site for pseudoaneurysm development is within the groin at the level of the femoral artery following a heart catheterization. Clinical findings include a pulsatile mass in the area of the puncture location. Sonographic findings of a pseudoaneurysm include a perivascular hematoma that contains swirling blood, producing a *yin–yang* sign, and has a neck connecting it to the vessel. Color Doppler demonstration of turbulent flow within the mass can be seen as well (Fig. 9-20). The historical treatment for pseudoaneurysms consisted of prolonged compression. However, ultrasound-guided thrombin injections can also be used to treat pseudoaneurysms.

🔊 SOUND OFF
A common site for pseudoaneurysm development is within the groin at the level of the femoral artery following a heart catheterization.

Abdominal Vasculature

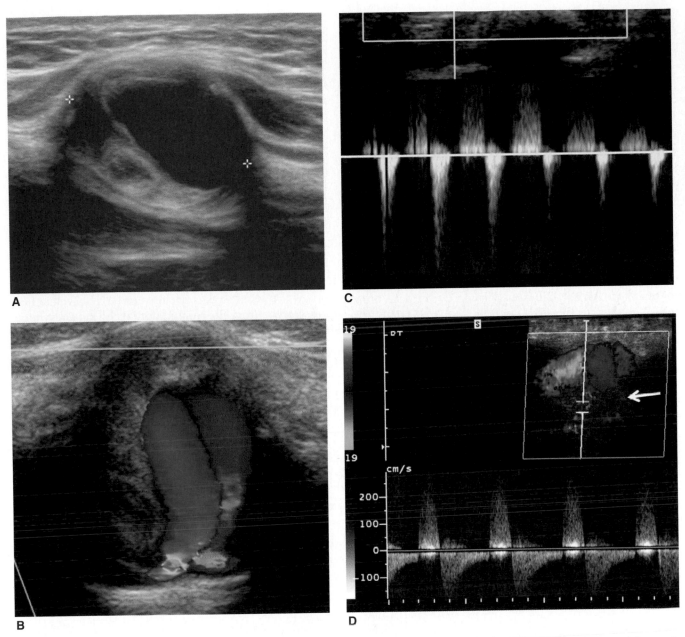

Figure 9-20 Pseudoaneurysm. Patient with a history of a femoral artery catheterization. **A.** Longitudinal scan of the groin shows a complex mass (*calipers*). **B.** Color Doppler image shows a swirling flow pattern (*yin–yang* sign) in the lumen of the pseudoaneurysm. **C.** Pulsed Doppler image shows the characteristic to-and-fro waveform. **D.** Doppler sonogram of the neck of the aneurysm in a different patient shows the to-and-fro waveform and also perivascular soft tissue vibrations (*arrow*).

CLINICAL FINDINGS OF A PSEUDOANEURYSM

1. Recent catheterization, surgical procedure, or trauma
2. Pulsatile mass in the area of the puncture location

SONOGRAPHIC FINDINGS OF A PSEUDOANEURYSM

1. Perivascular hematoma containing swirling blood (yin–yang sign) and has a neck connecting it to the vessel
2. Color Doppler demonstration of turbulent flow within the mass

ANATOMY AND PHYSIOLOGY OF THE INFERIOR VENA CAVA

The inferior vena cava (IVC) is the largest vein in the body. It is created by the union of the common iliac veins, usually near the level of the umbilicus. The wall of the IVC consists of three layers. Just like the abdominal aorta, the IVC has a tunica intima, tunica media, and tunica adventitia. However, as noted earlier, because the IVC is essentially a large vein, it has a smaller amount of smooth muscle within its tunica media compared with the abdominal aorta.

The IVC travels superiorly through the abdomen. It is considered retroperitoneal and located anterior to the spine and right lateral to the abdominal aorta (Fig. 9-21). The IVC travels through the vena caval foramen of the diaphragm and ultimately terminates in the right atrium of the heart. The IVC can be separated into four sections from superior to inferior: hepatic, prerenal, renal, and postrenal. The primary function of the IVC is to bring deoxygenated blood from the lower extremities, pelvis, and abdominal organs back to the heart.

Hepatic Veins

The most superior portion of the IVC, the segment just below the diaphragm, courses posterior to the caudate lobe of the liver and through the bare area. Within the liver, the three hepatic veins—right, middle, and left—can be seen connecting to the IVC. Variants of the hepatic veins include duplication and branching anomalies. With pulsed Doppler analysis, the hepatic veins will have a pulsatile, triphasic blood flow pattern secondary to their association with the right atrium (see Chapter 2).

The hepatic veins may become narrowed with **Budd–Chiari syndrome**. Budd–Chiari syndrome, which is further discussed in Chapter 2, is described as the occlusion of the hepatic veins with possible coexisting occlusion of the IVC. Budd–Chiari syndrome can be seen secondary to a congenital webbing disorder, coagulation abnormalities, tumor invasion from hepatocellular carcinoma, thrombosis, oral contraceptive use, pregnancy, and trauma. Enlargement of the hepatic veins and IVC is often seen with right-sided heart failure.

Renal Veins

The next main venous connections to the IVC, just below the hepatic veins, are the paired renal veins. They are derived from the termination of the smaller venous branches within the kidney and travel to the lateral aspect of the IVC. The left renal vein is much longer than the right renal vein. Its course takes it from the left renal hilum, anterior to the left renal artery and abdominal aorta, and posterior to the SMA, before entering the left side of the IVC. Compression of the left renal vein between the SMA and the abdominal aorta is referred to as the Nutcracker syndrome or renal vein entrapment syndrome (see Chapter 7). The left renal vein can also travel posterior to the aorta in some persons, which is termed a retroaortic left renal vein. The right renal vein is much shorter than the left renal vein, secondary to its

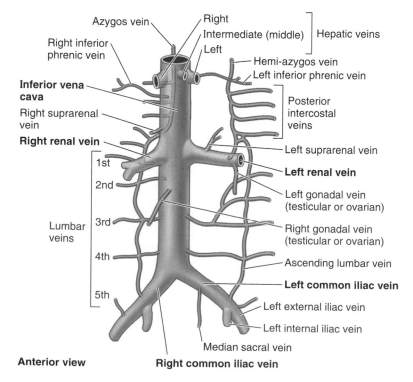

Figure 9-21 The inferior vena cava and its tributaries.

Abdominal Vasculature

proximity to the IVC. The renal veins characteristically have low-velocity, continuous flow. Pathology of the renal veins is discussed in Chapter 7.

Gonadal Veins

The gonadal veins are referred to as testicular veins in the male and ovarian veins in the female. These paired veins are different in their orientation to the IVC. The right gonadal vein connects to the anterior aspect of the IVC. Conversely, the left gonadal vein drains into the left renal vein, and is therefore much longer than the right gonadal vein.

 SOUND OFF
The left gonadal vein drains into the left renal vein, whereas right renal vein drains directly into the IVC.

Common Iliac Veins

The right and left common iliac veins combine to form the IVC near the umbilicus, typically just right of the midline.

SONOGRAPHY OF THE INFERIOR VENA CAVA

The hepatic section of the IVC can be recognized as an anechoic tube in the sagittal plane, marking the posterior border of the caudate lobe of the liver. In the transverse plane, the prerenal and renal IVC will be oval in shape and be seen to the right of the abdominal aorta. The postrenal segment of the IVC may be difficult to visualize. The size of the IVC is variable. Although its diameter should never exceed 2.5 cm, respiratory changes can alter the size of the IVC. Deep inspiration, sniffing, and the Valsalva maneuver will initially cause the IVC to collapse, whereas sustained inspiration will eventually lead to an enlargement of the IVC as blood begins to build up. The Doppler waveform of the IVC is pulsatile near the heart and more phasic near the common iliac veins.

 SOUND OFF
The diameter of the IVC should not exceed 2.5 cm.

PATHOLOGY OF THE INFERIOR VENA CAVA

Inferior Vena Cava Thrombosis and Inferior Vena Cava Filter

Thrombus may be seen within the IVC. The most common findings of IVC thrombosis are IVC enlargement, absence

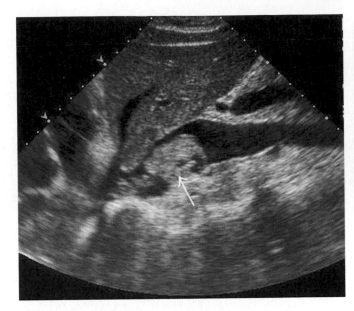

Figure 9-22 Inferior vena cava (*IVC*) thrombus. Longitudinal image of the IVC demonstrating echogenic clot (*white arrow*) within its walls.

of flow, and material noted within the IVC lumen. Acute thrombus may be completely anechoic and, therefore, may be overlooked initially. With time, thrombus will become more echogenic and may even calcify and produce acoustic shadowing (Fig. 9-22). Patients with the likelihood of having a pulmonary embolus often require the placement of an **IVC filter**, also referred to as the Greenfield inferior vena cava filter (Fig. 9-23). This filter is used to trap emboli that could be traveling upstream, potentially preventing a **pulmonary embolus**. Sonography can be used to evaluate the filter for proper placement and to assess for complications such as IVC perforation (Fig. 9-24).

Tumor Invasion of the Inferior Vena Cava

Tumor invasion of the IVC is often associated with renal cell carcinoma. The pediatric renal **Wilms tumor** and renal **transitional cell carcinoma** may also infiltrate the IVC. Tumors occupy the renal vein initially, move into the IVC, and may advance into the heart. This occurs more commonly on the right side, secondary to the short length of the right renal vein.

Enlargement of the Inferior Vena Cava

As stated earlier, the diameter of the IVC does not normally exceed 2.5 cm. Enlargement of the IVC, with subsequent enlargement of the hepatic veins, is seen in cases of right-sided heart failure. In fact, right-sided heart failure is the most common cause of IVC obstruction that leads to enlargement.

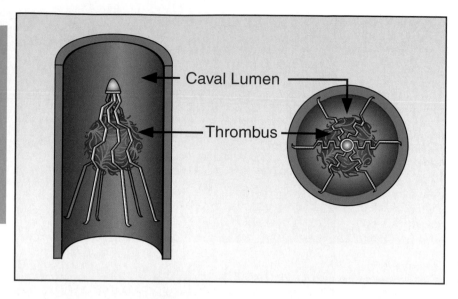

Figure 9-23 Inferior vena cava filter. The struts have hooked ends to anchor the filter to the wall of the vena cava, and the elongated, conical shape allows the filter to trap blood clots without obstructing blood flow.

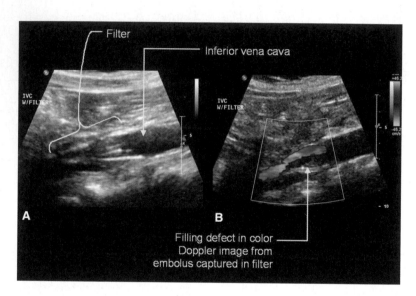

Figure 9-24 The inferior vena cava (*IVC*) can often be directly assessed, although obesity and overlying bowel gas may limit ultrasound imaging in some cases. Duplex scanning may be used to evaluate IVC patency. **A.** The presence of a conical-shaped IVC filter is apparent in this B-mode image. **B.** Color Doppler shows flow only around the periphery of the filter owing to the presence of a large captured thromboembolus in the center of the filter.

SOUND OFF
Right-sided heart failure is the most common cause of IVC enlargement.

ANATOMY AND PHYSIOLOGY OF THE PORTAL VENOUS SYSTEM

The main portal vein is created by the union of the superior mesenteric vein and splenic vein. A junction referred to as the portal splenic confluence or portal confluence is located posterior to the pancreatic neck. It consists of the splenic vein, superior mesenteric vein, and possibly the inferior mesenteric vein, although in some individuals the inferior mesenteric vein drains into the splenic vein (see Chapter 2). The confluence lies within the midabdomen and collects blood from the intestines and spleen. It is not connected directly to the IVC.

The main portal vein travels right lateral to the liver and enters the liver at the porta hepatis. From there, it branches into right and left portal veins, supplying blood to the respective lobes of the liver. Normal flow within the portal veins should be hepatopetal and monophasic, with some variation noted with respiratory changes and after meals. The diameter of the portal vein can vary with respiration, although typically it is less than 13 mm.

🔊 **SOUND OFF**
The normal flow pattern in the main portal vein is hepatopetal and monophasic, and it should not exceed 13 mm in diameter.

The splenic vein is located posterior to the pancreatic body and tail. Flow within it should be toward the midline. Other smaller vessels that contribute to the portal venous system include the inferior mesenteric vein and the coronary vein, although these are not typically seen with sonography. Pathology of the portal venous system is discussed in Chapter 2.

Arteriovenous Fistulas and Arteriovenous Malformations

The abnormal connection between an artery and vein is referred to as an arteriovenous fistula (Fig. 9-25). These may result from a simultaneous puncture of a vein and an artery. A connection between the vein and artery may be noted with color Doppler sonography. Arteriovenous fistulas can result from trauma or biopsy. Arteriovenous malformations (AVMs) are direct communications between arteries and veins as well. An AVM may be congenital or caused by surgery, malignancy, biopsy, or trauma. Turbulent flow and focal accumulation of vascular structures will often be noted in the area of an AVM.

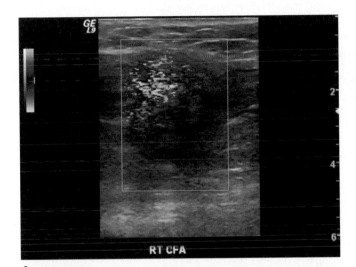

A

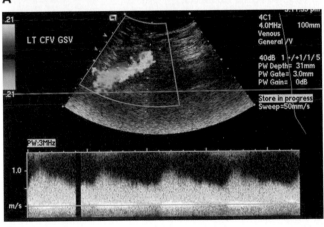

C

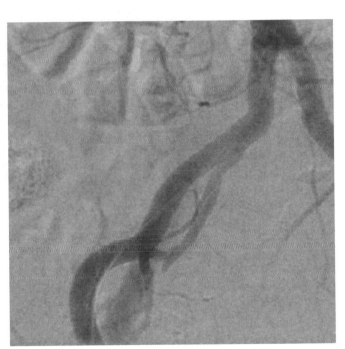

B

Figure 9-25 Arteriovenous fistula. **A.** Color bruit of a common femoral artery arteriovenous fistula. **B.** An angiography demonstrating filling of the venous system via the common femoral artery arteriovenous fistula. **C.** The arterialized Doppler signal present within the common femoral vein at the saphenofemoral junction.

REVIEW QUESTIONS

1. What is Figure 9-26 demonstrating?
   a. Yin–yang sign
   b. Corkscrew sign
   c. Milkleg sign
   d. Greenfield sign

2. What abnormality yields the sign in Figure 9-26?
   a. AAA
   b. IVC thrombus
   c. Arteriovenous fistula
   d. Pseudoaneurysm

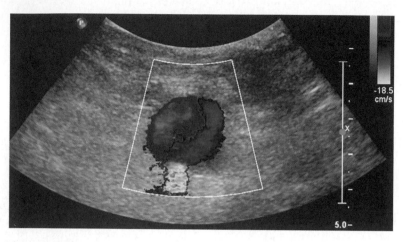

Figure 9-26

3. The IVC is located anterior and:
   a. to the left of the midline.
   b. to the right of the midline.
   c. within the midline.
   d. just left lateral to the abdominal aorta.

4. Which of the following is a common cause of a femoral artery pseudoaneurysm?
   a. Marfan syndrome
   b. Stenosis of the femoral vein
   c. Heart catheterization
   d. Abdominal aortic dissection

5. The diameter of the common iliac arteries should not exceed:
   a. 3 mm.
   b. 1 cm.
   c. 1.5 cm.
   d. 2.0 cm.

6. Which of the following abdominal aortic branches supplies blood to the transverse colon, descending colon, and rectum?
   a. Common iliac artery
   b. Superior mesenteric artery
   c. IMA
   d. Lumbar artery

7. Which of the following is true concerning the left renal vein?
   a. It is longer than the right renal vein.
   b. It passes posterior to the abdominal aorta.
   c. It enlarges as it passes between the SMA and abdominal aorta.
   d. It may be seen posterior to the inferior vena cava in some individuals.

8. The enlargement of a vessel that involves all three layers is termed a:
   a. false aneurysm.
   b. berry aneurysm.
   c. true aneurysm.
   d. saccular aneurysm.

9. Which of the following would be least likely noted sonographically secondary to its diminutive size?
   a. Splenic vein
   b. Superior mesenteric artery
   c. Left gastric artery
   d. Proper hepatic artery

10. The image in Figure 9-27 is:
    a. normal.
    b. abnormal.

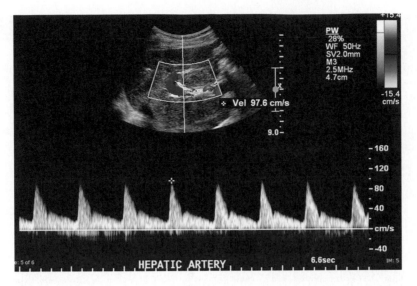

Figure 9-27

11. Which of the following would not yield a hepatopetal flow?
    a. Common hepatic artery
    b. Proper hepatic artery
    c. Main portal vein
    d. Middle hepatic vein

12. What pediatric renal tumor often invades the IVC?
    a. Nephroblastoma
    b. Morgagni tumor
    c. Hepatoblastoma
    d. Neuroblastoma

13. Nutcracker syndrome is described as the compression of the:
    a. right renal artery.
    b. left renal artery.
    c. right renal vein.
    d. left renal vein.

14. Which of the following can be noted in Figure 9-28?
    a. Dumbbell aneurysm
    b. Pseudoaneurysm
    c. Fusiform aneurysm
    d. Berry aneurysm

15. What are the findings consistent with in Figure 9-29?
    a. Fusiform aneurysm
    b. Dissecting aneurysm
    c. False aneurysm
    d. True aneurysm

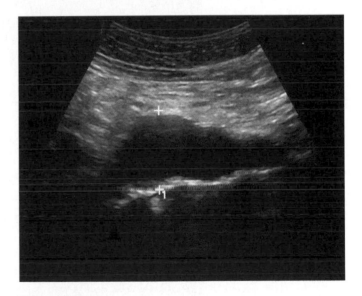

Figure 9-28

16. Which of the following is a finding noted in Figure 9-29?
    a. Intimal flap
    b. EVAR
    c. Mycotic aneurysm
    d. Tumor invasion of the abdominal aorta

17. What is the arrow in Figure 9-30 indicating?
    a. Abdominal aortic dissection
    b. IVC thrombosis
    c. Abdominal cystic dilatation
    d. Enlargement of the IVC

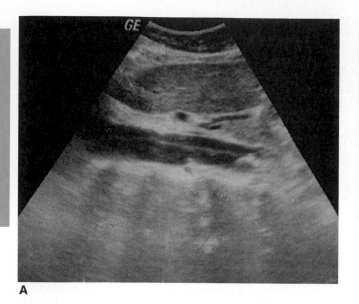

A   B

Figure 9-29

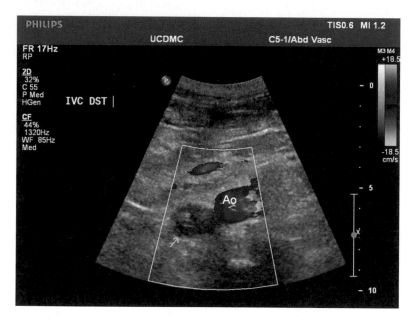

Figure 9-30

18. The right gonadal vein drains directly into the:
   a. splenic vein.
   b. IVC.
   c. right renal vein.
   d. left renal vein.

19. Which of the following section of the hepatic artery is located within the liver hilum?
   a. Inferior
   b. Medial
   c. Common
   d. Proper

20. Which vessel may be used to outline the posterior aspect of the pancreatic tail and body?
   a. Splenic vein
   b. Superior mesenteric vein
   c. Celiac artery
   d. Splenic artery

21. In the sagittal plane, you recognize a circular, anechoic vascular structure posterior to the IVC. Which of the following would this structure be most likely?
   a. Abdominal aorta
   b. Left renal vein
   c. Right renal artery
   d. SMA

22. A disorder of the connective tissue characterized by tall stature and aortic and mitral valve insufficiency is:
    a. Wilms syndrome
    b. Meckel–Gruber syndrome
    c. Marfan syndrome
    d. Kleinman syndrome

23. The inner wall layer of a vessel, closest to the passing blood, is the:
    a. tunica media.
    b. tunica intima.
    c. tunica rugae.
    d. Tunica adventitia.

24. What vessel can be often noted coursing between the SMA and the abdominal aorta in the transverse scan plane?
    a. Left renal vein
    b. Left renal artery
    c. Right renal vein
    d. Right renal artery

25. The first main visceral branch of the abdominal aorta is the:
    a. SMA.
    b. celiac artery.
    c. renal arteries.
    d. hepatic artery.

26. An aneurysm associated with infection is termed:
    a. recanalized.
    b. saccular.
    c. fusiform.
    d. mycotic.

27. Which of the following is not true about the abdominal aorta?
    a. The abdominal bifurcates into the common iliac arteries.
    b. The proximal aorta is situated more anterior than the distal aorta.
    c. The aorta has a thicker tunica media than the IVC.
    d. The third major branches of the abdominal aorta are the renal arteries.

28. All of the following are branches of the celiac axis except:
    a. right gastric artery.
    b. hepatic artery.
    c. splenic artery.
    d. left gastric artery.

29. The outer wall layer of a vessel is the:
    a. tunica media.
    b. tunica intima.
    c. tunica rugae.
    d. tunica adventitia.

30. What should the postprandial flow pattern be within the SMA?
    a. High resistance
    b. Low resistance

31. The second main branch of the abdominal aorta is the:
    a. SMA.
    b. celiac artery.
    c. renal arteries.
    d. hepatic artery.

32. Which of the following vessels show a different flow pattern after eating?
    a. Celiac artery
    b. Splenic artery
    c. Renal artery
    d. SMA

33. Which of the following vessels would most likely yield a high-resistance flow pattern?
    a. Celiac artery
    b. Common hepatic artery
    c. Renal artery
    d. Fasting SMA

34. What flow pattern would the postprandial SMA yield in small bowel ischemia?
    a. High resistance
    b. Low resistance

35. An AAA is present when the diameter of the abdominal aorta exceeds:
    a. 10 mm.
    b. 2.5 mm.
    c. 3 cm.
    d. 2 mm.

36. Occlusion of the hepatic veins describes:
    a. Marfan syndrome.
    b. Klinefelter syndrome.
    c. Morrison syndrome.
    d. Budd–Chiari syndrome.

37. The most common shape of an AAA is:
    a. saccular.
    b. bulbous.
    c. true.
    d. fusiform.

38. What branch and its tributaries of the abdominal aorta appears as a *seagull* in the transverse plane?
    a. SMA
    b. Hepatic artery
    c. Celiac artery
    d. Common iliac artery

39. Which vascular structure may be confused for the main pancreatic duct?
    a. Hepatic artery
    b. Left gastric artery
    c. SMA
    d. Splenic artery

40. The IVC terminates at the:
    a. common iliac veins.
    b. right atrium.
    c. left atrium.
    d. left ventricle.

41. A patient presents with unexplained abdominal pain for a vascular assessment of the SMA. Sonographically, you note that the patient's SMA yields a persistent high-resistive flow pattern. This is indicative of:
    a. Crohn disease.
    b. intussusception.
    c. bowel obstruction.
    d. small bowel ischemia.

42. The main portal vein is created by the union of the:
    a. splenic vein and superior mesenteric vein.
    b. superior mesenteric vein and inferior mesenteric vein.
    c. splenic vein and inferior mesenteric vein.
    d. splenic vein and gastroduodenal vein.

43. The veins seen attaching to the IVC just below the diaphragm are the:
    a. renal veins.
    b. superior mesenteric vein.
    c. hepatic veins.
    d. celiac axis.

44. The aorta originates at the:
    a. left atrium.
    b. right atrium.
    c. left ventricle.
    d. right ventricle.

45. Which of the following is not a section of the IVC?
    a. Postrenal
    b. Pancreatic
    c. Prerenal
    d. Hepatic

46. The hepatic artery should demonstrate:
    a. high-resistance flow.
    b. low-resistance flow.

47. Clinical findings of an AAA include all of the following except:
    a. lower extremity pain.
    b. back pain.
    c. abdominal bruit.
    d. elevated hematocrit.

48. An outpatient with a history of back pain and hypertension presents to the sonography department for an abdominal aortic sonogram. Sonographically, you visualize a 6 cm infrarenal aortic aneurysm with an echogenic linear structure noted gently swaying in the aortic lumen. What is the most likely diagnosis?
    a. Aortic rupture
    b. Chronic aortic aneurysm
    c. Aortic dissection
    d. Aortic rupture

49. The left gonadal vein drains directly into the:
    a. IVC.
    b. superior mesenteric vein.
    c. left renal vein.
    d. left iliac vein.

50. Which of the following would most likely yield a high-resistance flow pattern?
    a. Celiac artery
    b. Common iliac artery
    c. Splenic artery
    d. Right renal artery

51. What vessel may attach to the splenic vein before reaching the portal confluence?
    a. Left renal vein
    b. Inferior mesenteric vein
    c. Right renal vein
    d. Celiac vein

52. What vessel travels directly anterior to the left renal artery?
    a. Left renal vein
    b. Hepatic artery
    c. Right renal vein
    d. Superior mesenteric vein

53. What abnormality would the failure of an EVAR to isolate an aneurysm from circulation most likely results in?
    a. Endoleak
    b. Aortic dissection
    c. Pulmonary embolism
    d. Deep venous thrombosis

54. A patient presents to the sonography department with a history of Marfan syndrome. The sonographic evaluation reveals a linear echo within the aortic lumen that extends from the celiac axis to the iliac arteries. Color Doppler reveals flow throughout the aorta on both sides of the linear echo. The patient has had no surgeries, and there is no AAA. What does the linear echo most likely represent?
    a. Calcific thrombus
    b. Intimal flap
    c. EVAR
    d. Aortic filter

55. Which vessel would be the shortest in length?
    a. Right renal vein
    b. Right renal artery
    c. Left renal vein
    d. Left renal artery

56. Enlargement of the IVC, with subsequent enlargement of the hepatic veins, is seen in cases of:
    a. Budd–Chiari syndrome.
    b. Marfan syndrome.
    c. left-sided heart failure.
    d. right-sided heart failure.

57. Which of the following would have a pulsatile, triphasic blood flow pattern?
    a. Renal veins
    b. Hepatic veins
    c. Gonadal veins
    d. Common iliac veins

58. The diameter of the IVC should never exceed:
    a. 1.5 cm.
    b. 2.5 cm.
    c. 3.5 cm.
    d. 8 mm.

59. Which of the following statements about the IVC is not true?
    a. The diameter of the IVC is variable.
    b. Respiration can affect the size of the IVC.
    c. The IVC is located to the left of the abdominal aorta.
    d. The IVC is considered retroperitoneal in location.

60. Which of the following statements about the abdominal aorta is not true?
    a. Most aneurysms located within the abdominal aorta are false aneurysms.
    b. The abdominal aorta is located just left of the midline.
    c. The most common location of an AAA is infrarenal.
    d. The abdominal aorta is considered to be retroperitoneal in location.

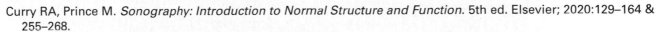

SUGGESTED READINGS

Curry RA, Prince M. *Sonography: Introduction to Normal Structure and Function.* 5th ed. Elsevier; 2020:129–164 & 255–268.

Hagen-Ansert SL. *Textbook of Diagnostic Sonography.* 7th ed. Elsevier; 2012:165–204.

Henningsen C, Kuntz K, Youngs D. *Clinical Guide to Sonography: Exercises for Critical Thinking.* 2nd ed. Elsevier; 2014:113–122.

Hertzberg BS, Middleton WD. *Ultrasound: The Requisites.* 3rd ed. Elsevier; 2016:218–227.

Kawamura DM, Nolan TD. *Diagnostic Medical Sonography: Abdomen and Superficial Structures.* 4th ed. Wolters Kluwer; 2018:59–100.

Kupinski AM. *Diagnostic Medical Sonography: The Vascular System.* Lippincott Williams & Wilkins; 2013:1–34 & 277–344.

Radiology Key (PSV ranges). Accessed October 9, 2021, from https://radiologykey.com/anatomy-and-normal-doppler-signatures-of-abdominal-vessels-3/

Rumack CM, Wilson SR, Charboneau JW, et al. *Diagnostic Ultrasound.* 4th ed. Elsevier; 2011:447–485.

Sanders RC, Hall-Terracciano B. *Clinical Sonography: A Practical Guide.* 5th ed. Wolters Kluwer; 2016:381–389, 488–494, & 536–538.

Zweibel W, Pellerito J. *Introduction to Vascular Ultrasonography.* 5th ed. Elsevier Saunders; 2005:513–552.

BONUS REVIEW!

Nutcracker Syndrome with Duplex Sonography (Fig. 9-31)

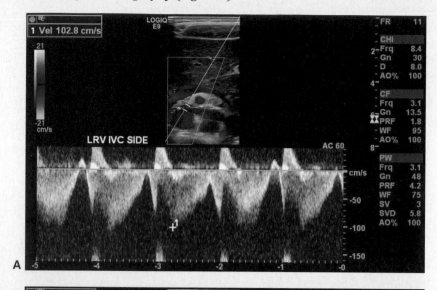

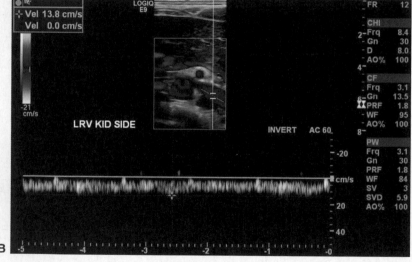

Figure 9-31 Nutcracker syndrome. Peak left renal vein velocities are measured (**A**) at the point of compression beneath the superior mesenteric artery and (**B**) in the proximal renal vein (kidney side). A velocity ratio greater than 5 is suggestive of aortomesenteric compression (nutcracker syndrome). In this case, the velocity ratio is 102.8/13.8 = 7.45. LRV, left renal vein; IVC, inferior vena cava; KID, kidney

BONUS REVIEW! (*continued*)

MRI Coronal View of a Tortuous Abdominal Aortic Aneurysm (Fig. 9-32)

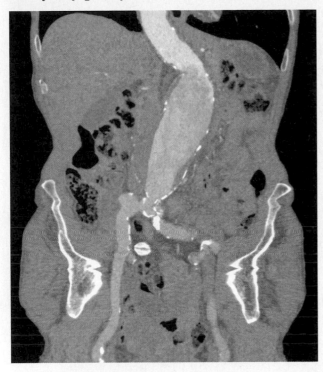

Figure 9-32 Magnetic resonance imaging coronal view of a tortuous abdominal aortic aneurysm.

Aortic Dissection on MRI (Fig. 9-33)

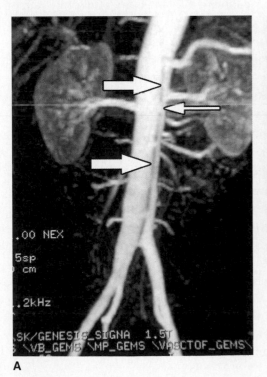

A

Aortic Occlusion on CT (Fig. 9-34)

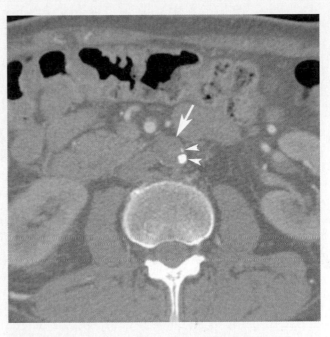

Figure 9-34 Aortic occlusion on computed tomography (*CT*). Coned view of the abdominal aorta at the level of the kidneys on axial slice from abdominal CT demonstrates complete occlusion of the infrarenal abdominal aorta (*arrow*). Foci of atherosclerotic calcification are noted (*arrowheads*).

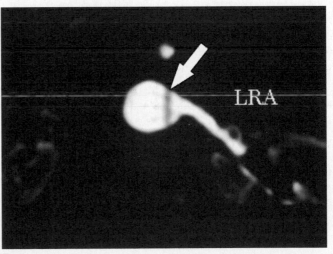

B

Figure 9-33. Aortic dissection on magnetic resonance imaging. **A.** Maximum intensity projection image from three-dimensional gadolinium-enhanced magnetic resonance imaging (MRA) of abdominal aorta shows dissection flap (*arrows*). **B.** Flap (*arrow*) is clearly demonstrated on axial reformation at level of left renal artery. LRA, left renal artery

The Gastrointestinal Tract and Abdominal Wall

Introduction

Although sonography may not always be the modality of choice for the detection of all gastrointestinal abnormalities, it does provide a noninvasive, nonionizing diagnostic instrument. This chapter provides an overview of gastrointestinal structures often analyzed with sonography. It also discusses abnormalities of the abdominal wall. The "Bonus Review" section includes radiographic images of pyloric stenosis and diverticulitis and computed tomography (CT) images of appendicitis and intussusception.

Key Terms

acute appendicitis—inflammation of the appendix

adenocarcinoma—cancer originating in glandular tissue

appendicolith—a dense, calcified stone within the appendix

autoimmune disorder—a disorder in which the immune system attacks normal tissue

bezoars—masses of various ingested materials that may cause an intestinal obstruction

cervix sign—a sonographic sign associated with pyloric stenosis in the long axis

cinnamon-bun sign—a sonographic sign associated with the appearance of intussusception

compression sonography—operator-applied transducer pressure on a structure during a sonographic examination

Crohn disease—an autoimmune disease characterized by periods of inflammation of the gastrointestinal tract

direct groin hernia—acquired inguinal hernia; result from the weakening of the transversalis fascia

diverticulitis—the inflammation of a diverticulum or multiple diverticuli within the digestive tract, most often in the sigmoid colon

diverticulosis—the development of small outpouchings termed diverticuli in the digestive tract, most often in the sigmoid colon

doughnut sign—a sonographic sign associated with pyloric stenosis in the short axis

duodenal bulb—the proximal portion of the duodenum closest to the stomach

endometriosis—functional endometrial tissue located outside the uterus

fecalith—a stone that consists of feces

gastroesophageal junction—the junction between the stomach and the esophagus

gastroesophageal reflux—an abnormality in which fluid is allowed to reflux out of the stomach back into the esophagus

hypertrophic pyloric stenosis—a defect in the relaxation of the pyloric sphincter that leads to the enlargement of the pyloric muscles and closure of the pyloric sphincter

indirect groin hernia—occurs when the abdominal contents protrude through the deep inguinal ring, lateral to the inferior epigastric vessels and anterior to the spermatic or round ligament

inflammatory bowel disease—chronic inflammation of the gastrointestinal tract; used as an umbrella term for both Crohn disease and ulcerative colitis

intussusception—the telescoping of one segment of bowel into another; most often the proximal segment of the bowel inserts into the distal segment

intussusceptum—the proximal segment of the bowel with intussusception

intussuscipiens—the distal segment of the bowel with intussusception

invaginate—to insert

keyboard sign—sign of small bowel obstruction representing the plicae circulares surrounded by fluid within distended loops of bowel

lactobezoar—a bezoar that consists of powdered milk

McBurney point—a point halfway between the anterior superior iliac spine and the umbilicus; the area of pain and rebound tenderness in patients suffering from acute appendicitis

mechanical obstruction—a situation in which bowel is physically blocked by something

Meckel diverticulum—a common congenital outpouching of the wall of the small intestine

melanoma—a malignant form of cancer found most often on the skin

midgut malrotation—abnormal rotation of the bowel that leads to a proximal small bowel obstruction

nonbilious—not containing bile

nonmechanical obstruction—a situation in which bowel is blocked because of the lack of normal peristalsis of a bowel segment or segments; also referred to as a paralytic ileus

olive sign—when the pyloric sphincter muscle is enlarged and palpable on physical examination of the abdomen; often indicative of pyloric stenosis

paralytic ileus—see key term nonmechanical obstruction

perienteric fat—fat around the intestines

peristalsis—contractions that move in a wavelike pattern to propel a substance

plicae circulares—the mucus membrane folds within the inner wall of the small bowel

projectile vomiting—vomiting with so much force that the vomit can travel for quite a distance

phytobezoars—a bezoar that consists of vegetable matter

pseudomyxoma peritonei—an intraperitoneal extension of mucin-secreting cells that result from the rupture of a malignant mucinous ovarian tumor or possibly a malignant tumor of the appendix

pylorospasm—a temporary spasm and thickening of the pyloric sphincter that can replicate the sonographic appearance of pyloric stenosis

rebound tenderness—pain encountered after the removal of pressure; a common clinical finding in patients suffering from acute appendicitis

red currant jelly stool—feces that contains a mixture of mucus and blood; a common clinical finding in patients suffering from intussusception

Rovsing sign—pain elicited in the right lower quadrant after the left lower quadrant has been palpated; associated with appendicitis

thyroid in the belly sign—the sonographic appearance of the hyperechoic edematous connective tissue that surrounds the inflamed appendix

trichobezoars—a bezoar that consists of matted hair

Valsalva technique—performed by attempting to forcibly exhale while keeping the mouth and nose closed

vermiform appendix—a blind-ended tube that is connected to the cecum of the colon

volvulus—a situation in which a loop of bowel twists upon itself

ANATOMY OF THE GASTROINTESTINAL TRACT

The gastrointestinal tract, or alimentary canal, consists of the mouth, pharynx, esophagus, stomach, the small intestines, and colon (Fig. 10-1). The mouth is the most proximal portion of the gastrointestinal tract. The pharynx lies distal to the mouth and unites it to the esophagus. The esophagus travels inferiorly within the thorax and through an opening in the diaphragm called the esophageal hiatus. The distal esophagus attaches to the stomach. This area, the **gastroesophageal junction**, can be identified with sonography and will appear as a bull's-eye structure between the left lobe of the liver and the abdominal aorta in the sagittal imaging plane (Fig. 10-2).

After the cecum, the colon is termed the *ascending colon* as it travels superiorly toward the liver, within the right side of the abdomen. A bend in the colon, the hepatic flexure or right colic flexure, marks the beginning of the transverse colon, which travels across the abdomen. Another bend, the splenic flexure or left colic flexure, located inferior to the spleen, marks the beginning of the descending colon, which is located within the left side of the abdomen. The colon travels inferiorly and becomes the sigmoid colon and subsequently the rectum. The anus, the external opening of the rectum, marks the termination point of the alimentary canal. Most gastrointestinal tract parts are considered intraperitoneal, with the exception of the duodenum and ascending and descending colon, which are regarded as retroperitoneal in location.

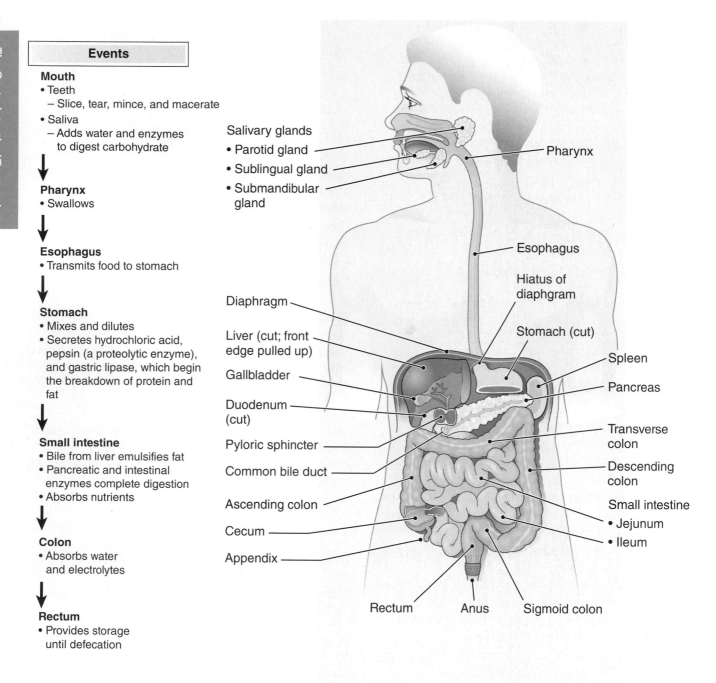

Events

Mouth
- Teeth
  - Slice, tear, mince, and macerate
- Saliva
  - Adds water and enzymes to digest carbohydrate

↓

Pharynx
- Swallows

↓

Esophagus
- Transmits food to stomach

↓

Stomach
- Mixes and dilutes
- Secretes hydrochloric acid, pepsin (a proteolytic enzyme), and gastric lipase, which begin the breakdown of protein and fat

↓

Small intestine
- Bile from liver emulsifies fat
- Pancreatic and intestinal enzymes complete digestion
- Absorbs nutrients

↓

Colon
- Absorbs water and electrolytes

↓

Rectum
- Provides storage until defecation

Salivary glands
- Parotid gland
- Sublingual gland
- Submandibular gland

Pharynx

Esophagus

Hiatus of diaphgram

Diaphragm

Liver (cut; front edge pulled up)

Stomach (cut)

Spleen

Gallbladder

Pancreas

Duodenum (cut)

Transverse colon

Pyloric sphincter

Descending colon

Common bile duct

Small intestine
- Jejunum
- Ileum

Ascending colon

Cecum

Appendix

Rectum   Anus   Sigmoid colon

Figure 10-1 Anatomy and events of the gastrointestinal tract.

SONOGRAPHY OF THE GASTROINTESTINAL TRACT

Sonography of the gastrointestinal tract may be indicated in the setting of several clinical conditions, including **hypertrophic pyloric stenosis** (HPS), **intussusception**, and **acute appendicitis**. Most gastrointestinal tract sonographic studies are performed using a high-frequency linear-array transducer, although some studies may require a curved-array transducer. Though scanning for specific gastrointestinal pathology is often regional, scanning for possible small bowel and colon pathology, such as bowel obstructions, may be performed via the global view. The global or panoramic view includes an assessment of the abdominal cavity from the bottom up, using vertical probe movements, starting from the right iliac fossa, followed by horizontal movements from the right to the left. During the examination, normal "gut signature" should be noted with sonography. The gastrointestinal tract consists of

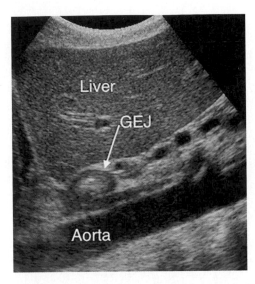

Figure 10-2 Gastroesophageal junction (*GEJ*). The GEJ can be noted in the sagittal plane posterior to the left lobe of the liver and anterior to the abdominal aorta.

TABLE 10-1 Layers of the gut identified with sonography and their associated echogenicities

Layers of Gut Identified with Sonography	Echogenicity
Superficial mucosa (innermost layer)	Echogenic
Deep mucosa	Hypoechoic
Submucosa (muscularis propria interface)	Echogenic
Muscularis propria	Hypoechoic
Serosa (outermost layer)	Echogenic

five histologic layers that sonographically appear as alternating echogenic and hypoechoic segments (Table 10-1; Fig. 10-3). However, not all of these are consistently identified with sonography. The alternating echogenicities of the bowel wall layers should produce the classic "target" or "bull's-eye" appearance.

The stomach consists of a fundus, body, and pyloric region. Within the distal stomach lies the pyloric sphincter, a muscle that controls the emptying of the contents of the stomach into the duodenum. The proximal duodenum is C-shaped; thus, it is referred to as the C-loop of the duodenum. Distal to the duodenum are the jejunum and ileum of the small intestines. The ileum meets the cecum, or proximal colon, at the ileocecal valve within the right lower quadrant of the abdomen. At this level, a blind-ended tube, the **vermiform appendix**, is connected to the cecum.

A sonographic examination of much of the gastrointestinal tract should include graded compression or **compression sonography** to differentiate normal from anomalous bowel. Specifically, normal bowel should be compressible and should have observable **peristalsis**. Compression of the bowel will also move intraluminal

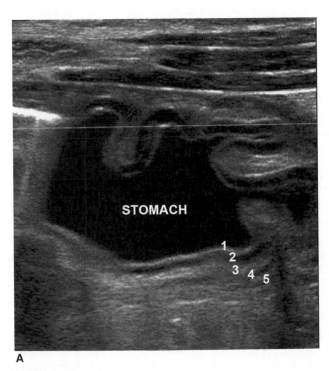

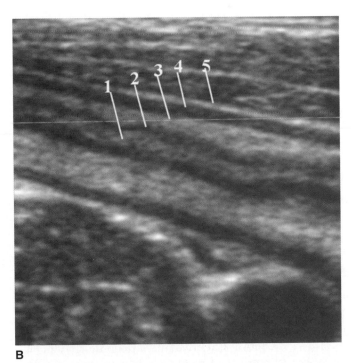

Figure 10-3 Gut signature. **A** and **B.** *1*, Echogenic superficial mucosa. *2*, Hypoechoic deep (muscularis) mucosa. *3*, Echogenic submucosa. *4*, Hypoechoic muscularis propria. *5*, Echogenic serosa.

fluid and/or gas out of the area of interest, which aids in the visualization of pathology. In addition, the wall of the involved bowel segment(s) should be closely analyzed. Generally, the normal small bowel wall thickness is between 1.5 and 3 mm in thickness, with small bowel distention defined as 2.5 cm or greater from outer wall to outer wall. The colon wall should measure between 4 and 9 mm in thickness in the nondistended state. *Colon distention* has been defined as the diameter of a segment that exceeds 6 cm. The bowel walls should appear thin in the distended state. Wall thickness should be measured from the central hyperechoic lumen to the outer hyperechoic margin.

A normal bowel wall segment produces little to no color Doppler. Consequently, color Doppler can be beneficial because inflammatory changes and neoplasms within the gastrointestinal tract will often reveal evidence of hyperemia. In addition, transvaginal imaging has proven to be useful in identifying the inflamed appendix in some women and may also prove valuable for analyzing the rectum and sigmoid colon for irregularities. Although rarely used, a water enema technique can be integrated during the examination to assess the rectum and sigmoid colon for suspected pathology.

> ### 🔊 SOUND OFF
> Sonography utilizes compression to analyze bowel. In many situations, normal bowel is compressible, whereas abnormal bowel is noncompressible.

GASTROINTESTINAL PATHOLOGY

Acute Appendicitis

The appendix, or vermiform appendix, is a long, narrow, blind-ended tube. Although its location may be variable, it is commonly located within the right lower quadrant, at the level of the cecum. Appendicitis, inflammation of the appendix, has been cited as the most common cause of acute abdominal pain, resulting in surgery.

Acute appendicitis may be the result of some form of obstructive process, such as an **appendicolith**, **fecalith**, lymph node, tumor, foreign body, seeds, or parasite. Clinically, patients may present with a history of epigastric pain, periumbilical pain, or general abdominal pain that, with time, is eventually restricted to the right lower quadrant or directly over the inflamed appendix. Patients will also suffer from **rebound tenderness** over the **McBurney point** in the right lower quadrant, which is referred to as McBurney sign (Fig. 10-4). **Rovsing sign** may also be present with acute appendicitis, and is explained as pain elicited in the right lower quadrant when the left lower quadrant is palpated. Therefore, if

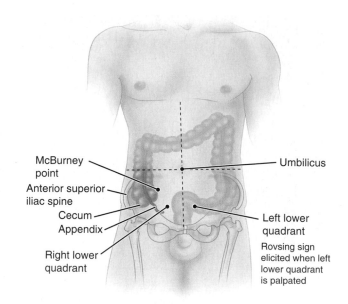

Figure 10-4 McBurney sign. Pain and tenderness over McBurney point (under the middle finger on this drawing) is associated with acute appendicitis. The point is located about 2 inches from the right anterior superior iliac spine, on a line between the iliac spine and the umbilicus. Pain at this point is referred to as McBurney sign.

possible, it is helpful to have the patient point to the most painful region. Laboratory tests, such as white blood cell count, are helpful as well because many patients with acute appendicitis will have evidence of leukocytosis.

> ### 🔊 SOUND OFF
> Patients with appendicitis will suffer from rebound tenderness over the McBurney point in the right lower quadrant.

Graded compression is used to sonographically investigate the abdomen for signs of appendicitis. The inflamed appendix will appear as a noncompressible, blind-ended tube that measures more than 6 mm in diameter (Fig. 10-5). This measurement is taken from outer wall to outer wall. Careful exploration is further warranted for the presence of an obstructive etiology, such as an appendicolith. An appendicolith will appear as an echogenic, shadowing structure within the lumen of the appendix. There may also be evidence of a periappendiceal fluid collection, fat stranding around the appendix, and hyperemic flow within the wall of the irritated appendix. The **thyroid in the belly** sign has been used to describe the sonographic appearance of the hyperechoic edematous connective tissue that surrounds the inflamed appendix because

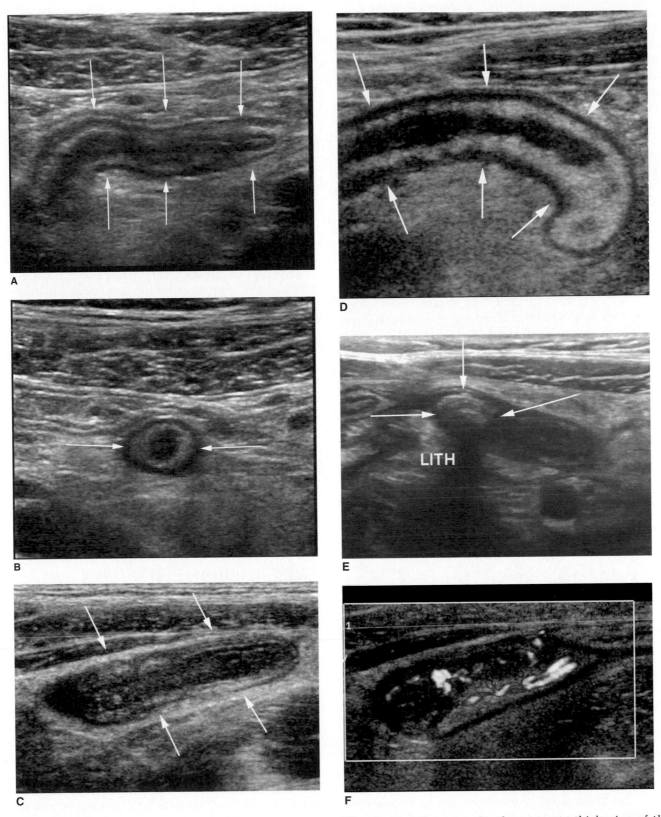

Figure 10-5 Appendicitis. Longitudinal (**A**) and transverse (**B**) images of the appendix demonstrate thickening of the wall (*arrows*) consistent with appendicitis. **C** and **D**. Longitudinal images of two different patients with a dilated, inflamed appendix (between *arrows*), with a thickened wall and dilatation of the appendiceal lumen. **E**. Longitudinal image of an inflamed appendix containing an echogenic appendicolith (*arrows*). **F**. Longitudinal image demonstrates hyperemia within an inflamed appendix consistent with appendicitis. Lith, appendicolith

the echogenicity of this tissue appears much like that of the normal thyroid. Complications of appendicitis include perforation, peritonitis, abscess formation, and, possibly, even death. A normal appendix may be perceived sonographically, especially in children and thin patients, and therefore, a comprehensive assessment, which includes both clinical findings and sonographic criteria, should be performed.

> ### 🔊)) SOUND OFF
> Appendicitis is indicative when inflamed appendix is noncompressible and measures greater than 6 mm. Occasionally, an appendicolith will be identified within the abnormal appendix.

CLINICAL FINDINGS OF ACUTE APPENDICITIS

1. Initial epigastric or general abdominal pain that, with time, is eventually restricted to the right lower quadrant or over the inflamed appendix
2. Acute abdominal pain
3. Rebound tenderness (McBurney sign)
4. Nausea and vomiting
5. Possible leukocytosis
6. High fever (with abscess formation)
7. Rovsing sign

SONOGRAPHIC FINDINGS OF ACUTE APPENDICITIS

1. Noncompressible, blind-ended tube that measures more than 6 mm in diameter from outer wall to outer wall
2. Echogenic structure within the lumen of the appendix (appendicolith)
3. Hyperemic flow within the wall of the inflamed appendix
4. Periappendiceal fluid collection

Hypertrophic Pyloric Stenosis

The pylorus is the distal region of the stomach. The pyloric channel is located at the distal portion of the pylorus, between the stomach and the proximal **duodenal bulb**. In this region, a group of muscles, called the pyloric sphincter, controls gastric emptying and prevents undigested food products, or chyme, from refluxing back into the stomach from the duodenum. HPS is a defect in the relaxation of the pyloric sphincter. This leads to the enlargement, or hypertrophy, of the

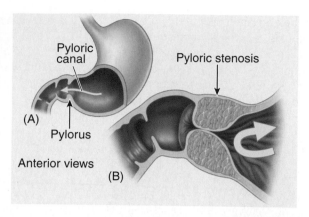

Figure 10-6 Pyloric stenosis. **A.** Normally fluid and food products are allowed to travel freely through the pyloric canal (*arrow*) and into the proximal duodenum. **B.** With pyloric stenosis, the pyloric sphincter muscles are thickened and produce a gastric outlet obstruction, preventing the fluid and food products from exiting the stomach.

pyloric muscles, effectively causing a persistent closure of the pyloric sphincter. Ultimately, HPS causes a gastric outlet obstruction (Fig. 10-6).

Although HPS can occur in adults, it is most commonly encountered in infants between 2 and 6 weeks old. First-born, white male infants are more likely to suffer from HPS. The patient with HPS often presents clinically with **nonbilious**, **projectile vomiting**, dehydration, weight loss, constipation, and an insatiable appetite. The enlarged pyloric muscle may be palpable during a physical examination of an infant with pyloric stenosis. This is referred to as the **olive sign**.

> ### 🔊)) SOUND OFF
> The clinical finding where the enlarged pyloric muscle can be palpated is referred to as the olive sign.

In the past, the customary diagnostic modality used to evaluate infants with clinical findings consistent with pyloric stenosis was radiography. Now, sonography has become the modality of choice. To examine the pyloric region of the stomach, the infant is placed in the right lateral decubitus position. If the stomach is completely empty, a small amount of glucose solution may be given to the infant to drink to better visualize the pylorus. However, care should be taken to not over distend the stomach with fluid, because this may prevent adequate visualization of the pylorus.

In the longitudinal plane, the pylorus will be noted within the epigastrium, slightly right of the midline, near the gallbladder. The pylorus is normally positioned transversely in the abdomen. Thus, a longitudinal image of the abdomen will often yield a short-axis image of the stenosis, whereas a transverse image of the abdomen will often yield a long-axis image of the stenosis. The abnormal pylorus appears as a "target" or "doughnut" (**doughnut sign**) in the short axis and as a cervix (**cervix sign**) in the long axis (Figs. 10-7 and 10-8). If pyloric stenosis is present, the wall of the pyloric muscle will measure 3 mm or greater in thickness, whereas the length of the abnormal pyloric channel will measure 17 mm or greater. It is important to note that the thickness of the muscle appears to be the more specific sonographic measurement. Furthermore, with real-time sonography, the fluid will be noted to initially collect within the pyloric antrum and then as peristalsis moves the fluid toward the sphincter, the sphincter will open. The sonographer should observe the fluid traveling from the pylorus into the duodenum. This dynamic

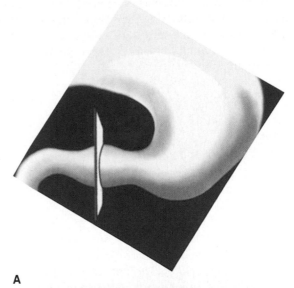

A

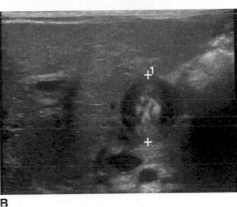

B

Figure 10-8 Transverse pyloric stenosis. **A.** Transverse view of the pylorus is often accomplished with a longitudinal abdominal image. **B.** Transverse sonogram of an enlarged pyloric sphincter (between *plus signs*).

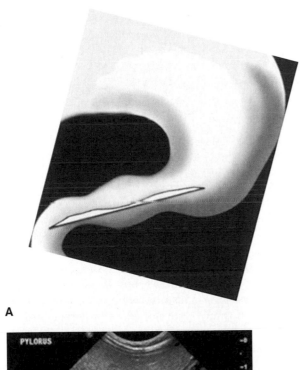

A

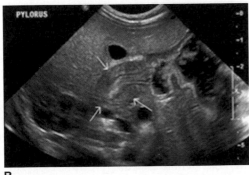

B

Figure 10-7 Longitudinal pyloric stenosis. **A.** Longitudinal view of the pylorus is often accomplished with a transverse abdominal image. **B.** Longitudinal sonogram of an enlarged pyloric sphincter (between *arrows*).

mechanism should be noted during the examination to eliminate the diagnosis of pyloric stenosis.

> **🔊 SOUND OFF**
> The pylorus is transversely oriented within the abdomen. Therefore, pyloric stenosis yields a cervix appearance when the transducer is placed transverse to the abdomen, whereas in the longitudinal plane to the abdomen, the enlarged pylorus yields a doughnut appearance.

Three additional causes of nonbilious vomiting in the infant are **pylorospasm**, **gastroesophageal reflux**, and malrotation of the midgut. These abnormalities should be excluded in those patients who present with clinical findings consistent with pyloric stenosis.

Pylorospasm is a common cause of delayed gastric opening as well. Unlike HPS, the measurements tend to be within normal limits, and eventually, during follow-up examinations, some fluid is noted traveling through the pyloric channel.

> ### 🔊 SOUND OFF
> The abnormal pyloric channel will measure greater than 17 mm in length, and the muscle will measure greater than 3 mm.

Gastroesophageal reflux is another cause of nonbilious projectile vomiting in the infant. Sonography can be used to evaluate infants for gastroesophageal reflux. For this examination, a transverse section of the gastroesophageal junction can be obtained in most persons posterior to the left lobe of the liver and anterior to the abdominal aorta in the sagittal scan plane of the abdomen. After identifying the gastroesophageal junction, the transducer is manipulated to obtain a longitudinal image of the esophagus. Fluid mixed with gas bubbles can be observed traveling retrograde up the esophagus in cases of gastroesophageal reflux.

Midgut malrotation, with or without **volvulus**, has a presentation that is clinically similar to that of HPS, although patients most often suffer from bilious vomiting rather than nonbilious vomiting as seen with HPS. With malrotation, the small bowel mesentery rotates around the superior mesenteric artery (SMA). The sonographic diagnosis of malrotation is confirmed by identifying the relationship of the SMA with the superior mesenteric vein (SMV). The SMA is typically located to the left of the SMV. With malrotation, the position of the two vessels will be reversed. With color Doppler, a whirlpool appearance of the vasculature may be noted (Fig. 10-9). An upper gastrointestinal radiographic series is typically used to verify the diagnosis of malrotation.

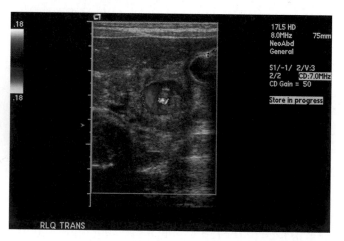

Figure 10-9 Color Doppler of whirlpool appearance of the circumferential orientation of superior mesenteric vein around the superior mesenteric artery in an infant with intestinal malrotation and midgut volvulus.

> ### CLINICAL FINDINGS OF PYLORIC STENOSIS
> 1. First-born (white) male infant (most often)
> 2. Nonbilious, projectile vomiting
> 3. Weight loss
> 4. Constipation
> 5. Dehydration
> 6. Insatiable appetite
> 7. Palpable olive sign

> ### SONOGRAPHIC FINDINGS OF PYLORIC STENOSIS
> 1. Abnormal pylorus appears as a target or doughnut in the short-axis view
> 2. Abnormal pylorus appears as a cervix in the long-axis view
> 3. Wall of pylorus will measure 3 mm or greater in thickness
> 4. Length of pyloric channel will measure 17 mm or greater

Intussusception

Sonography has become the modality of choice for evaluating pediatric patients with clinical symptoms suggestive of intussusception. Intussusception is the telescoping of one segment of bowel into another (Fig. 10-10). Specifically, the **intussusceptum**, the proximal portion of the bowel, is allowed to **invaginate** into the next distal segment, the **intussuscipiens**. The most common type of intussusception, the ileocolic intussusception, occurs within the right lower quadrant at the level of the ileocecal valve. Intussusception, which is often idiopathic, occurs more often in male patients, and it has been cited as the most common cause of intestinal obstructions in children less than 2 years of age. Conversely, it rarely occurs in those under 3 months and over 3 years of age. In patients older than 2 years, there may be a lead point. This lead point may be an intestinal polyp, **Meckel diverticulum**, lymphoma, or intraluminal hematoma. In adults, intussusception can be caused by a neoplasm.

Clinically, patients present with intermittent, severe abdominal pain, vomiting, and a palpable abdominal mass. Their stool often contains a mixture of blood and mucus. This is referred to as a **red currant jelly stool**, and it is a hallmark clinical finding of intussusception. Laboratory tests may reveal anemia, dehydration, and/or leukocytosis as well.

> ### 🔊 SOUND OFF
> A key clinical finding of intussusception is red currant jelly stool.

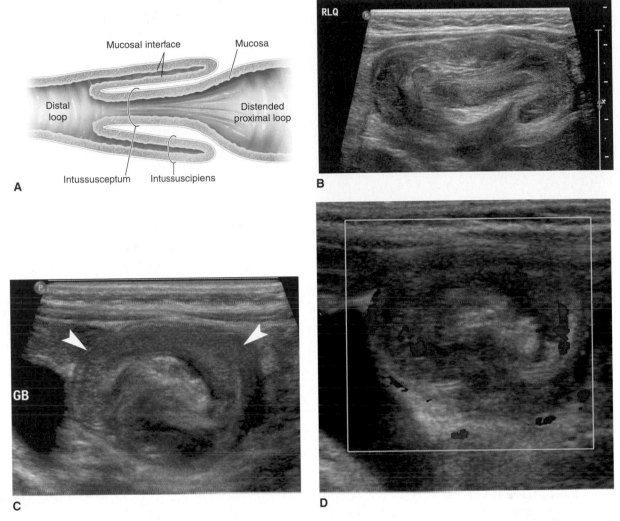

Figure 10-10 Diagram of intussusception. **A.** Longitudinal diagram of intussusception. **B.** Longitudinal sonogram of an intussusception revealing the "pseudokidney" sign. **C.** Transverse diagram of intussusception (*arrowheads*). **D.** Transverse sonogram of intussusception with color Doppler employed. RLQ, right lower quadrant, *GB*, gallbladder.

Graded compression sonography should be used to evaluate the pediatric patient who has clinical findings suspicious for intussusception. With sonography, an intussusception will appear as a "target" mass in the transverse plane or a "pseudokidney" in the longitudinal plane to the mass. The intussusception will have alternating rings of echogenicity representing the edematous layers of the bowel wall. Therefore, intussusception may also resemble a **cinnamon-bun sign** in the transverse plane as a result of the alternating echogenicity and the elliptical shape of the mass. The intussusception will also maintain its shape when compression is applied. The diameter of the intussuscepted bowel will exceed 3 cm.

This condition can lead to ischemia and gangrene of the bowel. Consequently, color Doppler may be utilized to determine whether blood flow is present within the intussusception (Fig. 10-11). Flow is often present within the bowel wall with higher gain settings. If gangrene is suspected, surgical intervention is warranted. However,

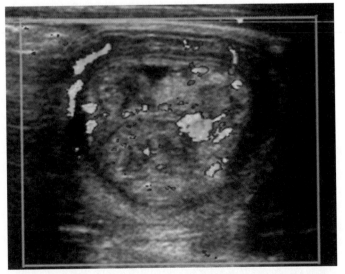

Figure 10-11 Intussusception. Color Doppler sonogram shows flow in the intussuscepted loop of bowel. This intussusception was reduced by air-contrast enema.

treatment for intussusception is typically by means of a therapeutic enema via radiography or hydrostatic reduction. Sonographic reduction has been performed with some success.

CLINICAL FINDINGS OF INTUSSUSCEPTION

1. Intermittent, severe abdominal pain
2. Vomiting
3. Palpable abdominal mass
4. Red currant jelly stools
5. Leukocytosis

SONOGRAPHIC FINDINGS OF INTUSSUSCEPTION

1. Noncompressible, target-shaped or pseudokidney-shaped mass that consists of alternating rings of echogenicity (cinnamon-bun sign)
2. The diameter of the intussuscepted bowel will exceed 3 cm

Intestinal Obstruction

Although sonography is not typically the diagnostic modality of choice, an intestinal or a bowel obstruction may be incidentally noted during a sonographic examination of the abdomen. Patients with bowel obstructions can present with abdominal distention, intermittent abdominal pain, constipation, and nausea and vomiting. There are two types of intestinal obstructions: mechanical and nonmechanical. A **mechanical obstruction** results from the bowel being physically blocked by something, including adhesions, volvulus, herniations, intussusception, tumors, and **inflammatory bowel disease** (Fig. 10-12). A **nonmechanical obstruction** or **paralytic ileus** is when the bowel lacks normal peristalsis. Sonographically, an intestinal obstruction appears as distended fluid-filled loops of bowel (Fig. 10-13). As mentioned earlier, with obstruction, the small bowel diameter will measure 2.5 cm or greater from outer wall to outer wall. The **plicae circulares** will also be clearly identified when the bowel is distended with fluid. This may be referred to as the **keyboard sign**. The colon diameter will exceed 6 cm. Occasionally, an abrupt termination point of the distended bowel may be identified with sonography, although bowel gas may inhibit this finding. Peristaltic motion may also be increased in cases of mechanical obstruction, with signs of to-and-fro motion of the intraluminal contents.

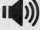

SOUND OFF
A mechanical obstruction results from the bowel being physically blocked by something,

whereas a nonmechanical obstruction or paralytic ileus is when the bowel lacks normal peristalsis.

Although rarely identified sonographically, masses of various ingested materials may cause intestinal obstructions. These are referred to as **bezoars**. Bezoars that are more often found in pediatric patients, **trichobezoars**, consist of ingested hair. Pediatric patients may also suffer from **lactobezoars**, which are bezoars that consist of powdered milk that has not been adequately mixed with water. Bezoars that consist of vegetable material are called **phytobezoars** and are more often found in older patients. Sonographically, bezoars will appear as complex masses with varying degrees of acoustic enhancement and posterior shadowing, depending on their structure.

CLINICAL FINDINGS OF AN INTESTINAL OBSTRUCTION

1. Abdominal distention
2. Intermittent abdominal pain
3. Constipation
4. Nausea and vomiting

SONOGRAPHIC FINDINGS OF AN INTESTINAL OBSTRUCTION

1. Small bowel diameter measures 2.5 cm or greater from outer wall to outer wall
2. Distended fluid-filled loops of bowel (keyboard sign)
3. An abrupt termination point of the distended bowel may be identified
4. Increased peristaltic motion with to-and-fro motion of intraluminal contents (mechanical obstruction only)
5. Colon diameter will exceed 6 cm

Crohn Disease

Crohn disease is an **autoimmune disorder** characterized by periods of inflammation of the gastrointestinal tract. Although it is the most common inflammatory disease of the small intestine, its cause is unknown. This disease usually involves the terminal ileum or proximal colon, although it can affect any part of the gastrointestinal tract. Patients can present with episodes of diarrhea, abdominal pain, weight loss, and rectal bleeding. Once more, like other bowel abnormalities discussed in this chapter, the sonographic appearance of Crohn disease resembles a target and will not be compressible (Fig. 10-14). Sonographically, the affected bowel wall will measure greater than 3 mm and will reveal hyperemia with color Doppler interrogation.

Adhesions

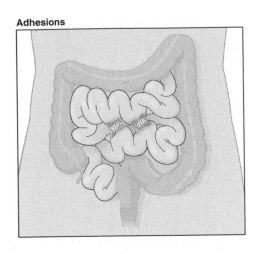

Intussusception

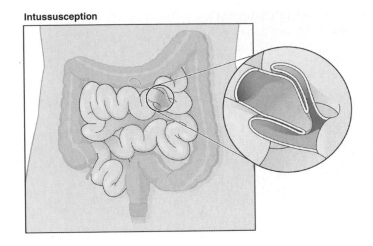

Volvulus

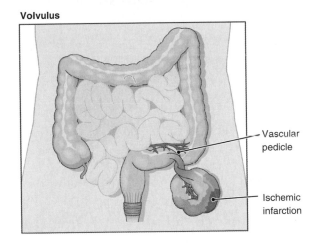

Vascular pedicle

Ischemic infarction

Herniation

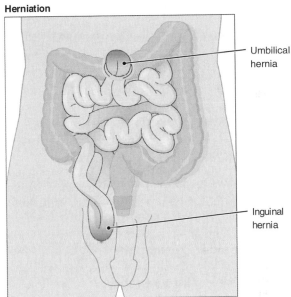

Umbilical hernia

Inguinal hernia

Figure 10-12 Some causes of mechanic bowel obstruction.

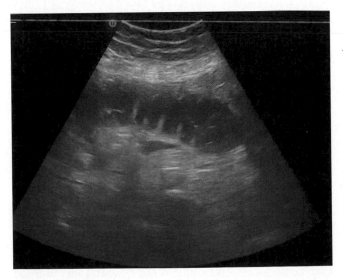

Figure 10-13 Small bowel obstruction is evident when the plicae circulares can be noted projecting into the lumen of the small bowel.

CLINICAL FINDINGS OF CROHN DISEASE

1. Episodes of diarrhea
2. Abdominal pain
3. Weight loss
4. Rectal bleeding

SONOGRAPHIC FINDINGS OF CROHN DISEASE

1. Bowel wall thickening
2. Affected bowel will be noncompressible and have a target appearance
3. Hyperemic wall

Diverticulitis

Diverticulosis is the development of small outpouchings termed diverticuli in the digestive tract, most often the sigmoid colon. Inflammation resulting from infection of

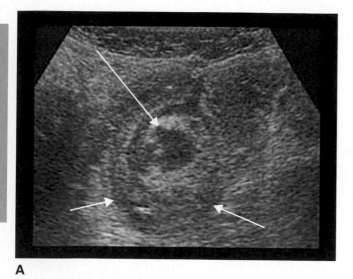

A

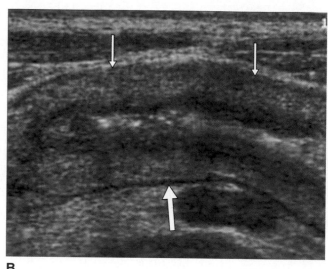

B

Figure 10-14 Crohn disease. **A.** A transverse view of the bowel demonstrates the "target" sign with wall thickening (*short arrows*) and abscess (*long arrow*). **B.** Note the thickened bowel wall of the longitudinal distal ileum (*arrows*).

those outpouching is termed **diverticulitis**. Clinically, patients with diverticulitis can present with constipation or diarrhea, fever, nausea and vomiting, and cramping abdominal pain, especially in the left lower quadrant, where the sigmoid colon is found.

Sonographically, diverticulitis appears as segmentally thickened bowel with evidence of an inflamed diverticula and inflamed **perienteric fat**. The bowel segment will typically reveal hyperemia, and the inflamed diverticula may appear as echogenic projections from the bowel that produce shadowing or ring-down artifact (Fig. 10-15). A close evaluation of the quadrant should also ensue for signs of fistula or abscess formation.

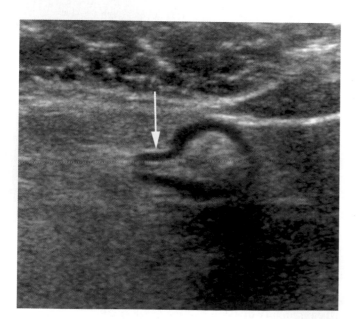

Figure 10-15 Diverticulitis. An inflamed outpouching (*arrow*) of the intestine is noted in this image.

CLINICAL FINDINGS OF DIVERTICULITIS
1. Constipation or diarrhea
2. Fever
3. Nausea and vomiting
4. Cramping, left lower quadrant pain

SONOGRAPHIC FINDINGS OF DIVERTICULITIS
1. Segmentally thickened bowel with evidence of an inflamed diverticula and inflamed perienteric fat
2. Affected bowel segment will typically reveal hyperemia
3. Inflamed diverticula may appear as echogenic projections from the bowel that produce shadowing or ring-down artifact

🔊 **SOUND OFF**
Diverticulitis typically presents with constipation or diarrhea, fever, nausea and vomiting, and cramping abdominal pain, especially in the left lower quadrant, where the sigmoid colon is found.

Colitis

Colitis is the inflammation of the colon. There are several different forms of colitis, including pseudomembranous, ulcerative, ischemic, and infectious. Watery and/or bloody diarrhea is a common feature of colitis. Pain and fever also occur. Pseudomembranous colitis, which is more often associated with watery diarrhea, can result from the use of antibiotic therapy that destroys the healthy flora of the intestines and leads to the subsequent proliferation of *Clostridium difficile* (*C. difficile*). Sonographically, colitis will yield bowel thickening of the colon wall with an increase in echogenicity, and, especially with infectious colitis, hyperemia can be depicted with color Doppler.

CLINICAL FINDINGS OF COLITIS

1. Bloody or watery diarrhea
2. Fever
3. Abdominal pain
4. Previous use of antibiotic therapy

SONOGRAPHIC FINDINGS OF COLITIS

1. Thickened, hypoechoic colon wall
2. Hyperemia within the colon wall

Gastric Cancer, Colon Cancer, and Metastatic Disease of the Bowel

Gastric cancer (stomach cancer) is most often in the form of **adenocarcinoma**. Patients typically present with weight loss, abdominal pain, anorexia, and vomiting. Occasionally, gastric carcinoma may be identified with sonography. Colon cancer, which is the third leading cause of death in Western countries after lung and breast, is typically found in the rectosigmoid colon. For these lesions, endorectal sonography is more effective than transabdominal imaging, especially for staging purposes.

Most often, a malignancy of the alimentary tract will appear as a hypoechoic, irregularly shaped, bulky mass that can measure up to 10 cm in size. The mass may have a "target" or "pseudokidney" appearance as well. Adenocarcinoma of the appendix can lead to rupture with the subsequent development of a gelatinous ascites referred to as **pseudomyxoma peritonei**. Sonographically, this form of ascites may appear as a multiseptated cystic mass within the pelvis. Lastly, malignant **melanoma** and primary tumors of the lungs and breast are the most commonly encountered metastatic tumors to the bowel. Their sonographic appearance may be similar to that of primary adenocarcinoma.

CLINICAL FINDINGS OF GASTROINTESTINAL CARCINOMA

1. Weight loss
2. Abdominal pain
3. Anorexia
4. Vomiting

SONOGRAPHIC FINDINGS OF GASTROINTESTINAL CARCINOMA

1. Hypoechoic, irregularly shaped, bulky mass
2. Could appear as a target or have a pseudokidney appearance

SOUND OFF
Colon cancer is typically found in the rectosigmoid colon.

ANTERIOR ABDOMINAL WALL PATHOLOGY

Rectus Sheath Hematoma

The rectus sheath forms a covering for the paired rectus abdominis muscles. The rectus abdominis muscles are found on both sides of the midline of the anterior abdomen. They are divided by a band of connective tissue, the linea alba, which is located in the midline of the abdomen (Fig. 10-16). A rupture in the muscle or associated vasculature can lead to a rectus sheath hematoma. Blood accumulation within the muscle or under the sheath can be the result of abdominal trauma or may occur spontaneously. Abdominal contractions that result from child birth, sneezing, coughing, defecation, urination, and intercourse have been shown to result in a rectus sheath hematoma. Clinically, patients present with abdominal pain, palpable abdominal mass, discoloration of the skin in the area of the hematoma, and a decreased hematocrit. Sonographically, a rectus sheath hematoma can appear anechoic, hypoechoic, complex, or hyperechoic depending on the stage of development (Fig. 10-17).

CLINICAL FINDINGS OF A RECTUS SHEATH HEMATOMA

1. Abdominal pain
2. Palpable abdominal mass
3. Discoloration of the skin in the area of the hematoma
4. Decreased hematocrit

SONOGRAPHIC FINDINGS OF A RECTUS SHEATH HEMATOMA

1. Blood can appear hypoechoic, hyperechoic, complex, and/or anechoic depending on the stage of development

Endometriosis of the Abdominal Wall

The most common site for endometriosis outside the female pelvis region is the anterior abdominal wall. **Endometriosis** is ectopic, functional endometrial tissue. The ectopic tissue is typically located within the scar of a previous cesarean section and is thus termed *scar endometriosis*. The mass may be palpable. And because the endometrial tissue is reactive to the hormones of the menstrual cycle, patients may complain of cyclical pain in the region. Sonographically, a linear transducer

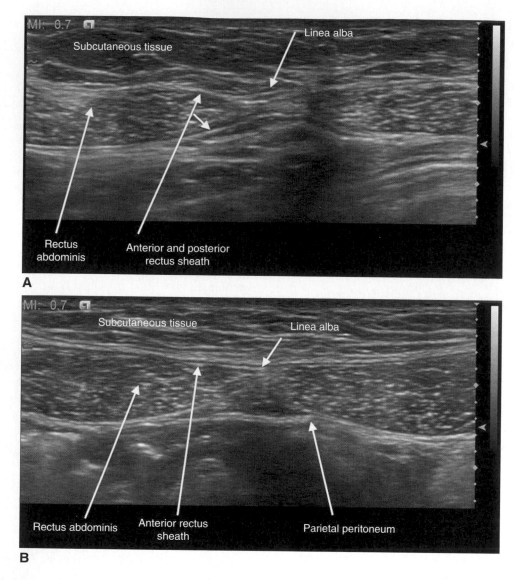

Figure 10-16 Anterior abdominal wall. **A.** Superior to the umbilicus. **B.** Inferior to the umbilicus.

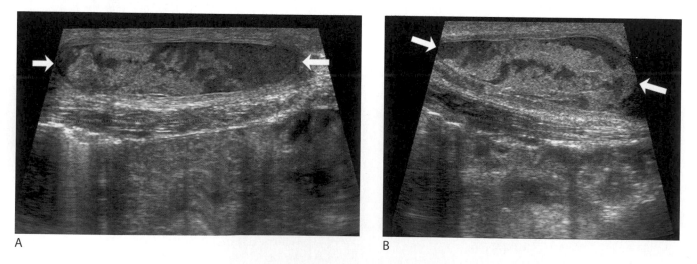

Figure 10-17 Rectus sheath hematoma. **A.** A heterogeneous fluid collection is noted within the midline of the abdomen in the sagittal plane (between *arrows*). **B.** The same mass is noted in transverse (between *arrows*).

should be utilized. Scar endometriosis within the abdominal wall can be well defined, lobulated, or infiltrative and will most likely appear hypoechoic or heterogeneous. Cystic changes may be seen within the mass as well. A biopsy is typically warranted.

CLINICAL FINDINGS OF ENDOMETRIOSIS OF THE ABDOMINAL WALL

1. History of endometriosis
2. Prior cesarean section
3. Pain at the area of the cesarean section scar (possible pain that correlates with the menstrual cycle)
4. Palpable mass

SONOGRAPHIC FINDINGS OF ENDOMETRIOSIS OF THE ABDOMINAL WALL

1. Well-defined, lobulated, or infiltrative mass
2. Hypoechoic to the adjacent tissue

Abdominal Wall Hernias

The abdominal wall can be sonographically interrogated for various abdominal wall hernias. There are several different types of hernias (Table 10-2; Fig. 10-18). Inguinal hernias are further discussed in Chapter 13. A high-frequency linear transducer and standoff pad should be utilized during the examination. Sonography of abdominal wall hernias can be difficult. Often, the **Valsalva technique** is utilized to show movement and the change in size of the hernia. Hernias should be carefully examined for bowel content and the peristaltic motion of the potentially trapped bowel (Fig 10-19). Abdominal wall hernias can have different sonographic appearances because the contents of the hernia can vary. Complications of abdominal wall hernias include incarceration, strangulation, and ischemia of the affected bowel.

TABLE 10-2 Types of abdominal hernias

Type of Hernia	Description and Important Facts	Location
Femoral hernia	Hernia that allows abdominal contents to protrude through the femoral canal	Medial to the femoral vein and inferior to the inguinal ligament
Inguinal hernia	Can be further described as **direct groin hernia** or **indirect groin hernia**; bowel protrudes into the groin; makes up 75% of all hernias	Groin Scrotum or labia
Incisional hernia	Type of ventral hernia where bowel protrudes into a surgical incision site; parastomal hernia is a type of incisional hernia adjacent to a stoma	Surgical incision site
Linea alba hernia	Bowel protrudes through the fascia of the linea alba; may be referred to as an epigastric hernia	Midline of the abdomen between the sternum and umbilicus
Spigelian hernia	Bowel protrudes into a weakened area in the lower one-fourth of the rectus muscle through the spigelian fascia	Midline of the abdomen Between the umbilicus and the symphysis pubis
Umbilical hernia	Type of ventral hernia where bowel protrudes into the umbilicus; most common type of ventral hernia and may be referred to as paraumbilical hernias in adults	Umbilicus

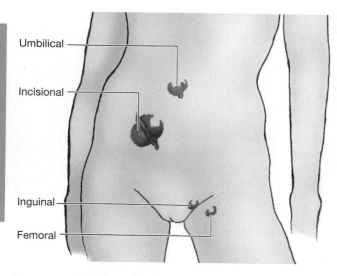

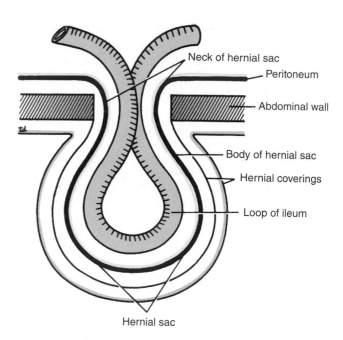

Figure 10-18 Common sites of hernia. These are four of the most common sites of hernia: umbilical, incisional, inguinal, and femoral.

Figure 10-19 Component of a hernia. Abdominal wall hernias consist of three parts: the sac, the contents of the sac, and the structures contained within the sac.

REVIEW QUESTIONS

1. The measurement identified by the *arrows* in Figure 10-20 should not exceed:
   a. 2 mm.
   b. 3 mm.
   c. 3.5 mm.
   d. 6 mm.

2. What is the most common age range at which the abnormality occurs in Figure 10-20?
   a. 5 to 10 years of age
   b. 1 to 4 weeks of age
   c. 3 months to 3 years of age
   d. 2 to 6 weeks of age

3. What is the sonographic sign noted in Figure 10-20?
   a. Doughnut sign
   b. Pyloric sign
   c. Cervix sign
   d. Cinnamon-bun sign

4. What would be the least likely clinical finding associated with Figure 10-20?
   a. Weight gain
   b. Olive sign
   c. Projectile vomiting
   d. Dehydration

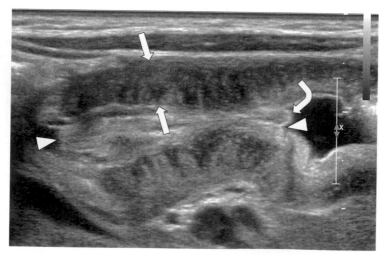

Figure 10-20

5. The patient in Figure 10-21 presented with right lower quadrant pain and nausea. The anteroposterior measurement of this structure in this image should not exceed:
   a. 4 mm.
   b. 3 mm.
   c. 10 mm.
   d. 6 mm.

6. Which of the following would be another common clinical finding for the patient in Figure 10-21?
   a. Thyroid in the belly sign
   b. Leukocytosis
   c. Kernicterus
   d. Hypernatremia

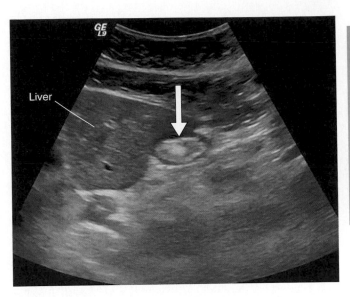

Figure 10-22

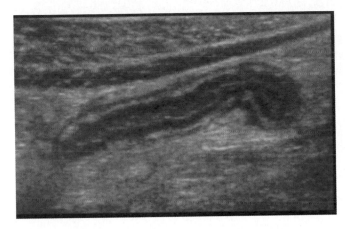

Figure 10-21

7. What is the thyroid in the belly sign?
   a. Anechoic fluid surrounding an inflamed bowel segment
   b. Hypoechoic material adjacent to a distended pyloric stenosis
   c. Enlargement of the distal colon in the presence of diverticulitis
   d. Hyperechoic edematous connective tissue surrounding an inflamed appendix

8. What does the large white arrow in Figure 10-22 indicate?
   a. Esophagus
   b. Transverse colon
   c. Stomach
   d. Pyloric stenosis

9. What is another name for the right colic flexure?
   a. Splenic flexure
   b. Hepatic flexure
   c. Ascending flexure
   d. Descending flexure

10. What is the term that denotes twisting of the bowel?
    a. Intussusception
    b. Reflux
    c. Volvulus
    d. Ileus

11. What is the most common type of ventral hernia?
    a. Paraumbilical hernia
    b. Spigelian hernia
    c. Incisional hernia
    d. Linea alba hernia

12. Where is the most common location of endometriosis in the abdominal wall?
    a. Paraumbilical
    b. Cesarean section scar
    c. Rectus sheath
    d. Mesentery

13. Which of the following would be among the most commonly encountered metastatic diseases of the bowel?
    a. Brain cancer
    b. Diverticulitis
    c. Splenic carcinoma
    d. Melanoma

14. What bowel segment is most often affected by diverticulitis and what is the most common location?
    a. Sigmoid colon in the left lower quadrant
    b. Cecum in the right lower quadrant
    c. Ascending colon in the right upper quadrant
    d. Splenic flexure in the left upper quadrant

15. Which of the following statements is true of a rectus sheath hematoma?
    a. It may occur during defecation.
    b. It is best seen with the Valsalva technique.
    c. It is often located adjacent to the proximal duodenum.
    d. It presents with general abdominal pain that eventually shifts to the left upper quadrant.

16. Which of the following is typically found in older patients and may lead to a bowel blockage?
    a. Lactobezoar
    b. Trichobezoar
    c. Mycobezoar
    d. Phytobezoar

17. The diameter of intussuscepted bowel will exceed:
    a. 1 cm.
    b. 5 mm.
    c. 9 cm.
    d. 3 cm.

18. The finding in Figure 10-23 was discovered in the right lower quadrant of an 18-month-old patient with a history of intermittent, severe abdominal pain, and vomiting. What is the most likely diagnosis?
    a. Appendicitis
    b. Colitis
    c. Mechanical obstruction
    d. Intussusception

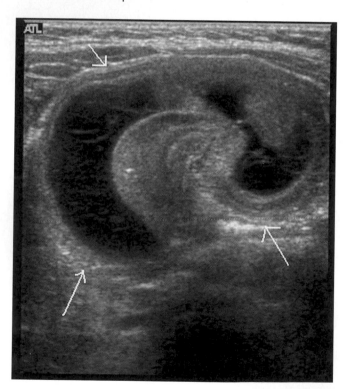

Figure 10-23

19. What does the arrow demonstrate in the patient in Figure 10-24 who complained of focal right lower quadrant pain?
    a. Appendicolith
    b. Thyroid in the belly
    c. Olive sign
    d. McBurney sign

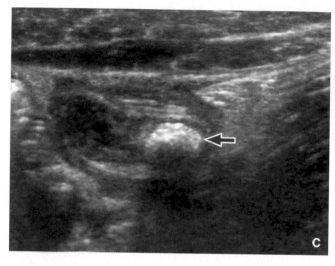

Figure 10-24

20. Which of the following gut layers would yield an echogenic pattern?
    a. Deep mucosa
    b. Superficial mucosa
    c. Muscularis propria
    d. Perimucosa propria

21. A patient presents to the sonography department with bilious vomiting. While investigating the pediatric patient for pyloric stenosis, you note that while the pyloric sphincter appears normal, the SMA is abnormally located to the right of the SMV. What is the most likely diagnosis?
    a. Pylorospasm
    b. Intussusception
    c. Crohn disease
    d. Midgut malrotation

22. What anatomic structure may be noted as a bull's-eye structure anterior to the abdominal aorta and posterior to the left lobe of the liver in the sagittal scan plane?
    a. Pyloric sphincter
    b. Duodenal antrum
    c. Gastroesophageal junction
    d. Distal jejunum

23. Which of the following is not a layer of gut identified with sonography?
    a. Visceral
    b. Serosa
    c. Submucosa
    d. Mucosa

24. All of the following are true of normal intestinal findings with sonography except:
    a. normal bowel does not compress.
    b. normal bowel should have observable peristalsis.
    c. colon wall should measure less than 9 mm.
    d. normal bowel has little to no color Doppler signals.

25. Upon sonographic evaluation of the right lower quadrant in a patient complaining of focal abdominal pain in that area, you visualize a hyperemic blind-ended, tubular structure that contains a shadowing focus. What is the most likely etiology of the shadowing focus?
    a. Ureteral stone
    b. Appendicolith
    c. Gallstone
    d. Herniated omentum

26. All of the following are sonographic criteria in the diagnosis of pyloric stenosis except:
    a. wall of the pylorus is focally thinned.
    b. length of the pylorus measures more than 17 mm.
    c. doughnut appearance in transverse.
    d. cervix appearance in longitudinal.

27. All of the following are sonographic findings of acute appendicitis except:
    a. appendicolith.
    b. compressible, blind-ended tube.
    c. periappendiceal fluid collection.
    d. hyperemic flow.

28. Clinical findings of acute appendicitis include all of the following except:
    a. leukocytosis.
    b. right lower quadrant pain.
    c. constipation.
    d. rebound tenderness.

29. All of the following are common clinical findings in infants who present with pyloric stenosis except:
    a. weight loss.
    b. dehydration.
    c. olive sign.
    d. first-born female.

30. Pseudomyxoma peritonei can result from:
    a. intussusception.
    b. pyloric stenosis.
    c. Crohn disease.
    d. appendix cancer.

31. A patient presents to the sonography department with a painful, superficial abdominal mass located within a prior cesarean scar. What clinical feature would be most consistent with scar endometriosis?
    a. Hematuria
    b. Chronic headaches
    c. Cyclical pain
    d. Bloody diarrhea

32. What abnormality associates red currant jelly stools?
    a. Diverticulosis
    b. Appendicitis
    c. Intussusception
    d. Pyloric stenosis

33. Other abnormalities that can present much like pyloric stenosis include all of the following except:
    a. midgut malrotation.
    b. pylorospasm.
    c. gastroesophageal reflux disease.
    d. intussusception.

34. Which of the following would be the most likely clinical feature of colitis?
    a. Inguinal herniation of the bowel
    b. Right shoulder pain
    c. Watery diarrhea
    d. Midline hematoma

35. Gastric cancer is most often in the form of:
    a. cystadenocarcinoma.
    b. adenocarcinoma.
    c. rhabdomyocarcinoma.
    d. angiosarcoma.

36. Pediatric patients could suffer from bowel obstructions that are caused by a buildup of ingested hair. The mass associated with this type of obstruction is termed a:
    a. phytobezoar.
    b. lactobezoar.
    c. trichobezoar.
    d. permabezoar.

37. An autoimmune disease characterized by periods of inflammation of the gastrointestinal tract describes:
    a. Crohn disease.
    b. intussusception.
    c. pyloric stenosis.
    d. Meckel diverticulitis.

38. The telescoping of one segment of bowel into another is referred to as:
    a. volvulus.
    b. Crohn disease.
    c. intussusception.
    d. pyloric stenosis.

39. Which of the following types of obstruction refers to the bowel being physically blocked by something?
    a. Mechanical
    b. Nonmechanical
    c. Obstreperous
    d. Bezoarine

40. Which of the following would be useful to employ during a sonographic evaluation of a suspected abdominal wall hernia?
    a. Upright positioning
    b. Prone positioning
    c. Graded compression
    d. Valsalva

41. The situation when bowel protrudes into the groin is referred to as a(n):
    a. inguinal hernia.
    b. linea alba hernia.
    c. umbilical hernia.
    d. spigelian hernia.

42. The situation when bowel protrudes into a weakened area in the lower one-fourth of the rectus muscle is referred to as a(n):
    a. inguinal hernia.
    b. linea alba hernia.
    c. umbilical hernia.
    d. spigelian hernia.

43. The area of pain and rebound tenderness with acute appendicitis is most likely at:
    a. Meckel point.
    b. McBurney point.
    c. Murphy point.
    d. Olive point.

44. Which of the following best describes the location of McBurney point?
    a. Left lateral to the umbilicus and medial to the left iliac crest
    b. Halfway between the anterior superior iliac spine and the umbilicus
    c. Midway between the umbilicus and the symphysis pubis
    d. Medial to the superior iliac spine

45. The olive sign is best described as:
    a. the palpation of the inflamed appendix with rebound tenderness.
    b. an area of pain halfway between the anterior superior iliac spine and the umbilicus.
    c. an enlarged palpable pyloric sphincter.
    d. the sonographic appearance of pyloric stenosis.

46. Rebound tenderness is associated with:
    a. appendicitis.
    b. intussusception.
    c. diverticulitis.
    d. gastric carcinoma.

47. The most common location of the vermiform appendix is in the area of the:
    a. jejunum.
    b. descending colon.
    c. cecum.
    d. sigmoid colon.

48. Which of the following is the development of small outpouchings within the sigmoid colon?
    a. Diverticulitis
    b. Crohn disease
    c. Diverticulosis
    d. Midgut malrotation

49. Which of the following is not associated with a rectus sheath hematoma?
    a. Palpable abdominal mass
    b. Increased hematocrit
    c. Childbirth
    d. Sneezing

50. Which of the following is not a sonographic finding consistent with Crohn disease?
    a. Bowel wall thickening
    b. Noncompressible bowel that has a target appearance
    c. Increased peristalsis
    d. Hyperemic wall

51. All of the following are common clinical findings in infants who present with intussusception except:
    a. vomiting.
    b. first-born male infant.
    c. red currant jelly stools.
    d. leukocytosis.

52. The sonographic finding of fluid-filled, distended loops of bowel is consistent with:
    a. Meckel diverticulum.
    b. diverticulitis.
    c. gastroesophageal reflux disease.
    d. intestinal obstruction.

53. Traditionally, treatment for intussusception is by means of:
    a. surgery.
    b. external manipulation.
    c. compression sonography.
    d. therapeutic enema.

54. The most common cause of intestinal obstruction in children less than 2 years of age is:
    a. intussusception.
    b. midgut malrotation.
    c. pyloric stenosis.
    d. acute appendicitis.

55. What abnormality may be diagnosed by observing fluid mixed with gas bubbles traveling from the stomach to the esophagus with sonography?
    a. Pylorospasm
    b. Pyloric stenosis
    c. Gastroesophageal reflux disease
    d. Midgut malrotation

56. In what position is the infant often placed for better sonographic visualization of the pyloric sphincter?
    a. Right lateral decubitus
    b. Left lateral decubitus
    c. Prone
    d. Upright

57. An adult patient presents to the sonography department with left lower quadrant pain, fever, and bouts of both constipation and diarrhea. Which of the following would be the most likely etiology?
    a. Diverticulitis
    b. Intussusception
    c. Midgut malrotation
    d. Appendicitis

58. What are the diagnostic criteria for pyloric stenosis?
    a. 17 mm in thickness and 2 mm in length
    b. 17 mm in thickness and 3 mm in length
    c. 3 mm in thickness and 10 mm in length
    d. 3 mm in thickness and 17 mm in length

59. Clinical findings of a patient with Crohn disease include all of following except:
    a. palpable abdominal mass.
    b. rectal bleeding.
    c. abdominal pain.
    d. weight loss.

60. Which of the following would be most likely a cause of colitis?
    a. Gastroesophageal reflux disease
    b. Antibiotic therapy
    c. Dehydration
    d. Rectus sheath hematoma

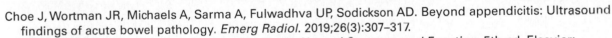

SUGGESTED READINGS

Choe J, Wortman JR, Michaels A, Sarma A, Fulwadhva UP, Sodickson AD. Beyond appendicitis: Ultrasound findings of acute bowel pathology. *Emerg Radiol.* 2019;26(3):307–317.

Curry RA, Tempkin BB. *Sonography: Introduction to Normal Structure and Function.* 5th ed. Elsevier; 2020:307–330.

Federle MP, Jeffrey RB, Woodward PJ, et al. *Diagnostic Imaging: Abdomen.* 2nd ed. Amirsys; 2010:II-5-2–II-6-81.

Henningsen C, Kuntz K, Youngs D. *Clinical Guide to Sonography: Exercises for Critical Thinking.* 2nd ed. Elsevier; 2014:123–140.

Hertzberg BS, Middleton WD. *Ultrasound: The Requisites.* 3rd ed. Elsevier; 2016:204–216.

Justice FA, Auldist AW, Bines JE. Intussusception: trends in clinical presentation and management. *J Gastroenterol Hepatol.* 2006;21:842–846.

Kawamura DM, Nolan TD. *Diagnostic Medical Sonography: Abdomen and Superficial Structures.* 4th ed. Wolters Kluwer; 2018:13–40 & 247–270.

Khurana B, Ledbetter S, McTavish J, Wiesner W, Ros PR. Bowel obstruction revealed by multidetector CT. *Am J Roentgenol.* 2002;178(5):1139–1144.

Rapp CL, Stavros T, Kaske TI. Ultrasound of abdominal wall hernias. *J Diagn Med Sonogr.* 1999;15:231–235.

Rosano N, Gallo L, Mercogliano G, et al. Ultrasound of small bowel obstruction: a pictorial review. *Diagnostics.* 2021;11(4):617.

Rumack CM, Wilson SR, Charboneau JW, et al. *Diagnostic Ultrasound.* 4th ed. Elsevier, 2011:261–316 & 486–523.

Sanders RC, Hall-Terracciano B. *Clinical Sonography: A Practical Guide.* 5th ed. Wolters Kluwer; 2016:479–487 & 605–625.

Siegel MJ. *Pediatric Sonography.* 5th ed. Wolters Kluwer; 2019:346–395.

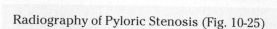

Radiography of Pyloric Stenosis (Fig. 10-25)

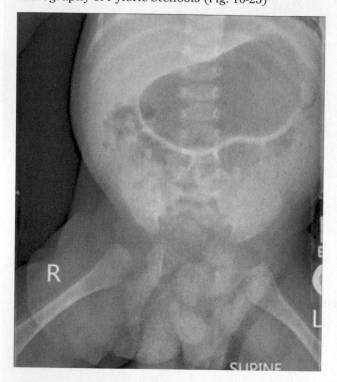

Figure 10-25 Plain radiograph demonstrating distended stomach in a patient with pyloric stenosis.

Radiograph of Diverticulitis (Fig. 10-27)

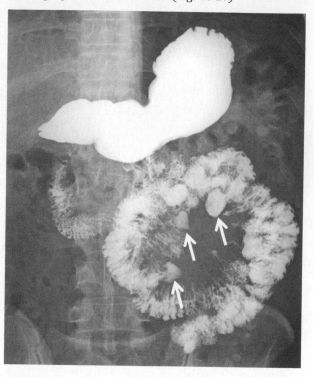

Figure 10-27 Barium examination reveals multiple diverticula of the small bowel (*arrows*).

Computed Tomography of Appendicitis (Fig. 10-26)

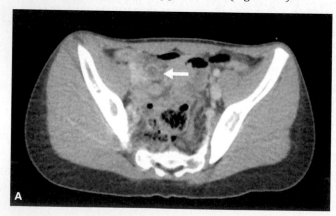

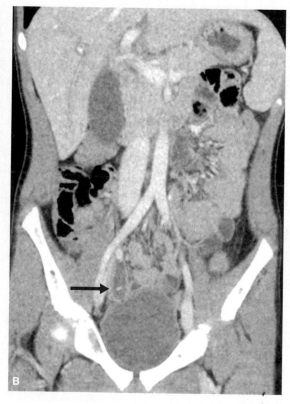

Figure 10-26 Acute appendicitis on computed tomography (*CT*). **A.** Axial contrast-enhanced CT image showing a dilated appendix (*arrow*) with adjacent inflammatory fat stranding consistent with acute appendicitis. **B.** Coronal contrast-enhanced CT image in a different patient with acute appendicitis showing a dilated fluid-filled appendix with a small intraluminal calcification consistent with an appendicolith (*arrow*).

Noncardiac Chest and Retroperitoneum

Introduction

This brief chapter provides a summary of relevant material pertaining to sonographic analysis of the noncardiac chest and retroperitoneum. The "Bonus Review" section contains two helpful computed tomography (CT) images.

Key Terms

barcode sign—abnormal M-mode tracing that indicates the presence of a pneumothorax

congenital cystic adenomatoid malformation—a mass consisting of abnormal bronchial and lung tissue that develops within the fetal chest

crura of the diaphragm—paired linear muscular sections of the diaphragm that attach to the anterolateral surfaces of the upper lumbar vertebrae

hemophiliac—an inherited bleeding disorder that inhibits the control of blood clotting

lung consolidation—the replacement of normal air-filled alveoli with fluid, inflammation, blood, or neoplastic cells

mediastinum—the central portion of the chest cavity between the pleural sacs of the lungs that contains all of the chest organs but the lungs, including the heart, thymus gland, part of the trachea, esophagus, and many lymph nodes

mesentery—a double fold of peritoneum that attaches the intestines to the posterior abdominal wall

parapneumonic effusion—pleural effusion associated with pneumonia

pericardial effusion—the accumulation of fluid around the heart in the pericardial cavity

pleural effusion—the abnormal accumulation of fluid in the pleural space

pneumothorax—free air within the chest outside the lungs that can lead to lung collapse

pulmonary sequestration—a separate mass of nonfunctioning lung tissue with its own blood supply

retroperitoneal fibrosis—a disease characterized by the buildup of fibrous tissue within the retroperitoneum; this mass may involve the abdominal aorta, inferior vena cava, ureters, and sacrum

retroperitoneal hematoma—a bloody tumor located within the retroperitoneum

retroperitoneal lymphadenopathy—the enlargement of the abdominal lymph nodes located within the abdomen

sandwich sign—the sign associated with abnormal abdominal lymph node enlargement that leads to the compression of the aorta and inferior vena cava

seashore sign—normal M-mode tracing of lung sliding

thoracentesis—a procedure that uses a needle to drain fluid from the pleural cavity for either diagnostic or therapeutic reasons

transversalis fascia—the fascia that lines the anterolateral abdominal wall and is located between the transversus abdominis muscle and the peritoneum

NONCARDIAC CHEST

The noncardiac chest, though not typically scanned often in the general sonography department, may be assessed nonetheless if needed, and sonographers should have a basic understanding of the anatomy, especially that of the lungs and pleurae. The left lung typically has a superior and inferior lobe, whereas the right lobe typically has three lobes—superior, middle, and inferior (Fig. 11-1). Each lung has a thin covering that is closely applied to its surface referred to as the visceral pleura. The inner lining of the chest is also covered by this tissue, and it is referred to as the parietal pleura. A normal amount of fluid is located between these layers, an area referred to as the plural space, allowing the lungs to slide freely with respiration.

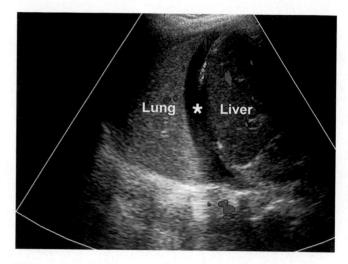

Figure 11-2 Right-sided pleural effusion. Fluid (*) is noted between the lung and the liver in this patient, representing a right pleural effusion.

> ### 🔊 SOUND OFF
> Each lung has a thin covering that is closely applied to its surface referred to as the visceral pleura. The inner lining of the chest is also covered by this tissue, and it is referred to as the parietal pleura.

Pleural Effusion, Pericardial Effusion, and Pneumothorax

Excessive fluid accumulation around the lung within the pleural space, referred to as a **pleural effusion**, may be noted during a sonographic examination of the abdomen (Fig. 11-2). Therefore, during abdominal sonogram studies, the lower chest should be evaluated for signs of pleural effusion. Simple pleural fluid tends to fall to the dependent side and is anechoic in appearance. The lungs will be noted

floating in the pleural fluid. A pleural effusion may be described as transudate or exudate. Transudate results from an imbalance in oncotic and hydrostatic pressure, whereas exudate typically results from inflammation or a reduction in lymphatic drainage. A pleural effusion associated with pneumonia is referred to as a **parapneumonic effusion**. A pleural effusion containing pus is referred to as empyema.

Complex fluid within the chest may indicate malignancy, infection, or blood. A **thoracentesis** is often performed either to determine the origin of the fluid (diagnostic thoracentesis) or for therapeutic reasons (therapeutic thoracentesis). The patient is typically placed in an upright position, and access to the fluid is obtained posteriorly. One complication of the thoracentesis is the development

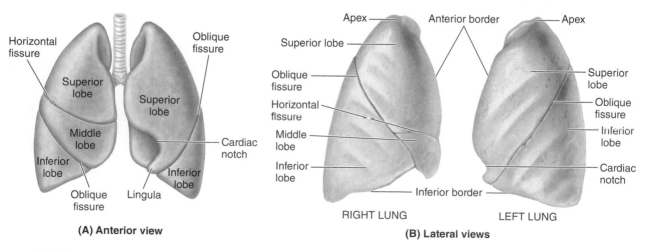

Figure 11-1 Lung anatomy. The lungs are shown in isolation in anterior (**A**) and lateral views (**B**), demonstrating lobes and fissures.

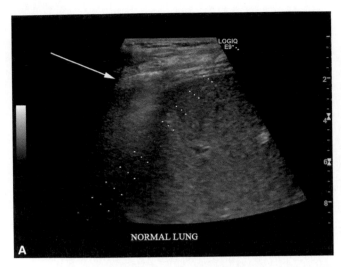
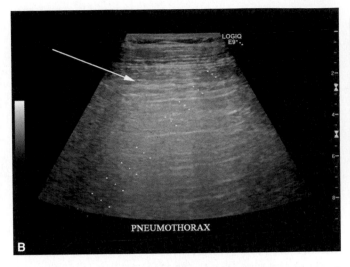

NORMAL LUNG

PNEUMOTHORAX

Figure 11-3 Pneumothorax. Procedural acute pneumothorax during ultrasound guidance. **A.** Consolidated lung (*arrow*) preprocedure. Markers show proposed needle path. **B.** Large pneumothorax (*arrow*) seen on ultrasound postprocedure.

of a **pneumothorax**. Occasionally, a pneumothorax may be noted with sonography (Fig. 11-3). B-mode assessment with real-time evaluation is aimed at identifying normal lung sliding. The pneumothorax air separates the two pleural layers, preventing imaging of normal lung sliding. M-mode has also been used by some to demonstrate evidence of a pneumothorax with sonography. With M-mode, the **barcode sign** is an indicator of a pneumothorax, whereas the **seashore sign** is a normal finding (Fig. 11-4). The barcode sign may also be referred to as the stratosphere sign. A pneumothorax is an abnormality better diagnosed with a chest radiograph. A **pericardial effusion** may also be noted during an abdominal sonogram. Fluid around the heart will most often appear anechoic (Fig. 11-5).

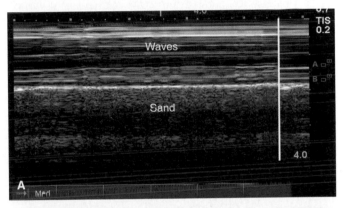

Waves

Sand

> ### SOUND OFF
> M-mode has also been used by some to demonstrate evidence of a pneumothorax with sonography. With M-mode, the barcode sign is an indicator of a pneumothorax, whereas the seashore sign is a normal finding.

Lung and Chest Masses

Superficial lung masses may be noted with sonography. Lung masses such as large lung cancers and surface irregularities may be further evaluated and biopsied with the assistance of sonography. Pediatric patients may be evaluated for **pulmonary sequestration** or **congenital cystic adenomatoid malformation**. Tumors of the **mediastinum**, such as lymphomas and thymomas, may be analyzed sonographically as well. The normal thymus may be noted in the pediatric patient posterior to the sternum and will appear as an echogenic mass of

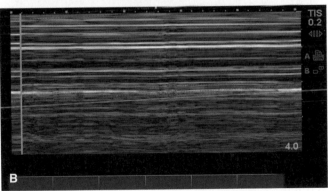

Figure 11-4 Barcode sign versus seashore sign. **A.** Normal M-mode of lung. Commonly referred to as "seashore" sign with "waves" and "sand." **B.** Pneumothorax, known as the "barcode" sign.

tissue that contains linear and punctuate echogenicities. Before puberty, the thymus gland is vital for the development of T cells, which are specialized lymphocytes. Following puberty, the thymus slowly begins to atrophy, ultimately being replaced by fat in adults.

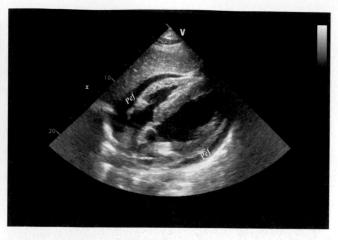

Figure 11-5 Pericardial effusion. This pericardial effusion (*perf*) can be seen surrounding the heart.

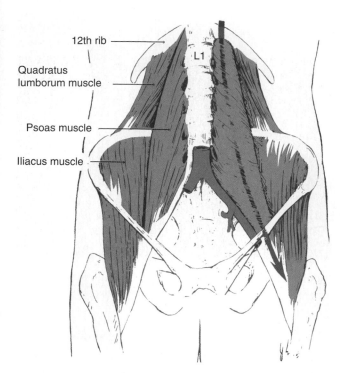

Figure 11-6 Coronal drawing depicting the location of the psoas, iliacus, and quadratus lumborum muscles.

Lung Consolidation

Lung consolidation is the replacement of normal air-filled alveoli with fluid, inflammation, blood, or neoplastic cells. Causes include pneumonia, pulmonary edema, hemorrhage, and carcinoma. Sonographically, lung consolidation may appear similar to the liver or spleen tissue, but typically contains several internal echoes that radiate in a linear pattern because of air within the bronchi. Pleural effusion is often seen with lung consolidation.

> 🔊 **SOUND OFF**
> Causes of lung consolidation include pneumonia, pulmonary edema, hemorrhage, and carcinoma.

RETROPERITONEUM

Retroperitoneal Overview

The retroperitoneum is the region that is located posterior to the parietal peritoneum and anterior to the **transversalis fascia**. Superiorly, the retroperitoneum is bounded by the diaphragm, whereas inferiorly, it is bounded by the pelvic brim. A list of retroperitoneal organs is provided in Chapter 1. Besides the abdominal aorta and inferior vena cava, there are some other smaller vascular structures located in the retroperitoneum as well, including the superior mesenteric artery, hepatic artery, splenic artery, and splenic vein.

Retroperitoneal Muscles and the Crura of the Diaphragm

There are several prominent muscles that may be seen on an abdominal sonogram adjacent to the kidneys, including the psoas muscles and the quadratus

lumborum (Figs. 11-6 and 11-7). On a transverse image of the kidney, the quadratus lumborum may be noted posterior to the kidney and lateral on the image, whereas the psoas muscle will be noted posterior to the kidney and closer to the spine. In addition, the paired **crura** (singular is crus) **of the diaphragm**, which are linear muscular sections of the diaphragm that attach to the anterolateral surfaces of the upper lumbar vertebrae, may be seen on sonography as hypoechoic structures in the longitudinal plane extending caudally into the abdomen anterior to the spine (Fig. 11-8).

> 🔊 **SOUND OFF**
> The quadratus lumborum may be noted posterior to the kidney and lateral, whereas the psoas muscle will be noted posterior to the kidney and closer to the spine.

Retroperitoneal Fibrosis

The development of a fibrous mass that covers the abdominal aorta, inferior vena cava, ureters, and sacrum is referred to as **retroperitoneal fibrosis**. Its cause is typically unknown. However, it has been linked with infections, migraine headache medication, malignant disease, and aneurysm rupture or leakage. Clinical symptoms include back or flank pain, weight loss, nausea, vomiting, and malaise. Sonographically, retroperitoneal fibrosis appears as a large, hypoechoic mass surrounding the abdominal aorta (Fig. 11-9).

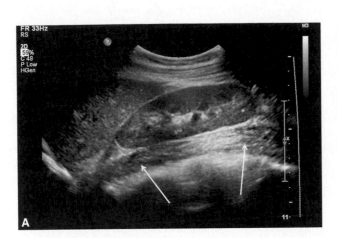

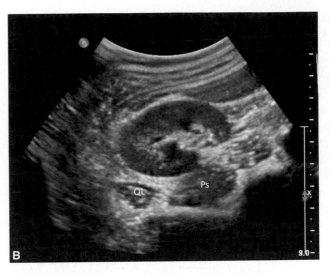

Figure 11-7 Psoas muscle and quadratus lumborum muscle. **A.** Longitudinal view of the psoas muscle (*arrows*). **B.** Transverse view of the psoas (*Ps*) and quadratus lumborum (*QL*) muscles.

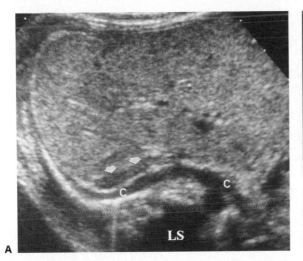

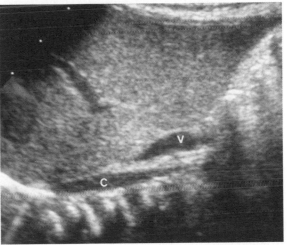

Figure 11-8 Crus of the diaphragm. **A.** Transverse view of the crura (*C*) of the diaphragm seen anterior to the lumbar spine (*LS*) and posterior to the adrenal gland (*arrowheads*). **B.** Longitudinal image of the right crus of the diaphragm (*C*) appearing as a linear, hypoechoic structure anterior to the spine and posterior to the inferior vena cava (*V*).

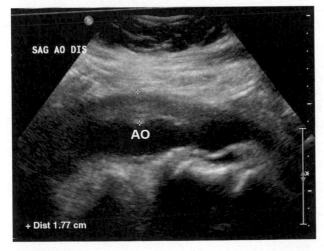

Figure 11-9 Retroperitoneal fibrosis. Longitudinal image of the abdomen demonstrating a hypoechoic region adjacent to the distal aorta (*AO*).

CLINICAL FINDINGS OF RETROPERITONEAL FIBROSIS

1. Migraine medication use
2. Back pain
3. Flank pain
4. Weight loss
5. Nausea
6. Vomiting
7. Malaise

SONOGRAPHIC FINDINGS OF RETROPERITONEAL FIBROSIS

1. Large, hypoechoic mass surrounding the abdominal aorta

🔊 SOUND OFF
Retroperitoneal fibrosis has been linked with infections, migraine headache medication, malignant disease, and aneurysm rupture or leakage.

Retroperitoneal Hematoma

The most common location for a **retroperitoneal hematoma**, especially in the **hemophiliac** patient, is within the psoas muscles. Clinical findings include hemophilia, trauma, and surgery. Laboratory findings include a drop in hematocrit and pain. Depending on the stage of the blood, hematomas may appear hypoechoic, complex, or hyperechoic.

CLINICAL FINDINGS OF A RETROPERITONEAL HEMATOMA

1. Hemophilia
2. Trauma
3. Recent surgery
4. Low hematocrit

SONOGRAPHIC FINDINGS OF A RETROPERITONEAL HEMATOMA

1. Depending on the stage of the blood, hematomas may appear hypoechoic, complex, or hyperechoic

🔊 SOUND OFF
Retroperitoneal hematoma has been linked with hemophilia.

Retroperitoneal Lymphadenopathy

Retroperitoneal lymphadenopathy is the enlargement of the abdominal lymph nodes located within the abdomen. Normal abdominal lymph nodes are typically not seen and measure less than 1 cm. Within the abdomen, lymph nodes are located in the **mesentery**, renal hilum, and along the length of the abdominal aorta. The enlargement of abdominal lymph nodes greater than 1 cm in diameter can indicate infection or malignancy such as lymphoma. The **"sandwich" sign** denotes abdominal nodes surrounding and compressing the aorta and inferior vena cava (Fig. 11-10). Enlarged nodes will also deviate from their normal sonographic appearance and become more hypoechoic or, possibly, anechoic.

🔊 SOUND OFF
Within the abdomen, lymph nodes are located in the mesentery, renal hilum, and along the length of the abdominal aorta.

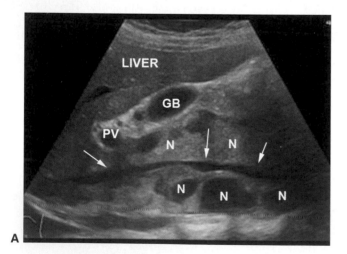
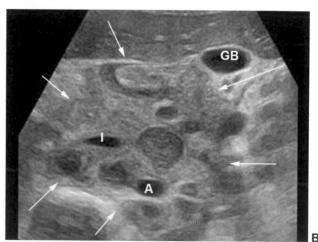

Figure 11-10 Retroperitoneal lymphadenopathy. **A.** Longitudinal image of the abdomen demonstrating compression of the inferior vena cava (*arrows*) by lymphadenopathy (*N*) seen anterior and posterior to the vessel. *PV*, portal vein, *GB*, gallbladder. **B.** Transverse midline image demonstrating an echogenic mass (*arrows*) encompassing and compressing the aorta (*A*) and inferior vena cava (*I*).

REVIEW QUESTIONS

1. What does the arrow in Figure 11-11 indicate?
   a. Ascites
   b. Hemoperitoneum
   c. Pleural effusion
   d. Pericardial effusion

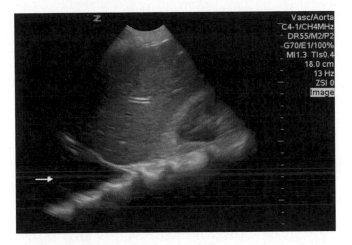

Figure 11-11

2. Which of the following muscles would be situated closest to the spine?
   a. Rectus abdominis
   b. Psoas muscle
   c. Quadratus lumborum
   d. Iliacus

3. Which of the following forms of pleural effusion is associated with an imbalance in oncotic and hydrostatic pressure?
   a. Parapneumonic effusion
   b. Exudate effusion
   c. Serous effusion
   d. Transudate effusion

4. Which of the following is included in the clinical findings of retroperitoneal fibrosis?
   a. Hematuria
   b. Migraine medication use
   c. Diabetes mellitus
   d. Diarrhea

5. Which of the following forms of pleural effusion is associated with inflammation?
   a. Parapneumonic effusion
   b. Exudate effusion
   c. Serous effusion
   d. Transudate effusion

6. A 45-year-old patient presents to the sonography department with chest pain and shortness of breath. During the sonographic examination of the abdomen, an anechoic fluid collection is noted superior to the diaphragm. What is the most likely diagnosis?
   a. Congenital cystic adenomatoid malformation of the lung
   b. Pulmonary sequestration
   c. Pleural effusion
   d. Cystic adenomatoid malformation

7. A pleural effusion that contains pus is referred to as:
   a. pneumonia.
   b. pleuritis.
   c. empyema.
   d. transudate.

8. The "sandwich" sign denotes:
   a. pyloric stenosis.
   b. intussusception.
   c. retroperitoneal fibrosis.
   d. abdominal lymphadenopathy.

9. Abnormal lymph nodes typically measure more than:
   a. 10 mm.
   b. 7 mm.
   c. 8 mm.
   d. 1 mm.

10. Where is the thymus located?
    a. Within the neck
    b. Within the mediastinum
    c. Superior to rectum
    d. Anterior to the abdominal aorta

11. Fluid located around the lungs is termed:
    a. ascites.
    b. pleural effusion.
    c. lung consolidation.
    d. pericardial effusion.

12. Normal lung sliding is demonstrated on M-mode with the:
    a. barcode sign.
    b. seashore sign.
    c. sandwich sign.
    d. sliding sign.

13. What is the most common location of a retroperitoneal hematoma in hemophiliac patients?
    a. Rectum
    b. Anterior abdominal wall
    c. Psoas muscle
    d. Rectus abdominis muscle

14. Which of the following is not located within the mediastinum?
    a. Heart
    b. Thymus
    c. Esophagus
    d. Lungs

15. How many lobes does the left lung have?
    a. Two
    b. Four
    c. Three
    d. Five

16. The replacement of normal air-filled alveoli with fluid, inflammation, blood, or neoplastic cells is referred to as:
    a. pneumothorax.
    b. congenital cystic adenomatoid malformation.
    c. pulmonary sequestration.
    d. lung consolidation.

17. How many lobes does the right lung have?
    a. Two
    b. Four
    c. Three
    d. Five

18. Free air within the chest outside the lungs is referred to as:
    a. pneumothorax.
    b. congenital cystic adenomatoid malformation.
    c. pulmonary sequestration.
    d. lung consolidation.

19. A separate mass of nonfunctioning lung tissue with its own blood supply describes:
    a. pneumothorax.
    b. congenital cystic adenomatoid malformation.
    c. pulmonary sequestration.
    d. lung consolidation.

20. What does the thymus create in the prepubescent individual?
    a. T cells
    b. Phagocytes
    c. Red blood cells
    d. Platelets

21. A mass consisting of abnormal bronchial and lung tissue that develops within the fetal chest best describes:
    a. pneumothorax.
    b. congenital cystic adenomatoid malformation.
    c. pulmonary sequestration.
    d. lung consolidation.

22. The diagnostic or therapeutic procedure where fluid is removed from the pleural space is referred to as:
    a. thoracentesis.
    b. pneumothorax.
    c. paracentesis.
    d. pericardiocentesis.

23. What do the arrows in Figure 11-12 indicate?
    a. Pleural effusion
    b. Pericardium
    c. Pericardial effusion
    d. Myocardial thickening

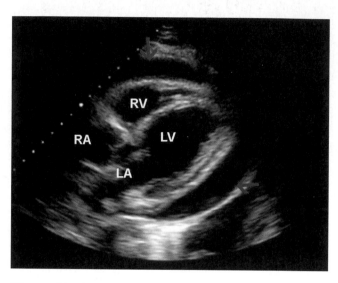

Figure 11-12

24. Which of the following could result from undergoing a thoracentesis?
    a. Deep venous thrombosis
    b. Pneumothorax
    c. Pericardial effusion
    d. Ascites

25. Typically, a hematoma appears:
    a. hyperechoic.
    b. hypoechoic.
    c. complex.
    d. all of the above.

26. The diagnosis of a pneumothorax is typically via a(n):
    a. upright sonogram.
    b. thoracentesis.
    c. chest radiograph.
    d. nuclear medicine chest perfusion study.

27. What is the term for a pleural effusion associated with pneumonia?
    a. Exudate
    b. Serous
    c. Intrapleural
    d. Parapneumonic

28. Fluid located around the heart is termed:
    a. ascites.
    b. pleural effusion.
    c. lung consolidation.
    d. pericardial effusion.

29. Which of the following is the most likely sonographic appearance of the thymus in the pediatric patient?
    a. Echogenic mass that contains linear and punctuate echogenicities
    b. Anechoic structure anterior to the sternum
    c. Complex mass anterior to the iliac crest
    d. Homogeneous mass with posterior shadowing containing anechoic cystic structures

30. Which of the following is the most common sonographic appearance of retroperitoneal fibrosis?
    a. Hypoechoic mass surrounding the aorta
    b. Multiple small lymph nodes anterior to the abdominal aorta
    c. Anechoic mass in the lower abdomen
    d. Echogenic mass posterior to the kidneys

31. A 74-year-old patient presents to the sonography department for an abdominal sonogram. The patient has a history of pneumonia and congestive heart failure. While scanning in the midline, you angle the transducer superiorly to evaluate the left lobe of the liver. Incidentally, you note a small amount of fluid adjacent to the heart. What is the most likely diagnosis?
    a. Ascites
    b. Cancer
    c. Pleural effusion
    d. Pericardial effusion

32. Which of the following can be seen posterior and lateral to the kidney?
    a. Rectus abdominis
    b. Psoas muscle
    c. Quadratus lumborum
    d. Iliacus

33. Which of the following is not typically involved in retroperitoneal fibrosis?
    a. Rectum
    b. Abdominal aorta
    c. Inferior vena cava
    d. Sacrum

34. Which of the following would not be a typical clinical finding of a patient with retroperitoneal hematoma?
    a. Low hematocrit
    b. Trauma
    c. Weight loss
    d. Hemophilia

35. Enlargement of the abdominal lymph nodes is referred to as:
    a. retroperitoneal fibrosis.
    b. retroperitoneal lymphadenopathy.
    c. abdominal consolidation.
    d. retroperitoneal sequestration.

36. Which of the following is a linear muscular section of the diaphragm that attaches to the anterolateral surfaces of the upper lumbar vertebrae?
    a. Crus of the diaphragm
    b. Psoas muscle
    c. Iliacus
    d. Quadratus lumborum

37. All of the following are potential causes of lung consolidation except:
    a. pneumonia.
    b. hemorrhage.
    c. carcinoma.
    d. pulmonary sequestration.

38. One complication of a thoracentesis that may require a chest radiograph for diagnosis is the development of a:
    a. pneumothorax.
    b. sequestration.
    c. cystic adenomatoid malformation.
    d. rib fracture.

39. Common locations for abdominal lymph nodes include all of the following except:
    a. mesentery.
    b. renal hilum.
    c. along the length of the abdominal aorta.
    d. within the subhepatic space.

40. Lung consolidation typically appears sonographically as:
    a. several internal echoes that radiate in a linear pattern because of air within the bronchi.
    b. an anechoic mass with posterior enhancement.
    c. an echogenic mass with posterior shadowing.
    d. a large, hypoechoic mass surrounding the pericardial space.

41. A 65-year-old patient presents to the sonography department with a history of abdominal pain and weight loss. Sonographically, you visualize multiple hypoechoic masses that extend along the anterior border of the abdominal aorta. Which of the following would be most likely?
    a. Pulmonary sequestration
    b. Retroperitoneal hematoma
    c. Retroperitoneal lymphadenopathy
    d. Encapsulated ascites

42. What patient position is typically required for a thoracentesis?
    a. Upright
    b. Prone
    c. Supine
    d. Trendelenburg

43. A 35-year-old female patient presents to the sonography department with a history of migraine headache medication use, weight loss, nausea, and malaise. Sonographically, you visualize a 15-cm hypoechoic mass within the abdomen. Which of the following would be most likely?
    a. Volvulus
    b. Retroperitoneal fibrosis
    c. Intussusception
    d. Retroperitoneal lymphadenopathy

44. All of the following are true of abnormal lymph nodes except:
    a. they tend to lose their echogenic hilum.
    b. enlargement may be associated with infection or malignancy.
    c. they tend to measure less than 1 cm.
    d. the "sandwich" sign denotes abdominal nodes surrounding and compressing the aorta and inferior vena cava.

45. Which of the following most often accompanies lung consolidation?
    a. Ascites
    b. Retroperitoneal fibrosis
    c. Retroperitoneal hematoma
    d. Pleural effusion

46. A 63-year-old male patient presents to the sonography department for an examination of the abdomen. He has a history of lung cancer and is suffering from shortness of breath. Sonographically, the liver and gallbladder appear normal. However, you visualize a heterogeneous fluid collection superior to the right hemidiaphragm. What is the most likely diagnosis?
    a. Pulmonary sequestration
    b. Complex pleural effusion
    c. Pneumothorax
    d. Cystic adenomatoid malformation

47. A 38-year-old female patient presents to the sonography department with a history of femoral artery puncture and back pain. What laboratory value would be helpful to assess the patient for active bleeding?
    a. Hematocrit
    b. Blood urea nitrogen
    c. Alkaline phosphatase
    d. Creatinine

48. A pleural effusion that is associated with infection will sonographically appear:
    a. complex.
    b. anechoic.
    c. septated.
    d. in varying appearances.

49. Which of the following best describes a hemophiliac?
    a. A person who lacks hemoglobin and hematocrit clotting factors
    b. A person who has an inherited bleeding disorder that inhibits the control of blood clotting
    c. A person who has an inherited breathing disorder that causes the development of pulmonary sequestrations
    d. A person who has abnormally shaped red blood cells

50. The tissue comprising a lung consolidation can appear sonographically isoechoic to the:
    a. liver.
    b. inferior vena cava.
    c. aorta.
    d. rectus abdominis.

51. Enlarged, abnormal lymph nodes tend to deviate from their normal sonographic appearance and become more:
    a. isoechoic.
    b. anechoic.
    c. hypoechoic.
    d. anechoic or hypoechoic.

52. All of the following may be discovered sonographically within the chest except:
    a. bronchial infections.
    b. pleural effusion.
    c. lymphomas.
    d. thymomas.

53. What is the name for the fascia that lines the anterolateral abdominal wall and is located between the transverse abdominis muscle and the peritoneum?
    a. Rectus abdominis
    b. Linea alba
    c. Transversalis fascia
    d. Psoas lumborum

54. What is the name of the pleura that is closely applied to each lung?
    a. Parietal
    b. Visceral
    c. Intimal
    d. Transverse

55. What it the name of the pleura that is closely applied to the inner chest wall?
    a. Visceral
    b. Mesenteric
    c. Parietal
    d. Adventitia

56. A patient with a known cause of pleural effusion would likely require what type of thoracentesis to relieve breathing difficulty due to the excessive pleural fluid?
    a. Therapeutic
    b. Diagnostic
    c. Intracavitary
    d. Transudative

57. Which of the following is the most likely sonographic appearance of the thymus in the adult patient?
    a. Echogenic mass that contains linear and punctuate echogenicities
    b. Thymus is typically not seen in adults.
    c. Complex mass anterior to the iliac crest
    d. Homogeneous mass with posterior shadowing containing anechoic cystic structures

58. Which of the following vascular structures is not located within the retroperitoneum?
    a. Abdominal aorta
    b. Inferior vena cava
    c. Splenic artery
    d. Right portal vein

59. Which of the following is a double fold of peritoneum that attaches the intestines to the posterior abdominal wall?
    a. Retroperitoneal membrane
    b. Mediastinum
    c. Crus of the diaphragm
    d. Mesentery

60. Which of the following would be performed to determine the origin of pleural fluid?
    a. Chest radiography
    b. CT-guided paracentesis
    c. Magnetic resonance imaging
    d. Diagnostic thoracentesis

SUGGESTED READINGS

Hertzberg BS, Middleton WD. *Ultrasound: The Requisites.* 3rd ed. Elsevier; 2016:254–260.

Kline JP, Dionisio D, Sullivan K, Early T, Wolf J, Kline D. Detection of pneumothorax with ultrasound. *AANA J.* 2013;81(4):265–271.

Rumack CM, Wilson SR, Charboneau JW, et al. *Diagnostic Ultrasound.* 4th ed. Elsevier; 2011:447–485, 1768–1799.

Sanders RC, Hall-Terracciano B. *Clinical Sonography: A Practical Guide.* 5th ed. Wolters Kluwer; 2016:588–594, 704–712.

Siegel MJ. *Pediatric Sonography.* 5th ed. Wolters Kluwer; 2019:500–510.

BONUS REVIEW!

Retroperitoneal Lymphadenopathy on Computed Tomography (Fig. 11-13)

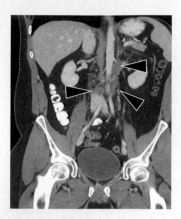

Figure 11-13 Coronal-enhanced soft-tissue window setting computed tomography image shows extensive retroperitoneal lymphadenopathy (*arrowheads*).

Pneumothorax on Radiograph and Computed Tomography (Fig. 11-14)

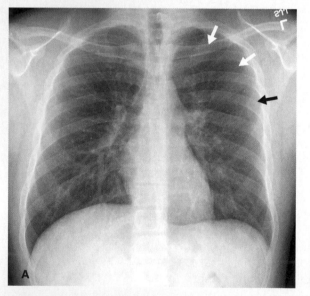
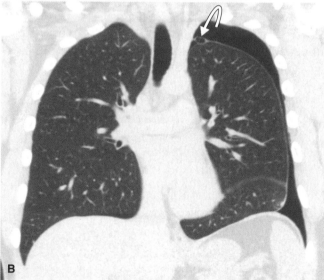

Figure 11-14 Pneumothorax on radiograph and computed tomography (CT). **A.** Upright frontal chest radiograph in a 28-year-old man shows a left pneumothorax with a visible visceral pleural line (*arrows*). **B.** Coronal CT scan shows the left pneumothorax (*curved arrow*).

The Face and Neck

Introduction

Sonography can provide a noninvasive image of the highly sensitive thyroid gland. This chapter presents anatomy, physiology, and sonography of the face and neck, including thyroid, parathyroid, the salivary glands, and lymph nodes. Pathology of these structures is also provided. The "Bonus Review" section contains a computed tomography (CT) image of a thyroid cancer.

Key Terms

branchial cleft cysts—benign congenital neck cysts found most often near the angle of the mandible

cervical lymphadenopathy—enlargement of the cervical lymph nodes

cold nodules—the hypofunctioning thyroid nodules seen on a nuclear medicine study that have malignant potential

colloid—the fluid produced by the thyroid that contains thyroid hormones

dysphagia—difficulty swallowing

dyspnea—difficulty breathing

exophthalmos—bulging eyes

fibromatosis colli—a rare, pediatric fibrous tumor located within the sternocleidomastoid muscle

goiter—an enlarged, hyperplastic thyroid gland

Graves disease—the most common cause of hyperthyroidism that produces bulging eyes, heat intolerance, nervousness, weight loss, and hair loss

Hashimoto thyroiditis—the most common cause of hypothyroidism in the United States

hot nodules—the hyperfunctioning thyroid nodules seen on a nuclear medicine study that are almost always benign

hypercalcemia—elevated serum calcium

hyperthyroidism—a condition that results from the overproduction of thyroid hormones

hypothyroidism—a condition that results from the underproduction of thyroid hormones

lymphangioma—pediatric neck mass that consists of lymphatic fluid secondary to the blockage of lymphatic channels; may also be referred to as a cystic hygroma; may occur in other regions of the body where lymphatic tissue exists

menorrhagia—abnormally heavy and prolonged menstruation

mucoepidermoid carcinoma—the most common malignancy of the salivary glands; typically starts in the parotid gland

oligomenorrhea—infrequent or light menstrual periods

papillary carcinoma—the most common form of thyroid cancer

pleomorphic adenoma—benign and most frequent tumor of the salivary glands; most commonly seen in the parotid gland

pretibial myxedema—clinical finding associated with Graves disease in which there is thickening of the skin and edema on the anterior legs

psammoma bodies—round, punctate calcific deposits

punctate—marked with dots

pyramidal lobe—a normal variant of the thyroid gland in which there is a superior extension of the isthmus

saliva—fluid produced by the salivary glands that aids in digestion

scintigraphy (thyroid)—nuclear medicine study in which a radiopharmaceutical is used to examine the thyroid gland

sialadenitis—inflammation of the salivary gland or glands

sialadenosis—benign, painless enlargement of a salivary gland or glands

sialolithiasis—salivary duct stones

Sjögren syndrome—an autoimmune disease that affects all glands that produce moisture, leading to dysfunction of the salivary glands and severe dryness of the eyes, nose, skin, and mouth

Stensen duct—the main duct of the parotid gland

thyroglossal duct—the embryonic duct that stretches the base of the tongue to the midportion of the anterior neck

thyroglossal duct cysts—benign congenital cysts located within the midline of the neck superior to the thyroid gland and near the hyoid bone

thyroid inferno—the sonographic appearance of hypervascularity demonstrated with color Doppler imaging of the thyroid gland

thyroidectomy—the surgical removal of the thyroid or part of the thyroid

torticollis—twisted neck

Wharton duct—the duct that drains the submandibular gland

THE FACE

Anatomy and Physiology of the Salivary Glands

Salivary glands are exocrine glands whose primary function is to produce **saliva** that is ultimately released into the oral cavity through ducts. Saliva, which aids in digestion, is mostly composed of water. However, it does contain electrolytes and digestive enzymes like amylase and lipase, which are also produced by the pancreas. There are three paired groups of salivary glands: the parotid glands, the submandibular glands, and the sublingual glands (Fig. 12-1).

The parotid glands are the largest of the salivary glands and are consequently the most likely to be analyzed with sonography. They are located bilaterally, anterior to the ears and extend inferiorly, where they are bounded anteriorly by the rami of the mandibles and posteriorly by the mastoid processes of the temporal

Oral Cavity

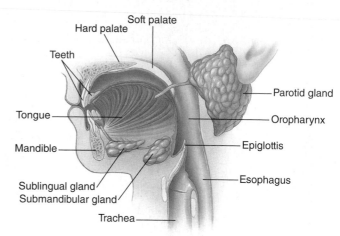

Figure 12-1 Oral cavity anatomy, including the salivary glands.

bones. The paired, bilateral sternocleidomastoid muscles are also located posterior to the parotid glands. The parotid gland can be separated into three anatomic lobes, and its main duct is referred to as the **Stensen duct**. The bilateral submandibular glands are located beneath the floor of the mouth and are bordered laterally by the body of the mandible and superiorly by musculature. The submandibular gland is drained by the **Wharton duct**. The bilateral sublingual glands are located just under the tongue and anterior to the submandibular glands.

Sonography and Pathology of the Salivary Glands

The salivary glands are most often imaged with a high-frequency linear transducer, although when the glands are enlarged, a lower frequency may be required. For superficial masses, a standoff device may be needed. When abnormalities of the salivary glands are suspected, it is best to image both sides for comparison because many diseases impact both glands.

The salivary glands are typically hyperechoic compared to the adjacent musculature (Fig. 12-2). Especially when dilated, the ducts of the glands may be recognized as anechoic tubular structures. Color flow should be used to delineate ducts from vasculature. The salivary glands should be imaged in both sagittal and transverse planes. The parotid gland will appear elliptical in the sagittal plane and round in the transverse plane. The sublingual glands are round as well, whereas the submandibular glands are more of a triangular shape. Pathology of the salivary glands includes **Sjögren syndrome**, **sialadenosis** (sialadenosis), **sialolithiasis**,

The Face and Neck

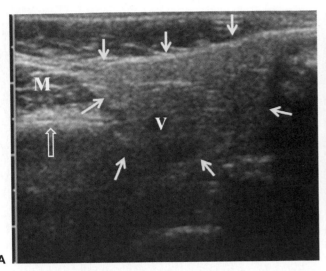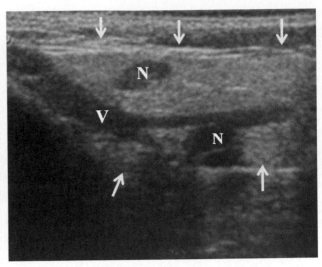

Figure 12-2 Normal parotid gland. **A.** In the transverse scan plane, which is perpendicular to the earlobe, the parotid gland (*arrows*) is ovoid in shape and hyperechoic to the adjacent muscle (*M*). **B.** In the longitudinal plane, the parotid gland is elliptical in shape. The mandibular vein (*V*) can be seen in both images, as well as several lymph nodes (*N*).

and **sialadenitis**. A brief summary of these pathologies and others is provided in Table 12-1. Especially when malignancy is suspected, an evaluation of the cervical lymphatic chain should be performed.

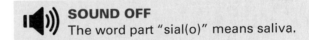 **SOUND OFF**
The word part "sial(o)" means saliva.

TABLE 12-1 Pathology of the salivary glands

Pathology	Explanation	Sonographic Appearance
Ranula	Mucus retention cyst in the floor of the mouth arising from an obstructed sublingual or minor salivary duct	Well-defined, homogeneous, hypoechoic, or anechoic mass. Infected cyst will appear complex
Sjögren syndrome	An autoimmune disease that affects all glands that produce moisture; leads to dysfunction of the salivary glands and severe dryness of the eyes, nose, skin, and mouth	Heterogeneous, hyperemic, visibly enlarged, and may contain diffuse hypoechoic regions
Slaladenitis	Inflammation of the salivary gland(s)	Heterogeneous, hyperemic, visibly enlarged, and may contain diffuse hypoechoic regions
Sialolithiasis	Salivary duct stones; most commonly located within the submandibular gland	Dilated duct containing a shadowing, echogenic focus or foci
Sialadenosis	Benign, painless enlargement of the salivary gland; usually affects both parotid glands	Enlarged gland without hypervascularity
Pleomorphic adenoma (see Fig. 12-3)	Benign and most frequent tumor of the salivary glands; most commonly seen in the parotid gland	Hypoechoic mass; biopsy is often warranted
Mucoepidermoid carcinoma (see Fig. 12-4)	Most common malignancy of the salivary glands; typically starts in the parotid gland	Hypoechoic or heterogeneous mass with moderate to marked internal vascularity; biopsy is often warranted

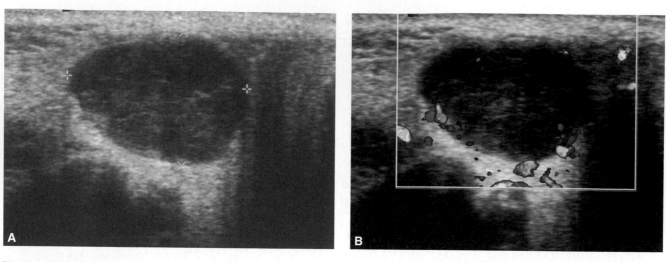

Figure 12-3 Pleomorphic adenoma. **A.** This hypoechoic mass (between *calipers*) was noted in the parotid gland and was diagnosed as a pleomorphic adenoma. **B.** Color Doppler image reveals flow around the mass, but not much within it.

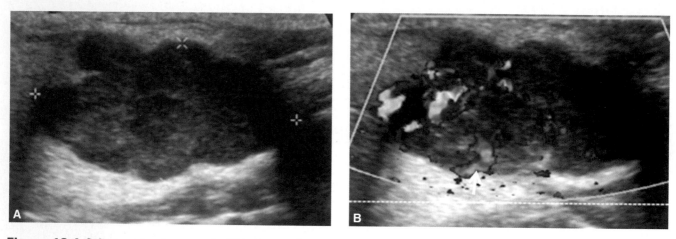

Figure 12-4 Salivary gland cancer. **A.** This hypoechoic mass has lobulated borders. It was identified as salivary gland cancer after biopsy. **B.** Color Doppler reveals extensive blood flow within the mass.

THE NECK

Anatomy and Physiology of the Thyroid Gland

The thyroid gland is a crucial endocrine gland that develops within the third week of gestation. In the embryo, the thyroid begins its initial development at the base of the tongue. It descends down the **thyroglossal duct** to ultimately rest anterior to the trachea. It is fully functional by the end of the first trimester. The thyroid consists of a right and a left lobe. A bridge of tissue, the isthmus, crosses over the midline of the neck anterior to the trachea, providing a link between the two thyroid lobes (Fig. 12-5). Occasionally, individuals may have a superior extension of the isthmus. This normal variant is termed a **pyramidal lobe**. Agenesis of a lobe may occur, and ectopic

thyroid tissue can occur as well. The hypothalamus, located within the brain, produces thyroid-releasing hormone, which, in turn, controls the release of thyroid-stimulating hormone (TSH) by the anterior pituitary gland. The thyroid consists of multiple follicles that contain a fluid called **colloid**. Colloid is composed of proteins and thyroid hormones. As a result of the TSH released by the pituitary gland, the thyroid, in turn, releases the hormones contained within its cells. These hormones are thyroxine (T_4), triiodothyronine (T_3), and calcitonin (Table 12-2).

> **SOUND OFF**
> The thyroid uses iodine to produce its hormones.

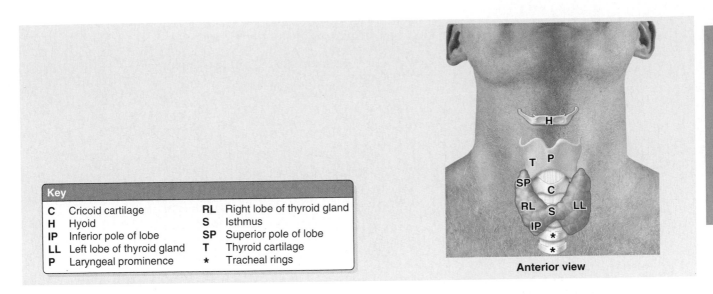

Figure 12-5 Thyroid anatomy.

Key

C	Cricoid cartilage	RL	Right lobe of thyroid gland
H	Hyoid	S	Isthmus
IP	Inferior pole of lobe	SP	Superior pole of lobe
LL	Left lobe of thyroid gland	T	Thyroid cartilage
P	Laryngeal prominence	*	Tracheal rings

Anterior view

TABLE 12-2 The three thyroid hormones and their functions

Thyroid Hormone	Function
Thyroxine (T_4)	Aids in the metabolism of fats, proteins, and carbohydrates
Triiodothyronine (T_3)	Aids in the metabolism of fats, proteins, and carbohydrates
Calcitonin	Responsible for removing calcium from the blood for storage in the bones

The thyroid utilizes iodine to manufacture its hormones. Iodine is found in some vegetables, seafood, and within many processed foods that contain iodized salt. Accordingly, the subscripted numbers "3" and "4" found in the thyroid hormones denote the number of iodine atoms contained within each hormone. Thyroxine is the most abundant hormone produced by the thyroid. However, each hormone is vital, and they work together to regulate metabolism, growth and development, and the activity of the nervous system. A surplus of these hormones will produce **hyperthyroidism**, and a reduction will cause **hypothyroidism**.

◀))) SOUND OFF
The most abundant hormone of the thyroid gland is thyroxine.

Vascular Anatomy of the Thyroid Gland and Neck

Two prominent vascular structures can be seen lateral to the thyroid gland: the common carotid artery and the internal jugular vein. The most medial vessel is the common carotid artery. The common carotid arteries branch into internal and external carotid arteries above the thyroid gland. The superior thyroid artery is the first branch of the external carotid artery. The inferior thyroid artery is a branch of the thyrocervical trunk of the subclavian artery. These arteries have corresponding thyroid veins that drain into the internal jugular vein. The jugular veins are located superior and lateral to the common carotid arteries.

Sonography of the Thyroid and Neck

A thyroid sonogram can be ordered for various clinical reasons, including a palpable mass found within the neck, abnormal laboratory findings, and as a follow-up examination from nuclear medicine studies and other diagnostic imaging studies. Before beginning the examination, the sonographer should determine whether there are any palpable nodules by standing behind the patient and palpating the thyroid gland. A thyroid and neck sonogram is performed with a high-frequency linear transducer. The patient should be in the supine position, with the neck

TABLE 12-3 Surrounding structures of the thyroid gland	
Structure	**Relationship to Thyroid Gland**
Strap muscles (sternohyoid, sternothyroid, thyrohyoid, and omohyoid)	Anterior to each lobe
Sternocleidomastoid muscles	Lateral to each lobe
Longus colli muscles	Posterior to each lobe
Common carotid artery	Lateral to each lobe
Internal jugular vein	Lateral to each lobe Superior and lateral to each common carotid artery
Esophagus	Most often seen on the left side posterior to the trachea and thyroid

extended. Normal thyroid tissue is homogeneous and consists of medium- to high-level echogenicities similar to that of the testes.

Images are obtained in both the sagittal and transverse planes of each lobe and of the isthmus. Each adult pear-shaped lobe measures approximately 4 to 6 cm in length, 2 to 3 cm in width, and 1 to 2 cm in thickness, with the right lobe typically being the largest. The isthmus normally measures between 2 and 6 mm in the anteroposterior dimension. A thyroid volume can be calculated using the following formula: length × width × thickness × 0.529. A sonographic examination of the entire neck should also be performed for enlarged lymph nodes or masses. Some institutions may require an analysis of various regions of the neck for classification, as suggested by the American Institute of Ultrasound in Medicine (see "Cervical Lymph Nodes and the Postsurgical Neck" section).

There are several prominent muscles and vascular structures that delineate the margins of the thyroid gland (Table 12-3; Fig. 12-6). The neck muscles, which appear more hypoechoic than the normal thyroid tissue, are easily seen with sonography. The thin infrahyoid or strap muscles, which include the sternohyoid, sternothyroid, thyrohyoid, and omohyoid, are found anterior to the thyroid gland. The much larger sternocleidomastoid muscles pass lateral to the thyroid lobes. The longus colli muscles are seen posterior to each lobe. The common carotid artery and internal jugular vein will be seen lateral to each lobe as anechoic tubes in the longitudinal plane and circles in the transverse plane. The esophagus lies posterior to the thyroid gland, most often on the left side, and can often resemble a mass. To differentiate the esophagus from a mass, one can have the patient swallow. Upon real-time observation of swallowing, the saliva can be visualized passing through the esophagus.

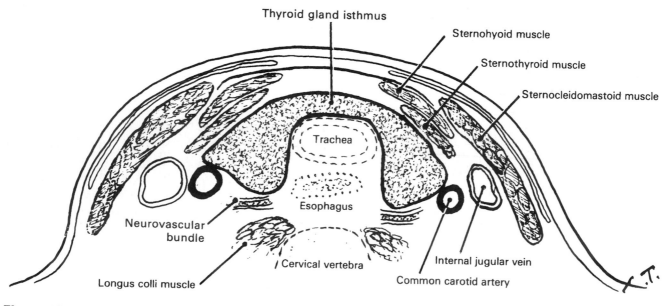

Figure 12-6 Neck anatomy. Transverse anatomy of the neck.

> **🔊 SOUND OFF**
> To differentiate the esophagus from a mass, have the patient swallow. Upon real-time observation of swallowing, the saliva can be visualized passing through the esophagus.

Each thyroid lobe should be evaluated using color Doppler because increased vascularity or hyperemia may be evident with **Graves disease** and **Hashimoto thyroiditis**, both of which are discussed further in this chapter. Identified thyroid nodules should be measured in two planes and further analyzed with color Doppler. Also, when technically pertinent, elastography may be performed as an adjunct to grayscale imaging to further characterize thyroid nodules based on stiffness properties. With elastography, a relative stiffness is obtained in relationship to the surrounding tissue. Softer nodules tend to be more likely benign, whereas harder nodules tend to be more likely malignant. Fine-needle aspiration (FNA) is a highly efficient way to determine the characteristics of clinically palpable and sonographically identifiable thyroid nodules. The use of sonographic guidance for FNA is especially beneficial. During this minimally invasive procedure, the tissue is identified with sonography, and a small needle is inserted into the nodule. An FNA is considered a low-risk procedure.

> **🔊 SOUND OFF**
> Both Graves disease and Hashimoto thyroiditis yield increased vascularity within the thyroid with color Doppler interrogation.

THYROID PATHOLOGY

Goiter

A **goiter** is a broad term that is defined as an enlarged or hyperplastic thyroid gland. It has many causes, including iodine deficiency, Graves disease, and thyroiditis. Clinically, patients with a goiter often have a palpable (and often visually) enlarged thyroid gland. The enlarged gland can cause a feeling of tightening in the throat, **dysphagia**, **dyspnea**, coughing, and hoarseness. Thyroid enlargement can be diagnosed by calculating volume measurements or by obtaining an anteroposterior thickness of the thyroid isthmus. An isthmus that measures greater than 1.0 cm may be indicative of thyroid enlargement (Fig. 12-7). Sonographically, the thyroid will appear enlarged and heterogeneous. The enlarged thyroid gland that contains multiple nodules with cystic and solid components may be referred to as a multinodular goiter or adenomatous goiter.

CLINICAL FINDINGS OF A GOITER

1. Palpable (and possibly visually) enlarged thyroid gland
2. Dyspnea
3. Dysphagia
4. Feeling of tightening in the throat
5. Coughing
6. Hoarseness

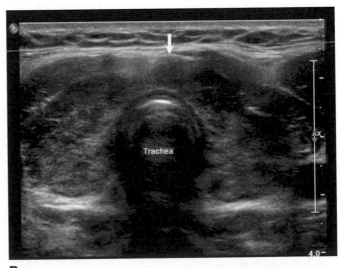

A **B**

Figure 12-7 Goiter and thyroid enlargement. **A.** Longitudinal image of the right thyroid lobe demonstrates diffuse enlargement and general heterogeneity indicative of a goiter. **B.** Transverse sonogram on the thyroid demonstrating a diffusely enlarged, heterogeneous thyroid. There is an increased anteroposterior (*AP*) diameter of the isthmus (*arrow*) measuring greater than 1 cm.

SONOGRAPHIC FINDINGS OF A GOITER

1. Enlarged thyroid gland (isthmus that exceeds 1 cm in the anteroposterior plane)
2. Diffusely heterogeneous echotexture
3. Multiple nodules with cystic and solid components

🔊 SOUND OFF
Goiter is the general term for thyroid enlargement that can result from inadequate iodine intake. However, there can be other underlying causes.

Graves Disease and Hyperthyroidism

Hyperthyroidism is a condition that results from the overproduction of thyroid hormones. Clinical findings in individuals suffering from hyperthyroidism include **exophthalmos**, heat intolerance, nervousness, weight loss with increased appetite, hair loss, tachycardia, palpitations, muscle wasting, fine tremors, **pretibial myxedema**, **oligomenorrhea**, and, possibly, high-output heart failure (Fig. 12-8). Graves disease, which may also be referred to as a diffuse toxic goiter, is the most common cause of hyperthyroidism. Sonographically, the thyroid may appear diffusely heterogeneous or hypoechoic (Fig. 12-9). Hypervascularity may be noted with color Doppler imaging within the thyroid gland. This is termed the "**thyroid inferno.**"

CLINICAL FINDINGS OF GRAVES DISEASE

1. Bulging eyes (exophthalmos)
2. Heat intolerance
3. Nervousness
4. Weight loss (with increased appetite)
5. Hair loss
6. Tachycardia, palpitations, high-output heart failure
7. Muscle wasting
8. Fine tremors
9. Oligomenorrhea
10. Pretibial myxedema

SONOGRAPHIC FINDINGS OF GRAVES DISEASE

1. Enlarged gland
2. Heterogeneous or diffusely hypoechoic echotexture
3. Thyroid inferno

🔊 SOUND OFF
Graves disease is the most common cause of hyperthyroidism. To recall this, remember that both Graves and hyperthyroidism both contain the letter "*e*."

Hashimoto Thyroiditis and Hypothyroidism

Hypothyroidism is a condition that results from the underproduction of thyroid hormones. Hashimoto thyroiditis is an autoimmune disease and is the most common cause of hypothyroidism in the United States. It may also be referred to as chronic autoimmune lymphocytic thyroiditis. With Hashimoto disease, the thyroid becomes inflamed, and as a result, the thyroid produces smaller amounts of thyroid hormones. In order to compensate, the pituitary gland releases more TSH, which causes the thyroid to become enlarged. Clinically, many patients are asymptomatic in the early stages of the disease. However, as the disease progresses, they may present with pallor, puffiness under the eyes, puffy face, dry skin, slight weight gain, depression, increased cold sensitivity, peripheral edema, muscle weakness, **menorrhagia**, slow pulse, and elevated blood cholesterol levels (Fig. 12-10). The end stage of the disease may lead to fibrosis and atrophy

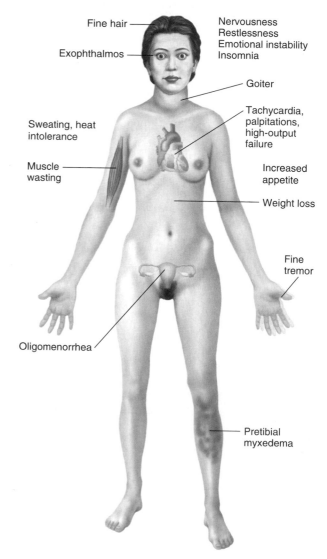

Figure 12-8 Several clinical findings of an overactive thyroid or hyperthyroidism.

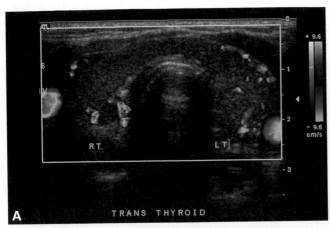
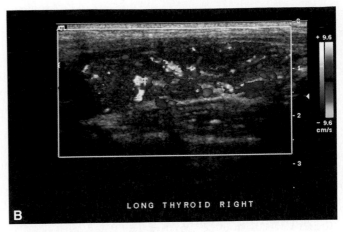

Figure 12-9 Graves disease. The transverse (**A**) and longitudinal (**B**) images of the right lobe image with color Doppler show markedly increased vascularity within a diffusely, enlarged heterogeneous thyroid gland.

of the gland. Sonographically, the thyroid will appear diffusely heterogeneous, coarse, and mildly enlarged with increased vascularity within the gland (Fig. 12-11). Oftentimes, multiple, ill-defined hypoechoic regions separated by fibrous hyperechoic tissue will be demonstrated with Hashimoto thyroiditis.

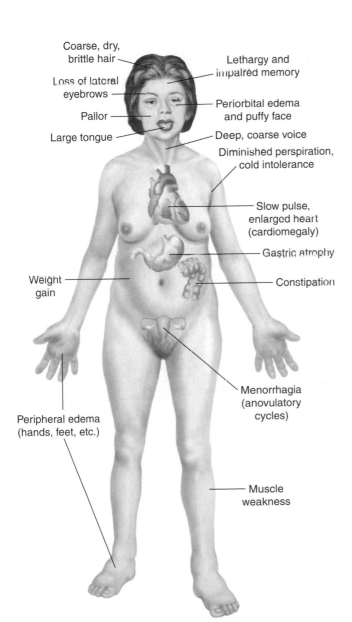

Figure 12-10 Several clinical findings of an underactive thyroid or hypothyroidism.

Labels on figure:
Coarse, dry, brittle hair
Loss of lateral eyebrows
Pallor
Large tongue
Weight gain
Peripheral edema (hands, feet, etc.)
Lethargy and impaired memory
Periorbital edema and puffy face
Deep, coarse voice
Diminished perspiration, cold intolerance
Slow pulse, enlarged heart (cardiomegaly)
Gastric atrophy
Constipation
Menorrhagia (anovulatory cycles)
Muscle weakness

CLINICAL FINDINGS OF HASHIMOTO THYROIDITIS

1. Depression
2. Increased cold sensitivity
3. Elevated blood cholesterol levels
4. Slight weight gain may occur
5. Puffy face and puffiness under the eyes
6. Menorrhagia
7. Pallor

SONOGRAPHIC FINDINGS OF HASHIMOTO THYROIDITIS

1. Mild enlargement of the thyroid gland (initially)
2. Heterogeneous echotexture
3. Multiple, ill-defined hypoechoic regions separated by fibrous hyperechoic tissue
4. Hypervascular gland

SOUND OFF
Hashimoto thyroiditis is the most common cause of hypothyroidism. To recall this, remember that both Hashim*o*to and hyp*o*thyroidism both contain the letter "*o*."

Benign Thyroid Nodules

Up to 68% of all adults have sonographically identifiable thyroid nodules, making them exceedingly common. Benign thyroid nodules are the most common masses identified within the thyroid gland with sonography. They

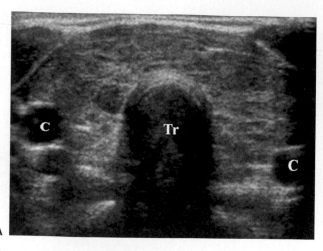 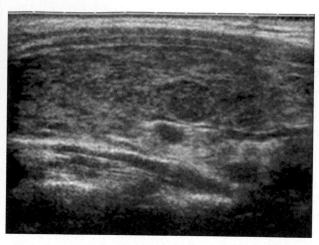

Figure 12-11 Hashimoto thyroiditis. **A.** Transverse image of the thyroid gland in a patient with hypothyroidism revealing a diffusely coarse, heterogeneous gland. The trachea (*Tr*) and carotid arteries (*C*) are also demonstrated. **B.** Longitudinal image of the same patient.

can be considered follicular adenomas or adenomatous or hyperplastic nodules, or colloid nodules.

Follicular adenomas are most often small, round, and can have varying sonographic appearances, including completely anechoic, isoechoic, or hyperechoic (Fig. 12-12). They may also have a surrounding halo. Nodular hyperplasia is the most common cause of thyroid nodules. Hyperplastic nodules, also referred to as adenomatous nodules, are almost always multiple and also have varying sonographic appearances.

Many benign thyroid nodules typically have cystic components. Within the cystic component of these nodules, especially colloid cysts, a hyperechoic focus or foci may be seen, which may produce comet-tail artifact (Fig. 12-13). Sonographic features of benign thyroid nodules are listed in Table 12-4, although benign and malignant features can overlap and no single feature can be used to delineate benign versus

malignant thyroid nodules. While many benign nodules are small and incidentally noted, large nodules may become palpable and impinge upon neighboring structures, consequently leading to dysphagia or general neck discomfort.

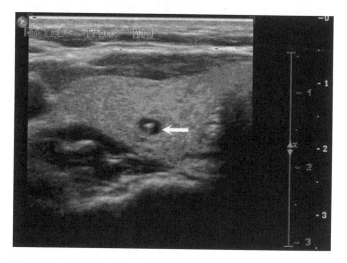

Figure 12-13 Colloid cyst. Transverse image of the thyroid revealing a small colloid cyst (*arrow*) with a small, hyperechoic focus contained within it that is producing comet-tail artifact.

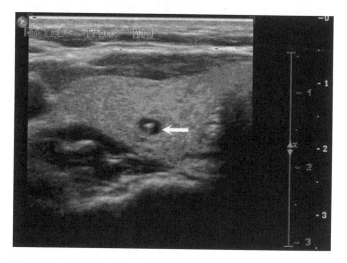

Figure 12-12 Benign thyroid nodule. Longitudinal image of a thyroid (*Th*) adenoma (*arrows*).

TABLE 12-4 Benign characteristics of thyroid nodules
Extensive cystic components
Cysts <5 mm
Hyperechoic mass
"Eggshell" calcifications
Spongiform composition
Wider-than-tall shape
"Hot" nodule (nuclear medicine finding)

Malignant Thyroid Nodules

Papillary carcinoma is the most common form of thyroid cancer. Other forms of thyroid malignancies include follicular carcinoma, medullary carcinoma, anaplastic carcinoma, lymphoma, and metastases of the thyroid. It is difficult to diagnose malignant thyroid nodules with sonography; however, there are some distinct features that increase the likelihood of the nodule being malignant (Table 12-5; Fig. 12-14). It is important to note that the presence of microcalcifications within a thyroid mass seems to increase the likelihood of a malignancy. These structures may be referred to as **psammoma bodies**, which are round calcific deposits that appear sonographically as **punctate**, hyperechoic foci

TABLE 12-5 Malignant characteristics of thyroid nodules

Hypoechoic mass
Taller-than-wide shape
Mass with internal microcalcifications (psammoma bodies)
Solitary mass
Marked vascularity within the central part of the nodule
Interrupted peripheral calcification
Extracapsular invasion
Lobulated margins
Enlargement of the cervical lymph nodes (metastasis)
"Cold" nodule (nuclear medicine finding)

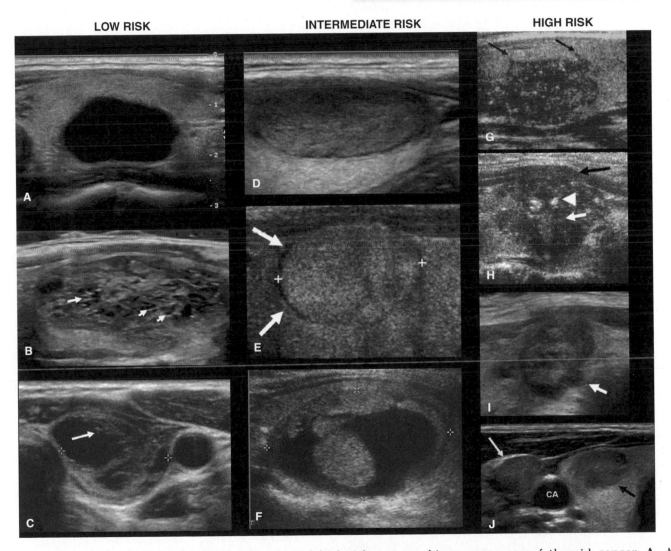

Figure 12-14 Nodules with low-, intermediate-, and high-risk sonographic appearances of thyroid cancer. **A.** A completely anechoic nodule. **B.** A nodule with both solid tissue and cystic areas (*arrows*). **C.** A complex cyst with echogenic foci that produce comet-tail artifact (*arrow*). **D.** A large hypoechoic mass. **E.** An isoechoic nodule with a hypoechoic halo (*arrows*). **F.** A large cystic nodule with solid mural or wall elements. **G.** A hypoechoic nodule that contains small echogenic foci and that is invading the surrounding tissue (*black arrows*). **H.** An invasive, hypoechoic nodule with varying size calcifications (*arrowhead*) that can produce acoustic shadows (*arrow*). **I.** A hypoechoic nodule that is taller than wide and has irregular borders (*arrow*). **J.** Hypoechoic nodule (*black arrow*) with metastasis to an area lymph node (*white arrow*).

without acoustic shadowing. A solitary, hypoechoic mass is also suspicious. Elastography can be used as an adjunct to grayscale imaging. With elastography, stiffer nodules, in comparison to the tissue around them, in general, have an increased risk for malignancy.

Thyroid Imaging Reporting and Data System

Because thyroid nodules are so common, and in order to prevent unnecessary follow-up, further imaging, and biopsies, the American College of Radiology worked to create a standardized reporting and description system of sonographically identified thyroid nodules. This system is referred to as Thyroid Imaging Reporting & Data System (TI-RADS). TI-RADS places thyroid nodule in five levels (TR1 to TR5) based on five ultrasound features: composition, echogenicity, shape, margin, and punctate echogenic foci (Fig. 12-15). Each feature is assigned points; thus, the more points a nodule is assigned, the higher the risk for malignancy. By analyzing the point system, one can decipher that the most worrisome nodules tend to contain punctate echogenic foci, are hypoechoic, have a taller-than-wide shape, and have irregular margins that may extend beyond the normal thyroid margins. Furthermore, the least worrisome nodules tend to be anechoic, have a wider-than-tall shape, have smooth margins, and either produce

a large comet-tail artifact or do not at all. The sum of all points results in the nodules being assigned a TI-RADS of 0 to 7 or more. The highest category is TR5, which is referred to as highly suspicious. In some clinical settings, sonographers may have to score sonographically identified thyroid nodules. A helpful online calculator can be found at http://tiradscalculator.com/.

> **◀))) SOUND OFF**
> The most worrisome thyroid nodules tend to contain punctate echogenic foci, are hypoechoic, have a taller-than-wide shape, and have irregular margins that may extend beyond the normal thyroid margins.

Nuclear Medicine and Thyroid Nodules

Nuclear medicine utilizes **scintigraphy** to classify thyroid nodules as either hyperfunctioning or hypofunctioning. This examination includes the injection of a radiopharmaceutical that is high in iodine. Because the thyroid utilizes iodine to create its hormones, the drug is absorbed by the thyroid gland. Images are obtained with a camera that detects radioactivity within the neck. The thyroid tissue, along with thyroid nodules, is displayed on the image obtained. Hyperfunctioning or "**hot nodules**" yield

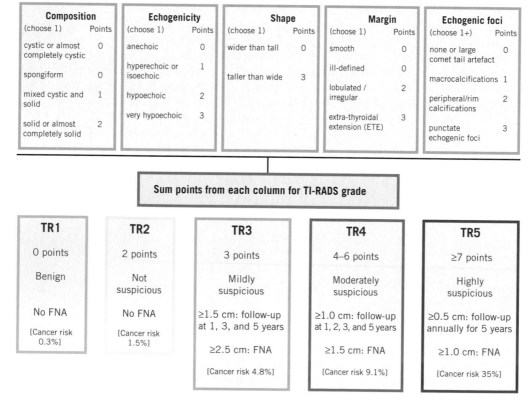

Figure 12-15 Thyroid Imaging Reporting & Data System (TI-RADS) places thyroid nodule in five levels (TR1 to TR5) based on five ultrasound features. *FNA*, fine-needle aspiration.

The Face and Neck

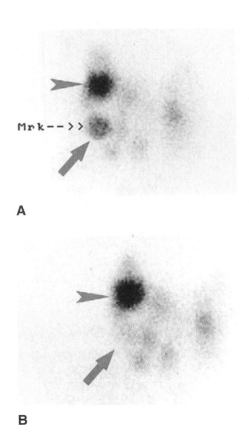

A

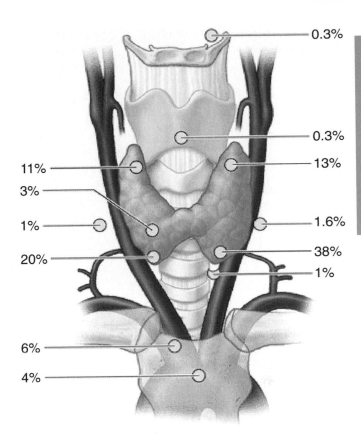

Figure 12-17 Parathyroid locations.

Figure 12-16 Nuclear medicine images of thyroid nodules. **A.** A radioactive marker (*Mrk*) was placed over a 2-cm palpable nodule (*arrow*) in the right thyroid lobe. **B.** The image on the right, without the marker, demonstrates the palpable nodule (*arrow*) to be cold. The second palpable nodule in the right upper lobe (*arrowhead*) is shown to be hot. A biopsy of the cold, palpable nodule demonstrated in (**B**) confirmed that the nodule was papillary thyroid cancer.

dark areas on a thyroid scan, whereas hypofunctioning or "**cold nodules**" yield light or blank areas on the scan. Most cancers are hypofunctioning nodules and will, therefore, appear as cold nodules, although not all cold nodules are malignant (Fig. 12-16). Although sonography and nuclear medicine can work together to establish the characteristics of a nodule, in almost all situations, an FNA is needed to obtain the most definitive diagnosis.

ANATOMY, PHYSIOLOGY, AND PATHOLOGY OF THE PARATHYROID GLANDS

There are typically two pairs of parathyroid glands, although some individuals may have a fifth gland. Their locations are variable. However, commonly one is located near the posterior aspect of the midportion of each lobe, and one is often positioned inferior to each lobe (Fig. 12-17). Normal parathyroid glands

will measure 5.0 mm × 3.0 mm × 1.0 mm, and their sonographic appearance is similar to the thyroid tissue. The parathyroid glands serve as calcium regulators for the body. The parathyroid glands control the release and absorption of calcium by producing parathyroid hormone (PTH). An elevated level of calcium is referred to as **hypercalcemia**, whereas a low level is hypocalcemia. Thus, hyperparathyroidism can cause hypercalcemia, and hypoparathyroidism can cause hypocalcemia.

Parathyroid Adenoma

A parathyroid adenoma is the most common cause of enlargement of a parathyroid gland. Patients with a parathyroid adenoma will present with elevated serum calcium levels and PTH (hyperparathyroidism). Sonographically, a parathyroid adenoma appears as a solid mass that will most likely be hypoechoic to the adjacent thyroid gland (Fig. 12-18).

◀)) SOUND OFF
If the patient has elevated serum calcium (hypercalcemia), analyze the neck carefully for signs of a parathyroid adenoma.

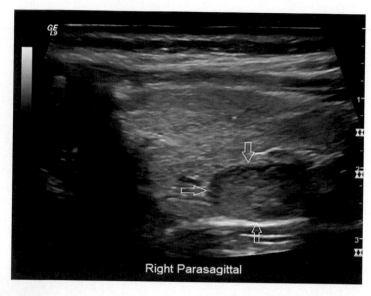

Figure 12-18 Parathyroid adenoma. This hypoechoic mass (*between arrows*) was identified as a parathyroid adenoma.

CLINICAL FINDINGS OF A PARATHYROID ADENOMA

1. Elevated serum calcium
2. Elevated PTH

SONOGRAPHIC FINDINGS OF A PARATHYROID ADENOMA

1. Hypoechoic mass adjacent to the thyroid

OTHER NECK PATHOLOGY

Cervical Lymph Nodes and the Postsurgical Neck

Enlargement of the cervical lymph nodes, or **cervical lymphadenopathy**, can be established sonographically. These structures, which normally measure less than 1 cm, are often recognized during a routine sonographic examination of the neck. They are typically oblong-shaped hypoechoic structures with a distinguishable echogenic hilum. Abnormal lymph nodes can result from infections and malignancy. Sonographically, abnormal lymph nodes will appear enlarged, measuring greater than 1 cm. They may also be more rounded in shape, lose their normal hilar feature, contain calcifications, or demonstrate abnormal vascular patterns (Fig. 12-19). The postsurgical neck sonogram—especially in those who require imaging following a **thyroidectomy** because of cancer—should include a thorough examination of the neck for lymphadenopathy (i.e., metastatic disease to the nodes). An analysis of the nodal levels and sublevels of the neck for classification may be required by some institutions (Fig. 12-20).

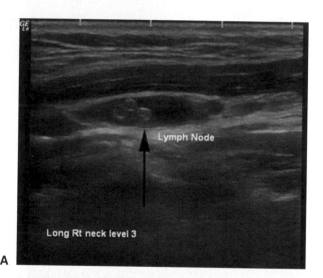

A

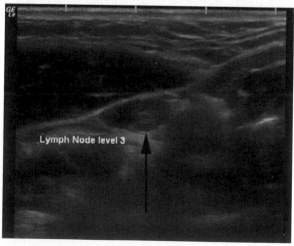

B

Figure 12-19 Abnormal-appearing lymph node. Sonographic examination of the right lateral cervical lymph nodes shows an abnormal right level III lymph node in the longitudinal (**A**) and transverse (**B**) images. The arrows denote the abnormal lymph node.

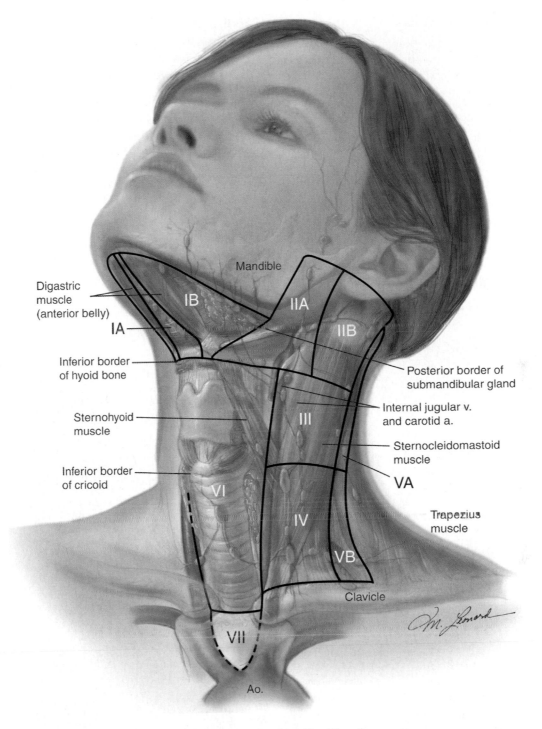

Digastric
muscle
(anterior belly)

IA

Inferior border
of hyoid bone

Sternohyoid
muscle

Inferior border
of cricoid

Mandible

IB

IIA

IIB

Posterior border of
submandibular gland

Internal jugular v.
and carotid a.

Sternocleidomastoid
muscle

VA

Trapezius
muscle

Clavicle

III

VI

IV

VB

VII

Ao.

Figure 12-20 Lymph node compartments separated into levels and sublevels.

CLINICAL FINDINGS OF ABNORMAL LYMPH NODES

1. Palpable neck mass (possibly)
2. Enlarged nodes may be painful

SONOGRAPHIC FINDINGS OF ABNORMAL LYMPH NODES

1. Enlargement of the node greater than 1 cm
2. Rounded shape
3. Loss of the echogenic hilum
4. Calcifications
5. May be hyperemic or demonstrate abnormal vascular patterns with color Doppler

Other Neck Masses

Thyroglossal duct cysts are benign congenital cysts located within the midline of the neck superior to the thyroid gland and are typically located below the level the hyoid bone. They are most often asymptomatic, although they may become painful when inflamed. Sonographically, a simple thyroglossal duct cyst will appear as an anechoic, well-defined, and unilocular cyst with posterior enhancement. Complicated or infected thyroglossal duct cysts will appear more complex (Fig. 12-21).

As the tissues of the neck develop in utero from the branchial apparatus, branchial clefts, which normally involute, may be maintained. **Branchial cleft cysts** are congenital neck cysts that result from this maldevelopment. They are found most often near the angle of the mandible, but may occur in the lower, lateral neck. They typically appear as an anechoic mass with posterior enhancement. A branchial cleft fistula can also occur in the same region. Fistulas may allow fluid to leak to the skin surface.

Fibromatosis colli is a rare, pediatric fibrous tumor located within the sternocleidomastoid muscle. Although the cause is unknown, it is speculated that perhaps malposition in utero or a traumatic birth leads to the development of fibrosis (scar tissue) within the muscle. Because of the mass within the sternocleidomastoid muscle, the muscle shortens, resulting in the twisting of the infant's chin toward the nonaffected side—termed congenital muscular **torticollis**. Sonographically, the mass will distort the normal shape of the muscle, often in a fusiform pattern, and may appear hypoechoic, hyperechoic, or even isoechoic to the adjacent tissue (Fig. 12-22). It may also contain calcifications and yield a hyperemic blood flow pattern with color Doppler.

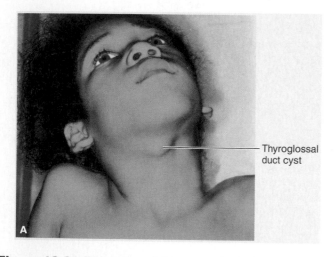
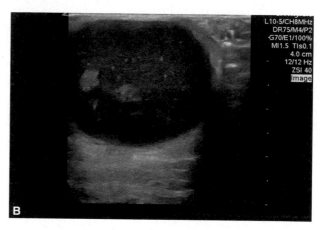

Figure 12-21 Thyroglossal duct cyst. **A.** A child with thyroglossal duct cyst. **B.** Sonographic appearance of an infected thyroglossal duct cyst.

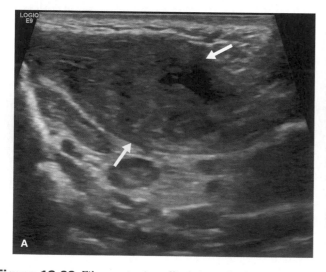
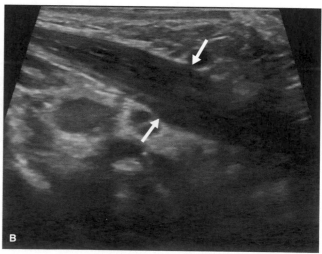

Figure 12-22 Fibromatosis colli. A 4-week-old girl with torticollis and firmness along the right aspect of her neck. Sagittal sonographic images of the right (**A**) sternocleidomastoid (*SCM*) muscles (*arrows*). There is fusiform thickening of the right SCM. Findings are compatible with fibromatosis colli. **B.** The left SCM (*arrows*) is normal.

A **lymphangioma**, also referred to as cystic hygroma, is a neck mass that may require sonographic evaluation. These masses are typically found in the posterior neck in utero or in the neonatal period. They consist of a buildup of lymphatic fluid. The sonographic appearance of a lymphangioma is often a thin-walled, hypoechoic or anechoic, septated mass. Clinically, they may be asymptomatic or painful with inflammation or hemorrhage.

CLINICAL FINDINGS OF A THYROGLOSSAL DUCT CYST

1. Palpable mass within the midline of the neck superior to the thyroid gland
2. Infected cysts may be painful

SONOGRAPHIC FINDINGS OF A THYROGLOSSAL DUCT CYST

1. Anechoic, well-defined, and unilocular cyst with posterior enhancement
2. May have internal components

CLINICAL FINDINGS OF A BRANCHIAL CLEFT CYST

1. Palpable neck mass located near the angle of the mandible
2. Infected cysts may be painful

SONOGRAPHIC FINDINGS OF A BRANCHIAL CLEFT CYST

1. Anechoic mass near the angle of the mandible

CLINICAL FINDINGS OF FIBROMATOSIS COLLI

1. Pediatric palpable neck mass
2. Torticollis (twisted neck with the chin angled to the nonaffected side)

SONOGRAPHIC FINDINGS OF FIBROMATOSIS COLLI

1. Fusiform-shaped mass within the sternocleidomastoid muscle that is hypoechoic, hyperechoic, or even isoechoic to the adjacent tissue
2. May also contain calcifications that shadow
3. May yield a hyperemic pattern with color Doppler

CLINICAL FINDINGS OF A LYMPHANGIOMA

1. Pediatric palpable neck mass
2. Asymptomatic or painful due to infection or hemorrhage

SONOGRAPHIC FINDINGS OF A LYMPHANGIOMA

1. Thin-walled, hypoechoic or anechoic, septated mass

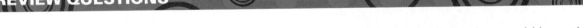

REVIEW QUESTIONS

1. What is another name for a cystic hygroma?
   a. Granuloma
   b. Lymphangioma
   c. Arteriovenous fistula
   d. Teratoma

2. What is the medical term for bulging eyes?
   a. Exophthalmos
   b. Exopglossia
   c. Exoccularia
   d. Exoglobia

3. Which of the following would be most likely associated with oligomenorrhea?
   a. Graves disease
   b. Parathyroid adenoma
   c. Hypothyroidism
   d. Cervical lymphadenopathy

4. Which of the following would have the clinical finding of pretibial myxedema?
   a. Hashimoto thyroiditis
   b. Addison disease
   c. Graves disease
   d. Pleomorphic carcinoma

5. Dysphagia is described as:
   a. difficulty speaking.
   b. difficulty eating.
   c. difficulty chewing.
   d. difficulty swallowing.

6. The patient in Figure 12-23 complained of weight gain, menorrhagia, and increased cold sensitivity. What is the most likely diagnosis?
   a. Parathyroiditis
   b. Graves disease
   c. Multiple intrathyroid parathyroid glands
   d. Autoimmune lymphocytic thyroiditis

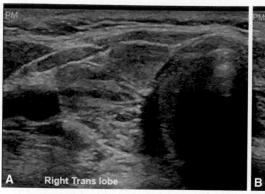
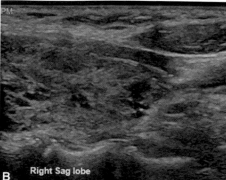

Figure 12-23

7. The transverse mid-neck image in Figure 12-24 is depicting a measurement that should not exceed:
   a. 5 mm.
   b. 10 mm.
   c. 3 mm.
   d. 15 mm.

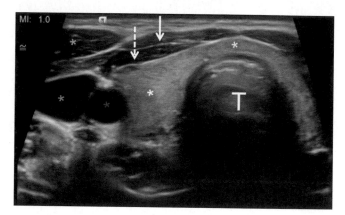

Figure 12-25

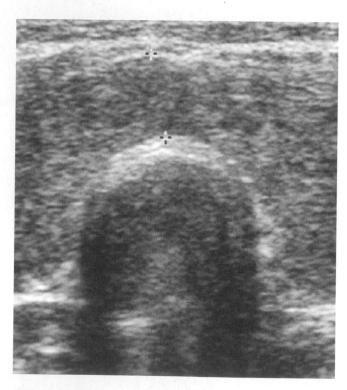

Figure 12-24

8. What does the red asterisk in Figure 12-25 indicate?
   a. Common carotid artery
   b. Internal carotid artery
   c. Internal jugular vein
   d. Subclavian vein

9. What does the blue asterisk in Figure 12-25 indicate?
   a. External carotid artery
   b. Internal carotid vein
   c. Common carotid artery
   d. Internal jugular vein

10. What does the orange asterisk in Figure 12-25 indicate?
    a. Right longus colli muscle
    b. Right sternocleidomastoid muscle
    c. Left longus colli muscle
    d. Left sternocleidomastoid muscle

11. The structures identified by the arrows in Figure 12-26 were discovered in the lateral neck of a patient with a history of thyroidectomy due to papillary carcinoma. What do these structures most likely represent?
    a. Parathyroid adenomas
    b. Parathyroid cystadenomas
    c. Metastatic disease within lymph nodes
    d. Normal lymph nodes

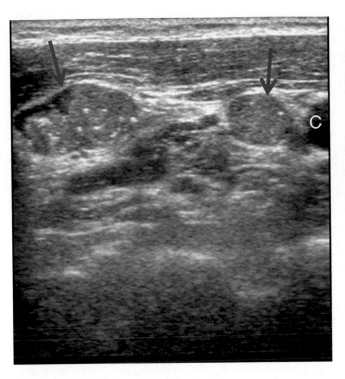

Figure 12-26

12. The structure that is measure in Figure 12-27 was discovered in an asymptomatic patient. Which of the following sonographic features is present and consequently most worrisome for malignancy?
    a. Anechoic echogenicity
    b. Internal microcalcifications
    c. Eggshell calcifications
    d. Colloid artifact

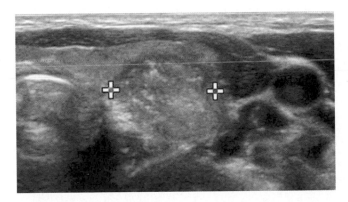

Figure 12-27

13. What does the structure noted in Figure 12-28 demonstrate?
    a. Colloid cyst
    b. Follicular carcinoma
    c. Papillary carcinoma
    d. Isoechoic thyroid nodule

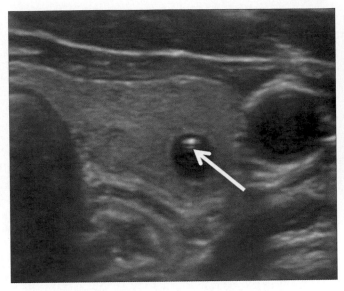

Figure 12-28

14. Which of the following represents the formula for thyroid volume?
    a. Length × width × thickness × 0.353
    b. Length × width × thickness × 0.459
    c. Length × width × thickness × 0.529
    d. Length × width × thickness × 0.642

15. The abnormality indicated in Figure 12-29 most likely represents a:
    a. benign thyroid nodule.
    b. papillary thyroid carcinoma.
    c. follicular thyroid carcinoma.
    d. medullary thyroid carcinoma.

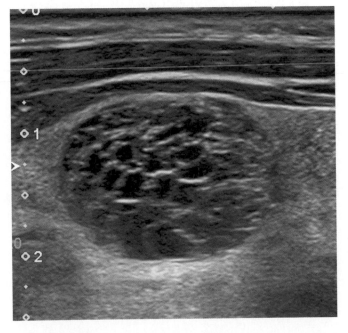

Figure 12-29

16. Which of the following would least likely indicative of a goiter?
    a. Dysphagia
    b. Dyspnea
    c. Hoarseness
    d. Hypercalcemia

17. Which of the following digestive enzymes is contained within saliva?
    a. Amylase
    b. Bile
    c. Sodium oxalate
    d. Acetaldehyde

18. What is the main duct of the parotid gland?
    a. Wharton duct
    b. Stenson duct
    c. Wirsung duct
    d. Sjögren duct

19. Which of the following is also referred to as diffuse toxic goiter?
    a. Hashimoto thyroiditis
    b. Adenomatous goiter
    c. Iodine deficiency syndrome
    d. Graves disease

20. You are performing a transverse scan through the right lobe of the thyroid. You note that there are two anechoic circles immediately adjacent to the thyroid representing vascular structures. What is the most lateral vessel?
    a. External jugular vein
    b. Internal jugular vein
    c. Internal carotid artery
    d. Common carotid artery

21. A patient with hypercalcemia presents to the sonography department for a neck sonogram. What abnormality in the neck should be suspected?
    a. Parathyroid adenoma
    b. Parotid gland enlargement
    c. Thyroid papillary carcinoma
    d. Hashimoto thyroiditis

22. Benign congenital cysts located superior to the thyroid gland near the hyoid bone are referred to as:
    a. branchial cleft cysts.
    b. follicular adenomas.
    c. thyroglossal duct cysts.
    d. parathyroid adenomas.

23. Normally, how many parathyroid glands are found within the adult neck?
    a. Three
    b. Four
    c. Six
    d. Eight

24. A cystic mass noted at the mandibular angle is most likely a:
    a. branchial cleft cyst.
    b. follicular adenoma.
    c. thyroglossal duct cyst.
    d. parathyroid adenoma.

25. Which of the following would more likely be a malignant thyroid nodule?
    a. Cold nodule
    b. Hot nodule

26. Parathyroid glands control the release and absorption of which nutrient?
    a. Thyroxine (T_4)
    b. Triiodothyronine (T_3)
    c. Calcitonin
    d. Calcium

27. A normal lymph node will not measure greater than:
    a. 8 mm.
    b. 5 mm.
    c. 12 mm.
    d. 10 mm.

28. With which of the following is elevated serum calcium associated?
    a. Graves disease
    b. Thyroglossal duct cyst
    c. Parathyroid adenoma
    d. Thyroid adenoma

29. Which of the following best describes the normal appearance of a cervical lymph node?
    a. A hypoechoic, oblong structure with a distinct echogenic hilum
    b. A rounded, echogenic structure with small calcifications
    c. A solid, hypoechoic mass that measures greater than 1 cm
    d. A solid, echogenic mass that measures less than 1 cm

30. Which abnormality is associated with the sonographic findings of a thyroid inferno?
    a. Hashimoto thyroiditis
    b. Graves disease
    c. Hyperparathyroidism
    d. Cervical lymphadenopathy

31. All of the following are sonographic findings of malignant thyroid nodules except:
    a. internal calcifications.
    b. hyperechoic mass.
    c. cervical node involvement.
    d. solitary mass.

32. All of the following are diagnostic findings of a likely benign thyroid nodule except:
    a. anechoic nodule.
    b. eggshell calcification.
    c. hyperechoic nodule.
    d. cold nodule.

33. Which of the following is the most common form of thyroid cancer?
    a. Follicular
    b. Anaplastic
    c. Lymphoma
    d. Papillary

34. What is the most common cause of hypothyroidism?
    a. Graves disease
    b. Hashimoto thyroiditis
    c. Papillary carcinoma
    d. Parathyroid adenoma

35. All of the following are sonographic findings of an abnormal lymph node except:
    a. rounded shape.
    b. echogenic hilum.
    c. calcifications.
    d. enlargement.

36. What is the most common cause of hyperthyroidism?
    a. Graves disease
    b. Hashimoto thyroiditis
    c. Papillary carcinoma
    d. Parathyroid adenoma

37. Which gland is located immediately anterior to the ear?
    a. Submandibular gland
    b. Sublingual gland
    c. Thyroid gland
    d. Parotid gland

38. Which muscle does fibromatosis colli mostly affect?
    a. Omohyoid
    b. Longus colli
    c. Sternocleidomastoid
    d. Infrahyoid

39. A 30-year-old patient presents to the sonography department for a thyroid sonogram with a history of weight loss, hair loss, and hyperthyroidism. You note that the patient has bulging eyes. What is the most likely diagnosis?
    a. Hashimoto thyroiditis
    b. Graves disease
    c. Hyperparathyroidism
    d. Cervical lymphadenopathy

40. The fluid produced by the thyroid gland that contains thyroid hormones is referred to as:
    a. thyroxine.
    b. calcitonin.
    c. colloid.
    d. triiodothyronine.

41. In the presence of Hashimoto thyroiditis, the thyroid produces:
    a. too many thyroid hormones.
    b. too much calcium.
    c. too few thyroid hormones.
    d. too much iodine.

42. A 45-year-old female patient presents to the sonography department with a palpable neck mass 6 months following a thyroidectomy for papillary carcinoma. Which of the following would be the most likely etiology of the palpable mass?
    a. Torticollis
    b. Lymphadenopathy
    c. Sialadenitis
    d. Graves disease

43. Which of the following is the duct that drains the submandibular gland?
    a. Stensen duct
    b. Wharton duct
    c. Seigel duct
    d. Partridge duct

44. Which of the following does the thyroid gland utilize to produce its hormones?
    a. Colloid
    b. Iodine
    c. Iron
    d. Calcium

45. Which muscles are located posterior to each thyroid lobe?
    a. Sternocleidomastoid
    b. Longus colli
    c. Sternohyoid
    d. Omohyoid

46. Which muscles are located lateral to each thyroid lobe?
    a. Sternocleidomastoid
    b. Longus colli
    c. Sternohyoid
    d. Omohyoid

47. Which of the following is associated with congenital muscular torticollis?
    a. Fibromatosis colli
    b. Branchial cleft cyst
    c. Pleomorphic adenoma
    d. Sialadenosis

48. What structure may be confused for a thyroid or parathyroid mass because of its relationship to the trachea and the posterior aspect of the left thyroid gland?
    a. Esophagus
    b. Common carotid artery
    c. Internal jugular vein
    d. Sternothyroid

49. Which vascular structure is located closest to the thyroid lobes?
    a. External carotid vein
    b. External carotid artery
    c. Internal jugular vein
    d. Common carotid artery

50. A thyroid isthmus that measures greater than _____ is indicative of thyroid enlargement.
    a. 8 mm
    b. 5 mm
    c. 12 mm
    d. 10 mm

51. Which of the following is the term for stones within the salivary duct?
    a. Sjögren syndrome
    b. Torticollis
    c. Cervical lymphadenopathy
    d. Sialolithiasis

52. Which muscles are located anterior to the thyroid gland?
    a. Sternocleidomastoid
    b. Longus colli
    c. Thyrocervical trunk
    d. Strap

53. What is the first branch of the external carotid artery?
    a. Internal carotid artery
    b. Optic artery
    c. Superior thyroid artery
    d. Inferior thyroid artery

54. Psammoma bodies are:
    a. hypoechoic structures.
    b. comet-tail artifacts emanating from inside as a colloid mass.
    c. punctate calcific deposits.
    d. mural or wall nodules within a solid mass.

55. All of the following are hormones produced by the thyroid except:
    a. thyroxine.
    b. iodine.
    c. triiodothyronine.
    d. calcitonin.

56. Which of the following is the hormone that is the most abundantly produced by the thyroid?
    a. Thyroxine
    b. Iodine
    c. Triiodothyronine
    d. Calcitonin

57. Which of the following is an autoimmune disease that affects the glands that produce moisture, leading to dysfunction of the salivary glands and dryness of the eyes, nose, skin, and mouth?
    a. Wharton syndrome
    b. Sjögren syndrome
    c. Stenson syndrome
    d. Sialadenosis syndrome

58. What type of gland is the thyroid gland?
    a. Endocrine
    b. Exocrine
    c. Both A and B
    d. Neither A nor B

59. The superior extension of the thyroid isthmus is referred to as the:
    a. thyroglossal duct.
    b. branchial cleft.
    c. Yodeler lobe.
    d. pyramidal lobe.

60. Which of the following is the most common form of salivary gland cancer?
    a. Mucoepidermoid carcinoma
    b. Papillary carcinoma
    c. Ancillary carcinoma
    d. Medullary carcinoma

SUGGESTED READINGS

American Institute of Ultrasound in Medicine. AIUM Practice Parameters for the performance of ultrasound examinations of the head and neck. Available at: https://www.aium.org/resources/guidelines/headNeck.pdf?__sw_csrfToken=f5c5cf00 Accessed August 30, 2021.

Curry RA, Tempkin BB. *Sonography: Introduction to Normal Structure and Function*. 5th ed. Elsevier; 2020:469–486.

Gritzmann N, Hollerweger A, Macheiner P, et al. Sonography of soft tissue masses of the neck. *J Clin Ultrasound*. 2002;30:356–373.

Hagen-Ansert SL. *Textbook of Diagnostic Sonography*. 7th ed. Elsevier; 2012:588–603.

Henningsen C, Kuntz K, Youngs D. *Clinical Guide to Sonography: Exercises for Critical Thinking*. 2nd ed. Elsevier; 2014:359–368.

Hertzberg BS, Middleton WD. *Ultrasound: The Requisites*. 3rd ed. Elsevier; 2016:229–247.

Hoang JK, Lee WK, Lee M, et al. US Features of thyroid malignancy: pearls and pitfalls. *Radiographics*. 2007;27(3):847–860.

Kawamura DM, Nolan TD. *Diagnostic Medical Sonography: Abdomen and Superficial Structures*. 4th ed. Wolters Kluwer; 2018:421–454.

Liu Y, Kamaya A, Desser TS, et al. A Bayesian network for differentiating benign from malignant thyroid nodules using sonographic and demographic features. *Am J Roentgenol*. 2011;196(5):W598–W605.

Penny SM. Sonographic diagnosis of fibromatosis colli. *J Diagn Med Sonogr*. 2006;22(6):399–402.

Rumack CM, Wilson SR, Charboneau JW, et al. *Diagnostic Ultrasound*. 4th ed. Elsevier; 2011:708–774.

Sanders RC, Hall-Terracciano B. *Clinical Sonography: A Practical Guide*. 5th ed. Wolters Kluwer; 2016:691 703.

Siegel MJ. *Pediatric Sonography*. 5th ed. Wolters Kluwer; 2019:112–155.

Tessler FN, Middleton WD, Grant EG. Thyroid Imaging Reporting and Data System (TI-RADS): a user's guide. *Radiology*. 2018; 287(1):29–36.

BONUS REVIEW!

Medullary Thyroid Cancer on Computed Tomography (Fig. 12-30)

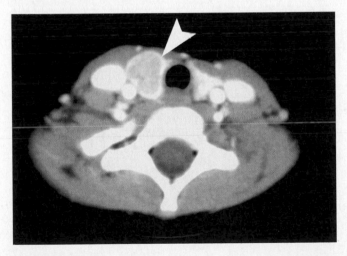

Figure 12-30 Medullary thyroid carcinoma in an 8-year-old girl. Axial contrast-enhanced computed tomography shows a mass within the left thyroid lobe, which enhances less than the surrounding thyroid gland (*arrowhead*).

The Male Pelvis

Introduction

The male pelvis and relevant pathology, including that of the penis, testicles, scrotum, prostate, and seminal vesicles, are discussed in this chapter. Reviewers should especially have a thorough understanding of the vastly different sonographic features of testicular torsion and epididymitis. Several helpful images can be found within "Bonus Review" section.

Key Terms

adrenal rest—mass of ectopic adrenal tissue within the testicle; are associated with congenital adrenal hyperplasia or Cushing syndrome

alpha-Fetoprotein—a protein produced by the fetal yolk sac, fetal gastrointestinal tract, and the fetal liver; may also be produced by some malignant tumors

appendix epididymis—the testicular appendage located at the head of the epididymis

appendix testis—the testicular appendage located between the head of the epididymis and the superior pole of the testis

appendix vas—the testicular appendage located between the body and tail of the epididymis

"bell-clapper" deformity—the condition in which the patient lacks the normal posterior fixation of the testis and epididymis to the scrotal wall

benign prostatic hyperplasia—the benign enlargement of the prostate gland

"blue-dot" sign—the appearance of a torsed testicular appendage that can be observed as a blue dot just under the skin surface

Buck fascia—deep layer of fascia that covers the corpora cavernosa and corpus spongiosum of the penis

bulbourethral gland—gland that secretes pre-ejaculate fluid that lubricates the penile urethra before ejaculation; also referred to as the Cowper gland

chlamydia—a sexually transmitted disease that can lead to infection of the genitals

corpora cavernosa—paired erectile tissues of the penis

corpus spongiosum—component of erectile tissue of the penis that contains the urethra

Cowper gland—see key term bulbourethral gland

cremaster muscle—the muscle that raises the testicle

cryptorchidism—the condition of having an undescended testis or testicles

digital rectal examination—the medical procedure that requires the insertion of the finger into the rectum to palpate the prostate gland and lower gastrointestinal tract

ductus (vas) deferens—the tube that connects the epididymis to the seminal vesicles

ecchymosis—subcutaneous spot of bleeding

epidermoid cyst—small benign mass within the testicle that contains keratin

epididymal cyst—a cyst located anywhere along the length of the epididymis

epididymis—a coiled structure that is attached to the testicle and the posterior scrotal wall that is responsible for storing sperm

epididymitis—inflammation of all or part of the epididymis

epididymo-orchitis—inflammation of the epididymis and testis

germ cell tumor—a type of neoplasm derived from germ cells of the gonads; may be found outside the reproductive tract

gonorrhea—sexually transmitted disease that leads to infection of the genitals

hematocele—a collection of blood within the scrotum

hematospermia—the presence of blood within the semen

human chorionic gonadotropin—hormone typically only produced by the trophoblastic cells of the early placenta; may also be used as a tumor marker in nongravid patients and males

hydrocele—a fluid collection within the scrotum; most often found between the two layers of the tunica vaginalis

idiopathic—from an unknown origin

inguinal canal—normal passageway in the lower anterior abdominal wall that allows for the passage of the spermatic cord into the scrotum

inguinal hernia—the protrusion of bowel or abdominal contents through the inguinal canal

Klinefelter syndrome—a condition in which a male has an extra X chromosome; characteristic features include small testicles, infertility, gynecomastia, long legs, and abnormally low intelligence

median raphe—the structure that separates the scrotum into two compartments externally

mediastinum testis—the structure that is formed by the tunica albuginea and contains the rete testis

nocturia—frequent urination at night

nutcracker syndrome—an anomaly where left renal vein entrapment occurs between the superior mesenteric artery and the abdominal aorta

omentum—a fold of peritoneum

orchiopexy—the surgery that moves and fixates an undescended testis into the scrotum

orchitis—inflammation of the testis or testicles

pampiniform plexus—the group of veins in the spermatic cord

peripheral zone—the largest zone of the prostate and most common location for prostatic cancer

Peyronie disease—the buildup of fibrous plaque (scar tissue) and calcifications within the penis that results in a painful curvature

polyorchidism—having more than two testicles

prostate-specific antigen—a protein produced by the prostate gland

prostatitis—inflammation of the prostate gland

pyocele—a pus collection within the scrotum

rete testis—a network of tubules that carry sperm from the seminiferous tubules to the epididymis

scrotal pearl—an extratesticular calculus

scrotum—sac of cutaneous tissue that holds the testicles

semen—a fluid that contains secretions from the testicles, seminal vesicles, and prostate gland

seminal vesicles—small glands located superior to the prostate gland and posterior to the base of the bladder, which secrete an alkaline-based fluid

seminiferous tubules—the location of spermatogenesis within the testicles

seminoma—the most common malignant neoplasm of the testicles

spermatic cord—the structure that travels through the inguinal canal and contains blood vessels, nerves, lymph nodes, and the cremaster muscle

spermatocele—a common cyst found most often in the head of the epididymis that is composed of nonviable sperm, fat, cellular debris, and lymphocytes

spermatogenesis—the production of sperm

supernumerary—having above the normal number of a structure; an extra

testicular torsion—a condition that results from the arterial blood supply to the testicle being cut off secondary to the twisting of the testicular axis

transitional zone—the prostatic zone that is the most common site for benign prostatic hyperplasia

transurethral resection of the prostate—surgical procedure performed to treat benign prostatic hyperplasia in which prostatic tissue is removed to relieve urinary complications

tubular ectasia of the rete testis—the cystic dilation and formation of cysts within the rete testis

tunica albuginea—the dense connective tissue that is closely applied to each testicle; it is also located within the penis

tunica albuginea cysts—cysts located within the tunica albuginea surrounding the testis

tunica dartos—the structure that separates the scrotum into two separate compartments internally

tunica vaginalis—the paired serous coatings of the testis; hydroceles are most often found between the two layers of the tunica vaginalis

undescended testis—testicles that do not descend into the scrotum; also referred to as cryptorchidism

Valsalva maneuver—performed by attempting to forcibly exhale while keeping the mouth and nose closed

varicocele—a dilated group of veins found within the scrotum

vasectomy—a form of male contraception in which the vas deferens is surgically interrupted to prohibit the flow of sperm from the testicles

verumontanum—an elevated area within the prostatic urethra at which the ejaculatory ducts meet the urethra

Zinner syndrome—syndrome that consists of unilateral renal agenesis, ipsilateral seminal vesicle cyst, and ejaculatory duct obstruction

ANATOMY AND PHYSIOLOGY OF THE SCROTUM, TESTICLES, AND EPIDIDYMIS

Sonography of the male pelvis is both common and crucial secondary to its ease of use and accuracy. The male pelvis consists of the lower ureters, urinary bladder, urethra, prostate, scrotum, testicles (testes), penis, and other accessory structures (Fig. 13-1).

The paired testicles begin to develop in the upper abdomen in the fetus and do not descend into the pelvis until the fourth week of gestation. By 28 weeks,

the testicles descend into the **scrotum**. They may become trapped anywhere along this path and consequently never completely descend into the scrotum. This condition is known as **cryptorchidism**. The normal adult testicles are located within a sac of cutaneous tissue called the scrotum. The scrotum is externally divided at the midline into two compartments by a structure known as the **median raphe**. Internally, it is divided by the **tunica dartos**. The scrotum provides a means for temperature control for the temperature-sensitive sperm. The **cremaster muscle**, a structure located within the **spermatic cord**, also alters the position of the testicle within the scrotum, which aids in their protection and temperature control.

The testes function as both endocrine glands and exocrine glands (Table 13-1). **Spermatogenesis** occurs within the **seminiferous tubules** that are found throughout each testicle. These tiny tubules converge into a structure called the **rete testis**, which is located within the **mediastinum testis**.

Each testis is surrounded by a double layer of tissue called the **tunica vaginalis**, which consists of a parietal and closely applied visceral covering (Fig. 13-2). **Hydroceles**, or scrotal fluid collections, are most commonly found between the two layers of the tunica vaginalis. Beneath the layers of the tunica vaginalis, the testis is also intimately surrounded by a dense fibrous layer of tissue called the **tunica albuginea**. The tunica albuginea extends posteriorly and enters each testicle to help form the previously described mediastinum testis.

> ◀))) **SOUND OFF**
> Hydroceles are most commonly located between the two layers of the tunica vaginalis.

The **epididymis** is a coiled structure. It is attached to the testicle and the posterior scrotal wall. It is divided into a head, body, and tail (Table 13-2). The epididymis is responsible for storing sperm in order for them to mature. It also transports sperm into the **ductus (vas) deferens**. The ductus (vas) deferens, also referred to as the deferent duct, is a tube that connects the epididymis to the **seminal vesicles**. Accordingly, the ductus (vas) deferens is the structure that is surgically interrupted in the surgical procedure referred to as a **vasectomy**.

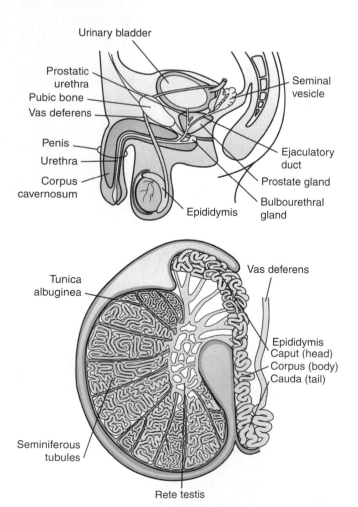

Figure 13-1 The male reproductive organs.

Labels: Urinary bladder; Prostatic urethra; Pubic bone; Vas deferens; Penis; Urethra; Corpus cavernosum; Epididymis; Seminal vesicle; Ejaculatory duct; Prostate gland; Bulbourethral gland; Tunica albuginea; Vas deferens; Epididymis Caput (head) Corpus (body) Cauda (tail); Seminiferous tubules; Rete testis

TABLE 13-1 Endocrine and exocrine functions of the testicles	
Endocrine function (released directly into bloodstream)	Produce testosterone: determines male characteristics
Exocrine function (released through ducts)	Produce sperm: permits reproduction

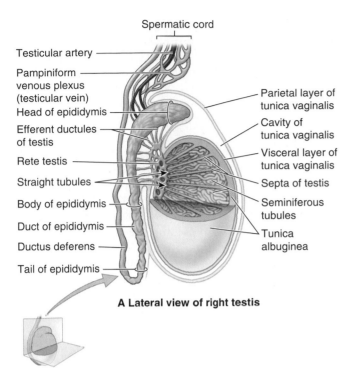

Figure 13-2 Structures of testis and epididymis in the sagittal plane.

Spermatic cord

Testicular artery

Pampiniform venous plexus (testicular vein)

Head of epididymis

Efferent ductules of testis

Rete testis

Straight tubules

Body of epididymis

Duct of epididymis

Ductus deferens

Tail of epididymis

Parietal layer of tunica vaginalis

Cavity of tunica vaginalis

Visceral layer of tunica vaginalis

Septa of testis

Seminiferous tubules

Tunica albuginea

A Lateral view of right testis

TABLE 13-2 Parts and location of the epididymis

Part of the Epididymis	Location
Head	Superior to the upper pole of the testis
Body	Posterior to the testicle
Tail	Inferior to the lower pole of the testis

From the vas deferens, sperm is transported to the paired seminal vesicles, which are located posterior to the male urinary bladder and above the prostate gland. These small glands secrete fluid that helps produce **semen**. At their junction, the seminal vesicles and the vas deferens combine to create the ejaculatory duct. The fluid is then passed through the prostatic urethra, where additional fluid from the prostate is added. The **bulbourethral gland**, also referred to as the **Cowper gland**, secretes pre-ejaculate (preseminal) fluid that lubricates the penile urethra before ejaculation. The anatomy, physiology, and pathology of the penis, prostate, and seminal vesicles are discussed later in this chapter.

Vascular Anatomy of the Male Pelvis

The spermatic cord enters the scrotum through the **inguinal canal** and contains essential structures,

TABLE 13-3 Components of the spermatic cord

Testicular artery
Pampiniform plexus
Lymph nodes
Nerves
Cremaster muscle

including the vascular supply and venous drainage for the testicles (Table 13-3; Fig. 13-3). The testicles receive most of their blood supply by means of the testicular arteries. These arteries emanate from the anterior abdominal aorta just below the level of the renal arteries. Venous drainage is performed through the **pampiniform plexus**, which empties into the testicular veins. The right testicular vein drains into the inferior vena cava, and the left testicular vein drains into the left renal vein.

SONOGRAPHY OF THE SCROTUM

Scrotal sonography is typically performed using a high-frequency linear transducer. The scrotal wall thickness ranges between 2 and 8 mm. Normal testicles appear isoechoic, and a small amount of extratesticular fluid is typically noted around each testicle. The echotexture of the testis is similar to that of the thyroid gland. The normal mediastinum testis will be noted as an echogenic linear structure within the testicle in the sagittal plane or as a triangular structure in the transverse plane. Adult testicles measure 3 to 5 cm in length, 2 to 4 cm in width, and 3 cm in thickness. The blood flow within each testicle and epididymis, which should be analyzed with color and pulsed Doppler, should be symmetric. Each part of the epididymis should be thoroughly analyzed for masses, hyperemic flow, and/or enlargement. Often, the head of each epididymis is measured, and its size compared to the size of the contralateral epididymal head. The normal head of the epididymis measures approximately 10 to 12 mm in size. The normal epididymis is either isoechoic or slightly more echogenic than the testis. Epididymal changes may be noted sonographically after a vasectomy, including enlargement of the epididymis, heterogeneous echotexture of the epididymis, and possibly cystic areas within the epididymis. Any intratesticular or extratesticular masses should be analyzed with color Doppler as well.

> **SOUND OFF**
> The normal mediastinum testis can be seen in the sagittal plane as an echogenic linear structure and in the transverse plane as an echogenic triangle.

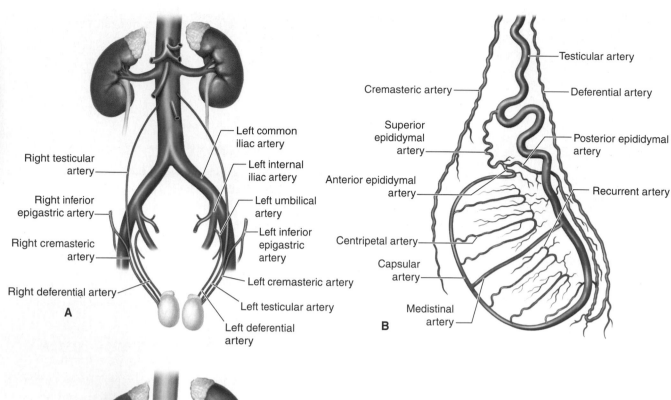

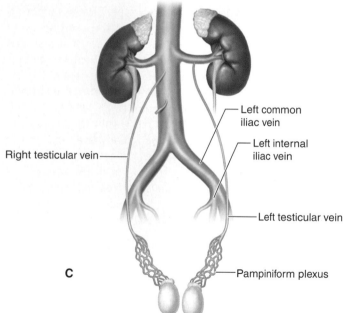

Figure 13-3 Vascular anatomy. Schematic illustration of normal arterial supply to the scrotum (**A**), intrascrotal arterial supply (**B**), and venous drainage form the scrotum (**C**).

PATHOLOGY OF THE SCROTUM

Polyorchidism

Although rare, a patient may have three or more testicles, a condition termed **polyorchidism**. Polyorchidism is most often located on the left side, and the **supernumerary** testicle does have an increased risk for developing testicular cancer. Patients may suffer from torsion of the supernumerary testicle as well. Though the condition is typically asymptomatic and often incidentally noted with sonography, the patient or his physician may palpate the extra testicle and thus consider it worrisome for a testicular mass. Sonographically, the extra testicle will appear smaller and have an isoechoic appearance to the normal testicle. It may have its own epididymis and vas deferens or share these structures with the ipsilateral testicle.

CLINICAL FINDINGS OF POLYORCHIDISM

1. Asymptomatic
2. Palpable extratesticular mass
3. Pain if torsion occurs

SONOGRAPHIC FINDINGS OF POLYORCHIDISM

1. Smaller, normal-appearing additional testicle
2. Doppler characteristics should be normal

CLINICAL FINDINGS OF CRYPTORCHIDISM

1. One or both testicles not palpable within the scrotum

SONOGRAPHIC FINDINGS OF CRYPTORCHIDISM

1. Testis located outside the scrotum (most likely in the inguinal canal)
2. The cryptorchid testis will appear hypoechoic to the normal testis

Cryptorchidism

Cryptorchidism describes the condition of having an **undescended testis**. Cryptorchidism, which is found in 3% to 4% of full-term births, is associated with infertility and an increase in the risk for malignancy in the involved testis. **Seminoma** is the most common cancer found in an undescended testis. Although they may be found within the abdomen, undescended testicles are most often found just above the scrotum or within the inguinal canal (Fig. 13-4). Surgical correction of an undescended testis is referred to as **orchiopexy**. Clinically, the affected testis will not be palpable within the scrotum. Sonographically, the undescended testis will typically appear hypoechoic to the normal testis.

> 🔊 **SOUND OFF**
> An undescended testis is most often found within the inguinal canal.

Testicular Torsion

Testicular torsion, which may also be referred to as spermatic cord torsion, occurs when the arterial blood supply to the testicle is cut off secondary to the twisting of the testicular axis. The degree of torsion can vary and can be intermittent. A 360-degree angle torsion will result in blocked venous drainage and arterial supply. This will lead to ischemia within the testis. Consequently, the amount of ischemic damage is directly related to the degree of the torsion. Testicular torsion occurs more often during adolescence, between 12 and 18 years of age. It is a true surgical emergency in which time is of the essence. In fact, salvage rates range from 80% to 100% if the patient is treated within 6 hours of symptom onset. After this time, the salvage rates drop considerably. The testicle is usually not salvageable after 24 hours.

Testicular torsion can be associated with trauma, strenuous exercise, and sexual activity. Often, patients

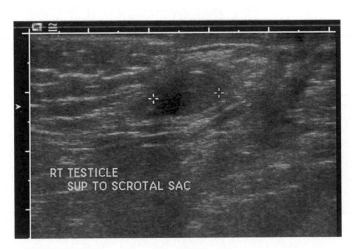

A Cryptorchidism

B

Figure 13-4 Cryptorchidism. **A.** Common locations of a cryptorchid testis. **B.** Sonographic appearance of a right testicle (*calipers*) within the inguinal canal.

who are predisposed to develop testicular torsion have a condition known as the **"bell-clapper" deformity**. This congenital abnormality describes the situation in which the patient lacks the normal posterior fixation of the testis and epididymis to the scrotal wall. **Bell-clapper deformity** is classically bilateral. It is part of what is termed intravaginal torsion, which is the most common form of testicular torsion. With intravaginal torsion, the testis, which is not affixed to the scrotal wall, is permitted to migrate and twist freely within the scrotum. The other form of torsion is extravaginal torsion, which occurs in the neonatal period or in utero and is related to torsion of the spermatic cord within the inguinal canal.

Patients suffering from testicular torsion complain of a sudden onset of testicular pain, often during sleep. The torsed testis will be swollen, and it may be positioned higher in the scrotum and have a horizontal orientation. Pain may radiate into the lower abdomen and inguinal region as well. Nausea and vomiting can result from the intense pain that occurs with this abnormality.

◄))) SOUND OFF
Patients suffering from testicular torsion are often awakened in the middle of the night by severe scrotal pain.

The sonographic appearance of the torsed testis depends on the duration of time that has passed since the first sign of symptoms. In the acute stage, the testis will often appear enlarged and hypoechoic or heterogeneous (Fig. 13-5). There will be no detectable intratesticular vascularity with Doppler interrogation when the testis is completely torsed. However, it is important to note that some intratesticular flow may be detectable with lesser degrees of torsion. For this reason, the sonographer should compare the flow within both testicles and should document both venous and arterial waveforms, if possible. In addition, the epididymis is often enlarged, and a reactive hydrocele

may be present. The scrotal wall may also appear thickened.

Chronic testicular torsion is torsion that has lasted for more than 10 days. The epididymis, testis, and spermatic cord will become enlarged and heterogeneous. Areas of necrosis may be noted within the testis, and there may be hyperemic flow around the testis.

◄))) SOUND OFF
Intratesticular flow between the testes should be compared. A torsed testis can either lack flow completely or have decreased flow compared to the normal testis.

CLINICAL FINDINGS OF ACUTE TESTICULAR TORSION

1. Acute onset of testicular pain (often during sleep)
2. Possible pain within the lower abdomen and inguinal region
3. Swollen testis/scrotum
4. Nausea and vomiting
5. Higher positioned, painful testis with a horizontal position

SONOGRAPHIC FINDINGS OF ACUTE TESTICULAR TORSION

1. Enlargement of the spermatic cord, epididymis, and testis
2. Thickened scrotal wall
3. Hypoechoic or heterogeneous testis
4. Reactive hydrocele
5. No intratesticular flow
6. Decreased intratesticular flow (as compared to the asymptomatic testis)

SONOGRAPHIC FINDINGS OF CHRONIC TESTICULAR TORSION

1. Enlargement of the spermatic cord, epididymis, and testis
2. No intratesticular flow
3. Hyperemic flow around the testis
4. Heterogeneous testis with areas of necrosis

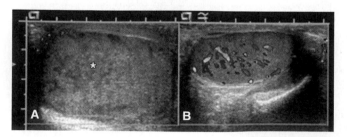

Figure 13-5 Testicular torsion. Longitudinal color Doppler sonogram of the right (**A**) and left (**B**) testicles demonstrates right testicular enlargement and heterogeneity (*asterisk*) as well as absent blood flow, consistent with testicular torsion. The left testicle is normal.

Torsion of the Testicular Appendages

Torsion of the **appendix testis** is the most common cause of acute scrotal pain in prepubertal boys. The appendix testis, **appendix epididymis**, and the **appendix vas** are appendages of the testis (Fig. 13-6).

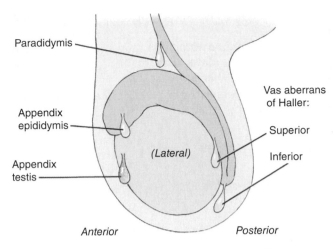

Figure 13-6 Locations of the testicular appendages.

These structures are said to be the embryologic remnants of the Müllerian duct, Wolffian duct, and mesonephric duct, respectively. The appendix testis is located between the head of the epididymis and the superior pole of the testis, whereas the appendix epididymis is located at the head of the epididymis. The appendix vas is positioned between the body and tail of the epididymis. During a normal sonographic examination, the appendages are not routinely identified as distinct structures. However, they may be seen in the presence of a hydrocele or other scrotal fluid collections. If visualized, the normal appendage

appears as a small, oval projection of tissue. After an appendage has undergone torsion, the appendage will likely become displaced and become mobile within the scrotum. The calcification of this free-floating structure will likely result in a **scrotal pearl**.

> ### SOUND OFF
> Torsion of the appendix testis is the most common cause of acute scrotal pain in prepubertal boys.

Clinically, torsion of the appendix testis presents much like testicular torsion. However, instead of general testicular pain, patients will present with focal testicular pain, often localized to the superior pole of the testis. Physicians can manually inspect the testis for evidence of the **"blue-dot" sign**. The blue-dot sign describes the appearance of the torsed appendage as a blue dot just under the skin surface. Sonographically, the torsed appendage will appear as a small, avascular, hypoechoic or hyperechoic mass adjacent to the superior pole of the testis (Fig. 13-7). There may also be evidence of scrotal wall thickening and a reactive hydrocele. Torsion of the appendix testis is treated with pain medication and bed rest.

> ### SOUND OFF
> The "blue-dot" sign is the observable clinical finding associated with torsion of the appendix testis.

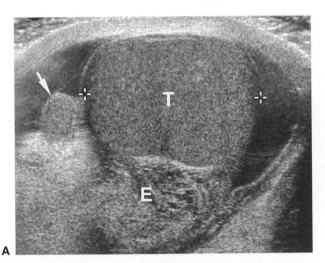

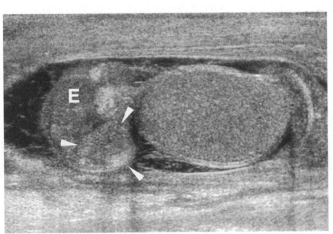

Figure 13-7 Torsion of testicular appendages. **A.** Torsed appendix testis in a 12-year-old boy with right scrotal pain and a paratesticular mass. Transverse sonogram shows an echogenic nodule (*arrow*) adjacent to the testis (*T*). There is epididymal swelling (*E*). **B.** Torsed appendix epididymis in a 10-year-old boy with left scrotal pain. Longitudinal scan shows a hypoechoic mass (*arrowheads*) contiguous with an enlarged right epididymis (*E*). There is scrotal skin thickening and a complex hydrocele indicative of inflammation.

CLINICAL FINDINGS OF TORSION OF THE TESTICULAR APPENDAGE

1. Acute testicular pain
2. Pain localized to the superior pole of the testis
3. "Blue-dot" sign

SONOGRAPHIC FINDINGS OF TORSION OF THE TESTICULAR APPENDAGE

1. Normal intratesticular flow
2. Small, avascular, hypoechoic or hyperechoic mass adjacent to the superior pole of the testis
3. Reactive hydrocele
4. Scrotal wall thickening

CLINICAL FINDINGS OF A HYDROCELE

1. Transilluminates light
2. Painless scrotal swelling
3. May present with pain when found in the presence of scrotal infections, testicular torsion, trauma, or a tumor

SONOGRAPHIC FINDINGS OF A HYDROCELE

1. Simple fluid anterior to the testis
2. Scrotal wall thickening
3. Chronic hydroceles may have internal debris and septations

Hydrocele

A few milliliters of extratesticular fluid is a normal sonographic finding. Scrotal enlargement that is thought to be caused by excessive fluid can be considered clinically because fluid within the scrotum will transilluminate light. A simple fluid collection within the scrotum is referred to as a hydrocele (Fig. 13-8). Hydroceles are found between the two layers of the tunica vaginalis and often displace the testicles posteriorly. They can be **idiopathic** or described as reactive hydroceles when found in the presence of scrotal infections, testicular torsion, trauma, or tumors. Hydroceles are often accompanied by scrotal wall thickening.

Extratesticular Cysts

A **spermatocele**, which is said to be the most common scrotal mass, is a cyst found most often in the head of the epididymis. It is composed of nonviable sperm, fat, cellular debris, and lymphocytes. Although it may be palpable during a physical examination, usually, it is not painful. The sonographic appearance of a spermatocele is that of a cyst in the head of the epididymis that may contain layering debris (Fig. 13-9). An **epididymal cyst** appears similar to a spermatocele and can be seen anywhere along the length of the epididymis. Lastly, **tunica albuginea cysts** are located anywhere along the periphery of the testicle, within the tunica albuginea.

> 🔊)) **SOUND OFF**
> The spermatocele is the most common scrotal mass.

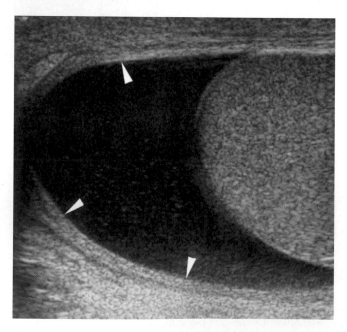

Figure 13-8 Hydrocele. Anechoic fluid can be noted surrounding the testicle. The scrotal wall (*arrowheads*) appears to be thickened as well.

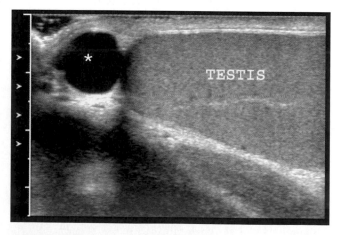

Figure 13-9 Spermatocele. A small spermatocele (*asterisk*) is noted superior to the testis.

CLINICAL FINDINGS OF A SPERMATOCELE, EPIDIDYMAL CYST, AND TUNICA ALBUGINEA CYST

1. If large enough, they may be palpable
2. Typically not painful

SONOGRAPHIC FINDINGS OF A SPERMATOCELE, EPIDIDYMAL CYST, AND TUNICA ALBUGINEA CYST

1. Round, anechoic mass with acoustic enhancement
2. May contain some layering debris

Varicocele

A dilated group of veins found within the scrotum is termed a **varicocele** (Fig. 13-10). Varicoceles are caused by incompetent or abnormal valves within the pampiniform plexus. Because of the increased heat released by excess blood within the scrotum, overheating of the fragile spermatozoa can occur. This overheating can influence the formation and mobility of sperm. In fact, varicoceles have been cited as the most common cause of correctable male infertility.

Varicoceles are usually painless, but if they become large, discomfort can result. There are two types of varicoceles: primary and secondary. Primary varicoceles are most often found on the left and are palpable during a physical examination. Their high incidence on the left is thought to be caused by the elevated vascular pressure on the left side or possibly as a result of the extended length of the left testicular vein (compared to the right testicular vein) and the sharp angle at which it enters the left renal vein. When found on the right side, this abnormality may be termed a secondary varicocele. Secondary varicoceles may be associated with a hepatic mass, marked hydronephrosis, hepatomegaly, or a retroperitoneal neoplasm like a right-sided renal mass. Therefore, a prompt investigation of the right upper quadrant and retroperitoneum may be warranted when a varicocele is discovered on the right. One predisposing factor for some patients for a varicocele is an anomaly where left renal vein entrapment occurs between the superior mesenteric artery and the abdominal aorta, which is termed the **"nutcracker" syndrome**.

> **SOUND OFF**
> Varicoceles are the most common causes of correctable male infertility and are most often located on the left side. Right-sided varicoceles

may be associated with right-sided pathology of the retroperitoneum, including hepatomegaly, a hepatic mass, or right-sided renal mass.

Sonographically, a varicocele commonly appears as a group of anechoic, tubular structures located outside the testis. However, varicoceles can be intratesticular in location. To diagnose a varicocele using color Doppler, the **Valsalva maneuver** can be performed. When the intra-abdominal pressure is increased with this maneuver, the veins should fill with blood and become enlarged. These dilated veins will measure greater than 2 mm. The patient may also stand while he is being scanned to simulate the Valsalva maneuver.

CLINICAL FINDINGS OF A VARICOCELE

1. Typically painless (large varicoceles can cause discomfort)
2. Palpable extratesticular mass
3. Possible infertility

SONOGRAPHIC FINDINGS OF A VARICOCELE

1. A group of anechoic, tubular structures located outside the testis
2. Distended veins that fill with color flow when the Valsalva maneuver is performed
3. Dilated veins that measure greater than 2 mm
4. Possibly associated with hydronephrosis, hepatomegaly, or a retroperitoneal neoplasm if found on the right

> **SOUND OFF**
> A varicocele can have an intratesticular location.

Scrotal Pearl

A scrotal pearl, also referred to as a scrotolith, is an extratesticular calculus. Scrotal pearls will be extremely echogenic and mobile and will produce a posterior acoustic shadow. They are often incidentally noted and thought to be remnants of a formerly torsed and displaced testicular appendage.

SONOGRAPHIC FINDINGS OF A SCROTAL PEARL

1. Extremely echogenic, mobile extratesticular structure that produces acoustic shadowing

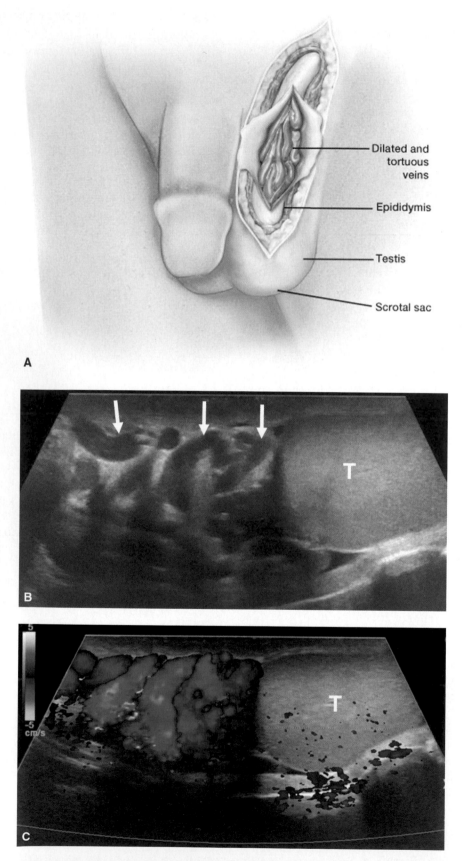

Figure 13-10 Varicocele. **A.** A varicocele is the abnormal dilation of the veins of the spermatic cord. It is usually asymptomatic, but it is important to identify and correct this condition because it is associated with infertility. **B.** Sonographic appearance of a varicocele represented by multiple tortuous dilated vessels (*arrows*) superior to the testicle (*T*). **C.** Color Doppler with the Valsalva maneuver reveals the vascular nature of these structures.

Epididymitis and Epididymo-orchitis

Inflammation of the epididymis is referred to as **epididymitis**. Epididymitis is the most common cause of acute testicular pain in adults. Patients with epididymitis can present with leukocytosis, fever, dysuria, urethral discharge, and scrotal wall edema. Infections that occur within the scrotum are ascending. Therefore, most infections start externally, or within the urinary tract or prostate, and then proceed into the vas deferens, epididymal tail, epididymal body, epididymal head, and perhaps into the testis. Inflammation of the testis is referred to as **orchitis**. Consequently, the combination of an infection within the epididymis and testis is termed **epididymo-orchitis**.

Although a frequent cause of epididymitis is the spread of bacteria from the prostate or urinary tract, it can be caused by trauma. Common causes of epididymitis in younger men are the sexually transmitted diseases **chlamydia** and **gonorrhea**. Epididymitis can be diffuse and involve the entire epididymis, or it may be focal and involve only one segment. Therefore, an analysis of the head, body, and tail of the epididymis is vital. Sonographically, the inflamed epididymis will appear enlarged, hypoechoic, or heterogeneous and have increased vascularity when interrogated with color or power Doppler. Orchitis will yield increased intratesticular vascularity with a low-resistance waveform pattern and is almost always accompanied by epididymitis (Fig. 13-11). Chronic epididymitis may appear as an enlarged, hyperechoic epididymis with calcifications.

🔊)) SOUND OFF
Common causes of epididymitis in younger men are the sexually transmitted diseases chlamydia and gonorrhea.

CLINICAL FINDINGS OF EPIDIDYMITIS AND EPIDIDYMO-ORCHITIS

1. Acute testicular pain
2. Leukocytosis
3. Fever
4. Dysuria
5. Urethral discharge
6. Scrotal wall edema
7. Possible sexually transmitted disease

SONOGRAPHIC FINDINGS OF EPIDIDYMITIS AND EPIDIDYMO-ORCHITIS

1. Enlargement of the entire epididymis (diffuse)
2. Enlargement of only part of the epididymis (focal)
3. Hypoechoic echotexture of the affected section(s) of the epididymis
4. Hypoechoic testis (with orchitis)
5. Hyperemia within the epididymis and/or testis
6. Thickened scrotal wall
7. Reactive hydrocele

Testicular Abscess and Pyocele

An abscess that occurs within the testicle is typically the result of untreated epididymo-orchitis. Patients will clinically present with a fever, leukocytosis, and a painful, swollen scrotum. With color Doppler imaging, a testicular abscess will appear as a complex intratesticular mass that has no flow centrally but increased flow around its margins (Fig. 13-12). A **pyocele** is a complex hydrocele that contains pus. It is often seen in the presence of a persistent scrotal infection or ruptured testicular abscess. Sonographically, a pyocele will appear as a complex fluid collection within the scrotum that may contain septations and loculations.

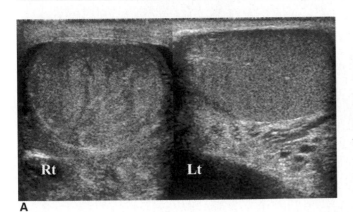

A

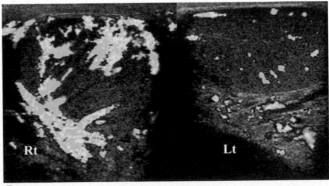

B

Figure 13-11 Epididymo-orchitis. **A.** Transverse grayscale sonogram of both testes in a patient with right (*Rt*) epididymitis shows an enlarged heterogeneous right testis with scrotal skin thickening and a small hydrocele. **B.** Color Doppler image shows increased right (*Rt*) testicular flow, indicating orchitis. The left testis (*Lt*) is normal.

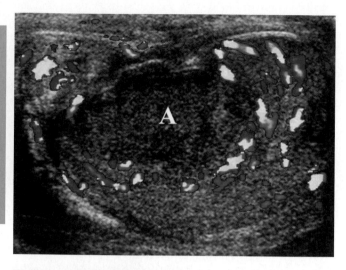

Figure 13-12 Testicular abscess. An abscess (*A*) is noted within this testicle. Note that there is increased flow detectable with color Doppler around the abscess, but there is absence of flow within the abscess itself.

Clinical history is extremely important to make the differentiation between a **hematocele**, pyocele, or complex hydrocele.

◀))) SOUND OFF
Although intratesticular abscesses lack detected flow within them, they are often surrounded by hyperemic flow.

CLINICAL FINDINGS OF A TESTICULAR ABSCESS

1. Painful, swollen scrotum
2. Fever
3. Leukocytosis

SONOGRAPHIC FINDINGS OF A TESTICULAR ABSCESS

1. Complex intratesticular mass
2. Mass that has no flow centrally but increased flow around its margins
3. May have a coexisting pyocele

SONOGRAPHIC FINDINGS OF A PYOCELE

1. Complex fluid collection within the scrotum
2. Scrotal wall thickening
3. May be seen in conjunction with rupture of a testicular abscess

Intratesticular Cyst and Testicular Microlithiasis

Intratesticular cysts are rarely large enough to be palpable. Multiple small intratesticular cysts are often seen along the mediastinum testis. These cysts are typically small and clinically insignificant and may be the result of **tubular ectasia of the rete testes** (Fig. 13-13). They are thought to represent cystic dilation of the rete testis. **Epidermoid cysts** may be noted within the testicle as well. Epidermoid cysts often appear to have a whorled or onion-skin appearance (Fig. 13-14).

◀))) SOUND OFF
Multiple small cysts located along the mediastinum testis represent cystic dilation of the rete testis, also referred to as tubular ectasia.

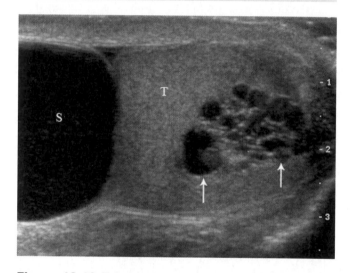

Figure 13-13 Tubular ectasia of the rete testis. Multiple cysts (*arrows*) are seen in the area of the mediastinum testes in this testicle (*T*). A large spermatocele (*S*) is also noted.

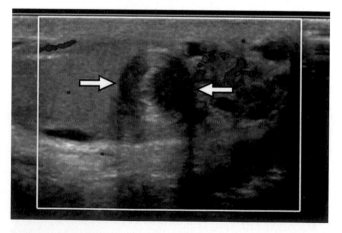

Figure 13-14 Longitudinal color Doppler ultrasound image demonstrates an avascular mass with a "whorled" or "onion-skin" appearance (*arrows*), consistent with an epidermoid cyst.

Testicular microlithiasis will appear as multiple echogenic foci with no acoustic shadowing within the testis (Fig. 13-15). These tiny calcifications have been associated with malignancies, infertility, **Klinefelter syndrome**, and cryptorchidism (Fig. 13-16). Screening of patients with intratesticular microlithiasis has been studied, and the cost-effectiveness has been questioned. However, there is a proven increased risk for cancer in patients who have microlithiasis in one testis and an identified intratesticular tumor in the contralateral testis. Therefore, a biopsy of the testis with microlithiasis may be warranted.

Adrenal Rests

Adrenal rests resemble a mass within the testicle and are associated with congenital adrenal hyperplasia or Cushing syndrome (see Chapter 8). Adrenal rests of the testis, which essentially consist of ectopic adrenal tissue, are caused by the migration of adrenal tissue with gonadal tissue during fetal development. Clinically, these patients will have evidence of increased levels of adrenocorticotropic hormone. Sonographically, adrenal rests appear as bilateral, round, hypoechoic, intratesticular masses, most commonly near the mediastinum testis.

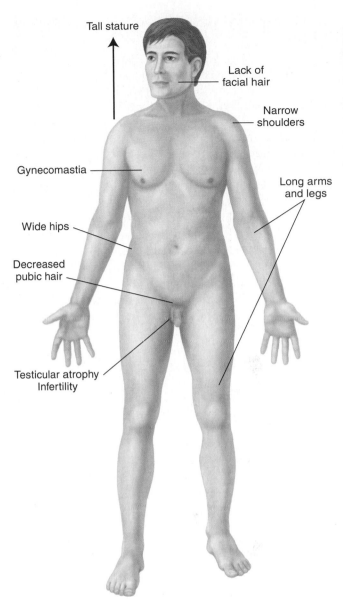

Figure 13-16 Clinical features of Klinefelter syndrome.

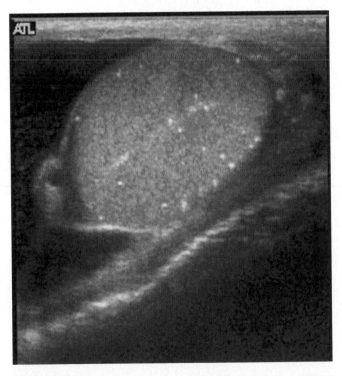

Figure 13-15 Intratesticular microlithiasis. Multiple echogenic foci with no acoustic shadowing are seen within this testis.

CLINICAL FINDINGS OF ADRENAL RESTS

1. History of congenital adrenal hyperplasia
2. Elevated adrenocorticotropic hormone
3. Cushing syndrome

SONOGRAPHIC FINDINGS OF ADRENAL RESTS

1. Bilateral, round, hypoechoic, intratesticular masses (most commonly near the mediastinum testis)

Malignant Testicular Tumors and Tumor Markers

As a rule, intratesticular masses are often considered malignant until proven otherwise, whereas the majority of extratesticular masses are typically benign. Most of the malignant intratesticular tumors are of germ cell origin (Table 13-4). Other, non–germ cell malignant tumors include sex cord–stromal tumors, lymphoma, leukemia, and metastases (Table 13-5). Lymphoma and leukemia can either appear as focal hypoechoic masses or produce diffuse involvement of the testicles. Metastatic disease to the testis is most commonly from melanoma, lung, kidney, and prostate cancer.

There are two laboratory values that are helpful to differentiate between benign and malignant intratesticular tumors, **human chorionic gonadotropin** (hCG) and **alpha-fetoprotein** (AFP). An elevation in hCG levels is found in conjunction with malignant intratesticular tumors in 60% of the time. hCG is produced by these masses because they contain syncytiotrophoblastic cells. These cells, also found in the developing placenta, produce hCG in the abnormal cells that comprise the testicular malignancy. AFP levels may also be evaluated to determine whether an intratesticular mass is malignant. An elevated AFP level is most often associated with embryonal cell carcinoma, teratomas, and yolk sac tumors. Lactate dehydrogenase (LDH) may also be used by some as a tumor marker for testicular cancer when a mass is detected, and it may be used to evaluate the effectiveness of treatment and to evaluate for recurrence as well, though its specificity is lacking. Consequently, a combination of an analysis of hCG, AFP, and LDH is often used in the clinical setting.

> **SOUND OFF**
> hCG and AFP are laboratory values used in pregnancy. Malignant tumors within the testicles may abnormally produce hCG or AFP as well. Thus, these can be used as tumor markers for testicular malignancies.

SEMINOMA

The seminoma is the most common malignant neoplasm of the testicles. The seminoma is a **germ cell tumor** that is typically found in males between 30 and 50 years of age. This type of malignant tumor is often found in patients suffering from cryptorchidism as well. Most seminomas are unilateral and may actually replace the entire testicle. Clinically, patients will present with a painless scrotal mass, hardening of the testis, and, possibly, elevated hCG level. A seminoma has an intratesticular location and will appear as a solid, hypoechoic mass (Fig. 13-17). Large seminomas may become heterogeneous.

> **SOUND OFF**
> The seminoma is the most common malignant neoplasm of the testicle.

TABLE 13-4 Germ cell tumors of the testicles

Pure seminoma
Teratoma
Embryonal cell carcinoma
Yolk sac tumor
Choriocarcinoma
Burned-out germ cell tumor

TABLE 13-5 Sex cord–stromal tumors of the testicles and unique features

Sex Cord–Stromal Tumor	Unique Features
Leydig cell tumor	Found in younger boys and produce increased levels of testosterone
Sertoli cell tumor	Found in younger boys and produce estrogens that results in gynecomastia
Granulosa cell tumor	Found in younger boys and are associated with chromosomal abnormalities

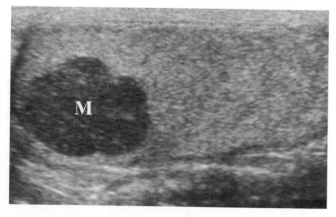

Figure 13-17 Seminoma. Longitudinal image of the testicle that contains a solid, hypoechoic mass (*M*), which was confirmed to be a seminoma.

CLINICAL FINDINGS OF A SEMINOMA

1. Painless scrotal mass
2. Hardening of the testis
3. Elevated hCG

SONOGRAPHIC FINDINGS OF A SEMINOMA

1. Solid, hypoechoic intratesticular mass
2. Large seminomas may become heterogeneous

Other Germ Cell Tumors of the Testicles

There are several different forms of nonseminomatous intratesticular tumors, including choriocarcinoma, embryonal cell carcinoma, teratomas, and yolk sac tumors. These noteworthy tumors and their clinical and sonographic findings are summarized in Table 13-6. It is important to note that a tumor can be composed of a mixture of these malignant tissues and thus referred to as a mixed germ cell tumor.

Scrotal Trauma and Hematocele

The testicle can be fractured as a result of trauma to the scrotum. Rarely, a fracture line may be seen. The testicular margins may be unclear, and a hematoma may be noted in or around the testis. Blood that is present within the scrotum is referred to as a hematocele. Although hematoceles are often associated with trauma to the scrotum, they may also be found after recent pelvic

surgery, scrotal surgery, or torsion. Sonographically, a hematocele will appear as a complex fluid collection within the scrotum that may contain septations and loculations. Clinical history is extremely important to make the differentiation between a hematocele, pyocele, or complex hydrocele.

CLINICAL FINDINGS OF SCROTAL TRAUMA

1. Trauma to the scrotum resulting in acute scrotal pain
2. Low hematocrit

SONOGRAPHIC FINDINGS OF SCROTAL TRAUMA

1. Possible fracture line
2. Indistinct testicular margins
3. Hematocele

CLINICAL FINDINGS OF A HEMATOCELE

1. Trauma to the pelvis or scrotum
2. Recent pelvic or scrotal surgery
3. Low hematocrit (possible)

SONOGRAPHIC FINDINGS OF A HEMATOCELE

1. Complex fluid collection within the scrotum
2. Scrotal wall thickening

TABLE 13-6 Nonseminomatous germ cell tumors with associated clinical and sonographic findings

Nonseminomatous Germ Cell Tumor	Malignant or Benign	Clinical Findings	Sonographic Findings
Choriocarcinoma	Malignant	May be palpable Elevated human chorionic gonadotropin (hCG)	Heterogeneous mass with areas of hemorrhage, necrosis, and calcifications
Embryonal cell carcinoma	Malignant	May be palpable Elevated alpha-fetoprotein (AFP) and hCG	Heterogeneous mass with cystic components
Yolk sac tumors	Malignant	May be palpable Elevated AFP (exclusively)	Heterogeneous mass with areas of hemorrhage and calcifications
Teratoma	Benign (with malignant potential)	May be palpable Elevated AFP and hCG (if malignant)	Heterogeneous with calcifications representing cartilage, bone, and fibrosis; may contain hair and teeth

Inguinal Hernia

An **inguinal hernia** may consist of intestine or **omentum**. Patients with an inguinal hernia often present with persistent or intermittent scrotal swelling (Fig. 13-18). Patients may also have abdominal pain and blood within their stool. Sonographically, an inguinal hernia will often show a mass that has peristalsis and that may contain air and fluid (Fig. 13-19). A hydrocele may also be an associated finding. The blood supply to the bowel can be lost when an inguinal hernia becomes incarcerated and strangulated. The Valsalva maneuver can be used to help demonstrate peristalsing bowel. Fluid or air within the loop of bowel may also be seen.

CLINICAL FINDINGS OF AN INGUINAL HERNIA

1. Persistent or intermittent scrotal swelling
2. May have abdominal pain and blood in stool

SONOGRAPHIC FINDINGS OF AN INGUINAL HERNIA

1. Heterogeneous mass within the scrotum that moves (peristalsis)
2. Mass may contain air and fluid
3. Hydrocele may be present

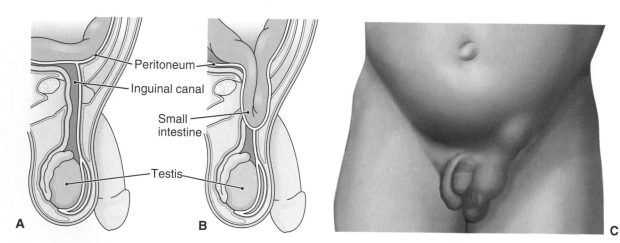

Figure 13-18 Inguinal hernia. **A.** Normal. **B.** Weakness in the abdominal wall allows the intestine or other abdominal contents to protrude into the inguinal canal. The hernial sac is a continuation of the peritoneum. **C.** An inguinal hernia can cause a visible bulge in the inguinal area and scrotum.

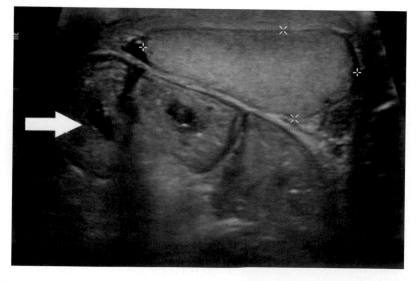

Figure 13-19 Inguinal hernia containing bowel. Sonogram shows bowel (*arrow*) within the inguinal hernia adjacent to the testicle (between *calipers*).

ANATOMY AND PHYSIOLOGY OF THE PENIS

The penis is a primary sex organ. It plays a vital role in both reproduction and urination. The penis is covered with skin and subsequently a dense fibrous tissue termed **Buck fascia**. The inner penis is composed of three cylindrical tissue components: a single **corpus** spongiosum and paired **corpora cavernosa** (singular form is cavernosum). These are composed of smooth muscle, erectile tissue, and vascular structures. The urethra is housed within the corpus spongiosum, which is situated ventrally. The paired cavernosa are situated dorsally. Tunica albuginea surrounds the corpora cavernosa and partially covers the corpus spongiosum. All three corpora are covered by Buck fascia (Fig. 13-20).

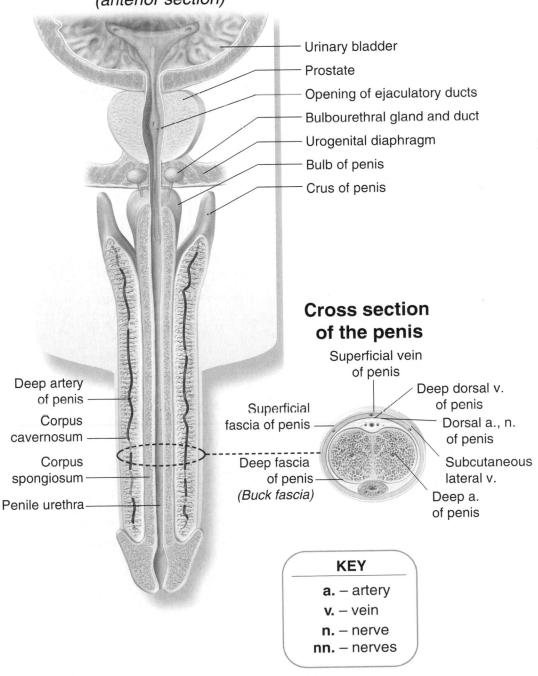

Penis in flaccid state
(anterior section)

- Urinary bladder
- Prostate
- Opening of ejaculatory ducts
- Bulbourethral gland and duct
- Urogenital diaphragm
- Bulb of penis
- Crus of penis

Deep artery of penis
Corpus cavernosum
Corpus spongiosum
Penile urethra

Cross section of the penis

Superficial vein of penis
Superficial fascia of penis
Deep fascia of penis (Buck fascia)
Deep dorsal v. of penis
Dorsal a., n. of penis
Subcutaneous lateral v.
Deep a. of penis

KEY

a. – artery
v. – vein
n. – nerve
nn. – nerves

Figure 13-20 Anatomy of the penis.

> 🔊 **SOUND OFF**
> The penis consists of two corpora cavernosa and one corpus spongiosum.

The vascular supply to the penis begins at the internal pudendal artery, which is a tributary of the internal iliac artery. The internal pudendal arteries branch into the deep artery of the penis or penile artery. The deep artery of the penis provides the blood supply to the corpora cavernosa. The cavernosal arteries are located within the corpora cavernosa bilaterally. When sexual arousal occurs, the arteries within the penis become engorged with blood, causing the compression of the adjacent veins, preventing venous drainage, and resulting in an erection.

SONOGRAPHY OF THE PENIS

The penis should be imaged using a high-frequency linear transducer. Most often, the patient is placed in the supine position, and the penis is allowed to rest upon the lower abdomen when flow assessment is warranted. This position will cause the dorsal surface of the penis to be placed alongside the abdomen, exposing the ventral surface (Fig. 13-21). Sonographically, the penis should be evaluated in both transverse and sagittal scan planes. In transverse, the singular corpus spongiosum, which contains the urethra, will be seen ventrally located, whereas the paired corpora cavernosa will be noted dorsally. The spongiosum will be elliptical in shape and consist of

medium- to low-level echoes, whereas the cavernosa will appear similar in echogenicity to the spongiosum, but have a more oval shape. The tunica albuginea, which is highly echogenic, can be seen separating and covering the corpora. Contained within each corpus cavernosum are the cavernosal arteries, which can be identified by their bright walls and apparent blood flow with color Doppler. In the sagittal plane, both the spongiosum and the cavernosa elongate, whereas the vascular channels can be seen stretching through the length of the cavernosa allowing for pulsed Doppler interrogation. The elongated penile urethra can be seen within the corpus spongiosum in the sagittal plane as well.

Sonography can aid in the detection of strictures of the penile urethra and vascular issues within the penis. For the identification of strictures of the urethra, the patient is often required to have a full bladder and to void during the examination. For vascular assessment, the penile flow is first analyzed in a flaccid state and then an injection of an erection-inducing drug into the penis may be required to evaluate the vascularity of the penis using color Doppler while the penis is erect (Fig. 13-22).

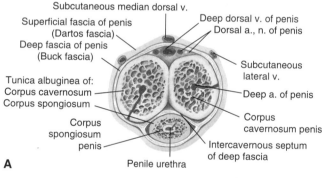

Cross section of the penis

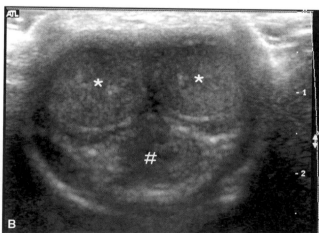

Figure 13-22 Transverse image of the penis. **A.** Cross section of the penis for comparison. **B.** In this image, the transducer has been placed on the dorsal aspect of the penis in order to perform Doppler evaluation, which allows for the assessment of the two corpora cavernosa (*asterisk*), with the corpus spongiosum noted ventrally (*hash*).

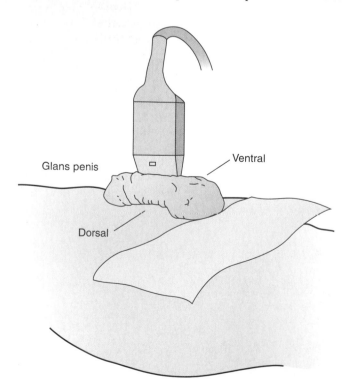

Figure 13-21 Positioning for penile sonogram.

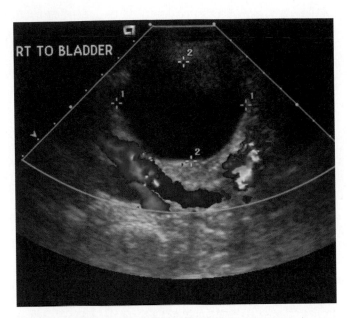

Figure 13-23 Penile inflatable prosthesis and reservoir in the pelvis. The well-defined, anechoic fluid structure (between *calipers*) was discovered to the right of the bladder during a pelvic sonogram.

Sonography can also be used to evaluate any palpable lesions of the penis, such as a benign fibroma or a malignant penile tumor, the latter of which is most often caused by human papillomavirus and is typically in the form of squamous cell carcinoma. Lastly, a penile inflatable prosthesis may be noted during a pelvic sonogram. Sonographically, the reservoir will appear as an anechoic round structure (Fig. 13-23).

PENILE PATHOLOGY

Vascular Impotence

Vascular impotence is caused by vascular compromise to or within the penis that results in the inability to obtain or maintain an erection. This disorder could be caused by diabetic neuropathy, in which case the tiny vessels within the penis are damaged. Upon pulsed Doppler interrogation in normal men, there is an increase in arterial flow to the cavernosal arteries that can be determined by evaluating the systolic velocities. In addition, normally, the venous outflow will become partially blocked, and the diastolic flow will greatly decrease. The diagnosis of venous incompetence can be made if the diastolic flow does not decrease. It is important to note that in healthy individuals, the cavernosal artery velocities measure 10 to 15 cm per second in the flaccid state.

Peyronie Disease

Peyronie disease is the buildup of fibrous plaque (scar tissue) and calcifications within the penis that results in a painful curvature. Patients typically have impotence

and poor arterial flow and complain of painful erections. Clinically, the area of scar tissue buildup can typically be palpated. Sonographically, the area will appear as thickening of the tunica albuginea, which may also contain areas of calcification.

CLINICAL FINDINGS OF PEYRONIE DISEASE

1. Impotence
2. Painful erections
3. Area of scar tissue can typically be palpated
4. Marked curvature of the penis

SONOGRAPHIC FINDINGS OF PEYRONIE DISEASE

1. Thickening of the tunica albuginea that may also contain areas of calcification

Penile Trauma

Fracture of the penis can occur with blunt sexual trauma. The audible sound of a popping or cracking sound is often heard because typically one of the corpora cavernosa snaps under the pressure. Although this disorder can be diagnosed clinically on the basis of history and evidence of **ecchymosis**—which is a subcutaneous spot of bleeding—sonography may be used to further analyze the penis for soft-tissue, urethral, and vascular damage. Sonographically, the area of hemorrhage within the penis can have the varying sonographic appearances associated with a new or aging hematoma, thus depending on the time of analysis. However, most likely, sonography will reveal an irregular hypoechoic or hyperechoic defect at the site of rupture. Careful assessment of the tunica albuginea for evidence of penile urethra is warranted because interruption to the urethra can lead to voiding complications. The damage, if not managed appropriately, can permanently disrupt penile function. Scar tissue development can result in the area of the fracture as well.

SOUND OFF
Careful assessment of the tunica albuginea for evidence of penile urethra damage is warranted because interruption to the urethra can lead to voiding complications.

CLINICAL FINDINGS OF PENILE TRAUMA

1. History of hearing an audible popping sound during intercourse
2. Subcutaneous bleeding area

SONOGRAPHIC FINDINGS OF PENILE TRAUMA

1. An irregular hypoechoic or hyperechoic defect at the site of rupture

ANATOMY, PHYSIOLOGY, AND PATHOLOGY OF THE PROSTATE GLAND AND SEMINAL VESICLES

The prostate is a retroperitoneal gland that produces and secretes an alkaline fluid that constitutes between 13% and 30% of the volume of semen. The gland is located inferior to the urinary bladder, between the symphysis pubis and the rectum. It is shaped like an inverted pyramid, with its base located superior and its apex positioned inferior. The prostate is divided into four zones. The prostatic urethra, which is used as the point of reference for the zones, travels through the center of the prostate. Zonal anatomy is described in Table 13-7 (Fig. 13-24). An additional area, the anterior fibromuscular stroma, is located anterior to the prostatic urethra and is of little clinical significance.

The paired seminal vesicles are located superior to the prostate gland and posterior to the base of the bladder. They secrete an alkaline-based fluid and empty into the paired ejaculatory ducts. The ejaculatory ducts are formed by the union of the seminal vesicles and ductus deferens. These tiny ducts travel through the prostate and empty into the urethra at an area called the **verumontanum**.

SONOGRAPHY OF THE PROSTATE GLAND AND SEMINAL VESICLES

Oftentimes, a patient will undergo a **digital rectal examination** before having a targeted sonogram of the prostate. The prostate can be imaged transabdominally or transrectally (Fig. 13-25). Transabdominal imaging

TABLE 13-7 Four prostatic zones: their locations and significant characteristics

Prostatic Zone	Location	Significance
Peripheral zone	Posterior lateral, apical gland	Largest prostatic zone Most common site for malignancy
Central zone	Base of prostate	Second largest prostatic zone
Transitional zone	On both sides of the proximal urethra	Site for benign prostatic hyperplasia Second most common site of malignancies
Periurethral glandular zone	Embedded in the muscle of the proximal urethra	Smallest prostatic zone

Zones of the prostate

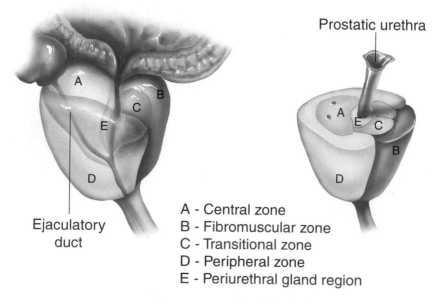

A - Central zone
B - Fibromuscular zone
C - Transitional zone
D - Peripheral zone
E - Periurethral gland region

Figure 13-24 Zonal anatomy of the prostate in the sagittal plane.

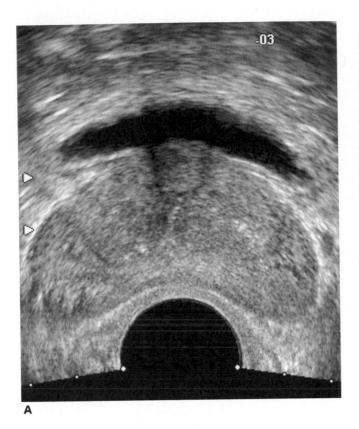

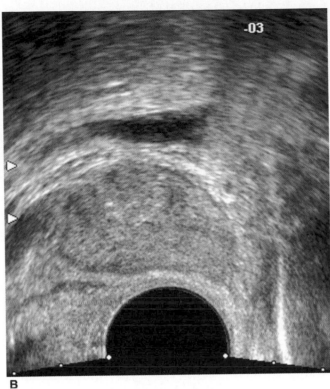

Figure 13-25 Prostate sonography. **A.** Transrectal ultrasound of the prostate: transverse view. **B.** Transrectal sonogram of the prostate: sagittal view.

is useful for measuring the overall size of the prostate, whereas transrectal imaging is used for biopsies and provides superior resolution. The patient is typically placed in the left lateral decubitus position with the knees flexed toward the chest or in the lithotomy position for transrectal imaging of the prostate. The prostate and seminal vesicles are examined in both coronal and sagittal planes. The prostatic zones are typically homogeneous and may be differentiated by visualizing landmarks such as the prostatic urethra and ejaculatory ducts. Patients may have benign calcification and simple-appearing cysts within the prostate as well.

The seminal vesicles appear as hypoechoic structures between the bladder and the prostate (Fig. 13-26). When the seminal vesicles are filled with fluid, they become enlarged and contain low-level echoes and anechoic fluid. The seminal vesicles can be imaged transabdominally or endorectally.

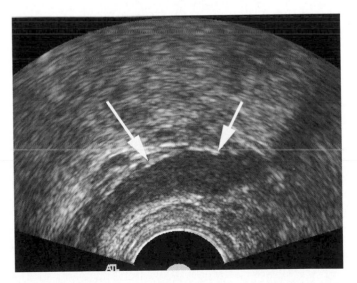

Figure 13-26 Transrectal image of a seminal vesicle (*arrows*).

PROSTATE PATHOLOGY

Prostate-Specific Antigen

Prostate-specific antigen (PSA) is a protein produced by the prostate gland. There are several methods currently used to evaluate PSA levels, including PSA velocity, volume-corrected PSA, age-adjusted PSA, and free and attached PSA. An elevation in this protein can be indicative of some disease processes, such as **benign prostatic hyperplasia (BPH)**, prostatic cancer, **prostatitis**, and prostatic infarcts. It has been claimed that the higher the PSA level, the more likely the patient will have prostate cancer. However, a normal PSA level can also be found in the presence of cancer.

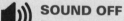
SOUND OFF
An elevated PSA is not specific for prostate cancer.

Prostate Cancer

Prostate cancer, in the form of adenocarcinoma, is the most common cancer in men. Patients with prostate cancer often present with blood in the urine or semen, back pain, pelvic pain, hip or thigh pain, impotence, and a decrease in the amount of ejaculated fluid. Prostate cancer may cause an enlarged prostate that can be determined with a digital rectal examination. Patients may also have elevated PSA values.

As mentioned earlier, the most common location for prostate cancer is within the **peripheral zone**. It may produce areas of hypervascularity, and it can have variable sonographic appearances. However, most prostate cancers will appear hypoechoic to normal adjacent prostatic tissue (Fig. 13-27). It is important to note that the sonographic appearance of prostatic cancer can mimic normal anatomy, prostatitis, and BPH. Therefore, experience is needed to perform these procedures correctly. Biopsy is warranted for a definitive diagnosis.

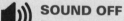
SOUND OFF
Prostate cancer is most commonly located within the peripheral zone.

CLINICAL FINDINGS OF PROSTATE CANCER

1. Elevated PSA
2. Enlarged prostate
3. Blood in the urine (hematuria) or semen (hematospermia)
4. Back pain, pelvic pain, hip or thigh pain
5. Impotence
6. Decrease in the amount of ejaculated fluid

SONOGRAPHIC FINDINGS OF PROSTATE CANCER

1. Varying sonographic appearances
2. Hypoechoic mass
3. May be hypervascular

Benign Prostatic Hyperplasia

The benign enlargement of the prostate gland is termed benign prostatic hyperplasia (BPH). BPH is most often located within the **transitional zone**. An enlarged prostate can obstruct the flow of urine through the urethra. Symptoms of BPH include **nocturia**, increased urinary frequency, a sense of urinary urgency, and a

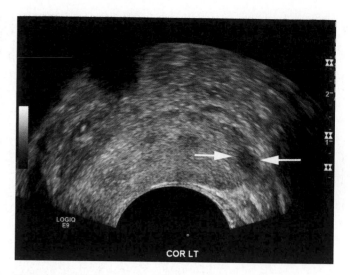

Figure 13-27 Prostate cancer. This transrectal image of the prostate reveals a small hypoechoic mass (between *arrows*) in the peripheral zone, which was eventually diagnosed as prostate carcinoma.

constant feeling of having a full bladder. Patients will also have elevated PSA. Sonographically, BPH will show an enlargement of the inner gland, and it can lead to hypoechoic areas within the prostate, calcifications, diffusely heterogeneous gland, and cystic changes (Fig. 13-28). Patients with BPH may undergo **transurethral resection of the prostate** to remove some of the hypertrophic prostatic tissue causing urinary complications.

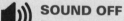
SOUND OFF
BPH is most commonly located within the transitional zone.

CLINICAL FINDINGS OF BENIGN PROSTATIC HYPERPLASIA

1. Nocturia
2. Increased urinary frequency
3. Sense of urinary urgency
4. Constant feeling of having a full bladder
5. Elevated PSA

SONOGRAPHIC FINDINGS OF BENIGN PROSTATIC HYPERPLASIA

1. BPH will show an enlargement of the inner gland
2. Can lead to hypoechoic areas within the gland
3. Calcifications within the gland
4. Diffusely heterogeneous gland
5. Cystic changes within the gland

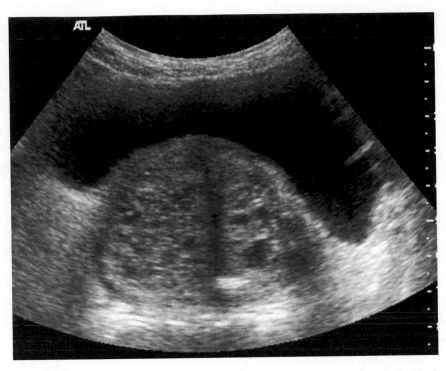

Figure 13-28 Transabdominal, transverse view of an enlarged, heterogeneous prostate gland secondary to benign prostatic hyperplasia.

Prostatitis

Prostatitis is inflammation of the prostate. Patients may complain of **hematospermia**, painful ejaculation, perineal pain, and dysuria. Sonographically, prostatitis appears as an enlarged, more hypoechoic prostate with evidence of hyperemia upon color Doppler interrogation.

CLINICAL FINDINGS OF PROSTATITIS

1. Hematospermia
2. Painful ejaculation
3. Perineal pain
4. Dysuria

SONOGRAPHIC FINDINGS OF PROSTATITIS

1. Enlarged, hypoechoic prostate
2. Hyperemia evident with color Doppler

Seminal Vesicle Cysts

Occasionally, seminal vesicle cysts may be identified as anechoic or complex cystic structures in the area of the seminal vesicles. Although seminal vesicle cysts are rare, they are said to be either congenital or acquired. Seminal vesicle cysts may be asymptomatic, but they can also be associated with **Zinner syndrome**. Zinner syndrome consists of unilateral renal agenesis, ipsilateral seminal vesicle cyst, and ejaculatory duct obstruction. Patients with Zinner syndrome present with perineal pain, recurrent prostatitis, painful ejaculation, and infertility.

CLINICAL FINDINGS OF SEMINAL VESICLE CYSTS

1. Asymptomatic
2. May be associated with Zinner syndrome (perineal pain, recurrent prostatitis, painful ejaculation, and infertility)

SONOGRAPHIC FINDINGS OF SEMINAL VESICLE CYSTS

1. Anechoic or complex cystic structures in the area of the seminal vesicles

The Male Pelvis

REVIEW QUESTIONS

1. Figure 13-29 is a sagittal image of the left hemiscrotum in a patient who had epididymo-orchitis and fever. What is the most likely diagnosis?
   a. Hematocele
   b. Hydrocele
   c. Pyocele
   d. Seminoma

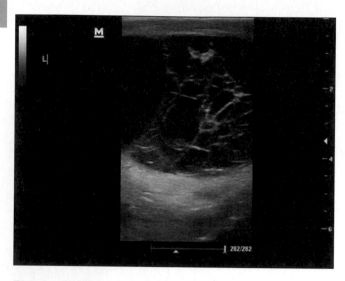

Figure 13-29

2. The patient in Figure 13-30 would least likely present with:
   a. testicular pain during sleep.
   b. nausea.
   c. lower positioning of the painful testis with a vertical position.
   d. swollen symptomatic testis.

3. Which of the following is not true concerning the condition in Figure 13-30?
   a. It is most common in the third or fourth decade of life.
   b. It is also referred to as spermatic cord torsion.
   c. It is associated with bell-clapper deformity.
   d. It is associated with strenuous exercise.

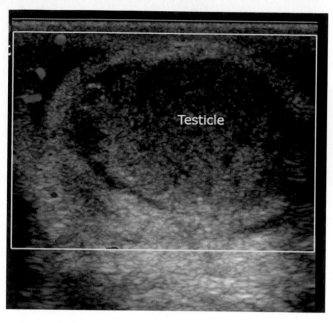

Figure 13-30

4. The patient in Figure 13-31 presented with a painful testicle and elevated AFP. Which of the following is the most likely etiology for this pathology?
   a. Testicular adenocarcinoma
   b. Yolk sac tumor
   c. Hamartoma
   d. Adrenal rest tumor

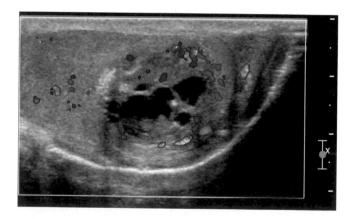

Figure 13-31

5. Which of the following is not typically used as a tumor marker for testicular cancer?
   a. hCG
   b. AFP
   c. LDH
   d. FSH

6. Which of the following covers the corpora cavernosa and corpus spongiosum of the penis?
   a. Tunica albuginea
   b. Tunica adventitia
   c. Buck fascia
   d. Tunica dartos

7. Which of the following is the dense fibrous layer of tissue that is closely applied to the testicle?
   a. Tunica dartos
   b. Tunica albuginea
   c. Tunica vaginalis
   d. Buck fascia

8. Which of the following is not a division of the epididymis?
   a. Head
   b. Body
   c. Tail
   d. Neck

9. What is another name for the Cowper gland?
   a. Bulbourethral gland
   b. Prostate gland
   c. Seminal vesicles
   d. Ejaculatory duct

10. What performs venous drainage of the testicles?
    a. Inguinal veins
    b. Vas deferens
    c. Pampiniform plexus
    d. Scrotal veins

11. A heterogeneous mass with calcifications is noted within the testicle. The mass was later determined to have cartilage, bone, and fibrotic tissue. What is the most likely diagnosis for this mass?
    a. Seminoma
    b. Embryonal cell tumor
    c. Sertoli cell tumor
    d. Teratoma

12. Which of the following would be most likely associated with hematospermia and painful ejaculation?
    a. Seminal vesicle cysts
    b. Zinner syndrome
    c. Prostatitis
    d. BPH

13. A 16-year-old patient presents to the sonography department for a scrotal sonogram with clinical features associated with Klinefelter syndrome. Which of the following is least likely associated with Klinefelter syndrome?
    a. Infertility
    b. Gynecomastia
    c. Cryptorchidism
    d. Long legs

14. A patient presents to the sonography department with a history of vasectomy 10 years earlier. What are the sonographic changes that may be noted after vasectomy?
    a. Enlargement of the epididymis
    b. Testicular atrophy
    c. Intratesticular calcifications
    d. Decreased intratesticular flow noted with color Doppler

15. Which of the following is noted in Figure 13-32?
    a. Tubular ectasia
    b. Intratesticular varicocele
    c. Seminoma
    d. Epididymitis

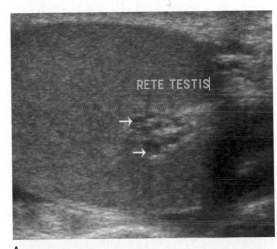

A

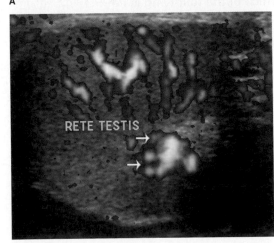

B

Figure 13-32

16. Which of the following is a protein produced by the prostate that can be evaluated in cases of suspected BPH and prostate cancer?
    a. LDH
    b. Testosterone
    c. PSA
    d. AFP

17. Which of the following testicular tumors are found in younger patients and are associated with high levels of estrogens and gynecomastia?
    a. Leydig cell tumor
    b. Seminoma
    c. Embryonal cell tumor
    d. Sertoli cell tumor

18. What is associated with the sonographic finding represented by the arrows in Figure 13-33?
    a. Testicular infarction
    b. Torsion of the appendix testis
    c. Sarcoidosis
    d. Adrenal hyperplasia

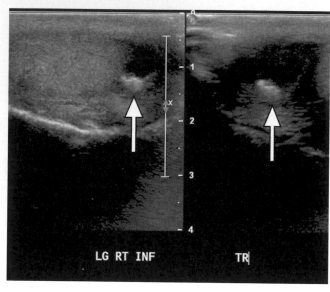

LG RT INF   TR

Figure 13-33

19. Upon sonographic investigation of a patient complaining of testicular pain, you note multiple, small nonshadowing foci scattered throughout both testicles. Which of the following has been associated with these findings?
    a. Chronic testicular torsion
    b. Calcification of the rete testis
    c. Infertility
    d. Chronic epididymitis

20. Epididymitis is associated with which of the following?
    a. Chlamydia
    b. Tuberculosis
    c. Prostatic cancer
    d. Elevated hCG

21. Which of the following is not a component of the spermatic cord?
    a. Epididymis
    b. Testicular artery
    c. Cremaster muscle
    d. Lymph nodes

22. What is the most common malignancy of the testicles?
    a. Embryonal cell carcinoma
    b. Seminoma
    c. Choriocarcinoma
    d. Spermatocele

23. Secondary varicoceles are most likely associated with all of the following except:
    a. left-sided location.
    b. right-sided location.
    c. hepatomegaly.
    d. renal mass.

24. The most common location of BPH is the:
    a. peripheral zone.
    b. transitional zone.
    c. central zone.
    d. verumontanum.

25. During a sonographic examination of the right testis, you visualize multiple small cysts located along the mediastinum testis. What is the most likely diagnosis?
    a. Epididymitis
    b. Tubular ectasia of the rete testis
    c. Multiple spermatoceles
    d. Epidermoid cysts

26. Enlargement of the prostate in older men is most often caused by:
    a. prostatitis.
    b. prostate cancer.
    c. BPH.
    d. Klinefelter syndrome.

27. Which of the following is a benign intratesticular mass that typically has a whorled or onion-skin sonographic appearance?
    a. Seminoma
    b. Teratoma
    c. Epidermoid cyst
    d. Adrenal rest

28. Which of the following best describes a spermatocele?
    a. The most common malignant neoplasm of the scrotum
    b. A benign intratesticular cyst
    c. A cyst, found within the head of epididymis, that may contain debris
    d. A dilated group of veins found within the scrotum

29. A dilated group of veins found within the scrotum is called a:
    a. varicocele.
    b. spermatocele.
    c. seminoma.
    d. hydrocele.

30. Which of the following would most likely resemble a solid intratesticular mass and be associated with Cushing syndrome?
    a. Choriocarcinoma
    b. Epidermoid cyst
    c. Intratesticular varicocele
    d. Adrenal rest

31. Primary varicoceles are associated with all of the following except:
    a. left-sided location.
    b. retroperitoneal mass.
    c. infertility.
    d. palpable extratesticular mass.

32. A common cyst most often seen in the head of the epididymis that contains nonviable sperm is the:
    a. epididymal cyst.
    b. tunica albuginea cyst.
    c. spermatocele.
    d. seminoma.

33. What scrotal abnormality is caused by incompetent valves within the pampiniform plexus?
    a. Testicular carcinoma
    b. Testicular microlithiasis
    c. Testicular torsion
    d. Varicocele

34. What laboratory value can be assessed as a tumor marker to evaluate a patient for testicular malignancy?
    a. Serum bilirubin
    b. Amylase
    c. Alpha-fetoprotein
    d. Adrenocorticotropic hormone

35. The blue-dot sign is indicative of:
    a. testicular torsion.
    b. epididymitis.
    c. orchitis.
    d. torsion of the testicular appendage.

36. A 23-year-old man presents to the sonography department with a history of infertility. Which of the following is associated with male infertility?
    a. Spermatocele
    b. Choriocarcinoma
    c. Varicocele
    d. Hydrocele

37. Which of the following houses the male urethra?
    a. Corpus spongiosum
    b. Buck fascia
    c. Bulbourethral gland
    d. Corpus cavernosum

38. All of the following are sonographic findings consistent with torsion of the testicular appendage except:
    a. no intratesticular flow.
    b. small hyperechoic mass adjacent to the testis.
    c. reactive hydrocele.
    d. scrotal wall thickening.

39. What is the most common correctable cause of male infertility?
    a. Varicocele
    b. Chlamydia
    c. Hydrocele
    d. Testicular torsion

40. A simple fluid collection surrounding the testis is referred to as a:
    a. hematocele.
    b. hydrocele.
    c. varicocele.
    d. spermatocele.

41. What is the most common malignancy of the penis?
    a. Cystadenocarcinoma
    b. Adenocarcinoma
    c. Follicular carcinoma
    d. Squamous cell carcinoma

42. A patient presents to the sonography department for a penile sonogram. He complains of a painful curvature of the penis and impotence. What is the most likely diagnosis?
    a. Squamous cell carcinoma
    b. Peyronie disease
    c. Zinner syndrome
    d. Testicular fracture

43. The exocrine function of the testicles is to produce:
    a. testosterone.
    b. hCG.
    c. AFP.
    d. sperm.

44. The most common location of a hydrocele is:
    a. superior to the testis.
    b. within the scrotal wall.
    c. between the two layers of the tunica vaginalis.
    d. between the tunica vaginalis and the tunica albuginea.

45. Acute onset of testicular pain at rest is a common clinical finding with:
    a. testicular carcinoma.
    b. hydrocele.
    c. testicular trauma.
    d. testicular torsion.

46. A 7-year-old boy presents to the emergency department with acute testicular pain localized to the superior pole of his right testis. What is the most likely diagnosis?
    a. Testicular torsion
    b. Hydrocele
    c. Torsion of the testicular appendage
    d. Yolk sac tumor

47. Zinner syndrome consists of unilateral renal agenesis, ejaculatory duct obstruction, and:
    a. prostate cancer.
    b. seminoma.
    c. bulbourethral stones.
    d. seminal vesicle cysts.

48. Dilated veins of a varicocele will measure:
    a. greater than 8 mm.
    b. greater than 4 mm.
    c. less than 2 mm.
    d. greater than 2 mm.

49. The lack of the normal fixation of the testis to the posterior scrotal wall is referred to as:
    a. Klinefelter syndrome.
    b. blue-dot sign.
    c. bell-clapper deformity.
    d. cryptorchidism.

50. Which of the following techniques is useful for providing sonographic evidence of a varicocele?
    a. Valsalva maneuver
    b. Sitting position
    c. Pulsed Doppler
    d. Right lateral decubitus position

51. The endocrine function of the testicles is to produce:
    a. testosterone.
    b. hCG.
    c. AFP.
    d. sperm.

52. All of the following are sonographic findings consistent with the diagnosis of testicular torsion except:
    a. hyperemic flow within the testis.
    b. hypoechoic testis.
    c. reactive hydrocele.
    d. decreased intratesticular flow (as compared with the asymptomatic testis).

53. Spermatogenesis occurs within the:
    a. tunica albuginea.
    b. seminiferous tubules.
    c. mediastinum testis.
    d. rete testis.

54. You have been asked to perform a study to rule out cryptorchidism. The term cryptorchidism denotes:
    a. one or both of the testicles have a malignancy.
    b. that the testicle has torsed.
    c. one or both of the testicles have not descended into the scrotum.
    d. the patient has been kicked in the scrotum.

55. The most common germ cell tumor of the testis is the:
    a. yolk sac tumor.
    b. seminoma.
    c. embryonal cell carcinoma.
    d. teratoma.

56. The most common location of a varicocele is:
    a. the right side of the scrotum.
    b. the left side of the scrotum.
    c. the inguinal canal.
    d. within the testis.

57. The most common location of prostatic cancer is the:
    a. peripheral zone.
    b. transitional zone.
    c. central zone.
    d. verumontanum.

58. Which of the following is consistent with the sonographic features of testicular abscess?
    a. Hyperemic flow around the abscess, but not within it
    b. Onion-skin sonographic appearance and hyperemic epididymis
    c. Hyperemic flow within an anechoic mass
    d. Hyperemic flow within the abscess, but not around it

59. What is the most common cancer found in men?
    a. Testicular cancer
    b. Lung cancer
    c. Liver cancer
    d. Prostate cancer

60. What would be the most likely sonographic appearance of a seminoma?
    a. Hyperechoic
    b. Anechoic
    c. Heterogeneous with calcifications
    d. Hypoechoic

SUGGESTED READINGS
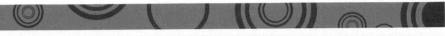

Bhatt S, Kocakoc E, Rubens DJ, et al. Sonographic evaluation of penile trauma. *J Ultrasound Med.* 2005;24:993–1000.

Cancer.org. Penile cancer. What is penile cancer? http://www.cancer.org/cancer/penilecancer/detailedguide/penile-cancer-what-is-penile-cancer. Accessed October 18, 2021.

Curry RA, Tempkin BB. *Sonography: Introduction to Normal Structure and Function.* 5th ed. Elsevier; 2020:501–516.

Hagen-Ansert SL. *Textbook of Diagnostic Sonography.* 7th ed. Elsevier; 2012:604–628.

Henningsen C, Kuntz K, Youngs D. *Clinical Guide to Sonography: Exercises for Critical Thinking.* 2nd ed. Elsevier; 2014:343–358.

Hertzberg BS, Middleton WD. *Ultrasound: The Requisites.* 3rd ed. Elsevier; 2016:146–178.

Kawamura DM, Nolan TD. *Diagnostic Medical Sonography: Abdomen and Superficial Structures.* 4th ed. Wolters Kluwer; 2018:511–550.

Murray, MJ, Huddart RA, Coleman N. The present and future of serum diagnostic tests for testicular germ cell tumours. *Nat Rev Urol.* 2016;13(12):715–725.

Nicholson BD, Jones NR, Protheroe A, et al. The diagnostic performance of current tumour markers in surveillance for recurrent testicular cancer: a diagnostic test accuracy systematic review. *Cancer Epidemiol.* 2019;59:15–21.

Radiopedia. Zinner syndrome. https://radiopaedia.org/articles/zinner-syndrome-1. Accessed May 25, 2017.

Rumack CM, Wilson SR, Charboneau WJ, et al. *Diagnostic Ultrasound.* 4th ed. Elsevier; 2011:840–877 & 1943–1961.

Sanders RC, Hall-Terracciano B. *Clinical Sonography: A Practical Guide.* 5th ed. Wolters Kluwer; 2016:735–762.

Siegel MJ. *Pediatric Sonography.* 5th ed. Wolters Kluwer; 2019:557–600.

BONUS REVIEW!

Varicocele and Hydrocele on Computed Tomography (Fig. 13-34)

Testicular Fracture (Fig. 13-35)

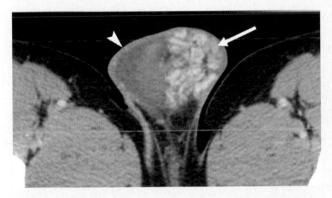

Figure 13-34 Varicocele and hydrocele. Axial post-contrast computed tomography through the scrotum reveals a large hydrocele (*arrowhead*) on the right and a very large enhancing varicocele (*arrow*) on the left.

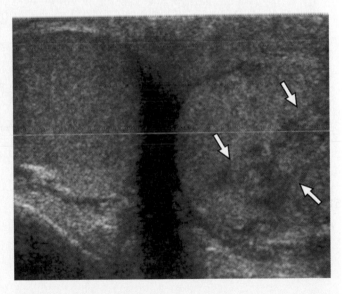

Figure 13-35 Side-by-side sonographic image of the testicles shows irregular linear areas of decreased echogenicity in the left testicle due to disruption of testicular parenchyma, consistent with fractures (between *arrows*). There was no disruption of the surrounding tunica albuginea to suggest testicular rupture.

(continued)

Penile Implants (Fig. 13-36)

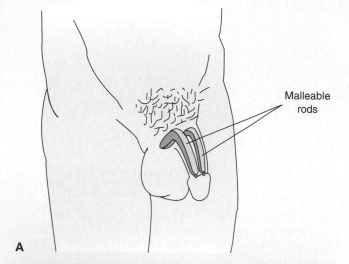

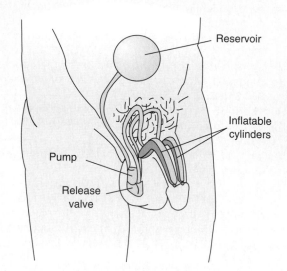

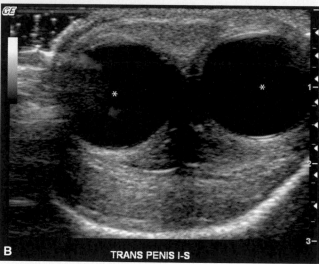

Figure 13-36 Penile implants. **A.** Semirigid. **B.** Inflatable. Transverse view through the penile shaft demonstrates paired, fluid-filled, inflatable cavernosal chambers (*asterisk*) surgically implanted to treat impotence.

14

Musculoskeletal Imaging, Breast, and Superficial Structures

Introduction

Because the certification examinations may contain some questions on musculo-skeletal specialty topics, this chapter is provided to offer a brief overview of musculoskeletal imaging, including infant hip and the Achilles tendon. Breast imaging may also be performed by the abdominal sonographer, especially in emergency situations or following surgical intervention. However, the aim of this chapter is not to prepare the sonographer for the breast sonographic certification examination, but rather to focus the information on basic anatomy of the breast and pathology that may arise in emergency situations. Imaging of superficial structures is also reviewed in this chapter.

Key Terms

acetabulum—the bowl-shaped surface of the pelvis where the head of femur normally rests

Achilles tendon—tendon located along the posterior ankle that connects the calf muscle to the posterior surface of the heel

angle of insonation—angle at which the sound beams interact with tissue

arthrogryposis—a congenital disorder associated with severe joint contractures

Baker cyst—a synovial cyst located within the popliteal fossa; may also be referred to as a popliteal cyst

Barlow test—clinical test for developmental hip dysplasia that is used to evaluate the hip for dislocation

cellulitis—inflammation and infection of the skin and subcutaneous tissues

developmental dysplasia of the hip—a congenital anomaly in which the ball of the hip is prohibited from resting appropriately in the natural socket provided for it on the pelvis

galactocele—a milk-filled breast cyst

ganglion cyst—a common cyst found adjacent to a joint or tendon; most often found along the dorsal aspect of the hand, wrist, ankle, or foot

Graf technique—a technique used to measure the relationship of the femoral head and acetabulum by evaluating the alpha and beta angles created by the relationships of these structures

gynecomastia—the benign enlargement of the male breast; typically located posterior to the areola

hemangioma—a benign tumor composed of blood vessels

hip joint effusion—buildup of fluid within the hip secondary to inflammation

ilium (pelvis)—the largest and most superiorly located pelvic bone

lactiferous ducts—the ducts of the breast used to transport milk to the nipple

lipoma—a benign, fatty tumor

mastitis—inflammation of the breast

meniscus—thin fibrocartilaginous tissue that is located between the surfaces of two joints

natal cleft—area located between the groove of the buttocks

occult—hidden

Ortolani test—clinical test for developmental hip dysplasia that is used to evaluate the hip for the reduction or relocation of a dislocated hip

pannus—a hanging flap of tissue

pilonidal cyst—cyst located along the natal cleft that is composed of loose hairs and skin debris

puerperal mastitis—inflammation of the breast that is related to pregnancy

radiolucent—transparent with radiography

refractive shadowing—acoustic shadowing caused by bending of a sound beam at the edge of a curved reflector; may be referred to as edge artifact or edge shadowing

subluxation—partial dislocation of the hip

superficial epidermal cyst—cysts commonly found in the scalp, face, neck, trunk, or back; they can be congenital, the result of trauma, or the result of an obstructed hair follicle

tendosynovitis—inflammation of the tendon and synovial tendon sheath

Thompson test—clinical test used to evaluate for a complete tear of the Achilles tendon

MUSCULOSKELETAL IMAGING

Sonographic Appearance of Muscles, Tendons, and Ligaments

As a sonographer, it is important to have a basic appreciation for the location of bones and superficial muscles of the body (Figs. 14-1 and 14-2). Musculoskeletal

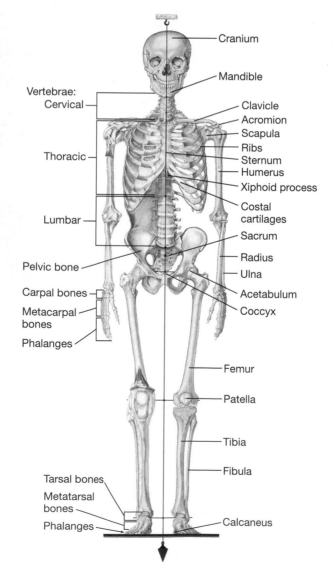

Figure 14-1 Anterior view of the skeleton.

structures are typically imaged with a linear array transducer for improved resolution. Muscles appear sonographically as hypoechoic tissue that contains linear, echogenic strands. Tendons may be noted as echogenic, fibrous structures connecting muscle to bone (Fig. 14-3). Although in most situations, the transducer must be placed perpendicular to the tendon for it to be appropriately imaged with sonography, occasionally altering the **angle of insonation** can help differentiate the tendon from adjacent fat (Fig. 14-4). Ligaments, which connect bones to other bones, appear echogenic as well.

Tendon Pathology

Tendonitis

Inflammation of a tendon, termed tendonitis, can be diffuse or focal. It may be caused by overuse or strain. Diffuse tendonitis appears as a thickened and hypoechoic tendon, whereas focal tendonitis will appear as a localized, enlarged hypoechoic area within the tendon. Hyperemic flow may be noted within the tendon as well (Fig. 14-5). Fluid within the synovial sheath is often indicative of **tendosynovitis**. Patients will present with pain, swelling, and, possibly, fever in the troubled area.

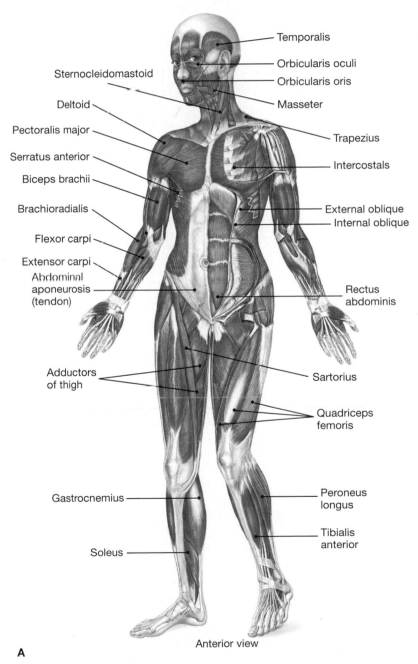

Temporalis
Orbicularis oculi
Orbicularis oris
Masseter
Sternocleidomastoid
Deltoid
Pectoralis major
Trapezius
Serratus anterior
Intercostals
Biceps brachii
Brachioradialis
External oblique
Internal oblique
Flexor carpi
Extensor carpi
Abdominal aponeurosis (tendon)
Rectus abdominis
Adductors of thigh
Sartorius
Quadriceps femoris
Gastrocnemius
Peroneus longus
Tibialis anterior
Soleus
Anterior view

A

Figure 14-2 Anterior (**A**) and posterior (**B**) views of the muscles.

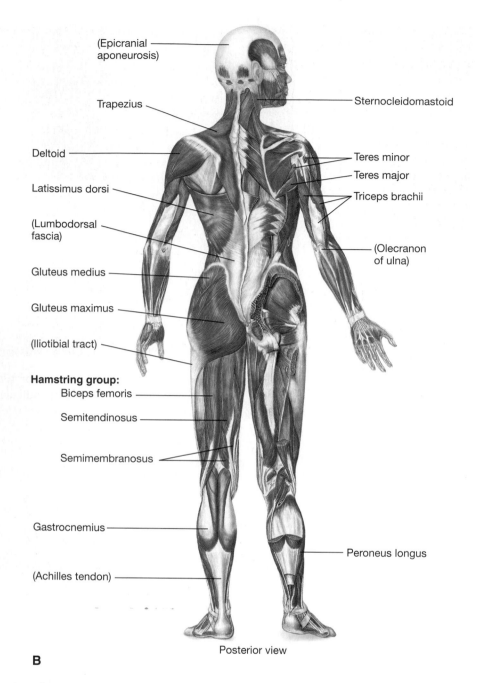

(Epicranial aponeurosis)

Trapezius

Sternocleidomastoid

Deltoid

Teres minor

Teres major

Latissimus dorsi

Triceps brachii

(Lumbodorsal fascia)

Gluteus medius

(Olecranon of ulna)

Gluteus maximus

(Iliotibial tract)

Hamstring group:

Biceps femoris

Semitendinosus

Semimembranosus

Gastrocnemius

Peroneus longus

(Achilles tendon)

Posterior view

B

Figure 14-2 (*continued*)

CLINICAL FINDINGS OF TENDONITIS

1. Pain
2. Painful region may be swollen
3. Painful region may be warm to touch

SONOGRAPHIC FINDINGS OF TENDONITIS

1. Diffuse: enlarged, hypoechoic tendon
2. Focal: localized, enlarged hypoechoic area within the tendon
3. Fluid may be noted
4. Hyperemic flow may be noted

SOUND OFF
Tendonitis may yield hyperemic flow with color Doppler.

Tendon Rupture

A tendon rupture may also be referred to as a tear, and it most likely results from some manner of recreational sport. Tendon tears can be partial or complete. Partial tears can appear as focal hypoechoic areas within the tendon, whereas complete tears are seen as an anechoic or heterogeneous area within the tendon, often indicative of a hematoma (Fig. 14-6). Complete ruptures may also be sonographically identified as **refractive**

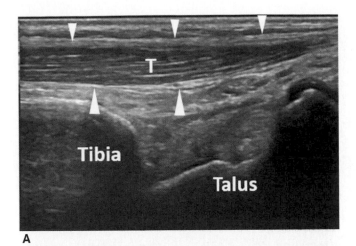

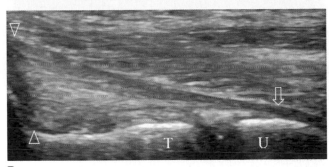

Figure 14-3 Normal tendon and ligament. **A.** Anterior tibialis tendon (*T*), longitudinal anterior image of the ankle. The normal tendon is echogenic with a fibrillated appearance and is surrounded by thin echogenic peritenon (*arrowheads*). Tendons connect muscle to bone. **B.** Longitudinal medial sonogram of the left elbow. The ligament has a normal fibrillar pattern and triangular shape with a broad-based attachment (*open arrowheads*) on the distal humerus and thinner tapered attachment (*open arrow*) on the sublime tubercle of the ulna (*U*). The ligament crosses the joint space between the ulna and the trochlea (*T*) of the humerus. There is echogenic fibrofatty material between the ligament and the humerus. Ligaments connect bone to bone.

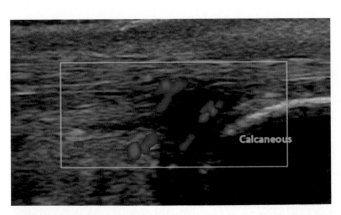

Figure 14-5 Tendonitis. Longitudinal color Doppler image of the Achilles tendon. Note the neovascularity, which suggests tendonitis.

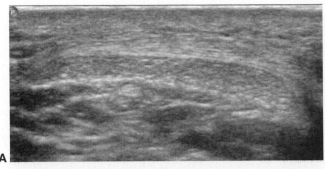

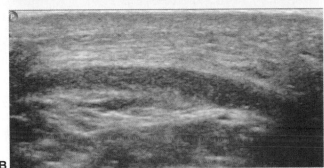

Figure 14-4 Angle of insonation for tendons. **A.** Image of the patellar tendon taken perpendicular to the tendon, resulting in the typical hyperechoic echogenicity of the normal tendon. **B.** Image slightly angled to cause the tendon to appear more hypoechoic, thus making it more distinguishable from the adjacent fat.

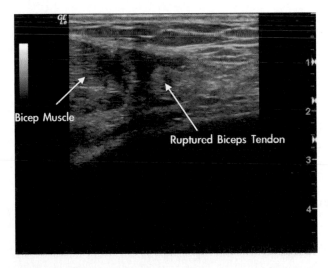

Figure 14-6 Tendon rupture. This biceps tendon has ruptured, with a resulting anechoic fluid collection that is most likely hemorrhage.

shadowing in the area of the separated tendon, with fat, a hematoma, or granulomatous material filling in the gap created by the tear. Surrounding the area of rupture will most likely be extensive edema, with corresponding fluid accumulation. A patient with a torn tendon will be suffering from edema and significant pain in the wounded region.

CLINICAL FINDINGS OF A TENDON RUPTURE

1. Pain
2. Edema
3. Audible snap may be heard

SONOGRAPHIC FINDINGS OF A TENDON RUPTURE

1. Partial tears: appear as focal hypoechoic areas within the tendon
2. Complete tears: seen as an anechoic or heterogeneous area within the tendon, often indicative of a hematoma; may also be sonographically identified as refractive shadowing in the area of the separated tendon, with fat, a hematoma, or granulomatous material filling in the gap created by the tear

Achilles Tendon Rupture

The **Achilles tendon** also referred to as the calcaneal tendon, is the most commonly injured ankle tendon. It is located along the posterior ankle and connects the calf muscle (gastrocnemius) to the posterior surface of the heel, or calcaneus (Fig. 14-7). To evaluate the Achilles tendon with sonography, the patient lies prone, with their feet hanging off the end of the bed. Both the symptomatic and asymptomatic Achilles tendons should be scanned for comparison. The entire tendon should be evaluated in sagittal and transverse scan planes. A landscape image of the entire length of the painful tendon may be useful.

The Achilles tendon should be assessed for the sonographic signs of tendonitis and rupture, as described in this chapter (Figs. 14-8 and 14-9). Patients will present with posterior ankle and leg pain, and they may state that they heard an audible snap as the tendon ruptured. Clinically, the **Thompson test** can be performed to see if there is a complete tear of the tendon. The Thompson test is conducted with the patient prone as well and can be performed before the sonographic examination. The calf is squeezed and the foot should plantarflex in a patient who does not have a complete tear of the Achilles tendon (Fig. 14-10).

CLINICAL FINDINGS OF ACHILLES TENDON RUPTURE

1. Audible snap may be heard
2. Posterior ankle and leg pain
3. Positive Thompson test

SONOGRAPHIC FINDINGS OF ACHILLES TENDON RUPTURE

1. Partial tears: appear as focal hypoechoic areas within the tendon
2. Complete tears: seen as an anechoic or heterogeneous area within the tendon, often indicative of a hematoma; may also be sonographically identified as refractive shadowing in the area of the separated tendon, with fat, a hematoma, or granulomatous material filling in the gap created by the tear

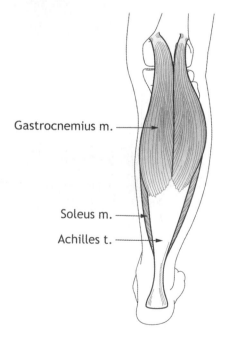
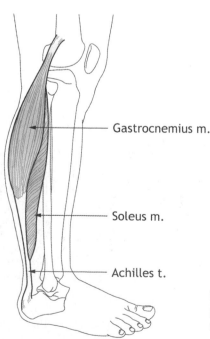

Gastrocnemius m.

Soleus m.

Achilles t.

Posterior aspect

Gastrocnemius m.

Soleus m.

Achilles t.

Lateral aspect

Figure 14-7 The anatomy of the gastrocnemius muscle, soleus muscle, and location of the Achilles tendon. m, muscle; t, tendon.

SOUND OFF
Patients with a torn Achilles tendon may have heard an audible snap when the tendon ruptures.

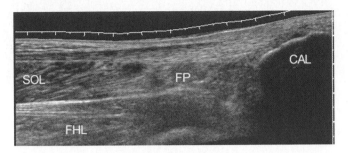

Figure 14-8 Normal Achilles tendon. Longitudinal image of the normal Achilles tendon demonstrating the fat pad (*FP*), soleus muscle (*SOL*), flexor hallucis longus tendon (*FHL*), and the calcaneus (*CAL*).

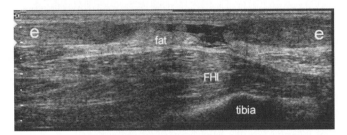

Figure 14-9 Ruptured Achilles tendon. Longitudinal image of a complete rupture of the Achilles tendon. The two ends (*e*) of the tendon, the flexor hallucis longus tendon (*FHL*), fat (*fat*), and the tibia (*tibia*) are all seen. A hypoechoic fluid gap in the area of the rupture is seen separating the two ends of the tendon.

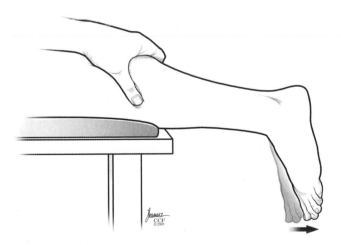

Figure 14-10 Thompson test. The Thompson test is conducted with the patient prone and can be performed before the sonographic examination. The calf is squeezed and the foot should plantarflex in a patient who does not have a complete tear of the Achilles tendon.

Developmental Dysplasia of the Infant Hip

Sonographers should have a basic understanding of the anatomy of the infant hip (Fig. 14-11). **Developmental dysplasia of the hip** (DDH) is a congenital anomaly that may be described as a shallow hip socket. With DDH, the ball of the hip—the femoral head—is prohibited from resting appropriately in the natural socket—the **acetabulum**—which is provided for it on the pelvis. DDH is thought to be caused by abnormal fetal ligament development within the hip that is intensified by the excessive levels of circulating maternal estrogen. Fetal malposition, such as breech and oligohydramnios, greatly increases the risk for developing DDH as well. DDH is more common in female patients and most often affects left side. It has been linked with spina bifida and **arthrogryposis**, and there is a familial link as well. These young patients are recommended to be screened between 4 and 6 weeks after birth. Clinically, patients will have asymmetric skinfolds on the legs, leg length discrepancy, and limited limb abduction (Fig. 14-12). There are two clinical tests that can be performed to evaluate an infant for DDH—the **Barlow test** and the **Ortolani test** (Fig. 14-13).

SOUND OFF
Clinically, patients with DDH will have asymmetric skinfolds on the legs, leg length discrepancy, and limited limb abduction.

The Barlow test is used to evaluate the hip for dislocation. For the Barlow test, the hip is flexed and adducted, and the knee is pushed posteriorly and superiorly. The Ortolani test, which evaluates for the reduction or relocation of a dislocated hip, is performed by abducting and lifting the thigh, essentially relocating the hip back into the acetabulum. During the Ortolani test, an audible "click" may be heard and a palpable "clunk" felt as the head of the femur passes over the acetabulum.

During sonographic imaging of the infant hip, several important landmarks should be evaluated while the hip is examined in both flexion and at rest. Specifically, the femoral head and its relationship to the acetabulum should be examined in both stress and relaxed states. The position of the head of the femur, as it relates to the acetabulum, can be described as normal, subluxed, or dislocated (Fig. 14-14). **Subluxation** is a term used to denote partial dislocation of the hip. Sonographically, the infant hip is examined in both coronal and transverse in either the supine or lateral decubitus position. Although protocols may vary, it is recommended that both hips be examined, and a neutral or resting coronal view and a transverse view of the flexed hip with and without stress be obtained. In the coronal plane, the femoral

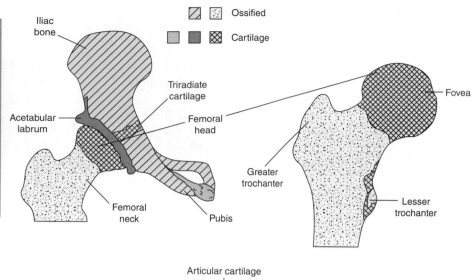

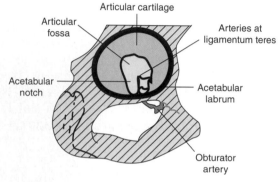

Figure 14-11 Parts of the infant hip.

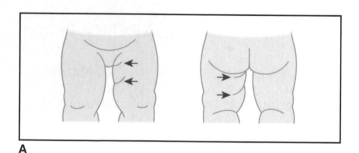

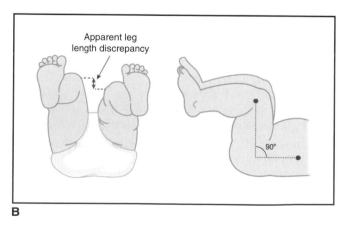

Figure 14-12 Developmental dysplasia of the hip physical findings. **A.** Asymmetric skin folds. **B.** Leg length discrepancy.

head appears as a hypoechoic rounded structure that contains echogenic stripes throughout. The **ilium** can be noted appearing to extend from the femoral head as an echogenic linearly structure producing an acoustic shadow. The acetabulum is the recessed region of the pelvis where the femoral head should rest.

> 🔊 **SOUND OFF**
> The Barlow test requires for the leg to be adducted, whereas the Ortolani test requires the leg to be abducted.

Sonographic imaging of the infant hip, which offers a dynamic analysis, should include both coronal and transverse images using a high-frequency linear transducer. The sonographic diagnosis of DDH can be definitive when the femoral head rests clearly outside the acetabulum, denoting dislocation. Whereas a normal hip rests centrally within the acetabulum, a subluxed hip will rest more laterally, although it is partially covered by the acetabulum. Because several techniques have been suggested, the interpretation results may depend upon the criteria utilized by the physician for the diagnoses of DDH. For example, in the coronal view, the **Graf technique** can be obtained (Fig. 14-15). This technique is used to measure the relationship of

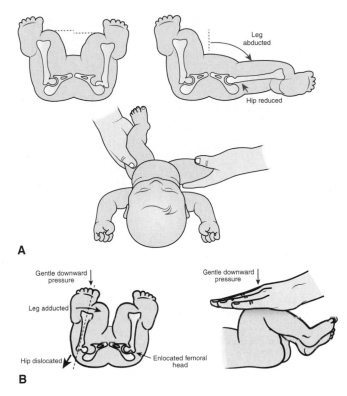

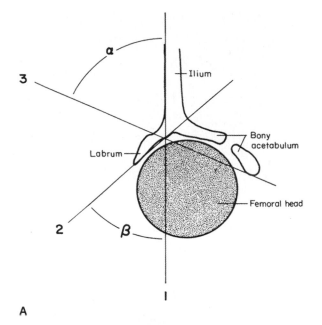

Figure 14-13 Clinical assessment for DDH. **A.** The Ortolani maneuver. From a flexed and adducted position, the hip is abducted; the examiner feels a clunk as the femoral head moves into the socket. The examiner's other hand stabilizes the infant's pelvis. **B.** The Barlow test. The examiner holds the infant's hip in flexion and slight abduction. The infant's hip is adduced while applying pressure in a posterior direction. Dislocation of the femoral head with pressure indicates an unstable hip.

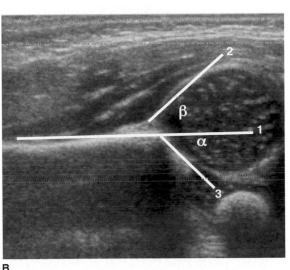

Figure 14-15 The Graf technique. Drawing of the coronal view of the hip (**A**) and coronal sonogram (**B**) delineate the femoral head, bony acetabulum, and labrum. A horizontal baseline is drawn along the ilium (*1*), along with lines along the labrum (*2*) and bony acetabulum (*3*). The alpha angle measures the acetabulum and is 60 degrees or greater in infants with seated hips and less than 50° in patients with dysplasia.

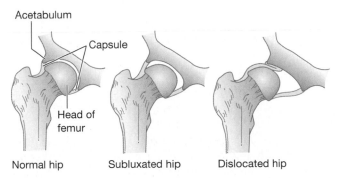

Figure 14-14 Developmental dysplasia of the hip (*DDH*). Normally, the head of the femur should sit snuggly within the acetabulum (left image). With DDH, flattening of the acetabulum prevents the head of the femur from rotating properly. The acetabulum may be shallow. Subluxation (middle image) is partial dislocation of the hip. With complete dislocation, the femoral head is located outside the acetabulum (right image).

the femoral head and acetabulum by evaluating alpha and beta angles created by the relationships of these structures (Fig. 14-16). To assess the depth of the acetabulum, from the coronal view, a line can be drawn along the ilium and through the femoral head, with two other lines drawn along the acetabulum and adjacent to the femoral head, to obtain the two pertinent angles. Essentially, the smaller the alpha angle and the larger the beta angle, the more likely the infant is suffering from DDH. The hip is also assessed in the transverse plane (Fig. 14-17).

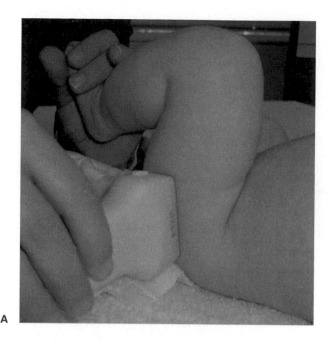

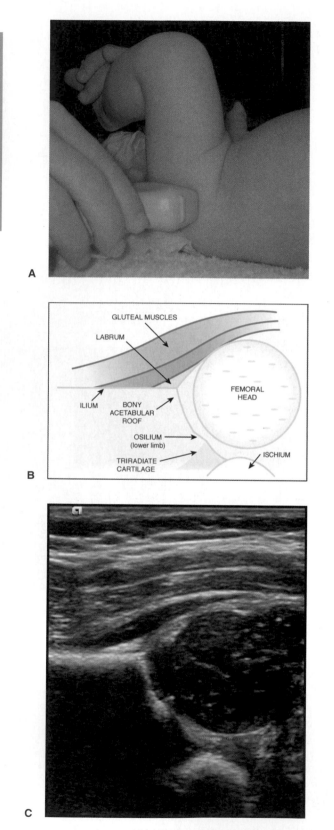

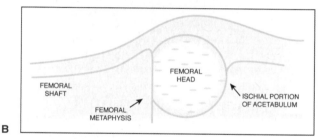

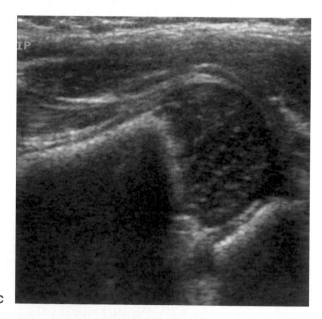

Figure 14-16 Coronal infant hip. **A.** Probe placement on an infant hip for the coronal flexion view. Note the infant's knee is bent at approximately 90 degrees. **B.** Anatomic drawing of the infant hip in coronal. **C.** Normal coronal sonogram of the infant hip in the coronal plane.

Figure 14-17 Transverse infant hip. **A.** Transducer placement for flexion transverse imaging of the infant hip. **B.** Drawing of the infant hip anatomy in the transverse flexion view. **C.** Sonogram of the normal infant hip in transverse.

Another test can be used to evaluate the amount of coverage of the femoral head by the acetabulum by obtaining a coronal image and drawing parallel lines along the ilium and the maximum depth and height of the femoral head. Coverage of the femoral head by the acetabulum of greater than 55% is said to be normal, whereas 50% or less is said to be shallow, and less than 45% is considered very shallow (Fig. 14-18). Nonsurgical treatment for DDH can be performed with casting or by means of a Pavlik harness. Sonography may be used as a follow-up imaging tool subsequent to treatment.

CLINICAL FINDINGS OF DEVELOPMENTAL DYSPLASIA OF THE INFANT HIP

1. History of breech birth
2. Family history of DDH
3. Asymmetric skinfolds on the legs
4. Leg length discrepancy
5. Limited limb abduction
6. Positive Barlow or Ortolani test

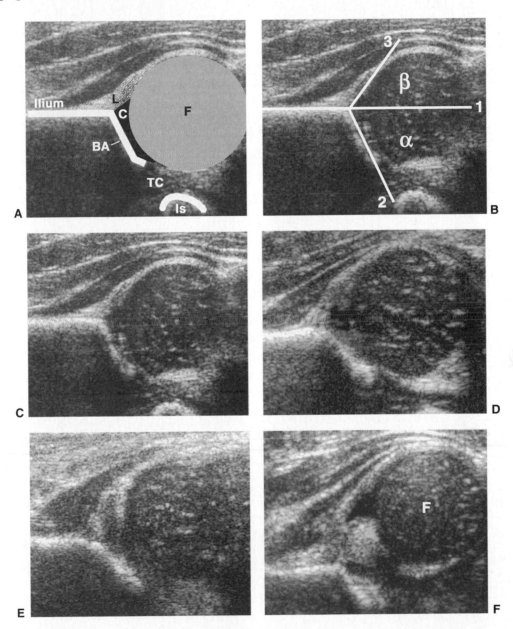

Figure 14-18 Sonographic anatomy of the hip evaluated by the Graf technique. **A.** Schematic representation of the coronal view of the hip: femoral head (*F*), bony acetabulum (*BA*), labrum (*L*). *C*, acetabular roof cartilage; *TC*, triradiate cartilage; *Is*, ischium. **B.** In the Graf technique, horizontal line is drawn along the ilium (*I*), and lines are drawn along the BA (*2*) and labrum (*3*) to obtain alpha (α) and beta (β) angles. The α angle is equal to or greater than 60 degrees in infants with seated hips and less than 50° in patients with dysplasia. The β angle increases proportionally with the degree of hip dysplasia and displacement. **C.** Normal hip. **D.** Slightly shallow acetabulum. **E.** Shallow acetabulum and the femoral head is minimally covered and displaced laterally. **F.** Dislocation.

SONOGRAPHIC FINDINGS OF DEVELOPMENTAL DYSPLASIA OF THE INFANT HIP

1. Femoral head located completely outside the acetabulum (complete dislocation)
2. Partially coverage of the femoral head by the acetabulum (subluxation)
3. Evidence of a shallow acetabulum (<50% coverage of femoral head)
4. Small alpha angle (Graf technique)
5. Large beta angle (Graf technique)

SOUND OFF
The smaller the alpha angle and the larger the beta angle, the more likely the infant is suffering from DDH.

Infant Hip Joint Effusion—Transient Synovitis

A **hip joint effusion**, which is the buildup of fluid within the hip secondary to inflammation, typically occurs in children between 5 and 10 years of age and is most likely the result of **transient synovitis**—also referred to as toxic synovitis or irritable hip. Transient synovitis is the most common cause of a painful hip and joint effusion in children. The cause is unknown, although viral causes, trauma, and an allergic reaction have been suspected. Patients typically present with leg and knee pain, a reluctance to walk, irritability, low-grade fever, and mild leukocytosis. The sonographic appearance of a joint effusion is that of anechoic or hypoechoic fluid that elevates the anterior capsule of the joint. Often, the abnormal joint capsule width exceeds 5 mm (Fig. 14-19). A sonographic analysis of the asymptomatic hip first can provide the sonographer with a valid baseline before

the symptomatic hip is analyzed. An ultrasound-guided hip aspiration may be performed to relieve pain and to differentiate the disorder from the more worrisome diagnosis of septic arthritis.

CLINICAL FINDINGS OF HIP JOINT EFFUSION

1. Leg and knee pain
2. Reluctance to walk
3. Irritability
4. Low-grade fever
5. Mild leukocytosis

SONOGRAPHIC FINDINGS OF HIP JOINT EFFUSION

1. Anechoic or hypoechoic fluid that elevates the anterior capsule of the joint
2. Width of the abnormal hip joint capsule typically exceeds 5 mm

SOUND OFF
A sonographic analysis of the asymptomatic hip first can provide the sonographer with a valid baseline before the symptomatic hip is analyzed.

BREAST

Though mammography is the gold standard for breast imaging, sonographers should have a fundamental appreciation of breast anatomy (Fig. 14-20). Sonographic annotation of the breast is typically based on the quadrant or clockface (Fig. 14-21). However,

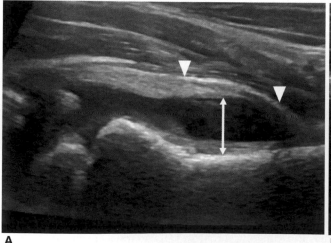
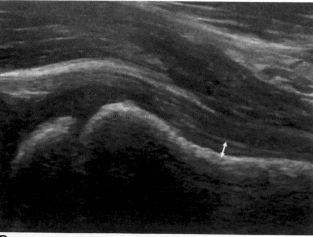

Figure 14-19 Joint effusion. **A.** Longitudinal image of the left hip shows fluid distending the joint capsule, which has a convex anterior contour (*arrowheads*). The double-headed arrow yields a fluid amount that exceeds 10 mm. **B.** Normal right hip.

Musculoskeletal Imaging, Breast, and Superficial Structures

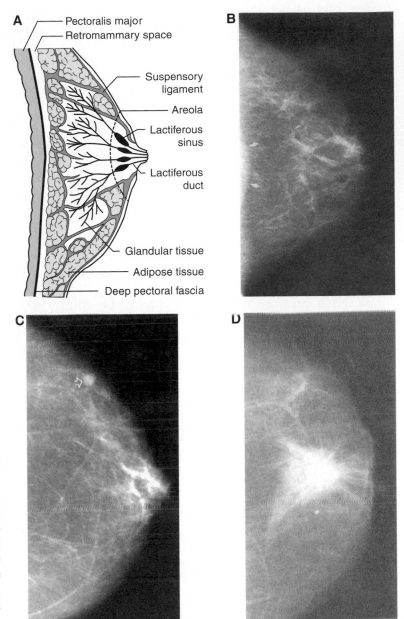

Figure 14-20 Diagram and mammograms of the breast. **A.** A sagittal diagram of the breast. **B.** A craniocaudal (*CC*) mammogram of a normal left breast. The pectoralis major muscle (*arrows*) is seen. **C.** A CC mammogram of a benign mass (*arrow*). A benign mass has the following characteristics: shape is round/oval, margins are well circumscribed, density is low-medium contrast, it becomes smaller over time, and calcifications are large, smooth, and uniform. D: A CC mammogram of a malignant mass. A malignant mass has the following characteristics: shape is irregular with many lobulations, margins are irregular or spiculated, density is medium-high, breast architecture may be distorted, it becomes larger over time, and calcifications (not shown) are small, irregular, variable, and found within ducts.

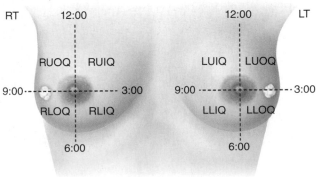

Figure 14-21 Quadrants and clockface annotation. RUOQ, right upper outer quadrant; RUIQ right upper inner quadrant; RLOQ, right lower outer quadrant; RLIQ, right lower inner quadrant; LUIQ, left upper inner quadrant; LUOQ, left upper outer quadrant; LLIQ, left lower inner quadrant; LLOQ, left lower outer quadrant

QUADRANT AND CLOCKFACE ANNOTATION

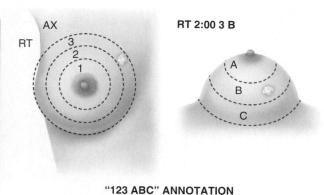

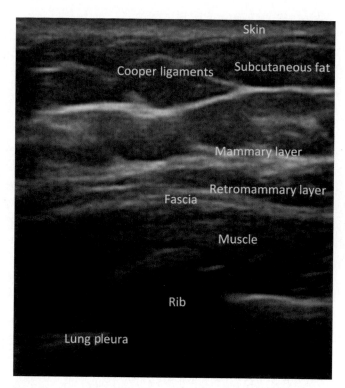

Figure 14-22 123 and ABC annotation. AX, axilla

some institutions may also employ the 123 and ABC annotation, which are used to further describe the breast tissue based on distance from the nipple and depth, respectively (Fig. 14-22). In addition, some institutions may use fingers from the nipple or use a measuring device to be precise in the localization of breast pathology.

Using a linear transducer, the breast may be imaged with the patient in a slight posterior oblique position to evenly distribute the breast tissue over the chest. Superficial pathology can be better visualized with a standoff device or a large amount of mounded gel. Images may be obtained in both the transverse and longitudinal planes. However, because of the radial arrangement of the **lactiferous ducts**, radial and antiradial imaging planes may be used by some institutions as well.

The normal sonographic appearance of the breast tissue layers should be appreciated by sonographers. The three layers of breast tissue from superficial to deep are the subcutaneous layer, the mammary layer, and the retromammary layer (Fig. 14-23). The subcutaneous layer is typically hypoechoic and is composed mostly of fat. The mammary layer, which is typically hyperechoic and contains the ducts and glandular tissue, is the functional layer of the breast. The sonographic appearance of the mammary layer can vary based on many factors, including the age of the patient and the distribution of the various functional elements. The retromammary layer is typically hypoechoic and contains fat as well.

BREAST PATHOLOGY

Mastitis and Breast Abscess

Breast infection—termed **mastitis**—is most often associated with lactation, but it may be encountered following trauma or surgery. Specifically, the type of mastitis associated with breastfeeding is referred to as **puerperal mastitis**. The infection is characteristically

Figure 14-23 Sample sonographic anatomy of the normal breast in sagittal.

caused by the *Staphylococcus* or *Streptococcus* organisms. Patients with mastitis will suffer from pain, swelling, and warmth and redness in the area. The patient may also suffer from fever and leukocytosis. The primary role of sonography is to determine the presence of a focal abscess within a breast that is affected with mastitis. Sonographically, mastitis will appear as ill-defined areas of echogenicity with diffuse edema and hypoechoic fluid within the subcutaneous tissue that may outline the fat lobules (Fig. 14-24). The affected skin may measure

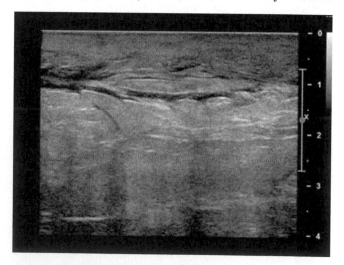

Figure 14-24 Mastitis. As seen in this image, mastitis may appear as ill-defined areas of echogenicity with diffuse edema and hypoechoic fluid within the subcutaneous tissue that outlines the fat lobules.

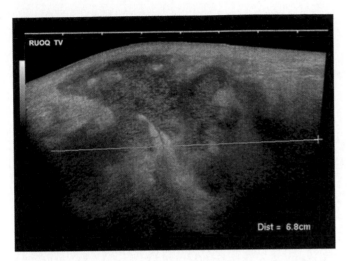

Figure 14-25 Breast abscess. This 6.8-cm complex mass was diagnosed as a breast abscess and was noted in a patient with coexisting mastitis. RUOQ, right upper outer quadrant; TV, transverse

greater than 2 mm in thickness. Reactive, enlarged lymph nodes may be seen as well.

A breast abscess is a focal area of pus. The patient will present clinically much like someone suffering from mastitis. Where diffuse pain may be seen more with mastitis, with an abscess, the patient may have a palpable, painful lump. Sonographically, an abscess is typically a focal, complex fluid collection that can contain debris (Fig. 14-25). Color Doppler will be increased around the abscess as opposed to within the mass, a sign of peripheral hyperemia. As with mastitis, enlargement of the lymph nodes may be evident as well in the presence of a breast abscess.

◀))) SOUND OFF
Mastitis is most often associated with breastfeeding.

CLINICAL FINDINGS OF MASTITIS

1. Pain
2. Swelling
3. Warmth and redness in the area (erythema)
4. Fever
5. Leukocytosis

SONOGRAPHIC FINDINGS OF MASTITIS

1. Ill-defined areas of echogenicity
2. Diffuse edema
3. Hypoechoic fluid within the subcutaneous tissue that outlines the fat lobules
4. Breast skin thickening greater than 2 mm
5. Enlarged lymph nodes may be present

SONOGRAPHIC FINDINGS OF A BREAST ABSCESS

1. Palpable, tender lump
2. Complex, focal mass that contains debris
3. Peripheral hyperemia

Postsurgical Breast

The postsurgical breast can suffer from various complications that may require investigation with sonography. Following surgery or an invasive procedure, the breast could certainly develop mastitis or, possibly, an abscess, both of which were mentioned earlier. However, other complications could include a hematoma, seroma, and lymphedema.

A breast hematoma should especially be considered following trauma or surgery. A hematoma will often appear complex and, with time, will disappear as it is reabsorbed by the body, though occasionally scar tissue and calcifications may remain (Fig. 14-26). The patient will likely have pain in the region and skin discoloration. A seroma typically results from surgery as well, as in the case of a lumpectomy or complete mastectomy, when simple serous fluid fills the vacated region. Serous fluid is sterile and contains no red blood cells. A seroma will likely appear as an anechoic fluid collection (Fig. 14-27).

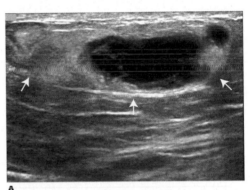

A

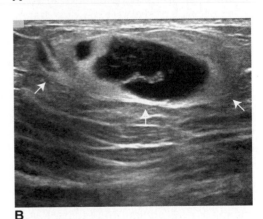

B

Figure 14-26 Breast hematoma. Views of a focal fluid collection (both **A** and **B** *arrows*) representing a hematoma following trauma.

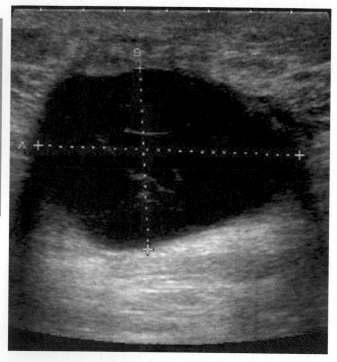

Figure 14-27 Breast seroma following a lumpectomy. An anechoic mass lesion with good through transmission consistent with a seroma (between *calipers*).

Galactocele

Lactating patients may present to the emergency department with a palpable mass that may be painful. A **galactocele** is a milk-filled cyst that can develop after an abrupt termination to breastfeeding or result from an obstruction to the lactiferous duct or ducts. The mass is typically palpable and located near the areola. These cysts can be painful and can become infected as well. Sonographically, a galactocele will appear as a round mass with good borders. They may appear complex or contain a fluid-fluid level.

CLINICAL FINDINGS OF A GALACTOCELE

1. Palpable, periareolar mass
2. Possible pain

SONOGRAPHIC FINDINGS OF GALACTOCELE

1. Round, complex mass
2. May contain a fluid-fluid level

Gynecomastia

Gynecomastia is the benign enlargement of the male breast. Gynecomastia can occur at any time but is most commonly encountered just after birth, during puberty, and during mid-to-late adulthood between 50 and 80 years of age. Gynecomastia can be bilateral and can be associated with high levels of human

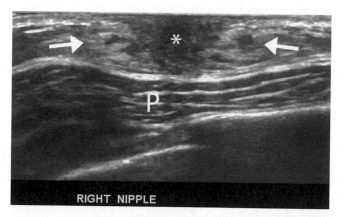

RIGHT NIPPLE

Figure 14-28 Gynecomastia. A 13-year-old body with right breast development. Longitudinal image reveals echogenic breast tissue (*arrows*) and a subareolar hypoechoic nodule (*asterisk*). *P*, pectoralis muscle.

chorionic gonadotropin, which may be produced by some testicular tumors, high levels of estrogen, adrenal tumors, hepatoblastoma, **Klinefelter syndrome** (see Fig. 13-16), and with some drugs, including steroids and marijuana. Patients most often present with a tender, palpable retroareolar breast mass that is firm to touch. Sonographically, gynecomastia most likely appears as a triangular hypoechoic mass posterior to the areola (Fig. 14-28).

CLINICAL FINDINGS OF GYNECOMASTIA

1. Tender, palpable retroareolar breast mass that is firm to touch

SONOGRAPHIC FINDINGS OF GYNECOMASTIA

1. Hypoechoic mass posterior to the areola
2. May have a triangular shape

SONOGRAPHY OF SUPERFICIAL STRUCTURES

Soft-tissue sonography typically requires the use of a high-frequency linear transducer, although if the area of interest lies deeper than expected, a lower frequency transducer may be utilized. Sonographers should have an appreciation of the anatomy and the sonographic appearance of the skin, subcutaneous tissue, fascia, and muscle (Fig. 14-29). The skin consists of two layers—the epidermis and the dermis. These two layers are indistinguishable and appear collectively as a hyperechoic linear structure. The subcutaneous layer appears hypoechoic, with interspersed hyperechoic linear echoes representing connective tissue septa. Fascia appears as a hyperechoic layer of varying thickness.

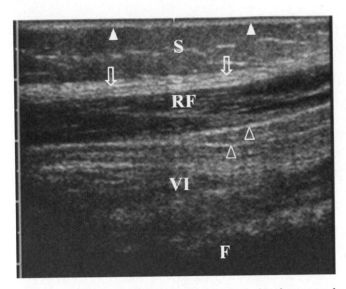

Figure 14-29 Sonographic appearance of skin layers and muscle in the thigh. Longitudinal image of the epidermis and dermis (*white arrowheads*), the subcutaneous fat (*S*), the rectus femoral muscle (*RF*), connective tissue (*open arrowheads*), the vastus intermedius muscle (*VI*), and the femur (*F*).

PATHOLOGY OF SUPERFICIAL STRUCTURES

Superficial Epidermal Cyst

A **superficial epidermal cyst** may also be referred to as an epidermal inclusion cyst, an epidermoid cyst, or, possibly, a sebaceous cyst, although a sebaceous cyst implies that the cyst is sebaceous in origin, which is not always true. True sebaceous cysts are uncommon. Superficial epidermal cysts are most likely found in the scalp, face, neck, trunk, or back. These cysts, which can be congenital or the result of trauma, are potentially the result of an obstructed hair follicle. Clinically, the patient will have a palpable mass that raises the skin and is most likely asymptomatic. However, infection can result in pain and oozing of fluid or solid material from the cyst. An epidermal cyst can have varying sonographic appearances, including anechoic, hypoechoic, complex, or hyperechoic (Fig. 14-30). They have been described as having a pseudotestis appearance. To better visualize the cyst, a standoff device can be utilized.

> **CLINICAL FINDINGS OF A SUPERFICIAL EPIDERMAL CYST**
> 1. Visible, palpable mass just under the skin
> 2. Pain and redness in the area

> **SONOGRAPHIC FINDINGS OF A SUPERFICIAL EPIDERMAL CYST**
> 1. Anechoic, hypoechoic, complex, or hyperechoic cyst or mass
> 2. Pseudotestis appearance

> 🔊 **SOUND OFF**
> Superficial epidermal cysts are most likely found in the scalp, face, neck, trunk, or back.

Ganglion Cyst

A **ganglion cyst** is a common mass found along the dorsal aspect of the hand and wrist, although they can arise from any joint and are thus discovered in the knee, foot, and ankle as well (Fig. 14-31). Large ganglion cysts in the wrist have been referred to as Bible bumps, because individuals in the past have used large books—like the Bible—to reduce the cyst by slamming the large book against it. This practice is not a recommended course of treatment, however. Ganglion cysts within the wrist may be referred to as dorsal ganglion cysts, which are most common, whereas those located near the radial artery are referred to as volar ganglion cysts. Clinically, it may be hard to touch and painful. It is often treated with an injection of corticosteroids, or it may have to be surgically removed. Sonographically, it typically appears as a noncompressible, anechoic mass with acoustic enhancement (Fig. 14-32). However, they may contain debris and septations.

> **CLINICAL FINDINGS OF A GANGLION CYST**
> 1. Palpable mass most often located along the dorsal aspect of the hand or wrist
> 2. Can be painful

> **SONOGRAPHIC FINDINGS OF A GANGLION CYST**
> 1. Noncompressible, anechoic mass with acoustic enhancement
> 2. May contain debris or septations

> 🔊 **SOUND OFF**
> Large ganglion cysts in the wrist have been referred to as Bible bumps, because individuals in the past have used large books—like the Bible—to reduce the cyst by slamming the large book against it.

Superficial Lipoma and Hemangioma

A **lipoma** is a benign, fatty tumor. Superficial lipomas are typically oval in shape and isoechoic to the surrounding fat, but they can appear hypoechoic or hyperechoic (Fig. 14-33). Lipomas are usually compressible and may be observed during a physical examination. Patients are typically asymptomatic but may complain of an unsightly bulging of the skin in the area of the lipoma.

A superficial **hemangioma** is a benign mass that is composed of vascular channels. They are typically

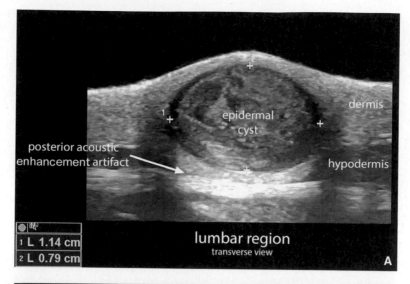

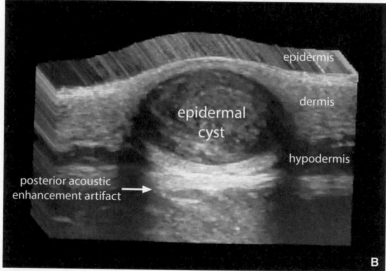

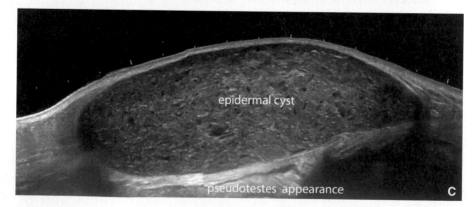

Figure 14-30 Epidermal cyst. **A.** Grayscale; **B.** 3D reconstruction; **C.** Panoramic view. **A** and **B** demonstrate a 1.1-cm (transverse) × 0.8-cm (thickness), well-defined, oval-shaped, hypoechoic dermal and hypodermal structure that produces posterior acoustic enhancement, while. **C** demonstrates the pseudotestis appearance.

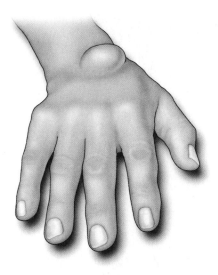

Figure 14-31 A common location for a ganglion cyst is within the wrist.

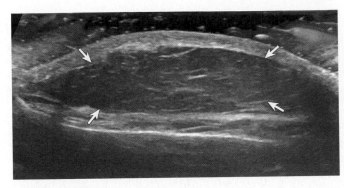

Figure 14-33 Lipoma. Sonographic image reveals an oval hypoechoic subcutaneous lipoma (*arrows*) with internal linear hyperechoic fibrous tissue. Note the use of a standoff mechanism (likely mounded gel) to better visualize the superficial mass.

asymptomatic and appear as a raised, red or reddish purple mass on the skin. Blood flow may be detectable with color Doppler, and superficial hemangiomas are typically sonographically hypoechoic in appearance.

Meniscal Cyst

A **meniscus** is thin, fibrocartilaginous tissue between the surfaces of some joints, like the knee. Meniscal cysts are most often thought to occur because of a fluid collection following a meniscal tear in the knee (Fig. 14-34). A meniscal tear is typically the result of trauma or degenerative changes within the knee. Patients tend to present with focal knee pain, swelling, and, possibly, a palpable mass within the knee joint. The patient may also suffer from joint popping, stiffness, or locking. Sonographically, these cysts typically appear anechoic or hypoechoic (Fig. 14-35).

CLINICAL FINDINGS OF A SUPERFICIAL LIPOMA

1. Asymptomatic
2. Obvious mass under the skin
3. Compressible

SONOGRAPHIC FINDINGS OF A SUPERFICIAL LIPOMA

1. Most likely an hypoechoic or isoechoic mass as compared to the surrounding tissues
2. Typically have an oval shape

CLINICAL FINDINGS OF A SUPERFICIAL HEMANGIOMA

1. Asymptomatic
2. Red or reddish purple, raised mass on the skin

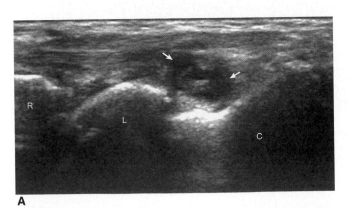

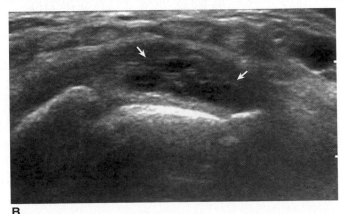

Figure 14-32 Sonographic appearance of a ganglion cyst within the dorsal wrist. Sonographic images long axis (**A**) and short axis (**B**) to dorsal extensor tendons of wrist show multilobular hypoechoic ganglion cyst (*arrows*) with increased through transmission. *R*, radius; *L*, lunate; *C*, capitate.

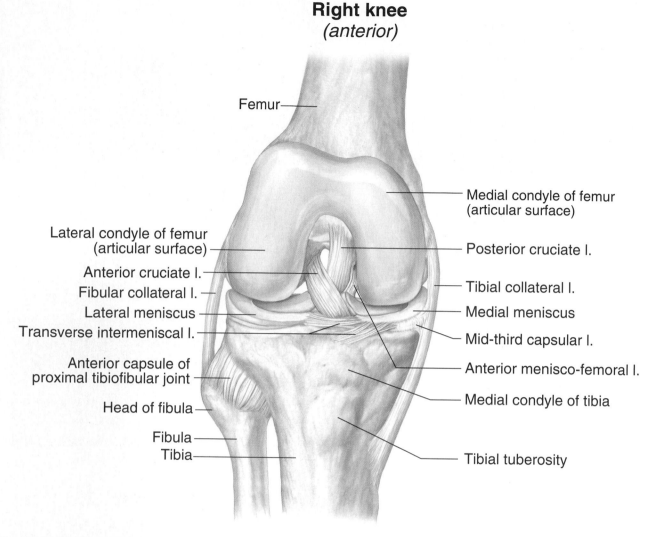

Figure 14-34 Anterior view of the knee.

SONOGRAPHIC FINDINGS OF A SUPERFICIAL HEMANGIOMA

1. Hypoechoic
2. Blood flow may be detectable with color Doppler

CLINICAL FINDINGS OF A MENISCAL CYST

1. Previous trauma
2. Focal knee pain
3. Knee swelling
4. Palpable mass within the knee joint
5. Popping, stiffness, or locking knee joint

SONOGRAPHIC FINDINGS OF A MENISCAL CYST

1. Anechoic or hypoechoic mass with posterior enhancement

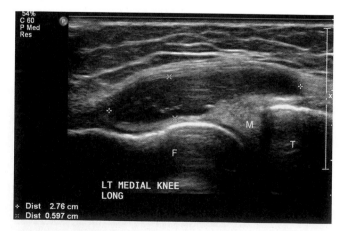

Figure 14-35 Meniscal cyst. Longitudinal image of the medial knee demonstrating a meniscal cyst (*calipers*). Note the close proximity of the cyst and meniscus. *F*, femur; *T*, tibia; *M*, meniscus.

Baker Cyst

A **Baker cyst**, also referred to as a popliteal cyst or synovial cyst, is located in the popliteal fossa, behind the knee (Fig. 14-36). These cysts are common and a result from the accumulation of synovial fluid from a weakening in the joint capsule of the knee, as seen in conditions such as rheumatoid arthritis or osteoarthritis. A channel or tract may be seen connecting the cyst to the joint space.

Baker cysts may be asymptomatic. However, they may also present with focal tenderness secondary to hemorrhage, rupture, or impingement on adjacent structures. Clinical findings of a Baker cyst may mimic those of a deep venous thrombosis. Sonographically, a Baker cyst appears as an anechoic mass with posterior enhancement in the popliteal fossa (Fig. 14-37). Complicated Baker cysts may contain echogenic fluid, debris, **pannus**, or septations. Baker cysts can be aspirated under sonographic guidance, corticosteroid injection, arthroscopic cystectomy, or arthroscopic enlargement of unidirectional valvular slits.

> ### SOUND OFF
> A Baker cyst may be seen in the presence of rheumatoid arthritis or other knee joint issues.

CLINICAL FINDINGS OF A BAKER CYST

1. Asymptomatic
2. Focal tenderness in the popliteal fossa

SONOGRAPHIC FINDINGS OF A BAKER CYST

1. Anechoic mass with posterior enhancement
2. Complicated Baker cysts may contain echogenic fluid, debris, or septations

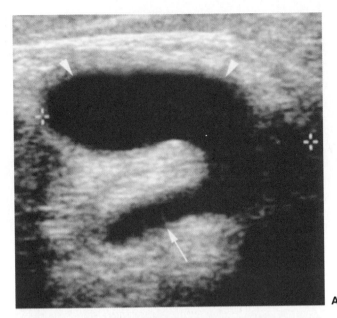

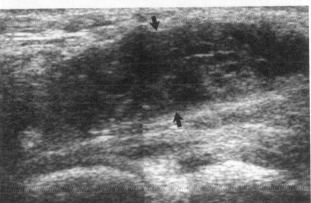

Figure 14-37 Baker cysts. **A.** An uncomplicated Baker cyst (between *calipers* and *arrows*) appears as an anechoic mass in the popliteal fossa. **B.** A large Baker cyst (*arrows*) in a patient with rheumatoid arthritis contains some echogenic debris and pannus.

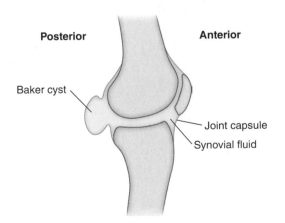

Figure 14-36 A common location for a Baker cyst in the knee.

Pilonidal Cyst

A **pilonidal cyst** is most often found within the **natal cleft**, which is also referred to as the intergluteal cleft or gluteal cleft, and is located between the buttocks. However, pilonidal cysts may also be referred to as pilonidal sinus and may also be seen within the fingers or toes. Pilonidal means "nest of hair." Consequently, these cysts are composed of loose hairs and skin debris. Some pilonidal cysts are asymptomatic, but they can become infected and develop into an abscess that requires intervention. Patients will present with skin edema, warmth, and pain in the area of the cyst that may produce bloody drainage. Patients who are more prone to pilonidal cyst include those who sit for an extended amount of time and hairdressers. During World War II, the cysts were linked with soldiers who

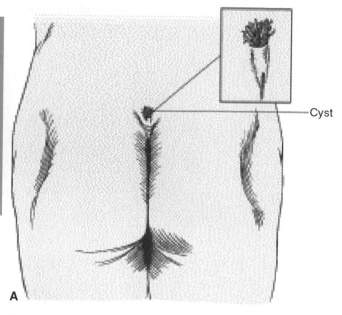
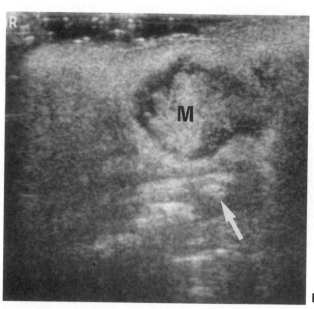

Cyst

Figure 14-38 Pilonidal cyst and sinus. **A.** A pilonidal cyst is typically located in the midline, superficial to the coccyx or the lower sacrum. It is clinically identified by the opening of a sinus tract. This opening may exhibit a small tuft of hair and be surrounded by a halo of erythema. **B.** This pilonidal cyst appeared as a complex mass (*M*) at the tip of the distal spine (*arrow*) in this infant.

had to endure long, bumpy jeep rides; thus, they were termed "jeep disease." Sonographically, pilonidal cysts are identified as a complex mass, and a hypoechoic tract may be noted extending from the cyst to the external surface of the skin (Fig. 14-38). Color Doppler can be used to confirmed hyperemia secondary to infection. A standoff device of some sort can be utilized for better visualization.

CLINICAL FINDINGS OF A PILONIDAL CYST

1. Edema, warmth, and pain in the area of the cyst
2. Bloody drainage from the cyst may be present

SONOGRAPHIC FINDINGS OF A PILONIDAL CYST

1. Complex, subcutaneous mass
2. Hyperemia around the mass
3. Hypoechoic tract may be seen extending from the cyst to the skin surface

Cellulitis and Superficial Abscess

Cellulitis is infection and subsequent inflammation of the skin and subcutaneous tissue. It is most often caused by *Staphylococcus aureus* and *Streptococcus pyogenes*. Often, the skin is red, tender, and warm. There may be evidence of leukocytosis as well, especially if an

abscess is present. Sonographically, cellulitis appears as hypoechoic, edematous strands within the soft tissue and has been described as a cobblestone appearance (Fig. 14-39). When cellulitis is identified, a thorough investigation for a focal abscess should ensue. A hidden abscess is termed an **occult** abscess. Abscesses can have a wide range of sonographic features. They are focal fluid collections that are often complex and have a peripheral rim of hyperemia that can be detected with color Doppler.

🔊 SOUND OFF
When cellulitis is identified, the sonographer should look carefully for a complex focal fluid collection that may represent abscess development.

CLINICAL FINDINGS OF CELLULITIS

1. Red, tender, warm area of the skin
2. Possible elevated white blood cell count (especially with abscess development)

SONOGRAPHIC FINDINGS OF CELLULITIS

1. Hypoechoic, edematous strands within the soft tissue (cobblestone appearance)

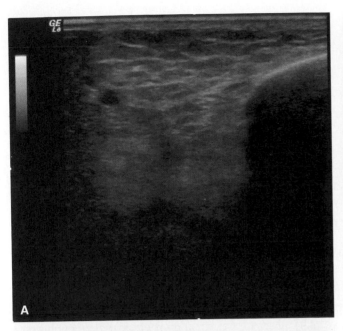

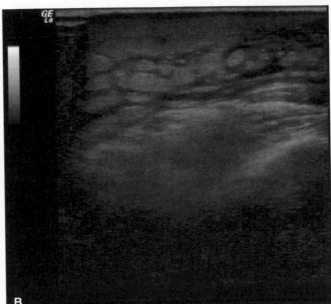

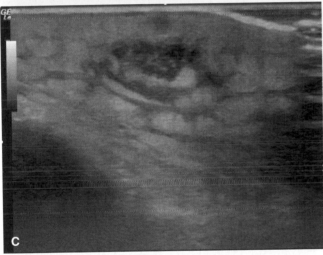

Figure 14-39 Cellulitis and superficial abscess. **A.** Sonogram of normal superficial soft tissue. **B.** Sonogram of cellulitis demonstrating the cobblestone appearance of the soft tissue when induration if present. **C.** Sonogram demonstrating a well-circumscribed fluid collection with surrounding cobblestoning seen in a patient with cellulitis with underlying abscess.

SONOGRAPHIC FINDINGS OF A SUPERFICIAL ABSCESS

1. Hypoechoic, edematous strands within the soft tissue (cobblestone appearance)
2. Focal fluid collection that is often complex, denoting the abscess
3. A peripheral rim of hyperemia may be detectable with color Doppler

Primary and Metastatic Melanomas

Malignant melanoma accounts for up to 11% of skin cancers. Primary melanoma classically appears hypoechoic, with increased vascular flow noted with color Doppler. Melanoma is also the most likely primary tumor to metastasize to the subcutaneous fat. It will most often appear sonographically as a solid, vascular hypoechoic mass as well.

SONOGRAPHIC FINDINGS OF METASTATIC MELANOMA

1. Solid, vascular hypoechoic mass

FOREIGN BODIES

Sonographic Assessment of Foreign Bodies

A high-frequency linear array transducer is utilized to image for foreign bodies. Foreign bodies just below the skin surface may require the aid of a standoff pad for improved visualization. Sonography can aid in the localization and removal of some objects, particularly wooden fragments, or other **radiolucent** objects, which may not be recognized with radiography. Most foreign bodies appear as hyperechoic structures with some

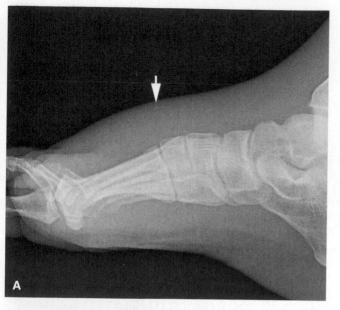
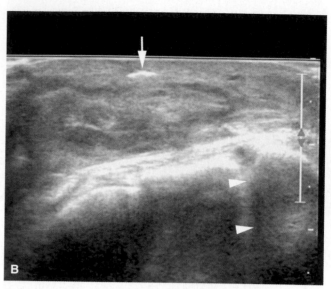

Figure 14-40 Foreign body. Foreign body in the dorsum of the foot. Concern for foreign body after the patient cut his foot with glass 1 month earlier. **A.** Lateral radiograph of the foot shows soft-tissue swelling over the dorsum of the foot and a small radio-opaque foreign body (*arrow*). **B.** Sonogram of this area clearly shows the glass fragment as an echogenic line in the subcutaneous tissues (*arrow*). The arrowheads indicate the location of the tarsometatarsal joint.

degree of posterior shadowing. Bullets, shrapnel, and other metallic objects may cause ring-down or comet-tail artifact as well. Inflammation around a foreign body will appear as a hypoechoic area adjacent to the structure. It is important to note that air at the site of a foreign body may produce bright echoes and, therefore, cause some ambiguity about the correct orientation of the object. To aid in the removal of the object, a distance can be obtained from the surface of the skin to the foreign object by using electronic calipers (Fig. 14-40).

REVIEW QUESTIONS

1. Which of the following is a common cause of cellulitis?
   a. *Staphylococcus*
   b. Cytomegalovirus
   c. Histoplasmosis
   d. Toxoplasmosis

2. What color Doppler finding is common with an abscess?
   a. Hypoemic flow surrounding the abscess
   b. Hyperemic flow surrounding the abscess
   c. Lack of blood flow within or around the abscess
   d. Reversed Doppler signals with spectral imaging

3. What is another name for a Baker cyst?
   a. Pilonidal cyst
   b. Articular cyst
   c. Ganglion cyst
   d. Popliteal cyst

4. Which of the following is a clinical finding that is common for a meniscal cyst?
   a. Ankle swelling
   b. Previous trauma
   c. Valvular slits
   d. Abscess formation

5. Which of the following would be better imaged with sonography rather than radiography?
   a. Radiolucent objects
   b. Radiopaque objects
   c. Hairline fractures
   d. Shrapnel

6. What is described as a congenital condition in which an individual suffers from severe joint contractors?
   a. Arthritis
   b. Subluxation
   c. Arthrogryposis
   d. Tendosynovitis

7. The masses in Figure 14-41 were discovered in lactating patients who were suffering from focal breast erythema, swelling, fever, and pain. What is the most likely diagnosis?
   a. Galactocele
   b. Ganglion cyst
   c. Intraductal carcinoma
   d. Breast abscess

8. What lab would most likely be elevated in the patients in Figure 14-41?
   a. Red blood cell count
   b. Platelets
   c. White blood cell count
   d. Hemoglobin

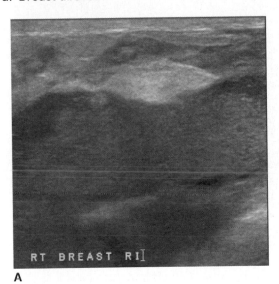

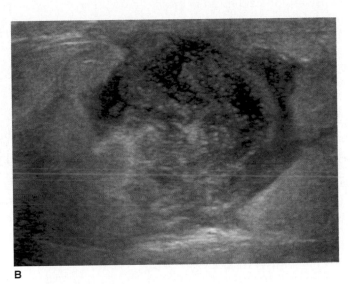

A

B

Figure 14-41

9. Which of the following would be most likely noted in a patient following the surgical removal of a malignant breast lesion?
   a. Hemangioma
   b. Hamartoma
   c. Fibroma
   d. Seroma

10. In Figure 14-42, Figure A is without stress, whereas Figure B is with stress. What disorder can be noted?
    a. Infantile traumatic dislocation
    b. Normal hip
    c. Developmental dislocation
    d. Subluxation

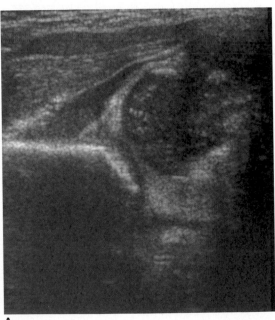

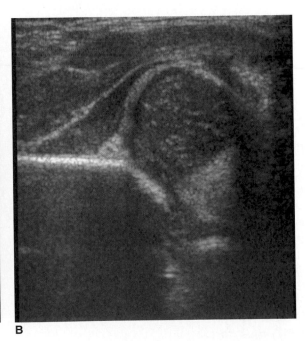

A

B

Figure 14-42

11. What is the painless abnormality noted in the wrist of the patient in Figure 14-43?
    a. Baker cyst
    b. Ganglion cyst
    c. Pilonidal cyst
    d. Lipoma

12. If the abnormality in Figure 14-43 was noted in the region of the radial artery, it would be referred to as:
    a. dorsal.
    b. anterior.
    c. posterior.
    d. volar.

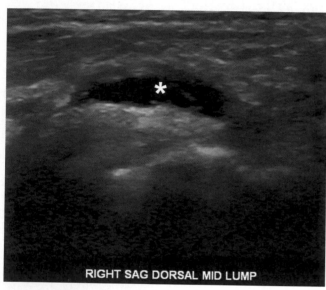

RIGHT SAG DORSAL MID LUMP

Figure 14-43

13. What is a thin fibrocartilaginous tissue that is located within the knee joint that may suffer from tearing?
    a. Tuberosity
    b. Synovial
    c. Meniscus
    d. Condyle

14. Which of the following circulating maternal hormones may be responsible for the development of DDH?
    a. Progesterone
    b. Human chorionic gonadotropin
    c. Estrogen
    d. Follicle-stimulating hormone

15. What is another name for the calf muscle?
    a. Gastrocnemius
    b. Peroneus
    c. Gluteus maximus
    d. Latissimus dorsi

16. A sonographer is asked to analyze a palpable, painful mass within the lateral shoulder muscle following an injection. What is the name of this muscle?
    a. Trapezius
    b. Pectoralis major
    c. Biceps brachii
    d. Deltoid

17. Why are radial and antiradial sonographic scanning useful for the analysis of the breast?
    a. Because they better demonstrate the pattern of the ducts
    b. Because they better demonstrate pathology
    c. Because they better determine what tissue layers are involved in the disease
    d. Because they limit the amount of tissue to thickness

18. What is the medical term for the wrist bones?
    a. Metacarpals
    b. Tarsals
    c. Metatarsals
    d. Carpals

19. Which of the following is not typically a cause of gynecomastia?
    a. Klinefelter syndrome
    b. Marijuana use
    c. Hepatoblastoma
    d. Renal adenocarcinoma

20. The arrow in Figure 14-44 indicates hemorrhage within a mass noted behind the knee. Which of the following would be the least helpful task that the sonographer should perform in this case?
    a. Apply color Doppler.
    b. Perform the Thompson test.
    c. Inquire if the patient has a history of rheumatoid arthritis.
    d. Analyze the cyst for evidence of channel leading to the joint.

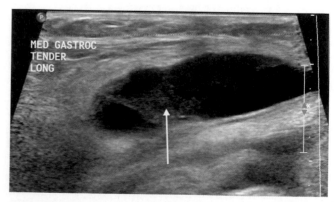

MED GASTROC TENDER LONG

Figure 14-44

21. Which of the following techniques is used to measure the relationship of the femoral head and acetabulum by evaluating the alpha and beta angles?
    a. Graf
    b. Ortolani
    c. Barlow
    d. Thompson

22. Inflammation and infection of the skin and subcutaneous tissue is termed:
    a. ascites.
    b. retroperitoneal fibrosis.
    c. cellulitis.
    d. subcutaneous edema.

23. Clinical findings of tendonitis include all of the following except:
    a. itching in the area of the tendon.
    b. pain.
    c. edema.
    d. the area is warm to touch.

24. Which of the following is a clinical test for developmental hip dysplasia that is used to evaluate the hip for the reduction or relocation of a dislocated hip?
    a. Graf
    b. Ortolani
    c. Barlow
    d. Thompson

25. What test can be performed to determine a torn Achilles tendon?
    a. McBurney test
    b. McDonald test
    c. Thompson test
    d. Baker test

26. A cystic mass located within the popliteal fossa is most likely a:
    a. Baker cyst.
    b. Thompson cyst.
    c. ganglion cyst.
    d. lipoma.

27. A patient presents with a palpable, oozing mass at the level of the natal cleft. What is the most likely etiology of this mass?
    a. Pannus cyst
    b. Epidermoid
    c. Hemangioma
    d. Pilonidal cyst

28. A common mass found along the dorsal aspect of the hand and wrist is the:
    a. Baker cyst.
    b. Thompson cyst.
    c. ganglion cyst.
    d. lipoma.

29. The Achilles tendon connects the:
    a. ankle to the knee.
    b. heel to the ankle.
    c. heel to the calf muscle.
    d. knee to the calf muscle.

30. In what position should the patient placed to better evaluate the Achilles tendon?
    a. Prone
    b. Supine
    c. Right lateral decubitus
    d. Left lateral decubitus

31. Inflammation of the breast that is related to pregnancy is referred to as:
    a. puerperal mastitis.
    b. retromammary mastitis.
    c. chronic mastitis.
    d. emphysematous mastitis.

32. Which of the following best describes the Thompson test?
    a. The patient lies prone and performs plantarflexion.
    b. The patient lies prone while the symptomatic calf is squeezed.
    c. The patient lies supine and performs plantarflexion.
    d. The patient lies prone and performs dorsiflexion.

33. Which of the following is true about patients with a lipoma?
    a. They often complain of pain in the area of the mass.
    b. They are often obese.
    c. They are only slightly tender in the area of the mass.
    d. They feel no pain in the area of the mass.

34. Subluxation denotes:
    a. synovial joint obstruction.
    b. partial hip dislocation.
    c. rupture of the bursa.
    d. inflammation of the acetabulum.

35. All of the following are keys to identifying foreign bodies with sonography except:
    a. most foreign bodies appear hypoechoic.
    b. a linear array transducer should be used.
    c. most foreign bodies are better visualized using a standoff pad.
    d. comet-tail artifact may be seen posterior to metallic objects.

36. A 6-year-old female patient presents to the sonography department for a hip sonogram with irritability, unwillingness to walk, and low-grade fever. Sonographically, you visualize a hypoechoic fluid collection that elevates the joint capsule. What is the most likely diagnosis?
    a. Developmental hip dysplasia
    b. Subluxation
    c. Joint effusion
    d. Hip dislocation

37. Which of the following would be best described as a benign tumor comprised of fat?
    a. Hemangioma
    b. Lipoma
    c. Hamartoma
    d. Oncocytoma

38. What is the most likely cause of a hip joint effusion in infants?
    a. Tendonitis
    b. Bursitis
    c. Developmental hip dysplasia
    d. Transient synovitis

39. Which of the following would be best described as a benign tumor composed of blood vessels?
    a. Hemangioma
    b. Lipoma
    c. Hamartoma
    d. Oncocytoma

40. Which of the following transducers would be best suited to sonographically assess for a splinter in a patient's hand?
    a. High-frequency linear array transducer
    b. Low-frequency curved array transducer
    c. High-frequency sector transducer
    d. Low-frequency linear array transducer

41. The accumulation of synovial fluid from a weakening in the joint capsule of the knee, as seen in conditions such as rheumatoid arthritis, can result in a:
    a. hemangioma.
    b. lipoma.
    c. Baker cyst.
    d. ganglion cyst.

42. Fluid within the synovial sheath is indicative of:
    a. hyperemic flow.
    b. tendosynovitis.
    c. cartilaginous inflammation.
    d. cartilaginous extension.

43. Which of the following best describes the most common sonographic appearance of gynecomastia?
    a. Hypoechoic, retroareolar mass
    b. Hyperechoic, exophytic mass
    c. Anechoic, retroareolar mass
    d. Hyperechoic, areolar mass

44. Acoustic shadowing caused by bending of a sound beam at the edge of a curved reflector is referred to as:
    a. mirror image artifact.
    b. indirect artifact.
    c. reflective shadowing.
    d. refractive shadowing.

45. Inflammation of the tendon and synovial tendon sheath is referred to as:
    a. tendosynovitis.
    b. tendonitis.
    c. cellulitis.
    d. pannus.

46. A patient presents to the sonography department with a history of cellulitis on his abdomen. The patient has fever, edema, and complains of focal tenderness in a specific region affected by the cellulitis. Sonographically, you identify a localized complex collection of fluid. What is the most likely diagnosis?
    a. Superficial hemangioma
    b. Subcutaneous carcinoma
    c. Mastitis
    d. Superficial abscess

47. A complicated Baker cyst may contain a thin flap of tissue referred to as:
    a. pannus.
    b. plica.
    c. septation.
    d. lipoma.

48. Which of the following is also referred to as a Bible bump?
    a. Ganglion cyst
    b. Superficial endodermal cyst
    c. Superficial epidermal cyst
    d. Epidermoid

49. Clinical findings of a Baker cyst may mimic those of a(n):
    a. arteriovenous malformation.
    b. deep venous thrombosis.
    c. knee fracture.
    d. ganglion cyst.

50. Sonographically, normal muscle appears as:
    a. hyperechoic tissue that contains linear, echogenic strands.
    b. complex tissue that contains linear, hypoechoic strands.
    c. hypoechoic tissue that contains linear, echogenic strands.
    d. echogenic tissue that contains linear, hypoechoic strands.

51. All of the following are true of ganglion cysts except:
    a. a ganglion cyst is a common mass found along the superior aspect of the hand and wrist, between the tarsals.
    b. ganglion cysts typically appear sonographically as an incompressible, anechoic mass with acoustic enhancement.
    c. clinically, ganglion cysts may be hard to touch and painful.
    d. ganglion cysts are often treated with an injection of corticosteroids.

52. A partial tear of a tendon typically appears as:
    a. a focal hypoechoic area within the tendon.
    b. a focal echogenic area within the tendon.
    c. a diffusely heterogeneous area within the tendon.
    d. edema and refractive shadowing in the area of the divided tendon.

53. Tendons sonographically appear as:
    a. echogenic, fibrous structures connecting muscles to bone.
    b. echogenic, fibrous structures connecting bone to bone.
    c. hypoechoic, linear arrangements within hyperechoic tissue.
    d. hyperechoic tissue that contains linear, echogenic strands.

54. A standoff pad is most useful in imaging:
    a. deep structures that produce acoustic enhancement.
    b. deep structures that produce acoustic shadowing.
    c. structures that produce refractive shadowing.
    d. superficial structures.

55. Hyperemic flow within or around a structure is often indicative of:
    a. malignancy.
    b. benignancy.
    c. inflammation.
    d. rupture.

56. All of the following will aid in the sonographic assessment of an Achilles tendon except:
    a. the patient lies prone, with their feet hanging off the end of the bed.
    b. both the symptomatic and asymptomatic Achilles tendons should be scanned for comparison.
    c. the entire tendon should be evaluated in sagittal and transverse scan planes.
    d. the patient is scanned standing, with a small amount of pressure placed on the symptomatic side.

57. Which of the following best describes the Thompson test?
    a. The calf is squeezed and the foot should plantarflex in a patient who does not have a complete tear of the Achilles tendon.
    b. The calf is squeezed and the foot should not plantarflex in a patient who does not have a complete tear of the Achilles tendon.
    c. The Achilles tendon is squeezed and the foot should plantarflex in a patient who does not have a complete tear of the Achilles tendon.
    d. The Achilles tendon is squeezed and the foot should not plantarflex in a patient who does not have a complete tear of the Achilles tendon.

58. Superficial lipomas may appear as all of the following except:
    a. hypoechoic to the surrounding tissue.
    b. isoechoic to the surrounding tissues.
    c. hyperechoic to the surrounding tissue.
    d. anechoic to the surrounding tissue.

59. Bullets, shrapnel, and other metallic objects may cause:
    a. acoustic enhancement.
    b. comet-tail artifact.
    c. edge enhancement.
    d. mirror image artifact.

60. Which of the following at the site of a foreign body may produce bright echoes and, therefore, cause some ambiguity about the correct orientation of the object?
    a. Fluid
    b. Enhancement
    c. Dust
    d. Air

SUGGESTED READINGS

American Institute of Ultrasound in Medicine. AIUM practice parameter for the performance of an ultrasound examination for detection and assessment of developmental dysplasia of the hip. http://www.aium.org/resources/guidelines/hip.pdf. Accessed October 3, 2021.

Artul S, Jabaly-Habib H, Artoul F, Habib G. The association between Baker's cyst and medial meniscal tear in patients with symptomatic knee using ultrasonography. *Clin Imaging*. 2015;39(4):659–661.

Beggs I. *Musculoskeletal Ultrasound*. Wolters Kluwer: 2014:178–220 & 292–301.

Conley S. Sonographic evaluation of a pilonidal cyst: a case study. *J Diagn Med Sonogr*. 2016;32(5):279–282.

Euerle B. American College of Emergency Physicians: soft tissue ultrasound. https://www.acep.org/sonoguide/basic/soft-tissue-ultrasound/. Accessed October 3, 2021.

Gibbs RS, Haney AF, Karlan BY, et al. *Danforth's Obstetrics and Gynecology*. 10th ed. Wolters Kluwer; 2008:943.

Hamilton C. Diagnosis and treatment of a lateral meniscal cyst with musculoskeletal ultrasound. *Case Rep Orthop*. 2015;2015:1–3.

Henningsen C, Kuntz K, Youngs D. *Clinical Guide to Sonography: Exercises for Critical Thinking*. 2nd ed. Elsevier; 2014:378–386.

Hertzberg BS, Middleton WD. *Ultrasound: The Requisites*. 3rd ed. Elsevier; 2016:263–276.

Huang CC, Ko SF, Huang HY, et al. Epidermal cysts in the superficial soft tissue. *J Ultrasound Med*. 2011;30:11–17.

Rumack CM, Wilson SR, Charboneau JW, et al. *Diagnostic Ultrasound*. 4th ed. Elsevier; 2011:773–839 & 1982–2005.

Sanders RC, Hall-Terracciano B. *Clinical Sonography: A Practical Guide*. 5th ed. Wolters Kluwer; 2016: 670–690 & 775–792.

Siegel MJ. *Pediatric Sonography*. 5th ed. Wolters Kluwer; 2019:601–652.

BONUS REVIEW!

Magnetic Resonance Imaging of an Achilles Tendon Tear (Fig. 14-45)

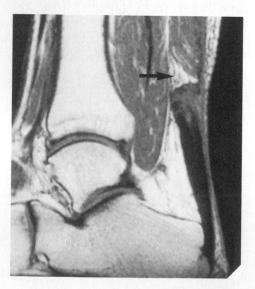

Figure 14-45 Magnetic resonance imaging (*MRI*) of an Achilles tendon tear. Sagittal T1-weighted MRI shows a complete rupture of the Achilles tendon near the musculotendinous junction (*arrow*).

BONUS REVIEW! (*continued*)

Mammogram and Sonogram of a Breast Abscess with Needle Aspiration (Fig. 14-46)

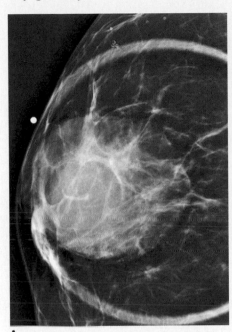

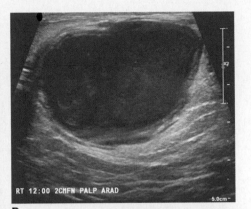

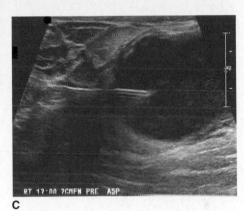

Figure 14-46 Abscess on mammogram (**A**), sonography (**B**), and sonographic drainage with needle noted in the abscess (**C**).

Gynecologic Sonography Overview

Introduction

A synopsis of gynecologic sonography practice is provided in this chapter. Accordingly, the subsequent chapters will build upon the foundation established in it. It is important for the sonographer to obtain and recognize vital clinical information from patients, including laboratory results and other data that are obtained through patient inquiry. This chapter offers relevant laboratory findings, imaging artifacts, a brief overview of physics and instrumentation, and infection control and serves as a gynecologic sonography imaging guide. Lastly, cross-referencing of potential information that may be encountered on the obstetrics and gynecology certification examination offered by the American Registry for Diagnostic Medical Sonography (ARDMS) (www.ardms.org) and the gynecology portion of the examination offered by the American Registry of Radiologic Technologists (www.arrt.org) has been performed to establish this chapter. In "Bonus Review" section, you will find examples of venous and arterial waveforms and several computed tomography (CT) images of the female pelvis.

Key Terms

adnexa—the area located posterior to the broad ligaments, adjacent to the uterus, which contains the ovaries and fallopian tubes

alpha-fetoprotein—a protein produced by the fetal yolk sac, fetal gastrointestinal tract, and the fetal liver; may also be produced by some malignant tumors

ambiguous genitalia—birth defect in which the external genitalia appear recognizably neither male nor female

amenorrhea—the absence of menstruation

ascites—a collection of abdominal fluid within the peritoneal cavity

CA-125—a tumor marker in the blood that can indicate certain types of cancers such as cancer of the ovary, endometrium, breast, gastrointestinal tract, and lungs; stands for cancer antigen 125

computed tomography—a diagnostic modality that utilizes ionizing radiation to produce images of the human body in cross-sectional and reconstructed 3D formats

dysmenorrhea—difficult or painful menstruation

dyspareunia—painful sexual intercourse

dysuria—painful or difficult urination

echotexture—the sonographic appearance of a structure

ectopic pregnancy—a pregnancy located outside the endometrial cavity of the uterus

endoscopy—a means of looking inside the human body by utilizing an endoscope

fluid–fluid level—the distinct layering of fluids within a cyst or cystic structure that is caused by the presence of at least two different fluid compositions

Foley catheter—a catheter placed into the urinary bladder via the urethra that is used to drain urine; it can also be clamped and used to temporarily distend the bladder for pelvic sonography

hematocrit—a laboratory value that indicates the amount of red blood cells in blood

hirsutism—excessive hair growth in women in areas where hair growth is normally negligible

human chorionic gonadotropin—a hormone produced by the trophoblastic cells of the early placenta; may also be used as a tumor marker in nongravid patients and males

hydronephrosis—the dilation of the renal collecting system resulting from the obstruction of the flow of urine from the kidney(s) to the bladder; also referred to as pelvocaliectasis, pelviectasis, or pyelectasis

hypomenorrhea—decreased or scant menstrual flow; regular timed menses but light flow

incontinence—inability to control urination

infertility—inability to conceive a child after 1 year of unprotected intercourse

intrauterine device—a common form of birth control in which a small device is placed within the endometrium to prevent pregnancy; also referred to as an intrauterine contraceptive device

lactate dehydrogenase—an enzyme found within the blood that may be used to monitor renal function; may also be used as a tumor marker for some ovarian tumors

leukocytosis—an elevated white blood cell count

magnetic resonance imaging—a diagnostic modality that utilizes electromagnetic radiation to produce images of the human body in cross-sectional and reconstructed 3D formats

Meigs syndrome—ascites and pleural effusion in the presence of some benign ovarian tumors

menometrorrhagia—excessive or prolonged bleeding between periods

menorrhagia—abnormally heavy and prolonged menstruation

metrorrhagia—irregular menstrual bleeding between periods; intermenstrual bleeding

multiloculated—having multiple chambers or compartments

mural nodules—growth or masses attached to the wall of a structure, most likely a cyst

neoplasm—a mass of tissue that contains abnormal cells; also called a tumor

nuclear medicine—a diagnostic imaging modality that utilizes the administration of radionuclides into the human body for an analysis of the function of organs, or for the treatment of various abnormalities

ovarian torsion—an abnormality that results from the ovary twisting on its mesenteric connection, consequently cutting off the blood supply to the ovary

pelvic inflammatory disease—an infection of the female genital tract that may involve the ovaries, uterus, and/or the fallopian tubes

pelvic kidney—kidney located within the pelvis

pleural effusion—the abnormal accumulation of fluid in the pleural space

polycystic ovary syndrome—a syndrome characterized by anovulatory cycles, infertility, hirsutism, amenorrhea, and obesity; may also be referred to as Stein–Leventhal syndrome

pseudomyxoma peritonei—an intraperitoneal extension of mucin-secreting cells that result from the rupture of a malignant mucinous ovarian tumor or, possibly, a malignant tumor of the appendix

radiography—a diagnostic imaging modality that uses ionizing radiation for imaging bones, organs, and some soft-tissue structures

septations—separations; structures that divide something into separate sections

simple cyst—an anechoic, round mass that has smooth walls and demonstrates through transmission (acoustic enhancement)

sliding sign—sonographic sign obtained during an endovaginal sonogram when gentle probe pressure is used to assess whether the anterior rectum and sigmoid colon glides freely across the posterior aspect of the uterus, cervix, and vaginal wall

sonohysterogram—a sonographic procedure that uses saline instillation into the endometrial cavity and fallopian tubes to evaluate for internal abnormalities; also referred to as saline infusion sonohysterography

tamoxifen—a breast cancer drug that inhibits the effects of estrogen in the breast

translabial sonogram—sonogram that requires the transducer be placed against the labia; often used for imaging of the cervix

Turner syndrome—a chromosomal aberration where one sex chromosome is absent; may also be referred to as monosomy X

unilocular—having one chamber or compartment

virilization—changes within the female that are caused by increased androgens; may lead to deepening of the voice and hirsutism

von Willebrand disease—an inherited bleeding disorder that is characterized by low levels of a specific clotting protein in the blood referred to as von Willebrand factor; results in excessive bleeding and specifically vaginal bleeding in women

SONOGRAPHIC TERMINOLOGY AND PRACTICE GUIDELINES

Before beginning your studies or performing a review, you must have a fundamental appreciation of sonographic terminology and commonly used sonographic descriptive terms (Table 15-1). Chapter 1 in this text also provides an overview of sonographic terminology that would be beneficial for review. Female pelvic sonograms may be requested for various reasons. The American Institute of Ultrasound in Medicine (AIUM) publishes the practice guidelines for a pelvic sonogram on their website at www.aium.org (Table 15-2). It also provides a valuable image resource that can be found at https://aium.s3.amazonaws.com/guidelines/femalePelvis/imageResources.pdf

SONOGRAPHIC DESCRIPTION OF ABNORMAL FINDINGS

The appreciation and recognition of sonographic pathology is vital for the sonographer. Not only should the sonographer be able to recognize the normal echogenicity of organs and structures, they must be capable of identifying abnormalities. Pathology is often described sonographically, relative to surrounding or adjacent tissue. For example, a uterine mass may be described as hypoechoic compared to the surrounding **echotexture** of the uterus (Fig. 15-1). Solid tumors may be hyperechoic (occasionally described as echogenic), hypoechoic, homogeneous, heterogeneous, complex, isoechoic, cystic, or a combination of terms. For example, an ovarian mass may be described as a complex mass that contains both cystic and solid components.

Lastly, a cyst must meet certain criteria to be referred to as a **simple cyst**. Simple cysts have *s*mooth walls or borders, demonstrate *t*hrough transmission (acoustic

TABLE 15-2 AIUM indications for female pelvic sonogram[a]

- Evaluation of pelvic pain
- Evaluation of pelvic masses
- Evaluation of endocrine abnormalities, including polycystic ovaries
- Evaluation of **dysmenorrhea** (painful menses)
- Evaluation of **amenorrhea**
- Evaluation of abnormal bleeding (e.g., **menorrhagia, metrorrhagia, menometrorrhagia**)
- Evaluation of delayed menses
- Follow-up of a previously detected abnormality
- Evaluation, monitoring, and/or treatment of infertility patients
- Evaluation in the presence of a limited clinical examination of the pelvis
- Evaluation for signs or symptoms of pelvic infection
- Further characterization of a pelvic abnormality noted on another imaging study
- Evaluation of congenital uterine and lower genital tract anomalies
- Evaluation of excessive bleeding, pain, or signs of infection after pelvic surgery, delivery, or abortion
- Localization of an intrauterine contraceptive device
- Screening for malignancy in high-risk patients
- Evaluation of **incontinence** or pelvic organ prolapse
- Guidance for interventional or surgical procedures
- Preoperative and postoperative evaluation of pelvic structures

AIUM, American Institute of Ultrasound in Medicine.
[a]This is an edited and limited list of indications. Other indications exist.

enhancement), are *a*nechoic, and are *r*ound in shape (*STAR* criteria). Occasionally, with higher frequency transducers with superior resolution, a diminutive amount of internal debris may be noted within a simple

TABLE 15-1 Sonographic descriptive terms

Sonographic Descriptive Term	Definition	Example
Anechoic	Without echoes	Simple ovarian cyst
Complex	Having both cystic and solid components	Pelvic abscess
Echogenic	Structure that produces echoes	Pelvic ligaments
Heterogeneous	Of differing composition	Irregular endometrium
Homogeneous	Of uniform composition	Normal uterus
Hyperechoic	Having many echoes	Endometrium in the secretory phase
Hypoechoic	Having few echoes	Leiomyoma
Isoechoic	Having the same echogenicity	Normal ovaries (in comparison to each other)

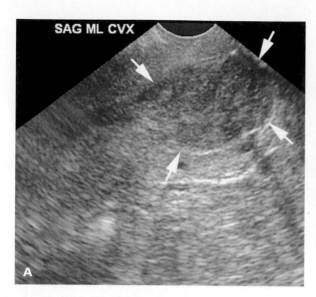

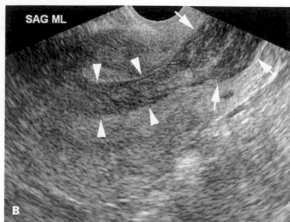

Figure 15-1 Hypoechoic mass within the uterus. **A.** Sagittal midline view of the cervix (*SAG ML CVX*) demonstrating a hypoechoic mass (*arrows*) within the cervix. **B.** Sagittal midline view of the uterus shows that the cervical mass (*arrows*) extends from the body of the uterus via a stalk (*arrowheads*).

cyst. However, cysts that have a large amount of internal debris, **septations**, **mural nodules**, **fluid–fluid level**, or other components may be described as complex cysts (see Fig. 1-4). Cysts may also be referred to as **multiloculated** or **unilocular**. Whereas simple cysts may not be worrisome, complex cysts may be followed with frequent sonograms, further analyzed with another imaging modality, or biopsied.

> 🔊 **SOUND OFF**
> A simple cyst should have *s*mooth walls, demonstrate *t*hrough transmission (acoustic enhancement), be completely *a*nechoic, and be *r*ound in shape (STAR criteria).

PATIENT PREPARATION FOR PELVIC SONOGRAPHY

Transabdominal imaging of the female pelvis requires the patient to have a full bladder. Patients are typically required to drink approximately 32 ounces of water before the examination. Whether the bladder is retrofilled via a **Foley catheter** or filled by drinking fluids, it must be distended adequately to visualize the entire uterus and **adnexa**. This practice will provide an acoustic window via the bladder and also displace bowel from the field of view. Sonography can be performed using both transabdominal and endovaginal, also referred to as transvaginal, techniques (Figs. 15-2 and 15-3). If possible, a pelvic sonogram should be performed before studies that require the administration of barium.

One of the chief advantages of transabdominal imaging of the pelvis is that this technique provides a global view of the entire pelvis. A disadvantage of transabdominal imaging is that it lacks the detail of endovaginal imaging because the transducer is much farther away from the organs that are being investigated. Obese patients and patients with a retroverted or retroflexed uterus present a unique challenge to the transabdominal technique as well.

Some facilities perform endovaginal imaging of the pelvis exclusively for certain indications, without the need for transabdominal imaging. Sonograms following a **computed tomography (CT)** or **magnetic resonance imaging** study may only need endovaginal imaging for sonographic correlation. Endovaginal imaging does not require a full bladder. Consequently, endovaginal imaging leads to reduced waiting time for the patient and quicker medical management. Another advantage of endovaginal imaging is that it offers improved resolution of the endometrium, uterus, and ovaries, especially in the obese patient. Dynamic imaging during an endovaginal sonogram can be performed as well. Gentle probe presssure during scanning can be assistive and the normal "**sliding**" **sign** may be noted. If negative, endometriosis may be suspected. The disadvantages of endovaginal imaging include the possibility of unintentionally omitting pathology that is not within the field of view. A thorough explanation of the endovaginal sonogram procedure should be provided to the patient before proceeding, and the patient must grant consent. Some institutions may require written consent for endovaginal sonograms. It is also recommended, and indeed required by some institutions, that sonographers utilize a chaperone while performing an endovaginal sonogram, **translabial sonogram**, or transperineal sonogram.

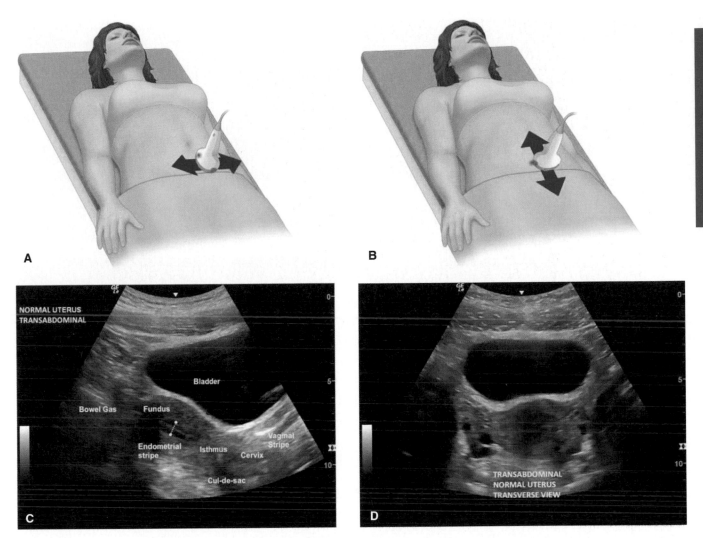

Figure 15-2 Transabdominal pelvic scanning. Note the locations of the index or notch in the drawings (*red dot*). **A.** Patient positioning with probe in the sagittal plane. Fan through the structures in the direction of the red arrows using the urinary bladder as an acoustic window (side-to-side). **B.** Patient positioning with probe in the transverse plane. Fan through the structures in the direction of the red arrows (superior to inferior). **C.** Transabdominal sagittal view of normal anteverted uterus. **D.** Transverse view of normal uterus (right ovary also visible).

> 🔊 **SOUND OFF**
> An advantage of endovaginal imaging is that it offers improved resolution of the endometrium, uterus, and ovaries, especially in the obese patient.

GATHERING A CLINICAL HISTORY AND LABORATORY FINDINGS

Sonographers should strive to offer high-quality, patient-centered health care, including, but not limited to, offering them a safe environment, effective and accurate examinations, and timely, equitable care. Consequently, protocols for patient engagement must be established by the organization to ensure that each patient is served impartially. As a consequence of these practices, patient confidence in the sonographer will be gained, thus leading to a more trustworthy environment where open communication can flourish.

A review of prior examinations should be performed by the sonographer before any interaction with the patient. This review includes an analysis of previous sonograms, CT scans, magnetic resonance imaging studies, **nuclear medicine** studies, **radiography** procedures, **endoscopy** examinations, and any additional related diagnostic reports available. Moreover, sonographers must be capable of analyzing the clinical history and complaints of their patients and also explore family history. Another important component of pelvic imaging is the act of inquiring about the patient's reproductive history. The sonographer should investigate the number of pregnancies—gravida—and inquire about how many of those pregnancies were carried to term—para. Further information about this procedure is provided in "Obstetric Sonography Overview" section

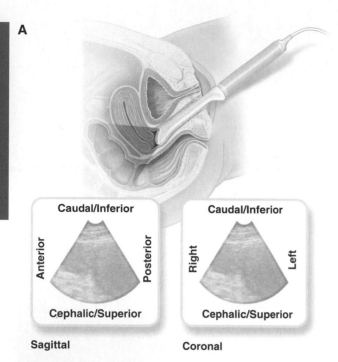

A

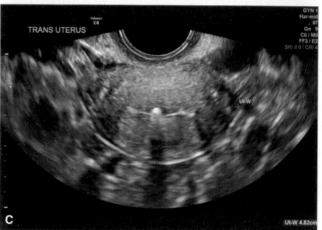

B

C

Figure 15-3 A. Orientation for endovaginal scan planes. Endovaginal imaging includes sagittal and coronal scan planes. Coronal may also be labeled transverse. **B.** Longitudinal (Long) transvaginal representation of a normal anteverted uterus. **C.** Transverse uterus. This patient also has an intrauterine device within the endometrium.

of Chapter 22. It is important to keep in mind that the optimal way to communicate with a patient who does not speak the same language as the sonographer is to obtain the assistance of a trained medical interpreter.

> **SOUND OFF**
> The number of pregnancies is gravida, whereas para is the number of those pregnancies that the patient carried to term.

Analyzing clinical history is vital. This practice will not only aid in clinical practice but also assist in answering complex certification examination questions. By correlating clinical findings with sonographic findings, the sonographer can directly impact the patient's outcome by providing the most targeted examination possible. Furthermore, when faced with a complicated, in-depth registry question, the registrant will be able to eliminate information that is not relevant to answer the question appropriately. Table 15-3 provides a review of common clinical indications for a pelvic sonogram and a list of differential gynecologic disorders.

LABORATORY FINDINGS RELEVANT TO GYNECOLOGIC SONOGRAPHY

Among the list of laboratory values that may warrant a pelvic sonogram are human chorionic gonadotropin, **hematocrit**, and white blood cell count. Although some rare ovarian tumors may cause an elevation in human chorionic gonadotropin, it is typically produced by a developing gestation and, therefore, most often indicates the existence of a pregnancy. It is important to note that simply having a positive human chorionic gonadotropin does not necessarily mean that the pregnancy is normal.

Hematocrit is a laboratory value that should be evaluated in cases of suspected **ectopic pregnancy**. Patients suffering from hemorrhage as a result of an ectopic pregnancy or pelvic trauma will have an abnormally low hematocrit level. Thus, a decrease in hematocrit indicates bleeding. Patients with **pelvic inflammatory disease** will often have an elevated white blood cell count, also referred to as **leukocytosis**. Patients who have some form of "itis" (such as salpingitis), or possibly even an abscess, will most likely

TABLE 15-3 Clinical indications and potential differential gynecologic disorders[a]

Clinical Findings	Potential Differential Gynecologic Diagnosis (Nongravid Patient)[b]
Abdominal distension	Ascites Leiomyoma (fibroid uterus) Ovarian hyperstimulation syndrome Ovarian malignancy
Acute pelvic pain	Ovarian mucinous cystadenocarcinoma Ovarian mucinous cystadenoma Ovarian serous cystadenocarcinoma Ovarian serous cystadenoma Ovarian torsion Pelvic inflammatory disease Ruptured ovarian hemorrhagic cyst Perforated intrauterine contraceptive device
Amenorrhea	Asherman syndrome **Polycystic ovary syndrome**
Chronic pelvic pain	Adenomyosis Endometriosis (endometrioma) Leiomyoma (fibroid uterus) Pelvic inflammatory disease
Constipation or painful bowel movements	Endometriosis (endometrioma) Leiomyoma (fibroid uterus) Leiomyosarcoma Ovarian mucinous cystadenocarcinoma Ovarian mucinous cystadenoma Ovarian serous cystadenocarcinoma Ovarian serous cystadenoma
Dysmenorrhea	Adenomyosis Endometriosis
Dyspareunia	Adenomyosis Endometriosis Pelvic inflammatory disease Vaginal disorders or masses
Dysuria	Leiomyoma (fibroid uterus) Leiomyosarcoma
Elevated **CA-125**	Endometriosis Leiomyoma (possibly) Ovarian carcinoma Pelvic inflammatory disease
Elevated serum **alpha-fetoprotein**	Ovarian yolk sac tumor
Elevated serum **human chorionic gonadotropin** (nongravid)	Ovarian dysgerminoma (possibly)
Elevated serum **lactate dehydrogenase**	Ovarian dysgerminoma
Elevated white blood cell count **(leukocytosis)**	Endometritis Pelvic inflammatory disease
Enlarged uterus	Adenomyosis Endometrial carcinoma Leiomyoma (fibroid uterus) Leiomyosarcoma
Fever	Endometritis Pelvic inflammatory disease
Hirsutism	Polycystic ovary syndrome Sertoli–Leydig cell tumor (androblastoma)

(continued)

TABLE 15-3 Clinical indications and potential differential gynecologic disorders[a] (*continued*)

Clinical Findings	Potential Differential Gynecologic Diagnosis (Nongravid Patient)[b]
Hypomenorrhea	Asherman syndrome
Infertility	Asherman syndrome (repeated pregnancy loss) Endometrial carcinoma Endometrial polyp Endometriosis (endometrioma) Leiomyoma (repeated pregnancy loss) Pelvic inflammatory disease (chronic) Polycystic ovary syndrome
Intermenstrual bleeding	Endometrial polyp
Lost intrauterine contraceptive device	Expelled intrauterine device Perforated myometrium/uterus
Meigs syndrome	Brenner tumor Fibroma (most often) and thecoma
Menometrorrhagia	Adenomyosis Endometrial polyp Pelvic inflammatory disease Perforated intrauterine device
Menorrhagia	Endometrial hyperplasia Endometriosis (endometrioma) Leiomyoma (fibroid uterus) Leiomyosarcoma **von Willebrand disease**
Nausea and vomiting	Ovarian hyperstimulation syndrome Ovarian torsion
Oliguria	Ovarian hyperstimulation syndrome
Ovarian enlargement	Ovarian hyperstimulation syndrome (cystic enlargement) Ovarian torsion
Palpable abdominal mass	Leiomyoma (fibroid uterus) Leiomyosarcoma
Palpable adnexal mass	Leiomyoma (pedunculated) Ovarian mass Pelvic inflammatory disease
Pelvic pressure and/or tenderness	Adenomyosis Endometritis Leiomyoma (fibroid uterus) Leiomyosarcoma Ovarian mucinous cystadenocarcinoma Ovarian mucinous cystadenoma Ovarian serous cystadenocarcinoma Ovarian serous cystadenoma Pediatric—hydrocolpos or hematocolpos Pelvic inflammatory disease
Post dilatation and post curettage	Asherman syndrome Endometritis Retained products of conception
Postmenopausal vaginal bleeding	Endometrial atrophy Endometrial hyperplasia Ovarian granulosa cell tumor Ovarian mucinous cystadenocarcinoma Ovarian mucinous cystadenoma Ovarian serous cystadenocarcinoma Ovarian serous cystadenoma Ovarian thecoma

TABLE 15-3 Clinical indications and potential differential gynecologic disorders[a] (*continued*)

Clinical Findings	Potential Differential Gynecologic Diagnosis (Nongravid Patient)[b]
Precocious puberty	Ovarian dysgerminoma Ovarian granulosa cell tumor
Right upper quadrant pain	Fitz-Hugh–Curtis syndrome
Tamoxifen therapy	Endometrial hyperplasia
Urinary frequency	Leiomyoma (fibroid uterus) Leiomyosarcoma
Vaginal discharge	Pelvic inflammatory disease
Virilization	Sertoli–Leydig cell tumor (androblastoma) Ovarian carcinoma

CA-125, cancer antigen 125.
[a] These abnormalities will be discussed in the following chapters.
[b] These listed differentials are for nongravid individuals and gynecologic-related pathology. Other possible abnormalities may be present, but for review purposes, these disorders should be initially considered.

have an abnormal white blood cell count with existing infection as well. Other labs and specific associated pathologies will be included in the following chapters.

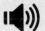 **SOUND OFF**
A decrease in hematocrit indicates bleeding.

BASIC PATIENT CARE DURING PELVIC IMAGING

Sonographers must be capable of providing basic patient care for every patient equitably and in a timely manner. Although we may spend a limited amount of time with each patient, we must also be prepared for emergency situations and how to respond. Basic patient care includes the assessment of body temperature, pulse, respiration, and blood pressure if needed (Table 15-4). Sonographers should be competent at transferring patients safely from wheelchairs and stretchers to the examination stretcher, being mindful of intravenous therapy, postsurgical, and urinary catheter needs. For

TABLE 15-4 Normal numbers or ranges for basic patient care assessment

Basic Patient Assessment	
Body temperature	98.6°F (oral)
Adult pulse	60–100 beats per minute
Adult blood pressure	<120/80
Adult respiration	12–20 breaths per minute

patients with intravenous therapy, the intravenous fluid bag should be continually elevated to prevent retrograde flow. For urinary catheter care, the urinary bag should be placed below the level of the urinary bladder to prevent retrograde urine flow that could result in a urinary tract infection. One of the most common causes of **nosocomial infections**, or hospital-acquired infections, is a urinary tract infection.

INFECTION CONTROL AND TRANSDUCER CARE

The cycle of infection may be depicted as a succession of steps (Fig. 15-4). Sonographers should continually employ the use of standard precautions and good hygiene to prevent the spread of infection. Standard precautions have been established to reduce the risk of microorganism transmission in the clinical setting. Standard precautions, formerly referred to as universal precautions, include (1) hand hygiene, (2) the use of personal protective equipment, (3) safe injection practices, (4) safe handling of potentially contaminated equipment and surfaces, and (5) respiratory hygiene and coughing etiquette. These precautions apply to blood, nonintact skin, mucous membranes, contaminated equipment, and all other body fluids, except for sweat.

The use of proper handwashing and hand cleaning techniques is one of the most effective means of preventing the spread of infection. The Centers for Disease Control and Prevention now recommends that health care workers employ the use of an alcohol-based hand rub as the primary mode of hand hygiene in the clinical setting. Traditional handwashing should be used as well when time permits, especially in situations when

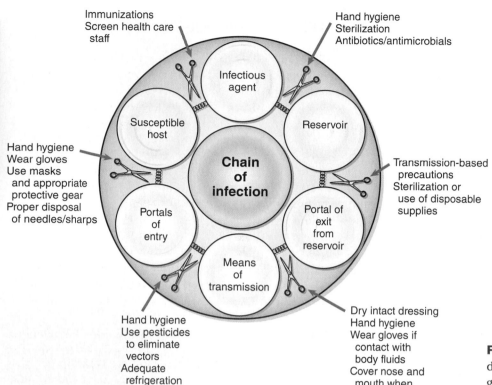

Immunizations
Screen health care
staff

Hand hygiene
Sterilization
Antibiotics/antimicrobials

Hand hygiene
Wear gloves
Use masks
and appropriate
protective gear
Proper disposal
of needles/sharps

Transmission-based
precautions
Sterilization or
use of disposable
supplies

Hand hygiene
Use pesticides
to eliminate
vectors
Adequate
refrigeration

Dry intact dressing
Hand hygiene
Wear gloves if
contact with
body fluids
Cover nose and
mouth when
sneezing

Figure 15-4 An infection cycle demonstrated as a chain. The goal is to break the links of the chain to end the cycle.

the hands are visibly soiled. Sonographers should also utilize personal protective equipment, such as gloves, gowns, face shields, and masks, when clinically applicable. Gloves, which are made of latex, nonlatex, or other synthetic material, should be worn during the sonographic examination and should be changed between patients. And although latex materials are rarely employed, be mindful of the potential for patient latex allergies, and adapt accordingly by using appropriate replacements.

Medical asepsis refers to the practices used to render an object or area free of pathogenic microorganisms. Although medical asepsis includes handwashing, it also includes the use of disinfectants in the clinical setting. The AIUM has an official statement on transducer care available online. Following each examination, the transducer, ultrasound machine, stretcher, and any other equipment used during the examination should be thoroughly disinfected. The transabdominal transducer should be cleaned with a disinfectant spray or wipe as recommended by the institution and manufacturer. Because endovaginal imaging requires the transducer to be placed into the vagina, a single-use cover should be placed on the transducer, and it should be inserted into the vagina using sterile gel as a lubricant (Fig. 15-5). Following the examination, the endovaginal transducer may be soaked in a high-level disinfectant—occasionally a glutaraldehyde-based solution—and the specified manufacturer's instructions should be followed. Some institutions may utilize a tabletop unit

that employs a hydrogen peroxide–based disinfection process. Regardless of the procedure, the transducer must undergo high-level disinfection.

◀)) SOUND OFF
Some institutions may utilize a tabletop unit that employs a hydrogen peroxide–based disinfection process for their endocavity transducers.

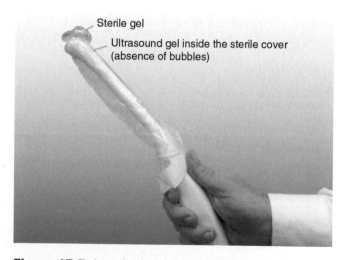

Sterile gel

Ultrasound gel inside the sterile cover
(absence of bubbles)

Figure 15-5 A probe cover is placed on the endovaginal transducer before inserting the transducer into the vagina. Ultrasound gel should be placed in the probe cover over the face of the transducer to reduce artifacts from air.

INVASIVE AND STERILE PROCEDURES

Patient preparation for invasive procedures varies among clinical facilities. However, informed consent from the patient and laboratory results are universally obtained. Laboratory findings, including an analysis of prothrombin time, partial thromboplastin time, international normalized ratio, fibrinogen, and platelets, are used to evaluate the patient for coagulopathies. Sterile field preparation is performed before the sterile procedure as well, and sterile asepsis, also referred to as surgical asepsis, must be maintained (Table 15-5). Of course, sterile asepsis is always practiced in the surgical suite. Some invasive procedures that are commonly performed in the sonography department include the **sonohysterogram**, which may also be referred to as saline infusion sonohysterography, organ biopsies, mass biopsies, and abscess drainages. Biopsies can be performed using a freehand technique or under sonographic guidance using a needle guide that attaches to the transducer. Transducers used during invasive procedures should be covered with a sterile probe cover, and sterile ultrasound gel should be utilized. Again, if a latex product is going to be utilized during the examination, the sonographer should inquire about latex allergies before the examination.

SOUND OFF
Transducers used during invasive procedures should be covered with a sterile probe cover, and sterile ultrasound gel should be utilized.

TABLE 15-5 Ten vital rules of surgical asepsis to remember

1. Always know which area and items are sterile and which are not.
2. If the sterility of an object is questionable, it is considered nonsterile.
3. If you recognize that an item has become nonsterile, act immediately.
4. A sterile field must never be left unmonitored. If a sterile field is left unattended, it is considered nonsterile.
5. A sterile person does not lean across a sterile field.
6. A sterile field ends at the level of the tabletop.
7. Cuffs of a sterile gown are not considered sterile.
8. The edges of a sterile wrapper are not considered sterile.
9. If one sterile person must pass another, they must pass back to back.
10. Coughing, sneezing, or excessive talking over a sterile field leads to contamination.

INSTRUMENTATION

Although a thorough physics review is beyond the scope of this book, there are several topics that must be addressed in preparation for the pelvic sonogram. Sonographic images are typically recorded and stored in a picture-archiving and communication system (PACS). PACS allows for both easy storage and comparison between sonographic findings and straightforward correlation between other imaging modality findings.

Pelvic imaging requires the use of a transducer that balances penetration with high-quality resolution. In general, the higher the frequency employed, the poorer the penetration abilities, but the better the resolution. Conversely, the lower frequencies provide better penetration with a sacrifice in resolution. Transducers that may be used for pelvic sonography include linear array, matrix array, curved or convex array, phased array, or the vector or sector array. Transabdominal transducers employ frequencies lower than 6 MHz, unless if the patient is thin. Endovaginal transducers also have varying frequencies but are typically 7.5 MHz or higher. Higher frequency linear array transducers (7.5 to 18 MHz or higher when appropriate) may be used for superficial structures, such as the ovaries if needed. A **standoff pad** or a mound of gel may be used for imaging some superficial structures, such as protruding masses just below the skin surface. When applicable, sonographers should utilize technology including power Doppler, color Doppler, spectral Doppler, harmonics imaging, compound imaging, extended field of view, elastography, and three-dimensional (3D) sonography to promote diagnostic accuracy.

SOUND OFF
↑Frequency = ↑Resolution = ↓Penetration
↓Frequency = ↓Resolution = ↑Penetration

THREE-DIMENSIONAL GYNECOLOGIC SONOGRAPHY

When used separately or as an addition to routine 2D sonography, 3D sonography provides enhanced imaging of the female pelvis. 3D sonography offers the ability to accurately obtain volumetric measurements of structures. 3D may also be combined with color and power Doppler sonography for improved blood flow assessment within pelvic organs. It is often used to assess or confirm the presence of a uterine malformation, to provide an accurate representation of the location of an **intrauterine device**, or to investigate the uterine cavity during sonohysterography (Fig. 15-6).

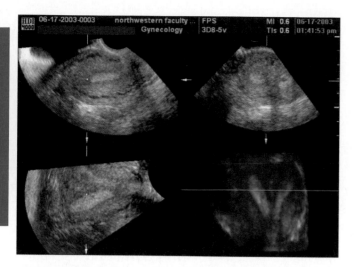

Figure 15-6 A 3D study revealing a complete septation of the uterus and cervix. The acquisition was performed endovaginally in the sagittal plane.

It may also be used during pregnancy to confirm a precise location of ectopic pregnancies that may be located within the cornu of the uterus (Fig. 15-7). For ovarian imaging, 3D sonography is useful for evaluating complex ovarian masses and may be employed during ovarian follicular assessment as part of fertility treatment. The physics associated with 3D is beyond the scope of this text, although the sonographer should be familiar with the manner in which 3D images are acquired by the ultrasound machine at their institution.

> **◄))) SOUND OFF**
> 3D sonography may be used to assess or confirm the presence of a uterine malformation or to provide an accurate representation of the location of an intrauterine device.

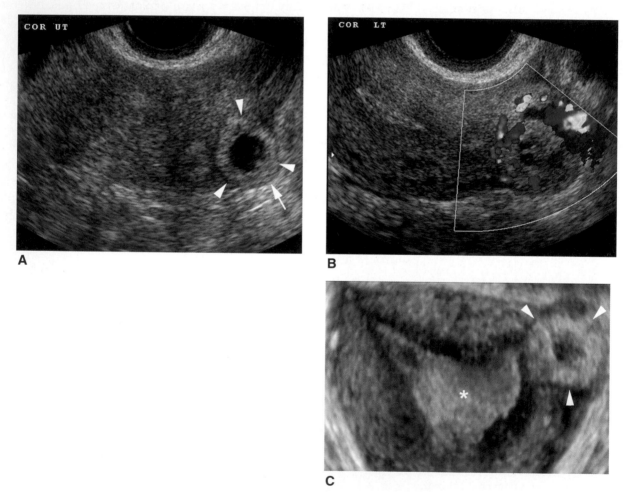

Figure 15-7 Cornual ectopic pregnancy with confirmatory 3D view. **A.** A gestational sac (*arrowheads*) is suspected in the left superolateral aspect of the uterus, a region corresponding to the left cornu. The sac bulges the external contour of the uterus, and there is little or no hypoechoic myometrium around the bulging portion of the sac (*arrow*). **B.** Color Doppler reveals a large amount of blood flow around the left cornual gestational sac. **C.** Coronal reformatting from 3D sonogram of the uterus clearly shows that the gestational sac (*arrowheads*) is located in the left cornu, separate from the endometrium in the body of the uterus (*asterisk*).

ARTIFACTS IN PELVIC IMAGING

There are a few artifacts that may be seen during a routine pelvic sonogram. It is important to know that artifacts exist and why they occur. Often, artifacts will be observed during real-time 2D and during Doppler imaging as well. A description of these artifacts can be found in Tables 15-6 and 15-7, and several representative figures can be found in Chapter 1 of this text.

PEDIATRIC GYNECOLOGIC SONOGRAPHY

Sonography is especially utilized in pediatric gynecologic imaging secondary to its ease of use, low cost, and lack of ionizing radiation. Other advantages of sonography over other imaging modalities for the pediatric patient include the ability of real-time imaging, lack of the need for sedation,

TABLE 15-6 Possible artifacts that may be noted during 2D pelvic sonography[a]

2D Artifact	Description	Example
Reverberation	Caused by a large acoustic interface and subsequent production of false echoes.	Echogenic region in the anterior aspect of the urinary bladder.
Mirror image	Produced by a strong specular reflector and results in a copy of the anatomy being placed deeper than the correct location.	May occur during endovaginal imaging and produce a (artificial) duplicate uterus (Fig. 15-8). Can also be seen in Doppler modes.
Shadowing	Caused by attenuation of the sound beam.	Seen posterior to pelvic bones or a tooth within a cystic teratoma.
Ring-down artifact	Artifact that appears as a solid streak or a chain of parallel bands radiating away from a structure.	Gas or air within the endometrium secondary to endometritis.
Dirty shadowing	Caused by air or bowel gas.	Most often seen emanating from bowel; may be seen posterior to gas within an abscess.
(Posterior) Acoustic enhancement	Produced when the sound beam is barely attenuated through a fluid or a fluid-filled structure. May occasionally be referred to as through transmission.	Posterior to the urinary bladder or simple ovarian cyst.

[a] Figures for these and other artifacts can be found in Chapter 1.

TABLE 15-7 Doppler artifacts[a]

Doppler Artifact	Explanation	Adjustment
Absent Doppler signal	Could be caused by low gain, low-frequency, high wall filter, or too high velocity scale.	• Decrease pulse-repetition frequency. • Turn up spectral gain. • Decrease the wall filter. • Open the sample gate.
Aliasing	Occurs when the Doppler sampling rate (pulse-repetition frequency) is not high enough to accurately display the Doppler frequency shift.	• Increase the pulse-repetition frequency. • Adjust the baseline. • Switch to a lower frequency. • Increase the angle of insonation to decrease Doppler shift.
Doppler noise	Caused by inappropriately high Doppler settings.	Reduce color gain setting.
Flow directional abnormalities	Caused by the sound beam striking a vessel at a 90-degree angle, producing an area void of color.	Change the angle of insonation.
Twinkle artifact	Occurs behind strong, granular, and irregular surfaces like crystals, calculi, or calcifications.	Artifact that is actually useful at identifying small kidney or biliary stones.

[a] Figures for some of these artifacts can be found in Chapter 1.

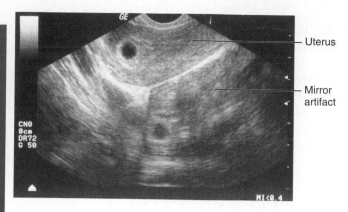

Figure 15-8 Mirror image noted during an endovaginal sonogram.

excellent resolution, and portability. Patient preparation for pediatric patients is similar for adults, although a smaller amount of water is warranted to distend the urinary bladder. Endovaginal imaging is contraindicated for virginal patients. Adolescent females may suffer from polycystic ovary syndrome, **ovarian torsion**, pelvic inflammatory disease, ectopic pregnancy, and, although rare, a malignant ovarian **neoplasm**. Although ovarian torsion has been known to occur in utero and in adulthood, it is much more common in adolescence. Adnexal or ovarian torsion can be associated with a large ovarian mass or cyst, or result from the excessive mobility of the adnexal structures. These topics are further discussed in subsequent chapters of this book (see Chapters 15–21).

Ambiguous genitalia, a condition in which the newborn's external genitalia are recognizably neither male nor female, is an indication for pelvic sonography for the newborn infant. The role of sonography for patients with ambiguous genitalia is to locate the gonads, to determine the presence or absence of the uterus, and to possibly assess the adrenal glands for masses or swelling. The most common disorder of sex development is **Turner syndrome**, also referred to as monosomy X. These patients suffer from gonadal dysfunction and have physical characteristics such as short stature and webbing of the skin on the neck. And although there is a separate certification offered by the ARDMS for *Pediatric Sonography*, various gynecologic pathologies of the pediatric patient will be discussed in the following chapters.

((•)) SOUND OFF
Adnexal or ovarian torsion can be associated with a large ovarian mass or cyst, or result from the excessive mobility of the adnexal structures.

EXTRAPELVIC PATHOLOGY ASSOCIATED WITH GYNECOLOGY

Ovarian and uterine masses may become large enough to obstruct the flow of urine from the kidney(s) to the bladder, resulting in **hydronephrosis**. Often, patients with pelvic disorders will have indistinct clinical findings suggestive of a bowel or renal disorder. For instance, a uterine leiomyoma—a benign tumor of the uterus that can grow fairly large—may cause clinical symptoms such as constipation, hydronephrosis, and lower back pain. Multiple leiomyomata could indeed do the same. A **pelvic kidney**, which is a kidney located within the pelvis, may also be discovered during a pelvic sonogram and can mimic pathology (Fig. 15-9).

A small amount of free fluid within the female pelvis is a common sonographic finding and is most often associated with a normal ovarian cycle. **Ascites** can collect in the pelvis in several peritoneal cavity spaces (Table 15-8; Fig. 15-10). Massive amounts of pelvic ascites may be associated with some ovarian tumors, ectopic pregnancy, cirrhosis, and portal hypertension. **Meigs syndrome** (pelvic ascites, **pleural effusion**, and a benign ovarian mass) may also be suspected if there is an extensive amount of free fluid in the pelvis. Malignant ovarian tumors may leak mucinous material, a condition known as **pseudomyxoma peritonei**, as in the case of a ruptured ovarian mucinous cystadenocarcinoma. Pelvic inflammatory disease, ovarian hyperstimulation syndrome, and Fitz-Hugh–Curtis syndrome are all associated with free fluid within the pelvis as well. The sonographic characterization of ascites is important. That is to say, the sonographer must not only note the presence of the pelvic ascites but also be able to assess the amount and describe whether there are septations, debris, or membranous components because these findings are more worrisome for blood, infection, or, possibly, malignancy.

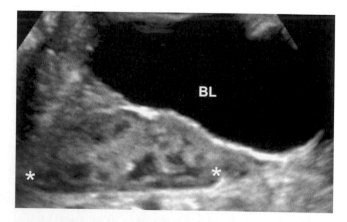

Figure 15-9 Pelvic kidney. Transverse sonogram shows an ectopic kidney (*asterisk*) posterior to the bladder (*BL*). Scans of the upper abdomen had not shown a right kidney.

Gynecologic Sonography Overview

TABLE 15-8 Location and significance of the peritoneal cavity spaces in the pelvis

Peritoneal Cavity Spaces	Location and Significant Points
Retropubic space	• Between the pubic bone and urinary bladder • Also referred to as the space of Retzius
Paracolic gutters	• Extend alongside the ascending and descending colon on both sides of the abdomen
Posterior cul-de-sac	• Male: between the urinary bladder and rectum; also referred to as the rectovesical pouch • Female: between the uterus and rectum; also referred to as pouch of Douglas and rectouterine pouch
Anterior cul-de-sac	• Between the urinary bladder and uterus • Also called the vesicouterine pouch in females

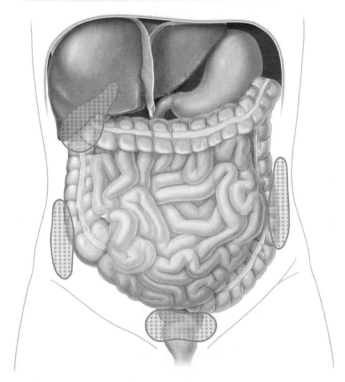

Figure 15-10 Diagrammatic view of the peritoneal cavity. Dotted areas represent the most common sites of ascites fluid collection.

🔊 SOUND OFF
A small amount of free fluid within the female pelvis is a common sonographic finding and is most often associated with a normal ovarian cycle.

ANALYZING A GYNECOLOGIC SONOGRAPHY REGISTRY QUESTION

Registry examinations can be intimidating. The following are a few steps that you can take to give you a better chance at answering these complex questions. Read the following question:

A 32-year-old multiparous patient presents to the sonography department with a history of abnormal uterine bleeding and dyspareunia. Sonographic findings include a diffusely enlarged uterus with notable thickening of the posterior myometrium. What is the most likely diagnosis?

A. Endometriosis
B. Adenomyosis
C. Posterior uterine leiomyoma
D. Endometrial carcinoma

Step 1: Read the question and try to answer it without looking at the answers provided.
The first step is to see if you know the answer without looking at the answers provided. If you have an idea, and your answer is one of the choices, then you are well on your way to answering the question correctly.

Step 2: If you do not know the answer right away, then break the question down.
Let us assume that you have no idea what the answer is. Then you move on to step 2, which is breaking the question down. This step is complicated, but it will help.

The first part of the question provides the age of the patient, which is 32 years. Look at the answers provided. Is there one that you can eliminate solely on the patient's age? There is one: 32-year-old women rarely get endometrial carcinoma. Mark it off the list! You now have a 33% chance of answering the question correctly. We now move on to the next part of the patient's history, which is the word "multiparous"; this means that the patient has had several children. Look at the answers and see if there are any that you can eliminate that are linked with infertility. There is one definite choice and one possible choice. Endometriosis is definitely linked with infertility, and leiomyoma could possibly be linked with repeated abortion, but remember this patient has several children. Mark off the one that you know for certain is linked with infertility, endometriosis. Now, you have a 50% chance of getting the question correct. We now move on to the two patient complaints (and this is where the following chapters will help). *You must know your clinical and sonographic findings to correctly answer these questions.* In our sample question, the patient is complaining of abnormal uterine bleeding, which is common with both of our remaining answers. So, we move on. Dyspareunia is the next complaint. This is where you must know your medical terminology. Dyspareunia is defined as painful intercourse, a common complaint with adenomyosis. So, there is your answer! Not convinced? Look at the sonographic findings. Does it fit? The question lists the sonographic findings as "thickening of the posterior myometrium," which is a distinctive sonographic finding consistent with the sonographic diagnosis of adenomyosis.

REVIEW QUESTIONS

1. Which of the following is an inherited bleeding disorder that is characterized by low levels of a specific clotting protein in the blood?
   a. Stein–Leventhal disease
   b. Fitz-Hugh–Curtis disease
   c. Meigs disease
   d. von Willebrand disease

2. The structure measure between the #2 calipers in Figure 15-11 is what echogenicity?
   a. Hypoechoic
   b. Hyperechoic
   c. Anechoic
   d. Isoechoic

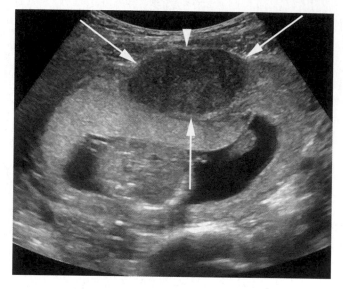

Figure 15-12

4. What is the term for elevated white blood cell count?
   a. Hematocrit
   b. Leukemia
   c. Leukocytosis
   d. Leukopenia

5. What artifact is demonstrated by the large arrow in Figure 15-13?
   a. Aliasing
   b. Reverberation
   c. Dirty shadowing
   d. Acoustic enhancement

6. What do the arrows in Figure 15-14 indicate?
   a. Anechoic mass in the posterior cul-de-sac
   b. Hypoechoic mass in the anterior cul-de-sac
   c. Anechoic fluid in the anterior cul-de-sac
   d. Anechoic fluid in the posterior cul-de-sac

7. What is another name for the anterior cul-de-sac?
   a. Vesicouterine pouch
   b. Pouch of Douglas
   c. Morison Pouch
   d. Rectouterine pouch

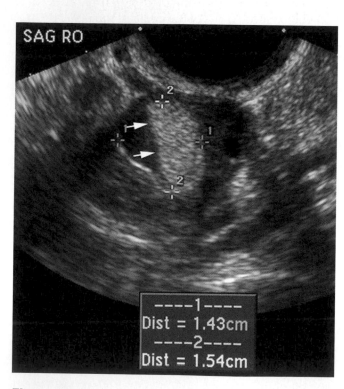

Figure 15-11

3. The structure noted between the arrows in Figure 15-12 is what echogenicity?
   a. Hypoechoic
   b. Hyperechoic
   c. Anechoic
   d. Isoechoic

8. Which of the following is also referred to as the space of Retzius?
   a. Paracolic gutters
   b. Retropubic space
   c. Anterior cul-de-sac
   d. Posterior cul-de-sac

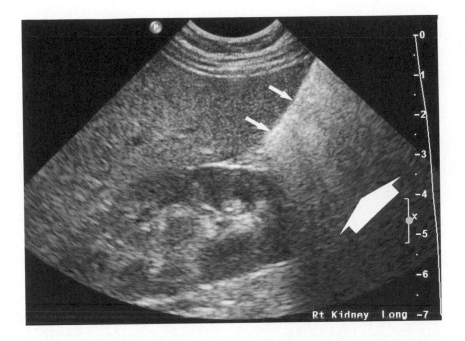

Figure 15-13

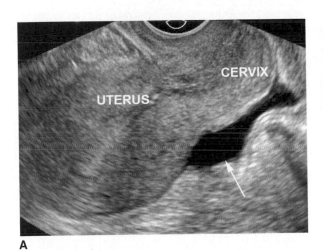

A

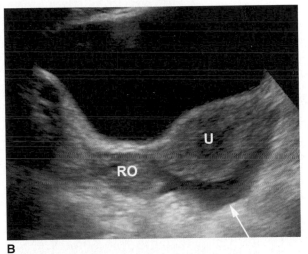

B

Figure 15-14

9. Which of the following is evident in Figure 15-15?
   a. Doppler noise
   b. Spectral broadening
   c. Mirror image
   d. Aliasing

10. Which of the following would not be a way the artifact in Figure 15-15 could be corrected?
    a. Switch to a higher frequency
    b. Increase the angle of insonation
    c. Increase the pulse-repetition frequency
    d. Adjust the baseline

11. What is the artifact identified by the arrows in Figure 15-16?
    a. Dirty shadowing
    b. Mirror image
    c. Reverberation
    d. Posterior shadowing

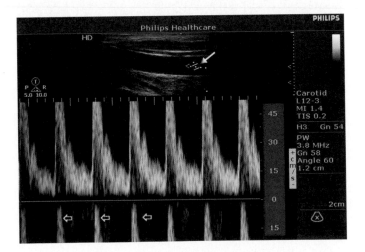

Figure 15-15

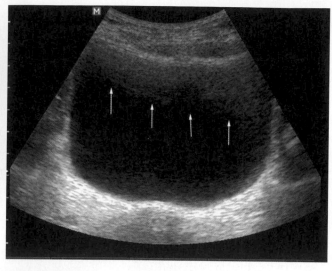

Figure 15-16

12. Which of the following would be the least likely indication for a pelvic sonogram?
    a. Diarrhea
    b. Palpable pelvic mass
    c. Amenorrhea
    d. Screening for malignancy

13. The patient in Figure 15-17 was found to have a benign ovarian neoplasm. What is the most likely diagnosis?
    a. Ovarian carcinoma
    b. Meigs syndrome
    c. von Willebrand disease
    d. Ascites

14. What does the arrow in Figure 15-17 letter "D" indicate?
    a. Pleural effusion
    b. Pericardial effusion
    c. Ascites
    d. Free fluid

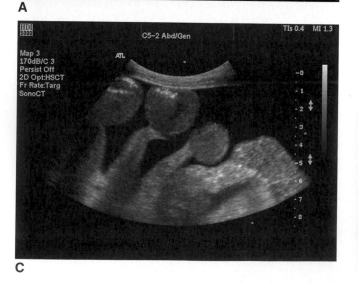

A

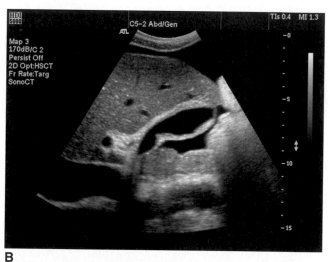

B

C

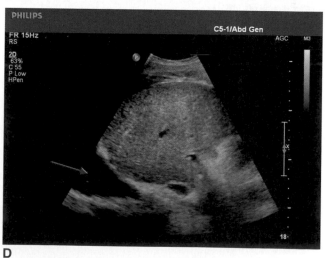

D

Figure 15-17

15. What does the image labeled "A" in Figure 15-17 depict?
    a. Pleural effusion
    b. Pericardial effusion
    c. Ascites
    d. Free fluid

16. Which of the following would be least likely associated with a palpable pelvic mass?
    a. Ovarian hyperstimulation syndrome
    b. Leiomyoma
    c. Ovarian cyst
    d. Endometrial hyperplasia

17. Which of the following is defined as painful or difficult urination?
    a. Dyspareunia
    b. Nocturia
    c. Dyspnea
    d. Dysuria

18. A linear structure coursing through an anechoic cyst separating it into two separate cavities may be referred to as a:
    a. mural nodule.
    b. septation.
    c. polyp.
    d. dringo.

19. Which of the following would least likely indicate the presence of a complex cyst?
    a. Septation
    b. Mural nodule
    c. Acoustic enhancement
    d. Internal debris

20. Which of the following is a protein produced by the fetal yolk sac, fetal gastrointestinal tract, fetal liver, and by some malignant tumors?
    a. Lactate dehydrogenase
    b. CA-125
    c. Alpha-fetoprotein
    d. Human chorionic gonadotropin

21. What term describes the echogenicity of a simple ovarian cyst?
    a. Anechoic
    b. Hypoechoic
    c. Echogenic
    d. Hyperechoic

22. The "S" in the STAR criteria stands for:
    a. Simple.
    b. Sound.
    c. Smooth walls.
    d. Septations.

23. Which of the following is defined as pain during intercourse?
    a. Dysuria
    b. Dysmenorrhea
    c. Dyspareunia
    d. Hirsutism

24. Which of the following is defined as excessive hair growth in women in areas where hair growth is normally negligible?
    a. Dyspareunia
    b. Hirsutism
    c. Meigs syndrome
    d. Polycystic ovary syndrome

25. Which of the following laboratory tests may be used as a tumor marker for an ovarian dysgerminoma?
    a. Lactate dehydrogenase
    b. Alpha-fetoprotein
    c. CA-125
    d. Tamoxifen

26. All of the following are associated with acute pelvic pain except:
    a. pelvic inflammatory disease.
    b. ruptured ovarian hemorrhagic cyst.
    c. perforated intrauterine contraceptive device.
    d. Asherman syndrome.

27. Which of the following is best defined as Intermenstrual bleeding?
    a. Dysmenorrhea
    b. Menorrhagia
    c. Menometrorrhagia
    d. Metrorrhagia

28. Having the same echogenicity means:
    a. anechoic.
    b. isoechoic.
    c. echogenic.
    d. hypoechoic.

29. Which of the following would typically not be associated with amenorrhea?
    a. Asherman syndrome
    b. Polycystic ovarian disease
    c. Pregnancy
    d. Adenomyosis

30. Which of the following is best defined as difficult or painful menstruation?
    a. Dysmenorrhea
    b. Dyspareunia
    c. Dysuria
    d. Menorrhagia

31. What term relates to the number of pregnancies a patient has had?
    a. Para
    b. Menarche
    c. Menorrhagia
    d. Gravida

32. Which of the following definitions best describes the term adnexa?
    a. The area posterior to the uterus, between the uterus and the rectum
    b. The area located posterior to the broad ligaments and adjacent to the uterus
    c. The area anterior to the uterus, between the uterus and the urinary bladder
    d. The area lateral to the iliac crest and posterior to the pubic symphysis

33. All of the following statements are true of endovaginal imaging except:
    a. endovaginal imaging requires a full urinary bladder.
    b. endovaginal imaging leads to reduced waiting time for the patient and quicker medical management.
    c. endovaginal imaging offers improved resolution of the endometrium, uterus, and ovaries, especially in the obese patient.
    d. endovaginal imaging is contraindicated for pediatric patients and for those with an intact hymen.

34. What laboratory value would be most useful to evaluate in a patient with suspected internal hemorrhage?
    a. White blood cells
    b. Lactate dehydrogenase
    c. Amylase
    d. Hematocrit

35. What abnormality results from the ovary twisting on its mesenteric connection?
    a. Pelvic inflammatory disease
    b. Fitz-Hugh–Curtis syndrome
    c. Ovarian torsion
    d. Ovarian hyperstimulation syndrome

36. Which of the following most often leads to an elevation of CA-125?
    a. Ovarian carcinoma
    b. Fitz-Hugh–Curtis syndrome
    c. Ovarian torsion
    d. Ovarian hyperstimulation syndrome

37. When does the Centers for Disease Control and Prevention recommend that alcohol-based hand rub be combined with hand washing?
    a. After performing a sonogram
    b. Before performing a sonogram
    c. When your hands are visibly soiled
    d. Between patients

38. The best way to communicate with a patient who speaks a language other than your own is to use:
    a. sign language.
    b. proper body cues.
    c. an online search engine.
    d. a trained medical interpreter.

39. What artifact would be seen posterior to a tooth within a cystic teratoma?
    a. Ring-down
    b. Reverberation
    c. Through transmission
    d. Shadowing

40. Which of the following is best described as an artifact that is produced by a strong reflector and results in a copy of the anatomy being placed deeper than the correct location?
    a. Reverberation
    b. Mirror image
    c. Acoustic shadowing
    d. Comet tail

41. Which of the following statements is not true concerning transabdominal pelvic imaging?
    a. Transabdominal imaging of the pelvis provides a global view of the entire pelvis.
    b. Transabdominal imaging lacks the detail of endovaginal imaging.
    c. Obese patients and patients with a retroverted or retroflexed uterus present a unique challenge to the transabdominal technique.
    d. Transabdominal imaging is contraindicated for pediatric patients.

42. Malignant ovarian tumors may leak mucinous material, and this condition is known as:
    a. Dandy–Walker syndrome.
    b. pseudomyxoma peritonei.
    c. Asherman syndrome.
    d. Fitz-Hugh–Curtis syndrome.

43. All of the following are proper techniques for providing patient care for patients during a pelvic sonogram except:
    a. all transducers and their cords should be cleaned before performing a pelvic sonogram.
    b. endovaginal transducers should be cleaned with a high-level disinfectant.
    c. a probe cover should be placed on the transducer for transabdominal imaging to prevent the spread of infection.
    d. a sterile jelly should be used as a lubricant for endovaginal imaging.

44. The breast cancer drug that inhibits the effects of estrogen in the breast is:
    a. CA-125.
    b. methotrexate.
    c. RA-916.
    d. tamoxifen.

45. Which of the following statements would be considered an acceptable disadvantage of endovaginal imaging?
    a. Endovaginal imaging has a limited field of view.
    b. The resolution of endovaginal imaging is reduced compared to transabdominal imaging.
    c. Endovaginal imaging is more time-consuming than transabdominal imaging.
    d. Endovaginal imaging can be performed only by female sonographers.

46. What artifact could be noted emanating from air or gas within the endometrium in a patient with endometritis?
    a. Ring-down
    b. Mirror image
    c. Posterior enhancement
    d. Dirty transmission

47. What Doppler artifact occurs when the Doppler sampling rate is not high enough to display the Doppler shift frequency?
    a. Doppler noise
    b. Aliasing
    c. Twinkle artifact
    d. Absent Doppler signal

48. Which of the following would be the least likely to cause abdominal distension?
    a. Ascites
    b. Multiple leiomyoma
    c. Ovarian hyperstimulation syndrome
    d. Polycystic ovarian disease

49. All of the following are common indications for a pelvic sonogram except:
    a. evaluation of congenital anomalies.
    b. evaluation of pelvic anatomy immediately following a motor vehicle accident.
    c. localization of an intrauterine contraceptive device.
    d. postmenopausal bleeding.

50. Precocious puberty is best defined as:
    a. pubertal development before the age of 8.
    b. pubertal development before the age of 13.
    c. excessive hair growth in girls in areas where hair growth is normally negligible.
    d. changes within the female that are caused by increased levels of alpha-fetoprotein.

51. Amenorrhea is defined as:
    a. the first menstrual cycle.
    b. excessive bleeding after the cycle.
    c. lack of menstrual flow.
    d. painful menstrual flow.

52. Which of the following would most likely be associated with hirsutism?
    a. Polycystic ovary syndrome
    b. Meigs syndrome
    c. Adenomyosis
    d. Adenomyomatosis

53. Which of the following would be caused by a large acoustic interface and subsequent production of false echoes?
    a. Posterior shadowing
    b. Acoustic enhancement
    c. Mirror image
    d. Reverberation

54. Which of the following would be best defined as abnormally heavy menstrual flow?
    a. Menometrorrhagia
    b. Menorrhagia
    c. Metrorrhagia
    d. Hypomenorrhea

55. Which of the following would be best defined as regularly timed menses but light flow?
    a. Menometrorrhagia
    b. Menorrhagia
    c. Metrorrhagia
    d. Hypomenorrhea

56. All of the following would be relevant laboratory tests to evaluate before performing a routine pelvic sonogram except:
    a. human chorionic gonadotropin.
    b. hematocrit.
    c. white blood cell count.
    d. lipase.

57. Which of the following could be described as an infection of the female genital tract that may involve the ovaries, uterus, and/or the fallopian tubes?
    a. Pseudomyxoma peritonei
    b. Pelvic inflammatory disease
    c. Polycystic ovarian disease
    d. Ovarian torsion

58. Which of the following diagnostic tests is used to evaluate emitted radiation from the patient to assess the function of organs?
    a. Magnetic resonance imaging
    b. Nuclear medicine
    c. Radiography
    d. CT

59. Endovaginal transducers may be disinfected by submerging in a(n) ___-based solution.
    a. glutaraldehyde
    b. ascites
    c. formaldehyde
    d. alcohol

60. Leukocytosis would most likely be associated with:
    a. multiple degenerating fibroids.
    b. ovarian teratoma.
    c. adenomyosis.
    d. pelvic inflammatory disease.

SUGGESTED READINGS

AIUM official statements: guidelines for cleaning and preparing external-and internal-use ultrasound transducers and equipment between patients as well as safe handling and use of ultrasound coupling gel. https://www.aium.org/officialStatements/57. Accessed November 7, 2021.

AIUM practice parameter for the performance of an ultrasound of the female pelvis. Retrieved on November 7, 2021, from AIUM Practice Parameter for the Performance of an Ultrasound Examination of the Female Pelvis – 2020 – https://www.aium.org/resources/guidelines/femalePelvis.pdf

Penny SM. *Introduction to Sonography and Patient Care.* 2nd ed. Wolters Kluwer; 2021:307–406.

Sanders RC, Hall-Terracciano B. *Clinical Sonography: A Practical Guide.* 5th ed. Wolters Kluwer; 2016:61–93 & 399.

Siegel MJ. *Pediatric Sonography.* 5th ed. Wolters Kluwer; 2019:1–39.

BONUS REVIEW!

Venous and Arterial Waveform Examples (Fig. 15-18)

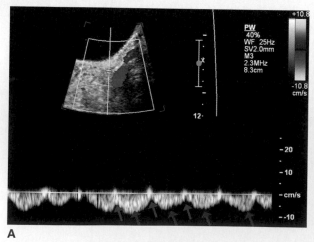
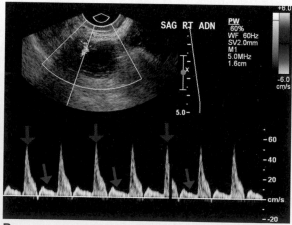

Figure 15-18 Venous and arterial waveforms. **A.** Venous waveform with continuous flow during both systole (*red arrows*) and diastole, with the relative reduction in diastolic flow (*blue arrows*). **B.** Arterial flow is typically distinguishable and distinct, with an alternating quick uptake systolic peak (*red arrows*) and a reduction in flow during diastole (*blue arrows*).

BONUS REVIEW! (*continued*)

Computed Tomography Transverse Axial of Female Pelvis (Fig. 15-19)

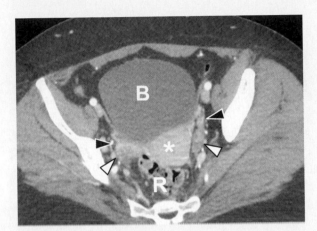

Figure 15-19 CT transverse axial enhanced soft tissue window setting CT image of the female pelvis demonstrates enhancement of the uterus (*asterisk*) and adjacent veins (*black arrowheads*). Bilateral ovaries are noted (*white arrowheads*). The uterus lies between the urinary bladder (*B*), containing uniformly hypodense urine, and the rectum (*R*).

Sagittal-Enhanced Soft-Tissue Window Setting Computed Tomography Image of the Pelvis (Fig. 15-20)

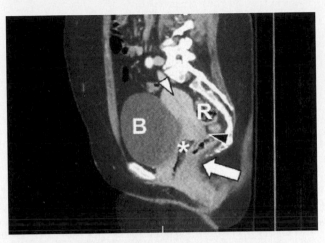

Figure 15-20 Sagittal-enhanced soft-tissue window setting computed tomography image of the pelvis. Both the endometrial lining (*white arrowhead*) and cervix (*black arrowhead*) are mildly hypoenhancing to the adjacent myometrium. The uterus is anteverted and lies between the urinary bladder (*B*) and the rectum (*R*). The rectum and vagina are supported by the puborectalis muscle (*arrow*). Hypoattenuating and air-containing longitudinal structure in the vagina is a tampon (*asterisk*).

Anatomy of the Female Pelvis

Introduction

This chapter offers an overview of normal structures and their location within the female pelvis. Anatomic landmarks are provided as well as the anatomy routinely visualized on a pelvic sonogram. Bony pelvis anatomy, pelvic muscles, ligaments, normal vascular anatomy, and extrauterine pelvic spaces are all discussed. This chapter also provides the reader with an overview of the location of these structures in relationship to the uterus and ovaries. More detailed chapters will follow concerning the uterus, ovaries, and fallopian tubes. In the *Bonus Review* section, further detailed magnetic resonance imaging (MRI) anatomy of the female pelvis is provided.

Key Terms

abdominal aorta—major abdominal artery responsible for supplying the abdomen, pelvis, and lower extremities with oxygenated blood

adnexa—the area located posterior to the broad ligaments, adjacent to the uterus, which contains the ovaries and fallopian tubes

anterior cul-de-sac—peritoneal outpouching located between the bladder and the uterus; also referred to as the vesicouterine pouch

arcuate arteries—peripheral arteries of the uterus that lie at the edge of the myometrium

broad ligament—pelvic ligament that extends from the lateral aspect of the uterus to the side walls of the pelvis

cardinal ligament—pelvic ligament that extends from the lateral surface of the cervix to the lateral fornix of the vagina and houses the uterine vasculature

coccygeus—pelvic muscle located posteriorly within the pelvis that helps support the sacrum

common iliac arteries—abdominal aortic bifurcation vessels

external iliac arteries—external branches of the common iliac arteries

false pelvis—superior portion of the pelvis

iliopsoas muscles—bilateral muscles located lateral to the uterus and anterior to iliac crest

innominate bones—pelvic bones that consist of the ilium, ischium, and pubic symphysis

internal iliac arteries—internal branches of the common iliac arteries

levator ani muscles—hammock-shaped pelvic muscle group located between the coccyx and the pubis consisting of the iliococcygeus, pubourethralis, pubococcygeus, pubovaginalis, and puborectalis

linea alba—the tendonous, fibrous structure that runs along the midline of the abdomen, separating the rectus abdominis muscles

linea terminalis—imaginary line that separates the true pelvis from the false pelvis

obturator internus muscles—paired pelvic muscles located lateral to the ovaries

ovarian ligaments—pelvic ligaments that provide support to the ovary extending from the ovary to the lateral surface of the uterus

pelvic diaphragm—group of pelvic muscles consisting of the levator ani and coccygeus muscles that provide support to the pelvic organs

piriformis muscles—paired pelvic muscles located posteriorly that extend from the sacrum to the femoral greater trochanter

posterior cul-de-sac—see key term rectouterine pouch

pouch of Douglas—see key term rectouterine pouch

prolapse—(uterine prolapse) a condition that results from the weakening of the pelvic diaphragm muscles and allows for the displacement of the uterus, often through the vagina

radial arteries—arteries that supply blood to the deeper layers of the myometrium

rectouterine pouch—peritoneal outpouching located between the uterus and the rectum; also referred to as the posterior cul-de-sac, pouch of Douglas, and the rectovaginal pouch

rectus abdominis muscles—paired anterior abdominal muscles that extend from the xiphoid process of the sternum to the pubic bone; separated by the linea alba

space of Retzius—extraperitoneal space located between the bladder and the symphysis pubis that contains fat

spiral arteries—tiny, coiled arteries that supply blood to the functional layer of the endometrium

straight arteries—uterine radial artery branch that supplies blood to the basal layer of the endometrium

suspensory ligament of the ovary—pelvic ligament that provides support to the ovary and extends from the ovaries to the pelvic side walls

true pelvis—inferior portion of the pelvis that contains the uterus, ovaries, fallopian tubes, urinary bladder, small bowel, sigmoid colon, and rectum

uterine arteries—branches of the internal iliac artery that supplies blood to the uterus, ovaries, and fallopian tubes

vesicouterine pouch—peritoneal outpouching located between the bladder and the uterus; also referred to as the anterior cul-de-sac

PELVIC STRUCTURE

Bony Pelvis and Location of the Female Genitalia

The bony pelvis consists of the sacrum, coccyx, and **innominate bones** (Fig. 16-1). These bones mark the boundaries of the pelvic cavity. The posterior border of the pelvic cavity is marked by the sacrum and coccyx. The innominate bones consist of the ilium, ischium, and pubic symphysis. The pelvic bones will produce an acoustic shadow when noted during a sonogram. For example, bilaterally, the iliac crest will be demonstrated, while in the midline, the pubic symphysis can be recognized.

The boundaries of the female pelvis are considered to be from the iliac crest to a group of muscles known as the **pelvic diaphragm**, located at the base of the pelvis. The pelvis can further be divided into a **true pelvis** (lesser pelvis) and **false pelvis** (major or greater pelvis) by an imaginary line known as the **linea terminalis** (Fig. 16-2). The false pelvis is located more superiorly than the true pelvis, the latter of which contains the

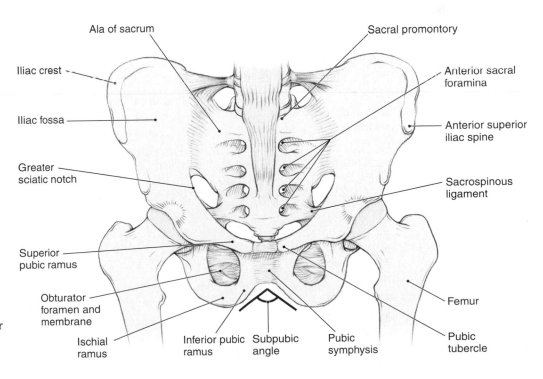

Figure 16-1 The anterior view of the female bony pelvis.

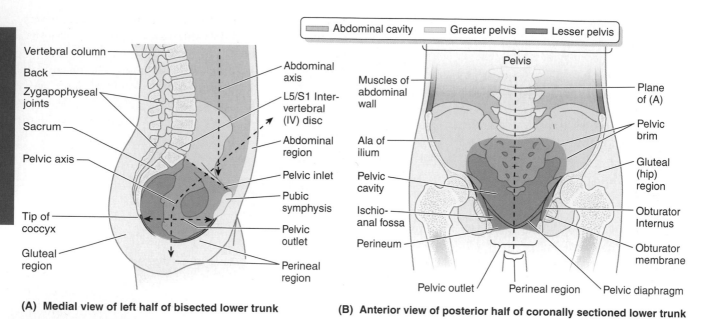

(A) **Medial view of left half of bisected lower trunk**

(B) **Anterior view of posterior half of coronally sectioned lower trunk**

Figure 16-2 Pelvis and perineum. **A** and **B.** The pelvis (*green*) is the space within the pelvic girdle, overlapped externally by the abdominal and gluteal regions, perineum, and lower back. Thus, the pelvis has no external surface area. The greater pelvis (*light green*) is pelvic by virtue of its bony boundaries, but is abdominal in terms of its contents. The lesser pelvis (*dark green*) provides the bony framework (skeleton) for the pelvic cavity and deep perineum.

urinary bladder, small bowel, sigmoid colon, rectum, ovaries, fallopian tubes, and uterus.

> 🔊)) **SOUND OFF**
> The true pelvis contains the urinary bladder, small bowel, sigmoid colon, rectum, ovaries, fallopian tubes, and uterus.

Within the pelvis, the nongravid uterus lies within the midline, posterior to the urinary bladder and anterior to the rectum (Fig. 16-3). The vagina extends inferiorly from the external os of the cervix to the external genitalia, where it is positioned posterior to the urethra. The fallopian tubes and ovaries are considered bilateral adnexal structures. However, the course of the fallopian tubes and location of the ovaries are relatively unpredictable.

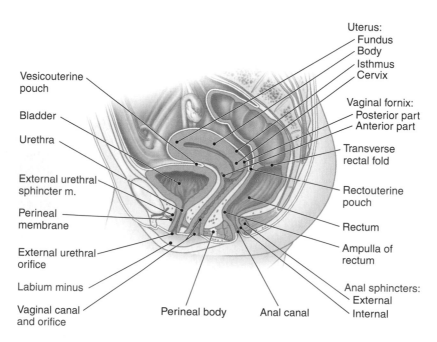

Figure 16-3 Female pelvic anatomy median section.

Pelvic Muscles and Bowel

Several pelvic muscles may be identified sonographically within the female pelvis (Table 16-1; Fig. 16-4). Muscles visualized on a sonogram include the **rectus abdominis muscles**, the **iliopsoas muscles**, **obturator internus muscles**, **piriformis muscles**, and a group of muscles known as the pelvic diaphragm, which is composed of the **levator ani** and **coccygeus** muscles (Figs. 16-5 to 16-7). The pelvic diaphragm muscles provide support to the pelvic organs. A weakening in the **levator ani muscles** could result in **prolapse** of the pelvic organs.

> **SOUND OFF**
> The weakening of the pelvic diaphragm, which includes the levator ani muscles, can lead to prolapse of the uterus.

Because pelvic muscles can be seen sonographically, sonographers must have an understanding of their locations and sonographic appearance in order to differentiate them from pelvic masses. For instance, the piriformis muscles or iliopsoas may be confused with the ovaries or adnexal masses because of their location within the pelvis. Pelvic muscles will appear as hypoechoic structures with varying degrees of hyperechoic, striated muscle fibers noted in the transverse and longitudinal scanning planes.

Segments of both the large and small bowels are located in the pelvis. These include part of the ileum, cecum, descending and ascending colon, sigmoid colon, and rectum (Fig. 16-8). Occasionally, normal bowel can be mistaken for an ovarian or pelvic mass or possibly even the ovary itself. In most instances, peristalsis may be noted within the bowel segments that are located within the female pelvis. However, peristalsis may not always be evident in the rectum, so

care must be taken in this regard. In some situations, a water enema may be administered during real-time sonography to differentiate the rectum from a pelvic mass, but often, another imaging modality, such as CT, is preferred.

> **SOUND OFF**
> Normal bowel can be mistaken for an ovarian or pelvic mass or possibly even the ovary itself.

Pelvic Ligaments

The ligaments of the pelvis provide support to the ovaries, uterus, and fallopian tubes (Table 16-2). The **broad ligaments** and **suspensory ligament of the ovary** are actually double folds of peritoneum. In addition to providing support, the suspensory ligament of the ovary contains the ovarian artery, ovarian vein, lymphatics, and ovarian nerves. Conversely, the **cardinal ligaments** house the vasculature of the uterus. The majority of pelvic ligaments are not identified during a routine sonographic examination of the pelvis. However, when surrounded by free fluid, the dense broad ligaments may be identified as echogenic structures extending from the lateral borders of the uterus bilaterally (Fig. 16-9).

> **SOUND OFF**
> The dense broad ligaments may be identified as echogenic structures extending from the lateral borders of the uterus bilaterally.

Pelvic Spaces

Pelvic ascites and free fluid may accumulate within potential spaces or recesses within the female pelvis. When filled with fluid, these regions can be easily identified sonographically. The **vesicouterine pouch**, or **anterior cul-de-sac**, is located anterior to the uterus and posterior to the urinary bladder. The **rectouterine pouch**, located between the rectum and the uterus, may also be referred to as the rectovaginal pouch, **posterior cul-de-sac**, or **pouch of Douglas** (Figs. 16-10 and 16-11). The rectouterine pouch is considered the most dependent part of the peritoneal cavity, making it the most likely place for fluid to collect in the pelvis. Between the anterior wall of the urinary bladder and the symphysis pubis lies the **space of Retzius**, or retropubic space, an area that contains extraperitoneal fat. Free fluid, when excessive, may also be noted within the **adnexa**, lower quadrants of the abdomen, and may serve the purpose of delineating the borders of pelvic organs. In addition, when free fluid is noted within the pelvis, a general assessment of the upper abdomen for additional fluid may be warranted.

TABLE 16-1 Sonographically identifiable pelvic muscles	
Sonographically Identifiable Pelvic Muscles	**Location**
Rectus abdominis muscle (2)	Anterior (separated by the **linea alba**)
Iliopsoas muscles (2)	Lateral and anterior to iliac crest
Obturator internus (2)	Lateral to ovaries
Piriformis (2)	Posterior
Pelvic diaphragm (levator ani and coccygeus muscles)	Inferior near the vagina in transverse

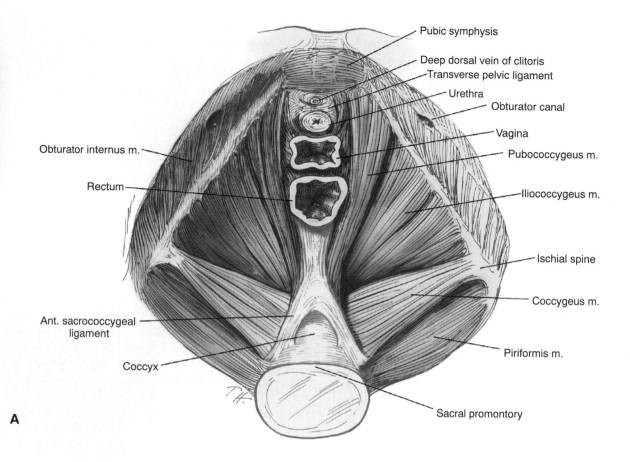

Pubic symphysis

Deep dorsal vein of clitoris

Transverse pelvic ligament

Urethra

Obturator canal

Obturator internus m.

Vagina

Pubococcygeus m.

Rectum

Iliococcygeus m.

Ischial spine

Coccygeus m.

Ant. sacrococcygeal ligament

Piriformis m.

Coccyx

Sacral promontory

A

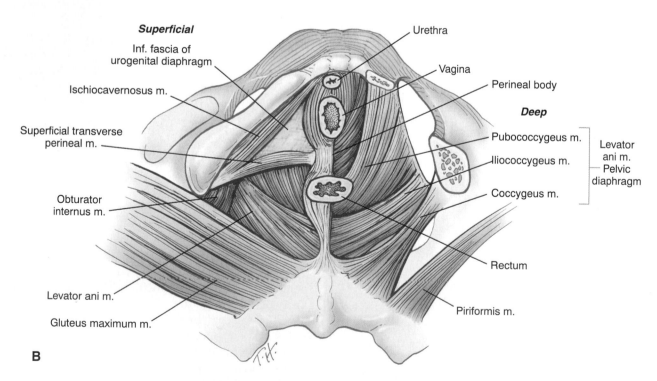

Superficial

Urethra

Inf. fascia of urogenital diaphragm

Vagina

Ischiocavernosus m.

Perineal body

Deep

Superficial transverse perineal m.

Pubococcygeus m.

Levator ani m. Pelvic diaphragm

Iliococcygeus m.

Obturator internus m.

Coccygeus m.

Rectum

Levator ani m.

Piriformis m.

Gluteus maximum m.

B

Figure 16-4 The muscles of the pelvic floor. **A** and **B.** Inferior views of the female of the pelvis. **A.** Superficial. **B.** Deep.

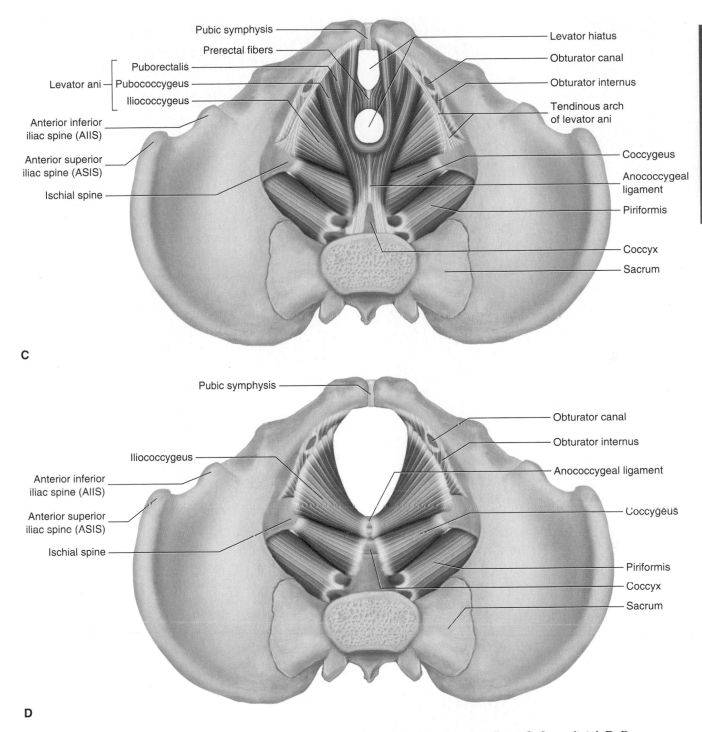

Figure 16-4 (*continued*) C and D. Superior views of the muscles of the female pelvic floor. **C.** Superficial. **D.** Deep.

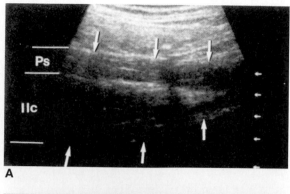

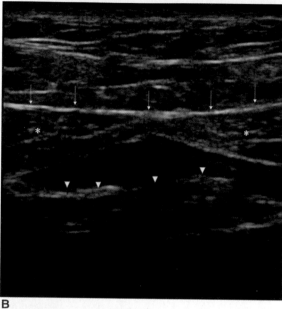

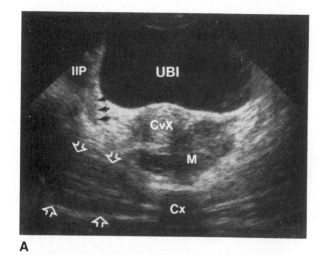

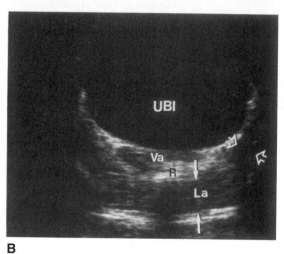

Figure 16-5 Psoas major and rectus abdominis muscles. **A.** Sagittal scan of the psoas major (*Ps*) and the iliac muscle (*Ilc*). **B.** Sonogram of the normal linea alba. The top layer of tissue is the dermis and subdermal fat. The rectus sheath fascial layer is seen below (*long arrows*). The two rectus abdominis muscles are below (*asterisk*). The area of meeting of the recuts sheath and two rectus abdominis muscles is the linea alba (*center long arrow*). The parietal peritoneum is below (*arrowheads*).

Figure 16-7 Pelvic muscles. **A.** Transverse scan of the pelvis demonstrates the obturator internus muscle as a thin, hypoechoic strip (*black arrows*) adjacent to the lateral pelvic wall. The upper margin of the muscle is just below the brim of the pelvis. The levator ani muscle group is also well seen (*open arrows*). *UBl*, urinary bladder; *CvX*, cervix; *Cx*, coccyx; *M*, mass adjacent to cervix; *Ilp*, iliopsoas muscle. **B.** Forming the floor of the true pelvic space is the levator ani muscle group (*arrows*), which attaches to the medial surface of the obturator internus muscle (*open arrows*). *UBl*, urinary bladder; *La*, levator ani muscle; *R*, rectum; *Va*, vagina.

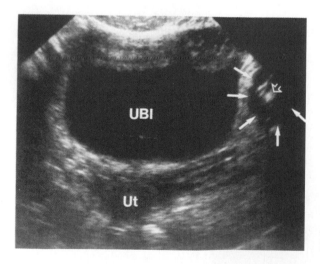

Figure 16-6 Transverse scan of the pelvis reveals the urinary bladder (*UBl*), uterus (*Ut*), and left iliopsoas muscle (*arrows*).

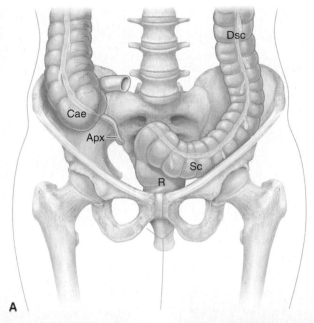

A

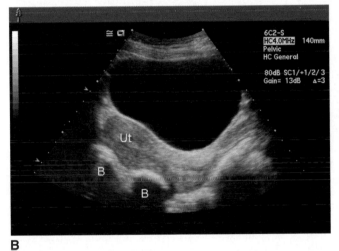

B

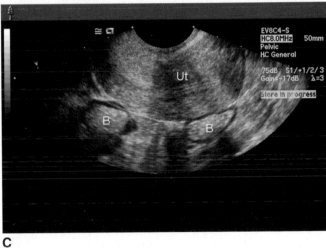

C

Figure 16-8 Large bowel and its relationship to the female pelvis. **A.** The cecum and appendix are found on the right side of the false pelvis, and the pelvic portion of the descending colon and the proximal (*upper*) part of the sigmoid colon are found on the left. *Apx*, appendix; *Cae*, cecum; *Dsc*, descending colon; *R*, rectum; *Sc*, sigmoid colon. **B.** A sagittal transabdominal image of the uterus demonstrating bowel (B) with typical "dirty" shadows. **C.** Endovaginal scan of the retroverted uterus. Loops of bowel (B) are seen posterior to the uterus (*Ut*).

TABLE 16-2 Location of pelvic ligaments and structures that they support

Pelvic Ligaments	Supports	Location
Broad ligaments	Uterus, tubes, ovaries	Extend from the lateral aspect of the uterus to the side walls of the pelvis
Round ligaments	Uterus (fundus)	Extend from uterine cornua to labia majora between the folds of the broad ligaments
Suspensory ligament of the ovaries (infundibulopelvic)	Ovaries and tubes	Extend from the ovaries to the pelvic side walls
Ovarian ligaments	Ovaries	Extend from ovary to lateral surface of the uterus
Cardinal ligaments	Cervix	Extend from the lateral surface of the cervix to the lateral fornix of vagina
Uterosacral ligaments	Uterus	Extend from the uterus to sacrum

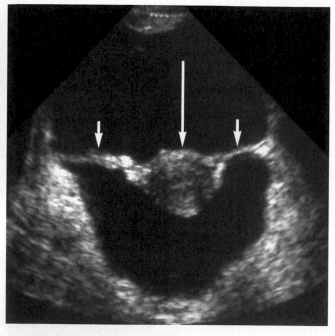

Figure 16-9 Broad ligament outlined by ascites. The bilateral broad ligaments (*short arrows*), outlined by ascites, are clearly noted in this transverse image. The longer arrow is indicating the uterus.

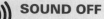

SOUND OFF
The most dependent part of peritoneal cavity is the posterior cul-de-sac or pouch of Douglas, making it the most likely place for free fluid to collect in the pelvis.

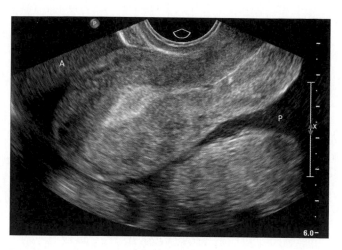

Figure 16-11 Anterior cul-de-sac versus posterior cul-de-sac. Sagittal endovaginal sonogram of the uterus surrounded by complex free fluid within both the anterior (*A*) and posterior (*P*) cul-de-sacs. Complex free fluid is worrisome for blood, especially in the setting of a suspected ectopic pregnancy.

PELVIC VASCULATURE

Arterial System of the Female Pelvis

Vascular structures can provide both important diagnostic information and landmarks during a sonographic examination of the female pelvis. The **abdominal aorta** supplies blood to the female genitalia. It branches into the paired **common iliac arteries**, typically near the umbilicus. The common iliac arteries then divide into the **external iliac arteries** and **internal iliac arteries** (Fig. 16-12). These vessels, along with their venous counterparts, provide useful landmarks for

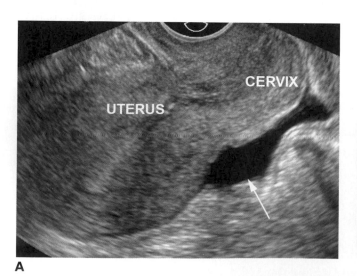

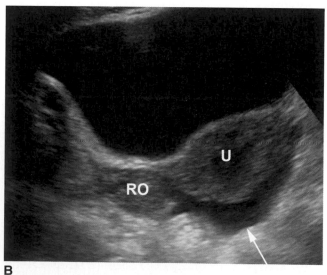

Figure 16-10 Posterior cul-de-sac (pouch of Douglas). **A.** Sagittal transvaginal image of the midline pelvis demonstrates free fluid in the posterior cul-de-sac (*arrow*). **B.** Transverse transabdominal image of the female pelvis demonstrates free fluid in the posterior cul-de-sac (*arrow*). *RO*, right ovary; *U*, uterus.

VASCULATURE OF UTERUS

```
                    ┌─────────────┐
                    │    AORTA    │
                    └─────────────┘
              ┌────────────┴────────────┐
    ┌──────────────────┐      ┌──────────────────┐
    │   branches of    │      │  INTERNAL ILIAC  │
    │     OVARIAN      │      │    ARTERIES      │
    │    ARTERIES      │      │                  │
    └──────────────────┘      └──────────────────┘
      anastomose              
      with uterine            
      arteries                
                    ┌──────────────────┐
                    │ UTERINE ARTERIES │
                    │ (wall of uterus) │
                    └──────────────────┘
                    ┌──────────────────┐
                    │     ARCUATE      │
                    │    ARTERIES      │
                    └──────────────────┘
                    ┌──────────────────┐
                    │     RADIAL       │
                    │    ARTERIES      │
                    └──────────────────┘
              ┌────────────┴────────────┐
    ┌──────────────────┐      ┌──────────────────┐
    │    STRAIGHT      │      │     SPIRAL       │
    │    (BASAL)       │      │    (COILED)      │
    │    ARTERIES      │      │    ARTERIES      │
    │                  │      │   -can slough    │
    └──────────────────┘      └──────────────────┘
    ┌──────────────────┐      ┌──────────────────┐
    │   BASAL LAYER    │      │  DECIDUAL LAYER  │
    └──────────────────┘      └──────────────────┘
```

A

ARTERIAL CIRCULATION
-Uterine artery runs medially off the internal iliac artery toward the cervix where it then ascends lateral to the uterus in the broad ligament to the cornua
-There it courses laterally toward the ovary to where it anastomoses with a branch of the ovarian artery

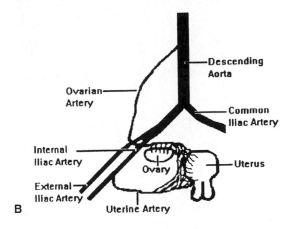

B

Figure 16-12 Arterial circulation within the female pelvis. **A.** Schematic of the arterial flow from the aorta to the uterus. **B.** Simple drawing of the branches of the abdominal aorta.

identifying the ovaries. The paired right and left **uterine arteries** are branches of the internal iliac arteries. They supply blood to the uterus, fallopian tubes, and ovaries and course along the lateral aspect of the uterus within the folds of the broad ligaments. Doppler sonography can be used to analyze the uterine arteries throughout the menstrual cycle. For example, the Doppler investigation of the uterine artery resistive index during the proliferative phase of the menstrual cycle is higher compared to just before ovulation and into the secretory phase.

Branches of the uterine artery include the **arcuate arteries**, which may be visualized with Doppler interrogation along the lateral aspect of the myometrium. The arcuate vessels progress further within the uterus and eventually become the **radial arteries**, which supply blood to the deeper layers of the myometrium. The radial arteries then divide into the **straight arteries** and **spiral arteries** (Fig. 16-13). The spiral arteries are the tiny, coiled vessels that supply blood to the functional or decidual layer of the endometrium. The ovarian arteries originate from the lateral aspect of the abdominal aorta. The ovaries have a dual blood supply. Each ovary

receives its nourishment from an ovarian artery and a branch of the uterine artery.

🔊 **SOUND OFF**
The spiral arteries are the tiny, coiled vessels that supply blood to the functional layer of the endometrium.

Venous System of the Female Pelvis

All venous structures mirror their arterial counterparts, with the exception of the left ovarian vein, which instead of returning blood to the inferior vena cava, drains directly into the left renal vein (Fig. 16-14). The common iliac veins unite at almost the same level as the common iliac artery bifurcation to help form the inferior vena cava.

🔊 **SOUND OFF**
The left ovarian vein drains into the left renal vein.

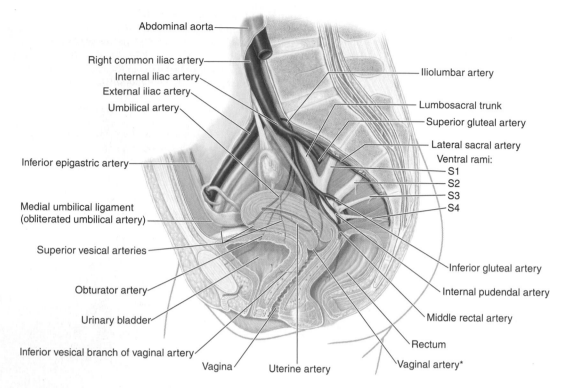

Abdominal aorta

Right common iliac artery

Internal iliac artery

External iliac artery

Umbilical artery

Inferior epigastric artery

Medial umbilical ligament (obliterated umbilical artery)

Superior vesical arteries

Obturator artery

Urinary bladder

Inferior vesical branch of vaginal artery

Vagina

Uterine artery

Iliolumbar artery

Lumbosacral trunk

Superior gluteal artery

Lateral sacral artery

Ventral rami:
S1
S2
S3
S4

Inferior gluteal artery

Internal pudendal artery

Middle rectal artery

Rectum

Vaginal artery*

A

*Vaginal artery arises from uterine artery in 11% of cases

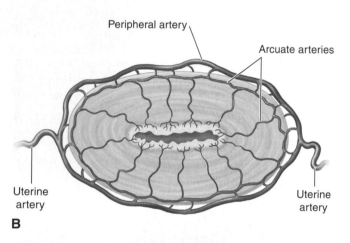

Peripheral artery

Arcuate arteries

Uterine artery

Uterine artery

B

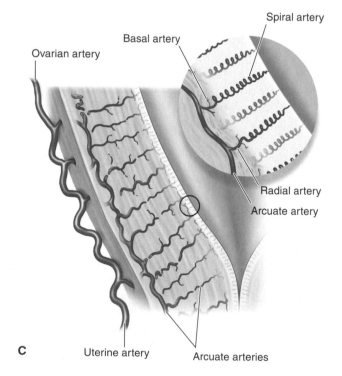

Ovarian artery

Basal artery

Spiral artery

Radial artery

Arcuate artery

Uterine artery

Arcuate arteries

C

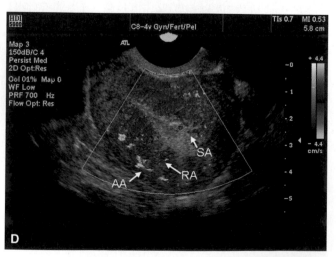

Figure 16-13 Uterine arteries. **A.** Sagittal diagram of the uterine vascular supply. **B.** Transverse diagram of the uterine vascular supply. **C.** Diagram of the uterine arterial branches in the longitudinal plane in more detail. **D.** Endovaginal color Doppler scan of the uterus demonstrating arcuate (*AA*), radial (*RA*), and spiral arteries (*SA*).

VENOUS CIRCULATION

Uterine Plexus

-situated along sides and cornua of uterus
-veins composing this plexus anastomose with each other and the ovarian veins
-are not tortuous like the arteries

Common Iliac Veins

-are formed by the union of the external and internal iliac veins
-ascend to join and form the inferior vena cava posterior and lateral to their corresponding artery
-right common iliac vein shorter and more vertical than the left

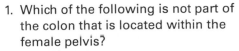

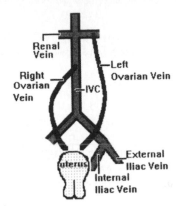

Figure 16-14 Venous circulation within the female pelvis. **A.** Schematic of the venous flow from the uterus to the inferior vena cava. **B.** Simple drawing of the venous return from the uterus and ovaries. Note the left ovarian vein attached to the left renal vein.

REVIEW QUESTIONS

1. Which of the following is not part of the colon that is located within the female pelvis?
   a. Ascending
   b. Descending
   c. Sigmoid
   d. Transverse

2. Which of the following is a pelvic ligament that extends from the lateral surface of the cervix to the lateral fornix of the vagina?
   a. Common iliac ligament
   b. Cardinal ligament
   c. Iliopsoas ligament
   d. Broad ligament

3. In Figure 16-15, what does the arrow indicate?
   a. Fluid within the rectouterine pouch
   b. Fluid within the vesicouterine pouch
   c. Fluid within the space of Retzius
   d. Fluid within the anterior cul-de-sac

4. The uterine vasculature is located within the:
   a. broad ligaments.
   b. cardinal ligaments.
   c. suspensory ligament of the ovary.
   d. obturator internus ligament.

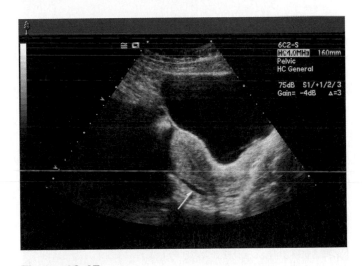

Figure 16-15

5. What do the arrows in Figure 16-16 indicate?
   a. Radial arteries
   b. Uterine arteries
   c. Spiral arteries
   d. Arcuate arteries

6. What is another name for the true pelvis?
   a. Greater pelvis
   b. Lesser pelvis
   c. Superior pelvis
   d. Major pelvis

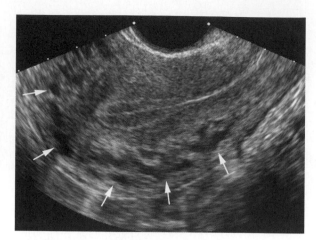

Figure 16-16

7. The patient in Figure 16-17 complained of right lower quadrant pain and presented for a transabdominal pelvic sonogram. Upon closer presentation with a linear transducer, you noted the structure identified by the arrow. What is the most likely etiology of this structure?
   a. Cecum
   b. Rectum
   c. Appendix
   d. Sigmoid colon

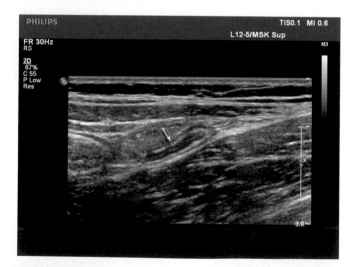

Figure 16-17

8. Which of the following muscles is located posteriorly within the pelvis and helps support the sacrum?
   a. Iliopsoas
   b. Coccygeus
   c. Obturator internus
   d. Piriformis

9. The arrow in Figure 16-18 indicates the:
   a. ovarian ligament.
   b. round ligament.
   c. uterosacral ligament.
   d. broad ligament.

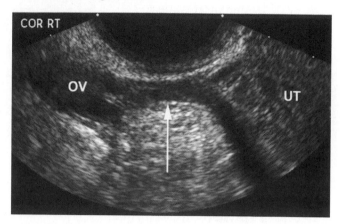

Figure 16-18

10. Which of the following is not supported by the broad ligaments?
    a. Pelvic diaphragm
    b. Uterus
    c. Uterine tubes
    d. Ovaries

11. Which of the following is not a levator ani muscle?
    a. Pubourethralis
    b. Pubovaginalis
    c. Puboileacus
    d. Iliococcygeus

12. What artery directly supplies blood to the basal layer of the endometrium?
    a. Spiral
    b. Arcuate
    c. Straight
    d. Radial

13. Which of the following is not true of the uterine plexus?
    a. They are tortuous like the arteries.
    b. They supply blood to the uterine tubes.
    c. They anastomose with each other and the ovarian vein.
    d. They are located along the sides of the cervix and the cornua.

14. What is the fibrous structure located along the midline of the abdomen that separates the rectus abdominis muscles?
    a. Linea terminalis
    b. Linea rectus
    c. Linea alba
    d. Linea aspera

15. What is the relationship of the lesser pelvis to the greater pelvis?
    a. It is located more inferiorly.
    b. It is located more laterally.
    c. It is located more anteriorly.
    d. It is located more superiorly.

16. What part of the cervix is closest to the vagina?
    a. Internal os
    b. Internal canal
    c. Adventitia
    d. External os

17. What midline, anterior pelvic structure may produce an acoustic shadow when scanning the female pelvis?
    a. Iliac crest
    b. Anterior superior iliac spine
    c. Pubic symphysis
    d. Ischial ramus

18. Figure 16-19 is a transverse sonogram of the female pelvis. Which of the following statements is not true of this image?
    a. The free fluid is noted within the right adnexa.
    b. The free fluid is noted within the rectouterine pouch.
    c. The free fluid is noted within the posterior cul-de-sac.
    d. The free fluid appears to be anechoic and simple.

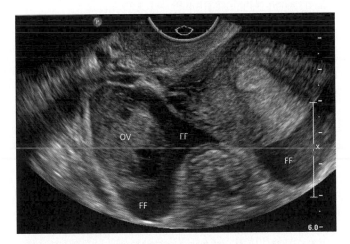

Figure 16-19

19. The common iliac veins combine to create the:
    a. inferior vena cava.
    b. external iliac vein.
    c. internal iliac vein.
    d. abdominal aorta.

20. You are performing a female pelvic sonogram and identify a solid mass adjacent to the right ovary, just right lateral to the uterus. What is the most likely location of this mass?
    a. Within the right adnexa
    b. Within the pouch of Douglas
    c. Within the pelvic diaphragm
    d. Within the space of Retzius

21. What structure within the female pelvis lies posterior to the urinary bladder and anterior to the rectum?
    a. Broad ligament
    b. Rectus abdominis muscle
    c. Space of Retzius
    d. Uterus

22. Fluid noted posterior to the uterus would most likely be located within the:
    a. space of Retzius.
    b. pouch of Douglas.
    c. anterior cul-de-sac.
    d. adnexa.

23. Both the straight and spiral arteries are branches of the:
    a. common iliac artery.
    b. radial artery.
    c. arcuate artery.
    d. external iliac artery.

24. The left ovarian vein drains directly into the:
    a. right renal vein.
    b. inferior vena cava.
    c. aorta.
    d. left renal vein.

25. Pelvic bones, when visualized on sonography, will produce:
    a. posterior shadowing.
    b. posterior enhancement.
    c. mirror image artifact.
    d. minimal enhancement.

26. The uterine arteries supply blood to all of the following except:
    a. fallopian tubes.
    b. rectum.
    c. ovaries.
    d. uterus.

27. The anterior cul-de-sac is also referred to as the:
    a. space of Retzius.
    b. rectouterine pouch.
    c. pouch of Douglas.
    d. vesicouterine pouch.

28. What is considered the most dependent part of the peritoneal cavity?
    a. Space of Retzius
    b. Anterior cul-de-sac
    c. Pouch of Douglas
    d. Rectovesical pouch

29. The right ovarian vein drains directly into the:
    a. right renal vein.
    b. aorta.
    c. inferior vena cava.
    d. common iliac vein.

30. The innominate bones of the pelvis consist of the:
    a. ischium, ilium, and pubic bones.
    b. ilium, sacrum, and coccyx bones.
    c. sacrum, coccyx, and pubic bones.
    d. sacrum, ischium, and ilium bones.

31. What other term is used to describe the space of Retzius?
    a. Posterior cul-de-sac
    b. Anterior cul-de-sac
    c. Murphy pouch
    d. Retropubic space

32. The true pelvis is delineated from the false pelvis by the:
    a. space of Retzius.
    b. adnexa.
    c. linea terminalis.
    d. linea alba.

33. The vagina is located __ to the uterus:
    a. anterior
    b. posterior
    c. inferior
    d. medial

34. The muscles that may be confused with the ovaries on a pelvic sonogram include the:
    a. rectus abdominis and obturator internus muscles.
    b. levator ani and coccygeus muscles.
    c. obturator internus and levator ani muscles.
    d. piriformis and iliopsoas muscles.

35. Which vessels supply blood to the deeper layers of the myometrium?
    a. Radial arteries
    b. Spiral arteries
    c. Straight arteries
    d. Arcuate arteries

36. Pelvic muscles appear:
    a. echogenic.
    b. anechoic.
    c. hypoechoic.
    d. complex.

37. The abdominal aorta bifurcates into the:
    a. internal iliac arteries.
    b. common iliac arteries.
    c. ovarian arteries.
    d. external iliac arteries.

38. Which of the following are the paired anterior abdominal muscles that extend from the xiphoid process of the sternum to the pubic bone?
    a. Iliopsoas muscles
    b. Rectus abdominis muscles
    c. Obturator internus muscles
    d. Piriformis muscles

39. Peritoneal spaces located posterior to the broad ligament are referred to as the:
    a. rectouterine spaces.
    b. anterior cul-de-sacs.
    c. lateral cul-de-sacs.
    d. adnexa.

40. The paired muscles that are located lateral to the uterus and anterior to the iliac crest are the:
    a. iliopsoas muscles.
    b. rectus abdominis muscles.
    c. obturator internus muscles.
    d. piriformis muscles.

41. Fluid noted anterior to the uterus would most likely be located within the:
    a. pouch of Douglas.
    b. vesicouterine pouch.
    c. space of Retzius.
    d. rectouterine pouch.

42. The bilateral muscles that are located posterior to and extend from the sacrum to the femoral greater trochanter are the:
    a. levator ani muscles.
    b. rectus abdominis muscles.
    c. obturator internus muscles.
    d. piriformis muscles.

43. The pelvic ligament that provides support to the ovary to the pelvic side wall is the:
    a. cardinal ligament.
    b. ovarian ligament.
    c. broad ligament.
    d. suspensory ligament of the ovary.

44. The pelvic muscle group that is located between the coccyx and the pubis is the:
    a. levator ani muscles.
    b. rectus abdominis muscles.
    c. obturator internus muscles.
    d. piriformis muscle.

45. The sonographic pelvic examination of a female patient reveals an extensive amount of ascites. In the transverse plane, you visualize two echogenic structures extending from the side walls of uterus to the pelvic side walls bilaterally. These structures are most likely the:
    a. broad ligaments.
    b. cardinal ligaments.
    c. ovarian ligaments.
    d. uterosacral ligaments.

46. The space of Retzius is located:
    a. between the uterus and the bladder.
    b. between the bladder and the ilium.
    c. along the lateral aspect of the uterus.
    d. between the bladder and the pubic bone.

47. The right ovarian artery branches off of the:
    a. aorta.
    b. right renal artery.
    c. uterine artery.
    d. internal iliac artery.

48. The muscle located lateral to the ovaries is the:
    a. iliopsoas muscle.
    b. rectus abdominis muscle.
    c. obturator internus muscle.
    d. piriformis muscle.

49. The arteries that directly supply blood to the functional layer of the endometrium are the:
    a. radial arteries.
    b. spiral arteries.
    c. straight arteries.
    d. arcuate arteries.

50. Another name for the rectouterine pouch is the:
    a. space of Retzius.
    b. pouch of Retzius.
    c. pouch of Douglas.
    d. anterior cul-de-sac.

51. A patient presents to the sonography department with a history of uterine prolapse. Which of the following best describes this disorder?
    a. A condition that results from the weakening of the pelvic diaphragm muscles and allows for the displacement of the uterus, often through the vagina.
    b. A congenital anomaly that results in the duplication of the uterus.
    c. A condition that results in the abnormal invasion of the myometrium through the bladder wall, leading to hematuria.
    d. An abnormality that describes the inversion of the myometrium and endometrium.

52. The pelvic ligament that extends from the lateral aspect of the uterus to the side walls of the pelvis is the:
    a. broad ligament.
    b. ovarian ligament.
    c. piriformis ligament.
    d. round ligament.

53. The uterine artery branches off of the:
    a. abdominal aorta.
    b. uterine plexus.
    c. internal iliac artery.
    d. external iliac artery.

54. The peripheral arteries of the uterus are the:
    a. radial arteries.
    b. spiral arteries.
    c. straight arteries.
    d. arcuate arteries.

55. The urinary bladder, uterus, and ovaries are located within the:
    a. true pelvis.
    b. false pelvis.

56. The pelvic ligament that provides support to the ovary and extends from the ovary to the lateral surface of the uterus is the:
    a. cardinal ligament.
    b. ovarian ligament.
    c. broad ligament.
    d. suspensory ligament of the ovary.

57. The surface of the pelvic bones, when visualized on sonography, will appear:
    a. anechoic.
    b. hypoechoic.
    c. dark.
    d. hyperechoic.

58. Which vessel is the longest?
    a. left ovarian vein
    b. left ovarian artery
    c. right ovarian vein
    d. right ovarian artery

59. The ovary is supplied blood by the:
    a. ovarian artery.
    b. ovarian artery and uterine artery.
    c. uterine artery.
    d. arcuate artery.

60. Prolapse of the pelvic organs most often involves the:
    a. rectus abdominis and obturator internus muscles.
    b. levator ani and coccygeus muscles.
    c. obturator internus and levator ani muscles.
    d. piriformis and iliopsoas muscles.

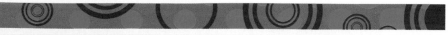

SUGGESTED READINGS

Curry RA, Tempkin BB. *Sonography: Introduction to Normal Structure and Function.* 5th ed. Elsevier; 2020:317–365.

Gibbs RS, Karlyn BY, Haney AF, et al. *Danforth's Obstetrics and Gynecology.* 10th ed. Wolters Kluwer; 2008:540–554.

Norton ME. *Callen's Ultrasonography in Obstetrics and Gynecology.* 6th ed. Elsevier; 2017:805–834.

Stephenson SR, Dmitrieva J. *Diagnostic Medical Sonography: Obstetrics and Gynecology.* 4th ed. Wolters Kluwer Health; 2018:75–126.

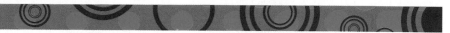

BONUS REVIEW!

Measurement of the Uterus (Fig. 16-20)

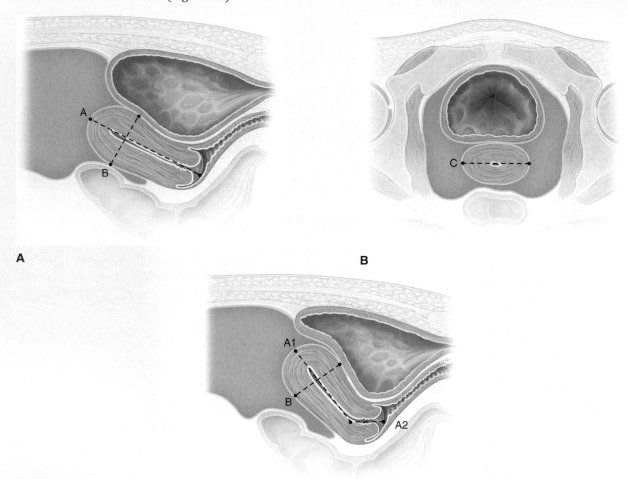

A

B

C

Figure 16-20 Measurement technique for the uterus. **A.** The long axis of the uterus should be measured from the fundus to the tip of the cervix (*line A*). On the same image, the greatest anteroposterior diameter of the uterus should be measured along a line perpendicular to line A at a point where the uterus appears widest (*B*). **B.** The transverse diameter (*line C*) is measured in the same plane as the anteroposterior diameter (*line B*), which increases accuracy and consistency of uterine measurements. **C.** If the uterus is strongly anteflexed, two measurements of the long axis (*lines A1* and *A2*) should be made and added together to obtain the true length.

BONUS REVIEW! (continued)

Midline MRI of the Female Pelvis (Fig. 16-21)

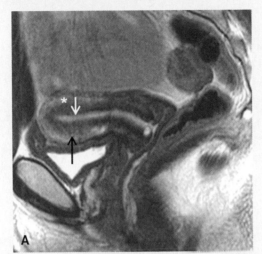

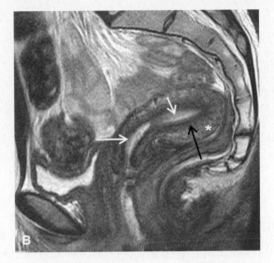

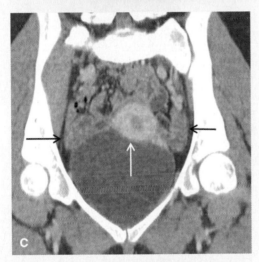

Figure 16-21 Midline MRI of the female pelvis. Normal uterus and ovary on MRI. Sagittal **(A, B)** and axial **(C)** MR images through the pelvis demonstrate normal uterus (anteverted in A, retroverted in B) and ovary. The uterine zonal anatomy is seen with the intermediate signal intensity outer myometrium (* in A, B), low signal intensity junctional zone (*black arrow* in A, B), and high signal intensity endometrium (*short white arrow* in A, B). Both ovaries (*black arrows* in C) are seen as soft-tissue attenuation ovoid structures adjacent to the uterus.

Pouch of Douglas on CT (Fig. 16-22)

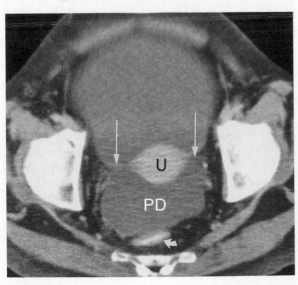

Figure 16-22 Pouch of Douglas. A computed tomography of the pelvis in a woman with abundant ascites demonstrates fluid distension of the pouch of Douglas (*PD*) posterior to the uterus (*U*) and anterior to the rectum (*curved arrow*). The broad ligament (*long arrows*) is outlined by fluid anteriorly and posteriorly.

The Uterus and Vagina

Introduction

This chapter provides the reader a review of both normal sonographic anatomy and pathology associated with the uterus and vagina. The discussion will continue in regard to endometrial pathology in upcoming chapters to include postmenopausal bleeding and also intracavitary masses that can lead to abnormal uterine bleeding. In the *Bonus Review* section, a three-dimensional image of a submucosal fibroid can be seen, as well as a schematic and image of a uterine artery embolization and an example of an arteriovenous fistula.

Key Terms

adenomyoma—a focal mass of adenomyosis

adenomyosis—the benign invasion of endometrial tissue into the myometrium of the uterus

agenesis—failure of an organ or a structure to grow during embryologic development

amenorrhea—the absence of menstruation

anteflexion—the uterine body tilts forward and comes in contact with the cervix, forming an acute angle between the body and the cervix

anteversion—the typical version of the uterus where the uterine body tilts forward, forming a 90-degree angle with the cervix

Bartholin duct cyst—a benign cyst that is located in one of the Bartholin glands in the region of the vulva

basal layer (endometrium)—the outer layer of the endometrium

bicornuate uterus—a common uterine anomaly in which the endometrium divides into two horns; also referred to as bicornis unicollis

boggy—limp

broad ligaments—pelvic ligament that extends from the lateral aspect of the uterus to the side walls of the pelvis

cervical polyp—an overgrowth of epithelial cells within the cervix resulting in a broad based or pedunculated mass of tissue

cervix—the rigid region of the uterus located between the isthmus and the vagina

congenital malformations—physical defects that are present in a person at birth; may also be referred to as congenital anomalies

cornua (uterus)—areas just inferior to the fundus of the uterus where the fallopian tubes are attached bilaterally

corpus (uterus)—the uterine body

dextroverted uterus—the long axis of the uterus deviating to the right of the midline

diethylstilbestrol (DES)—a drug administered to pregnant woman from the 1940s to the 1970s to treat threatened abortions and premature labor that has been linked with uterine malformation in the exposed fetus

dyschezia—difficult or painful defecation

dysmenorrhea—difficult or painful menstruation

dyspareunia—painful sexual intercourse

dysuria—painful or difficult urination

endometrial cavity—area that lies between the two layers of the endometrium; may also be referred to as the uterine cavity

endometrium—the inner mucosal layer of the uterus

external os—the inferior portion of the cervix that is in close contact with the vagina

fibroid—see key term leiomyoma

functional layer (endometrium)—the functional inner layer of the endometrium that is altered by the hormones of the menstrual cycle

fundus (uterus)—the most superior and widest portion of the uterus

Gartner duct cyst—a benign cyst located within the vagina

hematocolpos—blood accumulation within the vagina

hematometra—blood accumulation within the uterine cavity

hematometrocolpos—blood accumulation within the uterus and vagina

hydrocolpos—fluid accumulation within the vagina

hydrometrocolpos—fluid accumulation within the uterus and vagina

hysterectomy—the surgical removal of the uterus

hysterosalpingography—a radiographic procedure that uses a dye instilled into the endometrial cavity and fallopian tubes to evaluate for internal abnormalities

hysteroscopic uterine septoplasty—the surgical repair of a uterine septum in a septate uterus using hysteroscopy

imperforate hymen—a vaginal anomaly in which the hymen has no opening, therefore resulting in an obstruction of the vagina

internal os—the superior portion of the cervix closest to the isthmus

intracavitary (fibroid)—a leiomyoma located within the uterine cavity

intramural (fibroid)—location of leiomyoma within the myometrium of the uterus

isthmus (uterus)—area of the uterus between the corpus and the cervix

leiomyoma (uterine)—a benign, smooth muscle tumor of the uterus; may also be referred to as a fibroid or uterine myoma

leiomyosarcoma—the malignant manifestation of a leiomyoma

levoverted uterus—the long axis of the uterus deviating to the left of the midline

lower uterine segment—the term used for the isthmus of the uterus during pregnancy

magnetic resonance imaging–guided high-intensity–focused ultrasound—a fibroid treatment that utilizes focused high-frequency, high-energy ultrasound guided by magnetic resonance imaging to heat and destroy fibroid tissue

menometrorrhagia—excessive and prolonged bleeding at irregular intervals

menorrhagia—abnormally heavy and prolonged menstruation

Müllerian ducts—paired embryonic ducts that develop into the female urogenital tract

multiparous—having birthed more than one child

myomectomy—the surgical removal of a myoma (fibroid) of the uterus

myometrium—the muscular layer of the uterus

nabothian cysts—benign cysts located within the cervix

neonatal—the first 4 weeks (28 days) after birth

nulliparous—never given birth

parity—the total number of pregnancies in which the patient has given birth to a fetus at or beyond 20 weeks' gestational age or an infant weighing more than 500 g

pedunculated—something that grows off of a stalk

perimetrium—the outer layer of the uterus; may also be referred to as the serosal layer

precocious puberty—pubertal development before the age of 7; the early development of pubic hair, breast, or genitals

pseudoprecocious puberty—secondary sexual development induced by sex steroids or from other sources such as ovarian tumors, adrenal tumors, or steroid use

retroflexion—the uterine body tilts backward and comes in contact with the cervix, forming an acute angle between the body and the cervix

retroversion—the uterine body tilts backward, without a bend where the cervix and body meet

saline infusion sonohysterography—a sonographic procedure that uses saline instillation into the endometrial cavity and, possibly, the fallopian tubes to evaluate for internal abnormalities; also referred to as sonohysterography

septate uterus—common congenital malformation of the uterus that results in a single septum that separates two endometrial cavities

serosal layer (uterus)—the outermost layer of the uterus; may also be referred to as the perimetrium

submucosal (fibroid)—a leiomyoma that distorts the shape of the endometrium

subseptate uterus—congenital malformation of the uterus that results in a normal uterine contour with an endometrium that branches into two horns

subserosal (fibroid)—location of a leiomyoma in which the tumor grows outward and distorts the contour of the uterus

torsion—twisting

unicornuate uterus—congenital malformation of the uterus that results in a uterus with one horn

uterine artery embolization—procedure used to block the blood supply to a leiomyoma (fibroid)

uterine myoma—see key term leiomyoma

uterus didelphys—congenital malformation of the uterus that results in the complete duplication of the uterus, cervix, and vagina

vaginal atresia—occlusion or imperforation of the vagina; can be congenital or acquired

vaginal cuff—the portion of the vagina remaining after a hysterectomy

vaginal fornices—recesses of the vagina

vulva—collective term for the mons pubis, labia majora and labia minora, vestibule, Bartholin gland, and clitoris

EMBRYOLOGIC DEVELOPMENT OF THE FEMALE UROGENITAL TRACT

Though the two genders are initially indistinguishable, genetic gender is determined at fertilization or conception. Female development does not require estrogen but rather the absence of testosterone. It is the presence of the Y chromosome that supplies testis-determining factor, resulting in male gender development. Nonetheless, gender is not typically apparent until about the 12th week of embryonic life.

During the embryonic period, the uterus and kidneys develop at essentially the same time, hence the reason why they are included together as parts of the urogenital (genitourinary) system. Therefore, it is safe to assume that when there are congenital anomalies recognized on a routine sonogram of the uterus, coexisting anomalies may be present in the kidneys. In fact, about 10% of infants are born with an abnormality of the genitourinary system. For this reason, patients who present with uterine anomalies may also require a urinary tract sonogram. A list of renal anomalies is provided in Chapter 7 of this text, the most common being that of a duplicated or duplex renal collecting system.

The uterus, vagina, and fallopian tubes develop from the paired **Müllerian ducts** (paramesonephric ducts). Incomplete fusion, partial fusion, or agenesis of the Müllerian ducts will result in an anatomic variant of the uterus, cervix, and/or vagina that may be recognized sonographically. Thus, these anatomic variants may also be referred to as Müllerian anomalies or **congenital malformations**. Congenital malformations are discussed later in this chapter (see "Congenital Uterine Anomalies" section).

> 🔊 **SOUND OFF**
> Congenital anomalies of the kidneys and uterus often coexist.

ANATOMY AND PHYSIOLOGY OF THE UTERUS AND VAGINA

The uterus is a pear-shaped, retroperitoneal organ that lies anterior to the rectum and posterior to the urinary bladder and is bounded laterally by the **broad**

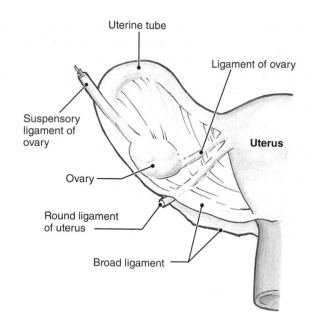

Figure 17-1 Schematic of the relationship of the uterus, ovary, and broad ligament.

ligaments (Fig. 17-1). Its primary function is to provide a place for the products of conception to implant and develop. The uterus can be divided into four major divisions: **fundus, corpus, isthmus,** and **cervix** (Fig. 17-2). The fundus is the most superior and widest portion of the uterus. Each fallopian tube attaches to the uterus at the level of the uterine horns called the **cornua**. The largest part of the uterus is the corpus, or body. The corpus is located inferior to the fundus. The isthmus is the area located between the corpus and the cervix. During pregnancy, the isthmus may be referred to as the **lower uterine segment**. The cervix is the rigid

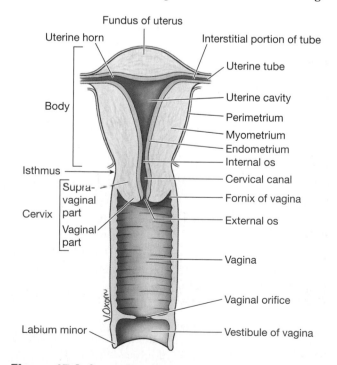

Figure 17-2 Coronal uterine anatomy.

component of the uterus that is located inferior to the isthmus, and it is the portion of the uterus that projects into the vagina. The cervix is marked superiorly by the **internal os**, which is in contact with the isthmus, and inferiorly by the **external os**, which is in close contact with the vagina.

> 🔊 **SOUND OFF**
> During pregnancy, the isthmus may be referred to as the lower uterine segment.

The vagina is a tubular organ that extends from the external os of the cervix to the external genitalia. The **vaginal fornices** (singular form is fornix) envelop the inferior aspect of the cervix. The vagina is composed of three layers: inner mucosal layer, middle muscular layer, and an outer layer that may be referred to as the adventitia. Sonographically, the divisions of the uterus can be demonstrated (Fig. 17-3).

The uterine wall consists of three layers (Fig. 17-4). The outermost layer is referred to as the **serosal layer** or **perimetrium**, which is continuous with the fascia of the pelvis. The middle layer is the **myometrium** or muscular layer, which constitutes the bulk of the uterine tissue, providing the area where contractile motion occurs. The inner mucosal layer of the uterus is referred to as the **endometrium**. The endometrium can be further divided into a deep or **basal layer** and a superficial or **functional layer** (Fig. 17-5).

The thickness of the basal layer is typically consistent, although minimal changes may occur throughout the menstrual cycle. The functional layer of the endometrium is the component that is shed during menstruation; thus, the thickness of the functional layer of endometrium will vary during the menstrual cycle

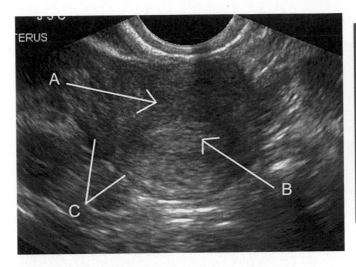

Figure 17-4 Endovaginal transverse image of the uterus demonstrating the myometrium (*A*), the endometrium (*B*), and the serosa (*C*).

as a result of hormonal stimulation. The **endometrial cavity**, also referred to as the uterine cavity, is located between the two functional layers of the endometrium. This cavity is contiguous with the lumen of the fallopian tubes laterally and the cervix inferiorly.

> 🔊 **SOUND OFF**
> The endometrial cavity, also referred to as the uterine cavity, is located between the two functional layers of the endometrium.

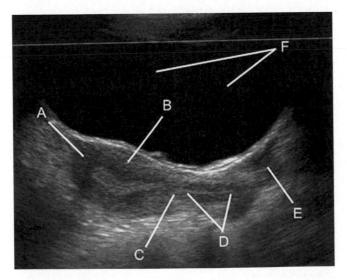

Figure 17-3 Sagittal transabdominal image of the uterus demonstrating posterior to the distended urinary bladder (*F*), the uterine fundus (*A*), uterine corpus (*B*), uterine isthmus (*C*), cervix (*D*), and vagina (*E*).

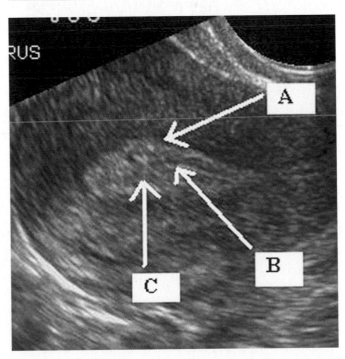

Figure 17-5 Sagittal endovaginal image of the endometrium demonstrating the outermost basal layer (*A*), the innermost echogenic stripe of the uterine cavity (*B*), and the functional layer (*C*).

Uterine Size and Shape

The size and shape of the uterus depends on the age of the patient, **parity**, and the presence of pathology or congenital anomalies that may alter its contour. The normal **neonatal** uterus is prominent and tubular in appearance and may exhibit distinct endometrial echoes in the first week of life as a result of maternal hormone stimulation (Fig. 17-6). Following the neonatal period, the cervical anteroposterior (AP) diameter is equal to or slightly greater than that of the uterine fundus. The normal prepubertal uterus has a cervix-to-uterus ratio of 2:1. The uterus grows minimally during prepubertal years, whereas after puberty, the uterine fundus becomes much larger than the cervix, consequently providing the pear-shaped appearance of the normal adult uterus. Uterine growth is secondary to an increase in circulating hormones both during and after puberty.

In the adult, the length of the uterus in the **nulliparous** individual is typically between 6 to 8.5 cm in length and 2 to 4 cm in AP diameter, whereas in the multiparous individuals, the uterus typically measures between 8 to 10.5 cm in length and 3 to 5 cm in AP diameter. Following menopause, the uterus typically becomes much smaller than the premenopausal uterus (Figs. 17-7 and 17-8). The postmenopausal uterus measures between 3.5 to 7.5 cm in length and 1.7 to 3.3 in AP diameter, with a thin endometrium (Fig. 17-9).

> **SOUND OFF**
> A newborn baby girl may have a thickened endometrium. This is caused by the stimulation of the baby's endometrium by maternal hormones.

Uterine Positions

The uterine position within the pelvis is variable (Fig. 17-10). Though the cervix is anchored at the angle of the bladder and is thus not typically highly mobile, the corpus and fundus are somewhat movable. The normal position of the uterus is considered to be **anteversion** or **anteflexion**. **Anteversion** describes the uterine position in which the body tilts forward or anteriorly, forming a 90-degree angle with the vagina. **Anteflexion** of the uterus denotes the position in which the uterine body folds forward, possibly coming in contact with the cervix. **Retroversion** of the uterus is the position in which the uterine body tilts backward or posteriorly, without a bend where the cervix and body meet (Fig. 17-11). **Retroflexion** is the uterine position that results in the uterine body tilting backward and actually coming in contact with the cervix (Fig. 17-12). The uterus may also be oriented more to the left or right of the midline, resulting in a variation between anatomic midline and functional midline. The uterus that is located more on the left is referred to as a **levoverted uterus**, whereas the uterus that is located on the right is referred to as **dextroverted uterus**.

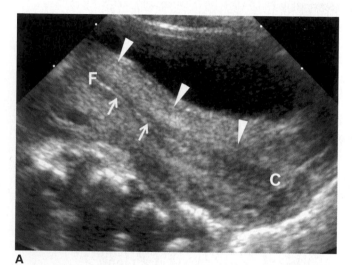

A

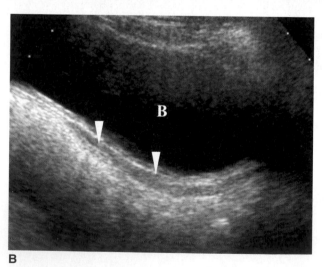

B

Figure 17-6 Variance in uterine size with age. **A.** Neonatal uterus. Longitudinal image shows a prominent uterus (*arrowheads*) with the cervix (*C*) and fundus (*F*) having a bulbous configuration and being of similar size. Note the thin echogenic endometrial stripe (*arrows*) as a result of maternal hormonal stimulation. **B.** An 8-year-old girl. The uterus (*arrowheads*) is smaller and still tubular in configuration with no differentiation between fundus and cervix. *B*, bladder.

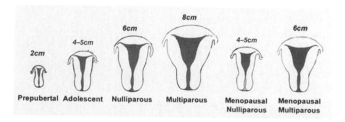

Figure 17-7 Changes in uterine size with age and parity.

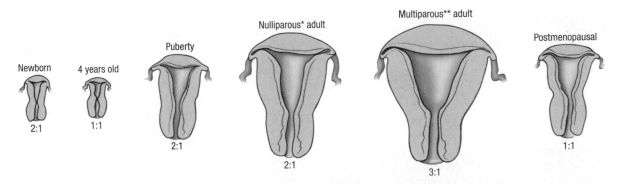

Figure 17-8 Lifetime changes in uterine body-to-cervical ratio.

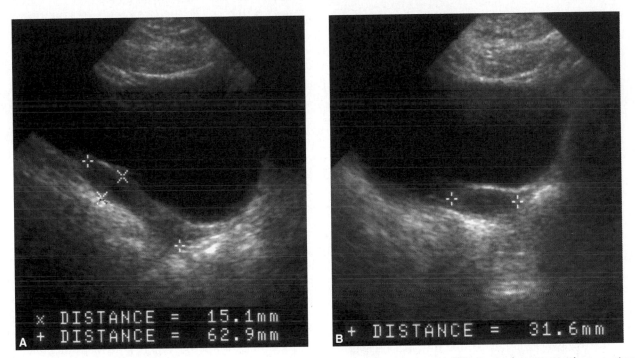

Figure 17-9 Postmenopausal uterus. Transabdominal sagittal (**A**) and transverse (**B**) views demonstrating an atrophic postmenopausal uterus (between *calipers*).

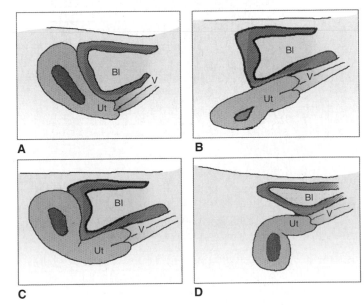

Figure 17-10 Various uterine positions. **A.** Anteverted. **B.** Retroverted. **C.** Anteflexed. **D.** Retroflexed. Note the septum where the uterus folds over on itself.

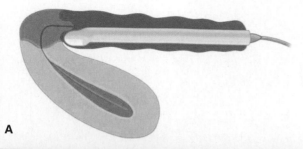

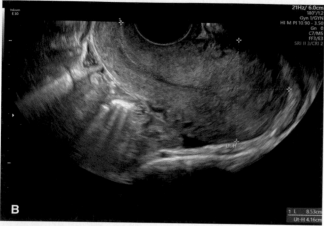

Figure 17-11 Retroverted uterus. **A.** Drawing of ultrasound transducer relative to retroverted uterus. **B.** Sagittal midline sonogram image of a retroverted uterus.

🔊 **SOUND OFF**
The normal position of the uterus is considered to be anteversion or anteflexion.

Congenital Uterine Anomalies

As stated earlier, uterine malformations are a result of fusion anomalies of the Müllerian ducts. For this reason, they may also be referred to as Müllerian ducts anomalies

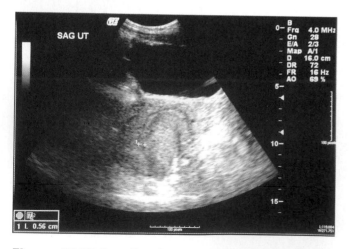

Figure 17-12 Retroflexed uterus. Transabdominal sagittal image of a retroflexed uterus. The endometrium is measured between the calipers.

(Fig. 17-13). **Agenesis** of the uterus is uncommon. A **bicornuate uterus**, also referred to as bicornis unicollis, is a common uterine anomaly that is present when the endometrium divides into two endometrial cavities with one cervix, with a prominent concavity noted in the outline of the uterine fundus (Fig. 17-14). The **unicornuate uterus** is present when the uterus has only one horn. The **septate uterus**, which is also a common Müllerian duct anomaly, describes a uterus that has two complete separate uterine cavities separated by an AP septum (Fig. 17-15). The **subseptate uterus**, which is characterized by an incomplete septum, has a normal uterine contour with an endometrium that branches into two horns. The arcuate uterus is a subtle variant in which the endometrium has a concave contour at the uterine fundus. The **uterus didelphys** is complete duplication of the vagina, cervix, and uterus (Fig. 17-16).

🔊 **SOUND OFF**
The word part "colli" refers to the neck or cervix of the uterus, whereas the word part "cornu" refers to the horn of the uterus. For example, bicornis unicollis is interpreted as two horns with a cervix, whereas bicornis bicollis is interpreted as two horns with a double cervix.

Some studies claim that intrauterine exposure to **diethylstilbestrol (DES)** has resulted in the formation of congenital malformation of the uterus (Fig. 17-17). DES was a drug administered to pregnant woman from the 1940s to the 1970s to treat threatened abortions and premature labor. The female fetus exposed to DES in utero had an increased likelihood of developing a congenital uterine malformation. Congenital malformations have been linked to menstrual disorders, infertility, and obstetric complications. Specifically, the septate uterus has an explicit connection with spontaneous abortion.

In the past, **hysterosalpingography**, which is a radiographic study that utilizes contrast to evaluate the uterine cavity and fallopian tubes, was often performed on women with suggested congenital uterine malformations or who are suffering from infertility (Fig. 17-18). But most recently, sonography has become a valuable tool as well. Two-dimensional (3D) ultrasound can be helpful in identifying the presence of possible uterine malformations that involve variants of the endometrium during routine examinations. However, 3D ultrasound, with an accuracy rate of greater than 90% for detecting uterine malformations, has become exceedingly useful (Fig. 17-19). **Saline infusion sonohysterography**, which may also be referred to as simply **sonohysterography**, can be used to provide additional helpful information in regard to congenital uterine malformations. For patients with a septate uterus, sonography can also aid in the resection of the septum during a **hysteroscopic uterine**

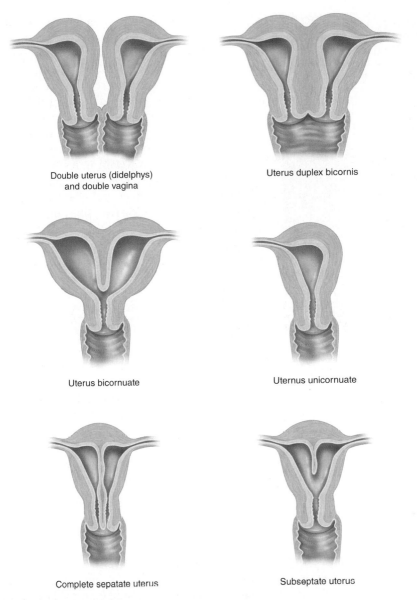

Double uterus (didelphys) and double vagina

Uterus duplex bicornis

Uterus bicornuate

Uternus unicornuate

Complete sepatate uterus

Subseptate uterus

Figure 17-13 Congenital uterine anomalies.

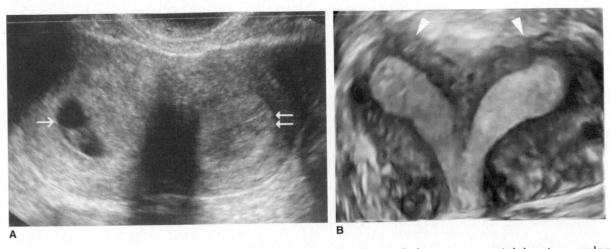

A

B

Figure 17-14 Bicornuate uterus. **A.** Transabdominal transverse image of the uterus containing two endometrial cavities, one without a gestational sac (*double arrows*) and one with a gestational sac (*single arrow*). **B.** Bicornuate uterus demonstrated by three-dimensional reconstruction. Coronal reconstructed image showing indentation of the uterine fundus, splaying the uterus and endometrial cavities into two horns (*arrowheads*).

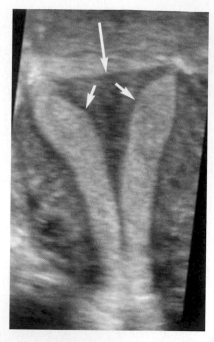

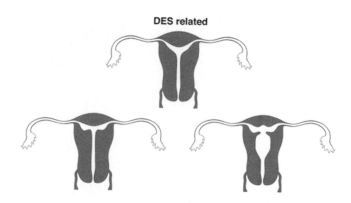

Figure 17-17 Diethylstilbestrol (*DES*) anomalies. Uterine anomalies associated with in utero DES exposure. The classic anomaly is a T-shaped uterus.

> 🔊)) **SOUND OFF**
> The septate uterus is said to be one of the most common Müllerian duct anomalies.

Figure 17-15 Septate uterus. Three-dimensional reformatting of a septate uterus in the coronal plane demonstrating the presence of two separate endometriums (*short arrows*) within the fundus (*long arrow*) of the uterus.

septoplasty. Other imaging modalities and techniques, such as computed tomography, magnetic resonance imaging (MRI), and laparoscopy, may be utilized to identify and further investigate evidence of congenital uterine malformations.

Congenital Malformation of the Vagina

Congenital malformations of the vagina can lead to the accumulation of fluid within the female genital tract secondary to an obstruction. The obstruction can be the result of **vaginal atresia**, a vaginal septum, or an **imperforate hymen**. The consequence of this obstruction could lead to the distension of the vagina, cervix, uterus, and fallopian tubes with fluid or blood.

Hydrocolpos describes the condition in which the vagina is distended with simple, anechoic fluid and is

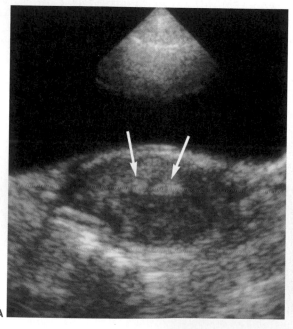

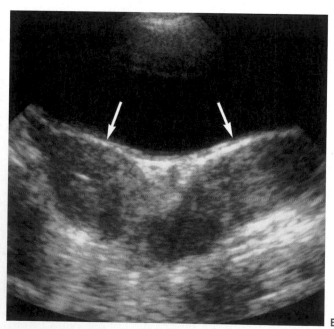

Figure 17-16 Didelphic uterus. **A.** Transverse transabdominal image of the cervix revealing two separate endocervical canals (*arrows*). **B.** Transverse transabdominal image of the upper uterus demonstrating a separate right and left uterine horn (*arrows*).

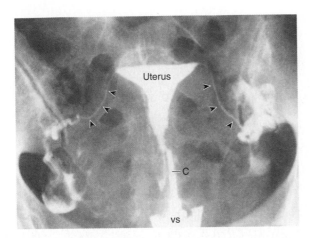

Figure 17-18 Hysterosalpingogram. A hysterosalpingogram is a radiographic (x-ray) procedure that requires the instillation of contrast media into the uterus and fallopian tubes. *Arrowheads*, uterine tubes; *c*, catheter in the cervical canal, *vs*, vaginal speculum.

seen more often in the neonatal period (Fig. 17-20). As the vagina distends with fluid, excessive amounts may lead to further accumulation of the fluid into the uterus, a condition known as **hydrometrocolpos**. Clinically, neonatal patients with vaginal obstructions present with a palpable pelvic or abdominal mass as a result of an excessive buildup of vaginal secretions in utero.

Patients may have blood components from menstruation retained in the uterine cavity or vagina, termed **hematometra** and **hematocolpos**, respectively (Figs. 17-21 and 17-22). They may also have **hematometrocolpos**, a condition when both the

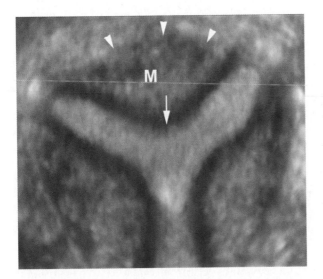

Figure 17-19 Three-dimensional (*3D*) sonography of arcuate uterus. True coronal view of the uterus, obtained by reconstruction using 3D sonography, demonstrating the myometrium (*M*) in the uterine fundus dips down with a rounded configuration (*arrow*) into the endometrium, indicating an arcuate uterus. The fundus had a normal shape (*arrowheads*).

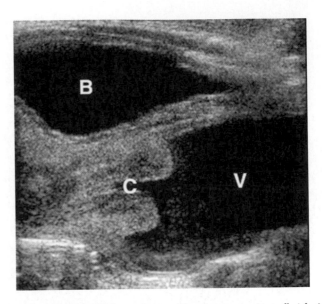

Figure 17-20 Hydrocolpos. Simple-appearing fluid is noted posterior to the urinary bladder (*B*) and inferior to the cervix (*C*) within the vagina (*V*) in this sagittal image of the neonatal pelvis.

uterine cavity and the vagina are filled with blood. This obstruction is frequently associated with the presence of an imperforate hymen in young girls. Clinically, these patients will present with **amenorrhea**, cyclic abdominal pain, an abdominal mass, enlarged uterus, and, possibly, urinary retention.

))) SOUND OFF
The word part "colpo" refers to the vagina, whereas the word part "metra" refers to the uterus. Thus, hydrocolpos is interpreted as fluid in the vagina, whereas hydrometrocolpos refers to fluid in both the uterus and the vagina.

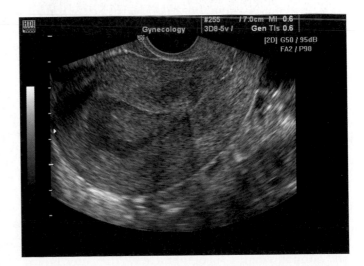

Figure 17-21 Hematometra. Sagittal endovaginal image of the endometrium. The uterus is distended with echogenic fluid representing blood.

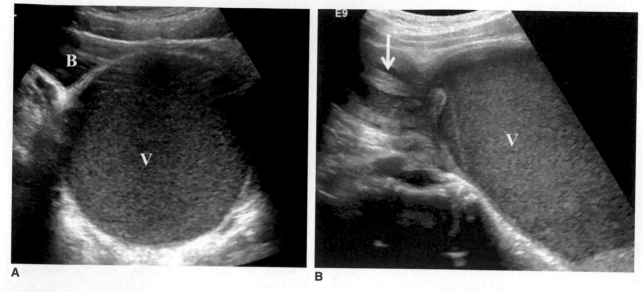

Figures 17-22 Hematocolpos in a 13-year-old girl with pelvic pain. **A.** Transverse and **B.** longitudinal images show a markedly distended vagina (*V*) and mildly dilated endometrial canal (*arrow*), both containing internal echoes representing blood. *B*, bladder.

CLINICAL FINDINGS OF VAGINAL OBSTRUCTIONS

1. Cyclic pelvic pain (often at the time of menses in adolescent girls)
2. Enlarged uterus
3. Abdominal pain
4. Urinary retention
5. Amenorrhea (adolescent girls)

SONOGRAPHIC FINDINGS OF VAGINAL OBSTRUCTIONS

1. Distension of the uterus or vagina or both with anechoic or complex fluid

UTERINE PATHOLOGY

Adenomyosis

Adenomyosis is the invasion of endometrial tissue into the myometrium and is a common cause of abnormal uterine bleeding. For unknown reasons, endometrial tissue is allowed to invade the myometrium (Fig. 17-23). The basal layer of the endometrium can often extend into the myometrium at depths of at least 2.5 mm. The involvement of adenomyosis may be either focal or diffuse and is typically found more often within the fundus and posterior portion of the uterus (Fig. 17-24). Focal adenomyosis in the form of a mass is termed an **adenomyoma**. Sonographically, the uterus will appear diffusely enlarged and heterogeneous. There may be indistinct hypoechoic or echogenic areas

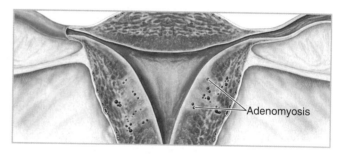

Figure 17-23 Adenomyosis. Adenomyosis occurs when endometrial cells grow within the wall of the uterus. This may cause heavy and painful menstrual cycles.

scattered throughout the myometrium, with small myometrial cysts noted as well (Fig. 17-25). Thickening of the posterior myometrium can also be recognized. Adenomyosis is often present in the uterus afflicted with **fibroid** tumors. Up to 20% of patients with adenomyosis suffer from endometriosis as well.

SOUND OFF
Adenomyosis is often present in the uterus afflicted with fibroid tumors.

The clinical presentation of adenomyosis is varied and nonspecific, with most women experiencing **dyschezia**, **dysmenorrhea**, **menometrorrhagia**, pelvic pain, and **dyspareunia**. They also typically have these symptoms up to 2 weeks before the onset of menstrual flow. Patients often have a **boggy**, enlarged, and tender uterus upon physical examination. Although sonography is steadily becoming a valuable diagnostic instrument in

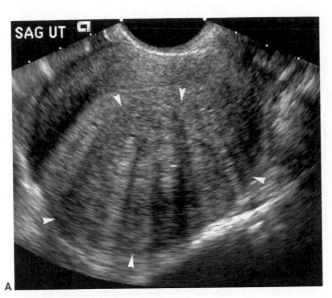
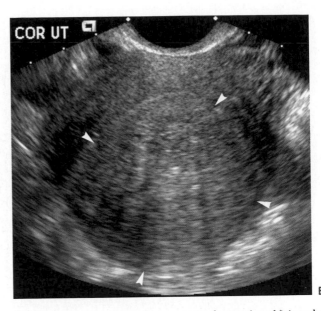

Figure 17-24 Adenomyosis. Sagittal (**A**) and coronal (**B**) of a uterus demonstrating adenomyosis (*arrowheads*) involving the posterior myometrium.

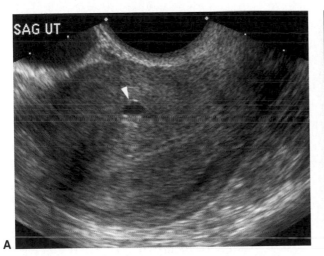
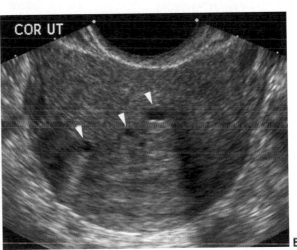

Figure 17-25 Adenomyosis and myometrial cysts. **A.** Myometrial cyst (*arrowhead*) associated with adenomyosis. **B.** Myometrial cysts (*arrowheads*) are noted throughout the uterus in a patient who is suffering from adenomyosis.

the diagnosis of adenomyosis, MRI appears to provide important diagnostic information (Fig. 17-26). Treatment for adenomyosis is hysterectomy or hormone therapy, with the latter often producing limited, if any, relief from symptoms. An important differentiation should be made between endometriosis and adenomyosis. Patients with endometriosis tend to be younger and have fertility troubles, whereas those with adenomyosis are often older (average age is older than 40) and **multiparous**. Other risk factors include increased early menarche and shorter menstrual cycles.

CLINICAL FINDINGS OF ADENOMYOSIS

1. Uterine enlargement
2. Boggy, tender uterus
3. Dysmenorrhea
4. Menometrorrhagia
5. Pelvic pain
6. Dyschezia
7. Dyspareunia
8. Multiparous

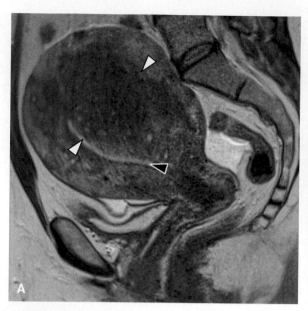
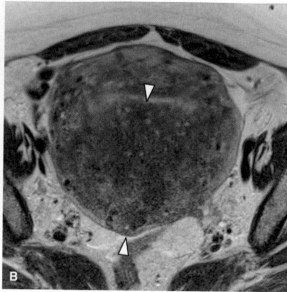

Figure 17-26 Adenomyosis on magnetic resonance imaging (*MRI*). **A.** Sagittal MRI demonstrates marked thickening of the posterior junctional zone of the uterus (*white arrowheads*), measuring up to 49 mm. There are associated foci noted that are typical of adenomyosis, which represent ectopic glandular foci. There is anterior displacement of the endometrium (*black arrowhead*). **B.** Axial MRI demonstrates marked thickening of the posterior junctional zone of the uterus (*arrowheads*) with evidence of glandular foci.

SONOGRAPHIC FINDINGS OF ADENOMYOSIS

1. Diffusely enlarged uterus
2. Hypoechoic or echogenic areas adjacent to endometrium
3. Heterogeneous myometrium
4. Myometrial cysts
5. Ill-defined interface between myometrium and endometrium
6. Thickening of the fundus or posterior myometrium

Uterine Leiomyoma

The **leiomyoma** is a benign, smooth muscle tumor of the uterus that may also be referred to as a fibroid or **uterine myoma**. Leiomyomas (leiomyomata) are the most common benign gynecologic tumors and the leading cause of hysterectomy and gynecologic surgery. These tumors can vary in size and may alter the shape of the uterus and have varying sonographic appearances. Those who are at greater risk for the development of fibroids are women who are obese, black, nonsmokers, and perimenopausal. There also appears to be a familial link, with first-degree relatives of women with fibroids having a 2.5 times greater risk of having fibroid themselves. Clinical findings include pelvic pressure, **menorrhagia**, palpable abdominal mass, enlarged uterus, urinary frequency, **dysuria**, constipation, and, possibly, infertility.

Sonographically, fibroids often appear as solid, hypoechoic masses that produce posterior shadowing.

Degenerating fibroids may have calcifications or cystic components, whereas multiple fibroids may cause diffuse uterine enlargement and heterogeneity. Fibroid degeneration occurs because as the fibroid enlarges, it outgrows its blood supply, possibly leading to pain. A uterus that is distorted by multiple leiomyomas may be referred to as a fibroid uterus. A fibroid uterus will be enlarged and have an irregular shape. Because fibroids are made up of smooth muscles fibers surrounded by a vascular pseudocapsule, color Doppler may be helpful to identify the borders of these tumors, thus aiding in measuring them appropriately.

> **SOUND OFF**
> Leiomyomas are the most common benign gynecologic tumors and the leading cause of hysterectomy and gynecologic surgery.

Fibroids are also described by their location (Figs. 17-27 and 17-28). The most common location for fibroids is **intramural**, or within the myometrium. A **subserosal** fibroid grows outward and distorts the contour of the uterus. Subserosal fibroids that are **pedunculated** (on a stalk), or those associated with the broad ligament, could resemble adnexal masses. Pedunculated fibroids may undergo **torsion** as well, thus cutting off the blood supply to the mass. This lack of blood supply results in necrosis, and clinically, the patient will present with acute, localized pelvic pain. **Submucosal** fibroids are located adjacent to the endometrial cavity and often

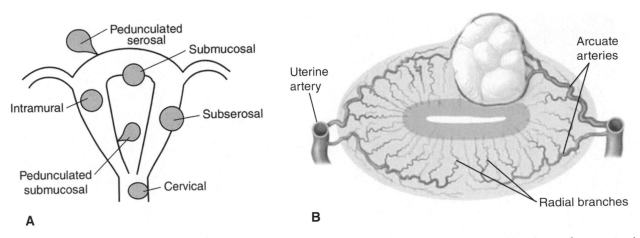

Figure 17-27 Location and blood supply to fibroids. **A.** Possible locations of fibroids. **B.** Blood supply to a typical, subserosal leiomyoma, with enlarged end vessels supplying the fibroid, with separate supply to the normal myometrium.

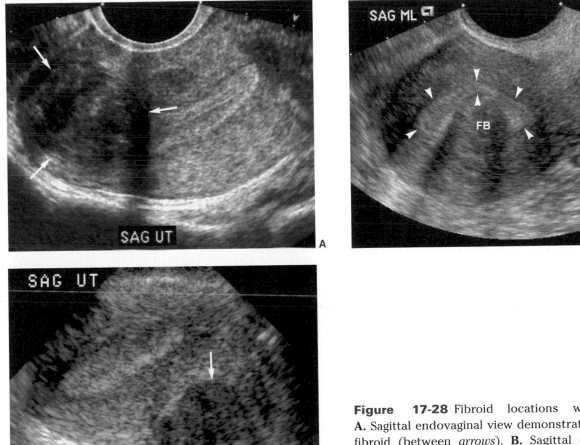

Figure 17-28 Fibroid locations with sonography. **A.** Sagittal endovaginal view demonstrating an intramural fibroid (between *arrows*). **B.** Sagittal endovaginal view demonstrating a submucosal fibroid (*FB*). Note the distortion of the endometrium (*arrowheads*). **C.** Sagittal endovaginal view showing a subserosal fibroid (*long arrows*).

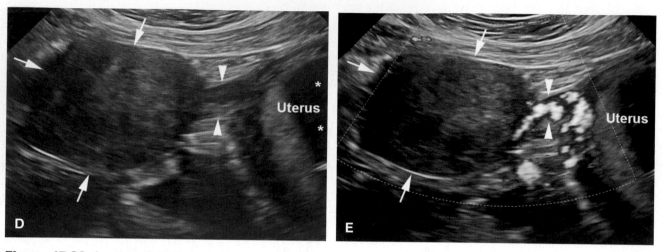

Figure 17-28 (*continued*) **D.** Pedunculated fibroid (between *arrows*) is demonstrated in this image connected to the uterus by a stalk (between *arrowhead*). **E.** Color flow is noted within the stalk (between *arrowheads*) connecting the fibroid (between *arrows*) to the uterus.

distort the shape of the endometrium. **Intracavitary** fibroids, the fibroids located within the uterine cavity, and submucosal fibroids usually lead to abnormal uterine bleeding because of their location in relationship to the endometrium. Some fibroids may also extend into the cervix when pedunculated and may prolapse into the vagina as well. Saline infusion sonohysterography may be utilized to better evaluate submucosal and intracavitary fibroids.

> **SOUND OFF**
> Pedunculated fibroids may undergo torsion, thus cutting off the blood supply to the mass. This lack of blood supply results in necrosis, and clinically, the patient will present with acute, localized pelvic pain.

Fibroid growth has been associated with estrogen stimulation, and consequently, their size may increase during pregnancy and reduce after menopause. A decrease in estrogen exposure secondary to smoking, exercise, and increased parity reduces the likelihood of developing fibroids.

Fibroids may also impact fertility if they are intracavitary or submucosal, because the location of these fibroids may result in a higher incidence of spontaneous abortion. Fibroids may also affect the contractile motion of the uterus, thus leading to interference with sperm migration. A concurrent intrauterine pregnancy and fibroid can be sonographically identified, although often this occurrence does not result in preterm labor or early pregnancy loss. Alternatively, fibroids may prevent cervical dilation during pregnancy, thus often requiring a cesarean section to be performed at the time of delivery.

> **SOUND OFF**
> Fibroids may impact fertility if they are intracavitary or submucosal, because the location of these fibroids may result in a higher incidence of spontaneous abortion.

The medical treatment for fibroids is hormone therapy and targeted drugs, which typically results in a reduction in tumor size. Surgical treatment may be either **hysterectomy** or **myomectomy**. Myomectomy is the surgical removal of a fibroid and may be performed abdominally or laparoscopically. Another alternative treatment for fibroids involves **uterine artery embolization**, which is used to obstruct the blood supply to the mass. Uterine artery embolization, which is performed under fluoroscopic guidance, results in a reduction in the size of the mass and also in a decline in the associated clinical symptoms. **Magnetic resonance imaging–guided high-intensity–focused ultrasound** offers an additional noninvasive management of fibroids that uses focused high-frequency, high-energy ultrasound guided by MRI to heat and destroy fibroid tissue.

CLINICAL FINDINGS OF A UTERINE LEIOMYOMA

1. Pelvic pressure
2. Menorrhagia
3. Palpable pelvic mass
4. Enlarged, bulky uterus (if multiple)
5. Urinary frequency
6. Dysuria
7. Constipation
8. Infertility

Leiomyosarcoma

Leiomyosarcoma was initially thought to be the malignant counterpart of the normally benign leiomyoma, though because of genetic differences and further investigation of the disease, leiomyosarcomas are now thought to be less likely the result of malignant degeneration of a benign fibroid. And though this pathway of disease can occur, it is exceedingly rare, occurring only between 0.13% and 0.81% of the time. African American women have a higher incidence of leiomyosarcoma. The median age of leiomyosarcomas is 54.

Although not specific, these masses are characterized by a rapid increase in growth over a short period of time (Fig. 17-29). They are also more commonly found in perimenopausal or postmenopausal woman. Their sonographic appearance is variable, and they may appear similar to a benign fibroid, with some evidence of degeneration. Clinically, patients with leiomyosarcoma may be initially asymptomatic or may present with the same symptoms as the benign leiomyoma, including pelvic pain and pressure. Treatment is typically in the form of a total hysterectomy, with postmenopausal women undergoing a bilateral salpingo-oophorectomy as well.

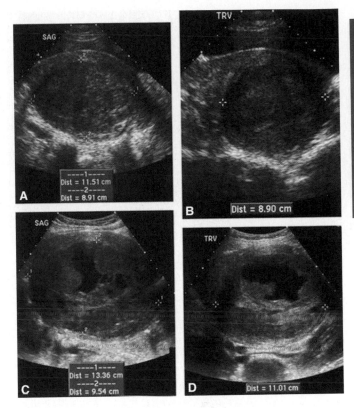

Figure 17-29 Leiomyosarcoma. Sagittal (*SAG*) (**A**) and transverse (*TRV*) (**B**) transabdominal views of the uterus in a postmenopausal woman demonstrating a hypoechoic mass (*calipers*) in the uterus. This mass was initially diagnosed as a benign fibroid. Sagittal (**C**) and transverse (**D**) views 5 months later showing the mass has grown substantially. Pathology following a hysterectomy revealed the diagnosis of leiomyosarcoma.

Nabothian Cyst

Nabothian cysts are common findings on routine sonographic examinations. These benign retention cysts are located within the cervix and may cause cervical enlargement on physical examination. Nabothian cysts are classically simple but may have some internal debris or septations, which may represent hemorrhage or infection. Nabothian cysts are typically asymptomatic and may be multiple (see Fig. 17-30).

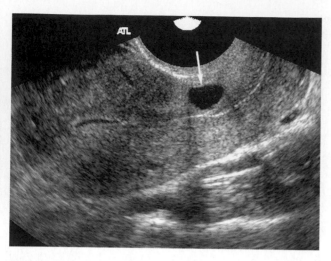

Figure 17-30 Nabothian cyst. Sagittal endovaginal view of the uterus revealing a cyst with the cervix (*arrow*), which is highly specific for a nabothian cyst.

PATHOLOGY OF THE CERVIX

Cervical Carcinoma, Cervical Stenosis, and Cervical Polyp

Cervical carcinoma is the most common female malignancy in women younger than 50 years. The greatest risk factor for cervical cancer is the human papillomavirus. Although cervical carcinoma is not routinely diagnosed with sonography, when seen, it may present as an inhomogeneous, bulky, enlarged cervix or as a focal mass within the cervix. Loss of the normal cervical canal may occur as well. The cervical width should not exceed 4 cm, and color Doppler typically demonstrated increased vascularity (Fig. 17-31).

Transvaginal and transrectal imaging are methods in which sonography can be used to better visualize the cervix. Masses may be large enough to obstruct the cervix, thus leading to hydrometra or hematometra. In patients who have had a hysterectomy, the cervical remnant should not exceed 4.4 cm in the AP plane and 4.3 cm in length. Patients who have undergone an abdominal hysterectomy may have no cervical remnant, but rather a **vaginal cuff** (Fig. 17-32). This cuff should not exceed 2 cm. Enlargement or a notable mass in the area of the cervical remnant or vaginal cuff will most likely lead to more imaging and possible a biopsy. Obtaining a thorough clinical history from patients is vital because sonographic findings will differ in relation to what type of hysterectomy was performed.

Cervical stenosis, which is the narrowing of the endocervical canal, often leads to an abnormal quantity of fluid in the endocervical or endometrial canals. It can be the result of a tumor in the cervix, cervical fibroid, **cervical polyp**, cervical infection, cervical atrophy, or scarring of the cervix following radiation treatment for cancer (Fig. 17-33). Clinically, women with cervical stenosis may be asymptomatic, whereas those who are still menstruating may present with absent menstrual flow when expected. In some women, an enlarged uterus may be noted during a physical examination as well. A cervical polyp is an overgrowth of epithelial cells within the cervix, resulting in a broad based or pedunculated mass of tissue. Patients with a cervical polyp may be asymptomatic; however, some may suffer from chronic inflammation, bleeding, or, possibly, infection.

> **SOUND OFF**
> Cervical stenosis can be the result of an obstructing tumor, fibroid, or polyp in the cervix. In addition, cervical infection, cervical atrophy, or scarring of the cervix following radiation treatment for cancer can result in stenosis of the cervix.

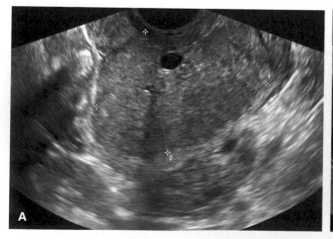
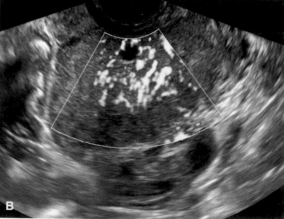

Figure 17-31 Cervical carcinoma. **A.** Transverse image of cervix in a 52-year-old patient with postmenopausal bleeding showing a large solid cervical mass (*calipers*). **B.** Color Doppler image of the mass showing abundant blood flow, a finding suggestive of malignancy.

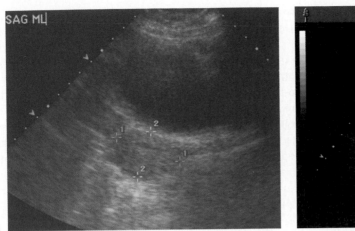

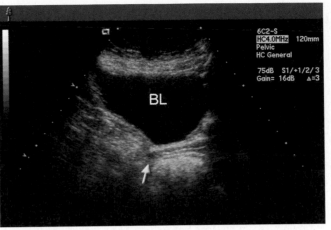

Figure 17-32 Hysterectomy appearance on sonography. **A.** Transabdominal sagittal sonogram of a patient who had a supracervical hysterectomy. This 72-year-old patient has a normal amount of prominent tissue (between *calipers*). **B.** Transabdominal image of a post-hysterectomy patient. The vaginal cuff (*arrow*) images posterior to the bladder (*BL*).

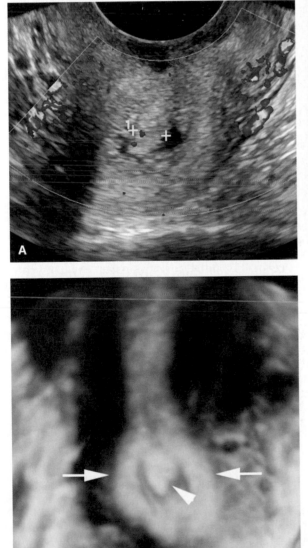

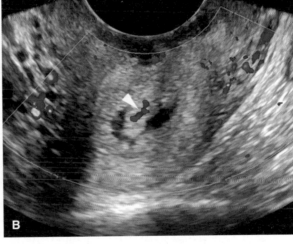

Figure 17-33 Cervical polyp. **A.** Coronal image of cervix showing a small echogenic mass (*calipers*) protruding into the cervical canal, representing a polyp. **B.** Color Doppler image shows a feeding vessel (*arrowhead*) to the cervical polyp. **C.** Three-dimensional image of cervix (*arrows*) showing polyp (*arrowhead*) within the cervical canal.

PATHOLOGY OF THE VAGINA

Gartner Duct Cyst

The vagina can be imaged well with transabdominal imaging. A **Gartner duct cyst** may be noted within the vagina. They are typically small and located along the wall of the vagina. **Gartner duct cysts** are often asymptomatic. Gartner duct cysts are thought to be remnants of the mesonephric or Wolffian duct. Sonographically, they may appear anechoic or complex (Fig. 17-34).

CLINICAL FINDINGS OF A GARTNER DUCT CYST

1. Asymptomatic

SONOGRAPHIC FINDINGS OF A GARTNER DUCT CYST

1. Anechoic or complex mass within the vagina

BARTHOLIN DUCT CYST AND BARTHOLIN DUCT ABSCESS

A **Bartholin duct cyst** is a benign cyst that is located in one of the Bartholin glands in the region of the **vulva**. There are two Bartholin ducts, which are essentially mucus-secreting glands, located on the posterolateral aspect of the vaginal orifice. It is obstruction of these glands that lead to a Bartholin duct cyst and possibly to a Bartholin duct abscess.

Sonography can be utilized to investigate these masses because of the modalities ease of use. A linear transducer should be employed, and possible a standoff pad, secondary to the superficial nature of the mass. Patients with a Bartholin cyst will present with painful

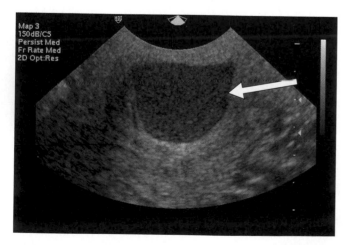

Figure 17-34 Gartner duct cyst. A complicated cyst is noted within the vagina representing a Gartner duct cyst.

swelling in the region of the vulva that may be fevered. They may also cause dysuria and dyspareunia.

A Bartholin duct cyst, if not infected, may appear sonographically simply and anechoic. However, when pain and fever is present, the sonographer must be concerned about the presence of a Bartholin duct abscess. These infected cysts will contain echogenic debris and, possibly, septations. Dirty shadowing may also be present. Color Doppler should be utilized. It may depict the presence of hyperemia secondary to infection.

CLINICAL FINDINGS OF A BARTHOLIN DUCT CYST OR ABSCESS

1. Painful swelling and enlargement in the area of the vulva
2. Fever
3. Dysuria
4. Dyspareunia

SONOGRAPHIC FINDINGS OF A BARTHOLIN DUCT CYST OR ABSCESS

1. Simple cyst
2. Abscess may contain debris and produce dirty shadowing
3. Color Doppler may provide evidence of hyperemia due to infection

---

PRECOCIOUS PUBERTY AND PUBERTAL DELAY

Precocious puberty is pubertal development before the age of 7 (Table 17-1). The diagnosis of precocious puberty typically constitutes an endocrinologic workup to evaluate gonadotropin levels, as well as gonadotropin-releasing hormone, which is a hormone produced by the hypothalamus. True precocious puberty, also referred to as central precocious puberty, may be associated with intracranial tumors, infection, congenital abnormality, or traumatic injury to the hypothalamus or may simply be idiopathic. The brain tumor most likely associated with central precocious puberty is the hypothalamic hamartoma.

Pseudoprecocious puberty, also referred to as peripheral pseudosexual precocity or gonadotropin-independent precocious puberty, has been linked with ovarian, adrenal, and liver tumors. Adrenal tumors may also lead to congenital adrenal hyperplasia. Therefore, patients who present with the indication of precocious puberty should perhaps be sonographically assessed for ovarian, hepatic, and adrenal gland tumors. The uterus may appear enlarged with a postpubertal shape and contain a prominent endometrial stripe. The ovary

TABLE 17-1 Terms associated with precocious puberty

Term	Description
Isosexual precocity	Early development of secondary sexual characteristics with menses, ovulation, and elevated gonadotropin levels
Premature adrenarche	Characterized by isolated pubic hair development and increased levels of adrenal androgens
Premature thelarche	Characterized by isolated breast development with normal prepubertal hormones
Secondary sexual characteristics	Body changes typically occurring at puberty, such as enlargement of breasts and growth of pubic hair
Virilization	A condition in which a female develops physical changes that are associated with male hormones (androgens), such as hair growth

or ovaries may be enlarged, and a functional ovarian cyst or ovarian mass may be seen.

Delayed puberty is described as absent or incomplete breast development after the age of 12. Turner syndrome, also referred to as monosomy X or gonadal dysgenesis, is the most common cause of delayed puberty in the presence of an elevation in follicle-stimulating hormone. Patients with Turner syndrome typically suffer several

conditions, including small stature, webbed neck, poor breast development, rudimentary ovaries, and primary amenorrhea (Fig. 17-35).

SOUND OFF
True precocious puberty may be associated with intracranial tumors or may simply be idiopathic. Pseudoprecocious puberty has been linked with ovarian, adrenal, and liver tumors.

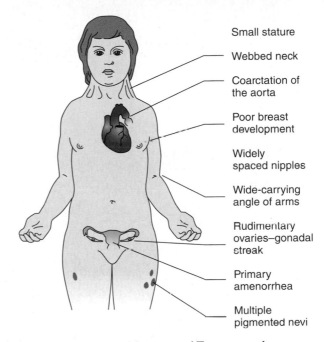

Small stature
Webbed neck
Coarctation of the aorta
Poor breast development
Widely spaced nipples
Wide-carrying angle of arms
Rudimentary ovaries–gonadal streak
Primary amenorrhea
Multiple pigmented nevi

Figure 17-35 Clinical features of Turner syndrome.

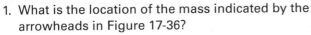

REVIEW QUESTIONS

1. What is the location of the mass indicated by the arrowheads in Figure 17-36?
   a. Submucosal
   b. Intramural
   c. Subserosal
   d. Subcervical

2. What is the location of the mass indicated by the arrows in Figure 17-37?
   a. Submucosal
   b. Intramural
   c. Subserosal
   d. Intracavitary

3. What is the location of the mass noted between the calipers in Figure 17-38?
   a. Submucosal
   b. Intramural
   c. Subserosal
   d. Pedunculated

4. What is the brain tumor that is most likely associated with central precocious puberty?
   a. Pituitary hematoma
   b. Hypothalamic hamartoma
   c. Pituitary adenoma
   d. Hypothalamic hemangioma

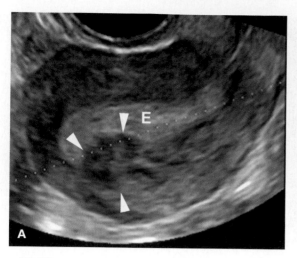
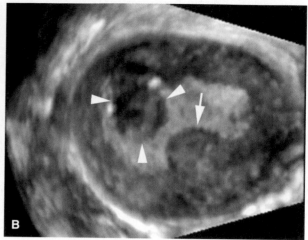

Figure 17-36

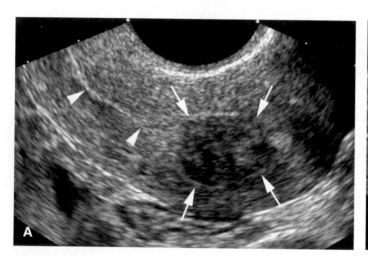
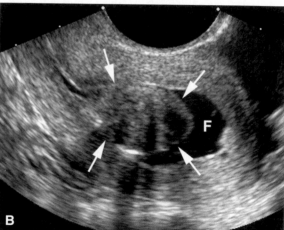

Figure 17-37

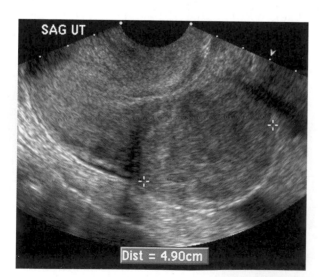

Figure 17-38

5. Which of the following would be found in the region of the vulva?
   a. Gartner duct cyst
   b. Nabothian cyst
   c. Cervical polyp
   d. Bartholin cyst

6. What is dyschezia?
   a. Painful menstruation
   b. Pain at ovulation
   c. Painful defecation
   d. Painful urination

7. What is another name for the perimetrium?
   a. Myometrium
   b. Serosal layer
   c. Endometrium
   d. Premetrium

8. Which of the following is the term for the accumulation of blood within the endometrium?
   a. Hydrometra
   b. Hydrocolpos
   c. Hematocolpos
   d. Hematometra

9. The patient in Figure 17-39 presented with a boggy, enlarged, tender uterus and complained of dyspareunia and dyschezia. What is the most likely diagnosis?
   a. Adenomyosis
   b. Submucosal adenoma
   c. Intramural fibroid
   d. Adenomyomatosis

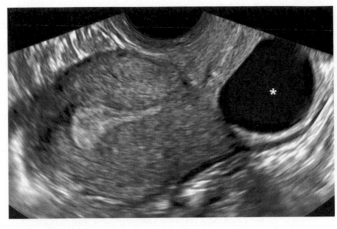

Figure 17-40

11. The patient in Figure 17-41 presented with pelvic fullness and left adnexal pain. What is the most likely diagnosis for the structure noted between the arrows?
    a. Adenomyoma
    b. Leiomyosarcoma
    c. Gartner duct cyst
    d. Degenerating leiomyoma

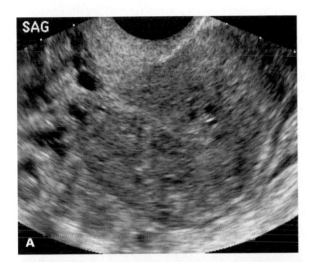

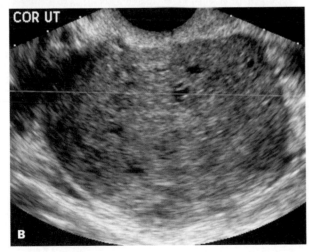

Figure 17-39

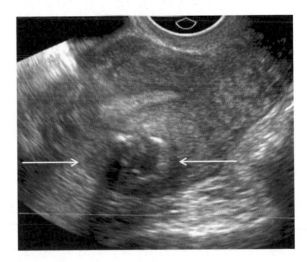

Figure 17-41

12. Which of the following may stimulate leiomyoma growth?
    a. Follicle-stimulating hormone
    b. Prolactin
    c. Estrogen
    d. Luteinizing hormone

10. What does the asterisk in Figure 17-40 most likely represent?
    a. Cervical polyp
    b. Nabothian cyst
    c. Cervical leiomyoma
    d. Bartholin cyst

13. What is the location of the mass noted in Figure 17-42?
    a. Intracavitary, anterior body
    b. Intramural, posterior body
    c. Intramural, anterior body
    d. Subserosal, posterior body

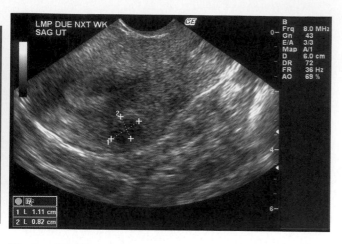

Figure 17-42

14. In postpubertal young girls, what is a likely cause of cyclic abdominal pain, amenorrhea, and an enlarged uterus?
    a. Hydrocolpos
    b. Imperforate hymen
    c. Cervical carcinoma
    d. Adenomyosis

15. What word part means horn?
    a. Colli
    b. Fornix
    c. Cornu
    d. Parity

16. Which of the following is characterized by an incomplete septum and a normal uterine contour with an endometrium that branches into two horns?
    a. Uterus didelphys
    b. Unicornuate uterus
    c. Subseptate uterus
    d. Septate uterus

17. What layer of the endometrium is typically affected by adenomyosis?
    a. Basal
    b. Uterine cavity
    c. Functional
    d. Myometrial

18. All of the following are parts of the uterus except:
    a. corpus.
    b. fundus.
    c. cervix.
    d. vagina.

19. What is the most common cause of delayed puberty in the presence of an elevation in follicle-stimulating hormone?
    a. Precocious puberty
    b. Pseudoprecocious puberty
    c. Gonadal dysgenesis
    d. Adrenal tumor

20. Which of the following is thought to be remnants of the Wolffian duct?
    a. Nabothian cyst
    b. Gartner duct cyst
    c. Bartholin duct cyst
    d. Leiomyoma

21. Which of the following fibroid locations would most likely result in abnormal uterine bleeding because of its relationship to the endometrium?
    a. Submucosal
    b. Intramural
    c. Subserosal
    d. Subserosal pedunculated

22. All of the following are sonographic findings consistent with adenomyosis except:
    a. diffuse, enlarged uterus.
    b. myometrial cysts.
    c. hypoechoic areas adjacent to the endometrium.
    d. complex adnexal mass.

23. The largest part of the uterus is the:
    a. corpus.
    b. isthmus.
    c. cervix.
    d. fundus.

24. Which of the following would be most indicative of a leiomyosarcoma?
    a. Vaginal bleeding
    b. Rapid growth
    c. Dysuria
    d. Large hypoechoic mass

25. The inferior portion of the cervix closest to the vagina is the:
    a. cornu.
    b. internal os.
    c. external os.
    d. inferior fornix.

26. The inner mucosal lining of the uterus is the:
    a. myometrium.
    b. endometrium.
    c. serosal layer.
    d. perimetrium.

27. Difficult or painful intercourse is referred to as:
    a. dysuria.
    b. dysmenorrhea.
    c. dyspareunia.
    d. hydrocolpos.

28. What congenital malformation of the uterus is common and has a clear association with an increased risk for spontaneous abortion?
    a. Anteflexed uterus
    b. Levoverted uterus
    c. Dextroverted uterus
    d. Septate uterus

29. Absence of a menstruation is referred to as:
    a. dysuria.
    b. dysmenorrhea.
    c. amenorrhea.
    d. menorrhagia.

30. The invasion of endometrial tissue into the myometrium of the uterus is referred to as:
    a. amenorrhea.
    b. endometriosis.
    c. adenomyomatosis.
    d. adenomyosis.

31. Pseudoprecocious puberty may be associated with all of the following except:
    a. ovarian tumor.
    b. adrenal tumor.
    c. liver tumor.
    d. brain tumor.

32. The layer of the endometrium that is significantly altered as a result of hormonal stimulation during the menstrual cycle is the:
    a. myometrium.
    b. endometrial cavity.
    c. functional layer.
    d. basal layer.

33. The most superior and widest portion of the uterus is the:
    a. corpus.
    b. isthmus.
    c. cervix.
    d. fundus.

34. A 24-year-old female patient presents to the sonography department for a pelvic sonogram with an indication of pelvic pain. Upon sonographic interrogation, the sonographer notes an anechoic mass within the vagina. This mass most likely represents a(n):
    a. nabothian cyst.
    b. Gartner duct cyst.
    c. Dandy–Walker cyst.
    d. ovarian cyst.

35. What section of the uterus is also referred to as the lower uterine segment?
    a. Cervix
    b. Isthmus
    c. Fundus
    d. Cornu

36. The outer layer of the endometrium is the:
    a. myometrium.
    b. endometrial cavity.
    c. functional layer.
    d. basal layer.

37. Which of the following would be considered the more common uterine anomaly?
    a. Bicornis univernus
    b. Bicornis bicollis
    c. Uterus didelphys
    d. Septate uterus

38. The rigid region of the uterus located between the vagina and the isthmus is the:
    a. cornu.
    b. corpus.
    c. cervix.
    d. fundus.

39. Upon sonographic evaluation of a patient complaining of abdominal distention, you visualize a large, hypoechoic mass distorting the anterior border of the uterus. What is the most likely location of this mass?
    a. Intramural
    b. Subserosal
    c. Submucosal
    d. Intracavitary pedunculated

40. A simple fluid accumulation within the vagina secondary to an imperforate hymen is:
    a. hydrometrocolpos.
    b. hydrocolpos.
    c. hematometra.
    d. hematocolpos.

41. The uterine position in which the corpus tilts forward and comes in contact with the cervix describes:
    a. anteflexion.
    b. anteversion.
    c. retroflexion.
    d. retroversion.

42. What leiomyoma location would have an increased risk to undergo torsion?
    a. Subserosal
    b. Intracavitary
    c. Pedunculated
    d. Submucosal

43. A 13-year-old girl presents to the sonography department with a history of cyclic pain, abdominal swelling, and amenorrhea. Sonographically, you visualize an enlarged uterus and a distended vagina that contains anechoic fluid with debris. What is the most likely diagnosis?
    a. Cervical stenosis
    b. Adenomyosis
    c. Endometriosis
    d. Hematocolpos

44. All of the following are clinical findings associated with leiomyoma except:
    a. myometrial cysts.
    b. infertility.
    c. palpable pelvic mass.
    d. menorrhagia.

45. The surgical removal of a fibroid is termed:
    a. hysterosonogram.
    b. total abdominal hysterectomy.
    c. myomectomy.
    d. uterine artery embolization.

46. Which of the following is typically not a clinical complaint of women who are suffering from adenomyosis?
    a. Amenorrhea
    b. Dysmenorrhea
    c. Dyspareunia
    d. Menometrorrhagia

47. The paired embryonic ducts that develop into the female urogenital tract are the:
    a. fallopian ducts.
    b. Wolffian ducts.
    c. Gartner ducts.
    d. Müllerian ducts.

48. Precocious puberty is defined as the development of pubic hair, breasts, and the genitals before the age of:
    a. 13.
    b. 7.
    c. 5.
    d. 10.

49. Abnormally heavy and prolonged menstrual flow between periods is termed:
    a. menometrorrhagia.
    b. menarche.
    c. menorrhagia.
    d. dysmenorrhea.

50. Leiomyomas that project from a stalk are termed:
    a. submucosal.
    b. intramural.
    c. subserosal.
    d. pedunculated.

51. Congenital malformation of the uterus that results in complete duplication of the genital tract is:
    a. unicornuate uterus.
    b. bicornis bicollis.
    c. uterus didelphys.
    d. subseptate uterus.

52. A 38-year-old female patient presents to the sonography department for a pelvic sonogram with an indication of pelvic pain. Upon sonography interrogation, the sonographer notes an anechoic mass within the cervix. This mass most likely represents a:
    a. nabothian cyst.
    b. benign follicular cyst.
    c. dermoid cyst.
    d. Gartner duct cyst.

53. Leiomyosarcoma of the uterus denotes:
    a. the benign invasion of endometrial tissue into the myometrium.
    b. the ectopic location of endometrial tissue in the adnexa.
    c. the malignant counterpart of a fibroid.
    d. an anechoic, simple cyst located within the cervix.

54. The location of a fibroid within the myometrium is termed:
    a. submucosal.
    b. intracavitary.
    c. subserosal.
    d. intramural.

55. The superior portion of the cervix is the:
    a. cornu.
    b. corpus.
    c. internal os.
    d. external os.

56. Anechoic fluid noted distending the uterus and vagina within a pediatric patient is termed:
    a. hydrocolpos.
    b. hydrometrocolpos.
    c. hydrometra.
    d. hematometrocolpos.

The Uterus and Vagina

57. The normal position of the uterus is:
a. retroverted.
b. retroflexed.
c. anteverted.
d. dysverted.

58. The area of attachment of the fallopian tubes to the uterus is the:
a. fundus.
b. corpus.
c. isthmus.
d. cornua.

59. The recesses of the vagina are the:
a. cornu.
b. isthmi.
c. fornices.
d. parity.

60. A patient presents to the sonography department for a pelvic sonogram with a history of adenomyosis that was diagnosed following an MRI of the pelvis. What are the most likely sonographic findings?
a. Complex, bilateral adnexal masses
b. Myometrial cysts with enlargement of the posterior uterine wall
c. Endometrial thinning and cervical dilation
d. Uterine atrophy with bilateral ovarian cysts

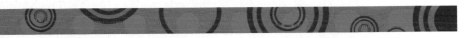

SUGGESTED READINGS

Beckmann CRB, Herbert W, Laube D, et al. *Obstetrics and Gynecology.* 7th ed. Wolters Kluwer; 2014:295–300, 349–354, & 423–434.

Berek JS, Berek DL. *Berek & Novak's Gynecology.* 16th ed. Wolters Kluwer; 2020:132–250, 381–408, & 1038–1076.

Callahan TL, Caughey AB. *Blueprints: Obstetrics & Gynecology.* 6th ed. Wolters Kluwer; 2013:187–196, 204–214, & 383–391.

Curry RA, Tempkin BB. *Sonography: Introduction to Normal Structure and Function.* 5th ed. Elsevier; 2020:317–365.

Doubilet PM, Benson CB. *Atlas of Ultrasound in Obstetrics and Gynecology: A Multimedia Reference.* 2nd ed. Wolters Kluwer; 2012:347–350 & 355–367.

Gibbs RS, Karlan BY, Haney AF, et al. *Danforth's Obstetrics and Gynecology.* 10th ed. Wolters Kluwer; 2008: 664–671, 916–931 & 971–1021.

Goldberg J, Pereira L. Pregnancy outcomes following treatment for fibroids: uterine fibroid embolization versus laparoscopic myomectomy. *Curr Opin Obstet Gynecol.* 2006;18(4):402–406.

Hagen-Ansert SL. *Textbook of Diagnostic Sonography.* 7th ed. Elsevier; 2012:978–1000.

Henningsen C, Kuntz K, Youngs D. *Clinical Guide to Sonography: Exercises for Critical Thinking.* 2nd ed. Elsevier; 2014:142–156.

Hertzberg BS, Middleton WD. *Ultrasound: The Requisites.* 3rd ed. Elsevier; 2016:527–564.

Norton ME, Scoutt LM, Feldstein VA. *Callen's Ultrasonography in Obstetrics and Gynecology.* 6th ed. Elsevier; 2017:835–920.

Parker W. Laparascopic myomectomy and abdominal myomectomy. *Clin Obstet Gynecol.* 2006;49(4):789–797.

Rumack CM, Wilson SR, Charboneau W, et al. *Diagnostic Ultrasound.* 4th ed. Elsevier; 2011:547–612.

Sanders RC, Hall-Terracciano B. *Clinical Sonography: A Practical Guide.* 5th ed. Wolters Kluwer; 2016:151–167.

Shah AB, Phatak SV, Parihar PS, Bisnoi L, Reddy GSN. Infected Bartholin cyst – ultrasonography Doppler, magnetic resonance evaluation. *J Evol Med Dental Sci.* 2021;10:1369–1371.

Siegel MJ. *Pediatric Sonography.* 5th ed. Wolters Kluwer; 2019:513–556.

Stephenson SR, Dmitrieva J. *Diagnostic Medical Sonography: Obstetrics and Gynecology.* 4th ed. Wolters Kluwer; 2018:25–126 & 145–220.

Timor-Tritsch IE, Goldstein SR. *Ultrasound in Gynecology.* 2nd ed. Elsevier; 2007:86–99 & 197–231.

BONUS REVIEW!

Three-Dimensional Sonogram Demonstrating a Submucosal Fibroid (Fig. 17-43)

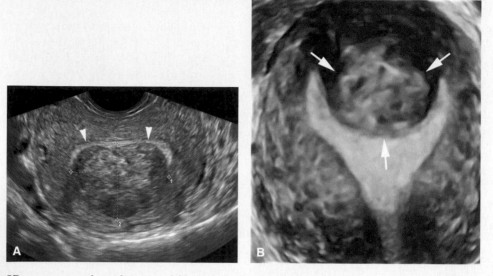

Figure 17-43 3D sonogram of a submucosal fibroid. **A.** Transverse transvaginal view of the uterus demonstrates a fibroid (*calipers*) indenting the endometrium (*arrowheads*). **B.** Coronal image of uterus reconstructed from 3D volume shows that the fibroid (*arrows*) is submucosal, projecting into the endometrium. The 3D image demonstrates the location of the fibroid with respect to the endometrium more precisely than does the 2D image.

Uterine Artery Embolization (Fig. 17-44)

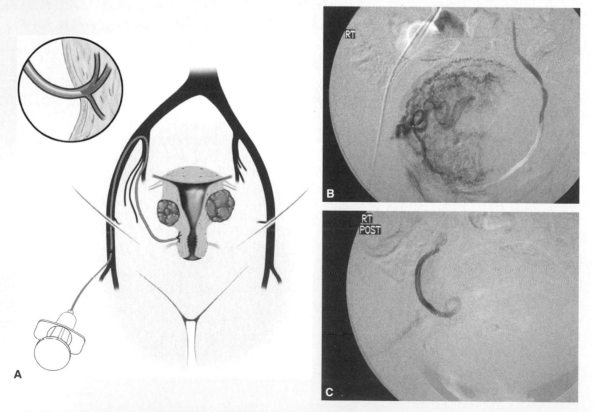

Figure 17-44 Uterine artery embolization (*UAE*). **A.** A catheter is threaded to the uterine arteries and embolic material injected to block off blood flow to the uterus. **B.** Contrast dye shows the vessels supplying the fibroid before UAE. **C.** Following UAE, embolic material blocks blood flow to the fibroid.

Arteriovenous Fistula (Fig. 17-45)

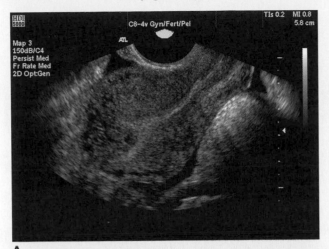

A

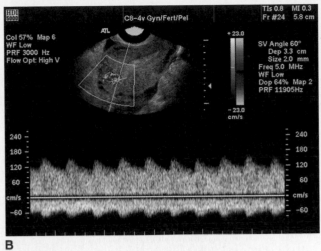

B

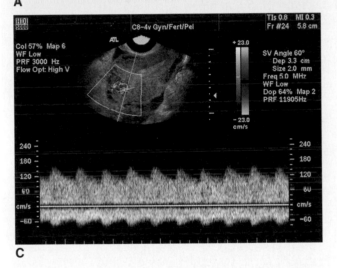

C

Figure 17-45 Arteriovenous (*AV*) fistula. **A.** An AV fistula found after an endometrial biopsy appears as a mass within the endometrium on the two-dimensional image. **B.** The color Doppler image demonstrates flow within the endometrial mass, whereas the spectral Doppler (**C**) shows the characteristic low-resistance flow seen with an AV fistula.

The Ovaries and Fallopian Tubes

Introduction

This chapter discusses the anatomy and physiology of the ovaries and fallopian tubes. Benign conditions of the ovary are the most frequently encountered processes during the sonographic examination of the female pelvis. It is important to note that sonographers must be capable of describing, in sonographic terminology, the characteristics of ovarian masses, because there are often overlapping benign and malignant sonographic signatures. Fallopian tube pathology is discussed in this chapter and revisited in Chapter 21. In the *Bonus Review* section, you will find a computed tomography (CT) of ovarian torsion, a radiograph of a dermoid, and a CT of ovarian carcinoma.

Key Terms

adnexa—the area located posterior to the broad ligaments and adjacent to the uterus, which contains the ovaries and fallopian tubes

ampulla—the longest and most tortuous segment of the fallopian tube

androblastoma—see key term Sertoli–Leydig cell tumor

anterior cul-de-sac—peritoneal outpouching located between the bladder and the uterus; also referred to as the vesicouterine pouch

ascites—excessive fluid in the peritoneal cavity

Brenner tumors—small benign ovarian tumors

CA 125—a protein that may be increased in the blood of women with ovarian cancer and other abnormalities

chocolate cysts—another name for endometriomas

cilia—hairlike projections within the fallopian tube

corpus albicans—the remaining structure of the corpus luteum after its deterioration

corpus luteum—temporary endocrine gland that results from the rupture of the Graafian follicle after ovulation

corpus luteum cyst—physiologic cyst that develops after ovulation has occurred

corpus luteum of pregnancy—the corpus luteum that is maintained during an early pregnancy for the purpose of producing estrogen and primarily progesterone

cumulus oophorus—structure that contains the developing oocyte

cystic teratoma—benign ovarian mass that is composed of the three germ cell layers; also referred to as a dermoid cyst

daughter cyst—a small cyst within a large cyst

dermoid cyst—another name for a cystic teratoma

dermoid mesh—mass of hair within a cystic teratoma

dermoid plug—part of a dermoid tumor that contains various tissues and may produce posterior shadowing during a sonographic examination

dyspareunia—painful sexual intercourse

ectoderm—the outer germ cell layer of the embryo that develops into the skin, hair, and nails, and other structures

endoderm—the germ cell layer of the embryo that develops into the gastrointestinal and respiratory tracts

endometrioid tumor—a typically malignant ovarian tumor that is often associated with a history of endometrial cancer, endometriosis, and endometrial hyperplasia

endometrioma—benign, blood-containing tumor that forms from the implantation of ectopic endometrial tissue; tumor associated with endometriosis

endometriosis—functional ectopic endometrial tissue located outside the uterus

fibroma—an ovarian sex cord–stromal tumor found in middle-aged women

fimbria—the fingerlike extension of the fallopian tube located on the infundibulum

follicle-stimulating hormone—hormone of the anterior pituitary gland that causes the development of multiple follicles on the ovaries

follicular cyst—ovarian cyst that forms as a result of the failure of the Graafian follicle to ovulate

germ cell tumor—a type of neoplasm derived from germ cells of the gonads; may also be found outside the reproductive tract

gestational trophoblastic disease—a disease associated with an abnormal proliferation of the trophoblastic cells during pregnancy; may also be referred to as a molar pregnancy

Graafian follicle—the name for the dominant follicle before ovulation

hematosalpinx—blood within the fallopian tube

hemorrhagic cyst—a cyst that contains blood

hirsutism—excessive hair growth in women in areas where hair growth is normally negligible

human chorionic gonadotropin—hormone produced by the trophoblastic cells of the early placenta; may also be used as a tumor marker in nongravid patients and males

hydrosalpinx—the abnormal accumulation of fluid within the fallopian tube

hyperemesis—excessive vomiting

hysterosalpingography—a radiographic procedure that uses a dye instilled into the endometrial cavity and fallopian tubes to evaluate for internal abnormalities

infundibulum—the distal segment of the fallopian tube

interstitial—the segment of the fallopian tube that lies within the uterine horn (cornu)

isthmus—tube: the segment of the fallopian tube that is located between the interstitial and ampulla; uterus: area of the uterus between the corpus and the cervix

Krukenberg tumor—malignant ovarian tumor that metastasizes from most likely the gastrointestinal tract

lysis—destruction or breaking down (i.e., hemolysis, the breaking down of blood components)

malignant degeneration—developing into cancer

Meigs syndrome—ascites and pleural effusion in the presence of a benign ovarian tumor

menorrhagia—abnormally heavy and prolonged menstruation

mesoderm—the germ cell layer of the embryo that develops into the circulatory system, muscles, reproductive system, and other structures

mittelschmerz—pelvic pain at the time of ovulation

multiloculated—having more than one internal cavity

nutcracker syndrome—an anomaly where left renal vein entrapment occurs between the superior mesenteric artery and the abdominal aorta

oogenesis—the creation of an ovum

oophorectomy—surgical removal of the ovary

ovarian cystectomy—the surgical removal of an ovarian cyst

ovarian hyperstimulation syndrome—a syndrome resulting from hyperstimulation of the ovaries by fertility drugs; results in the development of multiple, enlarged follicular ovarian cysts

ovarian torsion—an abnormality that results from the ovary twisting on its mesenteric connection, consequently cutting off the blood supply to the ovary

ovulation—the release of the mature egg from the ovary

papillary projections—a small protrusion of tissue

pedunculated uterine leiomyoma—leiomyoma (fibroid) that extends from the uterus on a stalk

pelvic congestion syndrome—a condition that is thought to result from the compression of the left renal vein at the origin of the superior mesenteric artery, a condition termed Nutcracker syndrome

pelvic inflammatory disease—infection of the female genital tract that may involve the ovaries, uterus, and/or the fallopian tubes

peristalsis—contractions that move in a wavelike pattern to propel a substance

peritonitis—inflammation of the peritoneal lining

pseudomyxoma peritonei—intraperitoneal extension of mucin-secreting cells that results from the rupture of a malignant mucinous ovarian tumor or, possibly, a malignant tumor of the appendix

pseudoprecocious puberty—secondary sexual development induced by sex steroids or from other sources like ovarian tumors, adrenal tumors, or steroid use

pyosalpinx—the presence of pus within the fallopian tube

salpingitis—inflammation of the fallopian tubes

sebum—an oily substance secreted by the sebaceous glands

septations—a partition separating two or more cavities

Sertoli–Leydig cell tumor—malignant sex cord–stromal ovarian neoplasm that is associated with virilization; also referred to as an androblastoma

serum lactate dehydrogenase—tumor marker that is elevated in the presence of an ovarian dysgerminoma and other abdominal abnormalities

sex cord–stromal tumors—ovarian tumors that arise from the gonadal ridges

sonohysterography—a sonographic procedure that uses saline instillation into the endometrial cavity and fallopian tubes to evaluate for internal abnormalities

theca lutein cysts—functional ovarian cysts that are found in the presence of elevated levels of human chorionic gonadotropin; also referred to as a theca luteal cyst

thecoma—benign ovarian sex cord–stromal tumor that produces estrogen in older women

"tip of the iceberg" sign—denotes the sonographic appearance of a cystic teratoma (dermoid) when only the anterior element of the mass is seen, while the greater part of the mass is obscured by shadowing

true pelvis—inferior portion of the pelvis that contains the uterus, ovaries, fallopian tubes, urinary bladder, small bowel, sigmoid colon, and rectum

unilocular—having only one internal cavity

venography—examination of the veins of the legs and pelvis that includes the use of contrast media; can be performed using radiography (fluoroscopy), computed tomography, and magnetic resonance imaging

virilization—(female) changes within the female that are typically associated with males; caused by increased androgens and may lead to deepening of the voice and hirsutism

"whirlpool" sign—an indicator of the torsed ovarian pedicle adjacent to the ovary, appearing as a round mass with concentric hypoechoic and hyperechoic rings that demonstrates a swirling color Doppler signature

yolk sac tumor—(ovary) malignant germ cell tumor of the ovary

ANATOMY AND PHYSIOLOGY OF THE OVARY

The ovaries form in the upper abdomen and descend into the pelvis in utero. They are paired, oval-shaped, intraperitoneal organs that have a dual blood supply from both the ovarian artery and ovarian branches of the uterine arteries (Fig. 18-1). It is important to remember that the ovarian arteries are the branches of the abdominal aorta. Also, whereas the right ovarian vein drains into the inferior vena cava, the left ovarian

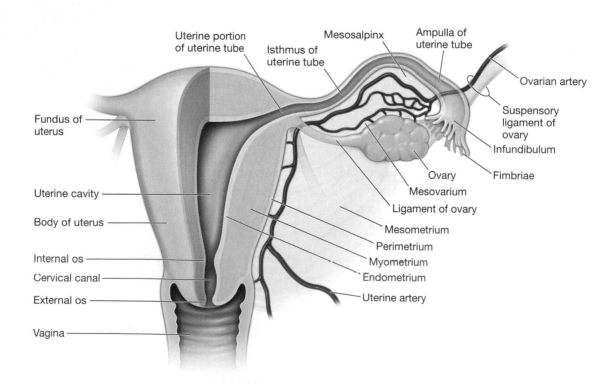

Figure 18-1 Posterior view of uterine adnexa and collateral circulation of uterine and ovarian arteries. Note that the Sampson artery is another name for the round ligament artery.

vein drains into the left renal vein. As endocrine glands, the ovaries are responsible for releasing estrogen and progesterone in varying amounts throughout the menstrual cycle. They may be located anywhere within the **true pelvis**, excluding the **anterior cul-de-sac** (Fig. 18-2). The ovarian fossa is located posterior to the ureter and internal iliac artery and superior to the external iliac artery.

Though the ovary has no peritoneal covering, it is covered by a layer of surface epithelium. Just below the epithelium lies the tunica albuginea, which serves as a protective layer for the ovary. The ovary essentially consists of an outer cortex and an inner medulla (Fig. 18-3). The medulla contains the ovarian vasculature and lymphatics, whereas the cortex, which is the parenchymal element, involves the mass of the ovary and is thus the site of **oogenesis**. The ovaries are stimulated by **follicle-stimulating hormone**, released by the anterior pituitary gland, to develop multiple follicles during the first half of the menstrual cycle (follicular phase). The cells surrounding the tiny follicles produce estrogen that stimulates the endometrium to thicken. Only one of these follicles will become the dominant follicle, or **Graafian follicle**, before **ovulation**, whereas all other follicles will undergo atrophy. A normal follicle measures 3 cm or higher in greatest diameter in the premenopausal patient.

> **SOUND OFF**
> Only one follicle will become the dominant follicle, or Graafian follicle, before ovulation, whereas all other follicles undergo atrophy.

The **ovum** is contained within the **cumulus oophorus** of the dominant follicle (Fig. 18-4). The cumulus oophorus may be seen within the ovary during a sonographic examination, with the sonographic appearance resembling that of a **daughter cyst**. At approximately day 14 of the menstrual cycle, ovulation occurs when the dominant follicle ruptures, releasing the mature ovum and a small amount of follicular fluid into the peritoneal cavity. **Mittelschmerz**, which means middle pain, describes pain at the time of ovulation, typically on the side of the dominant follicle.

The fluid from the ruptured follicle most often will settle in the rectouterine pouch (pouch of Douglas), the most dependent portion of the peritoneal cavity. After the Graafian follicle has ruptured, its structure is converted into the **corpus luteum**. During the second half of the menstrual cycle (luteal phase), the corpus luteum produces progesterone and, in small amounts, estrogen. If fertilization occurs, the corpus luteum is maintained and becomes the **corpus luteum of pregnancy**. If fertilization does not occur, the corpus luteum regresses and becomes the **corpus albicans**. The ovarian cycle is further discussed in Chapter 19.

> **SOUND OFF**
> After the Graafian follicle has ruptured, its structure is converted into the corpus luteum.

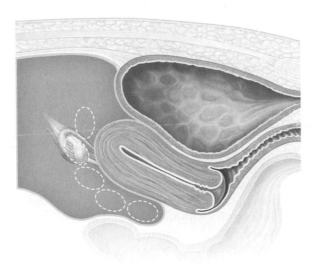

A

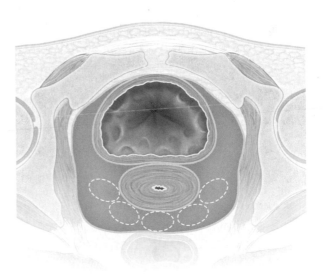

B

Figure 18-2 Positions of the ovary. **A.** Sagittal. **B.** Transverse. Because of its attachment to the posterior surface of the broad ligament, the ovary may be found in the posterior pelvic compartment or above the fundus of the uterus, in the adnexal spaces, or in the posterior cul-de-sac, but not in the anterior cul-de-sac or between the urinary bladder and the uterus.

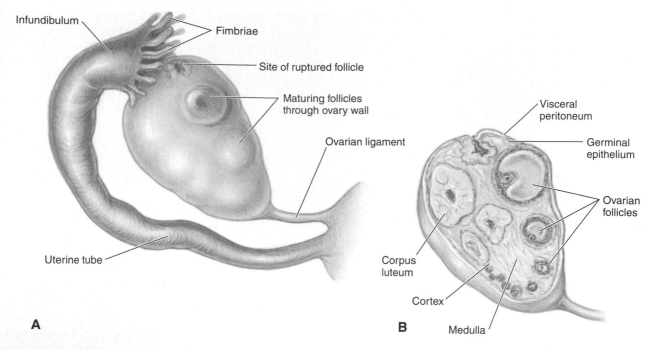

Figure 18-3 Ovarian anatomy. **A.** External structure of the ovary. **B.** Cross-sectioned ovary demonstrating the cortex, medulla, and ovarian follicle maturation.

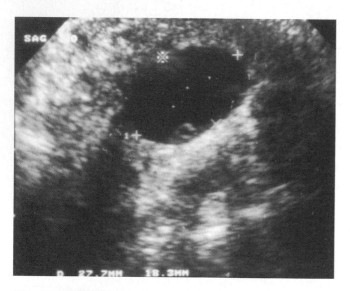

Figure 18-4 Mature follicle (between *cursors*) containing a small protrusion from the posterior wall representing the cumulus oophorus.

SONOGRAPHIC APPEARANCE OF THE OVARY

Sonographically, the normal ovary is homogeneous with a medium- to low-level echogenicity (Fig. 18-5). Multiple follicles may be noted with sonography during the neonatal and prepubertal ages. In addition, follicles on the ovaries, of varying sizes, may be seen throughout the normal menstrual cycle during reproductive years.

Color and spectral Doppler should be used to evaluate the ovaries. Typical ovarian flow varies throughout the menstrual cycle. During the early follicular phase and late luteal phase (days 0 to 7 and 18 to 28, respectively), the ovarian artery will demonstrate a high-resistive pattern, with increased impedance, and absent or low end-diastolic velocity. During the late follicular and early luteal phase (days 7 to 17), the ovary will demonstrate a low-resistive pattern, with low impedance and higher levels of diastolic flow (Fig. 18-6; Table 18-1). The size of the ovary depends on the physiologic state and age of the patient. Ovarian volume can be determined sonographically by utilizing the following formula: volume = length × width × height × 0.523 (Fig. 18-7). It can be provided in cm³ or milliliters (mL). The mean premenopausal ovarian volume is 9.8 cm³ (equivalent to 9.8 mL). There are several conditions that may increase ovarian volume (i.e., ovarian size), including **ovarian torsion**, **ovarian hyperstimulation syndrome**, and polycystic ovary syndrome. It is important to note that postmenopausal ovaries undergo atrophy and may be difficult to locate sonographically. The mean volume for postmenopausal ovaries is 5.8 cm³.

> **◀))) SOUND OFF**
> Typical ovarian flow is said to be high resistant during the early follicular phase and late luteal phase, and low resistant during the late follicular phase and early luteal phase.

The Ovaries and Fallopian Tubes

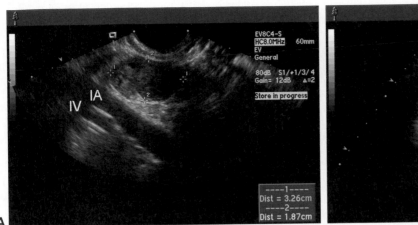
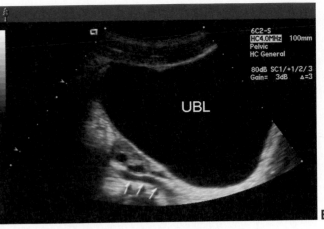

Figure 18-5 Normal sonographic appearance of the ovary. **A.** In this longitudinal endovaginal image of the pelvis, the ovary (between *calipers*) is noted adjacent to the iliac artery (*IA*) and iliac vein (*IV*). **B.** A normal ovary can be seen in this longitudinal transabdominal image of the pelvis between the urinary bladder (*UBL*) and prominent ureter (*arrows*).

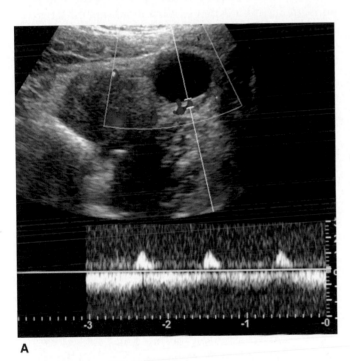
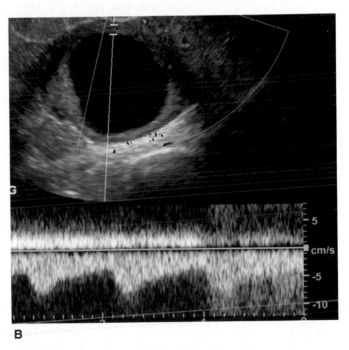

Figure 18-6 Doppler waveforms of the ovary. **A.** Transverse image in the early follicular phase (day 8) shows high impedance waveform and virtually no diastolic flow. **B.** Longitudinal sonogram in the late luteal phase (day 24) shows a low-resistance waveform with higher levels of diastolic flow. Also note monophasic venous flow on both images.

TABLE 18-1	Ovarian arterial flow throughout the menstrual cycle	
Early follicular phase	High impedance (resistance) with absent or low end-diastolic velocity	Resistive index = 1.0
Late follicular phase	Low impedance (resistance) with increased end-diastolic flow	Resistive index = 0.5
Early luteal phase	Low impedance (resistance) with increased end-diastolic flow	Resistive index = 0.5
Late luteal phase	High impedance (resistance) with absent or low end-diastolic velocity	Resistive index = 1.0

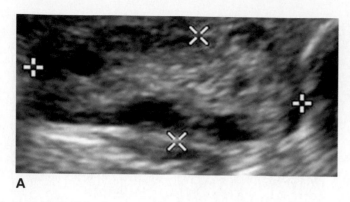
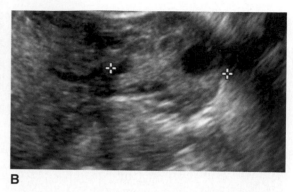

Figure 18-7 Calculating ovarian volume. The length and height measurements are taken on a sagittal scan (**A**), and the width is taken on a transverse scan (**B**). Ovarian volume is obtained using the formula: $L \times H \times W \times 0.523$.

PATHOLOGY OF THE OVARY

Ovarian-Adnexal Reporting and Data System

The ovarian-adnexal reporting and data system (O-RADS) was established by the American College of Radiology (ACR) and other medical organizations to standardize the ultrasound lexicon in gynecologic imaging in relation to adnexal pathology, such as ovarian cysts. These descriptive terms are placed in six categories: physiologic and lesion characteristics, size, solid or solid-appearing lesions, cystic lesions, vascularity, and general and extraovarian findings. Some organizations may require that their sonographers attempt to score ovarian cysts or other adnexal pathology. Though this practice is beyond the scope of this text, one can find more information if they visit ACR.org and search *O-RADS*.

Benign Ovarian Disease

Follicular Cysts

Should the Graafian follicle (dominant follicle) fail to ovulate, it could continue to enlarge and result in a **follicular cyst**. Follicular cysts range in size from 3 to 8 cm; however, larger cysts have been documented.

Their sonographic appearance is most often described as anechoic, thin walled, and **unilocular** (Fig. 18-8). Most follicular cysts regress and are asymptomatic, but some may lead to pain, resulting in frequent, follow-up sonographic examinations. In addition, surgical intervention or drainage may be warranted because a large cyst increases the risk for ovarian torsion. The surgical removal of an ovarian cyst is referred to as **ovarian cystectomy**. Fortunately, these cysts typically resolve within 6 weeks.

> **◄))) SOUND OFF**
> A large mass or cyst on the ovary increases the patient's risk for ovarian torsion.

Hyperstimulation of the ovaries, or ovarian hyperstimulation syndrome, from fertility treatment will also result in the development of multiple, enlarged follicular cysts. A follicular cyst that contains blood is referred to as a **hemorrhagic cyst**, and it most often appears complex or completely echogenic depending on the hemorrhagic component present and the stage of **lysis** (Fig. 18-9). The sonographic manifestation of a hemorrhagic cyst may be described as demonstrating a fluid–debris level, fishnet, weblike or lacy appearance.

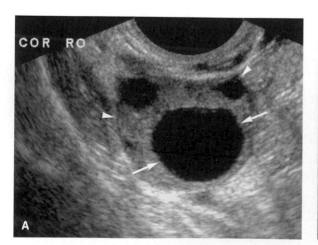
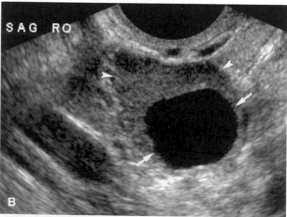

Figure 18-8 Simple ovarian cyst. Coronal (**A**) and sagittal (**B**) images of the right ovary demonstrating a simple ovarian cyst (*arrows*). Normal ovarian tissue (*arrowheads*) is noted around the cyst.

CLINICAL FINDINGS OF FOLLICULAR CYSTS

1. Asymptomatic
2. Pain associated with hemorrhage and enlargement of cyst

SONOGRAPHIC FINDINGS OF FOLLICULAR CYSTS

1. Simple cyst—anechoic, thin walled, unilocular, round, posterior enhancement
2. Hemorrhagic cyst—variable appearances, including complex components or entirely echogenic, depending on the amount of blood and the stage of lysis; may have a fluid–debris level, fishnet, weblike or lacy appearance as well

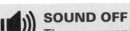 **SOUND OFF**
The sonographic manifestation of a hemorrhagic cyst may be described as demonstrating a weblike or lacy appearance.

Corpus Luteum Cysts (Corpus Luteal Cysts)

The **corpus luteum cyst** is a physiologic (functional) cyst that develops after ovulation has occurred. After the Graafian follicle ruptures, the structure hemorrhages and forms the corpus hemorrhagicum, but within hours, the corpus luteum develops (Fig. 18-10). The corpus luteum is primarily responsible for producing progesterone, thereby maintaining the endometrium during an early pregnancy in preparation for implantation.

Thus, the corpus luteum will normally regress if fertilization does not occur but may rarely be maintained and continue to enlarge. When regression takes place,

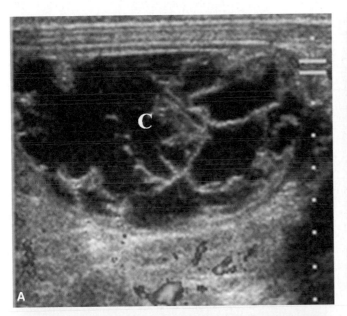

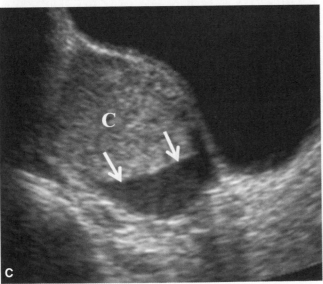

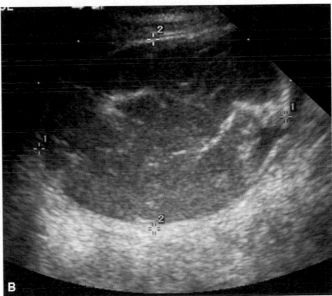

Figure 18-9 Hemorrhagic ovarian cysts, spectrum of sonographic appearances. **A.** Transverse color Doppler sonogram reveals a large complex cyst (*C*) with multiple septations creating a fishnet pattern. The cyst does not contain any Doppler signals. **B.** Transverse sonogram in shows a complex cyst (*calipers*) containing low-level echoes. **C.** Longitudinal sonogram of the right adnexa in a third patient demonstrates a cystic mass (*C*) with a fluid–debris level (*arrows*).

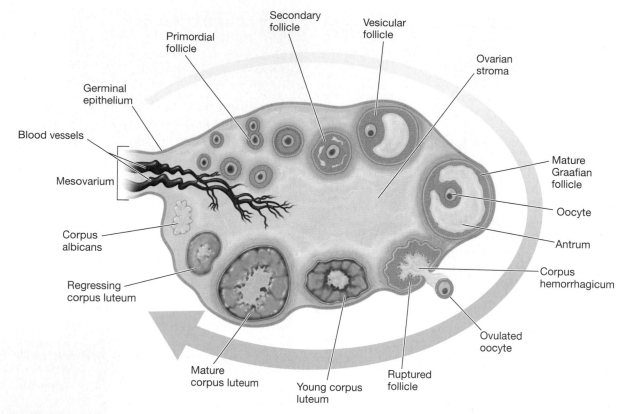

Figure 18-10 Schematic diagram of an ovary showing the sequence of events in the origin, growth, and rupture of an ovarian follicle and the formation and retrogression of a corpus luteum.

a small, echogenic structure may be noted within the ovary, representing the corpus albicans.

Corpus luteum cysts may reach sizes up to 8 cm, with resolution of the cyst taking place within 1 to 2 months in menstruating patients. Pain is associated with enlargement of the cyst, hemorrhage, and rupture. If the cyst is large, it increases the risk for ovarian torsion.

In the presence of a pregnancy, and thus the production of **human chorionic gonadotropin (hCG)** by the trophoblastic cells of the pregnancy, the corpus luteum is preserved. In this case, the cyst may be referred to as the corpus luteum of pregnancy. These cysts are considered the most common pelvic masses seen during a first-trimester sonographic examination. They may even reach sizes up to 10 cm, although, most often, they resolve by 16 weeks' gestation and do not exceed 3 cm. They tend to appear as simple cysts, although they may also have thick walls and may be difficult to differentiate from other solid and cystic adnexal masses (Fig. 18-11).

Patients with large corpus luteum cysts may present with pelvic pain if the cyst has ruptured or if hemorrhage within the cyst has occurred. Often, complex or thick-walled corpus luteum cysts can resemble an ectopic pregnancy, especially those that

display an obvious rim of color Doppler resembling the "ring of fire" often associated with an ectopic pregnancy (see Fig. 18-11 A). Consequently, precaution to establish the presence of an intrauterine pregnancy should be taken in this regard, as well as careful consideration of the entire clinical picture.

> **SOUND OFF**
> A complex or thick-walled corpus luteum cyst can resemble an ectopic pregnancy, so precaution to establish the presence of an intrauterine pregnancy should be taken in this regard, as well as careful consideration of the entire clinical picture.

CLINICAL FINDINGS OF CORPUS LUTEUM CYSTS AND CORPUS LUTEUM OF PREGNANCY

1. Asymptomatic
2. Pain associated with hemorrhage and enlargement of cyst
3. Corpus luteum of pregnancy accompanies a pregnancy

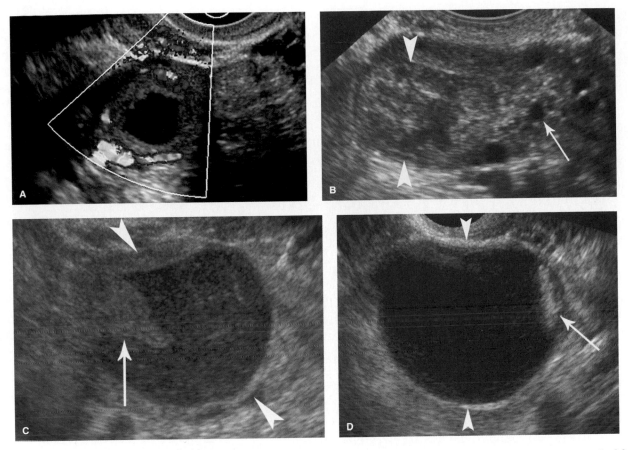

Figure 18-11 Corpus luteum. **A.** Transvaginal color Doppler image of the ovary reveals a 3-cm cyst surrounded by an intense ring of vascularity ("ring of fire") characteristic of the corpus luteum. **B.** Transvaginal image of the ovary reveals a collapsed cyst appearance of the corpus luteum (between *arrowheads*) that occurs just after ovulation. Note the follicles (*arrow*) that confirm the location of the structure on the ovary. **C.** The corpus luteum is prone to internal hemorrhage, creating a hemorrhagic ovarian cyst (between *arrowheads*). Note the echogenic fluid and clot (*arrow*) within the cyst. **D.** A hemorrhagic corpus luteal cyst (between *arrowheads*) may enlarge to become a prominent pelvic structure and be a source of adnexal pain in early pregnancy. Blood clots (*arrow*) within the cyst are also noted.

SONOGRAPHIC FINDINGS OF CORPUS LUTEUM CYSTS AND CORPUS LUTEUM OF PREGNANCY

1. Simple cyst appearance
2. May have a thick wall, be completely echogenic, and may be difficult to differentiate from other solid and cystic adnexal masses
3. Hemorrhagic components may appear complex or have a weblike or lacy appearance depending on the amount of blood and stage of lysis
4. "Ring of fire" around the cyst may be detected with color Doppler

Theca Lutein Cysts

Theca lutein cysts are the largest and least common of the functional cysts. They are found in the presence of elevated levels of hCG, occasionally exceeding 100,000 mIU per mL. Therefore, **gestational trophoblastic disease** (molar pregnancy) and ovarian

hyperstimulation syndrome are common conditions associated with theca lutein cysts. Certainly, multiple gestations would also have higher levels of hCG and, therefore, increase the likelihood of developing theca lutein cysts. Patients with such high levels of hCG may suffer from **hyperemesis** and complain of pelvic fullness. These large cysts are frequently bilateral and **multiloculated** and may reach sizes up to 15 cm (Fig. 18-12). Fortunately, they tend to regress after the high level of circulating hCG diminishes.

CLINICAL FINDINGS OF THECA LUTEIN CYSTS

1. Markedly elevated levels of hCG (as seen in cases of gestational trophoblastic disease, ovarian hyperstimulation, and twin gestations)
2. Nausea and vomiting
3. Pelvic fullness
4. Pain associated with hemorrhage, rupture, and ovarian torsion

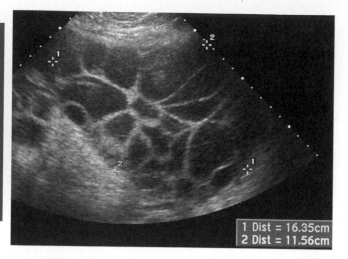

Figure 18-12 Theca lutein cysts. Transabdominal image of an enlarged ovary (between *calipers*) is seen in the patient with theca lutein cysts. This patient was undergoing infertility therapy and had a markedly elevated human chorionic gonadotropin blood level.

SONOGRAPHIC FINDINGS OF THECA LUTEIN CYSTS

1. Large, bilateral, multiloculated ovarian cystic masses
2. May contain hemorrhagic components

SOUND OFF

Theca lutein cysts are large, bilateral, multiloculated ovarian cystic masses that result from high levels of hCG as seen in patients with twins and those suffering from gestational trophoblastic disease or ovarian hyperstimulation syndrome.

Paraovarian Cysts

Paraovarian cysts are small cysts located adjacent to the ovary and most likely arise from the fallopian tubes or broad ligaments and are thought to be remnants of the Wolffian duct (Fig. 18-13). They may contain small amounts of hemorrhage and **septations**. Because these cysts can range in size from 1.5 to 19 cm, clinical presentation varies, with patients who have larger cysts presenting with pelvic pain and increased lower abdominal girth. Larger paraovarian cysts may cause ovarian torsion.

CLINICAL FINDINGS OF PARAOVARIAN CYSTS

1. Asymptomatic
2. If cyst is large, patients may present with pelvic pain and increased lower abdominal girth

SONOGRAPHIC FINDINGS OF PARAOVARIAN CYSTS

1. Simple cyst located adjacent, but not attached, to the ovary
2. If hemorrhagic, will appear complex

Cystic Teratoma (Dermoid)

The most common benign ovarian tumor is the ovarian **cystic teratoma**, also referred to as a **dermoid cyst**. Dermoids result from the retention of an unfertilized ovum that differentiates into the three germ cell layers. Therefore, these germ cell tumors are composed of **ectoderm**, **mesoderm**, and **endoderm**. As a result of the combination of these germ cells, a cystic teratoma

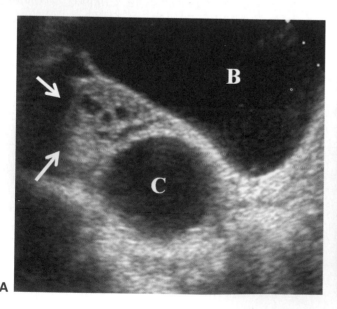
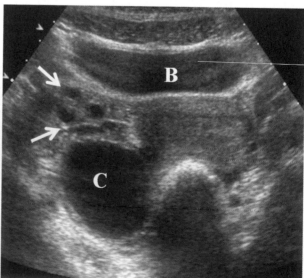

Figure 18-13 Paraovarian cyst. **A.** A simple appearing cyst (*C*) is noted adjacent to the ovary (*arrows*) and posterior to the urinary bladder (*B*) in this longitudinal image. **B.** The same patient in transverse.

may contain any number of tissues, including glandular thyroid components, bone, hair, **sebum**, fat, cartilage, and digestive elements (Fig. 18-14). They frequently will contain fully formed or rudimentary teeth as well. Dermoids are commonly found in the reproductive-aged group but may also be found in postmenopausal patients. Patients are most often asymptomatic but may suffer from pain associated with torsion or rupture of the mass, the latter of which can lead to **peritonitis**. Dermoids also have the capability of **malignant degeneration**, but this is rare.

> ◀))) **SOUND OFF**
> The most common benign ovarian tumor is the ovarian cystic teratoma, also referred to as a dermoid cyst.

The sonographic appearance of a cystic teratoma has been well documented, and it has most often been described as a complex or partially cystic mass in the ovary that includes one or more echogenic structures. These echogenic components may produce posterior shadowing (Fig. 18-15). The "**tip of the iceberg**" **sign** denotes the sonographic appearance of the mass when only the anterior element of the mass is seen, while the greater part of the mass is obscured by shadowing (Fig. 18-16). This occurs as a result of complete attenuation of the sound beam by the dense tissue components of the mass. Often, dermoid tumors contain

a "**dermoid plug**." The dermoid plug contains various tissues that will be a source of posterior shadowing. The "**dermoid mesh**" has been used to describe the visualization of hair within the mass. Hair will appear as numerous linear interfaces within the cystic area of a dermoid. A fluid–fluid level may also be visualized, in which case there is a clear demarcation between serous fluid and sebum.

CLINICAL FINDINGS OF A CYSTIC TERATOMA

1. Often asymptomatic
2. If torsion or rupture occurs, the patient may present with acute pelvic pain

SONOGRAPHIC FINDINGS OF A CYSTIC TERATOMA

1. Complex, partially cystic mass in the ovary that includes one or more echogenic structures that may shadow
2. "Tip of the iceberg" sign—only the anterior element of the mass is seen, while the greater part of the mass is obscured by shadowing
3. Dermoid plug—produces posterior shadowing
4. Dermoid mesh—produced by hair and will appear as numerous linear interfaces within the cystic area of the mass

Dermoid cyst

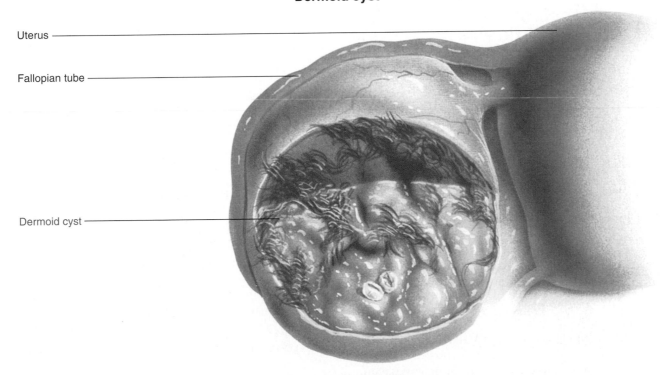

Uterus

Fallopian tube

Dermoid cyst

Figure 18-14 Dermoid cyst is a benign ovarian mass that consists of hair, teeth, fat, and other tissues.

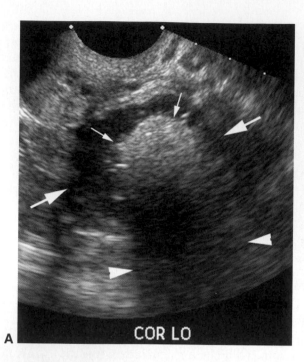
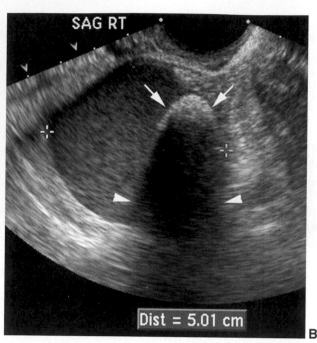

Figure 18-15 Cystic teratoma. **A.** A coronal image of the female pelvis demonstrating a complex ovarian mass (between *large arrows*) with several typical sonographic characteristics of a dermoid, including the dermoid plug (*small arrows*) and the posterior shadowing (between *arrowheads*) from the plug. **B.** In the sagittal plane, this dermoid (between *arrows*) reveals a solid (*arrows*) shadowing (between *arrowheads*) structure within its borders.

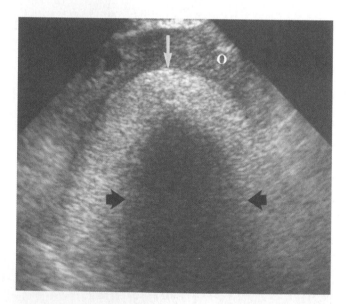

Figure 18-16 Cystic teratoma and the "tip of the iceberg" sign. The dermoid plug is seen as a highly echogenic mass (*white arrow*) attached to the ovary (*O*). Acoustic shadowing (*black arrows*) is produced as a result of the sound absorption.

Thecoma

A **thecoma** is a benign ovarian **sex cord–stromal tumor**. Thecomas are most often found in postmenopausal women and may be associated with **Meigs syndrome**. Meigs syndrome describes the condition of a having a benign ovarian tumor with **ascites** and pleural effusion. Thecomas are estrogen-producing tumors; therefore, patients often complain of postmenopausal vaginal bleeding associated with the unconstrained estrogen stimulation upon the endometrium. As the term denotes, these tumors are masses that are composed of multiple ovarian thecal cells. A thecoma will sonographically appear as a hypoechoic, solid mass with posterior attenuation. They are most often unilateral and may appear similar to a **pedunculated uterine leiomyoma**.

CLINICAL FINDINGS OF A THECOMA

1. May be asymptomatic
2. Postmenopausal vaginal bleeding or abnormal vaginal bleeding secondary to estrogen stimulation
3. Meigs syndrome (ascites and pleural effusion)

SONOGRAPHIC FINDINGS OF A THECOMA

1. Hypoechoic, solid mass with posterior attenuation
2. No posterior enhancement
3. If large, it may mimic a pedunculated leiomyoma

> 🔊 **SOUND OFF**
> A thecoma produces estrogen and can, therefore, lead to postmenopausal vaginal bleeding. It often appears as a hypoechoic mass, which can simulate the sonographic appearance of uterine fibroid.

Granulosa Cell Tumors

The granulosa cell tumor, also referred to as the granulose theca cell tumor, is considered to be the most common estrogenic tumor. It is also a sex cord–stromal tumor like the thecoma. These tumors typically occur unilaterally and are more commonly seen in the postmenopausal female, but they can also be found in younger patients. Because of its estrogen-producing potential, a granulosa cell tumor will present clinically much like the thecoma. Consequently, because of the estrogen interaction upon the endometrium, postmenopausal patients may present with vaginal bleeding, whereas adolescent patients may present with **pseudoprecocious puberty** findings. As a result of consistent estrogen stimulation, postmenopausal patients with granulosa cell tumors have approximately a 10% to 15% chance of developing endometrial carcinoma. The sonographic finding of a granulosa cell tumor is unpredictable, with appearances ranging from that of a solid, hypoechoic mass to one that has some cystic components (Fig. 18-17). Granulosa cell tumors can reach sizes up to 40 cm and do have malignant potential.

> **CLINICAL FINDINGS OF GRANULOSA CELL TUMORS**
>
> 1. Adolescence—pseudoprecocious puberty
> 2. Reproductive-aged and postmenopausal women will have abnormal vaginal bleeding

> **SONOGRAPHIC FINDINGS OF GRANULOSA CELL TUMORS**
>
> 1. Solid, hypoechoic mass
> 2. Complex or partially cystic mass

> 🔊 **SOUND OFF**
> In pediatric patients, the granulosa cell tumor is associated with pseudoprecocious puberty.

Fibroma

An ovarian **fibroma** is also considered a sex cord–stromal tumor. Unlike thecomas and granulosa cell tumors, however, fibromas are not associated with estrogen production. Fibromas are most often found in middle-aged women. They are benign ovarian masses that may be complicated by Meigs syndrome as well. The sonographic appearance of a fibroma is that of a hypoechoic, solid mass with posterior attenuation (Fig. 18-18). Often, fibromas, like thecomas, may mimic pedunculated uterine leiomyoma. The ascites and pleural effusions associated with Meigs syndromes usually resolve after resection of the tumor.

> **CLINICAL FINDINGS OF A FIBROMA**
>
> 1. May be asymptomatic
> 2. Meigs syndrome (ascites and pleural effusion)

> **SONOGRAPHIC FINDINGS OF A FIBROMA**
>
> 1. Hypoechoic, solid mass with posterior attenuation
> 2. No posterior enhancement
> 3. If large, it may mimic a pedunculated leiomyoma

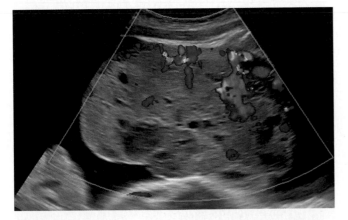

Figure 18-17 Granulosa cell tumor in a 13-year-old girl who presented with right lower quadrant pain. Midline pelvic color Doppler sonographic image demonstrates a large mass with both solid and cystic components and internal vascularity, a common appearance for pediatric granulosa cell tumor.

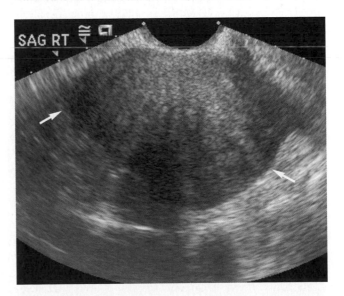

Figure 18-18 Ovarian fibroma. Sagittal image of the right ovary demonstrating a solid mass (*arrows*) with a homogeneous echotexture.

Brenner Tumor (Transitional Cell Tumor)

Brenner tumors, or transitional cell tumors, are most often small, solid, hypoechoic unilateral tumors that may contain calcifications. Consequently, their sonographic appearance may be similar to that of a uterine leiomyoma, thecoma, and fibroma. They are almost always benign, but they can undergo malignant degeneration. Patients may be asymptomatic or may present with a palpable mass or pain and, possibly, signs of Meigs syndrome.

CLINICAL FINDINGS OF A BRENNER TUMOR

1. May be asymptomatic
2. Meigs syndrome (ascites and pleural effusion)

SONOGRAPHIC FINDINGS OF A BRENNER TUMOR

1. Small, solid, hypoechoic mass
2. May contain calcifications

Endometrioma (Chocolate Cyst)

An **endometrioma** is a benign, blood-containing tumor that is associated with **endometriosis** and forms from the implantation of ectopic endometrial tissue. This ectopic endometrial tissue is functional. Therefore, the hormones of menstruation act on this tissue just as if it were located within the uterus, causing it to hemorrhage. It is this hemorrhage that forms into focal areas of bloody tumors—endometriomas. Consequently, they have been nicknamed "**chocolate cysts**" because they appear as dark, thick bloody masses during gross examination.

Endometriomas can be located anywhere outside the endometrial cavity, including on any other pelvic organ, such as the bladder and bowel, but are more commonly found on the ovary. Most often, these masses are multiple and seen more often in the reproductive years. Patients typically complain of pelvic pain, **menorrhagia**, **dyspareunia**, painful bowel movements (dyschezia), and, possibly, infertility.

The cause of endometriosis is still unknown; however, several hypotheses exist. One theory suggests that implantation of this ectopic tissue is a result of endometrial tissue being passed through the fallopian tubes during menstruation, whereas another proposes that scaring from surgery, such as a cesarean section, leads to endometriosis and the subsequent development of endometriomas. In fact, endometriomas can be found within the cesarean section scar and present as a palpable mass that may change shape throughout the menstrual cycle in relation to hormone alterations.

The sonographic appearance of an endometrioma is that of a predominately cystic mass with low-level echoes that resembles the sonographic appearance of a hemorrhagic cyst (Fig. 18-19). Endometriomas may also demonstrate a fluid–fluid level. They are discussed further in Chapter 21 of this text.

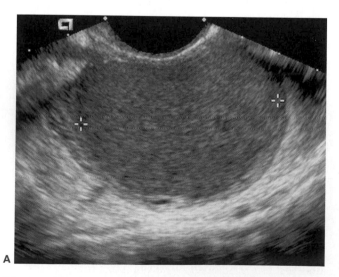

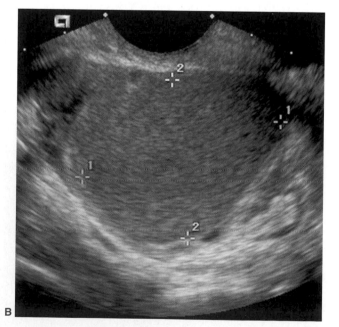

Figure 18-19 Endometrioma filled with homogeneous echoes. **A** and **B.** Images of cystic adnexal mass (*calipers*) filled with homogeneous echoes consistent with the sonographic findings of an endometrioma.

The Ovaries and Fallopian Tubes

CLINICAL FINDINGS OF ENDOMETRIOMAS

1. Patient may be asymptomatic
2. Pelvic pain
3. Infertility
4. Dysmenorrhea
5. Menorrhagia
6. Dyspareunia
7. Painful bowel movements (dyschezia)

SONOGRAPHIC FINDINGS OF ENDOMETRIOMAS

1. Predominantly cystic mass with low-level internal echoes (may resemble a hemorrhagic cyst)
2. Anechoic or complex, mostly cystic mass with posterior enhancement and may have a fluid–fluid level

🔊 **SOUND OFF**
Endometriomas are also referred to as "chocolate cysts."

Cystadenoma (Serous and Mucinous)

Together, serous cystadenomas and cystic teratomas comprise most neoplasms of the ovary. Approximately 50% to 70% of serous cystadenomas are benign, occurring more often in women in their forties and fifties as well as during pregnancy. Patients are often asymptomatic. These types of ovarian neoplasms are often large and bilateral. The sonographic appearance of a serous cystadenoma is that of a predominately anechoic lesion that contains septations and/or **papillary projections** (Fig. 18-20).

Mucinous cystadenomas are often larger than serous cystadenomas and can even reach sizes up to 50 cm. Mucinous cystadenomas also tend to have septations and papillary projections like serous cystadenomas, but are not as often bilateral. A supportive sonographic distinguishing factor is the presence of internal debris within the mucinous cystadenoma, secondary to the solid components of the material contained within it (Fig. 18-21).

The clinical presentation of these masses is unpredictable, with patients often complaining of pelvic pressure and swelling, secondary to the large size of the mass. Additional clinical symptoms include abnormal uterine bleeding, gastrointestinal symptoms, and acute abdominal pain secondary to rupture or ovarian torsion.

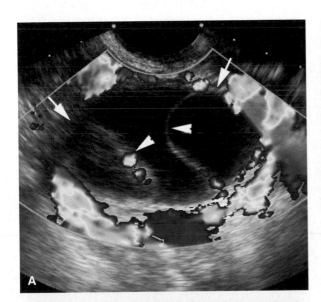

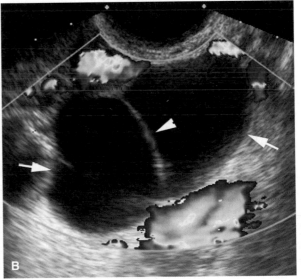

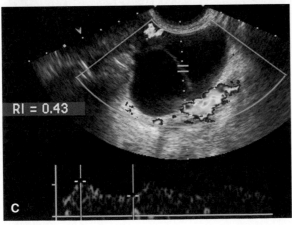

Figure 18-20 Ovarian serous cystadenoma. **A** and **B.** Transvaginal color Doppler images of cystic ovarian lesion (*arrows*) with anechoic fluid and a few thin septations (*arrowheads*). Color Doppler shows blood flow within the septations. **C.** Spectral Doppler demonstrating blood flow within a septation. An arterial waveform (*calipers*) is discovered with a resistive index (*RI*) of 0.43.

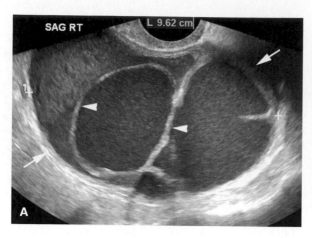
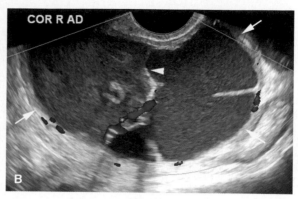

Figure 18-21 Ovarian mucinous cystadenoma. (**A**) Longitudinal and (**B**) color Doppler images of a right cystic mass (*calipers* and *arrows*) containing low-level echoes and a few thin septations (*arrowheads*). The fluid has different echogenicity in different components of the mass, typical of a mucinous cystadenoma.

🔊 **SOUND OFF**
Mucinous cystadenomas are often larger than serous cystadenomas, and they tend to contain echogenic material within their cystic components.

CLINICAL FINDINGS OF A SEROUS CYSTADENOMA

1. Patients are often asymptomatic

SONOGRAPHIC APPEARANCE OF A SEROUS CYSTADENOMA

1. Predominately anechoic lesion that contains septations and/or papillary projections

CLINICAL FINDINGS OF A MUCINOUS CYSTADENOMA

1. Pelvic pressure and swelling

SONOGRAPHIC APPEARANCE OF A MUCINOUS CYSTADENOMA

1. Large, predominately anechoic lesion that contains septations and/or papillary projections
2. May contain some recognizable internal, echogenic, layering debris

Malignant Ovarian Disease

Overview of Ovarian Cancer

Ovarian cancer is known as a silent killer because, most often, the disease manifests late clinically, with signs and symptoms that are vague. For example, these symptoms may simply be abdominal distention or bloating. Ovarian cancer may thus go undetected for a considerable amount of time, giving the disease the opportunity to grow and spread to other organs. Consequently, the survival rate for ovarian cancers that are discovered in the advanced stages is only around 15%. Ovarian cancer has a strong familial incidence, including those individuals who are known carriers of the *BRCA1*, *BRCA2*, and *HER2/neu* gene mutations. These patients will likely have a family history of breast cancer as well. Patients with these gene mutations may choose to undergo a prophylactic bilateral **oophorectomy** and, possibly, a hysterectomy as well.

Other risk factors for ovarian cancer include an age of over 50 years, nulliparity, delayed childbearing, early onset of menses, late menopause, and estrogen use for hormone replacement therapy following menopause for more than 10 years. Though there are several forms of ovarian cancer, the following section focuses primarily on the most common forms. The largest number of ovarian cancers are epithelial in origin (e.g., serous and mucinous cystadenocarcinomas). The epithelium is the covering of the ovary. Other ovarian cancers are referred to as malignant germ cell tumors, malignant sex cord–stromal tumors, or metastatic disease.

Cystadenocarcinoma (Serous and Mucinous)

Serous cystadenocarcinoma is the most common malignancy of the ovary. It is, like its benign counterpart the serous cystadenoma, frequently bilateral. In addition, a serous cystadenocarcinoma sonographically resembles a serous cystadenoma, with the exception that often with malignancy, there appears to be more prominent papillary projections and thicker septations (Fig. 18-22). Patients often complain of weight loss, pelvic pressure and swelling, abnormal vaginal bleeding, and gastrointestinal problems. Although not always specific, they may also have an elevated cancer antigen 125 (**CA 125**), a protein that may be increased in the blood of women with ovarian cancer and other abnormalities.

The Ovaries and Fallopian Tubes

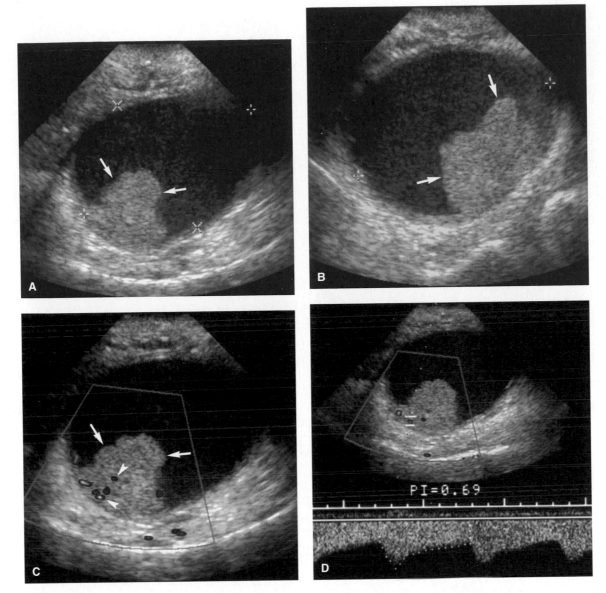

Figure 18-22 Ovarian papillary cystadenocarcinoma with solid nodule in wall. **A** and **B.** Images of an ovarian mass (*calipers*) with a solid nodule (*arrows*) projecting from the wall into the cystic portion. **C.** Color Doppler demonstrating blood flow (*arrowheads*) within the solid nodule (*arrows*) and wall of the tumor. **D.** Spectral Doppler of vessel within mass demonstrating low-resistance flow, with a pulsatility index (*PI*) of 0.69.

🔊 **SOUND OFF**
Patients with ovarian cancer may complain of weight loss, pelvic pressure and swelling, abnormal vaginal bleeding, and gastrointestinal problems. Although not always specific, they may also have an elevated CA 125.

Mucinous cystadenocarcinomas are malignant as well and are less often bilateral than serous cystadenocarcinomas. The mucinous cystadenocarcinoma is associated with a condition known as **pseudomyxoma peritonei**, which describes the intraperitoneal extension of mucin-secreting cells that result

from the rupture of this mucinous tumor. Often, the fluid escaping from the mass resembles ascites (Fig. 18-23).

CLINICAL FINDINGS OF SEROUS AND MUCINOUS CYSTADENOCARCINOMAS

1. Weight loss
2. Pelvic pressure and swelling
3. Abnormal vaginal bleeding
4. Gastrointestinal symptoms
5. Acute abdominal pain associated with torsion or rupture
6. Elevated CA 125

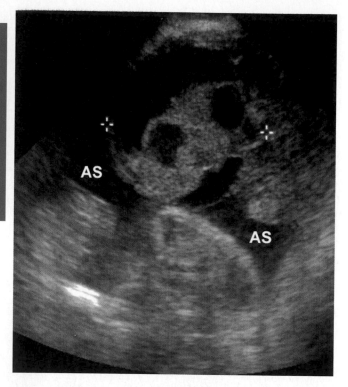

Figure 18-23 Ovarian mucinous cystadenocarcinoma. Transvaginal images of a large ovarian mass (between *calipers*) surrounded by malignant ascites (*AS*).

SONOGRAPHIC APPEARANCE OF SEROUS CYSTADENOCARCINOMA

1. Large, multilocular cystic masses
2. Papillary projections and septations are often noted within the mass
3. Ascites

SONOGRAPHIC APPEARANCE OF MUCINOUS CYSTADENOCARCINOMA

1. Large, multilocular cystic mass
2. Papillary projections and septations are often noted within the mass
3. Echogenic material within the cystic components of the mass
4. Pseudomyxoma peritonei (complex ascites)

Krukenberg Tumor

A **Krukenberg tumor** is a malignant ovarian tumor that has most likely metastasized from the gastrointestinal tract. The most frequent origin is the stomach (gastric cancer), although it may begin in the colon. In addition, some authors claim that Krukenberg tumors can originate from primary breast, lung, contralateral ovary, pancreas, or biliary tract cancers. The key to histologic diagnosis is the presence of "signet-ring" cells.

SOUND OFF
Krukenberg tumors are metastatic tumors to the ovary, most often from gastrointestinal cancers, like stomach cancer.

Krukenberg tumors appear sonographically as smooth-walled, hypoechoic, or hyperechoic tumors that are often bilateral and may be accompanied by ascites. The Krukenberg tumor may also be described as having a "moth-eaten" appearance in that it can be a solid mass containing scattered cystic spaces. Patients may be asymptomatic at the time of detection or may complain of weight loss and pelvic pain. They may also present with a history of gastric, colon cancer, or some other form of cancer.

CLINICAL FINDINGS OF A KRUKENBERG TUMOR

1. Asymptomatic
2. History of gastric or colon cancer
3. Possible weight loss
4. Pelvic pain

SONOGRAPHIC FINDINGS OF A KRUKENBERG TUMOR

1. Bilateral, smooth-walled, hypoechoic or hyperechoic ovarian masses
2. "Moth-eaten" appearance (solid mass containing cystic spaces)
3. May have ascites

SOUND OFF
Krukenberg tumors tend to have a "moth-eaten" sonographic appearance.

Sertoli–Leydig Cell Tumors (Androblastoma)

A **Sertoli–Leydig cell tumor**, or **androblastoma**, is a sex cord–stromal ovarian neoplasm that is associated with **virilization**; thus, patients may present with abnormal menstruation and **hirsutism** because of androgen production. Sertoli–Leydig tumors are found more often in women younger than 30 years but may be seen in older patients and may be malignant. Sonographically, a Sertoli–Leydig cell tumor may appear as a solid, hypoechoic ovarian mass or a complex, partially cystic mass.

CLINICAL FINDINGS OF SERTOLI–LEYDIG CELL TUMORS

1. Virilization
2. Abnormal menstruation
3. Hirsutism

SONOGRAPHIC FINDINGS OF SERTOLI–LEYDIG CELL TUMORS

1. Solid, hypoechoic ovarian mass
2. Complex or partially cystic mass

Dysgerminoma

A dysgerminoma is the most common malignant **germ cell tumor** of the ovary. Dysgerminomas arise more often in patients younger than 30 years and may be found in pregnancy. The dysgerminoma is the most frequent ovarian malignancy found in childhood. Children with ovarian dysgerminomas present with pseudoprecocious puberty and may have an elevation in serum hCG levels, although the tumor marker used for dysgerminoma is an elevation in **serum lactate dehydrogenase**. The testicular equivalent of an ovarian dysgerminoma is the seminoma.

CLINICAL FINDINGS OF DYSGERMINOMA

1. Children—pseudoprecocious puberty
2. Elevated serum lactate dehydrogenase
3. Possible elevated serum hCG

SONOGRAPHIC FINDINGS OF DYSGERMINOMA

1. Ovoid, solid echogenic mass on the ovary
2. May contain some cystic components

 SOUND OFF
The dysgerminoma is the most common malignant germ cell tumor of the ovary. It is the ovarian equivalent of the testicular seminoma.

Yolk Sac Tumor (Endodermal Sinus Tumor)

A **yolk sac tumor**, which may also be referred to as an endodermal sinus tumor, is the second most common malignant germ cell tumor of the ovary. It is characterized by rapid growth. A yolk sac tumor occurs in females younger than 20 years, is highly malignant, and carries a poor prognosis. Clinically, patients present with an elevation in serum alpha-fetoprotein (AFP). Sonographically, they have varying appearances.

CLINICAL FINDINGS OF YOLK SAC TUMOR

1. Elevation in serum AFP

SONOGRAPHIC FINDINGS OF YOLK SAC TUMOR

1. Homogeneous hyperechoic or complex mass
2. Varying sonographic appearances

SOUND OFF
The tumor marker for the yolk sac tumor is AFP.

Endometrioid Tumor (Endometrioid Carcinoma)

The **endometrioid tumor** (endometrioid carcinoma) is an ovarian tumor that has a high incidence of being malignant. It is most often seen in women in their fifth and sixth decades of life and is often associated with a history of endometrial cancer, endometriosis, or endometrial hyperplasia. It is the most common cancer to originate within an endometrioma. Sonographically, an endometrioid tumor appears as a complex mass with solid components or a cystic mass with papillary projections.

CLINICAL FINDINGS OF ENDOMETRIOID TUMOR

1. History of endometrial cancer or endometriosis

SONOGRAPHIC FINDINGS OF ENDOMETRIOID TUMOR

1. Complex mass with solid components
2. Cystic mass with papillary projections

Common Sonographic Findings and Doppler Findings of Ovarian Carcinoma

It is important to note that only about 10% of ovarian tumors are malignant in reproductive-age women, whereas 25% of tumors in postmenopausal women are malignant. Consequently, the sonographer must be able to appreciate the unique features of each sonographically identified ovarian mass. There are several grayscale indicators that are worrisome for ovarian carcinoma (Table 18-2). Doppler analysis of malignant ovarian masses often reveals higher diastolic flow velocities because of the abnormal vessels that are created with malignancy. These new vessels often lack smooth muscle within their walls and thus produce a less resistive waveform pattern (see Fig. 18-22). Specifically, malignant tumors tend to have resistive indices less than 0.4 and pulsatility indices less than 1.0. However, color-flow and spectral Doppler characteristic within a mass is not a specific finding and, therefore, is not typically used to determine the presence of malignancy.

Staging of Ovarian Carcinoma

The International Federation of Gynecology and Obstetrics (FIGO) recommends the proper staging of ovarian carcinoma. Table 18-3 is a summary of the FIGO staging of ovarian cancer.

TABLE 18-2 Sonographic findings that are worrisome for ovarian carcinoma

Worrisome Sonographic Findings for Ovarian Carcinoma[a]

- Complex ovarian mass
- Solid wall nodules within a cystic mass (the larger the solid component, the more likely for malignancy)
- Thick septations (>3 mm)
- Wall thickening
- Irregular wall or poorly defined margins
- Blood flow within the septations, wall, or nodules
- Ascites

[a] These findings may also be observed with benign tumors.

TABLE 18-3 Staging of ovarian carcinoma

Stage of Ovarian Carcinoma	Condition
Stage I	Tumor is confined to the ovary.
Stage II	Tumor involves one or both ovaries with pelvic extension.
Stage III	Tumor involves one or both ovaries with confirmed peritoneal metastasis outside the pelvis and/or regional lymph node involvement.
Stage IV	Distant metastasis beyond the peritoneal cavity.

Ovarian Torsion

Ovarian torsion, also referred to as adnexal torsion because it can involve the fallopian tube as well, results from the adnexal structures twisting on their mesenteric connection, consequently cutting off its blood supply. Ovarian torsion occurs most often on the right side, with the most common cause being an ovarian cyst or mass, such as the benign cystic teratoma or paraovarian cyst. Because of the cystic enlargement of the ovaries produced by ovarian hyperstimulation syndrome, this condition has also been recognized as a predisposing circumstance that can result in ovarian torsion. Torsion of the ovary has also been detected in the fetus and may even occur in normal ovaries. Patients most often present with slight leukocytosis, nausea, vomiting, and acute unilateral pelvic or abdominal pain. The sonographic appearance of the torsed ovary is that of an enlarged ovary, with or without multifollicular development (Fig. 18-24). In one study, the torsed ovary most often measured greater than 5 cm, with a mean of 9.5 cm. There may also be peripherally displaced small follicles secondary to edema. The **"whirlpool sign"** may be present as well. The "whirlpool sign" is an indicator of the torsed ovarian pedicle adjacent to the ovary, appearing as a round mass with concentric hypoechoic and hyperechoic rings that demonstrates a swirling color Doppler signature. An abnormal amount of free fluid in the pelvis is often seen as well.

> 🔊 **SOUND OFF**
> The sonographic appearance of the torsed ovary is that of an enlarged ovary, with or without multifollicular development.

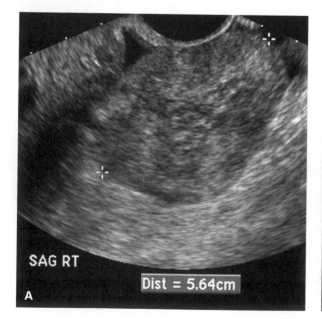
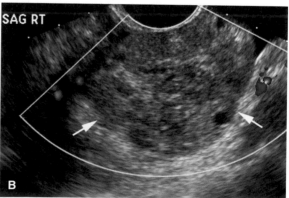

Figure 18-24 Ovarian torsion with no visible blood flow. **A.** Sagittal image of right ovary (SAG RT, *calipers*) showing enlargement, globular shape, and edema, all due to torsion. **B.** Sagittal view with color Doppler showing no flow in the torsed ovary (*arrows*).

Some debate exists over the effectiveness of color Doppler and flow analysis of the torsed ovary. As stated earlier, the ovary receives its blood supply from both the ovarian artery and a branch of the uterine artery. If one of these vessels has been occluded, thereby revealing a lack of arterial blood flow on spectral analysis, the other vessel may still be patent. That means, a lack of detectable arterial flow within an ovarian or uterine artery does not mean that there is occlusion of the entire blood supply. Venous flow should also be evaluated. As a result, a combination of clinical presentation and imaging findings is essential for the precise diagnosis of this urgent condition. Treatment for ovarian torsion typically involves laparoscopy with detorsion and the removal of the cause—most likely a large ovarian cyst.

CLINICAL FINDINGS OF OVARIAN TORSION

1. Acute unilateral abdominal or pelvic pain
2. Nausea and vomiting
3. Slight leukocytosis

SONOGRAPHIC FINDINGS OF OVARIAN TORSION

1. Enlarged ovary
2. Enlarged ovary in the presence of multifollicular development
3. Small peripherally located follicles on the enlarged ovary as a result of edema
4. Lack of or diminished flow patterns compared with the nonaffected ovary
5. "Whirlpool" sign
6. Excessive free fluid

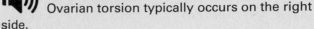

SOUND OFF
Ovarian torsion typically occurs on the right side.

ANATOMY AND PHYSIOLOGY OF THE FALLOPIAN TUBES

The fallopian tubes may be referred to as oviducts, uterine tubes, or salpinges. The primary purpose of the fallopian tube is to provide an area for fertilization (conception) to occur and to offer a means of transportation for the products of conception to reach the uterine cavity. The fallopian tubes consist of three layers: the outer serosa, middle muscular layer, and inner mucosal layer. Because the tube experiences **peristalsis**, within its lumen, small, hairlike structures referred to as **cilia** shift, thereby offering a mechanism for the transportation of the fertilized ovum.

The 7- to 12-cm paired fallopian tubes extend from the cornu of the uterus, travel within the broad ligaments, and are composed of five parts (Fig. 18-25). It is important to note that the proximal segment of the fallopian tube is located closest to the uterus, whereas the most distal part is within the **adnexa** or closer toward the ovary. Within the cornu of the uterus lies the intramural extension of the fallopian tube, known as the **interstitial** segment. The **isthmus**, which literally means bridge, is a short and narrow segment of the tube connecting the interstitial area to the ampulla. The **ampulla** is the longest and most tortuous segment of the tube. It is a significant portion of the tube because it is the most likely location of fertilization (conception) and the area

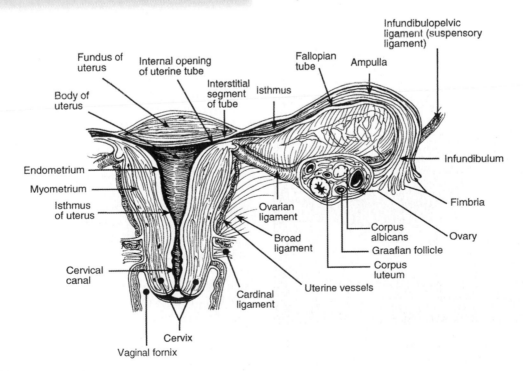

Figure 18-25 Fallopian tube anatomy.

where ectopic pregnancies often embed. The distal portion of the tube is termed the **infundibulum**, which provides an opening to the peritoneal cavity within the pelvis. The fingerlike projections that extend from the infundibulum are the **fimbriae**. The primary role of the fimbria is to draw the unfertilized egg into the tube.

> 🔊 **SOUND OFF**
> The ampulla is the longest and most tortuous segment of the tube. It is a significant portion of the tube because it is the most likely location of fertilization and the area where ectopic pregnancies often embed.

SONOGRAPHIC APPEARANCE OF THE FALLOPIAN TUBES

The fallopian tubes are not customarily identified on a transabdominal sonographic examination; however, some segments can be seen with today's high-resolution endovaginal transducers. Certainly, in cases in which the tube has been involved with an inflammatory process or is obstructed, the tubes, when distended with fluid, can be visualized with sonography. The inner cavity of the fallopian tubes can be visualized and evaluated for patency using **sonohysterography**, sonohysterosalpingography, or **hysterosalpingography** (see Chapter 20 for more details).

Abnormal Fallopian Tubes

Cancer of the fallopian tubes is rare and is typically in the form of adenocarcinoma. The sonographic appearance of fallopian tube carcinoma is that of a solid mass within the adnexa. The fallopian tubes may become distended secondary to obstruction or infection. The fluid

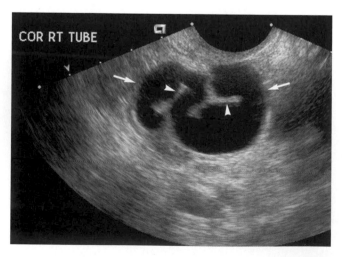

Figure 18-26 Hydrosalpinx. Coronal image of a dilated right fallopian tube (between *arrows*) filled with anechoic fluid. Note the folds (*arrowheads*) of the tortuous tube.

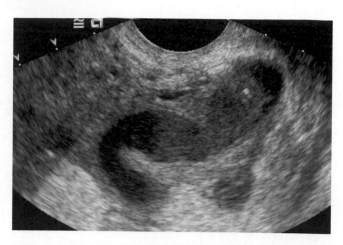

Figure 18-27 Pyosalpinx. Echogenic debris or pus is noted within this dilated and inflamed fallopian tube.

contained within the distended tubes could be simple serous fluid, blood, or pus. Simple serous fluid within the tube is termed **hydrosalpinx** (Fig. 18-26). Hydrosalpinx appears anechoic, whereas pus (**pyosalpinx**) and blood (**hematosalpinx**) have internal components and may appear echoic or have a fluid–fluid level (Fig. 18-27). The fallopian tubes may also become inflamed due to infection, which is termed **salpingitis**, a common issue caused by **pelvic inflammatory disease**. Fallopian tube pathology is further discussed in Chapter 21 of this text.

PELVIC CONGESTION SYNDROME

The etiology of **pelvic congestion syndrome** (PCS) may be multifactorial. One theory relates to a mechanic obstruction caused by the compression of the left renal vein at the origin of the superior mesenteric artery, a condition termed **Nutcracker syndrome**. Another hypothesis is that the combination of dysfunctional venous valves, estrogenic effects on vasodilation, or late pregnancy mechanical injury. Nonetheless, patient complaints vary and include persistent lower abdominal and back pain after standing for long periods of time; dull, chronic pelvic pain; dyspareunia; dysmenorrhea; abnormal uterine bleeding; chronic fatigue; and bowel issues. The diagnosis combines the need for evidence of uterine or ovarian varicose veins and chronic pelvic pain for more than 6 months. Patients also tend to have coexisting vulvar, perineal, gluteal, posterior thigh, and other lower extremity varices.

Though **venography** is the chosen imaging modality, sonography can be used to confirm PCS, and occasionally be the initial imaging tool where PCS is suspected. The sonographic findings of PCS include the demonstration of multiple tortuous and dilated venous structures adjacent to the uterus and ovaries that measure greater than 4 to 5 mm in diameter. The ovarian vein itself typically exceeds 6 mm. These dilated veins will yield a slow flow velocity with spectral imaging (Fig. 18-28).

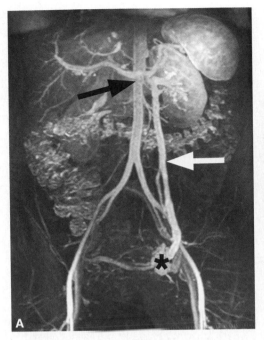
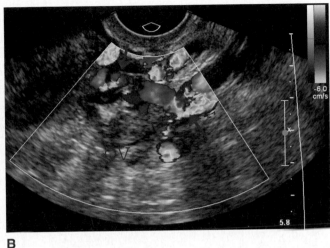

Figure 18-28 Pelvic congestion. **A.** Magnetic resonance venography of a woman with chronic pelvic pain and symptoms of pelvic congestion syndrome showed a dilated left gonadal (ovarian) vein (*white arrow*), left adnexal varices (*asterisk*), and poor enhancement of the central left renal vein (*black arrow*). **B.** Dilated venous vessels (*arrows*) adjacent to the ovary (*OV*), which is indicative of pelvic congestion syndrome.

CLINICAL FINDINGS OF PELVIC CONGESTION SYNDROME

1. Persistent lower abdominal and back pain after standing for long periods of time
2. Dull, chronic pelvic pain
3. Dyspareunia
4. Dysmenorrhea
5. Abnormal uterine bleeding
6. Chronic fatigue
7. Bowel issues
8. Coexisting vulvar, perineal, and lower extremity varices

SONOGRAPHIC FINDINGS OF PELVIC CONGESTION SYNDROME

1. Multiple tortuous and dilated venous structures adjacent to the uterus and ovaries
2. These dilated veins will yield measure greater than 4 to 5 mm in diameter and demonstrate a slow flow velocity with spectral imaging
3. Ovarian vein exceeds 6 mm in diameter

Ovarian Remnant Syndrome

Ovarian remnant syndrome (ORS) is a complication of bilateral salpingo-oophorectomy. Essentially, ORS results from ovarian tissue being left behind following this procedure, thus leading to stimulation of that tissue by circulating hormones. Patients often complain of chronic pelvic pain or cyclical pain and, possibly, a mass.

CLINICAL FINDINGS OF OVARIAN REMNANT SYNDROME

1. History of bilateral salpingo-oophorectomy
2. Chronic pelvic pain
3. Cyclic pelvic pain
4. Possible pelvic mass

SONOGRAPHIC FINDINGS OF OVARIAN REMNANT SYNDROME

1. Identifiable ovarian tissue
2. Possible ovarian/adnexal mass

REVIEW QUESTIONS

1. Which of the following would be least likely associated with PCS?
   a. Right renal vein entrapment
   b. Dysfunctional venous valves
   c. Abnormal uterine bleeding
   d. Chronic fatigue

2. Figure 18-29 shows sagittal and transverse images of the right adnexa. The patient complained of right adnexal tenderness. Which of the following is the most likely diagnosis?
   a. Right ovarian torsion
   b. Paraovarian cyst
   c. Hydrosalpinx
   d. Meigs syndrome

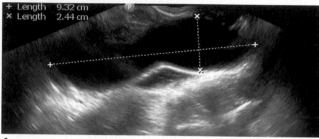

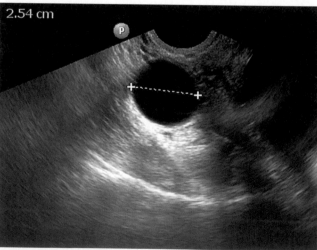

A

B

Figure 18-29

3. Which of the following would be least likely associated with an increase for developing ovarian cancer?
   a. Nulliparity
   b. Late menarche
   c. Delayed childbearing
   d. Age of over 50

4. What sign does the open arrow in Figure 18-30 indicate?
   a. Tip of the iceberg
   b. Whirlpool
   c. Plug
   d. Mesh

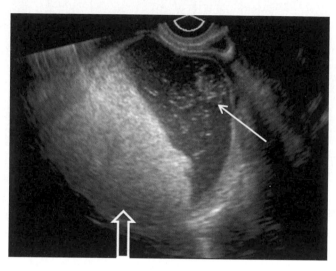

Figure 18-30

5. What sign does the long thin arrow in Figure 18-30 indicate?
   a. Tip of the iceberg
   b. Whirlpool
   c. Plug
   d. Mesh

6. What mass would least likely appear as a solid adnexal mass?
   a. Thecoma
   b. Fibroma
   c. Dermoid
   d. Brenner tumor

7. The 29-year-old patient in Figure 18-31 complained of adnexal pain, menorrhagia, and dyspareunia. What is the most likely diagnosis for the mass, given its sonographic appearance?
   a. Cystadenoma
   b. Endometrioma
   c. Cystic teratoma
   d. Fibroma

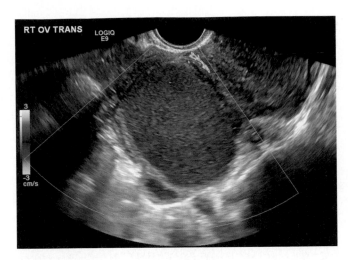

Figure 18-31

8. The finding in Figure 18-32 was noted in the presence of a triploid pregnancy at 13 weeks with thickened placenta. What is the most likely diagnosis?
   a. Endometrioid
   b. Surface epithelial inclusion cyst
   c. Polycystic ovary syndrome
   d. Theca lutein cyst

9. Which of the following clinical findings would be likely noted for the patient in Figure 18-32?
   a. Dyschezia
   b. Hirsutism
   c. Markedly elevated hCG
   d. Decreased lactate dehydrogenase

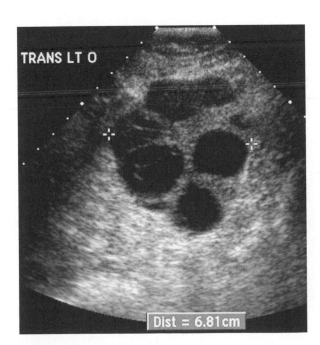

Figure 18-32

10. The finding in Figure 18-33 in the asymptomatic patient is most likely associated with a:
    a. corpus luteum cyst.
    b. thecoma.
    c. granulosa cell tumor.
    d. yolk sac tumor.

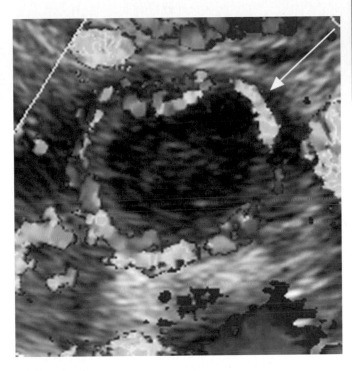

Figure 18-33

11. What is another name for the androblastoma?
    a. Granulosa cell tumor
    b. Krukenberg tumor
    c. Yolk sac tumor
    d. Sertoli–Leydig cell tumor

12. The patient in Figure 18-34 was initially diagnosed with colon cancer. A biopsy of the mass pictured revealed metastatic disease. What is the most likely diagnosis?
    a. Mucinous cystadenocarcinoma
    b. Krukenberg tumor
    c. Serous cystadenocarcinoma
    d. Dysgerminoma

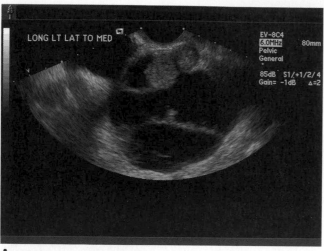

Figure 18-34

13. The 13-year-old patient in Figure 18-35 complained of severe, right lower quadrant pain, nausea, and vomiting. What is the most likely diagnosis?
    a. Brenner tumor
    b. Serous cystadenoma
    c. Ovarian torsion
    d. Meigs syndrome

14. What is the most common cancer to originate within an endometrioma?
    a. Yolk sac tumor
    b. Endometrioid tumor
    c. Androblastoma
    d. Serous cystadenocarcinoma

15. Intraperitoneal extension of mucin-secreting cells that results from the rupture of a mucinous tumor may be associated with ovarian carcinoma or cancer of the:
    a. appendix.
    b. rectum.
    c. stomach.
    d. fallopian tube.

16. Inflammation of the uterine tube is termed:
    a. pyosalpinx.
    b. hydrosalpinx.
    c. salpingitis.
    d. hematosalpinx.

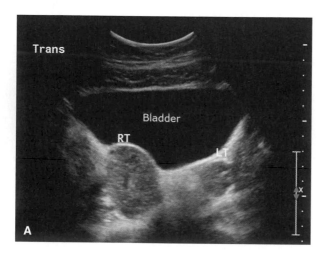

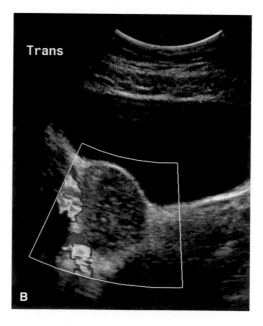

Figure 18-35

17. Which of the following would be associated with an elevated CA 125?
    a. Fibroma
    b. Thecoma
    c. Dysgerminoma
    d. PCS

18. Which of the following is not true concerning ovarian cancer?
    a. Patients tend to have ovarian cancer familial incidence.
    b. Patients tend to have a history of familial breast cancer.
    c. Patients tend to present early in the disease.
    d. Sonography does not serve as the best screening mechanism for ovarian cancer.

19. What germ cell tumor contains elements of the ectoderm, mesoderm, and endoderm?
    a. Brenner tumor
    b. Cystic teratoma
    c. Fibroma
    d. Theca cell tumor

20. The structure identified by the long arrow in Figure 18-36 was noted adjacent to the ovary. What is the most likely diagnosis?
    a. Cystadenocarcinoma
    b. Paraovarian cyst
    c. Endometrioid
    d. Cystadenoma

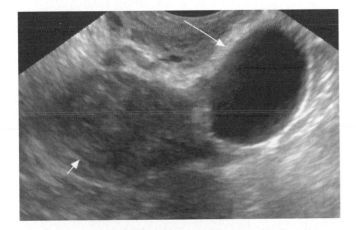

Figure 18-36

21. An endometrioma most likely appears as a:
    a. simple, anechoic mass with through transmission.
    b. complex mass with internal shadowing components.
    c. mostly cystic mass with low-level echoes.
    d. solid, hyperechoic shadowing mass.

22. With what ovarian tumor is Meigs syndrome most likely associated?
    a. Dysgerminoma
    b. Cystic teratoma
    c. Fibroma
    d. Yolk sac tumor

23. Sonographically, which of the following would most likely be confused for a pedunculated fibroid tumor because of its solid-appearing structure?
    a. Serous cystadenoma
    b. Mucinous cystadenoma
    c. Fibroma
    d. Theca lutein cyst

24. During a pelvic sonogram, you visualize a small cyst located adjacent to the ovary. What is the most likely etiology of this cyst?
    a. Dermoid cyst
    b. Ovarian cystadenoma
    c. Endometrioma
    d. Paraovarian cyst

25. The most common benign ovarian tumor is the:
    a. cystic teratoma.
    b. mucinous cystadenoma.
    c. fibroma.
    d. Sertoli–Leydig cell tumor.

26. The ovarian mass that contains fat, sebum, and teeth is the:
    a. dermoid.
    b. fibroma.
    c. mucinous cystadenoma.
    d. yolk sac tumor.

27. The ovarian cysts that are most often bilateral and are associated with markedly elevated levels of hCG are the:
    a. corpus luteum cysts.
    b. paraovarian cysts.
    c. granulosa cell cysts.
    d. theca lutein cysts.

28. The cystic mass commonly noted with a pregnancy is the:
    a. corpus luteum.
    b. dermoid cyst.
    c. dysgerminoma.
    d. serous cystadenoma.

29. The sonographic appearance of an ovarian dermoid tumor in which only the anterior elements of the mass can be seen, while the greater part of the mass is obscured by shadowing is consistent with:
    a. whirlpool sign.
    b. tip of the iceberg sign.
    c. dermoid mesh sign.
    d. dermoid plug sign.

30. The dominant follicle before ovulation is termed the:
    a. Graafian follicle.
    b. corpus albicans.
    c. corpus luteum.
    d. medulla.

31. After the Graafian follicle ruptures, the remaining structure is termed the:
    a. Graafian remnant.
    b. corpus albicans.
    c. corpus luteum.
    d. theca lutein cyst.

32. Which of the following is the correct formula for calculating ovarian volume?
    a. Length × width × height × 0.6243
    b. Length × width × height × 0.3899
    c. Length × width × height × 0.5233
    d. Ovarian volume cannot be calculated.

33. Which of the following sonographic findings would not increase the likelihood of an ovarian malignancy?
    a. Septation measuring greater than 3 mm in thickness
    b. Irregular borders
    c. Solid wall nodule
    d. Anechoic components with acoustic enhancement

34. Normal ovarian flow is said to be:
    a. low resistant during menstruation and high resistant during the proliferative phase.
    b. high resistant during menstruation and low resistant at the time of ovulation.
    c. low resistant.
    d. high resistant.

35. What would be a predisposing condition that would increase the risk for suffering from ovarian torsion?
    a. Hirsutism
    b. Excessive exercise
    c. Ovarian mass
    d. Sonohysterography

36. The malignant ovarian tumor with gastrointestinal origin is the:
    a. Brenner tumor.
    b. Krukenberg tumor.
    c. yolk sac tumor.
    d. granulosa cell tumor.

37. The malignant ovarian mass that is associated with pseudomyxoma peritonei is the:
    a. dysgerminoma.
    b. Sertoli–Leydig cell tumor.
    c. serous cystadenocarcinoma.
    d. mucinous cystadenocarcinoma.

38. All of the following adnexal masses may appear sonographically similar to a uterine leiomyoma except:
    a. thecoma.
    b. paraovarian cyst.
    c. fibroma.
    d. granulosa cell tumor.

39. Which of the following is also referred to as a chocolate cyst?
    a. Endometrioma
    b. Endometrioid
    c. Cystic teratoma
    d. Androblastoma

40. The ovarian tumor associated with an elevated serum lactate dehydrogenase is the:
    a. dysgerminoma.
    b. Sertoli–Leydig cell tumor.
    c. androblastoma.
    d. mucinous cystadenocarcinoma.

41. Which of the following is a tumor of ectopic endometrial tissue?
    a. Brenner tumor
    b. Cystic teratoma
    c. Yolk sac tumor
    d. Endometrioma

42. What ovarian mass is associated with virilization?
    a. Krukenberg tumor
    b. Cystic teratoma
    c. Serous cystadenoma
    d. Sertoli–Leydig cell tumor

43. A 24-year-old female patient presents to the emergency department with severe right lower quadrant pain, nausea, and vomiting. The sonographic examination reveals an enlarged ovary with no detectable Doppler signal. What is the most likely diagnosis?
    a. Ovarian cystadenocarcinoma
    b. Cystic teratoma
    c. Ovarian torsion
    d. Endometriosis

44. Which of the following is an estrogen-producing ovarian tumor?
    a. Cystic teratoma
    b. Fibroma
    c. Thecoma
    d. Endometrioma

45. What ovarian tumor will most likely have a moth-eaten appearance on sonography?
    a. Cystic teratoma
    b. Serous cystadenocarcinoma
    c. Krukenberg tumor
    d. Sertoli–Leydig cell tumor

46. A 55-year-old patient presents to the sonography department with a history of pelvic pressure, abdominal swelling, and abnormal uterine bleeding. A pelvic sonogram reveals a large, multiloculated cystic mass with papillary projections. What is the most likely diagnosis?
    a. Serous cystadenocarcinoma
    b. Cystic teratoma
    c. Androblastoma
    d. Dysgerminoma

47. A patient with an ovarian mass presents with an elevated serum AFP. Which of the following would be the most likely diagnosis?
    a. Ovarian fibroma
    b. Ovarian thecoma
    c. Cystic teratoma
    d. Yolk sac tumor

48. The ovarian cyst associated with gestational trophoblastic disease is the:
    a. corpus luteum cyst.
    b. theca lutein cyst.
    c. dermoid cyst.
    d. paraovarian cyst.

49. Pus within the fallopian tube is termed:
    a. hematosalpinx.
    b. pyosalpinx.
    c. hydrosalpinx.
    d. hemosalpinx.

50. Which of the following is the most common malignancy of the ovary?
    a. Cystic teratoma
    b. Serous cystadenocarcinoma
    c. Krukenberg tumor
    d. Sertoli–Leydig cell tumor

51. The short and narrow segment of the fallopian tube distal to the interstitial segment is the:
    a. ampulla.
    b. fimbria.
    c. infundibulum.
    d. isthmus.

52. The fingerlike extension of the fallopian tube is called:
    a. fimbria.
    b. infundibulum.
    c. cilia.
    d. ampulla.

53. The longest and most tortuous segment of the fallopian tube is the:
    a. fimbria.
    b. ampulla.
    c. isthmus.
    d. interstitial.

54. Blood within the fallopian tube is termed:
    a. hydrosalpinx.
    b. hematosalpinx.
    c. pyosalpinx.
    d. hemosalpinx.

55. Hairlike projections within the fallopian tube are called:
    a. interstitia.
    b. fimbriae.
    c. cilia.
    d. peristalsis.

56. The inner layer of the wall of the fallopian tube is the:
    a. muscular layer.
    b. mucosal layer.
    c. myometrial layer.
    d. serosal layer.

57. The most distal part of the fallopian tube is the:
    a. cornu.
    b. ampulla.
    c. interstitial.
    d. infundibulum.

58. The segment of the fallopian tube where fertilization typically occurs is the:
    a. cornu.
    b. fimbria.
    c. interstitial.
    d. ampulla.

59. What substance does hysterosalpingography utilize for the visualization of the uterine cavity and fallopian tubes?
    a. Saline
    b. Radiographic contrast
    c. Water
    d. Betadine

60. Which of the following is associated with the "whirlpool sign"?
    a. Ovarian torsion
    b. Hydrosalpinx
    c. Ovarian hyperstimulation syndrome
    d. Ovarian carcinoma

SUGGESTED READINGS

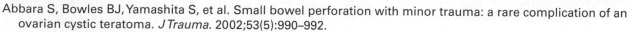

Abbara S, Bowles BJ, Yamashita S, et al. Small bowel perforation with minor trauma: a rare complication of an ovarian cystic teratoma. *J Trauma*. 2002;53(5):990–992.

Antignani, P. What's about pelvic congestion syndrome. *Vasc Invest Ther*. 2020;3(4):99.

Bartl T, Wolf F, Dadak C. Pelvic congestion syndrome (PCS) as a pathology of postmenopausal women: a case report with literature review. *BMC Womens Health*. 2021;21:1–5.

Curry RA, Tempkin BB. *Sonography: Introduction to Normal Structure and Function*. 5th ed. Elsevier; 2020: 317–365.

Doubilet PM, Benson CB. *Atlas of Ultrasound in Obstetrics and Gynecology: A Multimedia Reference*. 2nd ed. Wolters Kluwer; 2012:380–399.

Gibbs RS, Karlan BY, Haney AF, et al. *Danforth's Obstetrics and Gynecolgy*. 10th ed. Wolters Kluwer; 2008: 1022–1072.

Hagen-Ansert SL. *Textbook of Diagnostic Sonography*. 7th ed. Elsevier; 2012:1001–1038.

Henningsen C, Kuntz K, Youngs D. *Clinical Guide to Sonography: Exercises for Critical Thinking*. 2nd ed. Elsevier; 2014:183–200.

Hertzberg BS, Middleton WD. *Ultrasound: The Requisites*. 3rd ed. Elsevier; 2016:565–599.

Hurteau J. Gestational trophoblastic disease: management of a hydatidiform mole. *Clin Obstet Gynecol*. 2003;46(3):557–569.

Kinnear HM, Tomaszewski CE, Chang FL, et al. The ovarian stroma as a new frontier. *Reproduction*. 2020; 160(3):R25-R39. doi:10.1530/REP-19-0501

Norton ME, Scoutt LM, Feldstein VA. *Callen's Ultrasonography in Obstetrics and Gynecology*. 6th ed. Elsevier; 2017:883–890 & 919–951.

Penny SM. Ovarian cancer: an overview. *Radiol Technol*. 2020;91(6):561–577.

Rumack CM, Wilson SR, Charboneau W, et al. *Diagnostic Ultrasound*. 4th ed. Elsevier; 2011:547–612.

Sanders RC, Hall-Terracciano B. *Clinical Sonography: A Practical Guide*. 5th ed. Wolters Kluwer; 2016:168–205.

Siegel MJ. *Pediatric Sonography*. 5th ed. Wolters Kluwer; 2019:513–556.

Stephenson SR, Dmitrieva J. *Diagnostic Medical Sonography: Obstetrics and Gynecology*. 4th ed. Wolters Kluwer; 2018:161–240.

Timor-Tritsch IE, Goldstein SR. *Ultrasound in Gynecology*. 2nd ed. Elsevier; 2007:100–116.

BONUS REVIEW!

Ovarian Torsion on Computed Tomography and Sonography (Fig. 18-37)

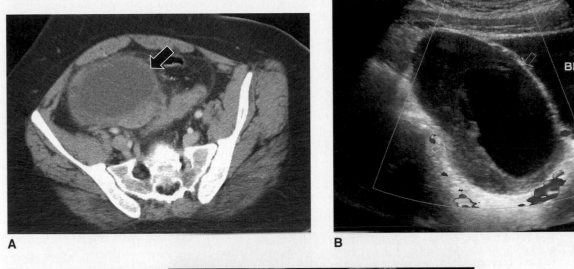

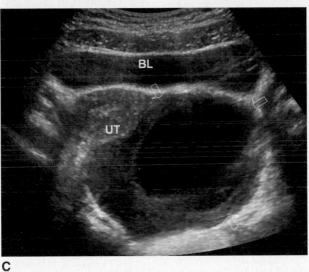

Figure 18-37 Ovarian torsion on computed tomography (*CT*) and sonography. **A.** Contrast-enhanced axial CT image shows a complex 10-cm ovarian mass (*arrows*) displacing the uterus to the right. **B.** Sagittal image of the pelvic mass shows a large anechoic cyst surrounded by ovarian tissue measuring 10.1 × 5.5 × 9.1 cm (*arrows*). Color Doppler imaging using the same imaging parameters used on the contralateral ovary demonstrates a lack of vascularity within the mass. **C.** Transverse image of the pelvis corresponding to the CT examination performed 1 week prior. A large mass containing a cystic structure is seen in the posterior left pelvis (*arrows*), resulting in deviation of the uterus anterior and to the right. The normal left ovary was noted. A normal right ovary was not identified; therefore, this mass most likely represents a torsed right ovary. At surgery, the ovary was black, necrotic, and torsed. *BL*, bladder; *UT*, uterus.

(*continued*)

BONUS REVIEW! (*continued*)

Radiograph of an Ovarian Dermoid (Fig. 18-38)

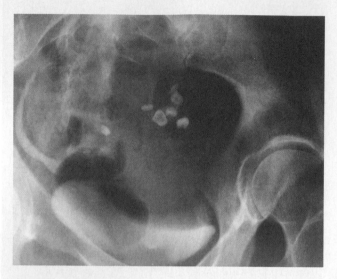

Figure 18-38 Ovarian dermoid. Several teeth are seen within the pelvis on this radiograph.

Ovarian Carcinoma on Computed Tomography (Fig. 18-39)

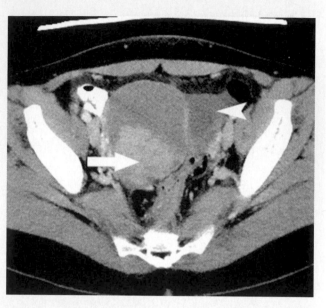

Figure 18-39 Ovarian carcinoma. Computed tomography (*CT*) shows a partially solid ovarian mass (*arrow*) displacing the bladder (*arrowhead*) to the left.

The Menstrual Cycle

Introduction

This chapter provides the reader with an overview of the menstrual cycle and the hormones that influence It. The variable sonographic appearance of the ovary and endometrium as they progress through the menstrual cycle is also presented. Lastly, the interruption of the cycle by pregnancy and causes of abnormal uterine bleeding (AUB) are discussed. In "Bonus Review" section, some useful diagrams are provided concerning patients who present with dysmenorrhea, menorrhagia, or hypomenorrhea.

Key Terms

abnormal uterine bleeding—a change in menstrual blooding patterns caused by either endocrine abnormalities or lesions within the uterus

adenomyosis—the benign invasion of endometrial tissue into the myometrium of the uterus

anovulatory—absence of ovulation

anterior pituitary gland—the anterior segment of the pituitary gland, which is responsible for releasing follicle-stimulating hormone and luteinizing hormone during the menstrual cycle

atresia (ovarian follicle)—degeneration of a follicle

blastocyst—the stage at which the conceptus implants within the decidualized endometrium

coagulopathy—blood clotting disorders

corpus albicans—the remaining structure of the corpus luteum after its deterioration

corpus hemorrhagicum—a temporary structure formed immediately following ovulation as the dominant follicle collapses and fills with blood; after the trauma heals, this becomes the corpus luteum

corpus luteum—the temporary endocrine gland that results from the rupture of the Graafian follicle after ovulation

corpus luteum of pregnancy—the corpus luteum that is maintained during early pregnancy for the purpose of producing estrogen and primarily progesterone

cumulus oophorus—the structure that contains the developing oocyte

endometrial atrophy—the degeneration of the endometrium with advancing age; most often seen in postmenopausal women

endometrial carcinoma—cancer of the endometrium

endometrial hyperplasia—an increase in the number of endometrial cells

endometrial polyps—small nodules of hyperplastic endometrial tissue

estrogen—the hormone released by the ovary during the proliferative phase that initiates the proliferation and thickening of the endometrium

fimbria—the fingerlike extension of the fallopian tube located on the infundibulum

follicle—small, round groups of cells

follicle-stimulating hormone—the hormone of the anterior pituitary gland that causes the development of multiple follicles on the ovaries

follicular phase—the first phase of the ovarian cycle

gonadotropin-releasing hormone—the hormone released by the hypothalamus that stimulates the pituitary gland to release the hormones that regulate the female menstrual cycle

Graafian follicle—the name for the dominant follicle before ovulation

human chorionic gonadotropin—the hormone produced by the trophoblastic cells of the early placenta; may also be used as a tumor marker in nongravid patients and males

hypothalamus—the area within the brain that is located just beneath the thalamus and controls the release of hormones by the anterior pituitary gland

hypothalamic–pituitary–gonadal axis—the complex interactions that take place between the hypothalamus, pituitary gland, and ovaries as part of the female reproductive cycle

imperforate hymen—a vaginal anomaly in which the hymen has no opening, resulting in an obstruction of the vagina

iatrogenic—a condition that is the result of medical treatment; may be due to exposure to a pathogen, toxin, or injury following a treatment or procedure

luteal phase—the second phase of the ovarian cycle

luteinizing hormone—the hormone of the anterior pituitary gland that surges around day 14 of the menstrual cycle, resulting in ovulation

menarche—the first menstrual cycle

menses—menstrual bleeding

mittelschmerz—pain at the time of ovulation

ovulation—the release of the mature egg from the ovary

periovulatory phase—another name for the late proliferative phase of the endometrial cycle, which occurs around the time of ovulation

primary amenorrhea—failure to experiencing menarche before age 16

progesterone—a hormone that prepares the uterus for pregnancy, maintains pregnancy, and promotes development of the mammary glands; primarily produced by the ovary and placenta

proliferation—the multiplication of similar forms

proliferative phase—the first phase of the endometrial cycle

secondary amenorrhea—the cessation of menstruation characteristically diagnosed in the postmenarchal woman who has had 3 to 6 months without a menstrual cycle

secretory phase—the second phase of the endometrial cycle

spiral arteries—coiled arteries that supply blood to the functional layer of the endometrium

syncytiotrophoblastic cells—the trophoblastic cells surrounding the blastocyst that are responsible for producing human chorionic gonadotropin

theca internal cells—cells of the follicle that produce estrogen

three-line sign—the periovulatory endometrial sonographic appearance in which the outer echogenic basal layer surrounds the more hypoechoic functional layer, with the functional layer separated by the echogenic endometrial stripe

THE MENSTRUAL CYCLE: DURATION AND DEFINITIONS

The last menstrual period relates to the onset of **menses**; therefore, the first day of the menstrual cycle is said to occur on the first day of bleeding. The average menstrual cycle lasts 28 days, with **ovulation** typically occurring around day 14. However, some menstrual cycles may last only 25 days, whereas others may last up to 45 days. Days 1 through 5 of the menstrual cycle correlate with menses, at which time the endometrium is shed.

> **))) SOUND OFF**
> The average menstrual cycle lasts 28 days, with ovulation occurring on day 14.

The first menstrual cycle is termed **menarche**. Menarche occurs at different ages and may be influenced by environment and diet. However, if an individual does not experience menarche before age 16, she is said to have **primary amenorrhea**. Primary amenorrhea may be caused by congenital abnormalities or congenital obstructions, such as an **imperforate hymen**. **Secondary amenorrhea** may be associated with endocrinologic abnormalities or pregnancy. Secondary amenorrhea that is not associated with pregnancy is characteristically diagnosed in the postmenarchal woman who has had 3 to 6 months without a menstrual cycle.

> **))) SOUND OFF**
> The first menstrual cycle is termed menarche.

THE ROLE OF THE HYPOTHALAMUS

The **hypothalamic–pituitary–gonadal axis** is the complex interactions that take place between the **hypothalamus**, pituitary gland, and ovaries as part of the female reproductive cycle. The hypothalamus is an area within the brain that is located just beneath the thalamus. The primary responsibility of the hypothalamus, as it relates to the menstrual cycle, is to regulate the release of hormones by the **anterior pituitary gland**. The hypothalamus achieves this function by releasing its own hormone, **gonadotropin-releasing hormone** (GnRH), which, in turn, stimulates the release of hormones by the anterior pituitary gland.

> **SOUND OFF**
> The hypothalamus releases GnRH, which, in turn, stimulates the release of hormones by the anterior pituitary gland.

HORMONES OF THE ANTERIOR PITUITARY GLAND

The pituitary gland, often referred to as the "master gland," is an endocrine gland located within the brain that consists of an anterior and a posterior lobe. The anterior lobe of the pituitary gland is responsible for the release of two chief hormones that influence the menstrual cycle: **follicle-stimulating hormone** (FSH) and **luteinizing hormone** (LH) (Fig. 19-1). Both of these hormones act upon the ovaries. FSH causes the development of multiple **follicles** on the ovaries, whereas LH surges around day 14 of the menstrual cycle, resulting in ovulation.

> **SOUND OFF**
> The hormones produced by the anterior pituitary gland (FSH and LH) both contain the word "hormone."

HORMONES OF THE OVARY

The ovary produces two hormones during the menstrual cycle, **estrogen** and **progesterone** (Fig. 19-2). Estrogen is produced throughout the menstrual cycle. It is initially produced by the **theca internal cells** of the secondary follicles during the first part of the menstrual cycle.

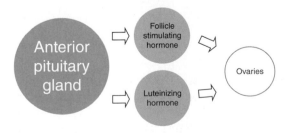

Figure 19-1 Hormones of the anterior pituitary gland influence the ovaries.

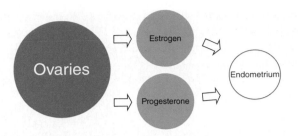

Figure 19-2 Hormones of the ovary influence the endometrium.

During this phase, estrogen initiates the **proliferation** and thickening of the endometrium by encouraging the growth and expansion of the **spiral arteries** and glands within the functional layer of the endometrium.

Estrogen has many other important functions, such as the regeneration of the endometrium after **menses** and the induction of salt and water retention. It also stimulates contractile motions within the uterine myometrium and the fallopian tubes. During the second half of the menstrual cycle, following ovulation, progesterone is produced by the **corpus luteum** of the ovary. Progesterone is responsible for maintaining the thickness of the endometrium and inducing its secretory activity as the endometrium prepares for the possible implantation of a pregnancy.

> **SOUND OFF**
> The hypothalamus releases GnRH, which influences the anterior pituitary gland. The anterior pituitary gland produces FSH and LH, which influence the ovary. The ovary produces estrogen and progesterone, which influence the endometrium.

THE PHYSIOLOGY OF THE OVARIAN CYCLE

The ovarian cycle consists of two phases: the **follicular phase** and the **luteal phase**. Consequently, the sonographic appearance of the ovaries will vary throughout the menstrual cycle. The follicular phase of the ovarian cycle is considered to begin on day 1 and lasts until day 14, thus, in effect, ending with ovulation. During the follicular phase, the anterior pituitary gland secretes FSH, which initiates the follicular development of the ovary. Many follicles are produced within the ovary. Whereas numerous follicles manifest, often, during this phase, only one follicle will progress from primordial follicle to primary follicle and then to become a secondary follicle. This secondary follicle will eventually mature to become the **Graafian follicle**

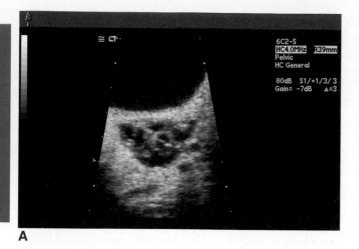

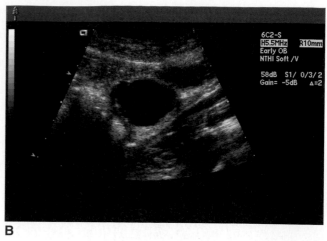

A

B

Figure 19-3 Varying sonographic appearance of the ovary during the menstrual cycle. **A.** Transabdominal transverse scan of a normal adult ovary on day 7 of the menstrual cycle. Several small follicles are seen within the ovary. **B.** Sagittal image of a dominant follicle immediately after its rupture at ovulation.

or dominant follicle before ovulation (Fig. 19-3). This Graafian follicle, which can grow as large as 2.7 cm, contains the developing oocyte (egg) within a region called the **cumulus oophorus** (Fig. 19-4).

Around day 14, LH, produced by the anterior pituitary gland, stimulates ovulation, at which time the Graafian follicle, which has grown to a size of 15 to 27 mm, ruptures and expels a small amount of fluid and the ovum into the peritoneum. At the time of ovulation, the individual may feel a twinge of pain, and this is termed **mittelschmerz**. The ovum that was expelled by the ovary is picked up by the **fimbria** of the fallopian tube and is propelled through the tube, either to be fertilized, resorbed by the body, or passed with menstruation. The fluid from the ruptured follicle mostly collects in the posterior cul-de-sac. Thus, a minimal amount of fluid within the pelvis may be detected with sonography.

The second phase of the ovarian cycle, days 15 to 28, is termed the luteal phase. After the Graafian follicle ruptures, bleeding occurs into that space, resulting in the **corpus hemorrhagicum**. That structure then rapidly converts into a temporarily endocrine gland in the form of the corpus luteum (Fig. 19-5). The corpus luteum, which is literally interpreted "yellow body," while producing estrogen in small amounts, primarily produces progesterone to maintain the thickness of the endometrium and prepares the endometrium for the (conceivably) fertilized ovum. All the other follicles undergo **atresia**.

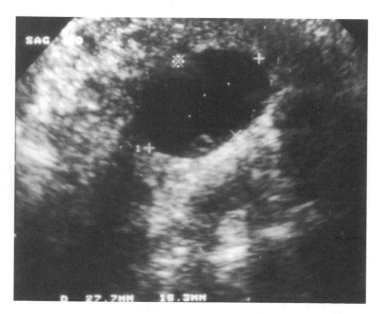

Figure 19-4 Sonographic appearance of the cumulus oophorus inside the dominant follicle before ovulation. The cumulus oophorus houses the oocyte.

The Menstrual Cycle

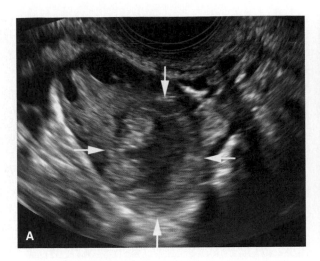

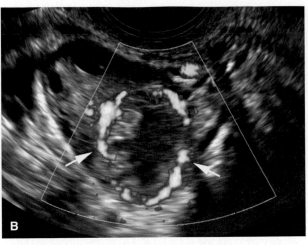

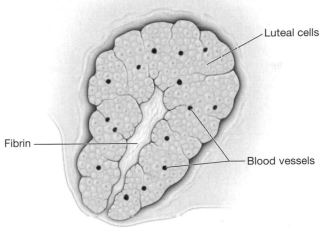

Luteal cells

Fibrin

Blood vessels

Corpus luteum

Figure 19-5 Sonographic appearance of the corpus luteum. **A.** Transvaginal image of right ovary after ovulation showing a thick-walled cyst (*arrows*) with internal echoes, representing a corpus luteum. **B.** Color Doppler showing the characteristic circumferential flow (*arrows*) of the corpus luteum. **C.** Drawing of the corpus luteum.

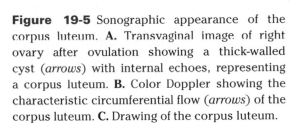

SOUND OFF
Remember this chain of events: primordial follicle > primary follicle > secondary follicle > Graafian (dominant) follicle > ovulation > corpus hemorrhagicum > corpus luteum > corpus albicans

While the corpus luteum depends on LH to be maintained, progesterone negatively inhibits the production of LH by the anterior pituitary gland, resulting in the regression of the corpus luteum. The remaining structure of the corpus luteum is now termed the **corpus albicans**, which can often be seen sonographically as a small echogenic scar on the ovary.

Ovarian blood flow varies throughout the cycle (Fig. 19-6). For example, during the early follicular phase and late luteal phase, the ovarian artery will demonstrate a high-resistive pattern, with increased impedance, and absent or low end-diastolic velocity. During the late follicular and early luteal phases, the

ovary will demonstrate a low-resistive pattern, with low impedance and higher levels of diastolic flow.

SOUND OFF
The corpus luteum primarily produces progesterone to maintain the thickness of the endometrium and prepares the endometrium for the (conceivably) fertilized ovum.

THE PHYSIOLOGY OF THE ENDOMETRIAL CYCLE

The endometrium has two basic layers. The innermost portion, the functional layer (stratum functionale), is the layer that is stimulated by the hormones of the ovary to undergo changes throughout the menstrual cycle. Thus, the functional layer provides an appropriate location

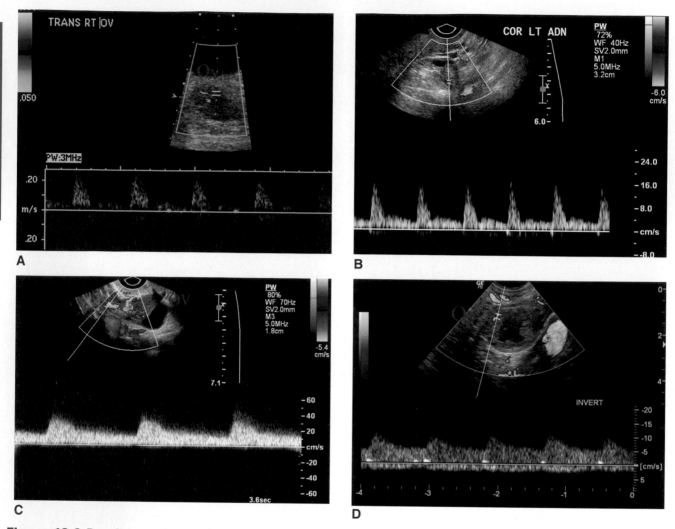

Figure 19-6 Doppler waveforms of the cyclic changes of the ovarian artery can be seen with these Doppler spectra. **A.** Intraovarian arterial flow during the follicular phase. **B.** Intraovarian arterial flow during the late luteal phase. **C.** Intraovarian arterial flow during the corpus luteal phase. **D.** Intraovarian flow during the corpus hemorrhagicum phase. *OV*, ovary.

for the implantation of the products of conception. The outermost portion, the basal layer (stratum basale), is only slightly altered during the menstrual cycle. It consists of dense, cellular stroma.

The endometrial cycle consists of two phases: the **proliferative phase** and the **secretory phase**. The proliferative phase occurs after menstruation and lasts until ovulation. Recall that the endometrium is influenced by estrogen and progesterone, which are produced by the ovary. During the first half of the menstrual cycle, the endometrium undergoes thickening as a result of estrogen stimulation. Thus, proliferation of the endometrium, which is described as the multiplication of similar forms, occurs during the proliferative phase of the endometrial cycle because the functional layer increases in thickness. The proliferative phase may be divided into two phases, early and late, with the late proliferative phase often being referred to as the **periovulatory phase**.

> **SOUND OFF**
> The proliferative phase may be divided into two phases, early and late, with the late proliferative phase often being referred to as the periovulatory phase.

The secretory phase of the endometrial cycle occurs after ovulation and is stimulated by progesterone. Progesterone maintains the thickness of the endometrium in preparation for implantation. Should fertilization not take place, menses begin on day 1 of the cycle, resulting from a lack of estrogen and progesterone. Conversely, if fertilization does occur, the endometrial thickness is maintained by the continual production of progesterone by the **corpus luteum of pregnancy** (see "Disruption of the Menstrual Cycle by Pregnancy" section).

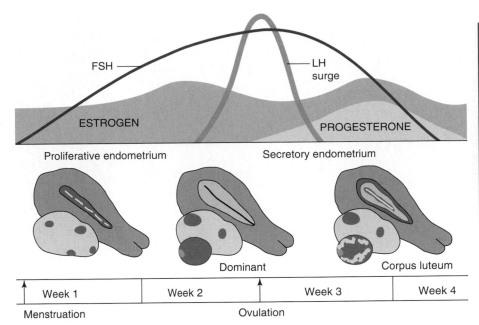

Figure 19-7 Sequence of events during a normal menstrual cycle. *FSH*, follicle-stimulating hormone; *LH*, luteinizing hormone.

CORRELATING THE PHASES OF THE MENSTRUAL CYCLE

It is significant for sonographers to have an understanding of what is concurrently taking place in the ovary and the endometrium throughout the menstrual cycle (Table 19-1). As stated earlier, days 1 through 5 of the menstrual cycle correlate with menses, at which time the endometrium is shed. Following menses, the ovary is in the follicular phase, whereas the endometrium is in the proliferative phase. Following ovulation, the ovary begins the luteal phase, whereas the endometrium enters the secretory phase (Fig. 19-7).

> 🔊 **SOUND OFF**
> Remember this mnemonic to recall the correlation of the menstrual cycle phases:

"Ovaries Freely Let Every Period Start"

Ovaries	**O**vary
Freely	**F**ollicular
Let	**L**uteal
Every	**E**ndometrium
Period	**P**roliferative
Start	**S**ecretory

TABLE 19-1 Correlation between the ovarian and endometrial phases

Structure	Days 1–14	Days 15–28
Ovary	Follicular phase	Luteal phase
Endometrium	Proliferative phase	Secretory phase

SONOGRAPHIC APPEARANCES OF THE ENDOMETRIUM

Because the hormones produced by the ovary act upon the endometrium, the thickness of the endometrium varies (Fig. 19-8). Consequently, the sonographic appearance of the endometrium changes (Table 19-2). During menses, the endometrium typically appears as a thin, echogenic line that can measure up to 4 mm (Fig. 19-9). During the early proliferative phase, the functional layer gradually increases in size and becomes more hypoechoic. It can measure between 4 and 8 mm. During the late proliferative phase or periovulatory phase, which is between days 5 and 14, the endometrial layers display a stark contrast and can measure between 6 and 10 mm. In the periovulatory phase, the outer echogenic basal layer of the endometrium will be seen surrounding the more hypoechoic functional layer, whereas the functional layer is separated by the echogenic uterine cavity (Fig. 19-10). This finding is referred to as the **three-line sign**. Following ovulation, the secretory endometrium is maintained by the production of progesterone because the endometrium becomes thickened and echogenic in appearance and measures between 7 and 14 mm (Fig. 19-11). The thickness measurement of the endometrium obtained with sonography should not include the adjacent hypoechoic myometrium and is considered accurate when the double-layer thickness measurement is performed. The double-layer thickness includes only the distance from basal layer to basal layer. If there is fluid within the endometrium, then the measurement of the two separate layers of the endometrium, excluding the fluid, should be obtained and then added together to obtain the true thickness (Fig. 19-12).

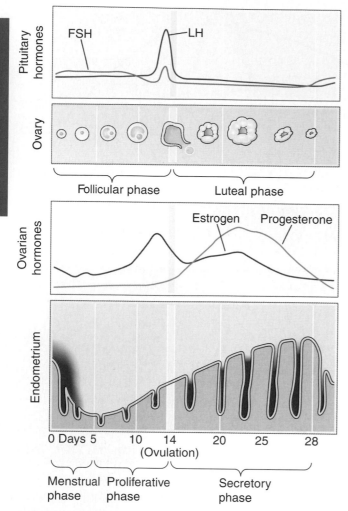

Figure 19-8 A diagram illustrating the relationship of the morphologic changes in the endometrium and ovary to the pituitary and ovarian blood hormone levels that occur during the menstrual cycle. The pituitary and ovarian hormones and their plasma concentrations are indicated in arbitrary units. *FSH*, follicle-stimulating hormone; *LH*, luteinizing hormone.

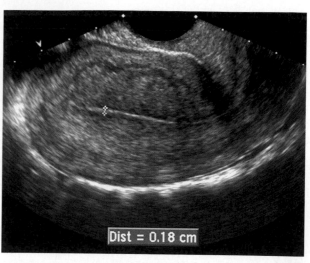

Figure 19-9 Sonographic appearance of the endometrium (between *calipers*) shortly after menses. Note how thin the endometrium appears in this image.

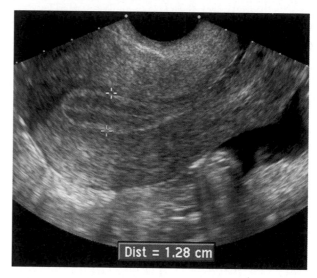

Figure 19-10 Sonographic appearance of the endometrium (between *calipers*) during the late proliferative (periovulatory) phase, also referred to as the "three-line" sign. The outer echogenic basal layer surrounds the more hypoechoic functional layer, whereas the functional layer is separated by the echogenic endometrial stripe.

TABLE 19-2 Review of endometrial thickness measurements and sonographic appearance

Phase of the Endometrial Cycle	Endometrial Thickness (mm)	Sonographic Appearance
During menses	Up to 4	Thin and echogenic
Early proliferative phase	4–8	Thickening hypoechoic functional layer
Periovulatory (late proliferative) phase	6–10	Distinct three-line sign
Secretory phase	7–14	Thick and echogenic

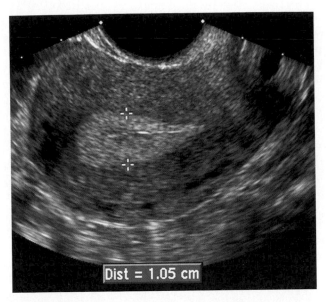

Figure 19-11 Sonographic appearance of the endometrium (between *calipers*) during the secretory phase. During this phase, the endometrium appears thick and echogenic.

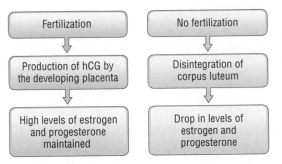

Figure 19-13 Menstrual cycle and fertility. When fertilization occurs, human chorionic gonadotropin is produced by the syncytiotrophoblastic cells around the blastocyst (developing placenta), and the corpus luteum is maintained in order to provide estrogen and progesterone until the second month of pregnancy. Once the placenta matures, it becomes the major source of estrogen and progesterone to maintain the pregnancy. No fertilization results in the disintegration of the corpus luteum.

Disruption of the Menstrual Cycle by Pregnancy

Fertilization, or conception, typically occurs on day 15, with the union of the egg and sperm in the fallopian tube. The cells that surround the **blastocyst**, the **syncytiotrophoblastic cells** (trophoblastic cells), then begin to produce **human chorionic gonadotropin** (hCG). The production of hCG maintains the corpus luteum. Thus, hCG allows the corpus luteum to continue to produce estrogen and progesterone, which, in turn, maintains the thickness of the endometrium so that implantation can take place and the pregnancy can continue to progress normally (Fig. 19-13).

Abnormal Uterine Bleeding

Dysfunctional uterine bleeding (DUB) has been referred to by some as an antiquated term, though it may still be utilized in the clinical setting. In this instance, when referring to unexplained vaginal bleeding, DUB may be idiopathic or possibly related to hormonal imbalances, resulting in endometrial changes with subsequent irregular bleeding. For example, polycystic ovary syndrome, which produces an **anovulatory** cycle, may be referred to by some as a cause of DUB.

Abnormal uterine bleeding (AUB) is a difference in frequency, duration, and amount of menstrual bleeding, and it may be caused by a number of complications (Table 19-3). Thus, the indication for patients who present with abnormal or absent uterine bleeding is variable, depending on their unique circumstances in the duration, amount, and frequency of

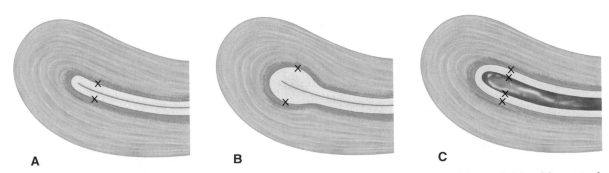

Figure 19-12 Measurement of the endometrium should be from basal layer to basal layer. It should not include the adjacent myometrium. **A.** Measurement of the thin uniform endometrium from a sagittal approach. **B.** Caliper placement for a focally thickened endometrium on a sagittal view. **C.** In the presence of intrauterine fluid, measure each endometrial layer on a sagittal plane. Those measurements can then be added together to obtain the true thickness of the endometrium.

TABLE 19-3 Causes of abnormal uterine bleeding

Causes of Abnormal Uterine Bleeding Can Be Structural or Nonstructural

Uterine fibroids (leiomyoma)
Adenomyosis
Cervical polyps
Endometrial polyps
Endometrial hyperplasia
Endometrial cancer
Hypothyroidism
Anovulation
Iatrogenic
Ovulatory dysfunction
Coagulopathy

menstruation (Table 19-4). One of the more common suspicious pathologies that results in AUB is the presence of fibroid tumors or leiomyomas within or abutting the uterine cavity. **Adenomyosis**, which is ectopic endometrial tissue within the myometrium of the uterus, is another etiology of AUB and painful menstruation. Other origins of AUB, including **endometrial hyperplasia**, **endometrial polyps**, and **endometrial carcinoma**, are primarily diagnosed in the perimenopausal or postmenopausal population but may be found in younger age groups. **Endometrial atrophy** is also a common occurrence in the postmenopausal patient who presents with vaginal bleeding. Postmenopausal sonography is further discussed in Chapter 20 of this text.

TABLE 19-4 Common terms related to abnormal uterine bleeding

Abnormal Uterine Bleeding Term	Definition
Amenorrhea	Absence of menstruation; can be classified as either primary amenorrhea or secondary amenorrhea
Cryptomenorrhea	Monthly symptoms of menstruation without bleeding
Dysmenorrhea	Painful or difficult menstruation
Menorrhagia (hypermenorrhea)	Abnormally heavy and prolonged menstruation
Metrorrhagia (intermenstrual bleeding)	Irregular menstrual bleeding between periods
Menometrorrhagia	Excessive or prolonged bleeding at irregular intervals
Oligomenorrhea	Irregular cycles >35 days apart
Polymenorrhea	Frequent regular cycles but <21 days apart
Hypomenorrhea	Regularly timed menses but light flow

REVIEW QUESTIONS

1. Based on Figure 19-14, what likely day of the menstrual cycle was this image obtained?
   a. 3
   b. 6
   c. 14
   d. 23

2. Based on Figure 19-15, what likely day of the menstrual cycle was this image obtained?
   a. 3
   b. 7
   c. 14
   d. 23

3. What is phase of the menstrual cycle depicted in Figure 19-15?
   a. Menstrual phase
   b. Early proliferative
   c. Late secretory phase
   d. Periovulatory phase

4. What would be the most likely sonographic appearance of the endometrium in the patient pictured in Figure 19-16?
   a. Thin and echogenic
   b. Thick and echogenic
   c. Three-line sign
   d. Thin and hypoechoic

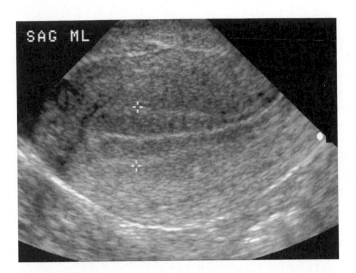

Figure 19-14

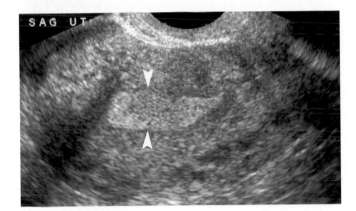

Figure 19-15

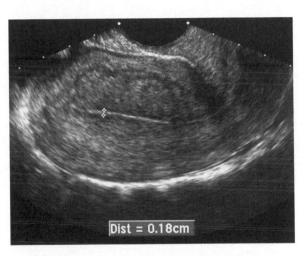

Figure 19-17

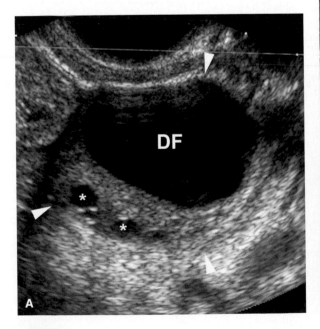

Figure 19-16

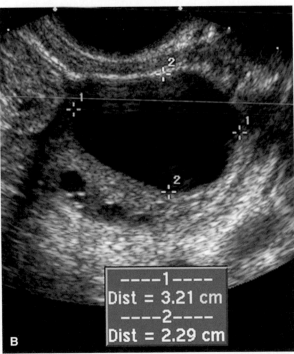

5. What is the most likely correlating ovarian phase for the patient in Figure 19-17?
   a. Follicular phase
   b. Late proliferative phase
   c. Menstrual phase
   d. Luteal phase

6. What is the most likely endometrial phase for the patient in Figure 19-17?
   a. Early proliferative
   b. Periovulatory
   c. Late secretory
   d. Late proliferative

7. What ovarian phase is depicted in Figure 19-18?
   a. Periovulatory
   b. Follicular
   c. Secretory
   d. Luteal

8. What endometrial phase would the ovarian finding occur in Figure 19-18?
   a. Early proliferative
   b. Menstrual
   c. Secretory
   d. Late proliferative

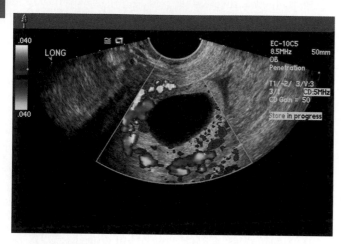

Figure 19-18

9. What hormone is produced by the theca internal cells of the ovary?
   a. Progesterone
   b. Estrogen
   c. FSH
   d. LH

10. What ovarian phase would the endometrium measure between 4 and 8 mm?
    a. Luteal
    b. Periovulatory
    c. Follicular
    d. Secretory

11. Which of the following is not a typical cause of AUB?
    a. Endometrial polyp
    b. Adenomyosis
    c. Endometrial hyperplasia
    d. Ovarian cystic teratoma

12. What is the term given to a condition that is the result of medical treatment?
    a. Exophytic
    b. Lexoprobal
    c. Iatrogenic
    d. Syncophatic

13. An individual who does not experience menarche before the age of 16 is said to be suffering from:
    a. primary amenorrhea.
    b. secondary amenorrhea.
    c. exophytic amenorrhea.
    d. inherent amenorrhea.

14. Monthly symptom of menstruation without bleeding is termed:
    a. hypomenorrhea.
    b. cryptomenorrhea.
    c. dysmenorrhea.
    d. imperforate hymen.

15. Which of the following stimulates the contractile motion within the uterine myometrium?
    a. LH
    b. Progesterone
    c. FSH
    d. Estrogen

16. You are performing a sonogram on a patient with an unknown last menstrual period. Sonographically, you note a thick, echogenic endometrium and a complex, mostly cystic mass on the right ovary. You also note a small amount of posterior cul-de-sac fluid. For this patient, which of the following would be most true?
    a. She is at midcycle.
    b. She is in the follicular phase of the ovarian cycle.
    c. She is in the proliferative phase of the ovarian cycle.
    d. She is in the luteal phase of the ovarian cycle.

17. Mittelschmerz is described as:
    a. painful menses.
    b. pelvic pressure associated with premenstrual syndrome.
    c. pain at the time of ovulation.
    d. false pregnancy.

18. What temporary structure develops before the corpus luteum?
    a. Corpus hemorrhagicum
    b. Corpus oophorus
    c. Corpus albicans
    d. Corpus functionalis

19. What phase occurs on day 3 of the menstrual cycle?
    a. Periovulatory phase
    b. Endometrial phase
    c. Early proliferative
    d. Luteal phase

20. Which layer of the endometrium appears hyperechoic during the periovulatory phase?
    a. Uterine cavity
    b. Basal layer
    c. Functional layer
    d. Myometrial layer

21. What hormone maintains the thickness of the endometrium after ovulation?
    a. LH
    b. Estrogen
    c. Progesterone
    d. FSH

22. Ovulation typically occurs on day _____ of the menstrual cycle.
    a. 12
    b. 14
    c. 16
    d. 1

23. What structure may be noted on the ovary just before ovulation?
    a. Corpus albicans
    b. Corpus luteum
    c. Graafian follicle
    d. Blastocyst

24. FSH is produced by the:
    a. ovary.
    b. endometrium.
    c. hypothalamus.
    d. anterior pituitary gland.

25. When the ovary is in the luteal phase, the endometrium is in the:
    a. early proliferative.
    b. periovulatory.
    c. late proliferative.
    d. secretory.

26. A change in menstrual bleeding associated with lesions within the uterus relates to:
    a. DUB.
    b. AUB.
    c. pelvic inflammatory disease.
    d. fibroids.

27. Painful and difficult menstruation is termed:
    a. menorrhagia.
    b. dysmenorrhea.
    c. metrorrhagia.
    d. amenorrhea.

28. The temporary endocrine gland that results from the rupture of the Graafian follicle is the:
    a. corpus albicans.
    b. corpus luteum.
    c. cumulus oophorus.
    d. trophoblastic cells.

29. Which hormone maintains the corpus luteum during pregnancy?
    a. FSH
    b. LH
    c. Progesterone
    d. hCG

30. What is the typical sonographic appearance of the endometrium during the secretory phase?
    a. Anechoic and thin
    b. Hyperechoic and thick
    c. Hypoechoic and thin
    d. Echogenic basil layer and hypoechoic functional layer

31. An increase in the number of endometrial cells is termed:
    a. endometrial hyperplasia.
    b. endometrial atrophy.
    c. endometrial carcinoma.
    d. polyps.

32. Which of the following is said to be a common cause of DUB?
    a. Hirsutism
    b. Polycystic ovary syndrome
    c. Fibroids
    d. Pelvic inflammatory disease

33. When the sonographic three-line sign is present, the functional layer of the endometrium typically appears:
    a. anechoic.
    b. echogenic.
    c. hypoechoic.
    d. complex.

34. The structure noted within the Graafian follicle containing the developing ovum is the:
    a. corpus luteum.
    b. corpus albicans.
    c. cumulus oophorus.
    d. theca internal cells.

35. Which of the following would not be a cause of AUB?
    a. Endometrial hyperplasia
    b. Hypothyroidism
    c. Adenomyosis
    d. Ovarian torsion

36. Which structure remains after the corpus luteum has regressed?
    a. Theca luteal cyst
    b. Corpus luteum of pregnancy
    c. Corpus albicans
    d. Cumulus oophorus

37. The hormone of the pituitary gland that stimulates follicular development of the ovary is:
    a. LH.
    b. estrogen.
    c. FSH.
    d. GnRH.

38. What structure produces hormones that directly act upon the endometrium to produce varying thicknesses and sonographic appearances?
    a. Hypothalamus
    b. Adrenal gland
    c. Ovary
    d. Uterus

39. The first phase of the ovarian cycle is the:
    a. luteal phase.
    b. secretory phase.
    c. proliferative phase.
    d. follicular phase.

40. The hormone produced by the hypothalamus that controls the release of the hormones for menstruation by the anterior pituitary gland is:
    a. FSH.
    b. estrogen.
    c. GnRH.
    d. LH.

41. The dominant follicle is also termed the:
    a. Graafian follicle.
    b. ovarian hyper follicle.
    c. corpus luteum.
    d. corpus albicans.

42. The hormone produced by the trophoblastic cells of the early placenta is:
    a. estrogen.
    b. FSH.
    c. LH.
    d. hCG.

43. The hormone that surges at ovulation is:
    a. GnRH.
    b. LH.
    c. aldosterone.
    d. progesterone.

44. The first phase of the endometrial cycle is the:
    a. secretory phase.
    b. follicular phase.
    c. luteal phase.
    d. proliferative phase.

45. What is defined as frequent regular cycles but less than 21 days apart?
    a. Hypomenorrhea
    b. Polymenorrhea
    c. Menorrhagia
    d. Cryptomenorrhea

46. Which hormone released by the ovary during the proliferative phase stimulates endometrial thickening?
    a. FSH
    b. LH
    c. Estrogen
    d. Progesterone

47. The periovulatory phase may also be referred to as the:
    a. early secretory phase.
    b. late proliferative phase.
    c. late secretory phase.
    d. early proliferative phase.

48. The corpus luteum primarily releases:
    a. estrogen.
    b. progesterone.
    c. LH.
    d. FSH.

49. Which of the following could also be described as intermenstrual bleeding?
    a. Metrorrhagia
    b. Polymenorrhea
    c. Menometrorrhagia
    d. Menorrhagia

50. Ectopic endometrial tissue within the uterus that leads to AUB is termed:
    a. endometriosis.
    b. adenomyosis.
    c. fibroids.
    d. endometrial hyperplasia.

51. The arteries within the functional layer of the endometrium that are altered by the hormones of the ovary and are shed with menstruation are the:
    a. arcuate arteries.
    b. radial arteries.
    c. straight arteries.
    d. spiral arteries.

52. During which phase of the endometrial cycle would the endometrium yield the three-line sign?
    a. Late proliferative
    b. Early proliferative
    c. Early secretory
    d. Late secretory

53. The second phase of the endometrial cycle is the:
    a. secretory phase.
    b. follicular phase.
    c. luteal phase.
    d. proliferative phase.

54. Which of the following hormones is released by the ovary during the second half of the menstrual cycle?
    a. LH
    b. FSH
    c. hCG
    d. Progesterone

55. LH is produced by the:
    a. ovary.
    b. endometrium.
    c. hypothalamus.
    d. anterior pituitary gland.

56. The average menstrual cycle lasts:
    a. 45 days.
    b. 24 days.
    c. 26 days.
    d. 28 days.

57. The first menstrual cycle is termed:
    a. amenorrhea.
    b. metrorrhagia.
    c. mittelschmerz.
    d. menarche.

58. The measurement of the endometrium during the early proliferative phase ranges from:
    a. 6 to 10 mm.
    b. 8 to 12 mm.
    c. 4 to 8 mm.
    d. 1 to 2 mm.

59. The second phase of the ovarian cycle is called the:
    a. follicular phase.
    b. luteal phase.
    c. secretory phase.
    d. proliferative phase.

60. The two hormones produced by the anterior pituitary gland that impact the menstrual cycle are:
    a. LH and FSH.
    b. LH and estrogen.
    c. progesterone and estrogen.
    d. FSH and progesterone.

SUGGESTED READINGS

AIUM practice parameters for the performance of an ultrasound examination of the female pelvis. *J Ultrasound Med*. 2020; 9999:1–7. https://www.aium.org/resources/guidelines/femalePelvis.pdf. Accessed December 16, 2021.

Beckmann C, Herbert W, Laube D, et al. *Obstetrics and Gynecology*. 7th ed. Wolters Kluwer; 2014:337–354.

Callahan TL, Caughey AB. *Blueprints: Obstetrics & Gynecology*. 6th ed. Wolters Kluwer; 2013:267–280.

Curry RA, Tempkin BB. *Sonography: Introduction to Normal Structure and Function*. 5th ed. Elsevier; 2020:317–365.

Gibbs RS, Karlyn BY, Haney AF, et al. *Danforth's Obstetrics and Gynecolgy*. 10th ed. Wolters Kluwer; 2008:648–671.

Henningsen C, Kuntz K, Youngs D. *Clinical Guide to Sonography: Exercises for Critical Thinking*. 2nd ed. Elsevier; 2014:142–156.

Norton ME, Scoutt LM, Feldstein VA. *Callen's Ultrasonography in Obstetrics and Gynecology*. 6th ed. Elsevier; 2017:805–834.

Rumack CM, Wilson SR, Charboneau JW, et al. *Diagnostic Ultrasound*. 4th ed. Elsevier; 2011:547–612.

Sanders RC, Hall-Terracciano B. *Clinical Sonography: A Practical Guide*. 5th ed. Wolters Kluwer; 2016:200–213.

Stephenson SR, Dmitrieva J. *Diagnostic Medical Sonography: Obstetrics and Gynecology*. 4th ed. Lippincott Williams & Wilkins; 2018:45–126.

BONUS REVIEW!

Possible Causes of Dysmenorrhea (Fig. 19-19)

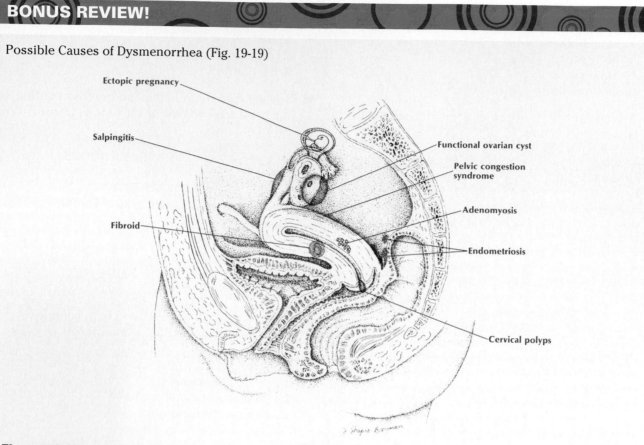

Figure 19-19

Possible Causes of Hypomenorrhea (Fig. 19-20)

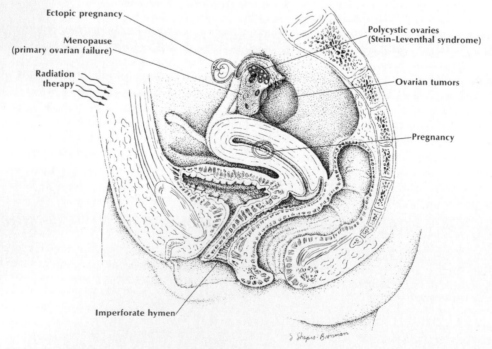

Figure 19-20 Hypomenorrhea.

BONUS REVIEW! (*continued*)

Possible Causes of Menorrhagia (Fig. 19-21)

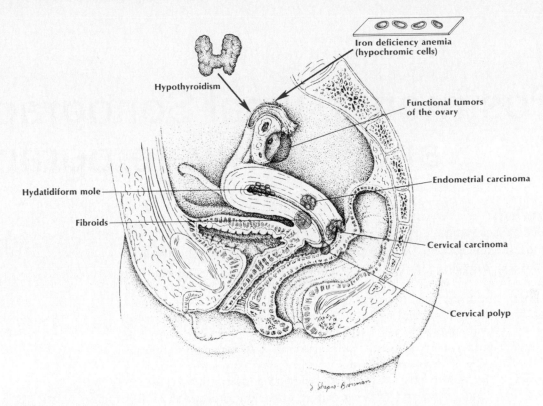

Figure 19-21 Menorrhagia.

Postmenopausal Sonography and Sonohysterography

Introduction

This chapter discusses the various causes of postmenopausal bleeding. Postmenopausal bleeding is a common clinical feature of endometrial carcinoma, and the sonographer should be aware of the sonographic findings associated with endometrial carcinoma and other causes of postmenopausal vaginal bleeding (PMB). This chapter also discusses the use of sonohysterography. Given that sonohysterography has begun to play an important role in the diagnosis and treatment of patients who present with abnormal uterine bleeding, a discussion on this essential diagnostic instrument is also provided in this chapter. In "Bonus Review" section, you will find endometrial carcinoma on magnetic resonance imaging (MRI), a positron emission tomography (PET) scan indicating ovarian metastasis, and Asherman syndrome depicted on a hysterosalpingogram.

Key Terms

adenocarcinoma—cancer that originates in glandular tissue

adhesions—irregular bands of tissue

amenorrhea—absence of menstruation

anovulation—lack of ovulation

Asherman syndrome—a syndrome characterized by endometrial adhesions that typically occur as a result of scar formation after some types of uterine surgery

atrophy—wasting away of a part of the body

bilateral salpingo-oophorectomy—the surgical removal of both ovaries and fallopian tubes

CA-125—a tumor marker in the blood that can indicate certain types of cancer, such as cancer of the ovary, endometrium, breast, gastrointestinal tract, and lungs; stands for cancer antigen-125

climacteric—another name for menopause

coronary heart disease—the buildup of plaque within the arteries that supply the myocardium of the heart

dilation and curettage—a procedure in which the cervix is dilated and the uterine cavity is scraped with a curette

double-layer thickness—measurement of the endometrium from basal layer to basal layer excluding both the adjacent hypoechoic myometrium and the intracavitary fluid (if present)

endometrial atrophy—the degeneration of the endometrium with advanced age; most often seen in postmenopausal women

endometrial carcinoma—cancer of the endometrium

endometrial hyperplasia—an increase in the number of endometrial cells

endometrial polyps—small nodules of hyperplastic endometrial tissue

estrogen—the hormone released by the ovary that initiates the proliferation and thickening of the endometrium

estrogen replacement therapy—hormone replacement therapy that involves the administration of synthetic estrogen

hematometra—blood accumulation within the uterine cavity

hormone replacement therapy—the medical treatment used to accommodate the reduction of estrogen and progesterone that occurs during menopause

hyperplasia—an increase in the number of cells of a tissue or an organ

hypertension—high blood pressure

hypomenorrhea—decreased or scant menstrual flow

hysteroscopy—endoscopy of the uterine cavity

intermenstrual bleeding—bleeding between periods; may be referred to as metrorrhagia

leiomyoma (uterine)—a benign, smooth muscle tumor of the uterus; may also be referred to as a fibroid or uterine myoma

menometrorrhagia—excessive and prolonged menstrual bleeding at irregular intervals

menopause—cessation of menstruation with advanced age

metastasis—the spread of cancer from a distant site

nulliparity—having birthed no children

osteopenia—a bone density that is lower than normal

osteoporosis—bone loss that predisposes the individual to fractures

pedunculated—something that grows off a stalk

pelvic inflammatory disease—infection of the female genital tract that may involve the ovaries, uterus, and/or the fallopian tubes

perimenopausal—the time before menopause

polycystic ovary syndrome—a syndrome characterized by anovulatory cycles, infertility, hirsutism, amenorrhea, and obesity; may also be referred to as Stein–Leventhal syndrome

polypectomy—the surgical removal of a polyp

polypoid—shaped like a polyp

postmenopause—the time after menopause

postmenopausal vaginal bleeding—vaginal bleeding after the onset of menopause

progesterone—a hormone that prepares the uterus for pregnancy, maintains pregnancy, and promotes development of the mammary glands; primarily produced by the ovary and placenta

progestogen therapy—a hormone replacement therapy that involves administering synthetic progesterone

pyometra—the presence of pus within the uterus

saline infusion sonography—see key term saline infusion sonohysterography

saline infusion sonohysterography—a sonographic procedure that uses saline instillation into the endometrial cavity and fallopian tubes to evaluate for internal abnormalities

Stein–Leventhal syndrome—see key term polycystic ovary syndrome

synechiae—adhesions

tamoxifen—a breast cancer drug that inhibits the effects of estrogen on the breast

thecoma—benign ovarian sex cord–stromal tumor that produces estrogen in older women

thromboembolism—the formation of a clot within a blood vessel with the potential to travel to a distant site and cause an occlusion

total abdominal hysterectomy—the removal of the uterus and cervix

MENOPAUSE

Menopause, or **climacteric**, is the cessation of menstruation with advanced age. The median age at which menopause occurs is 51, with a range in normal women between the ages of 42 and 58. As menopause approaches, the follicles that normally develop in the ovary are less responsive to the hormones produced by the anterior pituitary gland. During menopause, the follicles cease to mature, resulting in a considerable reduction in the amounts of **estrogen** and **progesterone**. Thus, the ovaries are typically more difficult to identify as menopause progresses.

REPERCUSSIONS OF MENOPAUSE

As discussed in Chapter 19, estrogen and progesterone are the hormones released by the ovary that facilitate menses. Without estrogen and progesterone, menstruation ceases, and the uterus and ovaries undergo **atrophy** or decrease in size. Although smaller, the uterus will maintain its adult shape. The ovaries also become more echogenic, during **postmenopause**, and lack follicles, thus making them more difficult to image with sonography.

The decrease production of estrogen by the ovaries has other physiologic consequences. Along with the decrease in uterine size, the mucosal layer of the uterus—the endometrium—begins to become atrophic as menstruation comes to an end. The vagina also becomes smaller and decreases in caliber. The breasts tend to accumulate more adipose or fat tissue within them. Patients undergoing menopause may also suffer from night sweats or hot flashes, mood changes, depression, dysparcunia, dysuria, and a decrease in libido. There are several long-term consequences of menopause that are a main concern. Because of the lack of circulating estrogen during and after menopause, there is a notable increased risk for **coronary heart disease** and an increase threat for developing **osteopenia** and **osteoporosis**.

HORMONE REPLACEMENT THERAPY

Hormone replacement therapy (HRT) is often used to combat the reduction of estrogen circulating in the female body after menopause and to prevent menopausal symptoms such as hot flashes and vaginal atrophy. **Estrogen replacement therapy** (ERT) has been shown to significantly reduce the risk of developing osteoporosis and coronary heart disease, with possible associated reduction in risk for developing colon cancer and Alzheimer disease. However, unopposed ERT (not combined with **progestogen therapy**) has been shown to increase the risk for developing **endometrial hyperplasia** and **endometrial carcinoma**. There may also be an increased risk of developing breast cancer, **thromboembolism**, **hypertension**, and, possibly, diabetes in patients who are on ERT. For this reason, many physicians attempt to thwart the risks of unopposed ERT with progestogen therapy (progestin therapy). This is referred to as estrogen–progestin therapy. These hormones, when used in conjunction, act upon the endometrium and in effect induce a menstrual cycle. Combined estrogen and progestogen therapy, when used consistently, can reduce the risk of developing endometrial carcinoma but cannot eliminate it entirely. The sonographic appearance and thickness of the endometrium is variable and comparable with the endometrium in the premenopausal female. Thus, before performing a postmenopausal pelvic sonogram, it is vital for the sonographer to inquire if the patient is undergoing HRT, because HRT will influence the sonographic appearance of the endometrium.

🔊 **SOUND OFF**
Unopposed estrogen exposure on the endometrium increases the risk for endometrial hyperplasia and endometrial carcinoma.

POSTMENOPAUSAL VAGINAL BLEEDING AND ENDOMETRIAL THICKENING

A common indication for postmenopausal sonography is **postmenopausal vaginal bleeding** (PMB). There are several complications that may lead to PMB.

Endometrial atrophy (59%), uncontrolled HRT, endometrial hyperplasia (10%), **endometrial polyps** (9%), submucosal or intracavitary **leiomyoma**, endometrial carcinoma (5% to 10%), and some ovarian tumors are among the differential abnormalities that can be linked to vaginal bleeding in the postmenopausal population.

🔊 **SOUND OFF**
Before performing a postmenopausal pelvic sonogram, it is vital for the sonographer to inquire if the patient is undergoing HRT, because HRT will influence the sonographic appearance of the endometrium.

Accurate sonographic endometrial thickness measurements are vitally important and are used in correlation with clinical findings in patients who present with PMB. Endometrial thickness cutoff measurements vary depending on the patient's clinical presentation (Table 20-1). The thickness measurement of the endometrium should not include the adjacent hypoechoic myometrium and is considered accurate only when the **double-layer thickness** measurement is performed without the inclusion of endometrial fluid in the measurement (Fig. 20-1). Transvaginal sonography has been reported to be highly effective for the detection of possible endometrial carcinoma when an endometrial thickness threshold of 4 to 5 mm is used for the patient with PMB. In fact, if the sonogram reveals a thin endometrium measuring 4 mm or less, endometrial cancer can nearly be completely excluded. Specifically, a 4 mm or less endometrial thickness in a patient with PMB yields a greater than 99% negative predictive value for endometrial cancer. If the endometrium measures less than 5 mm, the bleeding is typically caused by endometrial atrophy. Conversely, if the endometrium exceeds 5 mm, endometrial biopsy is typically warranted.

TABLE 20-1 Normal endometrial thickness measurements for the asymptomatic and symptomatic postmenopausal patient

Clinical Presentation	Normal Endometrial Thickness (mm)
Negative postmenopausal vaginal bleeding	≤8[a]
Positive postmenopausal vaginal bleeding	≤4

Any measurement over these thresholds would warrant further investigation.
[a]Some sources may utilize a cutoff of as high as 11 mm for the asymptomatic patient before biopsy is recommended.

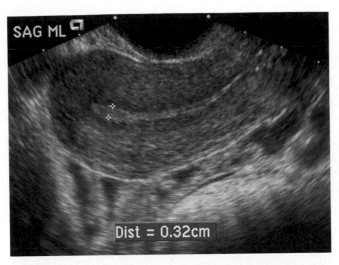

Figure 20-1 Normal sagittal postmenopausal endometrium. This endometrium (between calipers) appears thin and echogenic.

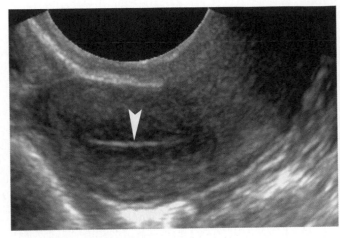

Figure 20-2 Endometrial atrophy. Longitudinal transvaginal sonogram revealing a thin endometrium (*arrowhead*) measuring only 2 mm in a postmenopausal woman with vaginal bleeding, which is indicative for endometrial atrophy.

The asymptomatic patient, or those with no vaginal bleeding, can have an endometrial thickness of up to 8 mm and, in some cases, 11 mm based on clinical presentation. It is significant to note that carcinoma has been found in patients with measurements below these thresholds too. Conversely, benign endometrial pathologies have been seen in patients with measurements above these thresholds. It may be that focal irregularity and myometrial distortion may be more specific findings than just endometrial thickness.

Endometrial Atrophy

In the postmenopausal patient, the endometrium often bleeds spontaneously secondary to atrophy. As a result, the most common cause of PMB is endometrial atrophy. The endometrium will appear thin and should not exceed 5 mm, although, with atrophy, the endometrium typically measures 4 mm or thinner (Fig. 20-2). The endometrium may also contain some intracavitary fluid. A thin endometrial stripe in the postmenopausal patient usually does not warrant endometrial biopsy, although the patient's clinical history should be closely analyzed.

> **SOUND OFF**
> The most common cause of PMB is endometrial atrophy.

Endometrial Hyperplasia

Endometrial **hyperplasia** is a common cause of abnormal vaginal bleeding, not only in the postmenopausal female but also in the reproductive years. Endometrial hyperplasia results from the unopposed stimulation of

estrogen on the endometrium. Secondary to continual estrogen stimulation, sonographically, the endometrium may contain small cystic spaces or appear diffusely echogenic (Fig. 20-3). Endometrial hyperplasia may also be caused by **polycystic ovary syndrome**, obesity, **tamoxifen** therapy for breast cancer, or estrogen-producing ovarian tumors, such as the ovarian **thecoma** or granulosa cell tumor. There seems to be an increased risk for one form of endometrial hyperplasia (atypical adenomatous hyperplasia) progressing into endometrial carcinoma more often in the postmenopausal woman. For this reason, an endometrial biopsy is typically warranted to rule out endometrial carcinoma.

> **CLINICAL FINDINGS OF ENDOMETRIAL HYPERPLASIA**
>
> 1. Abnormal uterine bleeding (any age)
> 2. Polycystic ovary syndrome
> 3. Obesity
> 4. Tamoxifen therapy

> **SONOGRAPHIC FINDINGS OF ENDOMETRIAL HYPERPLASIA**
>
> 1. Thickened echogenic endometrium
> 2. Small cystic spaces within the endometrium

> **SOUND OFF**
> Endometrial hyperplasia may also be caused by polycystic ovary syndrome, obesity, tamoxifen therapy for breast cancer, or estrogen-producing ovarian tumors, such as the ovarian thecoma or granulosa cell tumor.

Endometrial hyperplasia

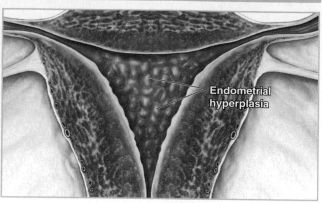

Endometrial hyperplasia is an abnormal overgrowth of the uterine lining (endometrium).

A

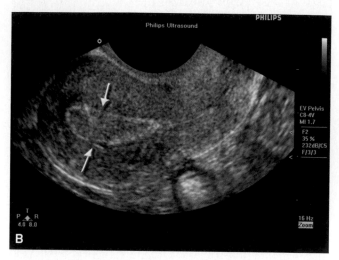

B

Figure 20-3 Endometrial hyperplasia. **A.** Endometrial hyperplasia drawing depicting an overabundance of hyperplastic endometrial tissue. **B.** A thickened endometrium (between *arrows*) is demonstrated in this patient with endometrial hyperplasia.

Endometrial Carcinoma

Endometrial carcinoma is the most common female genital tract malignancy, with PMB being the most common clinical presentation. Endometrial carcinoma is most often in the form of **adenocarcinoma**, and it has been linked with unopposed estrogen therapy, **nulliparity**, obesity, chronic **anovulation**, **Stein–Leventhal syndrome**, estrogen-producing ovarian tumors, and the use of tamoxifen. Peak incidence at the time of diagnosis is between 50 and 65 years of age. Tumors with penetration into the surrounding myometrium have a poorer prognosis than those confined to the endometrium.

The sonographic appearance of endometrial carcinoma is that of a thickened endometrium with variable echogenicity (Fig. 20-4). Sonographically, fluid and a **polypoid** mass may also be noted within the endometrium. Color Doppler should be applied to assess for vascularity within the thickened endometrium. Pulsed Doppler of the uterine cavity may indicate low-impedance flow in the presence of endometrial carcinoma. Suspicion of endometrial carcinoma typically leads to an endometrial biopsy, endocervical curettage, cancer antigen-125 (**CA-125**) testing, and, in most confirmed cases, the performance of a **total abdominal hysterectomy** with a **bilateral salpingo-oophorectomy**. Staging of the disease is performed surgically to determine the involvement of lymph nodes and the presence of extrauterine **metastasis** (Fig. 20-5). These tumors may obstruct the cervical canal, thus leading to an accumulation of blood or pus within the uterus termed **hematometra** or **pyometra**, respectively. It may also invade the urinary bladder and, therefore, may initially cause the patient to present with urinary symptoms.

CLINICAL FINDINGS OF ENDOMETRIAL CARCINOMA

1. Postmenopausal bleeding
2. Intermenstrual bleeding
3. Enlarged uterus
4. Elevation of CA-125

SONOGRAPHIC FINDINGS OF ENDOMETRIAL CARCINOMA

1. Thickened endometrium
2. Heterogeneous uterus
3. Enlarged uterus with lobular contour
4. Endometrial fluid
5. Polypoid mass within the endometrium

◀))) SOUND OFF
Pulsed Doppler of the uterine cavity may indicate low-impedance flow in the presence of endometrial carcinoma.

Endometrial Polyps

Endometrial polyps, which may be benign or malignant, are small nodules of hyperplastic endometrial tissue that may cause abnormal vaginal bleeding in both postmenopausal and **perimenopausal** woman. They have been linked with infertility during the reproductive period. Clinically, patients may present with **menometrorrhagia** and/or

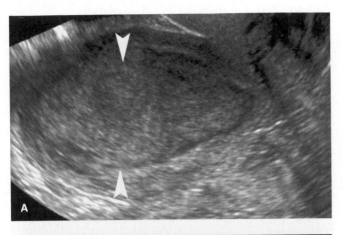

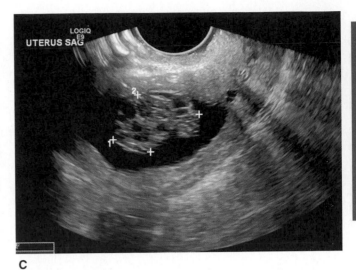

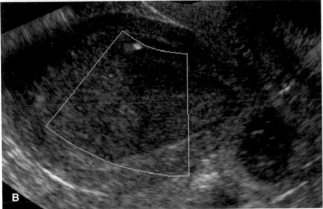

Figure 20-4 Endometrial carcinoma. **A.** Transvaginal sonogram (US) in a 72-year-old woman with vaginal bleeding reveals a markedly thickened endometrium measured at 29 mm between arrowheads. **B.** Color Doppler image shows blood flow within the heterogeneous endometrial tissue. US findings are highly indicative of malignancy. Biopsy confirmed endometrial carcinoma. **C.** Sagittal endovaginal sonogram demonstrating a complex mass within an endometrial cavity distended with fluid.

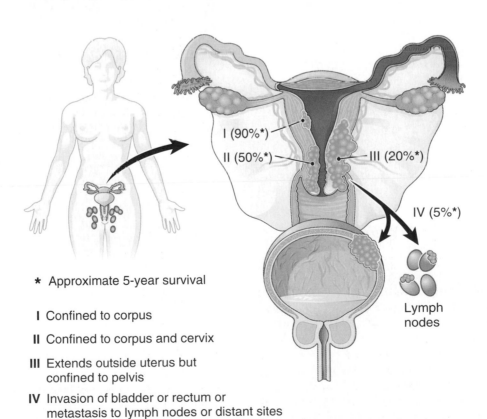

* Approximate 5-year survival

I Confined to corpus

II Confined to corpus and cervix

III Extends outside uterus but confined to pelvis

IV Invasion of bladder or rectum or metastasis to lymph nodes or distant sites

Figure 20-5 Staging of endometrial carcinoma. Approximately 5-year survival percentage (%) is shown for various stages.

intermenstrual bleeding, or may even be asymptomatic. Endometrial polyps can have many different shapes, including a broad base, or can be **pedunculated** and, if large, may prolapse through the cervix. The sonographic appearance of an endometrial polyp varies and can appear as a focal echogenic area of thickening within the endometrium if solitary or a diffuse thickening of the endometrium in the presence of multiple or large polyps. An endometrial polyp will most often contain a small vessel and have cystic areas within it. Polyps are better visualized with the use of **saline infusion sonohysterography** (SIS) (Fig. 20-6). Three-dimensional sonography can be used to better demonstrate polyps as well (Fig. 20-7). Treatment for endometrial polyps is typically a **polypectomy** with the use of **hysteroscopy**.

> ### 🔊 SOUND OFF
> A key clinical feature of patient with an endometrial polyp is intermenstrual bleeding.

CLINICAL FINDINGS OF ENDOMETRIAL POLYPS

1. Can be asymptomatic
2. Menometrorrhagia
3. Intermenstrual bleeding
4. Has been linked with infertility in reproductive-aged group

SONOGRAPHIC FINDINGS OF ENDOMETRIAL POLYPS

1. Focal thickening of the endometrium
2. Diffuse thickening of the endometrium

Ovarian Tumors and Postmenopausal Bleeding

Some functioning ovarian tumors and malignant ovarian neoplasms may in fact cause postmenopausal bleeding. For instance, estrogen-producing tumors such as the

Polyps

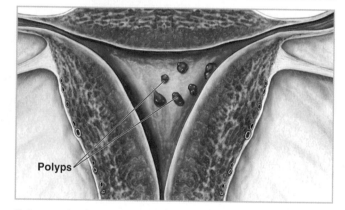

Polyps are benign growths of the endometrium that can cause irregular bleeding and spotting.

A

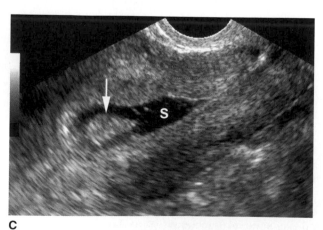

C

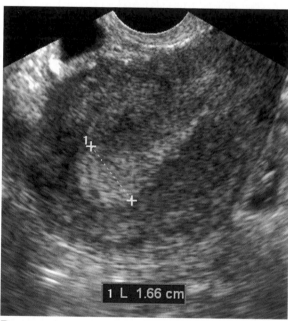

B

Figure 20-6 Endometrial polyp and saline infusion sonohysterography. **A.** Drawing of endometrial polyps. **B.** A polyp is suspected in a patient with focal thickening of the endometrium (between *calipers*). **C.** Saline (*S*) infusion sonohysterography better depicts the evidence of an endometrial polyp (*arrow*).

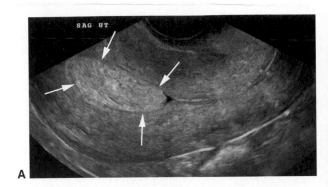

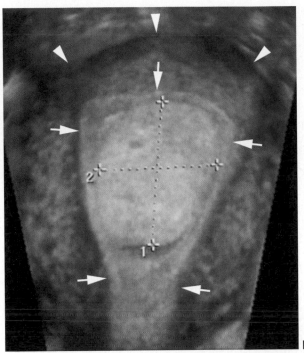

Figure 20-7 Three-dimensional endometrial polyp. **A.** Longitudinal image of a rounded mass (between *arrows*) within the endometrial cavity suggesting a polyp. **B.** Coronal reconstruction of the uterus (*arrowheads*) revealing the presence of a polyp (between *calipers*) within the endometrial cavity (*arrows*).

thecoma, which is mostly benign, have been shown to cause abnormal thickening of the endometrium with subsequent vaginal bleeding. In addition, the malignant serous and mucinous cystadenocarcinomas have been associated with vaginal bleeding.

CA-125

Serum levels of CA-125 are often elevated in women who have some forms of cancer. Elevation of this tumor marker has been linked with cancers of the ovary, endometrium, breast, gastrointestinal tract, and lungs. However, CA-125 may also be elevated in some benign conditions, such as endometriosis, **pelvic inflammatory disease**, fibroids, and even pregnancy. Therefore, it is not typically used as a screening tool but more as an adjunct to clinical examination and diagnostic imaging tests.

Tamoxifen

Tamoxifen is a breast cancer drug that inhibits the effects of estrogen on the breast, thus slowing the growth of malignant breast cells. Tamoxifen can also be used in the treatment of female infertility. Unfortunately, tamoxifen use has been linked with the development of endometrial hyperplasia, endometrial polyps, and endometrial carcinoma. Sonographically, tamoxifen will cause cystic changes to occur within the endometrium, and it produces a more heterogeneous and thickened endometrial appearance (Fig. 20-8).

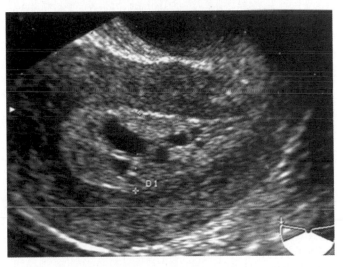

Figure 20-8 Tamoxifen effects on the endometrium. A 62-year-old woman with postmenopausal bleeding undergoing tamoxifen therapy. The sagittal view of the uterus revealing a thickened endometrial lining (between *calipers*) with cystic changes. A polyp was also confirmed.

SONOHYSTEROGRAPHY AND HYSTEROSALPINGO-CONTRAST SONOGRAPHY

SIS, or **saline infusion sonography** or sonohysterography, is a procedure in which sterile saline is instilled into the uterine cavity with a catheter under

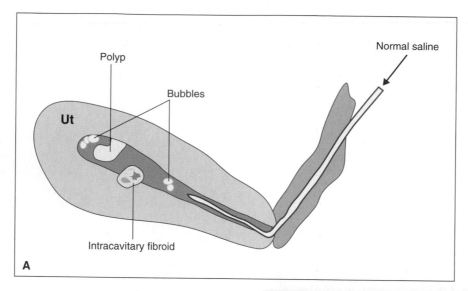

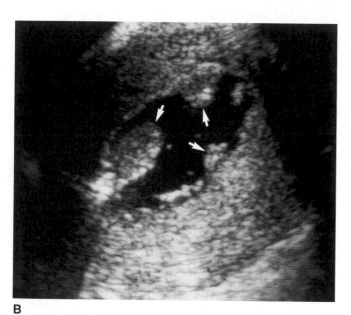

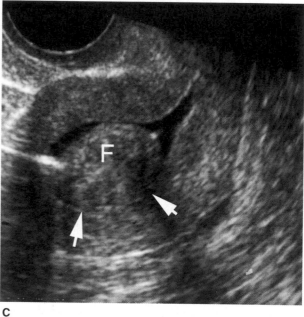

Figure 20-9 Sonohysterogram. **A.** A catheter is inserted into the endometrial cavity through which normal saline is infused. The catheter tip lies in the middle of the endometrial cavity and can be moved back or pushed forward under direct sonographic visualization. **B.** Polyps are typically on a stalk, mobile, and echogenic with irregular borders (*arrows*). **C.** Fibroids indent into the myometrium and are usually evenly echogenic with a well-defined border (*arrows*).

sonographic guidance (Fig. 20-9). Patients who present with abnormal uterine bleeding or have indications such as infertility, abnormally thickened endometrium, or a suspected intracavitary masses may be further evaluated with SIS (Table 20-2). A sonohysterogram can help determine whether the cause of the vaginal bleeding is intracavitary in origin, such as in the case of an endometrial polyp. It is also helpful in differentiating an endometrial polyp from a submucosal fibroid. Endometrial polyps will be outlined by the saline and seen projecting into the uterine cavity from the endometrium, whereas the submucosal fibroid will have a layer of endometrium overlying the mass and

TABLE 20-2 AIUM indications for saline infusion sonohysterography
Abnormal uterine bleeding
Uterine cavity evaluation for pathology
Focal or diffuse endometrial or intracavitary abnormalities
Congenital or acquired abnormalities of the uterus
Infertility
Recurrent pregnancy loss
Suboptimal visualization of the endometrium with routine sonography

AIUM, American Institute of Ultrasound in Medicine.

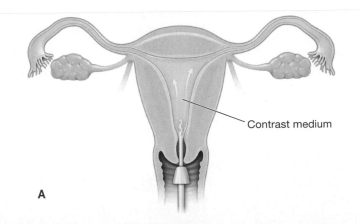

Contrast medium

A

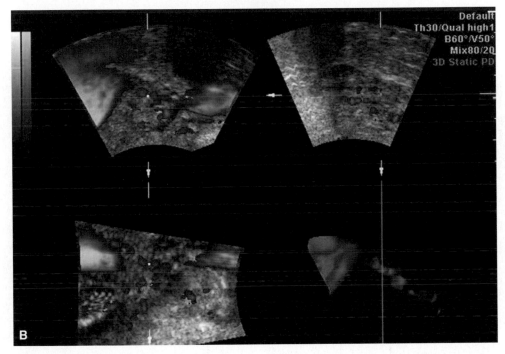

B

Figure 20-10 Sonohysterosalpingography. **A.** Insertion of a contrast medium for a sonohysterosalpingogram. The contrast medium outlines the uterus and fallopian tubes on the sonogram to demonstrate patency. **B.** Fallopian tube color Doppler saline infusion sonohysterosalpingography to assess tubal patency. Three-dimensional (3D) power Doppler scan of uterine cavity after injection of isotonic saline. 3D power Doppler rendering allows simultaneous assessment of triangular shape of uterine cavity and proximal part of tube (*lower right*).

originate in the myometrium. Contraindication for SIS includes patients who are pregnant or have known pelvic infections.

Hysterosalpingo-contrast sonography (HyCoSy), also referred to as sonohysterosalpingography, which further assesses for patency of the fallopian tubes, may also be used by some institutions for various reason (Fig. 20-10). HyCoSy is used to determine tubal patency in patients or to confirm tubal occlusion following a sterilization procedure. One major advantage of sonohysterosalpingography over hysterosalpingography is the lack of ionizing radiation

with sonography. Recall, hysterosalpingography is a radiographic procedure and thus uses a contrast agent and fluoroscopy to analyze the uterine cavity and fallopian tubes for patency.

Asherman Syndrome

Asherman syndrome is the presence of intrauterine **adhesions** or **synechiae** within the uterine cavity that typically occur as a result of scar formation after uterine surgery, especially after a **dilation and curettage** (D&C). The adhesions may cause

hypomenorrhea or **amenorrhea**, pregnancy loss, and/or infertility (for more about the infertility link with Asherman syndrome, see Chapter 21) (Fig. 20-11). Sonographic detection is difficult without the use of sonohysterography. Sonohysterography findings include bright bands of tissue traversing the uterine cavity.

CLINICAL FINDINGS OF ASHERMAN SYNDROME

1. History of D&C, trauma, and uterine surgery
2. Recurrent pregnancy loss
3. Amenorrhea or hypomenorrhea

SONOGRAPHIC FINDINGS OF ASHERMAN SYNDROME

1. Bright areas within the endometrium
2. Sonohysterography findings include bright bands of tissue traversing the uterine cavity

SOUND OFF
Remember, *Asherman* is associated with adhesions.

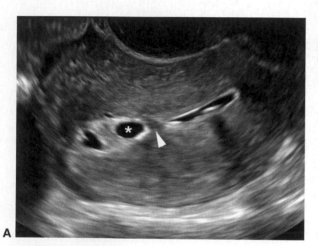

A

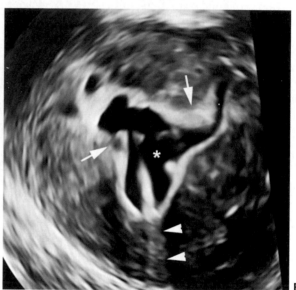

B

Asherman syndrome

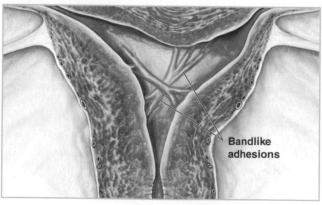

Bandlike adhesions

Asherman syndrome is the presence of bandlike adhesions that cross the lining of the uterus. This condition usually occurs after a surgical procedure such as dilatation and curettage (D&C).

C

Figure 20-11 Asherman syndrome. **A.** Sagittal image of the uterus during a saline infusion sonohysterography (SIS) showing poor dispensability of the cavity with fluid (*asterisk*) and an adhesion (*arrowhead*) interrupting the endometrial echo. **B.** Three-dimensional reconstructed coronal view during the SIS with the catheter (*arrowheads*) in the lower uterine segment and fluid in the cavity (*asterisk*) showing marked distortion of the cavity (*arrows*) from multiple adhesions. **C.** Drawing of Asherman syndrome. Note the bands crossing the endometrial cavity.

REVIEW QUESTIONS

1. The 65-year-old patient in Figure 20-12 presented
   with PMB. Which of the following must be
   initially suspected and ruled out given the
   sonographic findings?
   a. Endometrial polyp
   b. Intrauterine fibroid
   c. Submucosal fibroid
   d. Endometrial carcinoma

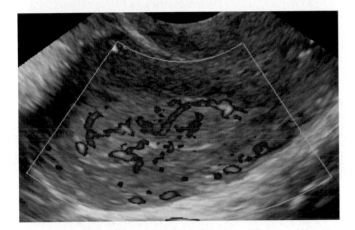

Figure 20-12

2. The 30-year-old patient in Figure 20-13 presented
   with a past history of dilatation and curettage
   and current amenorrhea. What is the most likely
   diagnosis?
   a. Endometrial hyperplasia
   b. Asherman syndrome
   c. Endometrial carcinoma
   d. Endometrial polyp

3. What do the arrows in Figure 20-13 indicate,
   given the patient's clinical history and
   sonographic findings?
   a. Synechia
   b. Endometrial hemorrhage
   c. Endometrial carcinoma
   d. Retained products of conception

4. For a patient suffering from the condition
   pictured in Figure 20-13, what other clinical
   finding would be most likely?
   a. Infertility
   b. Dyspareunia
   c. Metrorrhagia
   d. Endometriosis

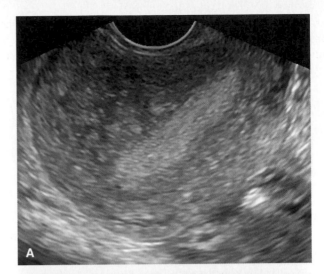

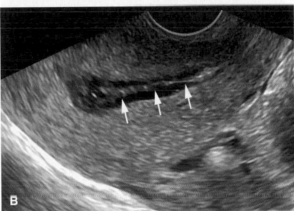

Figure 20-13

5. Which of the following utilizes fluoroscopy to
   analyze the uterine cavity and fallopian tubes?
   a. HyCoSy
   b. Hysteroscopy
   c. SIS
   d. Hysterosalpingography

6. The 46-year-old patient in Figure 20-14 is
   undergoing breast cancer treatment. She
   is taking tamoxifen. What is the most likely
   diagnosis?
   a. Endometrial carcinoma
   b. Endometrial hyperplasia
   c. Endometrial polyps
   d. Asherman syndrome

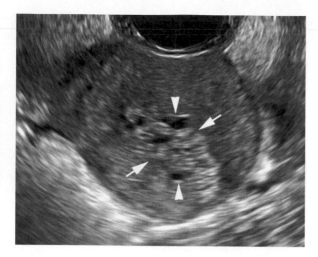

Figure 20-14

7. What does the arrow in Figure 20-15 indicate?
   a. Intramural fibroid
   b. Subserosal fibroid
   c. Endometrial polyp
   d. Synechia

8. What is the least likely clinical finding for the patient in Figure 20-15?
   a. Menometrorrhagia
   b. Infertility
   c. Asymptomatic
   d. Amenorrhea

9. If the structure identified in Figure 20-15 extended from a stalk, it would be said to be:
   a. pedunculated.
   b. hyperplastic.
   c. polypoid.
   d. hysteroplastic.

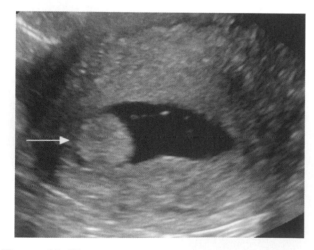

Figure 20-15

10. The 31-year-old patient in Figure 20-16 presented to the sonography department with excessive vaginal bleeding. Which of the following is the most likely diagnosis?
    a. Intramural leiomyoma
    b. Submucosal leiomyoma
    c. Endometrial carcinoma
    d. Endometrial hyperplasia

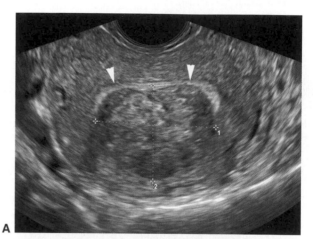

A

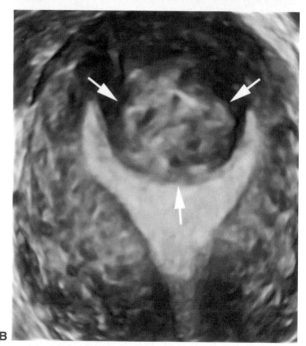

B

Figure 20-16

11. CA-125 has been shown to elevate in all of the following except:
    a. ovarian cancer.
    b. endometrial cancer.
    c. pelvic inflammatory disease.
    d. Asherman syndrome.

12. What contrast agent is used during sonohysterosalpingography?
    a. Iodine
    b. Water
    c. Saline
    d. Barium

13. What is defined as bone density lower than normal?
    a. Osteoarthritis
    b. Osteopenia
    c. Osteoporosis
    d. Osteogenesis

14. Why are the postmenopausal ovaries more difficult to visualize sonographically?
    a. They become more hypoechoic and lose their cystic appearance.
    b. They become more anechoic.
    c. They become enlarged but more hyperechoic.
    d. They become smaller and lose their follicles.

15. Which of the following is true concerning the uterus following menopause?
    a. The uterus enlarges.
    b. The uterus becomes more anechoic.
    c. The uterus becomes more hypoechoic.
    d. The uterus becomes atrophic.

16. What may be used to combat the reduction of estrogen circulating in the female body following menopause?
    a. HRT
    b. Thromboembolism
    c. Bilateral salpingo-oophorectomy
    d. SIS

17. Which of the following would be the least likely cause of PMB?
    a. Endometrial atrophy
    b. Endometrial enlargement
    c. Endometrial carcinoma
    d. Endometrial hyperplasia

18. In a menstruating patient, obstruction of the cervical canal by a large cervical mass could lead to:
    a. pyosalpinx.
    b. hydrosalpinx.
    c. hematometra.
    d. pyometra.

19. Synechiae within the uterus results from:
    a. scar tissue.
    b. leiomyoma.
    c. endometrial polyps.
    d. endometrial hyperplasia.

20. Which of the following is not an indication for SIS?
    a. Abnormal uterine bleeding
    b. Multiparity
    c. Recurrent pregnancy loss
    d. Diffuse endometrial thickening

21. What is the most likely pulsed Doppler characteristic of endometrial cancer?
    a. Low-impedance flow
    b. High-impedance flow
    c. Absent systolic flow
    d. Converse diastolic flow

22. The absence of menstrual bleeding is termed:
    a. amenorrhea.
    b. dysmenorrhea.
    c. oligomenorrhea.
    d. polymenorrhea.

23. Asherman syndrome is associated with:
    a. uterine leiomyoma.
    b. endometrial polyps.
    c. endometrial adhesions.
    d. ovarian fibroma.

24. What would increase a patient's likelihood of suffering from thromboembolism?
    a. Polycystic ovary disease.
    b. ERT.
    c. Endometrial carcinoma.
    d. Endometrial atrophy.

25. What is used as a tumor marker for endometrial carcinoma?
    a. CR-124
    b. CE-125
    c. CA-125
    d. CA-45

26. The removal of tissue from the endometrium by scraping is termed:
    a. dilatation.
    b. curettage.
    c. sonohysterography.
    d. hysteroscopy.

27. What is the most common form of endometrial carcinoma?
    a. Cystadenocarcinoma
    b. Krukenberg tumor
    c. Adenocarcinoma
    d. Squamous cell carcinoma

28. Measurement of the endometrium should include the:
    a. uterine cavity only.
    b. deep myometrial echoes and both basal layers.
    c. distance from the basal layer to the functional layer.
    d. measurement from the basal layer to the basal layer.

29. The most common cause of postmenopausal bleeding is:
    a. endometrial carcinoma.
    b. endometrial atrophy.
    c. endometrial leiomyoma.
    d. cervical carcinoma.

30. Which of the following is not associated with endometrial hyperplasia?
    a. Tamoxifen therapy
    b. Polycystic ovary syndrome
    c. Ovarian thecoma
    d. Asherman syndrome

31. The best description for endometrial polyps is:
    a. malignant nodules that cause bleeding.
    b. benign lesions associated with cervical stenosis.
    c. malignant nodules that are associated with endometrial atrophy.
    d. benign nodules of hyperplastic endometrial tissue.

32. Blood accumulation within the uterus is termed:
    a. hematometra.
    b. hydrometra.
    c. Asherman syndrome.
    d. endometrial carcinoma.

33. Which of the following would increase the risk of a patient developing endometrial cancer?
    a. Unopposed ERT
    b. Multiparity
    c. Osteoporosis
    d. Endometrial atrophy

34. What is a gynecologic procedure to remove an endometrial polyp?
    a. Hysterectomy with myomectomy
    b. Histogram with myomectomy
    c. Hysteroscopy with polypectomy
    d. Hysteroscopy with polyp myomectomy

35. Cessation of menstruation with advanced age is termed:
    a. Asherman disease.
    b. premenopausal syndrome.
    c. perimenopausal syndrome.
    d. menopause.

36. Stein–Leventhal syndrome is related to all of the following except:
    a. infertility.
    b. anovulatory cycles.
    c. hirsutism.
    d. ovarian hyperstimulation syndrome.

37. What hormone plays a major role in the symptoms associated with menopause?
    a. human chorionic gonadotropin
    b. LH
    c. Estrogen
    d. CA-120

38. The breast cancer treatment drug that may alter the sonographic appearance of the endometrium is:
    a. progestogen.
    b. estrogenate.
    c. tamoxifen.
    d. CA-125.

39. Possible benefits of ERT include all of the following except:
    a. reduction in osteoporosis risk.
    b. reduction in colon cancer risk.
    c. reduction in heart disease risk.
    d. reduction in endometrial cancer risk.

40. Which of the following does not occur as a result of menopause?
    a. Uterine atrophy
    b. Decreased sexual libido
    c. Accumulation of fat in the breasts
    d. Cystic enlargement of the ovaries

41. Unopposed estrogen therapy has been shown to increase the risk for developing:
    a. Alzheimer disease.
    b. colon cancer.
    c. coronary heart disease.
    d. endometrial carcinoma.

42. The sonographic appearance of a 59-year-old woman on HRT is:
    a. hypoechoic and thickened.
    b. hyperechoic and thickened.
    c. cystic areas within a thin endometrium.
    d. variable depending upon the menstrual cycle.

43. Tamoxifen has been linked with all of the following except:
    a. endometrial polyps.
    b. endometrial hyperplasia.
    c. endometrial leiomyoma.
    d. endometrial carcinoma.

44. Which of the following ovarian tumors would be most likely to cause postmenopausal bleeding?
    a. Cystic teratoma
    b. Endometrioma
    c. Thecoma
    d. Fibroma

45. Tamoxifen effects on the endometrium will sonographically appear as:
    a. cystic changes within a thickened endometrium.
    b. cystic areas within a thin endometrium.
    c. thin endometrium.
    d. no apparent effect on endometrial thickness or appearance.

46. Which of the following would most likely lead to the development of endometrial adhesions?
    a. Endometrial carcinoma
    b. D&C
    c. Pregnancy
    d. Adenomyomatosis

47. Causes of postmenopausal bleeding include all of the following except:
    a. Asherman syndrome.
    b. endometrial atrophy.
    c. endometrial hyperplasia.
    d. intracavitary fibroids.

48. An asymptomatic 65-year-old patient presents to the sonography department with pelvic pain but no vaginal bleeding. Her endometrial thickness should not exceed:
    a. 6 mm.
    b. 8 mm.
    c. 4 mm.
    d. 3 mm.

49. An 84-year-old patient presents to the sonography department with sudden onset of vaginal bleeding. Her endometrium should not exceed:
    a. 6 mm.
    b. 8 mm.
    c. 4 mm.
    d. 3 mm.

50. With endometrial atrophy, the endometrial thickness should not exceed:
    a. 6 mm.
    b. 3 mm.
    c. 8 mm.
    d. 4 mm.

51. A 68-year-old patient presents to the sonography department complaining of vaginal bleeding. The most likely cause of her bleeding is:
    a. endometrial carcinoma.
    b. endometrial polyps.
    c. endometrial atrophy.
    d. endometrial fibroids.

52. A 60-year-old patient presents to the emergency department with sudden onset of vaginal bleeding. The sonographic examination reveals an endometrium that measures 4 mm. There are no other significant sonographic findings. What is the most likely diagnosis?
    a. Endometrial atrophy
    b. Endometrial carcinoma
    c. Endometrial polyp
    d. Cervical stenosis

53. A 67-year-old patient on HRT presents to the sonography department with abnormal uterine bleeding. Sonographically, the endometrium is diffusely thickened, contains small cystic areas, and measures 9 mm in thickness. The most likely cause of her bleeding is:
    a. endometrial atrophy.
    b. Asherman syndrome.
    c. endometrial thecoma.
    d. endometrial hyperplasia.

54. Endometrial hyperplasia may be caused by all of the following except:
    a. HRT.
    b. ERT.
    c. endometrial atrophy.
    d. tamoxifen.

55. All of the following are clinical findings with endometrial hyperplasia except:
    a. obesity.
    b. polycystic ovary syndrome.
    c. abnormal uterine bleeding.
    d. thickened endometrium.

56. The sonographic findings of an endometrial polyp may include:
    a. diffuse thickening of the endometrium.
    b. menometrorrhagia.
    c. intermenstrual bleeding.
    d. infertility.

57. Endometrial polyps are associated with all of the following except:
    a. intermenstrual bleeding.
    b. tamoxifen therapy.
    c. prolapse through the cervix.
    d. coronary heart disease.

58. A 34-year-old patient presents to the sonography department for an endovaginal sonogram complaining of intermenstrual bleeding. The sonographic findings include a focal irregularity and enlargement of one area of the endometrium. The most likely diagnosis is:
    a. endometrial polyps.
    b. endometrial carcinoma.
    c. endometrial atrophy.
    d. intramural leiomyoma.

59. The most common female genital tract malignancy is:
    a. ovarian carcinoma.
    b. cervical carcinoma.
    c. endometrial carcinoma.
    d. pelvic inflammatory disease.

60. A 31-year-old patient presents to the sonography department for an SIS complaining of intermenstrual bleeding and infertility. Sonographically, a mass is demonstrated emanating from the myometrium and distorting the endometrial cavity. What is the most likely diagnosis?
    a. Endometrial polyp
    b. Endometrial carcinoma
    c. Endometrial hyperplasia
    d. Submucosal leiomyoma

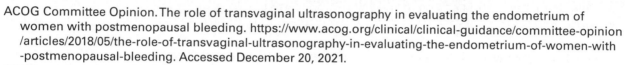

SUGGESTED READINGS

ACOG Committee Opinion. The role of transvaginal ultrasonography in evaluating the endometrium of women with postmenopausal bleeding. https://www.acog.org/clinical/clinical-guidance/committee-opinion/articles/2018/05/the-role-of-transvaginal-ultrasonography-in-evaluating-the-endometrium-of-women-with-postmenopausal-bleeding. Accessed December 20, 2021.

AIUM practice parameter for the performance of an ultrasound examination of the female pelvis. https://www.aium.org/resources/guidelines/femalePelvis.pdf. Accessed December 20, 2021.

AIUM practice parameter for the performance of sonohysterography and hysterosalpingo-contrast sonography. https://www.aium.org/resources/guidelines/sonohysterography.pdf. Accessed December 20, 2021.

Beckmann C, Herbert W, Laube D, et al. *Obstetrics and Gynecology.* 7th ed. Wolters Kluwer; 2014:363–354.

Callahan TL, Caughey AB. *Blueprints: Obstetrics & Gynecology.* 6th ed. Wolters Kluwer; 2013:273–276 & 383–391.

Doubilet PM, Benson CB. *Atlas of Ultrasound in Obstetrics and Gynecology: A Multimedia Reference.* 2nd ed. Wolters Kluwer; 2012:368–373 & 412–415.

Gibbs RS, Karlan BY, Haney AF, et al. *Danforth's Obstetrics and Gynecolgy.* 10th ed. Wolters Kluwer; 2008: 725–741 & 1002–1021.

Goldstein RB, Bree RL, Benson CB, et al. Evaluation of the woman with postmenopausal bleeding: Society of Radiologists in Ultrasound-Sponsored Consensus Conference statement. *J Ultrasound Med.* 2001;20:1025–1036.

Hagen-Ansert SL. *Textbook of Diagnostic Sonography.* 7th ed. Elsevier; 2012:978–1000.

Henningsen C, Kuntz K, Youngs D. *Clinical Guide to Sonography: Exercises for Critical Thinking.* 2nd ed. Elsevier; 2014:148–156.

Hertzberg BS, Middleton WD. *Ultrasound: The Requisites.* 3rd ed. Elsevier; 2016:541–547.

Mahoney S, Armstrong A. Accurate diagnosis of postmenopausal bleeding. *Nurse Pract.* 2005;30(8):61–63.

Mirsafi R, Attarha M. Postmenopausal pregnancy: a case report. *Iran J Nurs Midwifery Res.* 2020;25(3):260–262.

North American Menopause Society. Estrogen and progesterone use in peri- and postmenopausal women: March 2010 position statement of The North American Menopausal Society. *Menopause.* 2010;17(2):245–255.

Norton ME, Scoutt LM, Feldstein VA. *Callen's Ultrasonography in Obstetrics and Gynecology.* 6th ed. Elsevier; 2017:805–826 & 835–845.

Rumack CM, Wilson SR, Charboneau JW, et al. *Diagnostic Ultrasound.* 4th ed. Elsevier; 2011:547–612.

Sanders RC, Hall-Terracciano B. *Clinical Sonography: A Practical Guide.* 5th ed. Wolters Kluwer; 2016:206–213.

Stephenson SR. *Diagnostic Medical Sonography: Obstetrics and Gynecology.* 3rd ed. Wolters Kluwer; 2012: 175–185 & 213–220.

Endometrial Carcinoma on Magnetic Resonance Imaging (Fig. 20-17)

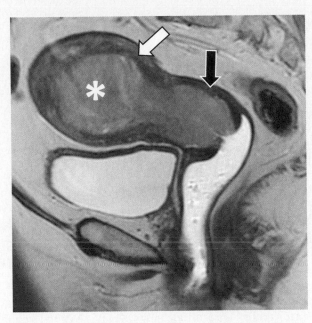

Figure 20-17 Endometrial carcinoma in a 54-year-old woman with postmenopausal bleeding. Surgical pathology confirmed high-grade endometrial carcinoma, endometrioid type. Sagittal T2-weighted magnetic resonance image with vaginal gel demonstrates a T2-hyperintense mass within the endometrial cavity (*asterisk*), invading the myometrium (*white arrow*), with loss of the normal junctional zone, and cervix (*black arrow*).

Ovarian Carcinoma on Computed Tomography and Positron Emission Tomography Scans (Fig. 20-18)

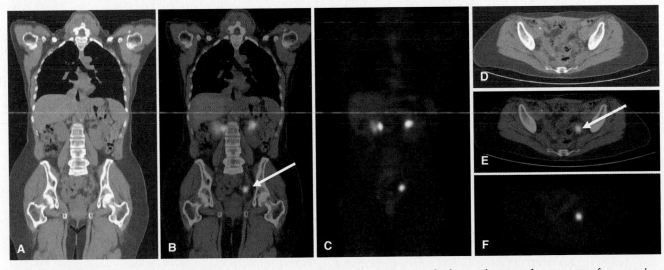

Figure 20-18 Recurrent ovarian carcinoma. This patient had surgery and chemotherapy 1 year ago for ovarian carcinoma. She now has an increasing serum CA-125 level. Coronal (A through C) and transaxial (D through F) computed tomography (CT) (**A, D**), positron emission tomography (PET)/CT (**B, E**) fusion, and PET (**C, F**) images demonstrate increased uptake within a left pelvic soft-tissue nodule (*arrows*). Fine-needle aspirate of this nodule was consistent with recurrent ovarian cancer.

(*continued*)

BONUS REVIEW! *(continued)*

Asherman on Hysterosalpingogram (Fig. 20-19)

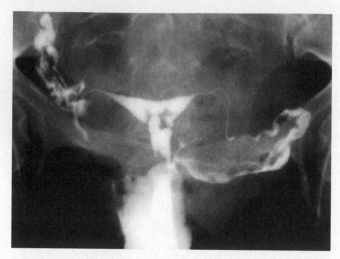

Figure 20-19 Intrauterine adhesion seen on hysterosalpingogram in a patient with Asherman syndrome.

Pelvic Inflammatory Disease and Infertility

Introduction

This chapter discusses the clinical manifestation and sonographic appearance of pelvic inflammatory disease (PID) and associated pathology. Given that there is a notable relationship between pelvic infections and infertility, this chapter also provides an overview of the causes and treatment of female infertility. A discussion on assisted reproductive technology (ART) and contraceptive use is also provided. The "Bonus Review" section includes endometritis and a pelvic abscess on computed tomography (CT).

Key Terms

acute respiratory distress syndrome—the buildup of fluid within the air sacs or alveoli within the lungs

amenorrhea—absence of menstruation

androgen—a hormone, such as testosterone, that is responsible for male characteristics

anovulation—lack of ovulation

Asherman syndrome—syndrome characterized by endometrial adhesions that typically occur as a result of scar formation after some types of uterine surgery

bicornuate uterus—a common uterine anomaly in which the endometrium divides into two horns; also referred to as bicornis unicollis

cervicitis—inflammation of the cervix

chlamydia—a sexually transmitted disease that can lead to an infection of the genital tract in both sexes

cholecystitis—inflammation of the gallbladder

Clomid or clomiphene citrate—fertility drug used to treat anovulation

dysmenorrhea—difficult or painful menstruation

dyspareunia—painful sexual intercourse

ectopic pregnancy—a pregnancy located outside the endometrial cavity of the uterus

endometriosis—functional ectopic endometrial tissue located outside the uterus

endometritis—inflammation of the endometrium

Essure device—a permanent form of birth control that uses small coils placed into the proximal isthmic segment of the fallopian tubes

Fitz-Hugh–Curtis syndrome—a perihepatic infection that results in liver capsule inflammation from pelvic infections such as gonorrhea and chlamydia

follicular aspiration—technique used for in vitro fertilization in which follicles are drained for oocyte retrieval

gamete intrafallopian tube transfer—infertility treatment in which oocytes and sperm are placed in the fallopian tube by means of laparoscopy

gonorrhea—a sexually transmitted disease that can lead to pelvic inflammatory disease

hepatorenal space—peritoneal space located between the liver and the right kidney; also referred to as Morison pouch

heterotopic pregnancy—coexisting ectopic and intrauterine pregnancies

hirsutism—excessive hair growth in women in areas where hair growth is normally negligible

hydrosalpinx—the abnormal accumulation of fluid within the fallopian tube

hyperandrogenism—excessive serum androgen levels; produces male characteristics in females

hyperemic—an increase in blood flow

hypomenorrhea—decreased or scant menstrual flow

hysterosalpingography—a radiographic procedure that uses a dye instilled into the endometrial cavity and fallopian tubes to evaluate for internal abnormalities

in vitro fertilization—fertility treatment that requires that a mature ovum be extracted from the ovary, with fertilization taking place outside the body

infertility—the inability to conceive a child after 1 year of unprotected intercourse

intracavitary (fibroid)—a leiomyoma located within the uterine cavity

intrauterine device—a common form of birth control in which a small device is placed within the endometrium to prevent pregnancy; also referred to as an intrauterine contraceptive device

leukocytosis—an elevated white blood cell count

luteal phase deficiency—when the endometrium does not develop appropriately in the luteal phase of the endometrial cycle as a result of reduced progesterone production

Mirena—a small plastic T-shaped intrauterine device

myometritis—inflammation of the myometrium, the muscular part of the uterus

obesity—overweight to the point of causing significant health problems and increased mortality

oliguria—scant or decreased urine output

oocyte retrieval—the removal of oocytes from ovarian follicles by aspiration

oophoritis—inflammation of the ovary

ovarian hyperstimulation syndrome—a syndrome resulting from hyperstimulation of the ovaries by fertility drugs; results in the development of multiple, enlarged follicular ovarian cysts

ovarian torsion—an abnormality that results from the ovary twisting on its mesenteric connection, consequently cutting off the blood supply to the ovary

ovulation induction—the stimulation of the ovaries by hormonal therapy in order to treat infertility

ParaGard—intrauterine contraceptive device that utilizes copper in its composition to inhibit sperm transport, or to prevent fertilization or transplantation

parametritis—inflammation of the connective tissue adjacent to the uterus

pelvic inflammatory disease—infection of the female genital tract that may involve the ovaries, uterus, and/or the fallopian tubes

Pergonal—infertility medicine used to stimulate the follicular development of the ovaries

polycystic ovary syndrome—syndrome characterized by anovulatory cycles, infertility, hirsutism, amenorrhea, and obesity; may also be referred to as Stein–Leventhal syndrome

postpartum—time directly after giving birth and extending to about 6 weeks

progestin—synthetic progesterone secreted by some intrauterine devices to regulate menstrual flow

purulent—an inflammatory reaction that leads to the formation of pus

pyometra—the presence of pus within the uterus

pyosalpinx—the presence of pus within the fallopian tube

ring-down artifact—artifact seen posterior to air or gas bubbles

salpingitis—inflammation of the fallopian tube

selective reduction—a method of reducing the number of pregnancies in a multiple gestation, whereby certain embryos/fetuses are terminated

septate uterus—congenital malformation of the uterus that results in a single septum that separates two endometrial cavities

sequela—an illness resulting from another disease, trauma, or injury

sonohysterography—a sonographic procedure that uses saline instillation into the endometrial cavity and fallopian tubes to evaluate for internal abnormalities; also referred to as a sonohysterogram

Stein–Leventhal syndrome—see key term polycystic ovary syndrome

"string of pearls" sign—sonographic finding that is described as the presence of 10 or more small cysts measuring 2 to 18 mm along the periphery of the ovary

submucosal (fibroid)—a leiomyoma that distorts the shape of the endometrium

synechiae—adhesion

theca lutein cysts—functional ovarian cysts that are found in the presence of elevated levels of human chorionic gonadotropin; also referred to as a theca luteal cyst

thromboembolism—the formation of clot within a blood vessel with the potential to travel to a distant site and cause an occlusion

tubal ligation—a permanent form of female sterilization in which the fallopian tubes are severed

tubal sterilization—see key term tubal ligation

tubo-ovarian abscess—a pelvic abscess involving the fallopian tubes and ovaries that is often caused by pelvic inflammatory disease

tubo-ovarian complex—when adhesions develop within the pelvis that leads to the fusion of the ovaries and dilated fallopian tubes as a result of pelvic inflammatory disease

upper genital tract—the uterus, ovaries, and fallopian tubes

uterine leiomyoma—a benign, smooth muscle tumor of the uterus; may also be referred to as a fibroid or uterine myoma

vaginitis—inflammation of the vagina

zygote intrafallopian transfer—infertility treatment where the zygote is placed into the fallopian tube

PELVIC INFLAMMATORY DISEASE

Pelvic inflammatory disease (PID) is an infection of the **upper genital tract** (Table 21-1). The origin of the majority of upper genital tract infections is ascension of an infection from the lower genital tract. Infections can travel into normally sterile areas such as the endometrium (**endometritis**) and fallopian tubes (**salpingitis**), resulting in inflammation of those regions. The myometrium (**myometritis**), cellular tissue adjacent to the uterus (**parametritis**),

and the ovary (**oophoritis**) are also often affected by PID. Previous history of PID, the utilization of an intrauterine contraceptive device (IUD or IUCD), postabortion, post childbirth, douching, multiple sexual partners, and early sexual contact have all been established as risk factors for developing PID. PID may manifest after pelvis surgery, accompany tuberculosis, or occur in association with an abscessed appendix or ruptured colonic diverticulum. A common cause of PID is sexually transmitted diseases like **chlamydia** and **gonorrhea** (Fig. 21-1). However, about half of PID cases have non–sexually transmitted disease causes, such as vaginal flora, anaerobic Gram-negative rods, and *Mycoplasma* bacteria. PID is characteristically a bilateral condition affecting not only the uterus but also both fallopian tubes and, possibly, the ovaries. The **sequela** of PID range from a negligible infection that is relatively easy to treat, to the development of a **tubo-ovarian abscess**. In some cases, PID may also lead to death. Potent antibiotic treatment is typically warranted.

TABLE 21-1 Evolution of PID

Vaginitis → Cervicitis → Endometritis → Salpingitis → Tubo-ovarian complex →Tubo-ovarian abscess

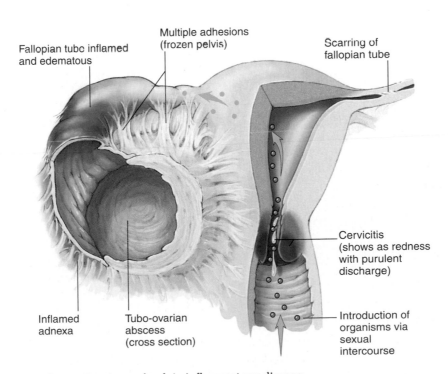

Fallopian tube inflamed and edematous

Multiple adhesions (frozen pelvis)

Scarring of fallopian tube

Cervicitis (shows as redness with purulent discharge)

Introduction of organisms via sexual intercourse

Inflamed adnexa

Tubo-ovarian abscess (cross section)

Figure 21-1 Progression and complications of pelvic inflammatory disease.

SOUND OFF
A common cause of PID is sexually transmitted diseases like chlamydia and gonorrhea.

Clinically, patients with PID tend to have complaints such as fever, chills, pelvic pain, cervical motion tenderness, **purulent** vaginal discharge with foul odor, vaginal itchiness, vaginal bleeding, and **dyspareunia**. **Leukocytosis** is also present. The sonographic findings of acute and chronic PID vary. The uterus involved with an acute infection may show signs of a thickened, irregular endometrium, which is often indicative of endometritis. The uterus can have ill-defined borders, and the fallopian tubes may contain fluid (Fig. 21-2). Echogenic material within the tubes can be evidence of **pyosalpinx**, whereas simple-appearing fluid may be referred to as **hydrosalpinx**. The sonographer should look for further signs of a tubo-ovarian abscess (see "**Tubo-ovarian Complex** and Tubo-ovarian Abscess" section). The possible evolution of PID is discussed in detail in the subsequent sections, but Table 21-1 provides a brief summary.

Chronic PID can lead to continual pelvic or abdominal pain, **infertility** (resulting from adhesions and scaring of the fallopian tubes), possible palpable adnexal mass, and irregular menses. Sonographically, the long-standing PID can reveal evidence of markedly distended fallopian tubes, the development of adhesion between the pelvic organs, and further findings consistent with tubo-ovarian complex and/or tubo-ovarian abscess.

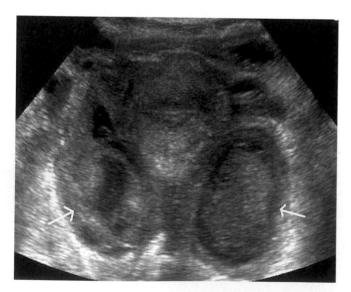

Figure 21-2 Pelvic inflammatory disease. Transverse transabdominal image of the female pelvis revealing bilateral complex adnexal masses (*arrows*) in the setting of an extensive pelvic infection.

CLINICAL FINDINGS OF ACUTE PELVIC INFLAMMATORY DISEASE

1. Possible history of a sexually transmitted disease (chlamydia or gonorrhea)
2. Fever
3. Chills
4. Pelvic pain and/or tenderness
5. Purulent vaginal discharge
6. Vaginal bleeding or itchiness
7. Dyspareunia
8. Leukocytosis

SONOGRAPHIC FINDINGS OF ACUTE PELVIC INFLAMMATORY DISEASE

1. Thickened, irregular endometrium (endometritis)
2. Ill-defined uterine borders
3. Tubular structures representing dilated fallopian tubes containing echogenic material (pyosalpinx)
4. Tubular structures representing dilated fallopian tubes containing simple-appearing, anechoic fluid (hydrosalpinx)
5. Cul-de-sac fluid
6. Multicystic and solid complex adnexal mass(es) (see "Tubo-ovarian Complex and Tubo-ovarian Abscess" section)

CLINICAL FINDINGS OF CHRONIC PELVIC INFLAMMATORY DISEASE

1. Continual pelvic or abdominal pain
2. Infertility (resulting from adhesions and scaring of the fallopian tubes)
3. Possible palpable adnexal mass
4. Irregular menses
5. Purulent vaginal discharge

SONOGRAPHIC FINDINGS OF CHRONIC PELVIC INFLAMMATORY DISEASE

1. Dilated fallopian tubes containing simple-appearing, anechoic fluid (hydrosalpinx)
2. Scars may be noted within the dilated tube and appear as echogenic bands within the tube
3. Development of adhesions may obliterate distinct borders of organs because they become fixated to each other
4. Multicystic and solid complex adnexal mass(es) (see "Tubo-ovarian Complex and Tubo-ovarian Abscess" section)

Vaginitis and Cervicitis

Vaginitis is the most common initial clinical presentation in the early stages of PID. Vaginitis can lead to excessive vaginal discharge, and in cases of PID, patient may present with a purulent, foul-smelling discharge. The progression of the infection into the cervix is termed **cervicitis**. Although vaginitis and cervicitis may not be apparent with sonography, sonography may be utilized to determine whether the infection has spread to the upper genital tract in patients with positive cultures. Infections that do ascend into the endometrium may lead to inflammation of the endometrium—termed endometritis.

Endometritis

Endometritis is the inflammation of the endometrium. It may occur **postpartum**, after a dilation and curettage (D&C), in the presence of PID, after surgery, and may be seen with an **intrauterine device** (IUD). Patients complain of pelvic tenderness and fever and will have evidence of leukocytosis. In some patients, **pyometra**, which is described as pus formation within the endometrium, may occur. Endometritis appears sonographically as a thickened echogenic or irregular-appearing endometrium that may contain some intraluminal fluid. Gas or air formation within the thickened endometrium, which is termed pneumouterus, may be seen and will produce a distinct **ring-down artifact** (Fig. 21-3). The gas formation within the endometrium results from the collection of bacteria. Color Doppler may yield an increase in vascularity (hyperemia) within the endometrium. Endometritis can be effectively treated with oral antibiotics and/or curettage.

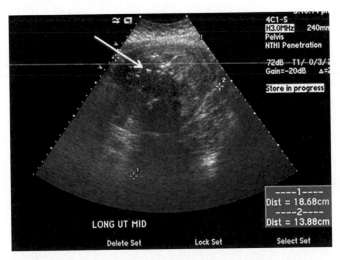

Figure 21-3 Endometritis. A transabdominal sonogram of the uterus in a patient with postpartum fever and sepsis demonstrates echogenic fluid distending the endometrium with shadowing echogenic foci suspicious for gas (*long arrow*).

SOUND OFF
Endometritis appears sonographically as a thickened or irregular-appearing endometrium that may contain some intraluminal fluid. Gas formation within the thickened endometrium may be seen and will produce a distinct ring-down artifact.

CLINICAL FINDINGS OF ENDOMETRITIS

1. History of recent abortion, postpartum, D&C, PID, surgery, or IUD
2. Pelvic tenderness
3. Fever
4. Leukocytosis

SONOGRAPHIC FINDINGS OF ENDOMETRITIS

1. Thickened echogenic or irregular-appearing endometrium
2. Endometrial fluid
3. Ring-down artifact from gas or air within the endometrium
4. Color Doppler may yield hyperemia

Pelvic Inflammatory Disease and the Fallopian Tubes

The fallopian tubes, often difficult to visualize with sonography, may be seen in the presence of PID. The spread of the infection beyond the endometrium can lead to inflammation of the fallopian tubes, commonly referred to as salpingitis. The tubes subsequently distend, thus allowing for visualization with sonography. Unfortunately, in cases where salpingitis is present and the tube is not distended, it may be difficult to determine whether salpingitis is present with sonography. In these instances, the sonographic evidence of salpingitis can be depicted by documenting **hyperemic** flow within or around the tube (Fig. 21-4). This is best demonstrated with the use of color Doppler. In addition, there may be signs of nodular thickening in the wall of the affected tube.

Patients suffering from salpingitis from PID may present clinically with symptoms resembling **cholecystitis**. Pelvic infections, such as chlamydia or gonorrhea, can actually lead to a perihepatic infection and the subsequent development of adhesions located between the liver and the diaphragm. As a result, the liver capsule can become inflamed, thus leading to a clinical presentation much like gallbladder disease. This event is called perihepatitis or **Fitz-Hugh–Curtis syndrome** (Fig. 21-5). Thus, right upper quadrant

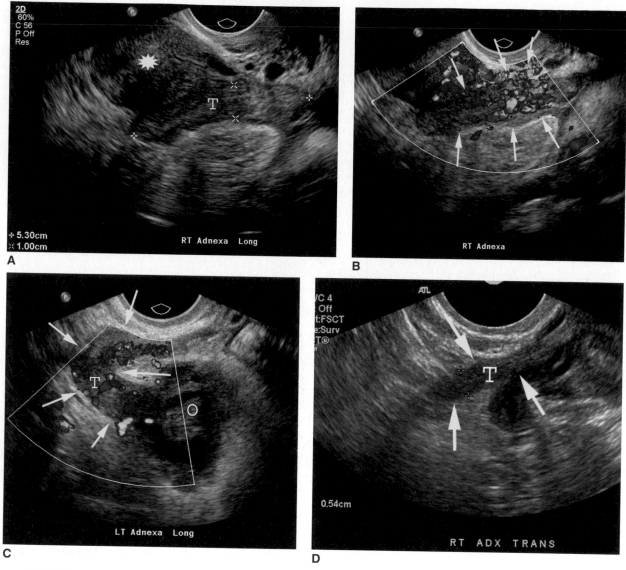

Figure 21-4 Salpingitis. **A.** Sagittal view of the right adnexa in a woman with pelvic pain. Note thick-walled, echogenic right fallopian tube (*T*). Portion of uterus (*asterisk*) are seen. **B.** Color Doppler image of same tube shows marked hyperemia (*arrows*) indicating acute inflammation. **C.** Color Doppler longitudinal image of left tube and ovary shows hyperemic (*arrows*), thickened tube (*T*) and adjacent ovary (*O*). **D.** After medical therapy, the image of the right adnexal region in transverse plane reveals marked improvement in the right fallopian tube (*T*), between *arrows*. Note the decreased width of the tube.

pain, free fluid within the **hepatorenal space** (Morison pouch), and elevated liver function tests may be noted with this condition.

> ### 🔊 SOUND OFF
> The liver capsule can become inflamed, thus leading to a clinical presentation much like gallbladder disease. This event is called Fitz-Hugh–Curtis syndrome.

Tubal infections often lead to fluid accumulation within the lumen of the tube. Pyosalpinx is the result of the tube becoming distended with purulent fluid (pus),

sonographically represented by a dilated fallopian tube filled with thick, echogenic material (Fig. 21-6). The accumulation of simple, anechoic, serous fluid within the dilated fallopian tube may also occur. This is referred to as hydrosalpinx.

PID has been linked with infertility and **ectopic pregnancy**. This is secondary to the formation of scarring within the formerly inflamed opening of the fallopian tube. Scar formation can disrupt the motility and function of the tube and/or inhibit the likelihood of conception. If conception does occur, the development of scar tissue within the fallopian tube increases the possibility of the pregnancy implanting in the tube, thus leading to an ectopic pregnancy.

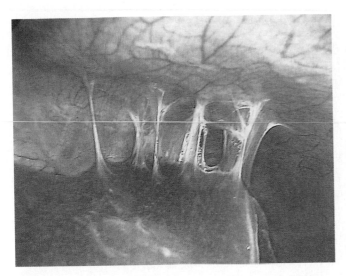

Figure 21-5 Fitz-Hugh–Curtis syndrome. Adhesions between the liver and the diaphragm are evidence of perihepatitis caused by pelvic inflammatory disease and chlamydia.

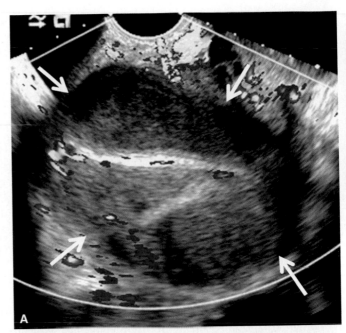

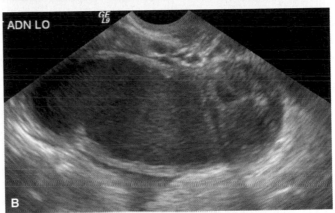

Figure 21-6 Pyosalpinx. **A.** Color Doppler transvaginal image shows a markedly dilated left fallopian tube (*arrows*) with echogenic debris and minimal flow. The tube has folded on itself, mimicking a solitary mass. **B.** Another patient with a distended tube containing echogenic debris, representing pyosalpinx.

> 🔊 **SOUND OFF**
> PID has been linked with infertility and ectopic pregnancy. This is secondary to the formation of scarring within the formerly inflamed opening of the fallopian tube. Scar formation can disrupt the motility and function of the tube and/or inhibit the likelihood of conception.

CLINICAL FINDINGS OF SALPINGITIS

1. Findings consistent with PID
2. Pelvic tenderness
3. Fever
4. Leukocytosis

SONOGRAPHIC FINDINGS OF SALPINGITIS

1. Distended fallopian tube filled with echogenic material (pus) or anechoic fluid
2. Hyperemic flow within or around the affected fallopian tube depicted with color Doppler
3. Nodular, thickened wall of the fallopian tube

Tubo-ovarian Complex and Tubo-ovarian Abscess

As PID progresses and reaches beyond the fallopian tubes, the ovaries and peritoneum become involved. Consequently, adhesions develop within the pelvis that lead to the fusion of the ovaries and the dilated tubes, a condition known as tubo-ovarian complex (Fig. 21-7). Further progression of PID beyond this stage leads to a tubo-ovarian abscess. The sonographic findings of these two processes are similar in that upon sonographic examination the pelvic structures are often indistinguishable, with a loss of discrete borders of the adnexal structures occurring more often when an abscess has developed (Fig. 21-8). Treatments for these two conditions differ in that drainage is required only when an abscess has developed. Consequently, it is important to understand the sonographic appearance of both abnormalities.

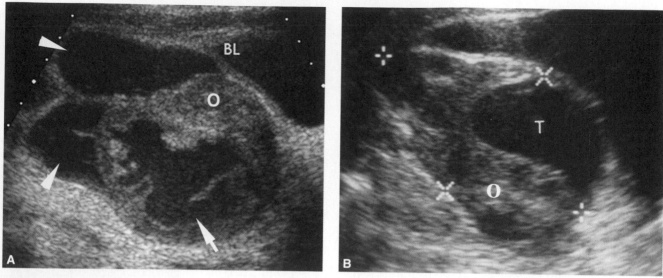

Figure 21-7 Tubo-ovarian complex. **A.** Longitudinal sonogram shows a complex adnexal mass resulting from fusion of a dilated fallopian tube (*arrowheads*), which contains a fluid–debris level (*arrow*), to the left ovary (*O*). *BL*, bladder. **B.** Longitudinal sonogram of the right adnexal region in a different patient shows another complex mass (*calipers*), representing the inflamed ovary (*O*) and fallopian tube (*T*) matted together.

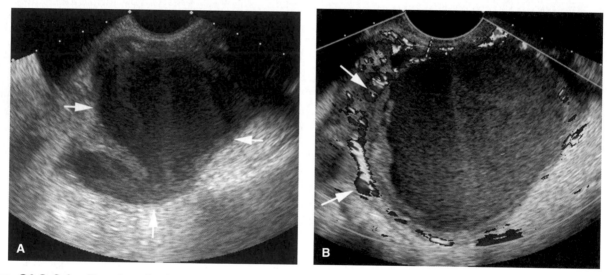

Figure 21-8 Color Doppler of tubo-ovarian abscess. **A.** Transvaginal sonogram showing large complex cystic mass (*arrows*), representing a tubo-ovarian abscess. **B.** Color Doppler image showing hypervascularity (*arrows*) in the wall of the abscess.

Sonographically, the tubo-ovarian complex has signs of PID progression that includes a thickened, irregular endometrium; pyosalpinx or hydrosalpinx; cul-de-sac fluid; and often bilateral complex adnexal masses. The distinguishing feature is that the ovaries and tubes are more readily recognized as distinct structures, but the ovaries will not be able to be separated from the tube by pushing with the vaginal probe. Conversely, when a tubo-ovarian abscess is present within the pelvis, there will be a complete loss of borders of all adnexal structures and the development of a conglomerated adnexal (possibly bilateral) mass.

◄)) SOUND OFF
With tubo-ovarian complex, the ovaries and tubes are more readily recognized as distinct structures, but the ovaries will not be able to be separated from the tube by pushing with the vaginal probe.

CLINICAL FINDINGS OF TUBO-OVARIAN COMPLEX AND TUBO-OVARIAN ABSCESS

1. Findings consistent with PID

SONOGRAPHIC FINDINGS OF TUBO-OVARIAN COMPLEX

1. Thickened, irregular endometrium
2. Pyosalpinx or hydrosalpinx
3. Cul-de-sac fluid
4. Multicystic and solid complex adnexal mass(es)
5. Ovaries and tubes recognized as distinct structures, but the ovaries will not be separated from the tube by pushing with the vaginal probe

SONOGRAPHIC FINDINGS OF TUBO-OVARIAN ABSCESS

1. Thickened, irregular endometrium
2. Pyosalpinx or hydrosalpinx
3. Cul-de-sac fluid
4. Multicystic and solid complex adnexal mass(es)
5. Complete loss of borders of all adnexal structures and the development of a conglomerated adnexal (possibly bilateral) mass

CAUSES OF FEMALE INFERTILITY

Infertility is defined as the inability to conceive a child after 1 year of unprotected intercourse. For females, there can be several different causes of infertility (Fig. 21-9). As noted in the beginning of this chapter, PID is a common cause of infertility. Congenital uterine malformations (especially **septate uterus**), **endometriosis**, **polycystic ovary syndrome (PCOS)**, tubal causes, **Asherman syndrome**, and **uterine leiomyomas**, and their impact on female infertility, are all topics of discussion in the following sections. Consequently, though other possible causes exist, the primary focus on the following sections is sonographically recognizable causes of female infertility.

Congenital Uterine Malformations and Infertility

Congenital uterine malformations, also referred to as Müllerian anomalies, have been linked with female infertility. Rather than preventing pregnancy from occurring, uterine malformations often lead

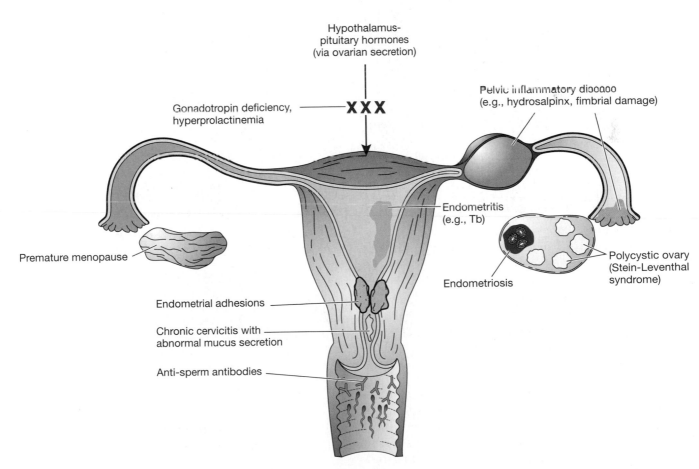

Figure 21-9 Acquired causes of female infertility.

to repeated abortions as a result of structural abnormalities within the uterus. The various types of uterine malformations are discussed in Chapter 17. **Bicornuate uterus** is a common structural defect of the uterus that could lead to fertility troubles. In addition, a septate uterus frequently requires surgical intervention to reduce the division of the uterine cavity. For patients with a septate uterus, sonography can also aid in the resection of the septum during a hysteroscopic uterine septoplasty. Specifically, transabdominal sonography can provide the proximity of the uterine repair to the subserosal surface to help prevent unnecessary bleeding.

Endometriosis

Endometriosis is defined as functional, ectopic endometrial tissue located outside the uterus (Fig. 21-10).

Implantation of ectopic endometrial tissue may be the result of endometrial tissue being passed through the fallopian tubes during menstruation or may result from scarring from surgery, such as after a cesarean section. This ectopic tissue does undergo physiologic changes as a result of stimulation by the hormones of the menstrual cycle. Hemorrhage of this tissue often occurs, resulting in focal areas of bloody tumors known as endometriomas or chocolate cysts. Endometriosis can be located anywhere throughout the pelvis, with the most common location being the ovaries. It has even been found within cesarean section scars, the appendix, lungs, liver, and extremities. The age of the patients at the time of diagnosis is typically between 25 and 35 years, with the common clinical findings being pelvic pain, dyspareunia, and infertility. Patient may also have **dysmenorrhea**, menorrhagia, or painful bowel movements or may be completely asymptomatic.

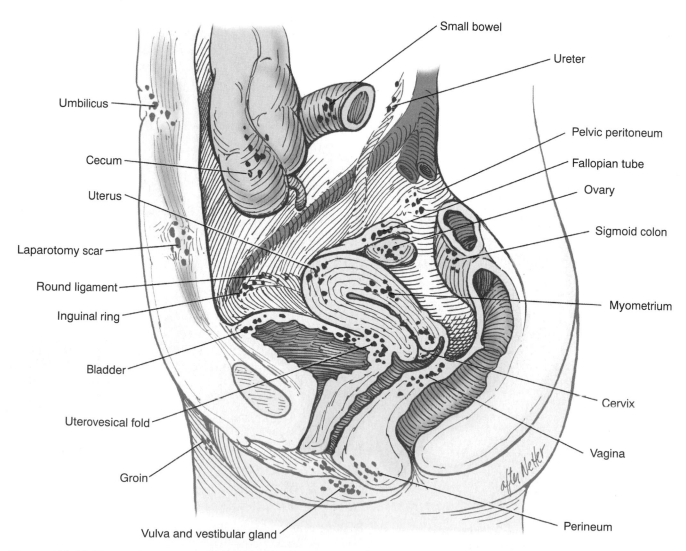

Figure 21-10 Various locations of endometriosis.

🔊 SOUND OFF
The most common location of endometriosis is the ovary.

The link between endometriosis and infertility is still being investigated. However, one valid argument states that infertility results from the development of pelvic adhesions that may alter normal anatomy, thus preventing ovum pickup or causing tubal obstruction. Sonography can be used to indicate the existence of endometriomas; however, smaller implants may be overlooked. Endometriomas are commonly cystic masses with low-level echoes that may or may not contain fluid–fluid levels (Fig. 21-11).

CLINICAL FINDINGS OF ENDOMETRIOSIS

1. Patient may be asymptomatic
2. Pelvic pain
3. Infertility
4. Dysmenorrhea
5. Menorrhagia
6. Dyspareunia
7. Painful bowel movements

SONOGRAPHIC FINDINGS OF AN ENDOMETRIOSIS

1. Predominantly cystic mass with low-level internal echoes (may resemble a hemorrhagic cyst)
2. Anechoic or complex mostly cystic mass with posterior enhancement and may contain a fluid–fluid level

Polycystic Ovary Syndrome

PCOS, also referred to as **Stein–Leventhal syndrome**, is an endocrinologic ovarian disorder linked with infertility. Patients suffer from chronic **anovulation** as a result of hormonal imbalances. The syndrome is characterized by **amenorrhea**, **hirsutism**, and **obesity**. Patients may present with oligomenorrhea and acne as well. PCOS has been cited as the most common cause of **androgen** excess, which is termed **hyperandrogenism**, and hirsutism in women. The established criteria for the diagnosis of PCOS include oligomenorrhea or amenorrhea, blood work indicative of hyperandrogenism, and sonographic findings consistent with PCOS. A patient must have two of the three criteria to be diagnosed with PCOS.

Sonographically, the ovaries are often enlarged and contain multiple, small follicles along the periphery or throughout the ovary, with prominent echogenic stromal

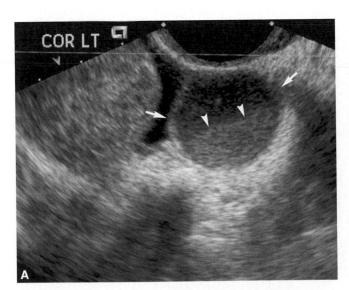

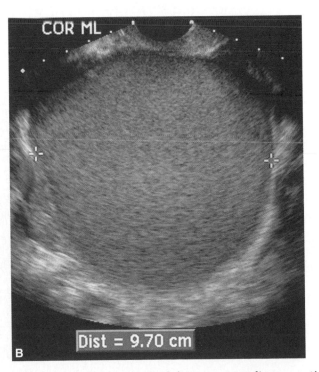

Figure 21-11 Endometrioma. **A.** Fluid–fluid level in an endometrioma. Coronal scan of the left ovary revealing a cystic adnexal mass (*arrows*) containing a fluid–fluid level (*arrowheads*). **B.** Transvaginal image of a homogeneous mass containing low-level echoes that was determined to be an endometrioma.

elements. The sonographic **"string of pearls" sign** or "necklace" sign denotes the presence of many small cysts *along the periphery of the ovary*, whereas another manifestation is many small cysts dispersed *throughout the ovary* (Fig. 21-12). Although clinical signs and symptoms are vital—for the imaging diagnosis of PCOS—it has been suggested that one or both ovaries should contain 12 or more follicles that measure between 2 and 9 mm in diameter, and the ovarian volume should exceed 10 mL. Another investigator suggested that a threshold of 25 small follicles should be used. Nonetheless, it is important to note that, although sonography can play an important confirmatory function, the diagnosis of PCOS is based more on clinical findings. Lastly, high levels of unopposed estrogen stimulation on the endometrium, as seen in patient suffering from PCOS, have also been linked to the subsequent development of endometrial and breast cancer.

> ◄))) **SOUND OFF**
> For the imaging diagnosis of PCOS, one or both ovaries should contain 12 or more follicles that measure between 2 and 9 mm in diameter, and the ovarian volume should exceed 10 mL. A threshold of 25 small follicles can also be used.

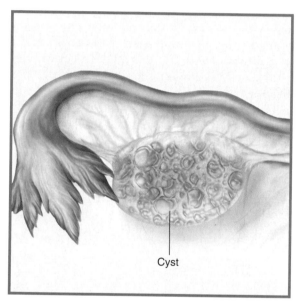

A Polycystic ovary syndrome

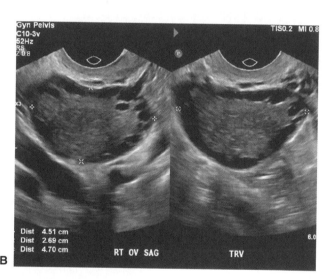

B

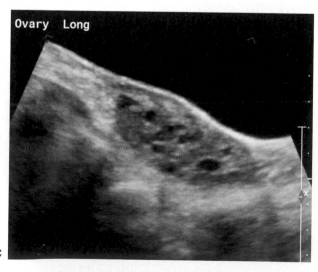

C

Figure 21-12 Polycystic ovary syndrome (*PCOS*). **A.** Drawing of PCOS. **B.** The right ovary is noted being mildly enlarged and exhibiting multiple tiny peripheral follicles. **C.** Although not arranged peripherally, numerous small follicles are present on this ovary. Observation of 12 or more follicles, or ovarian volume greater than 10 mL, supports the diagnosis of PCOS.

CLINICAL FINDINGS OF POLYCYSTIC OVARY SYNDROME

1. Stein–Leventhal syndrome (amenorrhea, hirsutism, and obesity)
2. Infertility
3. Oligomenorrhea
4. Hyperandrogenism

SONOGRAPHIC FINDINGS OF POLYCYSTIC OVARY SYNDROME

1. "String of pearls" sign or "necklace" sign describes the presence of many small cysts measuring along the periphery of the ovary
2. Many small cysts scattered throughout the ovary
3. Bilateral enlargement of the ovaries
4. Increased stroma and increased stromal echogenicity
5. One or both ovaries should contain 12 or more follicles that measure between 2 and 9 mm in diameter
6. Ovarian volume greater than 10 mL
7. Threshold of 25 small follicles can also be used

Tubal Causes of Infertility

As mentioned previously, hydrosalpinx is the accumulation of fluid within the fallopian tube. It is often the result of obstruction of the fimbriated end of the fallopian tube by adhesions. The presence of adhesions within the tube can prevent the normal peristaltic motion that typically occurs. Adhesion development can occur as a result of long-standing PID, endometriosis, and tubal surgery. **Hysterosalpingography** can be used to evaluate the patency of the fallopian tubes, as well as hysterosalpingosonography or hysterosalpingo-contrast sonography.

Endometrial Factors Contributing to Infertility

The endometrium may not develop appropriately in the luteal phase of the endometrial cycle as a result of reduced progesterone production by the ovary; this is termed "**luteal phase deficiency**." The sonographic appearance of the endometrium during the luteal phase can be analyzed. The endometrium becomes thickened and echogenic in appearance during the normal ovarian luteal phase (secretory phase of the endometrial cycle). However, this abnormality is typically diagnosed with endometrial biopsy.

Asherman Syndrome and Infertility

Asherman syndrome is the presence of intrauterine adhesions or **synechiae** within the uterine cavity that typically occur as a result of scar formation after uterine surgery, especially after a D&C. Adhesions within the uterine cavity often prevent implantation or lead to recurrent early pregnancy loss. Patients may suffer from amenorrhea or **hypomenorrhea**. Sonographic detection is difficult without the use of **sonohysterography** or saline infusion sonohysterography. Sonohysterography findings include bright bands of tissue traversing the uterine cavity. Asherman syndrome was also discussed in Chapter 20.

CLINICAL FINDINGS OF ASHERMAN SYNDROME

1. History of D&C, trauma, and uterine surgery
2. Recurrent pregnancy loss
3. Amenorrhea or hypomenorrhea

SONOGRAPHIC FINDINGS OF ASHERMAN SYNDROME

1. Bright areas within the endometrium
2. Sonohysterography findings include bright bands of tissue traversing the uterine cavity

🔊 SOUND OFF

Asherman syndrome is the presence of intrauterine adhesions or synechiae within the uterine cavity.

Uterine Leiomyomas and Infertility

A uterine leiomyoma is a benign, smooth muscular tumor of the uterus that may also be referred to as a fibroid or uterine myoma. Although women with fibroids can still become pregnant, fibroids that are **intracavitary** or **submucosal** in location may distort the endometrium, thus preventing implantation of the early products of conception. Implantation may also be located more inferiorly, lowering live birth rates. Fibroids are thought to impair tubal transport because of obstruction and they may also enlarge during pregnancy. Uterine leiomyomas are also discussed in Chapter 17.

CLINICAL FINDINGS OF A UTERINE LEIOMYOMA

1. Pelvic pressure
2. Menorrhagia
3. Palpable abdominal mass
4. Enlarged, bulky uterus (if multiple)
5. Urinary frequency
6. Dysuria
7. Constipation
8. Infertility

> **SONOGRAPHIC FINDINGS OF A UTERINE LEIOMYOMA**
>
> 1. Hypoechoic mass within the uterus
> 2. Posterior shadowing from mass
> 3. Degenerating fibroids may have calcifications or cystic components
> 4. Multiple fibroids appear as an enlarged, irregular shaped, diffusely heterogeneous uterus

ASSISTED REPRODUCTIVE TECHNOLOGY

Great advances in assisted reproductive technology (ART) have occurred since the 1970s. Sonography is often used to monitor ovulation and follicular growth and to assist during reproductive therapies such as **follicular aspiration** and **oocyte retrieval**. Oocyte retrieval may be performed via the endovaginal or transabdominal approach (Fig. 21-13). With ART, ovarian stimulation is often used to increase follicular development, thus allowing the opportunity to extract multiple oocytes during one procedure. **In vitro fertilization** requires that a mature ovum be extracted from the ovary. Fertilization takes place outside the body, and four to eight developing embryos are placed into the uterus by means of a catheter (Fig. 21-14). This often results in multiple gestations. **Selective reduction,** also referred to as multifetal pregnancy reduction, is the means by which twins, triplets, quadruplets, and quintuplet pregnancies are reduced.

Endovaginal sonography aids in both the initial follicular aspiration and providing guidance for catheter delivery into the uterus. An additional technique of ART, whereby fertilization takes place in the fallopian tube, is termed **gamete intrafallopian tube transfer** (GIFT). GIFT requires that oocytes and sperm be placed in the fallopian tube by means of laparoscopy. **Zygote intrafallopian transfer** is another method that requires the zygote to be inserted into the fallopian tube (Fig. 21-15). Sonographers should be aware that patients who are being treated with assisted reproductive therapy are an increased risk for ectopic pregnancy, **heterotopic pregnancy**, multiple gestations, and **ovarian hyperstimulation syndrome** (OHS).

Ovulation Induction

Ovulatory dysfunction can occur for many reasons, including thyroid disorders and diabetes mellitus. **Ovulation induction** is the stimulation of the ovaries by hormonal therapy to treat infertility. **Clomid,** or **clomiphene citrate**, is a drug that is used to stimulate the pituitary gland to secrete increased amounts of follicle-stimulating hormone (FSH). The increased level of FSH encourages the development of multiple follicles on the ovaries. **Pergonal** is also a fertility drug. It is a hormone extracted from the urine of postmenopausal women that is often used when Clomid administration is

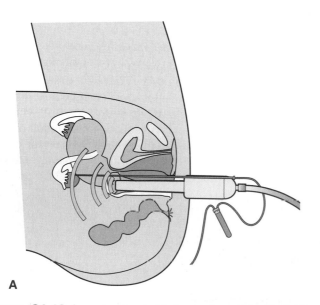

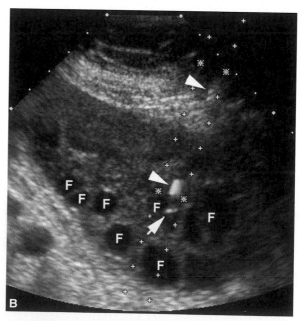

Figure 21-13 Sonography-guided oocyte retrieval. **A.** Endovaginal oocyte retrieval method. **B.** The transabdominal method may be used as well. This is a sagittal view (using a needle guide). The ovary is seen here containing multiple follicles (*F*) as a result of follicular-stimulating medication. A needle (*arrowheads*) has been inserted into the ovary, with its tip (*arrow*) in one of the follicles.

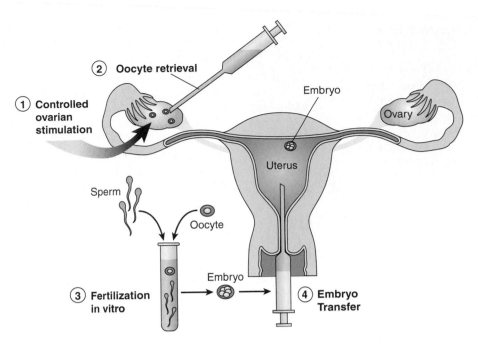

Figure 21-14 In vitro fertilization process.

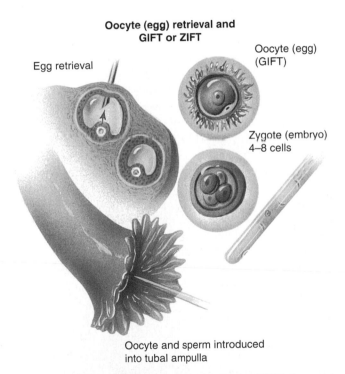

Figure 21-15 Gamete intrafallopian transfer (*GIFT*) (ova and sperm inserted into fallopian tube) or zygote intrafallopian transfer (*ZIFT*) (ova and sperm fertilized in vitro, and the zygote inserted into the fallopian tube). Both these procedures are rarely performed today. More commonly, embryos are transferred directly into the uterine cavity.

not successful. Pergonal consists of a mixture of FSH and luteinizing hormone and is often given in conjunction with human chorionic gonadotropin (hCG). Other infertility drugs include letrozole and gonadotropin

therapy. Nonetheless, there are many types of fertility drugs and combinations. It is important to note that ovulation induction dramatically increases the risk of multiple gestations and OHS.

> **SOUND OFF**
> Ovulation induction medications dramatically increase the risk of multiple gestations and OHS.

Ovarian Hyperstimulation Syndrome

Women who are undergoing ovulation induction by means of hormone administration are at an increased risk for developing OHS. The ovaries can enlarge, often measuring between 5 and 12 cm (Fig. 21-16). The ovary will also contain multiple large follicles known as **theca lutein cysts**. Remember that hCG is administered as part of ovulation induction, and theca lutein cysts occur as a result of high levels of hCG. As a result of these large cysts on the ovary, the patient could suffer from **ovarian torsion**, resulting in acute pelvic pain. In cases of severe OHS, patients have nausea, vomiting, abdominal distension, ovarian enlargement, an electrolyte imbalance, and **oliguria**, with sonographic signs of ascites and pleural effusions. OHS can initiate renal failure, **thromboembolism**, and **acute respiratory distress syndrome**.

> **SOUND OFF**
> Remember that hCG is administered as part of ovulation induction, and theca lutein cysts occur as a result of high levels of hCG.

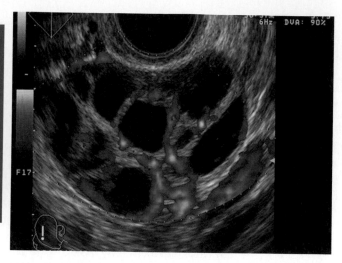

Figure 21-16 Power Doppler imaging of ovarian hyperstimulation.

CLINICAL FINDINGS OF OVARIAN HYPERSTIMULATION SYNDROME

1. Fertility treatment, including ovulation induction
2. Electrolyte imbalance
3. Oliguria
4. Nausea
5. Vomiting
6. Abdominal distension
7. Ovarian enlargement

SONOGRAPHIC FINDINGS OF OVARIAN HYPERSTIMULATION SYNDROME

1. Cystic enlargement of the ovaries greater than 5 cm
2. Ascites
3. Possible pleural effusion

🔊 **SOUND OFF**
OHS can initiate renal failure, thromboembolism, and acute respiratory distress syndrome.

FORMS OF CONTRACEPTION AND STERILIZATION

An IUD is a reversible form of contraception. An IUD is placed in the uterine cavity and prevents implantation of the fertilized ovum. There are several types of IUDs (Table 21-2). Some forms of IUDs also have **progestin**-releasing capabilities (Fig. 21-17). For

TABLE 20-2 Types of intrauterine devices and their sonographic findings	
Intrauterine Contraceptive Device	**Sonographic Findings**
Copper 7	Shadowing number "7"-shaped device
Copper T	Shadowing letter "T"-shaped device
Lippes loop	Five equally spaced shadowing structures
Dalkon shield	Shadowing ovoid shape device
Mirena (Liletta, Skyla, and Kyleena)	Shadowing letter "T"-shaped device
ParaGard	Shadowing letter "T"-shaped device

instance, the **Mirena**, a small plastic T-shaped IUD, distorts the uterine cavity and also releases small amounts of progestin to impede implantation and produce lighter menstrual bleeding. Other newer IUDs include Liletta, Skyla, and Kyleena, all of which are T shaped. The **ParaGard** is another T-shaped IUD, although it utilizes copper in its composition to inhibit sperm transport or to prevent fertilization or transplantation (Fig. 21-18).

IUDs create posterior shadowing and have been described as producing an "entrance and exit echo" on a sonogram (Figs. 21-19 and 21-20). A sonographic examination may be indicated when the string of an IUD cannot be found on physical examination. A sonographic description of these devices must include the location of the IUD in relation to the endometrium. IUDs should be located within the fundal portion of the endometrium. If the IUD is not located within

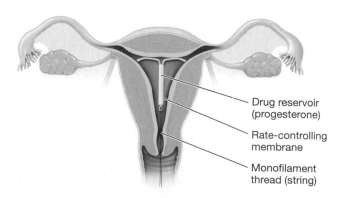

Drug reservoir (progesterone)

Rate-controlling membrane

Monofilament thread (string)

Figure 21-17 An intrauterine device in place in the uterus.

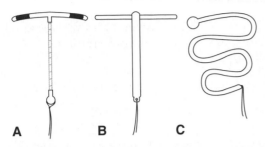

Figure 21-18 Intrauterine devices (IUD). **A.** The ParaGard is a copper-releasing IUD (approved life span, 10 years). **B.** The Mirena progestin-releasing IUD (approved life span, 5 years) is available in the United States. **C.** Although sonographers may encounter these devices, the flexible polyethylene Lippes loop is used throughout the world except in the United States.

the endometrium, then the existence of myometrial perforation should be explored. Three-dimensional (3D) sonography can be exceedingly helpful (Figs. 21-21 and 21-22). Patients who have an IUD that has perforated into the uterine wall will often complain of irregular or heavy bleeding and cramping. The use of IUDs has been linked with PID, ectopic pregnancy, and spontaneous abortions (Fig. 21-23).

> **SOUND OFF**
> IUDs create posterior shadowing and have been described as producing an "entrance and exit echo" on a sonogram.

The pill is a popular form of birth control, and it is highly successful if the manufacturer guidelines are strictly followed. Birth control pills produce an anovulatory cycle by suppressing, primarily, the secretion of luteinizing hormone by the anterior pituitary gland. Other forms of contraception include the formally utilized **Essure device**. The Essure device is no longer sold in the United States.

Female **tubal sterilization**, in the form of **tubal ligation**, and male sterilization, in the form of a vasectomy, offer permanent pregnancy prevention

Pelvic Inflammatory Disease and Infertility

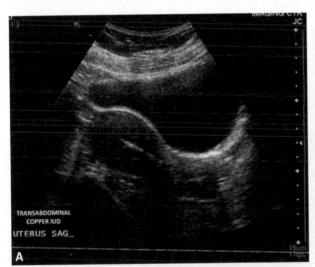

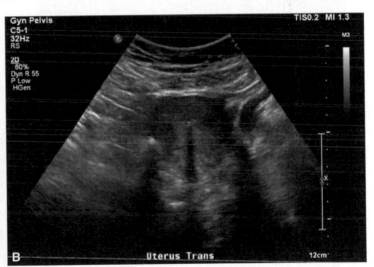

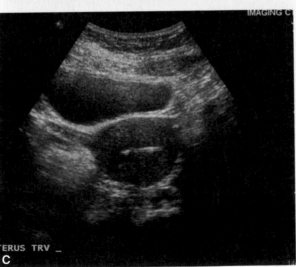

Figure 21-19 Transabdominal intrauterine device (*IUD*) images. **A.** A sagittal view of the uterus with a copper IUD. **B.** Transabdominal transverse view of the uterus with a copper IUD at the stem. **C.** Transabdominal transverse view of the uterus with a copper IUD at the crossbar.

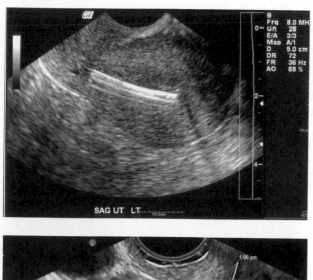

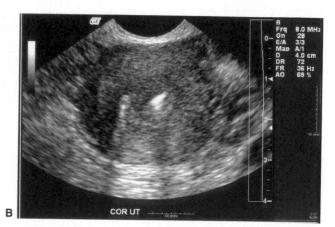

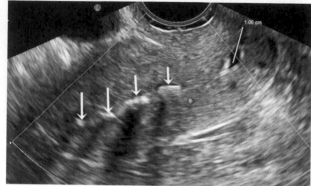

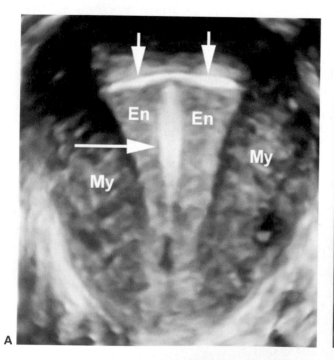

Figure 21-20 Transvaginal image of an intrauterine device (*IUD*) in sagittal (**A**) and coronal (**B**). **C.** Patient with Lippes loop IUD, represented by multiple, equally spaced shadowing foci (*arrows*).

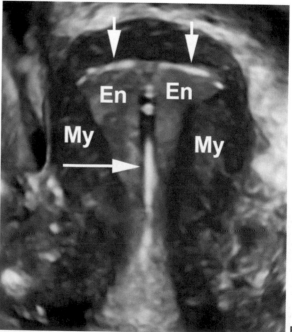

Figure 21-21 Intrauterine device (*IUD*) on three-dimensional (*3D*) ultrasound. **A** and **B.** Coronal planes of the uterus reconstructed from transvaginal 3D volumes in two patients, each displaying the shaft (*long arrow*) and arms (*short arrows*) of a normally positioned IUD. The entire IUD lies within the endometrium (*En*), which is brighter than the surrounding myometrium (*My*). The IUD appears brighter in **A** than **B**, with the difference in brightness due to different IUD types.

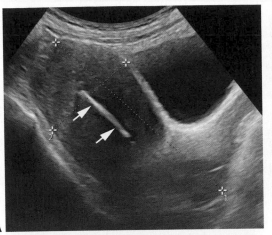

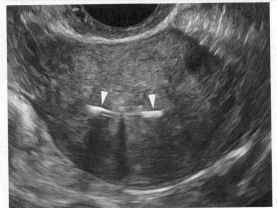

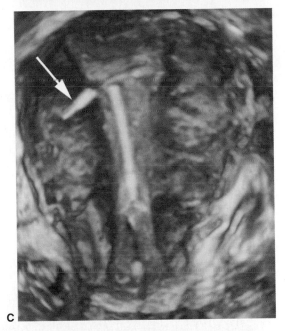

Figure 21-22 Abnormally located intrauterine device (*IUD*) proven with three dimension (*3D*). **A.** Transabdominal sagittal view of the uterus (*calipers*) showing the central location of the shaft of the IUD (*arrows*). **B.** Transvaginal transverse view showing the arms of the IUD (*arrowheads*) are also centrally located. The margins of the endometrial cavity are not visible. **C.** Coronal view reconstructed from a 3D volume demonstrates the endometrial cavity as well as the location of the IUD, showing that the right arm is embedded in the myometrium (*arrow*).

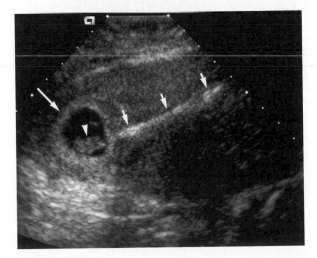

Figure 21-23 Intrauterine device and coexisting intrauterine pregnancy. Transabdominal image revealing an intrauterine device (*small arrows*) adjacent to an intrauterine gestational sac (*long arrow*) containing an embryo (*arrowhead*).

(Fig. 21-24). It is important to note that if a patient presents to the sonography department with a history of tubal ligation and a positive pregnancy test, an ectopic pregnancy should be highly suspected. That is to say, although rare, pregnancy can occur, even though the patient may have had a previous tubal ligation.

SOUND OFF
If a patient presents to the sonography department with a history of tubal ligation and a positive pregnancy test, an ectopic pregnancy should be highly suspected.

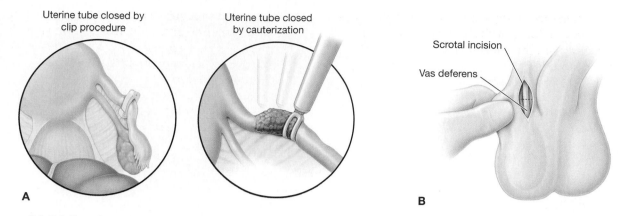

Uterine tube closed by clip procedure

Uterine tube closed by cauterization

Scrotal incision

Vas deferens

A

B

Figure 21-24 Female and male sterilization. **A.** Two different procedures for tubal ligation. **B.** The vas deferens is severed in a procedure referred to as a vasectomy.

REVIEW QUESTIONS

1. The 24-year-old patient in Figure 21-25 presented with hirsutism and obesity. What is the most likely clinical diagnosis based on these sonographic findings?
   a. Asherman syndrome
   b. PCOS
   c. Endometriosis
   d. Fitz-Hugh–Curtis syndrome

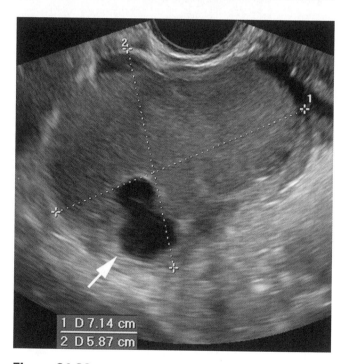

Figure 21-26

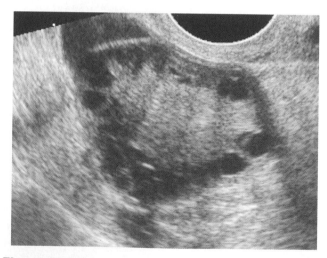

Figure 21-25

2. The patient in Figure 21-26 complained of dysmenorrhea and infertility. The structure between the calipers was noted in the right adnexa. What is the most likely diagnosis?
   a. Brenner tumor
   b. PCOS
   c. Endometrioma
   d. Endometrioid

3. What is the term for inflammation of connective tissue adjacent to the uterus?
   a. Myometritis
   b. Salpingitis
   c. PID
   d. Parametritis

4. Which of the following is not true concerning PID?
   a. PID often results in pelvic adhesions.
   b. PID often results in dyspareunia.
   c. PID often results in endometritis.
   d. PID often results in leukopenia.

5. Which of the following would be the likely cause of the production of artifactual echoes being produced from the endometrium in a patient with known PID?
   a. Dilated blood vessels
   b. Pneumouterus
   c. Endometriosis
   d. Pyosalpinx

6. What is inflammation of the ovary?
   a. Oophoritis
   b. Ovaritis
   c. Oogenesis
   d. Parametritis

7. Which of the following may require hysteroscopic uterine septoplasty in the case of infertility?
   a. Endometriosis
   b. Asherman syndrome
   c. PCOS
   d. Septate uterus

8. What is the most common location of endometriosis?
   a. Ovary
   b. Uterus
   c. Fallopian tube
   d. Bowel

9. Which of the following is an endocrinologic ovarian disorder?
   a. Asherman syndrome
   b. Ovulation induction
   c. Endometriosis
   d. PCOS

10. The patient in Figure 21-27 is undergoing ovulation induction. What type of ovarian cysts are noted in this image?
    a. Corpus luteal cysts
    b. Polycystic ovarian cysts
    c. Theca lutein cysts
    d. Nabothian cysts

11. The patient in Figure 21-27 is also suffering from electrolyte imbalance, oliguria, and nausea. The patient also has ascites. What other sonographic finding is most likely present?
    a. Pleural effusion
    b. Hepatic periportal cuffing
    c. Pancreatic enlargement
    d. Subhepatic adhesions

12. Which of the following may present like gallbladder disease in the patient suffering from PID?
    a. Ovarian torsion
    b. PCOS
    c. Fitz-Hugh–Curtis syndrome
    d. Endometriosis

13. The ovarian volume for the diagnosis of PCOS should not exceed:
    a. 4 mL.
    b. 5 mL.
    c. 8 mL.
    d. 10 mL.

14. Which of the following would least likely cause of the development of intrafallopian tube synechiae?
    a. Long-standing PID
    b. Endometriosis
    c. Tubal surgery
    d. Sonohysterography

15. Which of the following is not a way sonography assists in reproductive technology?
    a. Provides a definitive diagnosis for infertility
    b. Provides a way to monitor ovulation
    c. Provides imaging assistance during follicular aspiration
    d. Provides imaging assistance during oocyte retrieval

16. What blood disorder is associated with OHS?
    a. Sickle cell disease
    b. Hyperlipidemia
    c. Thromboembolism
    d. Polycythemia

17. What is inflammation of the muscular part of the uterus?
    a. Perimetritis
    b. Myometritis
    c. Cervicitis
    d. Endometritis

18. Which of the following would not appear as a "T" shaped IUD with sonography?
    a. Mirena
    b. Liletta
    c. Lippes loop
    d. Kyleena

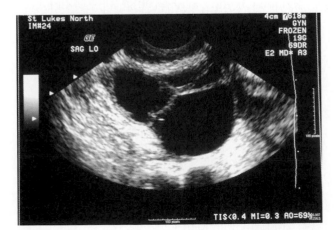

Figure 21-27

19. The patient in Figure 21-28 presented with a lost IUD string and vaginal bleeding. What is the most likely diagnosis?
    a. The IUD is located within the endometrium.
    b. The IUD is located within the myometrium.
    c. The IUD is located within both the endometrium and the myometrium.
    d. The IUD is located within the endometrium, myometrium, and through the perimetrium.

20. What would the patient also likely suffer from in Figure 21-28?
    a. Uterine synechiae
    b. PID
    c. Endometriosis
    d. Uterine cramping

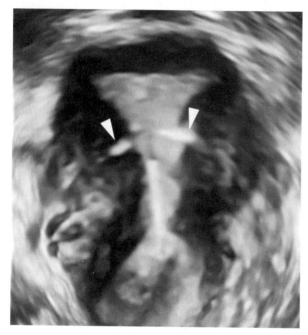

Figure 21-28

21. What is the radiographic procedure used to evaluate the patency of the fallopian tubes?
    a. Sonohysterography
    b. Hysterosalpingography
    c. Hysteroscopy
    d. Hysteroscopic fallopian septoplasty

22. The sonographic finding of a tubular, simple-appearing, anechoic structure within the adnexa is most consistent with:
    a. dyspareunia.
    b. hematometra.
    c. hydrosalpinx.
    d. endometritis.

23. All of the following are considered risk factors for PID except:
    a. IUD.
    b. multiple sexual partners.
    c. post childbirth.
    d. uterine leiomyoma.

24. Which of the following would be the least likely clinical finding for a patient with endometriosis?
    a. Pelvic pain
    b. Dysmenorrhea
    c. Painful bowel movements
    d. Hyperandrogenism

25. Which of the following is not a potential cause of PID?
    a. Intrauterine contraception use
    b. Postabortion
    c. Chlamydia
    d. Pyelonephritis

26. A patient presents to the sonography department with a fever, chills, and vaginal discharge. Sonographically, what findings would you most likely not encounter?
    a. Cul-de-sac fluid
    b. Uterine adhesions
    c. Dilated uterine tubes
    d. Ill-defined uterine border

27. A 26-year-old patient presents to the sonography department with a history of infertility and oligomenorrhea. Sonographically, you discover that the ovaries are enlarged and contain multiple, small follicles along their periphery, with prominent echogenic stromal elements. What is the most likely diagnosis?
    a. Ovarian torsion
    b. OHS
    c. PID
    d. PCOS

28. The most common initial clinical presentation of PID is:
    a. endometritis.
    b. tubo-ovarian abscess.
    c. vaginitis.
    d. pyosalpinx.

29. Sonographic findings of the endometrium in a patient with a history of PID, fever, and elevated white blood cell count would include all of the following except:
    a. ring-down artifact posterior to the endometrium.
    b. thin, hyperechoic endometrium.
    c. endometrial fluid.
    d. thickened, irregular endometrium.

30. What is another name for an endometrioma?
    a. Dermoid
    b. Teratoma
    c. Chocolate cyst
    d. String of pearl

31. Fitz-Hugh–Curtis syndrome could be described as:
    a. clinical findings of gallbladder disease as a result of PID.
    b. the presence of uterine fibroids and adenomyosis in the gravid uterus.
    c. coexisting intrauterine and extrauterine pregnancies.
    d. the presence of pyosalpinx, hydrosalpinx, and endometritis.

32. All of the following statements concerning PID are true except:
    a. PID is typically a unilateral condition.
    b. PID can be caused by douching.
    c. PID can lead to a tubo-ovarian abscess.
    d. dyspareunia is a clinical finding in acute PID.

33. A patient presents to the sonography department with complaints of infertility and painful menstrual cycles. Sonographically, you discover a cystic mass on the ovary consisting low-level echoes. Based on the clinical and sonographic findings, what is the most likely diagnosis?
    a. Cystic teratoma
    b. Endometrioma
    c. PID
    d. OHS

34. The development of adhesions between the liver and the diaphragm as a result of PID is termed:
    a. Fitz-Hugh–Curtis syndrome.
    b. Dandy–Walker syndrome.
    c. Stein–Leventhal syndrome.
    d. Asherman syndrome.

35. Assisted reproductive therapy can result in all of the following except:
    a. heterotopic pregnancy.
    b. multiple gestations.
    c. OHS.
    d. Asherman syndrome.

36. PCOS may also be referred to as:
    a. Fitz-Hugh–Curtis syndrome.
    b. Plateau syndrome.
    c. Stein–Leventhal syndrome.
    d. Asherman syndrome.

37. PID can lead to all of the following except:
    a. infertility.
    b. polycystic ovarian disease.
    c. ectopic pregnancy.
    d. scar formation in the fallopian tubes.

38. What term is used to describe painful intercourse?
    a. Dyspareunia
    b. Dysuria
    c. Dysmenorrhea
    d. Dysconception

39. The presence of functional, ectopic endometrial tissue outside the uterus is termed:
    a. adenomyosis.
    b. Asherman syndrome.
    c. Fitz-Hugh–Curtis syndrome.
    d. endometriosis.

40. All of the following are sonographic findings of a tubo-ovarian abscess except:
    a. the presence of 10 or more small cysts along the periphery of the ovaries.
    b. cul-de-sac fluid.
    c. thickened, irregular endometrium.
    d. fusion of the pelvic organs as a conglomerated mass.

41. A patient presents to the sonography department with a history of chlamydia and suspected PID. Which of the following would be indicative of the typical sonographic findings of PID?
    a. Enlarged cervix, thin endometrium, and theca lutein cysts
    b. Atrophic uterus, free fluid, and small ovaries
    c. Bilateral, cystic enlargement of the ovaries with no detectable flow
    d. Thickened irregular endometrium, cul-de-sac fluid, and complex adnexal masses

42. Causes of female infertility include all of the following except:
    a. previous IUD use.
    b. PCOS.
    c. Asherman syndrome.
    d. endometriosis.

43. Infertility is defined as:
    a. the inability to conceive a child after 2 years of unprotected intercourse.
    b. the inability to conceive a child after 5 years of unprotected intercourse.
    c. the inability to conceive a child after 1 year of unprotected intercourse.
    d. the inability to conceive a child after 3 months of unprotected intercourse.

44. A 25-year-old patient presents to the sonography department complaining of pelvic pain, dyspareunia, and oligomenorrhea. An ovarian mass, thought to be a chocolate cyst, is noted during the examination. Which of the following is consistent with the sonographic appearance of a chocolate cyst?
    a. Simple-appearing anechoic mass
    b. Echogenic mass with posterior shadowing
    c. Cystic mass with low-level echoes
    d. Anechoic mass with posterior shadowing

45. Amenorrhea, hirsutism, and obesity describe the clinical features of:
    a. Fitz-Hugh–Curtis syndrome.
    b. Stein–Leventhal syndrome.
    c. Asherman syndrome.
    d. endometriosis.

46. The sonographic evidence of a hyperemic fallopian tube is consistent with:
    a. pyosalpinx.
    b. hydrosalpinx.
    c. endometritis.
    d. salpingitis.

47. The sonographic "string of pearls" sign is indicative of:
    a. PCOS.
    b. tubo-ovarian disease.
    c. PID.
    d. OHS.

48. Complex-appearing fluid within the fallopian tubes seen with PID is most likely:
    a. pyosalpinx.
    b. pyometra.
    c. hydrosalpinx.
    d. hematometra.

49. Sonographic findings of OHS include all of the following except:
    a. cystic enlargement of the ovaries.
    b. ascites.
    c. pleural effusions.
    d. oliguria.

50. The development of adhesions within the uterine cavity is termed:
    a. Fitz-Hugh–Curtis syndrome.
    b. Dandy–Walker syndrome.
    c. Stein–Leventhal syndrome.
    d. Asherman syndrome.

51. OHS can cause multiple large follicles to develop on the ovaries termed:
    a. theca lutein cysts.
    b. chocolate cysts.
    c. corpus luteum cysts.
    d. dermoid cysts.

52. What is another name for adhesions within the endometrial cavity?
    a. Endometritis
    b. Synechiae
    c. Septation
    d. Mural nodules

53. A female patient presents to the sonography department with a clinical history of Clomid treatment. She is complaining of nausea, vomiting, and abdominal distension. What circumstance is most likely causing her clinical symptoms?
    a. Stein–Leventhal syndrome
    b. Polycystic ovarian disease
    c. Fitz-Hugh–Curtis syndrome
    d. OHS

54. A 35-year-old patient presents to the sonography department with a history of tubal ligation and positive pregnancy test. What condition should be highly suspected?
    a. Asherman syndrome
    b. Polycystic ovarian disease
    c. Endometriosis
    d. Ectopic pregnancy

55. Patients with OHS are at increased risk for:
    a. ovarian torsion.
    b. chlamydia.
    c. gonorrhea.
    d. vaginitis.

56. Which of the following would be described as functional cysts that are found in the presence of elevated levels of hCG?
    a. Theca lutein cysts
    b. Chocolate cysts
    c. Corpus luteum cysts
    d. Endometrial cysts

57. The presence of pus within the uterus defines:
    a. pyosalpinx.
    b. pyometra.
    c. pyocolpos.
    d. pyomyoma.

58. The occurrence of having both intrauterine and extrauterine pregnancies at the same time describes:
    a. PID.
    b. ectopic pregnancy.
    c. heterotopic pregnancy.
    d. molar pregnancy.

59. Excessive hair growth in women in areas where hair growth is normally negligible would be seen with:
    a. ectopic pregnancy.
    b. Fitz-Hugh–Curtis syndrome.
    c. Asherman syndrome.
    d. Stein–Leventhal syndrome.

60. What form of permanent birth control would be seen sonographically as echogenic, linear structures within the lumen of both isthmic portions of the fallopian tubes?
    a. Essure devices.
    b. ParaGard.
    c. Lippes loop.
    d. Mirena.

SUGGESTED READINGS

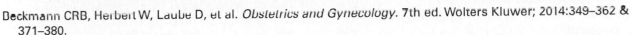

Deckmann CRB, Herbert W, Laube D, et al. *Obstetrics and Gynecology*. 7th ed. Wolters Kluwer; 2014:349–362 & 371–380.

Berek JS, Berek DL. *Berek & Novak's Gynecology*. 16th ed. Wolters Kluwer; 2020:942–1001.

Callahan TL, Caughey AB. *Blueprints: Obstetrics & Gynecology*. 6th ed. Wolters Kluwer; 2013:204–238 & 306–336.

Doubilet PM, Benson CB. *Atlas of Ultrasound in Obstetrics and Gynecology: A Multimedia Reference*. 2nd ed. Wolters Kluwer; 2012:395–399 & 416–419.

Gibbs RS, Haney AF, Karlan BY, et al. *Danforth's Obstetrics and Gynecology*. 10th ed. Wolters Kluwer; 2008:648–663 & 682–724.

Hagen-Ansert SL. *Textbook of Diagnostic Sonography*. 7th ed. Elsevier; 2012:978–1038.

Henningsen C, Kuntz K, Youngs D. *Clinical Guide to Sonography: Exercises for Critical Thinking*. 2nd ed. Elsevier; 2014:165–182.

Hertzberg BS, Middleton WD. *Ultrasound: The Requisites*. 3rd ed. Elsevier; 2016:527–600.

Kinnear HM, Tomaszewski CE, Chang FL, et al. The ovarian stroma as a new frontier. *Reproduction*. 2020;160(3):R25–R39. doi:10.1530/REP-19-0501

Norton ME, Scoutt LM, Feldstein VA. *Callen's Ultrasonography in Obstetrics and Gynecology*. 6th ed. Elsevier; 2017:891–897 & 934–965.

Rumack CM, Wilson S, Charboneau JW, et al. *Diagnostic Ultrasound*. 4th ed. Elsevier; 2011:547–612.

Sanders RC, Hall-Terracciano B. *Clinical Sonography: A Practical Guide*. 5th ed. Wolters Kluwer; 2016:151–167 & 200–220.

Siegel MJ. *Pediatric Sonography*. 5th ed. Wolters Kluwer; 2019:513–556.

Stephenson SR, Dmitrieva J. *Diagnostic Medical Sonography: Obstetrics and Gynecology*. 3rd ed. Wolters Kluwer; 2018:261–294.

Timor-Tritsch IE, Goldstein SR. *Ultrasound in Gynecology*. 2nd ed. Elsevier; 2007:212–231 & 293–306.

BONUS REVIEW!

Endometritis on Computed Tomography (Fig. 21-29)

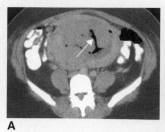
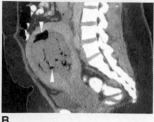

Figure 21-29 Endometritis on computed tomography (*CT*). Axial (**A**) and sagittal (**B**) contrast-enhanced CT in a different patient demonstrate an expanded endometrium filled with hyperdense material (*short arrow*) and large foci of gas (*arrowheads*), consistent with endometritis.

Pelvic Abscess on Computed Tomography (Fig. 21-30)

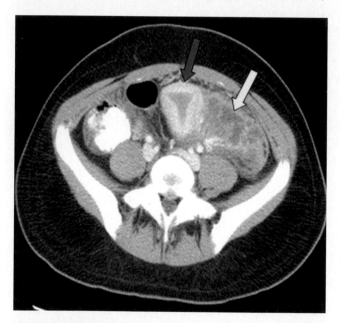

Figure 21-30 Axial computed tomography scan image shows the left lower quadrant pelvic abscess (*yellow arrow*) and surrounding inflammatory changes adjacent to the blood-filled uterus (*blue arrow*).

Low Positioned Intrauterine Contraceptive Device (Fig. 21-31)

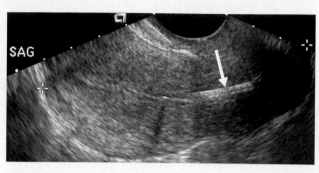

Figure 21-31 Low positioned intrauterine device (*IUD*). Sagittal transvaginal image of the uterus shows the IUD (*arrow*) abnormally positioned in the uterine isthmus. The IUD is seen as a bright linear echo with reverberation artifact. An IUD in this position is ineffective as a contraceptive.

Obstetric Sonography Overview

Introduction

A synopsis of obstetric sonography practice is provided in this chapter. The practice parameters, as prescribed by the American Institute of Ultrasound in Medicine and others, are provided in this chapter. Also, a brief summary of the importance of obtaining and recognizing significant clinical findings, relevant laboratory results, frequently identified artifacts, fetal biometry, biophysical profile scoring, fetal presentation, and extrauterine abnormalities should provide the analytical groundwork for a thorough preparation for the obstetric component of the registry provided by the American Registry for Diagnostic Medical Sonography and the obstetric portion of the registry offered by the American Registry of Radiologic Technologist. The outlines for each examination can be found at www.ardms.org and www.arrt.org, respectively. The "Bonus Review" section includes a novel way to determine fetal situs, a diagram of external cephalic version, and a magnetic resonance imaging (MRI) of a twin gestation.

Key Terms

acute appendicitis—inflammation of the appendix

adnexa—the area located posterior to the broad ligaments and adjacent to the uterus, which contains the ovaries and fallopian tubes

alpha-fetoprotein—a protein produced by the fetal yolk sac, fetal gastrointestinal tract, and the fetal liver; may also be produced by some malignant tumors

aneuploidy—a condition of having an abnormal number of chromosomes

corpus luteum cyst—a physiologic cyst that develops after ovulation has occurred

estriol—an estrogenic hormone produced by the placenta

estimated date of confinement—the due date of a pregnancy

external cephalic version—the manual manipulation by a physician of a fetus that is in breech or transverse position to a cephalic position in order to facilitate vaginal delivery

gestational diabetes—diabetes acquired as a result of pregnancy

gravid—pregnant

gravidity—the number of times that a woman has been pregnant

human chorionic gonadotropin—a hormone produced by the trophoblastic cells of the early placenta; may also be used as a tumor marker in nongravid patients and males

hydronephrosis—the dilation of the renal collecting system resulting from the obstruction of the flow of urine from the kidney(s) to the bladder; also referred to as pelvocaliectasis or pelvicaliectasis

idiopathic—from an unknown origin

inhibin A—a peptide hormone secreted by the placenta during pregnancy

meningocele—the herniation of the cranial or spinal meninges caused by an open cranial or spinal defect

myelomeningocele—mass that results from spina bifida that contains the spinal cord and the meninges

nonstress test—a noninvasive test performed on the fetus to evaluate fetal movement, heart rate, and reactivity of the heart rate to fetal movement; diagnostic use is to detect signs of fetal distress

nuchal translucency—the anechoic space along the posterior aspect of the fetal neck

ovarian torsion—an abnormality that results from the ovary twisting on its mesenteric connection, consequently cutting off the blood supply to the ovary; may be referred to as adnexal torsion

pallor—extreme paleness of the skin

parity—the number of pregnancies in which the patient has given birth to a fetus at or beyond 20 weeks' gestational age or an infant weighing more than 500 g

placenta previa—when the placenta covers or nearly covers the internal os of the cervix

placental abruption—the premature separation of the placenta from the uterine wall before the birth of the fetus

pregestational diabetes—diabetes that is preexisting to pregnancy

pregnancy-associated plasma protein A—a protein that is produced by the placenta

quadruple screen—a maternal blood test that includes an analysis of human chorionic gonadotropin, alpha-fetoprotein, estriol, and inhibin A

supine hypotensive syndrome—a reduction in blood return to the maternal heart caused by the gravid uterus compressing the maternal inferior vena cava

teratogen—something that can cause birth defects or abnormalities within an embryo or fetus; examples include medications, tobacco products, chemicals, alcohol, and certain infections

triple screen—a maternal blood test that typically includes an analysis of human chorionic gonadotropin, alpha-fetoprotein, and estriol

UNDERSTANDING THE TRIMESTERS AND PREGNANCY TERMS

A normal pregnancy lasts for 9 months, 40 weeks, or 280 days. However, it may last up to 42 weeks. As a result, typically, the first trimester is defined as conception to 12 weeks, the second trimester is defined as weeks 13 through 26, and the third trimester is defined as weeks 27 through 42. Fetal age is determined by the last menstrual period (LMP), which may be referred to as menstrual

age or gestational age. The date of the LMP is the last date at which the patient started menstruation. It can be used to determine the **estimated date of confinement** (EDC), or more commonly referred to as the "due date." The EDC will be calculated by the ultrasound machine once the LMP is entered into the machine's obstetric calculation package. It is important to note that not all patients are good historians; thus, the LMP may not be reliable, especially if the patient is clearly unsure about the beginning of her cycle.

From the time of conception to 10 weeks, the conceptus is referred to as an embryo, and after that point, it is then referred to as a fetus. A pregnancy that is considered term occurs between 37 and 42 gestational weeks. A pregnancy that is carried beyond 42 weeks is referred to as post-term, whereas one that is delivered between 24 and 37 weeks is referred to as preterm. Infants born before 24 weeks are often not sufficiently developed to survive outside the uterus, and those that do survive because of medical intervention often suffer from serious, lifelong health complications.

> **◄))) SOUND OFF**
> From the time of conception to 10 weeks, the conceptus is referred to as an embryo, and after that point, it is then referred to as a fetus.

CLINICAL INDICATIONS FOR AN OBSTETRIC SONOGRAM

An obstetric sonogram may be requested for various reasons. The American Institute of Ultrasound in Medicine publishes the practice parameters for an obstetric sonogram on their website at www.aium.org (Tables 22-1 to 22-4). Parameter suggestions now include those for the standard first and second/third trimester obstetric sonogram and detailed first and second/third trimester anatomy sonogram.

PATIENT PREPARATION FOR AN OBSTETRIC SONOGRAM, PATIENT CARE, AND TECHNICAL RECOMMENDATIONS

Both transvaginal (TV), also referred to as endovaginal, and transabdominal (TA) imaging may be utilized to evaluate the **gravid** uterus. Although both techniques have their limitations, they often work well in conjunction with each other. In the early first trimester, if TA imaging is used, the patient should have a distended urinary bladder to better visualize not only the uterus but also the **adnexa**. TV imaging is most often the technique used to image the early

TABLE 22-1 AIUM practice parameter for a standard first-trimester sonogram

Indications for a First-Trimester Sonogram[a]

Confirmation of the presence of an intrauterine pregnancy
Evaluation of a suspected ectopic pregnancy
Defining the cause of vaginal bleeding
Evaluation of pelvic pain
Estimation of gestational (menstrual) age
Diagnosis or evaluation of multiple gestations
Confirmation of cardiac activity
Imaging as an adjunct to chorionic villus sampling, embryo transfer, and localization and removal of an intrauterine device
Assessing for certain fetal anomalies, such as anencephaly
Evaluation of maternal pelvic masses and/or uterine abnormalities
Measuring the nuchal translucency (NT) when part of a screening program for fetal **aneuploidy**
Evaluation of suspected gestational trophoblastic disease

AIUM, American Institute of Ultrasound in Medicine.
[a]Other indications exist.

TABLE 22-2 AIUM practice parameter for a detailed first-trimester sonogram

AIUM Practice Parameter for a Detailed Diagnostic Obstetric Ultrasound Between 12 Weeks 0 Days and 13 Weeks 6 Days[a]

Previous fetus or child with a congenital, genetic, or chromosomal anomaly
Known or suspected fetal abnormality detected by ultrasound in the current pregnancy
Fetus at increased risk for a congenital anomaly based on the following:

35 years or older at delivery
Maternal pregestational diabetes
Pregnancy conceived via in vitro fertilization
Multiple gestation
Teratogen exposure
Enlarged nuchal translucency
Positive screening test results for aneuploidy, including cell-free DNA screening and serum
Only or combined first-trimester screening

Other conditions possibly affecting the pregnancy/fetus, including:

Maternal body mass index of $\geq$30 kg/m^2
Placental implantation covering the internal cervical os under a cesarean scar site or cesarean scar pregnancy diagnosed in index gestation

AIUM, American Institute of Ultrasound in Medicine.
[a]Other indications exist.

TABLE 22-3 AIUM practice parameter for a second- and third-trimester sonogram

AIUM Practice Parameter for a Second- and Third-Trimester Sonogram[a]

Screening for fetal anomalies
Evaluation of fetal anatomy
Estimation of gestational (menstrual) age
Evaluation of fetal growth
Evaluation of vaginal bleeding
Evaluation of abdominal or pelvic pain
Evaluation of cervical length

(continued)

TABLE 22-3 AIUM practice parameter for a second- and third-trimester sonogram (*continued*)

AIUM Practice Parameter for a Second- and Third-Trimester Sonogram[a]

Determination of fetal presentation
Evaluation of suspected multiple gestation
Adjunct to amniocentesis or other procedure
Evaluation of a significant discrepancy between uterine size and clinical dates
Evaluation of a pelvic mass
Evaluation of a suspected gestational trophoblastic disease
Suspected fetal death
Suspected uterine abnormalities
Evaluation of fetal well-being
Suspected amniotic fluid abnormalities
Suspected placental abruption
Adjunct to **external cephalic version**
Evaluation of premature rupture of membranes and/or premature labor
Follow-up evaluation of a fetal anomaly
Follow-up evaluation of placental location for suspected placenta previa, vasa previa, and abnormally adherent placenta

AIUM, American Institute of Ultrasound in Medicine.
[a] Other indications exist.

TABLE 22-4 AIUM practice parameter for a detailed second- and third-trimester diagnostic obstetric sonogram

AIUM Practice Parameter for the Performance of Detailed Second- and Third-Trimester Diagnostic Obstetric Ultrasound Examination[a]

Previous fetus or child with a congenital, genetic, or chromosomal abnormality
Known or suspected fetal anomaly or known or suspected fetal growth restriction in the current pregnancy

Fetus at increased risk for a congenital anomaly, such as the following:
 Maternal pregestational diabetes or gestational diabetes diagnosed before 24 weeks' gestation
 Pregnancy conceived via assisted reproductive technology
 Maternal body mass index of ≥ 30 kg/m^2
 Multiple gestations
 Abnormal maternal serum analytes
 Teratogen exposure
 First-trimester nuchal translucency measurement of ≥ 3.0 mm

Fetus at increased risk for a genetic or chromosomal abnormality, such as the following:
 Parental carrier of a chromosomal or genetic abnormality
 Maternal age of 35 years or older at delivery
 Positive screening test results for aneuploidy
 Aneuploidy marker noted on an ultrasound examination
 First-trimester nuchal translucency measurement of ≥ 3.0 mm

Other conditions affecting the fetus, including the following:
 Congenital infections
 Maternal drug use
 Alloimmunization
 Oligohydramnios
 Polyhydramnios
 Suspected placenta accrete spectrum or risk factors for placenta accrete spectrum such as
 Placenta previa in the third trimester or a placenta overlying a prior cesarean scar site

AIUM, American Institute of Ultrasound in Medicine.
[a] Other indications exist.

pregnancy because it offers superior resolution. An empty maternal bladder is needed for this examination. Second- and third-trimester sonographic examinations also require an empty maternal bladder.

First-trimester sonograms may require the use of a 5- to 10-MHz or higher TV transducer to better visualize intrauterine structures and the adnexa. Typically, a 3- to 5-MHz TA transducer will allow sufficient penetration in most pregnant patients, while providing sufficient resolution. These frequency ranges will vary among ultrasound equipment. While obese patients may require the use of lower frequency transducers for additional penetration, for some thin patients, especially in the first trimester, a linear transducer may be utilized to obtain high-resolution images.

Image optimization should always be pursued. Tools for image optimization include the use of harmonics, compound imaging, decreasing imaging depth when possible, narrowing the image sector, magnifying the region of interest, adjusting the focal zone, adapting the dynamic range, adjusting image resolution parameters, extended field-of-view, and the use of cine loops and three-dimensional imaging as needed (Fig. 22-1). Also, adjustments to color Doppler, spectral, and power Doppler should be made to portray accurate information.

All transducers and transducer cords should undergo disinfection after performing an obstetric sonogram to prevent the spread of disease. TV transducers should undergo high-level disinfection, and the manufacturer's specified instructions should be followed. Because TV imaging requires that the transducer be placed into the vagina, a probe cover should be placed on the transducer and it should be inserted into the vagina using sterile jelly as a lubricant.

🔊 **SOUND OFF**
TV transducers should undergo high-level disinfection, and the manufacturer's specified instructions should be followed.

There are several common maternal clinical issues and stressors that occur during pregnancy, including skin changes, postural changes, back pain, constipation, contractions, dehydration, edema, gastrointestinal reflux disease, hemorrhoids, round ligament pain, urinary frequency, varicose vein, and even an increase for cardiovascular issues exists in some situations (Fig. 22-2). The patient may have **pregestational diabetes** or develop **gestational diabetes** (see Chapter 32). The sonographer should be aware of these issues and try to provide a comfortable

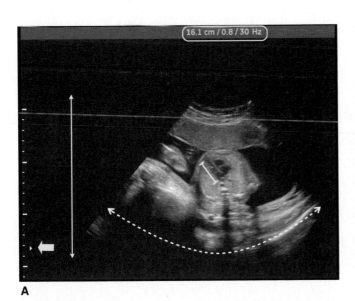

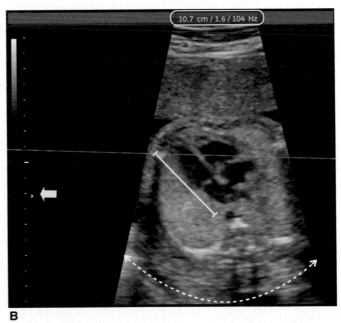

A   **B**

Figure 22-1 Four-chamber view of the fetal heart in the same fetus after image optimization. **A.** Note that the depth is high (*double straight arrow*), the angle is wide (*dashed arrow*), and the focal zone (*yellow arrow*) is not placed at the level of the region of interest (*four-chamber view*). The size of the heart within the whole image (*yellow line*) is so small that it does not allow for any reliable detailed analysis. **B.** The image is optimized by reducing the depth, magnifying the image, narrowing the sector width (*dashed arrow*), and placing the focal zone at the appropriate level (*yellow arrow*). These steps resulted in an image magnification with a high frame rate.

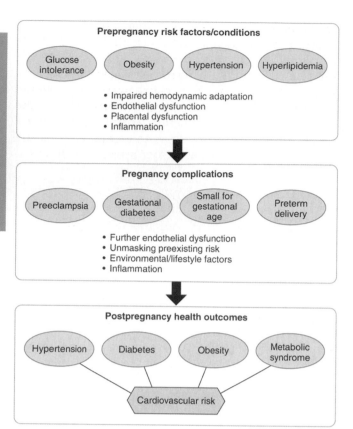

Figure 22-2 Risk factors and conditions associated with pregnancy complications and future cardiovascular risk.

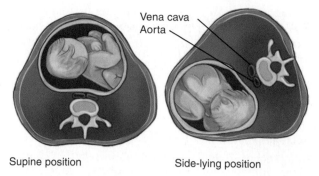

Supine position   Side-lying position

Figure 22-3 Supine hypotensive syndrome. When the pregnant woman lies flat on her back, the weight of the fetus and uterus can compress the aorta and inferior vena cava against the spine. Consequently, the amount of blood returning to the heart is compromised, pressure falls, and supine hypotensive syndrome occurs (image on the *left*). By placing the patient on her side (image on the *right*), the pressure is relieved, and the patient should feel better soon.

and safe environment for the patient. Some of these clinical issues increase in likelihood and severity with multiple gestations. The sonographer should also be ready to provide any emergency care to the pregnancy patient, including cardiopulmonary resuscitation (CPR), if needed.

While evaluating the gravid patient, the sonographer should be aware of a unique situation that may arise during the examination. Patients in their late second or third trimester may suffer from **supine hypotensive syndrome**, which is a reduction in blood return to the maternal heart caused by the gravid uterus compressing the maternal inferior vena cava. Patients can complain of tachycardia, sweating, nausea, and **pallor**. The sonographer can assist the patient into a right lateral or left lateral position to alleviate symptoms (Fig. 22-3).

GATHERING A CLINICAL HISTORY

A review of prior examinations should be performed by the sonographer before any interaction with the patient. This review includes previous sonograms and other imaging studies when applicable. For example, though computed tomography and radiography are rarely performed on the gravid patient, MRI is used in some situations. Gathering a clinical history includes a basic inquiry into the patients past obstetric history by documenting **gravidity** (G) and **parity** (P) (Table 22-5). Gravidity denotes the number of times a woman has been pregnant, whereas parity denotes the number of pregnancies that led to the birth of a fetus at or beyond 20 weeks' gestational age or of an infant who weighed at least 500 g. A more specific method can be further added using the *TPAL* (*T*erm, *P*remature, *A*bortions, *L*ive birth) description. These inquiries should include questions about previous pregnancies or fetal complications, diabetes, hypertension, infertility, and the general health of other children at the time of birth and currently. Moreover, sonographers must be capable of analyzing the clinical history and complaints of their patients. This practice will not only aid in clinical practice but will also assist in answering complex certification examination questions.

> **🔊 SOUND OFF**
> Patients in their late second or third trimester may suffer from supine hypotensive syndrome, which is a reduction in blood return to the maternal heart caused by the gravid uterus compressing the maternal inferior vena cava.

> **🔊 SOUND OFF**
> Gravidity denotes the number of times a woman has been pregnant, whereas parity denotes the number of pregnancies that led to the birth of a fetus at or beyond 20 weeks' gestational age or of an infant who weighed at least 500 g.

TABLE 22-5 Common clinical pregnancy terminology

Gravida (G) or gravidity	the number of pregnancies
Multigravida	has been pregnant more than once
Multiparous	has given birth more than once
Nulliparous	not given birth
Para (P) or parity	the number of pregnancies in which the patient has given birth to a fetus at or beyond 20 weeks' gestational age or an infant weighing >500 g
Primigravida	first pregnancy
Primiparous	has given birth once

By correlating clinical findings with sonographic findings, the sonographer can directly impact patient care by providing the most targeted examination possible. Furthermore, when faced with a complicated, in-depth registry question, the registrant will be able to eliminate information that is not relevant in order to answer the question appropriately. Although questions in the obstetric portion of these registries may have some clinical history, like laboratory findings, many are image-based questions that examine the reviewer's ability to discern sonographic anatomy and pathology. For this reason, crucial sonographic images and diagrams are provided throughout this section.

Determining the cause of vaginal bleeding is a common obstetrical dilemma. Although vaginal bleeding can be **idiopathic**, in the first trimester, the sonographer should be aware that there can be multiple reasons why a patient could present with vaginal bleeding, including ectopic pregnancy, gestational trophoblastic disease, miscarriage, blighted ovum, embryonic demise, and subchorionic hemorrhage. In the second trimester, *painless* vaginal bleeding is most often associated with **placenta previa**, whereas *painful* vaginal bleeding may occur as a result of **placental abruption**. More maternal complications can be found in Chapter 32. Furthermore, when maternal clinical findings are beneficial for the sonographer, they will be discussed with the associated pathology within the following chapters.

LABORATORY FINDINGS RELEVANT TO OBSTETRIC SONOGRAPHY

The Triple and Quadruple Screen

The **triple screen** is a maternal blood test performed between 15 and 20 gestational weeks. It includes **human chorionic gonadotropin** (hCG), maternal serum **alpha-fetoprotein** (MSAFP), and **estriol**. The **quadruple screen** adds an additional analysis of **inhibin A**. These hormones or proteins are made by various structures during pregnancy (Table 22-6). Atypical laboratory findings can be associated with abnormal pregnancies (Table 22-7).

Early First-Trimester Screening

A screening test is one that is used to assess for the possibility of disease. Some medical institutions provide an earlier test than the customary triple screen offered during the second trimester. This test can be performed between 11 and 14 gestational weeks. It is an analysis of maternal blood levels of hCG and **pregnancy-associated plasma protein A** (PAPP-A), combined with fetal **nuchal translucency** (NT) measurements obtained with sonography. Guidelines for the NT measurement can be found in Chapter 23.

TABLE 22-6 Biochemical markers in pregnancy

Biochemical Marker	Production	Detection
Alpha-fetoprotein	Protein produced by the fetal yolk sac and then the fetal liver	Maternal serum[a]
Cell-free DNA	Produced by the fetus	Maternal serum
Estriol	Hormone (estrogen) produced by the placenta	Maternal serum and urine
Human chorionic gonadotropin	Hormone produced by the placenta	Maternal serum and urine
Inhibin A	Hormone produced by the placenta	Maternal serum
Pregnancy-associated plasma protein A	Protein produced by the placenta	Maternal serum

[a] Serum = blood.

TABLE 22-7 Common abnormalities encountered during pregnancy and associated elevation (↑) or reduction (↓) in laboratory findings compared to a normal pregnancy

Abnormality	Triple Screen Findings	Additional Labs
Abortion (miscarriage)	↓ hCG	
Anembryonic pregnancy	↓ hCG	
Anencephaly	↑ MSAFP	
Cephalocele	↑ MSAFP	
Down syndrome (trisomy 21)	↑ hCG	↑ Inhibin A
	↓ Estriol	↓ PAPP-A
	↓ MSAFP	
Ectopic pregnancy	↓ hCG	↓ Hematocrit (with rupture)
Edwards syndrome (trisomy 18)	↓ Estriol	↓ Inhibin A
	↓ hCG	↓ PAPP-A
	↓ MSAFP	
Gastroschisis	↑ MSAFP	
Molar pregnancy	(markedly) ↑ hCG	
Omphalocele	↑ MSAFP	
Patau syndrome (trisomy 13)	(mildly) ↑ MSAFP	↑ Inhibin A
	↓ hCG	↓ PAPP-A
Spina bifida (**meningocele** or **myelomeningocele**)	↑ MSAFP	
Triploidy	↑ hCG (with molar)	
Turner syndrome	↓ Estriol	↓ Inhibin A (with hydrops)
	↓ hCG (with hydrops)	↓ PAPP-A
	↓ MSAFP	

Note that these listed laboratory findings are provided for narrowing the information for review purposes only. Additional fetal abnormalities may exist with these atypical laboratory findings.
hCG, human chorionic gonadotropin; MSAFP, maternal serum alpha-fetoprotein; PAPP-A, pregnancy-associated plasma protein A.

Another maternal blood test available is cell-free DNA (cfDNA) testing. This simple blood test can reveal gender and is also highly accurate in detecting chromosomal anomalies, including trisomies 21, 18, and 13 and sex chromosome abnormalities, as early as 9 to 10 weeks' gestation. There are limitations to cfDNA, including that up to 2% of cfDNA tests are inconclusive, it is limited to screening for only a few common aneuploidies. In addition, specific structural anomalies are not detected with cfDNA, and it loses its accuracy for obese patients. One author suggests that it may be most beneficial as an adjunct to first-trimester sonographic screening with NT measurement and additional biochemical markers.

SOUND OFF
Structural anomalies are not detected with cfDNA, and it loses its accuracy for obese patients.

FETAL BIOMETRY

Measurements obtained in the first trimester include yolk sac, gestational sac, crown rump length, and NT. These are discussed in the following chapters. Although standard fetal biometry of the second and third trimesters is also discussed in the following chapters of this book, Table 22-8 provides a brief synopsis for a rapid review (Fig. 22-4).

ARTIFACTS IN OBSTETRIC SONOGRAPHIC IMAGING

Obstetric sonography involves careful analysis of vital fetal and maternal structures. Often, artifacts will be observed during an obstetric sonogram. It is important to know that artifacts exist and why they

TABLE 22-8 Table of standard fetal measurements and explanation

Standard Fetal Measurement	Explanation
Abdominal circumference	Measured in an axial plane and taken around the abdomen at the level of the umbilical vein and fetal stomach. Other structures that may be seen, including the transverse thoracic spine, ribs, liver, right adrenal gland, and fetal gallbladder.
Head circumference	Measured with an ellipse at the outer perimeter of the skull at the level of the third ventricle, thalamus, cavum septum pellucidum, and falx cerebri.
Femur length	Measured at the long axis of the femoral diaphysis when the ultrasound beam is perpendicular to the shaft. The measurement is taken from the center of the femoral head and extends to the distal condyle.
Biparietal diameter	Measured from the outer edge of the proximal skull to the inner edge of the distal skull at the level of the third ventricle, thalamus, cavum septum pellucidum, and falx cerebri.

occur (Table 22-9). Also, it would be valuable to utilize the artifact review sections of both Chapter 1 and Chapter 15 of this text to optimize your understanding of sonographic imaging artifacts.

BIOPHYSICAL PROFILE SCORING

The purpose of biophysical profile scoring is to investigate for signs of fetal hypoxia and to assess overall fetal well-being. Each examination of the fetus lasts 30 minutes. The sonographic examination is scored

A Fetal gestational age (GA) measurements

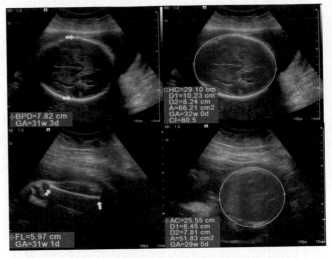

B Structured report with composite data

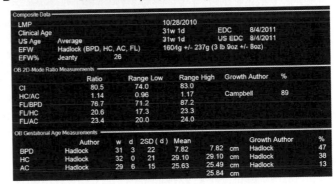

Figure 22-4 Fetal biometry in the second and third trimesters. **A.** Fetal age is often determined from measurements of biparietal diameter (*BPD*) (*top left*), circumference measurements (*top right*), and femur length (*FL*) (*bottom left*), abdominal circumference (*AC*) (*bottom right*). *HC*, head circumference. Based upon known correlation methods, the gestational age can be calculated for each of the measurements. **B.** The structured report captures and summarizes the data in a tabular format as part of the reporting mechanism. (FL is not noted on the report, but is calculated.)

TABLE 22-9 Artifacts frequently observed during an obstetric sonogram

Artifact	Description
Comet-tail artifact	Artifact caused by several small, highly reflective interfaces such as gas bubbles (Fig. 22-5)
(Posterior) Acoustic enhancement	Produced when the sound beam is barely attenuated through a fluid or a fluid-containing structure; formerly referred to as through transmission
Reverberation artifact	Caused by a large acoustic interface and subsequent production false echoes
Ring-down artifact	Artifact that appears as a solid streak or a chain of parallel bands radiating away from a structure
Shadowing	Caused by attenuation of the sound beam

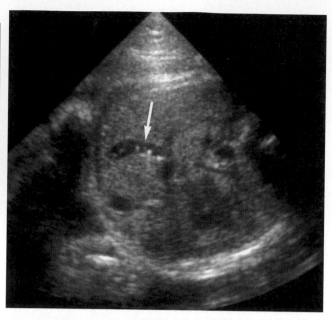

Figure 22-5 Comet-tail artifact. Transverse views of the fetal abdomen demonstrate nonshadowing echogenic material in the fetal gallbladder (*arrow*) producing the comet-tail artifact.

according to specific fetal movements (Table 22-10). The highest possible sonographic score is 8 points, or 2 points for each criterion accomplished. The nonstress test, also referred to as fetal cardiotocography, is worth 2 additional points. Therefore, if combined with a nonstress test, the highest possible score is 10 for a biophysical profile. It is important to note that different parameters may be utilized at some institutions.

◀))) SOUND OFF
A purpose of biophysical profile scoring is to investigate for signs of fetal hypoxia. Each examination of the fetus lasts 30 minutes.

FETAL PRESENTATION

Determining fetal lie and presentation is a significant element of an obstetric sonogram. Fetal lie can be described as longitudinal, transverse, or, possibly, oblique (Fig. 22-6). A longitudinal lie is present when the fetus lies along the longitudinal axis of the uterus, whereas transverse is when the fetus lies transversely within the uterus. Figure 22-7 provides some insight into how to determine fetal situs in the longitudinal lie (Fig. 22-7).

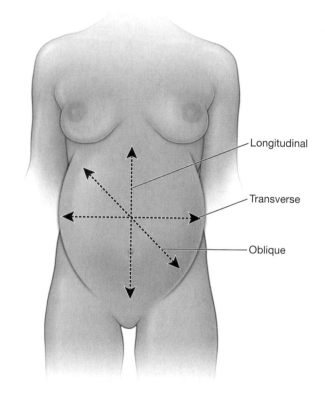

Figure 22-6 Fetal lie.

TABLE 22-10 Biophysical profile scoring		
Criteria	**Conditions for Normal Score in 30 min**	**Score**
Thoracic movements	At least one episode of simulated fetal breathing lasting at least 30 s (observed by watching the fetal diaphragm)	2 points
Fetal movements	At least three or more gross fetal body movements (simultaneous trunk and limb movement)	2 points
Fetal tone	At least one flexion to extension of a limb or one hand opening and closing	2 points
Amniotic fluid	At least one pocket of fluid that measures 1 cm in vertical diameter in two perpendicular planes	2 points
Nonstress test	At least two fetal heart accelerations (>15 beats/min and >15 s) together with one fetal movement	2 points

Adapted from Norton ME. *Callen's Ultrasonography in Obstetrics and Gynecology.* 6th ed. Elsevier; 2016:728.

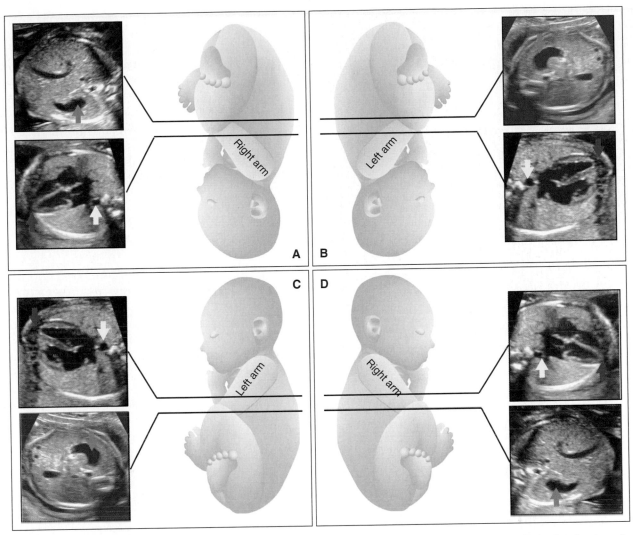

Figure 22-7 Determining fetal situs in longitudinal lie. **A.** The fetus is in a cephalic presentation with the fetal spine close to the left uterine wall, resulting in the right side being anterior and left side posterior. **B.** The fetus is in a cephalic presentation with the fetal spine close to the right uterine wall, resulting in the left side being anterior and right side posterior. **C.** The fetus is in a breech presentation with the fetal spine close to the left uterine wall, resulting in the left side being anterior and right side posterior. **D.** The fetus is in a breech presentation with the fetal spine close to the right uterine wall, resulting in the right side being anterior and left side posterior. Note the corresponding axial ultrasound planes of the chest and abdomen. *Blue arrows* point to the fetal stomach, *red arrows* to the apex of the heart, and *yellow arrows* to the descending aorta.

> **🔊)) SOUND OFF**
> A longitudinal lie is present when the fetus lies along the longitudinal axis of the uterus, whereas transverse is when the fetus lies transversely within the uterus.

Presentation of the fetus is determined by identifying the fetal anatomy that is closest to the internal os of the cervix. Cephalic presentation, or head first, is the most common presentation. A breech presentation can be further described as complete, incomplete (footling), or frank. A complete breech is when the fetal legs are flexed at the hips and there is flexion of the knees as well. Frank breech presentation

is when the fetal buttocks are closest to the cervix, whereas footling breech is when there is extension of at least one of the legs toward the cervix (Fig. 22-8). For the transverse lie, a sagittal orientation to the mother will yield a transverse image of the fetus, whereas a transverse orientation to the mother will yield a sagittal image of the fetus. Finally, an oblique lie is when the fetus is obliquely lying or slanted in comparison to the maternal longitudinal axis. At the time of delivery, the optional position of the fetus is a cephalic lie. If this is not indicated by imaging or palpation, external cephalic version may be used to place the fetus in the proper position. Sonography may be used to confirm that the fetus is in the proper position following this maneuver.

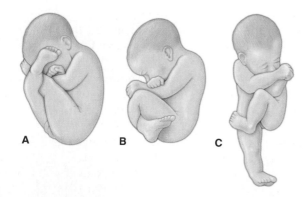

Figure 22-8 Types of breech. **A.** Frank breech, in which the feet are near the head. **B.** Complete breech, in which the legs are crossed. **C.** Incomplete (footling) breech, in which one or both feet are extended.

🔊)) SOUND OFF
Presentation of the fetus is determined by identifying the fetal anatomy that is closest to the internal os of the cervix.

EXTRAUTERINE ABNORMALITIES ASSOCIATED WITH OBSTETRIC SONOGRAPHY

During a sonographic examination of the gravid patient, the sonographer must not only be aware of the fetal findings but also cognizant of the surrounding maternal pelvic anatomy, including the ovaries and adnexa. The most common pelvic mass associated with pregnancy is the **corpus luteum cyst** of the ovary. These cysts can have a complex appearance, or a thick wall, and may, therefore, mimic an ectopic pregnancy. The corpus luteum cyst of pregnancy is further discussed in Chapter 23. Large ovarian cysts or masses can lead to **ovarian torsion**. If a patient presents with a large ovarian abnormality, further sonographic signs of ovarian torsion must be investigated. Ovarian torsion is discussed in Chapter 18, in the gynecologic section.

🔊)) SOUND OFF
The most common pelvic mass associated with pregnancy is the corpus luteum cyst of the ovary.

Pregnant patients who complain of right lower quadrant pain could be suffering from coexisting **acute appendicitis**. Signs of appendicitis are discussed in Chapter 10, in the abdominal section. The appendix may be visualized with endovaginal imaging as well.

Pregnant patients complaining of right upper quadrant pain could have gallstones. Gallbladder disease is further discussed in Chapter 3.

Maternal **hydronephrosis** is common during late pregnancy. Dilation of the renal collecting system is most often secondary to the large size of the uterus with subsequent transient asymptomatic obstruction of the ureters. However, some patients will often suffer from back pain. A thorough analysis for urinary calculi must be performed in these situations. Kidney stones are further discussed in Chapter 7.

ANALYZING AN OBSTETRIC REGISTRY QUESTION

Registry examinations can be intimidating. Unfortunately, clinical history during late pregnancy may not be helpful. For obstetric questions, laboratory findings and an accurate recognition of sonographic anatomy are vital to answering the question correctly. A couple of steps that you can use to give you a better chance at answering these complex questions are provided. Read the following question and look at the image (Fig. 22-9).

This is an image of the gravid uterus of a 39-year-old patient who presented to the ultrasound department with a history of elevated MSAFP. She states that the fetus appears to have been moving regularly, and she has had no pain or vaginal bleeding. What is the most likely diagnosis?

a. Spina bifida
b. Trisomy 18
c. Endometriosis
d. Anencephaly

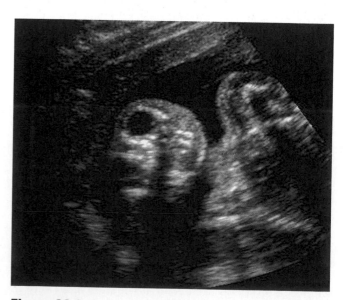

Figure 22-9

Step 1: Look at the Image and Try to Answer the Question Without Looking at the Answers Provided

As you study, you need to look at as many sonographic images as you can. There are images provided for quick reference. The more sonographic images you look at, the better prepared you will be to answer image-based questions. Try to determine what part of the fetus is being shown in the image. This step may eliminate some of the incorrect answers immediately.

Step 2: If You Do Not Know the Answer Right Away from the Image, Then Look at the Question, and Begin to Break It Down

Let us assume that you have no idea what the answer is from looking at the image. Then you move on to step 2, which is breaking the question down. This step is complicated, but it will help.

The first part of the question provides the age of the patient, which is 39 years. By simply knowing what advance maternal age is (35), we know that she is at increased risk for having a complicated pregnancy and that she is more likely to have a fetus with an abnormality.

Look at the answers provided. Is there one that you can eliminate solely on the patient's age or irrelevance? There is one, endometriosis does not make sense. Mark it off the list! You now have a 33% chance of answering the question correctly. We now move on to the next part of the patient's history, which is the elevated MSAFP. Look at the answers and see if there are any that you can eliminate that are not linked with elevated MSAFP. There is one choice that can be eliminated. Trisomy 18 is typically not linked with an elevated MSAFP. Now, you have a 50% chance at getting the question correct. This is where the following chapters will help. You must know your sonographic findings to correctly answer these questions. This is an image of the fetal head. The correct answer is anencephaly. The cranium is absent above the orbits with anencephaly, as seen in this image.

REVIEW QUESTIONS

1. What artifact can be noted posterior to the structure identified by the arrow in Figure 22-10?
   a. Comet-tail
   b. Reverberation
   c. Acoustic shadowing
   d. Acoustic enhancement

2. What artifact can be noted posterior to the structure identified by the arrows in Figure 22-11?
   a. Reverberation
   b. Anisotropy
   c. Acoustic shadowing
   d. Acoustic enhancement

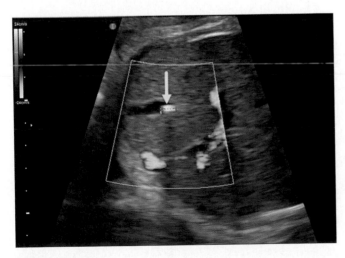

Figure 22-10

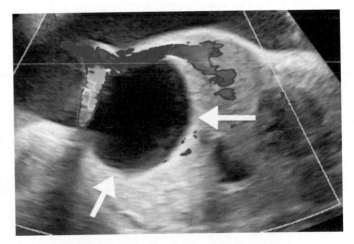

Figure 22-11

3. What artifact does the red arrow in Figure 22-12 indicate?
   a. Reverberation
   b. Comet-tail
   c. Refraction
   d. Edge artifact

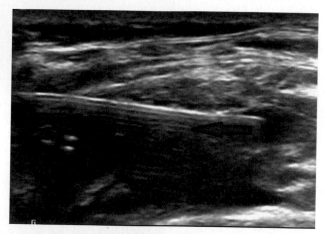

Figure 22-12

4. Which of the following is not a typical indication of a first-trimester sonogram?
   a. Confirmation of an intrauterine pregnancy
   b. Diagnosis of fetal gender
   c. Evaluation of pelvic pain
   d. Confirmation of fetal heart activity

5. The 33-year-old gravid patient in Figure 22-13 presented with left upper quadrant pain. Which of the following can be noted?
   a. Unilateral hydronephrosis
   b. Bilateral hydronephrosis
   c. Unilateral pyonephrosis
   d. Bilateral pyonephrosis

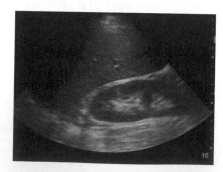

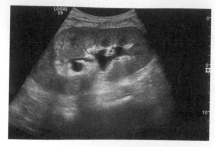

Figure 22-13

6. The 28-week gravid patient in Figure 22-14 complained of right lower quadrant pain. Which of following is demonstrated?
   a. Right ureteral stone
   b. Inflamed appendix
   c. Intussusception
   d. Colonic diverticulum

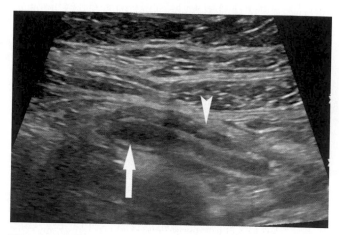

Figure 22-14

7. The conceptus is referred to as an embryo until after what week of gestation?
   a. 5
   b. 8
   c. 10
   d. 12

8. Figure 22-15 shows an amniocentesis. The arrow indicates the presence of an artifactual break in the needle. What artifact may lead to this finding?
   a. Side lobes
   b. Reverberation
   c. Anisotropy
   d. Refraction

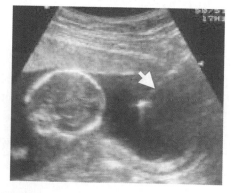

Figure 22-15

9. What imaging enhancement tool is demonstrated in Figure 22-16?
   a. Dynamic imaging
   b. Compound imaging
   c. Extended field-of-view imaging
   d. Three-dimensional imaging

11. What artifact is identified in Figure 22-18 by the arrows in both the bladder and the ovarian cyst?
    a. Side-lobe
    b. Noise
    c. Reverberation
    d. Ring-down

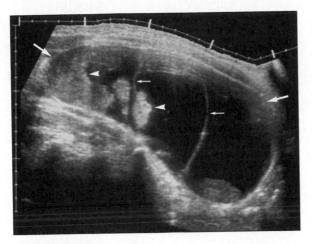

Figure 22-16

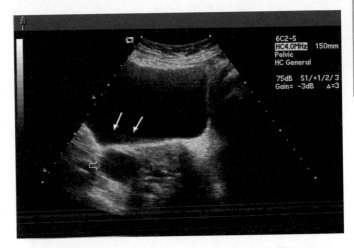

Figure 22-18

10. In Figure 22-17, which of the following would increase the visualization of the femur by highlighting the shades of white of the early ossified femur?
    a. Decreasing dynamic range
    b. Turning off harmonic imaging
    c. Increasing the imaging sector
    d. Decreasing frequency

12. Which of the following would be a way to fix the issue demonstrated in Figure 22-19A?
    a. Lower the baseline
    b. Decrease the scale
    c. Raise the baseline
    d. Increase the scale

13. Which of the following issue is demonstrated in Figure 22-19B?
    a. Improper transducer selection
    b. Improper dynamic range
    c. Improper gate size
    d. Improper baseline position

14. What artifact is identified by the arrow in Figure 22-20?
    a. Side-lobe
    b. Refraction
    c. Reverberation
    d. Ring-down

15. Which of the following likely resulted in color Doppler flow detection in the internal jugular vein in Figure 22-21B?
    a. Decreasing color Doppler gain
    b. Increasing the angle of incidence
    c. Reducing the scale
    d. Increasing the baseline

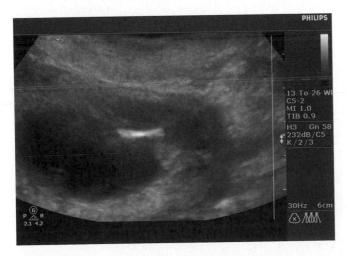

Figure 22-17

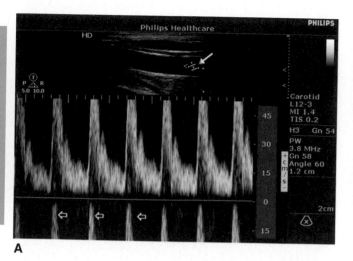
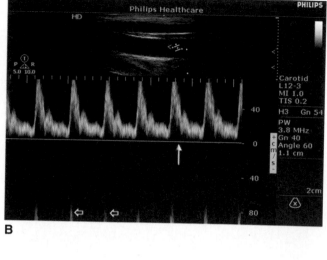

Figure 22-19

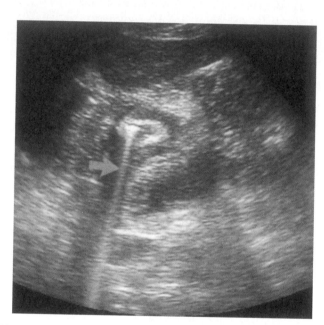

Figure 22-20

16. Which of the following is produced by the fetus?
    a. Estriol
    b. hCG
    c. Inhibin A
    d. cfDNA

17. What artifact appears as a solid streak or a chain of parallel bands radiating away from a structure?
    a. Shadowing
    b. Reverberation
    c. Ring-down
    d. Comet-tail

18. Which of the following would lead to an elevated MSAFP?
    a. Down syndrome
    b. Trisomy 18
    c. Molar pregnancy
    d. Omphalocele

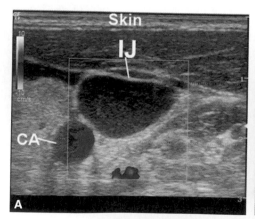
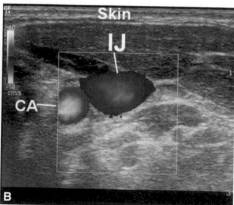

Figure 22-21

19. What is the term for something that can cause birth defects or abnormalities within an embryo or fetus, such as alcohol and certain infections?
    a. Teratogen
    b. Carcinogen
    c. Patrogen
    d. Exogen

20. What is another term for the "due" date of a pregnancy?
    a. Estimated date of conception
    b. Estimated date of confinement
    c. Estimated date of internment
    d. Estimated date of contractions

21. Which of the following is not part of the biophysical profile?
    a. Fetal swallowing
    b. Flexion of the limb
    c. Amniotic fluid
    d. Fetal breathing

22. For the normal biophysical profile, the amniotic fluid pocket should measure:
    a. greater than 4 cm in two perpendicular planes.
    b. at least 1 cm in two perpendicular planes.
    c. greater than 5 cm in two perpendicular planes.
    d. at least 3 cm in two perpendicular planes.

23. What is the term for the fetal presentation that is head down?
    a. Breech
    b. Crown
    c. Cephalic
    d. Vertical

24. Fetal presentation is determined by identifying the fetal part that is closest to the:
    a. placenta.
    b. external os of the cervix.
    c. maternal umbilicus.
    d. internal os of the cervix.

25. What is defined as the area located posterior to the broad ligaments and adjacent to the uterus, which contains the ovaries and fallopian tubes?
    a. Adnexa
    b. Paraovarian
    c. Pouch of Douglas
    d. Space of Retzius

26. All of the following may be visualized at the correct level of the head circumference except:
    a. third ventricle.
    b. thalamus.
    c. cavum septum pellucidum.
    d. falx cerebelli.

27. Typically, with a miscarriage, the serum hCG value will be:
    a. elevated.
    b. decreased.
    c. this laboratory finding is not helpful.
    d. unchanged.

28. Typically, with anencephaly, the MSAFP value will be:
    a. elevated.
    b. decreased.
    c. this laboratory finding is not helpful.
    d. unchanged.

29. Typically, with gastroschisis, the MSAFP value will be:
    a. elevated.
    b. decreased.
    c. this laboratory finding is not helpful.
    d. unchanged.

30. The quadruple screen includes an analysis of all of the following except:
    a. hCG.
    b. alpha-fetoprotein.
    c. inhibin A.
    d. PAPP-A.

31. The reduction in blood return to the maternal heart caused by the gravid uterus compressing the maternal inferior vena cava describes:
    a. Edwards syndrome.
    b. pulmonary obstructive syndrome.
    c. supine hypotensive syndrome.
    d. recumbent hypotensive syndrome.

32. Which of the following would be the least likely indication for a first-trimester sonogram?
    a. Evaluate pelvic pain
    b. Define the cause of vaginal bleeding
    c. Fetal lie
    d. Diagnosis of multiple gestations

33. All of the following would be an indication for a third-trimester sonogram except:
    a. evaluate nuchal translucency.
    b. evaluate fetal presentation.
    c. evaluate fetal growth.
    d. evaluate gestational age.

34. What is described as the number of pregnancies in which the patient has given birth to a fetus at or beyond 20 weeks' gestational age or an infant weighing more than 500 g?
    a. Gravidity
    b. Parity
    c. Primigravida
    d. Primiparous

35. The number of pregnancies is defined as:
    a. gravidity.
    b. parity.
    c. primigravida.
    d. primiparous.

36. In the TPAL designation, the "L" refers to:
    a. Living children.
    b. Lethal anomalies.
    c. Live births.
    d. Lost pregnancies.

37. The second trimester typically refers to weeks:
    a. 12 through 26.
    b. 13 through 26.
    c. 10 through 28.
    d. 26 through 42.

38. The clinical manifestations of supine hypotensive syndrome include all of the following except:
    a. proteinuria.
    b. tachycardia.
    c. nausea.
    d. pallor.

39. Painless second-trimester vaginal bleeding is most often associated with:
    a. placental abruption.
    b. ectopic pregnancy.
    c. miscarriage.
    d. placenta previa.

40. All of the following are observed during a biophysical profile except:
    a. fetal tone.
    b. thoracic movement.
    c. fetal breathing.
    d. fetal circulation.

41. Which of the following would not be decreased in the presence of Edwards syndrome?
    a. Estriol
    b. hCG
    c. Alpha-fetoprotein
    d. All would be decreased.

42. All of the following are produced by the placenta except:
    a. alpha-fetoprotein.
    b. hCG.
    c. PAPP-A.
    d. inhibin A.

43. A myelomeningocele is associated with:
    a. Down syndrome.
    b. spina bifida.
    c. Edwards syndrome.
    d. Patau syndrome.

44. The anechoic space along the posterior aspect of the fetal neck is the:
    a. nuchal fold.
    b. nuchal cord.
    c. nuchal translucency.
    d. rhombencephalon.

45. The premature separation of the placenta from the uterine wall before the birth of the fetus describes:
    a. placenta previa.
    b. placental abruption.
    c. ectopic cordis.
    d. subchorionic hamartoma.

46. Something that is idiopathic is said to be:
    a. caused by a functional abnormality.
    b. related to fetal development.
    c. from an unknown cause.
    d. found incidentally.

47. Which of the following forms of fetal presentation is the most common?
    a. Cephalic
    b. Complete breech
    c. Frank breech
    d. Transverse

48. Biophysical profile scoring is conducted:
    a. until the fetus cooperates.
    b. for 10 minutes.
    c. for 45 minutes.
    d. for 30 minutes.

49. What is the fetal presentation when the fetal buttocks are closest to the cervix?
    a. Footling breech
    b. Frank breech
    c. Complete breech
    d. Transverse

50. Which of the following would not typically produce an elevation in hCG?
    a. Down syndrome
    b. Anembryonic pregnancy
    c. Triploidy
    d. Molar pregnancy

51. The triple screen typically includes an analysis of:
    a. hCG, alpha-fetoprotein, and estriol.
    b. fetal NT, alpha-fetoprotein, and inhibin A.
    c. hCG, alpha-fetoprotein, and inhibin A.
    d. hCG, alpha-fetoprotein, and PAPP-A.

52. The dilation of the renal collecting system secondary to the obstruction of normal urine flow defines:
    a. nephrocalcinosis.
    b. hydronephrosis.
    c. renal calculi.
    d. urinary stasis.

53. The physiologic ovarian cyst that develops after ovulation has occurred is the:
    a. theca internal cyst.
    b. Graafian cyst.
    c. corpus luteum cyst.
    d. cystic teratoma.

54. The protein that is produced by the yolk sac, fetal gastrointestinal tract, and the fetal liver is:
    a. alpha-fetoprotein.
    b. hCG.
    c. PAPP-A.
    d. inhibin A.

55. Which of the following best describes the optimal instance to take the femur length measurement?
    a. When the epiphyseal plates are clearly identified, and the shaft is parallel to the sound beam
    b. When the diaphysis of the femur is parallel to the sound beam
    c. When the long axis of the femoral shaft is perpendicular to the sound beam
    d. When the femoral shaft is parallel to the sound beam

56. The abdominal circumference should include all of the following except:
    a. the fetal stomach.
    b. the fetal thoracic spine.
    c. the umbilical vein.
    d. the kidneys.

57. Which of the following artifacts is produced when the sound beam is barely attenuated through a fluid or a fluid-containing structure?
    a. Reverberation artifact
    b. Comet-tail artifact
    c. Posterior shadowing
    d. Acoustic enhancement

58. Which of the following artifacts is caused by attenuation of the sound beam?
    a. Reverberation artifact
    b. Comet-tail artifact
    c. Posterior shadowing
    d. Posterior enhancement

59. Which of the following would be least likely associated with an elevation in MSAFP?
    a. Anencephaly
    b. Turner syndrome
    c. Spina bifida
    d. Myelomeningocele

60. Which of the following is also referred to as trisomy 13?
    a. Down syndrome
    b. Edwards syndrome
    c. Turner syndrome
    d. Patau syndrome

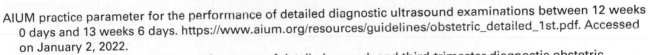

SUGGESTED READINGS

AIUM practice parameter for the performance of detailed diagnostic ultrasound examinations between 12 weeks 0 days and 13 weeks 6 days. https://www.aium.org/resources/guidelines/obstetric_detailed_1st.pdf. Accessed on January 2, 2022.

AIUM practice parameter for the performance of detailed second- and third-trimester diagnostic obstetric ultrasound examinations. https://www.aium.org/resources/guidelines/obstetric_detailed.pdf. Accessed on January 2, 2022.

AIUM-ACR-ACOG-SMFM-SRU practice parameter for the performance of standard diagnostic obstetric ultrasound examinations. https://www.aium.org/resources/guidelines/obstetric.pdf. Accessed on January 2, 2022.

Kline-Fath BM, Bulas DI, and Lee W. *Fundamental and Advanced Fetal Imaging: Ultrasound and MRI*. 2nd ed. Wolters Kluwer; 2021:9–29.

Penny SM. *Introduction to Sonography and Patient Care*. 2nd ed. Wolters Kluwer; 2021:307–350 & 462–464.

Sanders RC, Hall-Terracciano B. *Clinical Sonography: A Practical Guide*. 5th ed. Wolters Kluwer; 2016:61–93 & 399.

Siegel MJ. *Pediatric Sonography*. 5th ed. Wolters Kluwer; 2019:1–39.

BONUS REVIEW!

Determining Fetal Situs (Fig. 22-22)

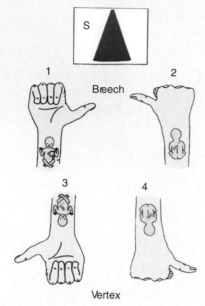

Figure 22-22 Determining fetal situs: a diagram of the fetus is presented in back posterior (*1* and *3*) and back anterior (*2* and *4*) positions. In transabdominal scanning, the sonographic beam (*S*) is directed from top to bottom. The palm of the right hand represents the face of the fetus, and the fetal heart and stomach are on the same side of the examiner's thumb.

Diagram of External Cephalic Version (Fig. 22-23)

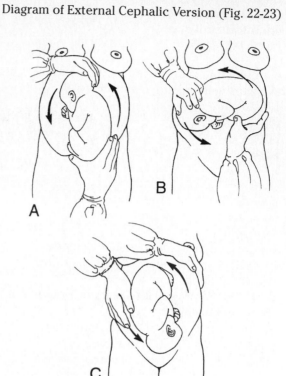

Figure 22-23 Diagram of external cephalic version.

Magnetic Resonance Imaging of Twins (Fig. 22-24)

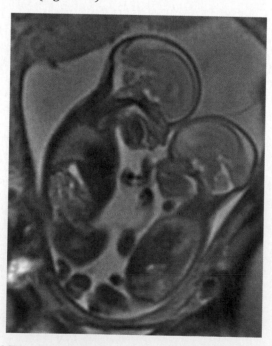

Figure 22-24 MRI of twins. This MRI is demonstrating asymmetry in the size of twins.

The First Trimester

Introduction

This chapter provides the normal progression of a singleton pregnancy and the sonographic findings consistent with an intrauterine pregnancy (IUP) during the first trimester. In addition, first-trimester pathology is also presented, with emphases on the specific sonographic and clinical findings of each abnormality. In "Bonus Review" section, figures of ductus venosus Doppler flow and tricuspid regurgitation in a fetus with trisomy 21 are provided, as well as a normal fetal profile with all intracranial anatomy labeled.

Key Terms

abortion—the complete expulsion or partial expulsion of the conceptus

adnexal ring sign—the sonographic sign that describes the appearance of an ectopic pregnancy within the fallopian tube; may be referred to as the tubal ring sign, bagel sign, or blob sign

amnion—the wall of the inner sac (amniotic cavity) that contains the embryo and amniotic fluid; echogenic curvilinear structure that may be seen during the first trimester within the gestational sac

amniotic cavity—the cavity that contains simple-appearing amniotic fluid and the developing embryo

ampulla (fallopian tube)—the longest and most tortuous segment of the fallopian tube; area of the tube in which fertilization takes place and a common location for ectopic pregnancies to implant

anembryonic gestation—an abnormal pregnancy in which there is no evidence of a fetal pole or yolk sac within the gestational sac; also referred to as a blighted ovum

aneuploid—a condition of having an abnormal number of chromosomes

blastocyst—the stage of the conceptus that implants within the decidualized endometrium

blighted ovum—see key term anembryonic gestation

bradycardia—a low heart rate

choriocarcinoma—the most malignant form of gestational trophoblastic disease with possible metastasis to the liver, lungs, and vagina

chorion—the outer membrane of a gestation that surrounds the amnion and the developing embryo

chorion frondosum—the part of the chorion, covered by chorionic villi, that is the fetal contribution of the placenta

chorionic cavity—the space between the chorionic sac and the amniotic sac that contains the secondary yolk sac; also referred to as the extraembryonic coelom

chorionic sac—the gestational sac; also see key term chorion

chorionic villi—fingerlike projections of gestational tissue that attach to the decidualized endometrium and allow the transfer of nutrients from the mother to the fetus

choroid plexus—specialized cells within the ventricular system responsible for cerebrospinal fluid production

conception—the combination of a female ovum with a male sperm to produce a zygote; also referred to as fertilization

corpus luteum cyst—physiologic ovarian cyst that develops after ovulation has occurred

corpus luteum of pregnancy—the corpus luteum that is maintained during an early pregnancy for the purpose of producing estrogen and primarily progesterone

crown rump length—the measurement of the embryo/fetus from the top of the head to the rump

decidua basalis—the endometrial tissue at the implantation site, and the maternal contribution of the placenta

decidual reaction—the physiologic effect on the endometrium in the presence of a pregnancy

discriminatory zone—the level of human chorionic gonadotropin beyond which an intrauterine pregnancy is consistently visible

double decidual sign—the normal sonographic appearance of the decidua capsularis and decidua parietalis, separated by the anechoic fluid-filled uterine cavity

double sac sign—see key term double decidual sign

eclampsia—a sequela of preeclampsia in which uncontrollable maternal hypertension and proteinuria lead to maternal convulsions and, possibly, fetal and maternal death

ectopic pregnancy—a pregnancy located outside the endometrial cavity of the uterus

embryo—term given to the developing fetus before 10 weeks' gestation

embryonic demise—the death of an embryo before 10 weeks' gestation

extraembryonic coelom—see key term chorionic cavity

falx cerebri—a double fold of dura mater located within midline of the brain

fimbria—the fingerlike extension of the fallopian tube located on the infundibulum

focal myometrial contraction—localized, painless contractions of the myometrium in the gravid uterus that should resolve within 20 to 30 minutes

gestational age—the way in which a pregnancy can be dated based on the first day of the last menstrual cycle; also referred to as menstrual age

gestational trophoblastic disease—a disease associated with an abnormal proliferation of the trophoblastic cells during pregnancy; may also be referred to as a molar pregnancy

Graafian follicle—the name for the dominant follicle before ovulation

hematocrit—the laboratory value that indicates the amount of red blood cells in blood

hematopoiesis—the development of blood cells

heterotopic pregnancy—coexisting ectopic and intrauterine pregnancies

human chorionic gonadotropin—hormone produced by the trophoblastic cells of the early placenta; may also be used as a tumor marker in nongravid patients and males

hydatidiform mole—the most common form of gestational trophoblastic disease in which there is excessive growth of the placenta and high levels of human chorionic gonadotropin; typically benign

hyperemesis gravidarum—excessive vomiting during pregnancy

idiopathic—from an unknown origin

implantation bleeding—a bleed that occurs at the time in which the conceptus implants into the decidualized endometrium

infundibulum—the distal segment of the fallopian tube

intradecidual sign—the appearance of a small gestational sac in the uterine cavity surrounded by the thickened, echogenic endometrium

intrauterine contraceptive device—a reversible form of contraception that is manually placed in the uterine cavity to prevent pregnancy; also referred to as an intrauterine device

invasive mole—a type of gestational trophoblastic disease in which a molar pregnancy invades into the myometrium and may also invade through the uterine wall and into the peritoneum

limb buds—early embryonic structures that will eventually give rise to the extremities

mean sac diameter—the measurement of the gestational sac to obtain a gestational age; achieved by adding the measurements of the length, width, and height of the gestational sac and dividing by 3

menstrual age—see key term gestational age

methotrexate—a chemotherapy drug used to attack rapidly dividing cells like those seen in an early pregnancy; this drug is often used to manage ectopic pregnancies

miscarriage—the spontaneous end of a pregnancy before viability

missed abortion—fetal demise with a retained fetus

Morison pouch—the space between the liver and right kidney; also referred to as the right subhepatic space or hepatorenal space

morula—the developmental stage of the conceptus following the zygote

multiloculated—having more than one internal cavity

multiparity—having birthed more than one child

nuchal translucency—the anechoic space along the posterior aspect of the fetal neck

pelvic inflammatory disease—infection of the female genital tract that may involve the ovaries, uterus, and/or the fallopian tubes

physiologic bowel herniation—the normal developmental stage when the midgut migrates into the base of the umbilical cord

preeclampsia—pregnancy-induced maternal high blood pressure and excess protein in the urine after 20 weeks' gestation

pseudogestational sac—the appearance of an abnormally shaped false gestational sac within the uterine cavity as a result of an ectopic pregnancy; this often corresponds with the accumulation of blood and secretions within the uterine cavity

rhombencephalon—the primary brain vesicle also referred to as the hindbrain; becomes the cerebellum, pons, medulla oblongata, and fourth ventricle

secondary yolk sac—the structure responsible for early nutrient transfer to the embryo; the yolk sac seen during a sonographic examination of the early gestation

subchorionic hemorrhage—a bleed between the endometrium and the gestational sac at the edge of the placenta

triploid—having three sets of each chromosome or 69 total

trisomy 18—chromosomal aberration in which there is a third chromosome 18; also referred to as Edwards syndrome

trisomy 21—chromosomal aberration in which there is a third chromosome 21; also referred to as Down syndrome

trophoblastic cells—the cells that surround the gestation that produce human chorionic gonadotropin

Turner syndrome—a chromosomal aberration where one sex chromosome is absent; may also be referred to as monosomy X

uterine leiomyoma—a benign, smooth muscle tumor of the uterus; may also be referred to as a fibroid or uterine myoma

vitelline duct—the structure that connects the developing embryo to the secondary yolk sac

zygote—the cell formed by the union of two gametes; the first stage of a fertilized ovum

NORMAL CONCEPTION AND THE FIRST 6 WEEKS

A mature ovum is released through ovulation at around day 14 of the menstrual cycle because the **Graafian follicle** ruptures and liberates the ovum into the peritoneal cavity. The **fimbria** of the fallopian tube transports the ovum into the distal portion of the tube, the **infundibulum**. **Conception**, also referred to as fertilization, is the union of an ovum and a sperm. A sperm, which can live up to 72 hours, unites with the egg in the distal one-third of the fallopian tube, most likely in the **ampulla**. Conception usually occurs within 24 hours after ovulation.

The combination of the sperm and ovum produces a structure referred to as the **zygote** (Fig. 23-1). The zygote undergoes rapid cellular division and eventually forms into a cluster of cells called the **morula**. The morula continues to differentiate and form a structure referred to as the **blastocyst**. The outer tissue layer of the blastocyst is composed of syncytiotrophoblastic tissue, also referred to as **trophoblastic cells**. The trophoblastic

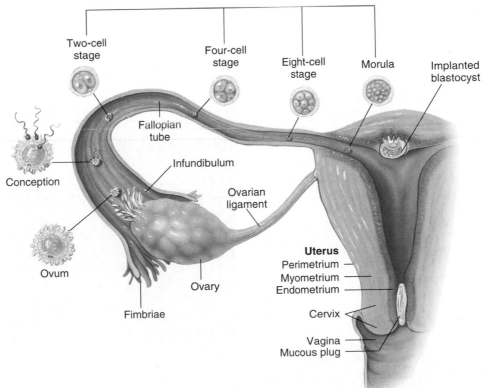

Early cell division of fertilized zygote

Two-cell stage · Four-cell stage · Eight-cell stage · Morula · Implanted blastocyst

Conception · Fallopian tube · Infundibulum · Ovarian ligament

Ovum · Fimbriae · Ovary

Uterus
Perimetrium
Myometrium
Endometrium
Cervix
Vagina
Mucous plug

Figure 23-1 Fertilization and implantation. Early cell division of fertilized zygote.

cells are the cells that produce the pregnancy hormone **human chorionic gonadotropin** (hCG). The inner part of the blastocyst will develop into the **embryo, amnion**, umbilical cord, and the primary and secondary yolk sacs. The outer part, the trophoblastic tissue, will develop into the placenta and **chorion**.

> 🔊 **SOUND OFF**
> The trophoblastic cells are the cells that produce the pregnancy hormone hCG.

On day 20 or 21 of the menstrual cycle, the blastocyst begins to implant into the decidualized endometrium at the level of the uterine fundus. By 28 days, complete implantation has occurred, and all early connections have been established between the gestation and the mother. The blastocyst makes these link with the maternal endometrium via small projections of tissue called **chorionic villi**. The implantation of the blastocyst within the endometrium may cause some women to experience a small amount of vaginal bleeding. This is referred to as **implantation bleeding**.

The fourth week of gestation is an extremely dynamic stage in the pregnancy. The primary yolk sac regresses during week 4, and two separate membranes are formed. The outer membrane is the **chorionic sac** or **gestational sac**. Within the gestational sac is the amnion or amniotic sac. By the end of week 4, the **secondary yolk sac** becomes wedged between these two membranes in an area called the **chorionic cavity** or **extraembryonic coelom**.

The developing embryo is located between the yolk sac and the amnion at 4 weeks. At this time, the alimentary canal is formed. It will become the foregut, midgut, and hindgut. The neural tube also begins to develop at this time. The neural tube will become the fetal head and spine. By 5 weeks, suspicion of pregnancy abounds, because the woman misses the scheduled onset of menses for the month. Within the developing gestation, the embryonic heart begins to beat for the first time. By 6 weeks, all internal and external structures are in the process of forming. Sonographic findings are additionally discussed in this chapter.

> 🔊 **SOUND OFF**
> The gestational sac is also referred to as the chorionic sac.

LAST MENSTRUAL PERIOD

Obtaining an accurate last menstrual period (LMP) can be a vital part of the sonographic examination of a pregnant patient. **Menstrual age** or **gestational age** is

used by obstetricians, radiologists, and sonographers to date a pregnancy. They are calculated using the LMP. An accurate LMP is significant in determining whether the pregnancy is progressing normally. The obstacle of an inaccurate LMP provided by the patient can be overcome by referencing the level of hCG found in the maternal circulation and relating those findings with sonographic findings.

HUMAN CHORIONIC GONADOTROPIN AND THE DISCRIMINATORY ZONE

The laboratory test used to detect pregnancy is hCG. This hormone is produced throughout pregnancy by the placenta. In the first trimester, hCG maintains the **corpus luteum cyst** of the ovary so that the corpus luteum can continue to produce progesterone (Fig. 23-2). The sustained production of progesterone maintains the thickness of the endometrium, thus allowing implantation to occur. Clinically, hCG can be detected in the maternal urine and serum (blood).

> 🔊 **SOUND OFF**
> In the first trimester, hCG maintains the corpus luteum of the ovary so that the corpus luteum can continue to produce progesterone.

Both blood, or serum, and urine tests can be qualitative, answering the question, "Is the patient pregnant?" But only blood can be quantitative, answering the question, "How pregnant is the patient?" hCG is detected in the maternal blood as early as 23 days' menstrual age. hCG can be detected in the urine at 20 mIU/mL or

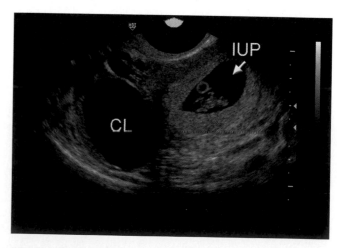

Figure 23-2 Corpus luteum of pregnancy. The normal finding of a corpus luteum cyst (*CL*) adjacent to an intrauterine pregnancy (*IUP*).

greater, whereas serum can detect levels greater than 5 mIU/mL.

hCG can be measured using several methods. Most assays for hCG are now calibrated against the Third International Standard, but some may still use the Second International Standard. The laboratory performing the test will provide the reference range. However, a gestational sac, the earliest definitive sign of an IUP, should generally be visualized between 1,000 and 2,000 mIU per mL with transvaginal sonography. The period given to describe the earliest sonographic detection of an IUP is termed the **discriminatory zone** or level.

> ### 🔊)) SOUND OFF
> A gestational sac, the earliest definitive sign of an IUP, should generally be visualized between 1,000 and 2,000 mIU per mL with transvaginal sonography.

Based on quantitative hCG levels, sonographers can utilize the discriminatory zone and determine whether an IUP should be visualized. Typically, a 5-mm gestational sac will be seen at approximately 5 menstrual weeks. Normal hCG levels double every 48 hours in the first trimester. High and low levels of hCG compared with LMP and sonographic findings can be indicative of an abnormal pregnancy (Table 23-1). The hCG level will continue to rise until the end of the first trimester, at which time it plateaus and slowly decreases with advancing gestation. However, research has shown that an hCG level above the discriminatory level in conjunction with a normal sonogram does not necessarily exclude the possibility of a normal IUP. Consequently, sequential hCG levels and sonograms may be warranted.

> ### 🔊)) SOUND OFF
> Normal hCG levels double every 48 hours in the first trimester.

TABLE 23-1 hCG levels compared with normal pregnancy

Nature of Pregnancy	hCG Level
Ectopic pregnancy	↓
Anembryonic pregnancy	↓
Abortion (miscarriage)	↓
Twin pregnancy	↑
Complete molar pregnancy	(markedly) ↑

hCG, human chorionic gonadotropin.

NORMAL SONOGRAPHIC FINDINGS DURING THE FIRST TRIMESTER

The following sections provide an analysis of the maternal uterus and fetus in the first trimester. The sonographer should be mindful of the potential biologic effect of ultrasound on the fetus. Specifically, the use of color Doppler exposure in the first trimester should be limited, and the ALARA principle (as-low-as-reasonably achievable) be practiced. The thermal index, which is the amount of energy required to raise tissue temperature 1°C, should be kept below 1 (Fig. 23-3). The mechanical index should also be kept below 1.

Decidual Reaction (Weeks 3 to 4)

The **decidual reaction** of the endometrium is essentially the first sonographically identifiable sign of a pregnancy. In essence, the endometrium is preparing itself for the implantation of the conceptus. The decidualized endometrium will appear thick and echogenic as a result of the continued production of progesterone by the corpus luteum. A decidual reaction is considered to be a nonspecific sonographic finding of pregnancy because the endometrium can also appear thick and echogenic during the secretory phase of the endometrial cycle and in the presence of an **ectopic pregnancy**. A correlation between hCG levels and sonographic findings should be performed.

Gestational Sac (Weeks 4 to 5)

The first definitive sonographic sign of an IUP is identification of the gestational sac within the decidualized endometrium. The blastocyst is the developmental stage of the conceptus that implants into the uterine cavity. The blastocyst gives rise to the gestational sac, or chorionic sac. The early gestational sac, which is first seen at 5 weeks, appears as a small, anechoic sphere within the decidualized endometrium. It will grow at a rate of 1 mm per day in early pregnancy.

> ### 🔊)) SOUND OFF
> The first definitive sonographic sign of an IUP is identification of the gestational sac within the decidualized endometrium.

The **intradecidual sign** denotes the appearance of the small gestational sac in the uterine cavity surrounded by the thickened, echogenic endometrium. The intradecidual sign can be misdiagnosed because it may resemble the **pseudogestational sac** of an ectopic pregnancy. To differentiate an intrauterine gestational sac from the pseudogestational sac, sonographers can assess the endometrium for evidence of the **double sac sign** or **double decidual sign** (Fig. 23-4).

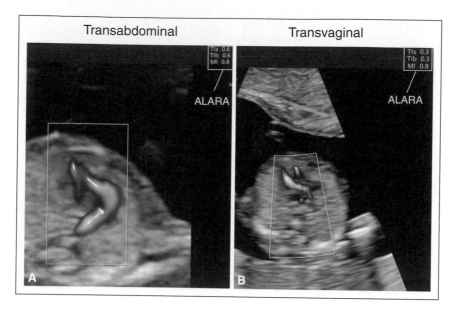

Figure 23-3 ALARA principle states that the lowest ultrasound energy should be used in sonography during pregnancy, especially in the first trimester. Note the display of the mechanical index (*MI*) and thermal index bone (*TIb*) and soft tissue (*TIs*) in transabdominal (**A**) and transvaginal (**B**) sonograms. Ideally, the TI should be kept below 1. *ALARA*, as-low-as-reasonably achievable.

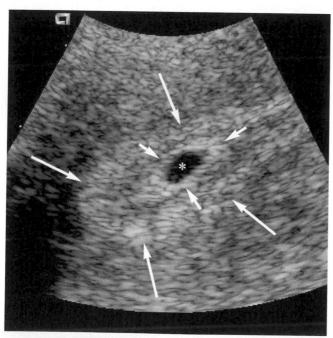

Figure 23-4 Gestational sac at 5.0 weeks' gestation. The gestational sac (*asterisk*) is seen as a round fluid collection within the endometrium, with no structures yet seen within it. The gestational sac is surrounded by two echogenic rings, an inner ring (*short arrows*) and an outer ring (*long arrows*), corresponding to the two layers of the decidua. This is referred to as the double sac sign or double decidual sign.

The double sac sign denotes the typical appearance of the two distinct layers of decidua, the decidua capsularis (inner layer) and decidua parietalis (outer layer), separated by the anechoic fluid-filled uterine

cavity. Table 23-2 and Figure 23-5 provide both a diagram and an explanation of the embryologic tissues present in the early gestation.

TABLE 23-2 A list of various embryologic tissues and their description

Embryologic Tissues	Description
Chorionic cavity	The space between the gestational sac and the amniotic sac. The location of the secondary yolk sac.
Chorion frondosum	The decidualized tissue at the implantation site containing the chorionic villi. The fetal contribution of the placenta.
Chorion laeve	The portion of the chorion that does not contain chorionic villi.
Chorionic villi	Fingerlike extension of trophoblastic tissue that invades the decidualized endometrium.
Decidua basalis	The endometrial tissue at the implantation site. The maternal contribution of the placenta.
Decidua capsularis	The portion of the decidua opposite the uterine cavity, across from the decidua basalis.
Decidua parietalis (vera)	The decidualized tissue along the uterine cavity adjacent to the decidua basalis.

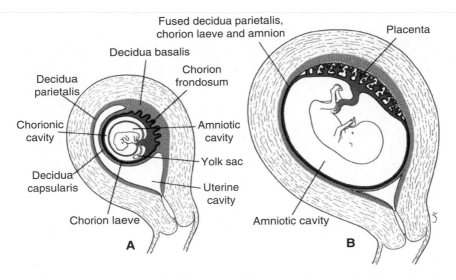

Figure 23-5 Relation of fetal membranes to wall of the uterus.

Both the intradecidual sign and double sac sign are sonographic findings that were initially discovered and relied upon in the past with transabdominal pelvic sonography. However, high-resolution transvaginal sonography can, in most cases, clearly depict the endometrium and its contents much more readily than transabdominal imaging. Therefore, it is safe to assume that a round or an oval-shaped fluid collection within the endometrium of a patient with a positive pregnancy test, and whose hCG level is above the discriminatory zone, is most likely a gestational sac. Nonetheless, it is vital that other clinical findings, such as vaginal bleeding and pain, be correlated with sonographic findings.

The measurement of the gestational sac is the earliest sonographic measurement that can be obtained to date the pregnancy. A **mean sac diameter** (MSD) is achieved by adding the measurements of the length,

width, and height of the gestational sac and dividing by 3 (Fig. 23-6). The gestational sac measurement is a relatively accurate form of dating that can be used until a **fetal pole** is sonographically recognized. Although modern sonography equipment calculates the MSD for sonographers, there is also a simple formula that can be used. By adding 30 to the MSD (measurement in millimeters), sonographers can obtain an estimate for the gestational age in days.

When the gestational sac seems visually disproportional to the size of the embryo, that is, too small or too large compared to the size of the embryo, an MSD measurement can be exceedingly beneficial in determining whether asymmetry truly exists. An irregularly shaped gestational sac and an MSD of greater than 25 mm that does not contain a fetal pole are both signs of potential pregnancy failure.

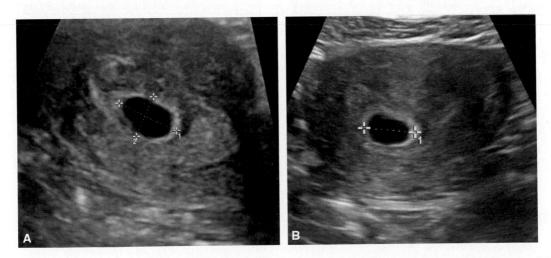

Figure 23-6 Measurement of the mean sac diameter (*MSD*). **A.** Sagittal and **B.** transverse measurements of the MSD of a gestational sac at 5 weeks.

> ◀)) **SOUND OFF**
> By adding 30 to the MSD (measurement in millimeter), sonographers can obtain an estimate for the gestational age in days.

Secondary Yolk Sac (5.5 Weeks)

The first structure seen with sonography within the gestational sac is the secondary yolk sac (Fig. 23-7). It appears within the gestational sac as a round, anechoic structure surrounded by a thin, echogenic rim. It is located within the chorionic cavity, between the amnion and the chorion. This cavity may also be referred to as the extraembryonic coelom or extracelomic space. The

yolk sac produces alpha-fetoprotein (AFP) and plays an important role in angiogenesis and **hematopoiesis** during early embryologic development. It is connected to the embryo by the **vitelline duct**, also referred to as the omphalomesenteric duct, which contains one artery and one vein. It may be visualized during a first-trimester sonographic examination. The yolk sac can be measured during the first trimester. It should be measured from the inner-to-inner aspects of the yolk sac wall (Fig. 23-8). The yolk sac should not exceed 7 mm, and it should also be evaluated for irregular shape and echogenicity. Abnormal appearances of the yolk sac are discussed further in this chapter (see "Embryonic Demise and Pregnancy Failure" section).

> ◀)) **SOUND OFF**
> The yolk sac is connected to the embryo by the vitelline duct, also referred to as the omphalo-mesenteric duct, which contains one artery and one vein.

Chorionic and Amniotic Cavities (5.5 Weeks)

The gestational sac consists of two cavities: the chorionic cavity and **amniotic cavity**. The chorionic cavity lies between the amnion and the chorion. It contains the yolk sac and fluid. The amniotic cavity contains simple-appearing amniotic fluid and the developing embryo. The amniotic membrane, or amnion, can be seen within the gestational sac as a thin, echogenic line loosely surrounding the embryo (Fig. 23-9). The amnion and chorion typically fuse around the middle of the first trimester, but may not be totally fused until 16 weeks' gestation.

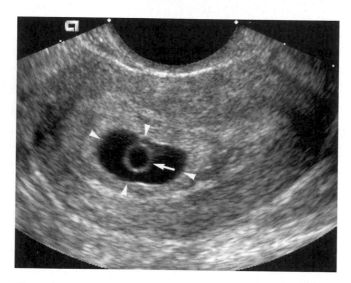

Figure 23-7 Gestational sac and secondary yolk sac at 5.5 weeks' gestation. The gestational sac (*arrowheads*) contains the secondary yolk sac (*arrow*). No embryo is seen at this time.

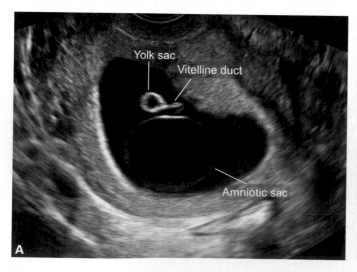
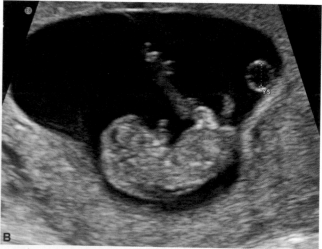

Figure 23-8 Measurement of the yolk sac and the vitelline duct. **A.** Gestational sac at 7 weeks of gestation. The amniotic sac is seen as a thin reflective circular membrane. The yolk sac and vitelline duct are seen as extra-amniotic structures. **B.** The yolk sac (*YS*) measurement should be obtained from the inner-to-inner aspects of the yolk sac wall (*calipers*).

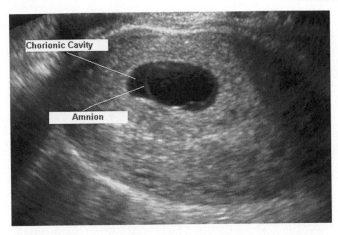

Figure 23-9 Chorionic cavity and amnion. The chorionic cavity and amnion are seen within this image of an early pregnancy.

> 🔊 **SOUND OFF**
> The yolk sac is located within the chorionic cavity.

Embryo (5 to 6 Weeks)

By 6 weeks, the embryo can be seen located within the amniotic cavity adjacent to the yolk sac, with transvaginal sonography (Fig. 23-10). The

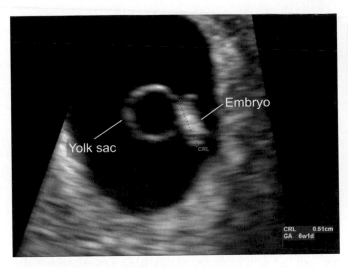

Figure 23-10 Early embryo. Gestational sac at 6 weeks with an embryo measuring 5.1 mm in crown rump length (*CRL*). Note the straight shape of the embryo, resembling a grain of rice. The yolk sac is seen adjacent to the embryo. *GA*, gestational age.

documentation of fetal heart activity is performed using motion mode (M-mode) (Fig. 23-11). Occasionally, a tiny heartbeat is often seen before an embryo can be measured, with sonographic documentation of heart activity being present between 5 and 6 weeks.

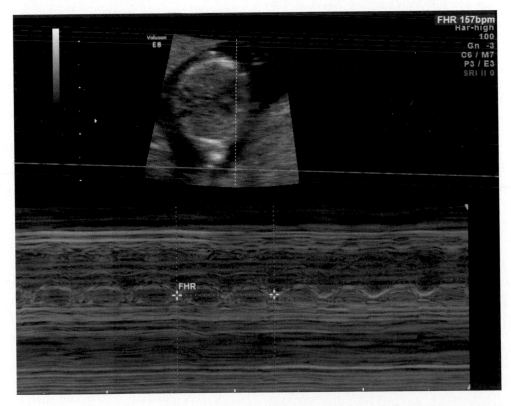

Figure 23-11 M-mode image of the fetal heart at 12 weeks. Note that the M-mode line intersects the heart and the cardiac activity, or the fetal heart rate (*FHR*) is displayed on the M-mode spectrum. Note that the FHR is measured at 157 beats per minute (bpm).

Heart motion can be detected in a 4-mm embryo, with motion certainly evident within the 5-mm embryo. The embryo will grow at a rate of 1 mm per day in the first trimester. Embryonic heart rate is considered normal at 100 to 110 bpm between 5 and 6 weeks. The heart rate increases to 150 bpm by 9 weeks. From the second trimester to term, the fetal heart rate is typically around 150 bpm, although it will vary with gestation age. **Bradycardia** is associated with a poor prognosis and is often the first sonographic sign of an eminent embryologic demise (see "Embryonic Demise and Pregnancy Failure" section).

The most accurate sonographic measurement of pregnancy is the **crown rump length (CRL)**. The CRL can be taken when a fetal pole is identified and should not include the yolk sac or fetal **limb buds** within the measurement (Fig. 23-12). This measurement can be taken throughout the first trimester, and typically until second-trimester biometric measurements can be obtained.

> 🔊 **SOUND OFF**
> The most accurate sonographic measurement of pregnancy is the CRL.

Embryo (7 to 8 Weeks)

Fetal limb buds are readily identified by 7 weeks. The fetal head at this time is proportionally larger than the body. Within the fetal head, a cystic structure may be noted. This most often represents the **rhombencephalon**, or hindbrain (Fig. 23-13). The rhombencephalon will eventually develop into the fourth ventricle and several other essential brain structures. As early as 8 weeks, the stomach may be visualized in the upper abdomen as well.

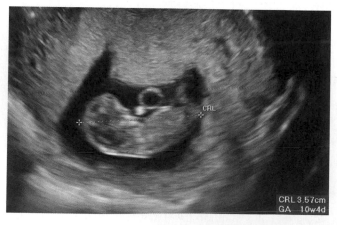

Figure 23-12 Crown rump length (*CRL*). The CRL at 10 weeks and 4 days.

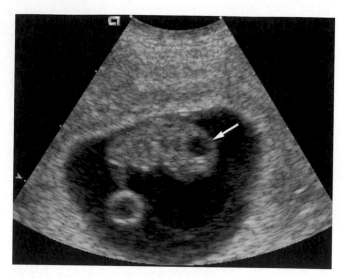

Figure 23-13 Rhombencephalon. The rhombencephalon (*arrow*) is seen within the head of this 8-week embryo, appearing as a cyst.

> 🔊 **SOUND OFF**
> Within the fetal head, a cystic structure may be noted. This most often represents the rhombencephalon, which will develop into the fourth ventricle and other essential brain structures.

Embryo (9 to 12 Weeks)

Physiologic bowel herniation begins at 8 weeks, which marks the developmental stage when the midgut migrates into the base of the umbilical cord (Fig. 23-14). This phenomenon is developmentally normal. The sonographer should determine the gestational age based on CRL and understand that physiologic herniation is normal during this early stage of maturity. Conversely, if physiologic bowel herniation does not resolve by 12 weeks, a follow-up examination is often warranted.

> 🔊 **SOUND OFF**
> If physiologic bowel herniation does not resolve by 12 weeks, a follow-up examination is often warranted.

At the end of the first trimester, the fetal limbs are much more readily identifiable with sonography. Inside the fetal head, the lateral ventricles may be noted, containing the echogenic **choroid plexus**. The cerebral hemispheres can also be separated by the echogenic, linear **falx cerebri**, which lies within the midline of the brain. Fetal movement, the heart chambers, the stomach, urinary bladder, umbilical cord, extremities, and spine can also be noted by the end of the first

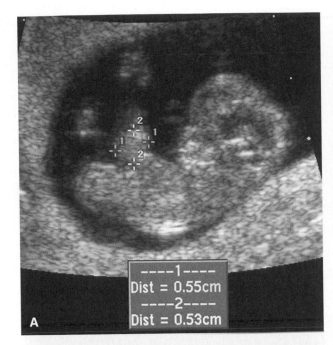

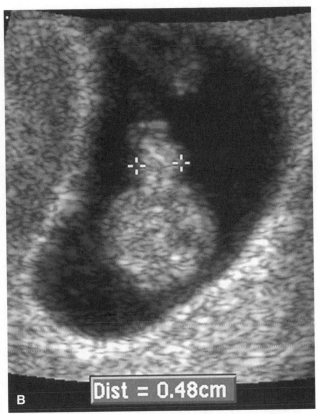

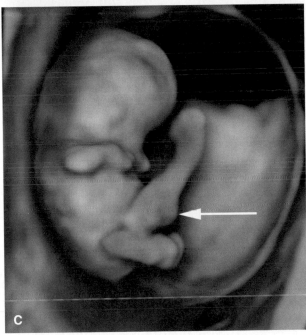

Figure 23-14 Physiologic bowel herniation. **A.** Sagittal and **B.** transverse views of the fetal abdomen at 10 weeks' gestation demonstrate echogenic tissue (*calipers*) projecting out of the anterior abdominal wall. **C.** Three-dimensional sonogram of another 10-week fetus demonstrates a bulge (*arrow*) in the umbilical cord at its insertion into the fetal abdomen. Both of these fetuses were normal on follow-up second-trimester scans.

trimester (Fig. 23-15). With transvaginal sonography, the fetal kidneys may be seen between 13 and 14 weeks. Fetal abnormalities, such as neural tube defects, abdominal wall defects, cardiac defects, facial features including the nasal bones and clefts, and disorders of the extremities, can be identified with high-resolution endovaginal sonography. However, in many institutions, a detailed examination of fetal anatomy is usually not performed at this time. Follow-up sonographic examinations and clinical correlation are warranted when fetal structural abnormalities are suspected during a first-trimester sonogram.

Placenta and Umbilical Cord

The developing placenta may be noted at the end of first trimester as a well-defined, crescent-shaped homogeneous mass of tissue, along the margins of the gestational sac (Fig. 23-16). The placenta is formed by the **decidua basalis**, the maternal contribution of the placenta, and the **chorion frondosum**, the fetal contribution. The umbilical cord is visible during the latter half of the first trimester as a tortuous structure connecting the fetus to the developing placenta.

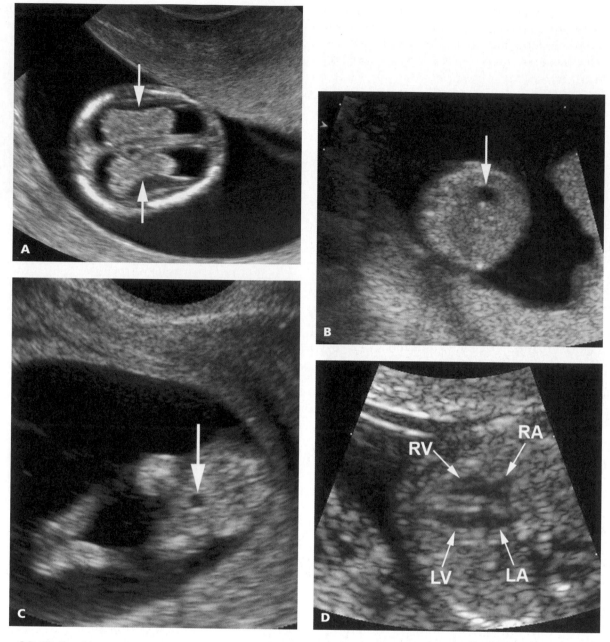

Figure 23-15 Fetal internal organs in the late first trimester. Anatomic structures identifiable in these 13-week fetuses include the following: **A.** choroid plexus (*arrows*); **B.** stomach (*arrow*); **C.** bladder (*arrow*); **D:** heart (*RV*, right ventricle; *LV*, left ventricle; *RA*, right atrium; *LA*, left atrium).

Nuchal Translucency, Nasal Bones, and Other First-Trimester Sonographic Screening Tools for Chromosomal Aneuploidies (11 to 14 Weeks)

The evaluation of the **nuchal translucency** (NT) has become a vital part of early first-trimester screening. The term *nuchal* refers to the neck. Thus, this translucency is represented by a thin membrane along the posterior aspect of the fetal neck, which can be measured sonographically (Fig. 23-17). The most common abnormalities associated with increased NT

are **trisomy 21**, **trisomy 18**, **Turner syndrome**, and congestive heart failure. When NT is combined with first-trimester laboratory findings, such as hCG and pregnancy-associated plasma protein A results, a high detection rate for these and other fetal abnormalities can be achieved.

The measurement of this area is performed in the sagittal plane to the fetus, with the fetus in a neutral position. The NT is optimally measured between 11 and 13 weeks 6 days' gestation, when the CRL measures between 45 and 84 mm based on recommendations by the Fetal Medicine Foundation, although laboratory specifications may vary. Care should be taken as to not confuse the amnion for a prominent NT, because the fetus may be resting on the amnion. The normal range of thickness of the NT is based on

the gestational age, although, most often, a measurement greater than 3 mm between 11 and 13 weeks 6 days is considered abnormal and warrants a follow-up examination, referral for fetal echocardiography, and fetal karyotyping. The cutoff measurement for NT screening for some institutions may be as high as 3.5 mm, however; thus, the sonographer should be aware of institutional protocols. The guidelines for obtaining the NT measurement have been established by the American Institute of Ultrasound in Medicine and can be found at www.aium.org. They are summarized in Table 23-3.

> **SOUND OFF**
> The NT is optimally measured between 11 and 13 weeks 6 days' gestation, when the CRL measures between 45 and 84 mm.

It has been recognized that with many Down syndrome fetuses, the nasal bone is either hypoplastic or absent between 11- and 13-weeks' gestation. Thus, the sonographic assessment of the nasal bone can be performed as part of a screening first-trimester protocol. There are specific guidelines for these images, including the task of obtaining a midsagittal plane view of the fetus and gently rocking the transducer to ensure that the nasal bone can be visualized separate from the overlying nasal skin (Fig. 23-18). In a normal fetus, this

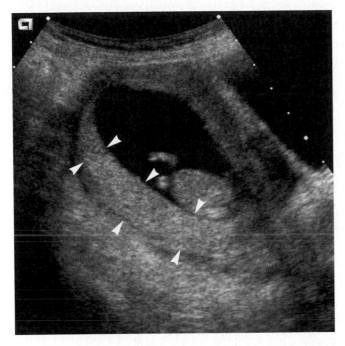

Figure 23-16 Placenta at 11 weeks. The developing placenta (*arrowheads*) is seen in this early pregnancy.

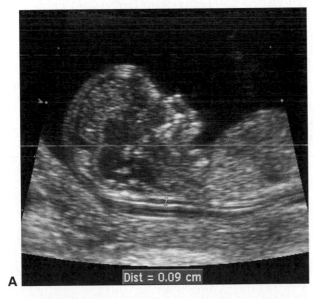

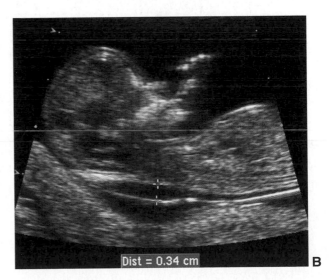

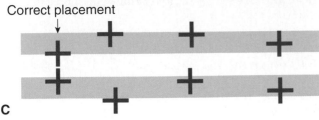

Figure 23-17 Nuchal translucency (NT). **A.** Normal NT. **B.** Abnormal NT. **C.** The first set of calipers is the correct placement for the NT measurement according to the American Institute of Ultrasound in Medicine.

TABLE 23-3 Sonographic guidelines for an NT measurement
Guidelines for NT Measurement
1. The margins of the NT edges must be clear enough for proper placement of the calipers.
2. The fetus must be in the midsagittal plane.
3. The image must be magnified so that it is filled by the fetal head, neck, and upper thorax.
4. The fetal neck must be in a neutral position, not flexed and not hyperextended.
5. The amnion must be seen as separate from the NT line.
6. The (+) calipers on the ultrasound must be used to perform the NT measurement.
7. Electronic calipers must be placed on the inner borders of the nuchal space with none of the horizontal crossbar itself protruding into the space.
8. The calipers must be placed perpendicular to the long axis of the fetus.
9. The measurement must be obtained at the widest space of the NT.

NT, nuchal translucency.

will provide an "equal sign" in the area of the nasal bone and overlying nasal skin.

Other detailed first-trimester sonographic screening tools exist, including ductus venosus assessment and tricuspid flow. Though these assessments are not performed on all pregnancies routinely, it may be beneficial for the sonographer to have a fundamental understanding of why these assessments are conducted. Ductus venosus flow is analyzed with color and pulsed Doppler to evaluate for signs of increased impedance in the fetal ductus venosus at 11 to 13 weeks' gestation. This increased impedance has been shown to be associated

with fetal aneuploidies and cardiac defects. It is the a-wave that is analyzed, and studies have revealed that the a-wave is normal when it is positive during atrial contraction and abnormal when the a-wave is absent or reversed. Tricuspid flow, which is again not a routine sonographic assessment in the low-risk population, is analyzed for signs of tricuspid regurgitation between 11 and 13 weeks, a common malady in fetuses with trisomies 21, 18, and 13 and those with cardiac defects. For more information and to obtain certification in these measurements, the sonographer can visit https://fetalmedicine.org/.

◄))) SOUND OFF
Sonographers can obtain certification in NT, nasal bone, ductus venosus flow, tricuspid flow, and other fetal and maternal assessments through the Fetal Medicine Foundation.

Corpus Luteum of Pregnancy

The most common pelvic mass associated with pregnancy is the ovarian corpus luteum cyst. The **corpus luteum of pregnancy** is a functional cyst that is maintained during the first trimester by hCG, which is produced by the developing placenta. As a result, the corpus luteum secretes progesterone and thereby maintains the thickness of the endometrium. Typically, the corpus luteum measures between 2 and 3 cm and regresses near the end of the first trimester, although it may continue to grow as large as 10 cm. The sonographic appearance of the corpus luteum is variable. It may appear as a simple cyst, as a complex cyst with hemorrhagic components, as a hypoechoic mass, or have a thick echogenic rim that display increased color flow seen with color Doppler. This circumferential

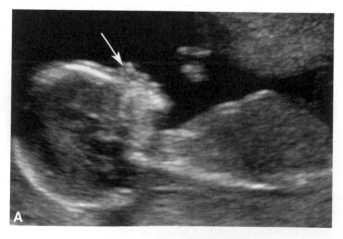
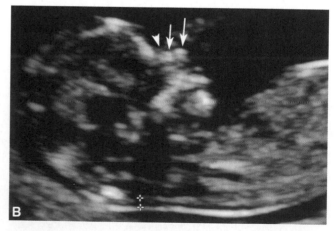

Figure 23-18 Nasal bone. **A.** Absent nasal bone (*arrow*). **B.** Normal nasal bone (*arrows*) and overlying skin (*arrowhead*). Note that calipers are measuring the normal nuchal translucency.

rim of vascularity often produces as low-resistance spectral Doppler waveform. For this reason, a corpus luteum cyst could be confused for an ectopic pregnancy because ectopic pregnancies can appear as an adnexal ring. Thus, a careful examination of the relationship of the cyst to the ovary and the components of the cyst should be undertaken. Images and additional information on corpus luteum cysts are provided in Chapter 18.

CLINICAL FINDINGS OF THE CORPUS LUTEUM OF PREGNANCY

1. Asymptomatic
2. Pain associated with hemorrhage and enlargement of cyst

SONOGRAPHIC FINDINGS OF THE CORPUS LUTEUM OF PREGNANCY

1. Simple cyst appearance
2. A cysts with a thick, echogenic rim around it (may be difficult to differentiate from other solid and cystic adnexal masses)
3. Hemorrhagic cyst appearance, including complex components or entirely echogenic depending on the amount of blood and stage of lysis

◄))) SOUND OFF
The most common pelvic mass associated with pregnancy is the ovarian corpus luteum cyst.

FIRST-TRIMESTER PATHOLOGY

Ectopic Pregnancy

An ectopic pregnancy, also referred to as an extrauterine pregnancy (EUP), is the most common cause of pelvic pain with a positive pregnancy test. It can lead to pregnancy loss and, in some cases, maternal death. An EUP is defined as a pregnancy located anywhere other than the endometrial or uterine cavity. Women with a history of assisted reproductive therapy (technology), fallopian tube scarring, and/or **pelvic inflammatory disease** are among the list of patients who are at high risk for an EUP (Table 23-4). The most common location of an EUP is within the fallopian tube, specifically the ampullary portion of the tube. Other locations for ectopic implantation include the isthmus of the tube, the fimbria, abdomen, interstitial portion of the fallopian tube (cornu of the uterus), ovary, and cervix, with the least common locations being the latter two (Fig. 23-19). Although rare, patients can have a coexisting EUP and

TABLE 23-4	Contributing factors for ectopic pregnancy

Previous ectopic pregnancy

Previous tubal surgery (including tubal sterilization)

History of pelvic inflammatory disease (salpingitis)

Undergoing infertility treatment

Previous or present use of an intrauterine contraceptive device

Multiparity

Advanced maternal age

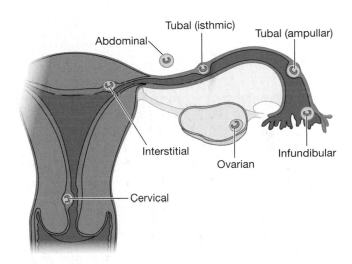

Figure 23-19 Possible ectopic pregnancy locations.

IUP. This is termed a **heterotopic pregnancy**. Patients who are undergoing assisted reproductive therapy are also at increased risks for heterotopic pregnancies.

◄))) SOUND OFF
The most common location of an EUP is within the fallopian tube, specifically the ampullary portion of the tube.

The classic clinical triad of an EUP includes pain, vaginal bleeding, and a palpable abdominal/pelvic mass. Other clinical findings include amenorrhea, positive pregnancy test, low hCG compared to a normal IUP based on the gestational age, shoulder pain (secondary to intraperitoneal hemorrhage with diaphragmatic irritation), low **hematocrit** (with rupture), and cervical motion tenderness. hCG can be helpful, because with a normal IUP, the hCG level should double every 48 hours, whereas with an EUP, the hCG will have a slower rise. Sonographically, an EUP may be obvious, offering evidence of an extrauterine gestational sac that contains a fetus and yolk sac (Fig. 23-20). Other sonographic

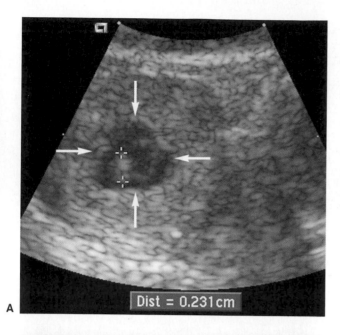

Dist = 0.231cm

A

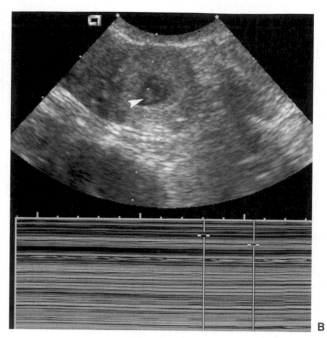

B

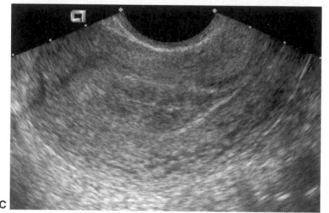

C

Figure 23-20 Ectopic pregnancy with an extrauterine gestational sac containing a live embryo. **A.** Transvaginal view of the right adnexa demonstrating an extrauterine gestational sac (*arrows*) containing an embryo (*calipers*). **B.** The embryo (*arrowhead*) does have cardiac activity documented by M-mode (*calipers*). **C.** Sagittal transvaginal image of the uterus revealing a thickened endometrium with no visible gestational sac.

findings include the **adnexal ring sign** with a possible "ring of fire," a complex adnexal mass located between the ovary and the uterus, a large amount of free fluid within the pelvis and in **Morison pouch** (with complex free fluid representing hemoperitoneum), a pseudogestational sac, and a poorly decidualized endometrium.

An EUP that implants within the intramural portion of the fallopian tube may be referred to as an interstitial pregnancy, and in the past, it was referred to as a cornual pregnancy. This portion of the uterus is highly vascular and is prone to excessive hemorrhage. Interstitial pregnancies are considered potentially life-threatening because the pregnancy may progress normally until spontaneous rupture occurs. In the presence of an interstitial pregnancy, sonography will yield a gestational sac that is located in the superolateral portion of the uterus. Care must be taken to assess for thinning of the myometrium surrounding the gestation that is located within the interstitial portion of the

fallopian tube. Three-dimensional (3D) imaging can be especially helpful if an interstitial location is suspected (Fig. 23-21).

> **🔊 SOUND OFF**
> The classic clinical triad of an EUP includes pain, vaginal bleeding, and a palpable abdominal/ pelvic mass.

Several treatment options exist when an ectopic pregnancy is identified. **Methotrexate** is a drug used to medically treat an EUP. It can be either injected into the ectopic pregnancy with sonographic guidance or taken intramuscularly. Methotrexate destroys rapidly dividing cells, such as those that comprise the developing EUP. This drug works well with many ectopic pregnancies when they are confined to the fallopian tube and are small in diameter, typically less than 4 or 5 cm. Some ectopic pregnancies, especially those that have ruptured or are advanced, require surgical intervention.

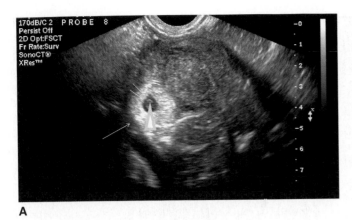

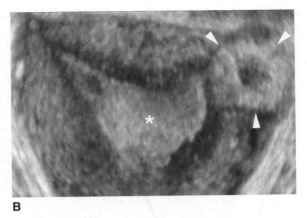

A B

Figure 23-21 Interstitial ectopic. **A.** Interstitial ectopic. Transvaginal transverse image through upper uterine fundus shows echogenic ring (*arrow*), gestational sac (*double arrow*), and yolk sac (*arrowhead*) of ectopic pregnancy within the interstitial portion of the fallopian tube. **B.** Coronal reformatting from three-dimensional sonogram of the uterus reveals that the gestational sac (*arrowheads*) is located in the left interstitial portion of the tube, separate from the endometrium in the body of the uterus (*asterisk*).

CLINICAL FINDINGS OF ECTOPIC PREGNANCY

1. Classic clinical triad—pain, vaginal bleeding, palpable abdominal/pelvic mass
2. Amenorrhea
3. Positive pregnancy test
4. Low beta-hCG compared with normal intrauterine gestation
5. Shoulder pain (secondary to intraperitoneal hemorrhage with diaphragmatic irritation)
6. Low hematocrit (with rupture)
7. Cervical motion tenderness

SONOGRAPHIC FINDINGS OF ECTOPIC PREGNANCY

1. Extrauterine gestational sac containing a yolk sac or an embryo
2. Adnexal ring sign (may be surrounded by rim of vascularity—"ring of fire")
3. Complex adnexal mass
4. Large amount of free fluid within the pelvis or in Morison pouch
5. Complex free fluid could represent hemoperitoneum
6. Pseudogestational sac
7. Poor decidual reaction
8. Endometrial cavity containing blood

Gestational Trophoblastic Disease

Benign **gestational trophoblastic disease** (GTD), often referred to as a molar pregnancy or a hydatidiform mole, is a group of disorders that result from an abnormal combination of male and female gametes (Table 23-5). The common forms of GTD can be described as either a

TABLE 23-5 Classification of gestational trophoblastic disease and important details to remember

Classification of Gestational Trophoblastic Disease	Important Facts
Hydatidiform molar pregnancy: complete	Most common form of gestational trophoblastic disease Characterized by hydropic chorionic villi Absence of the fetus and amnion Benign with malignant potential Markedly elevated hCG
Hydatidiform molar pregnancy: partial or incomplete	May be accompanied by a coexisting **triploid** fetus, parts of fetus, or amnion Minimal malignant potential Normal or minimally elevated hCG
Invasive molar pregnancy (chorioadenoma destruens)	Molar pregnancy that invades into the myometrium and may also invade through the uterine wall and into the peritoneum Result of malignant progression of hydatidiform moles
Choriocarcinoma	Most malignant form of trophoblastic disease with possible metastasis Result of malignant progression of a hydatidiform molar pregnancy Most common sites for metastasis are the liver, lungs, and vagina

hCG, human chorionic gonadotropin.

complete molar pregnancy or partial (incomplete) molar pregnancy, with complete being the most common. The term *trophoblast* in the title of this disease relates to the cells that surround the developing gestation. As stated earlier, trophoblastic cells are those cells that produce hCG. GTD results in the excessive growth of the trophoblastic cells. Therefore, there are excessive amounts of hCG in the maternal circulation. Although the cause of molar pregnancy is unknown, it has been speculated that perhaps in these situations, a normal sperm fertilizes an empty ovum.

> **SOUND OFF**
> The most common form of GTD is the complete molar pregnancy.

Although most molar pregnancies are typically benign, they do have malignant potential. The complete molar pregnancy has a higher malignant potential compared to the partial molar pregnancy. The most common forms of malignant GTD are the **invasive mole** and **choriocarcinoma**. Because this disease has malignant potential, other imaging modalities and hCG monitoring are typically warranted. The most common sites of metastatic involvement are the lungs, liver, and vagina. However, other organs may be affected. Patients who present with the diagnosis of molar pregnancy are commonly referred for chest radiographs or other studies for further evaluation of metastasis. Treatment for GTD includes dilation and curettage, hCG monitoring, hysterectomy, and, possibly, chemotherapy.

Clinical findings of GTD include **hyperemesis gravidarum**, a markedly elevated hCG level (potentially >100,000 mIU per mL), heavy vaginal bleeding with the possible passage of grape-like molar clusters, hypertension, uterine enlargement, and even hyperthyroidism and possible **preeclampsia** or **eclampsia**. Sonographic findings of a complete molar pregnancy include a large complex mass within the uterus with a "vesicular, snowstorm appearance" containing multiple cystic spaces, representing hydropic chorionic villi (Fig. 23-22).

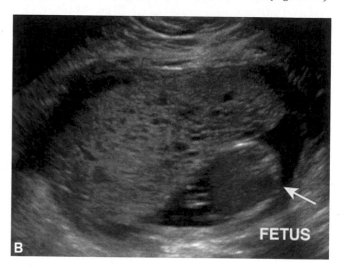

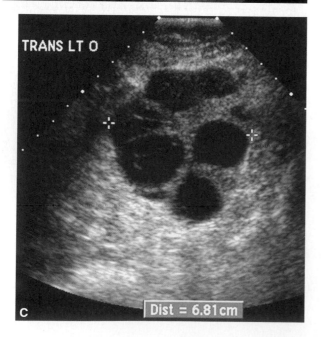

Figure 23-22 Complete and partial hydatidiform mole. **A.** Transverse image of the uterus demonstrating the uterine cavity filled with an echogenic mass (*arrow, calipers*) that contains small cystic spaces representing hydropic chorionic villi. **B.** Partial molar pregnancy demonstrating a hydropic placenta with a coexisting fetus. **C.** Example of theca lutein cyst. Transverse sonogram of an enlarged ovary (*arrows*) representing a theca lutein cyst because of gestational trophoblastic disease.

Color Doppler interrogation of the abnormal placental tissue often reveals hypervascularity around the tissue, but not within it. The ovarian mass associated with a molar pregnancy and elevated hCG is the **theca lutein cyst**. These masses are typically bilateral and appear as large, multiloculated ovarian masses.

CLINICAL FINDINGS OF MOLAR PREGNANCY

1. Hyperemesis gravidarum
2. Markedly elevated hCG level (potentially >100,000 mIU per mL)
3. Heavy vaginal bleeding (with the possible passage of grape-like molar clusters)
4. Enlarged uterus
5. Possible preeclampsia or eclampsia
6. Hypertension
7. Hyperthyroidism

SONOGRAPHIC FINDINGS OF COMPLETE MOLAR PREGNANCY

1. Complex mass within the uterus
2. Color Doppler may reveal hypervascularity around the mass, but not within it
3. "Vesicular snowstorm appearance" secondary to placental enlargement
4. Multiple, variable-sized cysts replacing the placental tissue (hydropic chorionic villi)
5. Bilateral ovarian theca lutein cysts (large, bilateral, multiloculated ovarian masses)

CLINICAL FINDINGS OF PARTIAL MOLAR PREGNANCY

1. Normal physical examination
2. Normal or slightly evaluated hCG level
3. Smaller-than-normal uterus or, possibly, normal-sized uterus based on gestational age
4. Possible vaginal bleeding

SONOGRAPHIC FINDINGS OF PARTIAL MOLAR PREGNANCY

1. Complex mass within the uterus partially filling the uterine cavity adjacent to the gestational sac
2. "Vesicular snowstorm appearance" secondary to placental enlargement
3. Multiple, variable-sized cysts replacing the placental tissue (hydropic chorionic villi)
4. Triploid fetus

🔊 **SOUND OFF**
The ovarian mass associated with a molar pregnancy and elevated hCG is the theca lutein cyst.

Blighted Ovum or Anembryonic Gestation

A **blighted** ovum or **anembryonic gestation** is diagnosed when there is no evidence of a fetal pole or yolk sac within the gestational sac at the appropriate time of development (Fig. 23-23). Although empty, the gestational sac often has an irregular shape with a poor decidual reaction. Patients present with vaginal bleeding, a low hCG, and reduction in pregnancy symptoms.

CLINICAL FINDINGS OF BLIGHTED OVUM

1. Vaginal bleeding
2. Reduction of pregnancy symptoms
3. Low hCG

SONOGRAPHIC FINDINGS OF BLIGHTED OVUM

1. Large, irregular gestational sac without an embryo or a yolk sac
2. Absent or minimal gestational sac growth
3. Poor decidual reaction

Embryonic Demise and Pregnancy Failure

Embryonic demise, sometimes referred to as fetal demise, is defined as the death of the embryo or fetus. With transvaginal imaging, cardiac activity should be detected in the pole that measures 4 to 5 mm. The causes of embryonic death are often **idiopathic** but may be linked with chromosomal abnormalities. Clinically, patients present small for dates and typically have vaginal bleeding with a closed cervix.

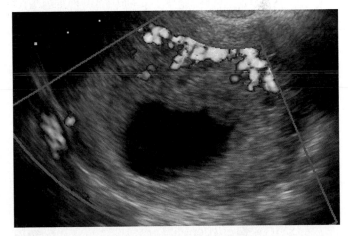

Figure 23-23 Anembryonic pregnancy. An empty gestational sac measuring 27 mm in mean sac diameter is demonstrated within the uterus with transvaginal sonography. The margin of the sac is irregular in contour, and the decidual reaction is poorly defined and only weakly echogenic. In a normal intrauterine pregnancy, a yolk sac should always be demonstrable by transvaginal sonography at this time.

The normal embryonic heart rate at 6 weeks is typically between 100 and 110 beats per minute (bpm). By 7 weeks, the rate should be at least 120 bpm. Between 8 and 9 weeks, the rate can increase slightly and then plateau at approximately 150 bpm. Sonography provides a definitive diagnosis of embryonic demise when there is no detectable fetal heart motion with real-time imaging. Absent cardiac activity when the CRL is below 7 mm is suspicious for pregnancy failure. An impending embryonic demise is associated with embryonic bradycardia. A heart rate that is less than 90 bpm at around 6 weeks is considered abnormal. In addition, the majority of pregnancies with less than 80 bpm will eventually go on to miscarry.

It is important to evaluate the appearance of the yolk sac during the first-trimester sonographic examination, because a yolk sac that is echogenic, large, abnormally shaped, or calcified carries an increased risk for ensuing embryonic demise (Fig. 23-24). Specifically, a yolk sac that measure over 7 mm in diameter has been linked with a high rate of pregnancy failure. The sonographer should also closely analyze the appearance of the gestational sac. For example, an abnormally small gestational sac, in relation to the CRL, is also an indicator of a poor prognosis. Furthermore, a gestational sac that has an MSD of between 16 and 24 mm with no evidence of an embryo can be a suspicious sign of early pregnancy failure. A follow-up sonogram in 7 to 10 days is often recommended to confirm viability.

CLINICAL FINDINGS OF EMBRYONIC OR FETAL DEMISE

1. Vaginal bleeding
2. Small for dates
3. Closed cervix
4. Low (based on LMP) hCG

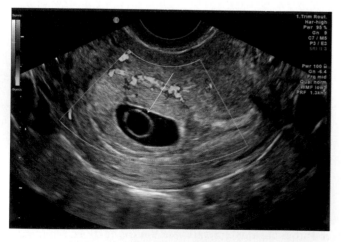

Figure 23-24 Abnormally enlarged yolk sac (*arrow*) measuring greater than 5 mm in diameter associated with early demise.

SONOGRAPHIC FINDINGS OF EMBRYONIC OR FETAL DEMISE

1. No detectable fetal heart activity in a pole that measures 4 to 5 mm
2. Irregularly shaped fetus
3. Irregularly sized or shaped gestational sac
4. Irregular-appearing yolk sac (misshapen, calcified, large, or echogenic)

🔊 SOUND OFF
The normal embryonic heart rate at 6 weeks is typically between 100 and 110 beats per minute. A heart rate that is less than 90 bpm at around 6 weeks is considered abnormal.

Miscarriage and Abortion

The termination of a pregnancy before viability is termed a **miscarriage** or an **abortion**. There are several categories of abortions, including threatened, complete, incomplete, missed, inevitable, septic, and elective (Table 23-6). Clinical findings consistent with a miscarriage include vaginal bleeding, pelvic cramping, and the passage of the products of conception. Many miscarriages are idiopathic. However, first-trimester miscarriages have been linked with ovarian abnormalities, **aneuploid** fetuses, maternal infections, physical abuse, trauma, drug abuse, maternal endocrine abnormalities, and anatomic factors. Often, hCG levels are lower than normal with miscarriage compared to those in a normal IUP. The sonographic findings of a miscarriage are variable, although if a fetus is present, careful analysis must be made to determine the presence of a fetal heartbeat (Fig. 23-25). If the fetus has demised but retained in the uterus, as seen with a **missed abortion**, it may appear to be irregular in appearance as the body attempts to break down fetal tissues.

Subchorionic Hemorrhage

Small, benign **subchorionic hemorrhages** can be seen during a routine first-trimester sonogram. A subchorionic hemorrhage is essentially a bleed between the endometrium and the gestational sac and, therefore, may be referred to as a perigestational hemorrhage. A subchorionic hemorrhage results from the implantation of the fertilized ovum into the uterus with subsequent low-pressure bleeding or spotting. The patient may complain of uterine cramping as well. Sonographically, a subchorionic hemorrhage appears as an anechoic, crescent-shaped area adjacent to the gestational sac at the margin of the placenta (Fig. 23-26). Recent bleeds are often hyperechoic or isoechoic to the placenta, whereas older bleeds may appear anechoic or even hypoechoic depending on the age of the hemorrhage. A subchorionic

TABLE 23-6 Types of abortion, a description, and typical sonographic findings

Types of Abortion	Description	Sonographic Findings
Threatened abortion	Vaginal bleeding before 20 weeks' gestation; closed cervical os	Low fetal heart rate
Complete (spontaneous) abortion	All products of conception expelled	No intrauterine products of conception identified Prominent endometrium, which may contain hemorrhage
Incomplete abortion	Part of the products of conception expelled	Thickened and irregular endometrium Enlarged uterus
Missed abortion	Fetal demise with retained fetus	No detectable fetal heart motion detected Abnormal fetal shape
Inevitable abortion	Vaginal bleeding with dilated cervix	Low-lying gestational sac Open internal os of cervix

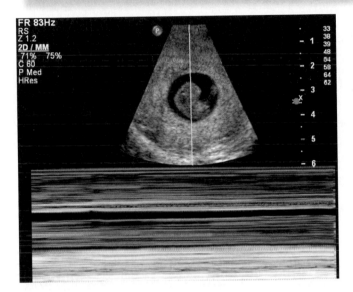

Figure 23-25 First-trimester embryonic demise. M-mode is used to document an absent heartbeat.

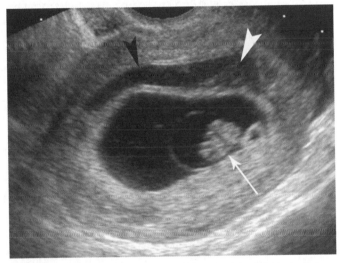

Figure 23-26 Subchorionic hemorrhage. Hemorrhage (*black arrowhead*) is seen in the uterine cavity between the decidua capsularis and the decidua vera. Some of the blood is clotted and appears more echogenic (*white arrowhead*) than the liquid blood. A live embryo (*arrow*) was present within its amniotic sac.

hemorrhages can be confused for a twin gestational sac. Although large bleeds may be associated with miscarriage and stillbirth, fetal activity is often a reassuring sign that the pregnancy will progress normally.

CLINICAL FINDINGS OF SUBCHORIONIC HEMORRHAGE

1. Vaginal bleeding or spotting
2. Uterine cramping
3. Closed cervix

SONOGRAPHIC FINDINGS OF SUBCHORIONIC HEMORRHAGE

1. Crescent-shaped anechoic, echogenic, or hypoechoic area adjacent to the gestational sac (depends on the age of the hemorrhage)
2. May resemble a second gestational sac

UTERINE LEIOMYOMA AND PREGNANCY

A **uterine leiomyoma**, also referred to as a fibroid, is a common benign pelvic mass that can often be identified during a first-trimester sonographic examination. These tumors, although benign, have been associated with an increased risk for early pregnancy failure, especially in women who are pregnant with multiple gestations. The two most important sonographic findings of fibroids during pregnancy are location and size. The location of a fibroid is easily identified with sonography, with cervical and lower uterine fibroids being of most relevance, because they may pose a dilemma at delivery. Fibroids are stimulated by estrogen and can consequently experience rapid growth during pregnancy, although this does not always occur. Thus, sonography can also be used to assess the size of these masses and provide important data for follow-up examinations.

> **SOUND OFF**
> Fibroids are stimulated by estrogen and can consequently experience rapid growth during pregnancy.

The most common sonographic appearance of a fibroid is that of a solid, hypoechoic, myometrial mass. Fibroids must be differentiated from **focal myometrial contractions**, which are smooth muscle contractions that can be noted during a sonographic examination. Fibroids will consistently alter the shape of the myometrium, whereas true myometrial contractions typically disappear within 20 to 30 minutes. Leiomyomas are also discussed in Chapter 17 of this text.

CLINICAL FINDINGS OF A UTERINE LEIOMYOMA (WITH PREGNANCY)

1. Positive pregnancy test
2. Pelvic pressure
3. Menorrhagia
4. Palpable pelvic mass
5. Enlarged, bulky uterus (if multiple)
6. Urinary frequency
7. Dysuria
8. Constipation

SONOGRAPHIC FINDINGS OF UTERINE LEIOMYOMA

1. Hypoechoic mass within the uterus
2. Posterior shadowing
3. Degenerating fibroids may have calcifications or cystic components
4. Multiple fibroids appear as an enlarged, irregularly shaped, diffusely heterogeneous uterus

Intrauterine Contraceptive Device and Coexisting Pregnancy

Occasionally, an **intrauterine contraceptive device** (IUCD) may not be effective and thus allow pregnancy to occur and implant within the uterus. If this occurs, the IUCD will be seen as an echogenic structure within the uterine cavity adjacent to the gestational sac. The IUCD will often produce acoustic shadowing. Its location to the gestational sac should be reported. IUCDs are also discussed in Chapter 21 of this text.

REVIEW QUESTIONS

1. Which of the following is present in Figure 23-27?
   a. Anembryonic gestation
   b. Molar pregnancy
   c. Miscarriage
   d. Ectopic pregnancy

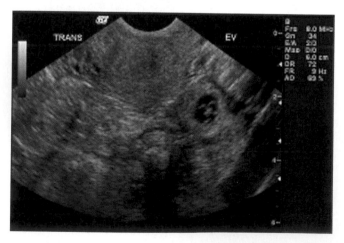

Figure 23-27

2. The patient in Figure 23-28 presented to the sonography department with nausea and vomiting, and a markedly elevated hCG level. What is the most likely diagnosis?
   a. Miscarriage
   b. Partial molar pregnancy
   c. Complete molar pregnancy
   d. Ectopic pregnancy

3. What do the arrows in Figure 23-28 A indicate?
   a. Uterine fibroid
   b. Subchorionic hemorrhage
   c. Hydropic placenta
   d. Miscarriage

4. Which of the following would be the most likely aneuploidy noted in the fetus in Figure 23-28?
   a. Triploidy
   b. Trisomy 13
   c. Turner syndrome
   d. Trisomy 18

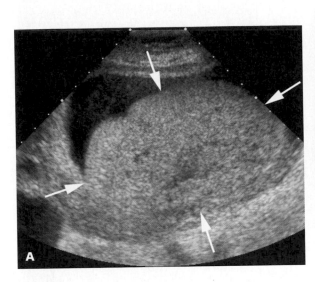
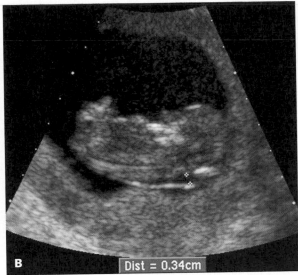

Figure 23-28

5. What does the arrow in the 11-week fetus in Figure 23-29 indicate?
   a. Omphalocele
   b. Physiologic bowel herniation
   c. Gastroschisis
   d. Ectopia cordis

7. What is the likely outcome of Figure 23-30?
   a. Normal pregnancy
   b. Ectopic pregnancy
   c. Anembryonic gestation
   d. Abortion

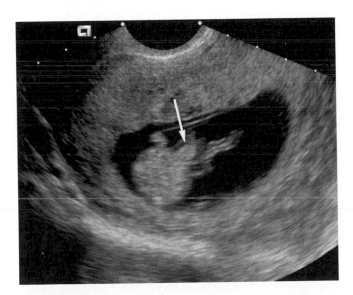

Figure 23-29

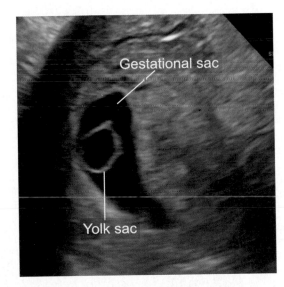

Figure 23-30

6. Which abnormality can be noted in Figure 23-30?
   a. Subchorionic hemorrhage
   b. Normal yolk stalk
   c. Enlarged yolk sac
   d. Enlarged chorionic sac

8. What does the arrow in Figure 23-31 indicate?
   a. Chorionic cavity
   b. Thickened NT
   c. Amnion
   d. Yolk sac

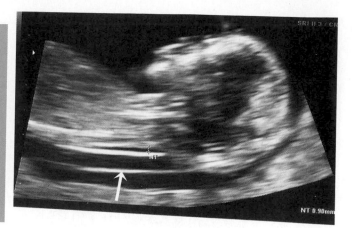

Figure 23-31

9. What does the arrow in Figure 23-32 indicate?
   a. Cephalic cyst
   b. Thickened NT
   c. Fourth ventricle
   d. Choroid plexus cyst

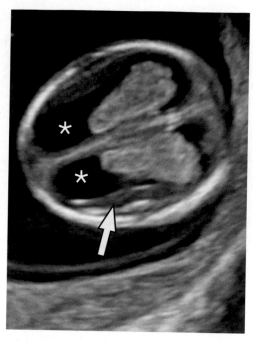

Figure 23-33

11. The adnexal finding in Figure 23-34 was discovered in a patient with a live 8-week IUP. She did not complain of pain or vaginal bleeding. What is the most likely diagnosis?
    a. Corpus luteum
    b. Ectopic pregnancy
    c. Heterotopic pregnancy
    d. Blighted ovum

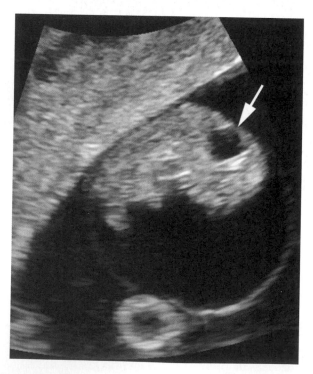

Figure 23-32

10. What do the "*" in Figure 23-33 indicate?
    a. Choroid plexus
    b. Lateral ventricles
    c. Cebocephaly
    d. Anencephaly

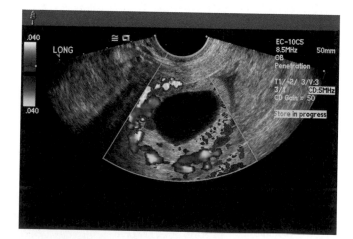

Figure 23-34

12. The patient in Figure 23-35 complained of vaginal bleeding and hyperemesis. What is the most likely diagnosis?
    a. Complete molar pregnancy
    b. Anembryonic gestation
    c. Miscarriage
    d. Pseudogestational sac associated with an ectopic pregnancy

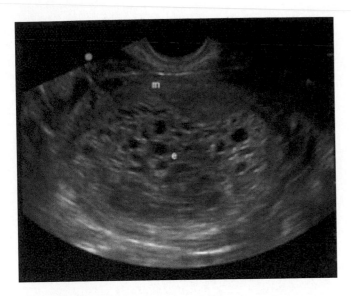

Figure 23-35

13. What do the multiple anechoic spaces within the endometrium (e) in Figure 23-25 represent?
    a. Subchorionic hemorrhage
    b. Demised fetus
    c. Hydropic chorionic villi
    d. Endometrial hyperplasia

14. In Figure 23-25, what adnexal finding is likely present?
    a. Cystic teratoma
    b. Theca lutein cyst
    c. Ovarian torsion
    d. Hydrosalpinx

15. What abnormality is noted in Figure 23-36?
    a. Increased nuchal fold
    b. Increased NT
    c. Enlarged chest
    d. Absent nasal bone

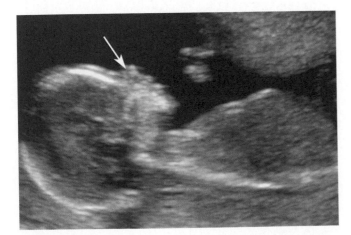

Figure 23-36

16. What abnormality is associated with Figure 23-36?
    a. Trisomy 21
    b. Beckwith–Wiedemann syndrome
    c. Triplexity
    d. Monosomy Y

17. What does the white arrow in Figure 23-37 indicate?
    a. Amnion
    b. Yolk stalk
    c. Gestational sac
    d. Yolk sac

18. What does the white arrowhead in Figure 23-37 indicate?
    a. Chorion
    b. Chorionic cavity
    c. Amnion
    d. Gestational sac

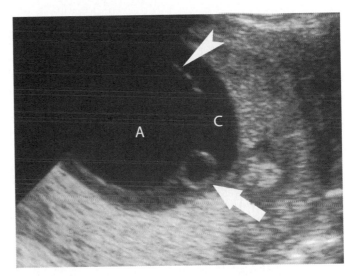

Figure 23-37

19. What is the outer membrane of the gestation?
    a. Chorionic sac
    b. Yolk sac
    c. Chorionic space
    d. Yolk sac cavity

20. What membrane in the early gestation is located across from the decidua basalis?
    a. Chorion frondosum
    b. Decidua vera
    c. Chorion laeve
    d. Decidua capsularis

21. What structure connects the embryo to the yolk sac?
    a. Vitelline duct
    b. Yolk stalk
    c. Amnion
    d. Chorionic stalk

22. What is the name of the dominant follicle before ovulation?
    a. Graafian
    b. Corpus luteum
    c. Morula
    d. Corpus albicans

23. Fertilization typically occurs within ____ after ovulation.
    a. 40 hours
    b. 12 hours
    c. 24 hours
    d. 56 hours

24. The most common site of fertilization is within the:
    a. isthmus of the uterine tube.
    b. uterine fundus.
    c. cornu of the uterine tube.
    d. ampulla of the uterine tube.

25. With a normal pregnancy, the first structure noted within the decidualized endometrium is the:
    a. yolk sac.
    b. chorionic sac.
    c. amniotic cavity.
    d. embryo.

26. The structure created by the union of sperm and egg is the:
    a. blastocyst.
    b. zygote.
    c. morula.
    d. ampulla.

27. The trophoblastic cells produce:
    a. estrogen.
    b. progesterone.
    c. follicle-stimulating hormone.
    d. hCG.

28. Sonographically, a normal-appearing 7-week IUP is identified. Within the adnexa, an ovarian cystic structure with a thick, hyperechoic rim is also discovered. What does this ovarian mass most likely represent?
    a. Theca lutein cyst
    b. Corpus luteum cyst
    c. Corpus albicans
    d. Ectopic pregnancy

29. What is the stage of the conceptus that implants within the decidualized endometrium?
    a. Blastocyst
    b. Morula
    c. Zygote
    d. Ovum

30. Another name for the chorionic sac is the:
    a. chorionic cavity.
    b. extraembryonic coelom.
    c. amniotic sac.
    d. gestational sac.

31. What is often used to medically treat an ectopic pregnancy?
    a. Dilatation and curettage
    b. Dilatation and evacuation
    c. Open surgery
    d. Methotrexate

32. What structure lies within the extraembryonic coelom?
    a. Gestational sac
    b. Embryo
    c. Yolk sac
    d. Amnion

33. What hormone, produced by the corpus luteum, maintains the thickened endometrium?
    a. Estrogen
    b. Progesterone
    c. hCG
    d. Luteinizing hormone

34. What is the most common form of GTD?
    a. Complete molar pregnancy
    b. Partial molar pregnancy
    c. Invasive mole
    d. Choriocarcinoma

35. In the first trimester, normal hCG levels will:
    a. double every 48 hours.
    b. triple every 24 hours.
    c. double every 24 hours.
    d. double every 12 hours.

36. Compared with a normal IUP, the ectopic pregnancy will have a:
    a. high hCG.
    b. low hCG.
    c. markedly elevated hCG.
    d. high AFP.

37. Which of the following locations for an ectopic pregnancy would be least likely?
    a. Isthmus of the tube
    b. Ampulla of the tube
    c. Ovary
    d. Interstitial of the tube

38. The first sonographically identifiable sign of pregnancy is the:
    a. amnion.
    b. yolk sac.
    c. decidual reaction.
    d. chorionic cavity.

39. The first structure noted within the gestational sac is the:
    a. yolk sac.
    b. embryo.
    c. decidual reaction.
    d. chorionic sac.

40. NT measurements are typically obtained between:
    a. 1 and 5 weeks.
    b. 5 and 8 weeks.
    c. 8 and 11 weeks.
    d. 11 and 14 weeks.

41. The normal gestational sac will grow:
    a. 2 mm per day.
    b. 3 mm per day.
    c. 1 cm per day.
    d. 1 mm per day.

42. During a first-trimester sonogram, you note a round, cystic structure within the fetal head. This most likely represents the:
    a. prosencephalon.
    b. mesencephalon.
    c. rhombencephalon.
    d. proencephalon.

43. The migration of the embryologic bowel into the base of the umbilical cord at 9 weeks is referred to as:
    a. physiologic bowel herniation.
    b. pseudo-omphalocele.
    c. omphalocele.
    d. gastroschisis.

44. During a 12-week sonogram, bilateral echogenic structures are noted within the lateral ventricles of the fetal cranium. These structures most likely represent:
    a. cerebral tumors.
    b. cerebral hemorrhages.
    c. anencephalic remnants.
    d. choroid plexuses.

45. The most common pelvic mass associated with pregnancy is the:
    a. uterine leiomyoma.
    b. dermoid cyst.
    c. theca luteum cyst.
    d. corpus luteum cyst.

46. All of the following are associated with an abnormal NT except:
    a. trisomy 21.
    b. Dandy-Walker malformation.
    c. trisomy 18.
    d. Turner syndrome.

47. What hormone maintains the corpus luteum during pregnancy?
    a. Estrogen
    b. Progesterone
    c. Follicle-stimulating hormone
    d. hCG

48. The most common cause of pelvic pain with pregnancy is:
    a. ectopic pregnancy.
    b. heterotopic pregnancy.
    c. missed abortion.
    d. molar pregnancy.

49. The most common location of an ectopic pregnancy is the:
    a. ovary.
    b. interstitial portion of the uterine tube.
    c. cornual portion of the uterine tube.
    d. ampullary portion of the uterine tube.

50. All of the following are contributing factors for an ectopic pregnancy except:
    a. pelvic inflammatory disease.
    b. assisted reproductive therapy.
    c. IUCD.
    d. advanced paternal age.

51. All of the following are clinical features of an ectopic pregnancy except:
    a. pain.
    b. vaginal bleeding.
    c. shoulder pain.
    d. adnexal ring.

52. In the early gestation, where is the secondary yolk sac located?
    a. Chorionic cavity
    b. Base of the umbilical cord
    c. Embryonic cranium
    d. Amniotic cavity

53. All of the following are sonographic findings consistent with ectopic pregnancy except:
    a. decidual thickening.
    b. complex free fluid within the pelvis.
    c. bilateral, multiloculated ovarian cysts.
    d. complex adnexal mass separate from the ipsilateral ovary.

54. All of the following are consistent with a complete hydatidiform mole except:
    a. heterogeneous mass within the endometrium.
    b. bilateral theca lutein cysts.
    c. hyperemesis gravidarum.
    d. low hCG.

55. A malignant form of GTD is:
    a. choriocarcinoma.
    b. hydatidiform mole.
    c. anembryonic.
    d. hydropic villi.

56. A sonographic examination was performed on a pregnant patient who complained of vaginal bleeding. Sonographically, a crescent-shaped anechoic area was noted adjacent to the gestational sac. The gestational sac contained a 6-week single live IUP. What is the most likely diagnosis?
    a. Ectopic pregnancy
    b. Molar pregnancy
    c. Subchorionic hemorrhage
    d. Anembryonic gestation

57. All of the following would be associated with a lower-than-normal hCG level except:
    a. ectopic pregnancy.
    b. molar pregnancy.
    c. blighted ovum.
    d. spontaneous abortion.

58. All of the following are clinical findings consistent with a complete molar pregnancy except:
    a. vaginal bleeding.
    b. hypertension.
    c. uterine enlargement.
    d. small for dates.

59. Which of the following is the most likely metastatic location for GTD?
    a. Rectum
    b. Pancreas
    c. Spleen
    d. Lungs

60. All of the following may be sonographic findings in the presence of an ectopic pregnancy except:
    a. pseudogestational sac.
    b. corpus luteum cyst.
    c. adnexal ring.
    d. low beta-hCG.

SUGGESTED READINGS

Abuhamad A, Chaoui R. *First Trimester Ultrasound Diagnosis of Fetal Abnormalities.* Wolters Kluwer; 2018:51–96.

Beckmann CRB, Herbert W, Laube D, et al. *Obstetrics and Gynecology.* 7th ed. Wolters Kluwer; 2014:79–92 & 179–188.

Callahan TL, Caughey AB. *Blueprints: Obstetrics & Gynecology.* 6th ed. Wolters Kluwer; 2013:1–39.

Curry RA, Prince M. *Sonography: Introduction to Normal Structure and Function.* 5th ed. Elsevier; 2020:367–383.

Doubilet PM, Benson CB. *Atlas of Ultrasound in Obstetrics and Gynecology: A Multimedia Reference.* 2nd ed. Wolters Kluwer; 2012:3–14, 253–258, & 274–276.

Gibbs RS, Haney AF, Karlan BY, et al. *Danforth's Obstetrics and Gynecology.* 10th ed. Wolters Kluwer; 2008:60–87 & 137–138.

Henningsen C, Kuntz K, Youngs D. *Clinical Guide to Sonography: Exercises for Critical Thinking.* 2nd ed. Elsevier; 2014:201–204, 232–245, & 269–285.

Hertzberg BS, Middleton WD. *Ultrasound: The Requisites.* 3rd ed. Elsevier; 2016:322–354 & 512–515.

Kline-Fath BM, Bulas DI, and Lee W. *Fundamental and Advanced Fetal Imaging: Ultrasound and MRI.* 2nd ed. Wolters Kluwer; 2021:1–78.

Norton ME, Scoutt LM, Feldstein VA. *Callen's Ultrasonography in Obstetrics and Gynecology.* 6th ed. Elsevier; 2017:57–117 & 966–1000.

Nyberg D, McGaham J, Pretorius D, et al. *Diagnostic Imaging of Fetal Anomalies.* Lippincott Williams & Wilkins; 2003:815–859.

Rumack CM, Wilson SR, Charboneau JW, et al. *Diagnostic Ultrasound.* 4th ed. Elsevier, 2011:1072–1118.

Sanders RC, Hall-Terracciano B. *Clinical Sonography: A Practical Guide.* 5th ed. Wolters Kluwer; 2016:221–231 & 233–240.

Stephenson SR, Dmitrieva J. *Diagnostic Medical Sonography: Obstetrics and Gynecology.* 4th ed. Wolters Kluwer; 2018:333–370.

The Fetal Medicine Foundation. Ductus venosus. https://fetalmedicine.org/ductus-venosus-flow. Accessed January 29, 2022.

The Fetal Medicine Foundation. Nasal bone. https://fetalmedicine.org/fmf-certification-2/nasal-bone. Accessed January 29, 2022.

The Fetal Medicine Foundation. Nuchal translucency. https://fetalmedicine.org/fmf-certification-2/nuchal-translucency-scan. Accessed January 29, 2022.

BONUS REVIEW!

Ductus Venosus Doppler Flow (Fig. 23-38)

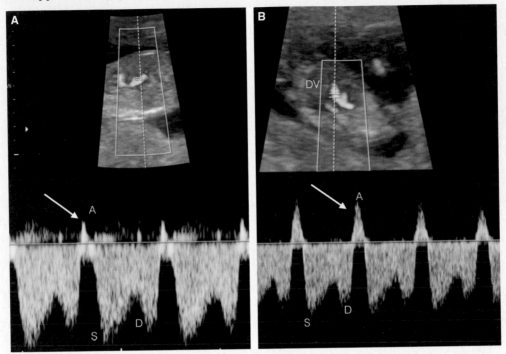

Figure 23-38 Ductus venosus (*DV*) Doppler flow assessment in two fetuses (**A** and **B**) with trisomy 21 at 13 weeks of gestation. Note the presence of reverse flow during the atrial contraction phase (**A**) of the cardiac cycle (*arrow*). Fetus A had no associated cardiac defect, whereas fetus B had a cardiac defect, which may explain the more severe reverse flow of the *A*-wave (*arrow* in **B**). Normal Doppler waveforms of the DV show antegrade flow throughout the cardiac cycle with low impedance. *S*, systolic flow; *D*, diastolic flow.

Fetus with Trisomy 21 and Tricuspid Regurgitation in the First Trimester (Fig. 23-39)

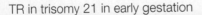

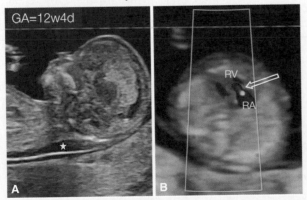
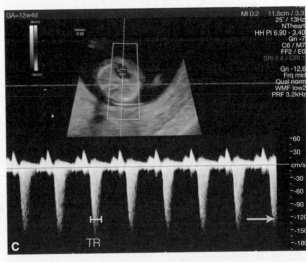

Figure 23-39 Fetus with trisomy 21 and tricuspid regurgitation (*TR*) at 12 weeks of gestation. **A.** The thickened nuchal translucency (*star*), raising the suspicion for aneuploidy. **B.** A four-chamber view in color Doppler in systole and demonstrates the presence of *TR* with the TR jet (*open arrow*) from the right ventricle (*RV*) into the right atrium (*RA*). **C.** This image confirms, with spectral Doppler, the presence of *TR*, and shows that the *TR* lasts through half of systole (*double bars*) and has peak velocities around 140 cm/s (*arrow*).

(*continued*)

BONUS REVIEW! (continued)

Midsagittal Plane View of the Fetal Face and Intracranial Contents Labeled (Fig. 23-40)

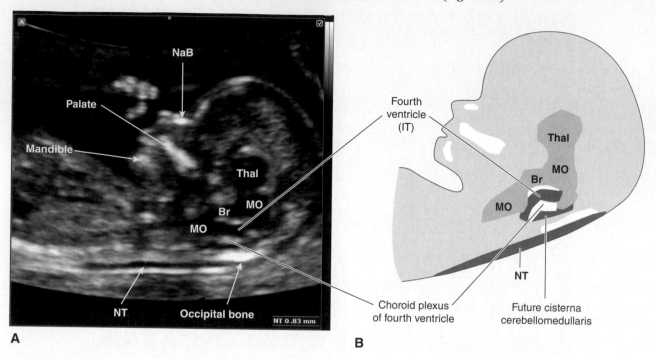

Figure 23-40 First trimester anatomy on a sonographic image (**A**) and diagram (**B**). Sonogram and diagram showing the intracranial translucency in a normal fetus. Midsagittal plane view of the fetal face showing the nasal bone (*NaB*), palate, mandible, nuchal translucency (*NT*), thalamus (*Thal*), midbrain (*Mb*), brainstem (*Br*), and medulla oblongata (*MO*). The fourth ventricle is noted as an intracranial translucency (*NT*) between the Br and the choroid plexus. The intracranial translucency is absent if spina bifida is present.

The Fetal Head and Brain

Introduction

It is vital for the sonographer to have a thorough understanding of both cranial and intracranial anatomy. This chapter provides a summary of the significant anatomy of the cranium and brain. It also provides the information pertaining to abnormalities of the fetal head and brain. In the "Bonus Review" section, a diagram of normal midline brain anatomy is offered as well as a three-dimensional sonogram case of anencephaly that was caused by amniotic band syndrome.

Key Terms

acrania—the absence of the cranial vault above the bony orbits

agenesis of the corpus callosum—the congenital absence of corpus callosum; may be partial or complete

alobar holoprosencephaly—the most severe form of holoprosencephaly

anencephaly—a neural tube defect that is described as the absence of the cranium and cerebral hemispheres

anophthalmia—the absence of the eye(s)

Apert syndrome—genetic disorder that includes craniosynostosis, midline facial hypoplasia, and syndactyly

aperture(s)—an opening in a structure

aqueduct of Sylvius—see key term cerebral aqueduct

aqueductal stenosis—the abnormal narrowing of the cerebral aqueduct

arachnoid cyst(s)—benign cysts within the brain that do not communicate with the ventricular system

arachnoid granulations—nodular structures located along the falx cerebri that reabsorb cerebrospinal fluid into the venous system

arachnoid membrane—the middle layer of the meninges

arachnoid villi—see key term arachnoid granulations

Arnold–Chiari II malformation—a group of cranial abnormalities associated with spina bifida

basal ganglia—a group of nuclei within the brain that function in several ways, including information processing and emotional response

Beckwith–Wiedemann syndrome—a growth disorder syndrome associated with enlargement of several organs, including the skull, tongue, and liver

brachycephalic—round skull shape

brainstem—the lower part of the brain composed of the pons, midbrain, and medulla oblongata

cavum septum pellucidum—a normal midline brain structure identified in the anterior portion of the brain between the frontal horns of the lateral ventricles

cebocephaly—close-set eyes (hypotelorism) and a nose with a single nostril

cephalic index—the ratio used for assessing fetal head shape

cerebellar vermis—the portion of the cerebellum, located within the midline of the brain, that connects its two hemispheres

cerebral aqueduct—the duct that connects the third ventricle of the brain to the fourth ventricle; also referred to as the aqueduct of Sylvius

cerebral peduncles—paired structures located anterior to the cerebral aqueduct

cerebrospinal fluid—the protective and nourishing fluid of the brain and spinal cord produced by the cells of the choroid plexus

choroid plexus—specialized cells within the ventricular system responsible for cerebrospinal fluid production

cistern—a prominent space within the skull that contains cerebrospinal fluid; a cistern is created by the separation of the arachnoid membrane and pia mater

cisterna magna—the largest cistern in the skull; located in the posterior portion of the skull

colpocephaly—the abnormal lateral ventricle shape in which there is a small frontal horn and enlarged occipital horn

communicating hydrocephalus—the obstruction of cerebrospinal fluid from a source outside the ventricular system

corpus callosum—a thick band of white matter that provides communication between the right and left halves of the brain

corrected-BPD—represents the biparietal diameter of a standard-shaped fetal head with the same cross-sectional area

craniosynostosis—the premature closure of the cranial sutures with subsequent fusion of the cranial bones

cyclopia—fusion of the orbits

Dandy–Walker complex—a spectrum of posterior fossa abnormalities that involves the cystic dilatation of the cisterna magna and fourth ventricle

Dandy–Walker malformation—congenital brain malformation in which there is enlargement of the cisterna magna, agenesis of the cerebellar vermis, and dilation of the fourth ventricle

dangling choroid sign—a sonographic sign associated with ventriculomegaly when the choroid plexus is noted hanging freely within the dilated lateral ventricle

dilatation—an enlargement or expansion of a structure

dolichocephaly—an elongated, narrow head shape; may also be referred to as scaphocephaly

dura mater—the dense, fibrous outer layer of the meninges

ependyma—the lining of the ventricles within the brain

exencephaly—a form of acrania in which the entire cerebrum is located outside the skull

facies—the features or appearance of the face

falx cerebri—a double fold of dura mater located within midline of the brain

folate—a vitamin that has been shown to significantly reduce the likelihood of neural tube defects; also referred to as folic acid

foramen magnum—the opening in the base of the skull through which the spinal cord exits

gastroschisis—herniation of abdominal contents through a right-sided, periumbilical abdominal wall defect

germinal matrix—a group of thin-walled blood vessels and cells within the subependymal layer of the fetal brain responsible for brain cell migration during fetal development

glomus (of choroid plexus)—the largest part of the choroid plexus

gyri—folds in the cerebral cortex

holoprosencephaly—a group of brain abnormalities consisting of varying degrees of fusion of the lateral ventricles, absence of the midline structures, and associated facial anomalies

hydranencephaly—a fatal condition in which the entire cerebrum is replaced by a large sac containing cerebrospinal fluid

hydrocephalus—the dilatation of the ventricular system caused by an increased volume of cerebrospinal fluid, resulting in increased intraventricular pressure

hydrops (fetal)—an abnormal accumulation of fluid in at least two fetal body cavities

hypoplasia—incomplete growth of a structure or an organ

hypotelorism—reduced distance between the orbits

hypoxia—a shortage of oxygen or decreased oxygen in the blood

interhemispheric fissure—groove within the midline of the brain that divides the two cerebral hemispheres

interthalamic adhesion—the mass of tissue, located in the third ventricle within the midline of the brain, which connects the two lobes of the thalamus; also referred to as the massa intermedia

intracranial hemorrhage—hemorrhage within the cranium

intraventricular hemorrhage—hemorrhage located within the ventricles of the brain

lissencephaly—"smooth brain"; condition where there is little to no gyri or sulci within the cerebral cortex

lobar holoprosencephaly—the least severe form of the holoprosencephaly

macrocephaly—an enlarged head circumference

massa intermedia—see key term interthalamic adhesion

Meckel–Gruber syndrome—a fetal syndrome associated with microcephaly, occipital encephalocele, polydactyly, and polycystic kidneys

median cleft lip—a subdivision within the middle of the lip

mega cisterna magna—an enlargement of the cisterna magna as defined by a depth of more than 10 mm

meninges—the coverings of the brain and spinal cord

meningocele—herniation of the cranial or spinal meninges because of an open cranial or a spinal defect

mesencephalon—the primary brain vesicle also referred to as the midbrain; it eventually becomes the cerebral peduncles, quadrigeminal plate, and cerebral aqueduct

mesocephalic—normal head shape

microcephaly—small head

monoventricle—one large ventricle within the brain associated with holoprosencephaly

myelomeningocele—mass that results from spina bifida that contains the spinal cord and the meninges

neural plate—the early embryologic structure that develops into the central nervous system

neural tube—embryologic formation that results from fusion of the two folded ends of the neural plate

noncommunicating hydrocephalus—the obstruction of cerebrospinal fluid from a source within the ventricular system

omphalocele—an anterior abdominal wall defect where there is herniation of the fetal bowel and other abdominal organs into the base of the umbilical cord

parenchyma—the functional part of an organ

Patau syndrome—a chromosomal aberration in which there is a third chromosome 13; also referred to as trisomy 13

pia mater—the innermost layer of the meninges

porencephaly—a condition in which a cyst, most often caused by an intraparenchymal hemorrhage, communicates with a lateral ventricle

proboscis—fleshy, tongue-like appendage that is typically located within the midline above the orbits in association with cyclopia and holoprosencephaly

prosencephalon—the primary brain vesicle also referred to as the forebrain; it eventually becomes the lateral ventricles, cerebral hemispheres, third ventricle, thalamus, hypothalamus, pineal gland, and pituitary gland

rhombencephalon—the primary brain vesicle also referred to as the hindbrain; it eventually becomes the cerebellum, pons, medulla oblongata, and fourth ventricle

scalloping (frontal bones)—indentations on a normally smooth margin of a structure

scaphocephaly—see key term dolichocephaly

schizencephaly—a cerebral malformation associated with the development of fluid-filled clefts

spinal dysraphism—a group of neural tube defects that describe some manifestation of incomplete closure of the spine

subarachnoid space—an area located between the arachnoid membrane and the pia mater

subependymal (layer)—the area just beneath the ependymal lining the lateral ventricles

sulci—grooves within the brain

suture (skull)—a flexible, connective tissue that lies between the cranial bones

thalamus—a brain structure that allows communication between the senses; also performing many other functions

thanatophoric dysplasia—the most common lethal skeletal dysplasia characterized by a cloverleaf skull with frontal bossing and hydrocephalus

TORCH infections—an acronym that stands for toxoplasmosis, other infections, rubella, cytomegalovirus, and herpes simplex virus; this group of infections may be acquired by a woman during pregnancy

triploidy—a fetus that has three of every chromosome

trisomy 8—chromosomal aberration in which there is a third chromosome 8; also referred to as Warkany syndrome 2

trisomy 13—chromosomal aberration in which there is a third chromosome 13; also referred to as Patau syndrome; often associated with holoprosencephaly

trisomy 18—chromosomal aberration in which there is a third chromosome 18; also referred to as Edwards syndrome

trisomy 21—chromosomal aberration in which there is a third chromosome 21; also referred to as Down syndrome

vein of Galen aneurysm—an arteriovenous malformation that occurs within the fetal brain and is associated with congestive heart failure

EMBRYOLOGIC DEVELOPMENT OF THE FETAL BRAIN

By 4.5 weeks, the **neural plate**, the structure that will form the central nervous system, has developed. The neural plate will give rise to the **neural tube**, which will become the spine and the brain. Initially, the brain is divided into three primary vesicles termed the **prosencephalon** (forebrain), **mesencephalon** (midbrain), and **rhombencephalon** (hindbrain) (Fig. 24-1). These vesicles will continue to develop and form critical brain structures. For example, the prosencephalon will continue to mature into two other vesicles, the telencephalon and diencephalon. The telencephalon will form the cerebral hemispheres, lateral ventricles, and third ventricle. The diencephalon will become the thalamus and hypothalamus. The mesencephalon will become the midbrain, including the superior parts of the brainstem. As noted in Chapter 23, the rhombencephalon, which separates into two other vesicles, will become the fourth ventricle, as well as the medulla oblongata and cerebellum.

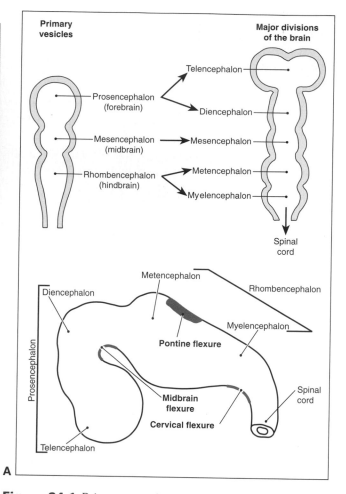

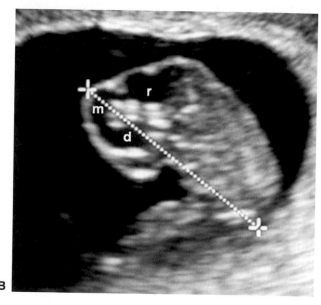

Figure 24-1 Primary vesicles. **A.** Drawing of the lateral view of the vesicles of the early brain. **B.** Sagittal view of an 8-week gestation. *Calipers*, crown-rump length measurement; *d*, diencephalon; *m*, mesencephalon; *r*, rhombencephalon.

NORMAL FETAL SKULL AND BRAIN ANATOMY

The skull consists of eight cranial bones (Table 24-1). These bones are connected by structures known as **sutures** (Table 24-2). Fetal sutures may be noted during a

TABLE 24-1 Cranial bones and their locations

Cranial Bone(s)	Location
Frontal bone	Anterior
Parietal bones	Superior and lateral
Temporal bones	Inferior and lateral
Occipital bone	Posterior
Sphenoid bone	Lateral (helps form the base of the skull)
Ethmoid bone	Anterior (between the orbits)

TABLE 24-2 Fetal sutures and their locations

Suture	Location
Coronal suture	Between the frontal and two parietal bones
Sagittal suture	Between the two parietal bones
Lambdoidal suture	Between the parietal bones and occipital bone
Squamosal sutures	Between the parietal bones and temporal bones
Metopic suture	Located within the frontal bone along the midline of the forehead

routine sonographic examination as hypoechoic spaces between the bones. Because of the flexibility of sutures, the fetal cranial bones remain slightly mobile until delivery to facilitate the passage of the skull through the birth canal. Premature fusion of the sutures is termed **craniosynostosis**. Consequently, craniosynostosis leads to an irregular-shaped skull.

> ### 🔊 SOUND OFF
> Premature fusion of the sutures is termed craniosynostosis.

Spaces that exist between the forming fetal bones are referred to as fontanelles or "soft spots" (Table 24-3). Several fontanelles persist in the postnatal period and into infancy. Fontanelles are often utilized as sonographic windows during neurosonographic examinations to evaluate newborns for intracranial hemorrhage or suspected brain anomalies. The anterior fontanelle, when completely filled with bone, is referred to as the bregma, whereas the posterior fontanelle is referred to as the lambda. The **foramen magnum** is the opening in the base of the cranium through which the spinal cord travels.

Midline fetal brain anatomy and those structures that lie on both sides of the midline should be routinely evaluated during an obstetric sonogram (Table 24-4). These structures are discussed in the following sections.

The Cerebrum

The brain can be divided into two main parts, the cerebrum and the cerebellum. The cerebrum is the largest part of the brain. The normal cerebrum contains multiple **sulci** and **gyri**. There are six cerebral lobes: the frontal lobe, two temporal lobes, two parietal lobes, and the occipital lobe.

The cerebrum can be further divided into a right and left hemisphere by the **interhemispheric fissure**.

TABLE 24-3 Locations of the fontanelles and when they close

Fontanelle	Location	Closure
Anterior or frontal	Bordered by the frontal and parietal bones	By 18 mo
Posterior or occipital	Bordered by the occipital and parietal bones	By 6 mo
Anterolateral or sphenoidal	Bordered by the frontal, parietal, and sphenoid bones	By 2 yr
Posterolateral or mastoid	Bordered by the mastoid and occipital bones	By 2 yr

TABLE 24-4 Brain structures located within the midline (left column) and those that are located on both sides of the midline (right column)

Midline Brain Anatomy	Bilateral Brain Structures
Falx cerebri	Hemispheres of the cerebellum
Interhemispheric fissure	Hemispheres of the cerebrum
Corpus callosum	Lobes of the thalamus
Cavum septum pellucidum	Foramen of Monro (interventricular foramina)
Third ventricle	Lateral ventricles
Aqueduct of Sylvius (cerebral aqueduct)	Choroid plexus (within lateral ventricles)
Fourth ventricle	
Cerebellar vermis	
Cisterna magna	
Interthalamic adhesion (massa intermedia)	
Brainstem (pons, midbrain, and medulla oblongata)	

The **falx cerebri**, a double fold of **dura mater**, is located within the interhemispheric fissure and can readily be noted on a fetal sonogram as an echogenic linear formation coursing through the midline of the fetal brain. The cerebral hemispheres are linked in the midline by the **corpus callosum**, a thick band of tissue that provides communication between the right and left halves of the brain (Fig. 24-2).

> ### 🔊 SOUND OFF
> The falx cerebri separates the cerebral hemispheres, whereas the corpus callosum connects the cerebral hemispheres and allows communication between the two lobes.

The **meninges** are three protective tissues layers that cover the brain and the spinal cord. The innermost layer of the meninges is the **pia mater**, the middle layer is the **arachnoid membrane**, and the dense, outermost layer is the dura mater.

The Corpus Callosum

The corpus callosum forms late in gestation, but should be completely intact between 18 and 20 weeks. As stated earlier, the corpus callosum connects the

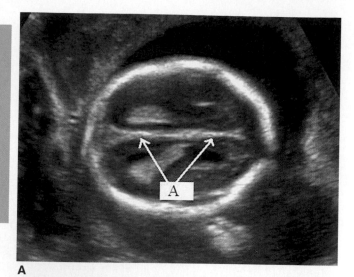

A

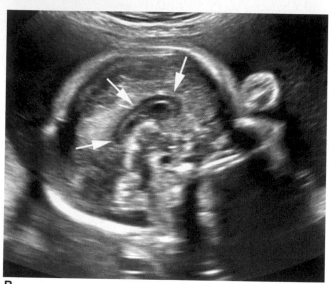

B

Figure 24-2 Falx cerebri and corpus callosum. **A.** Transaxial view of the fetal cranium demonstrating the echogenic falx cerebri (*A*). **B.** Sagittal image through the fetal head demonstrating the entire corpus callosum (*arrows*) from anterior to posterior.

two lobes of the cerebrum (see Fig. 24-2). The corpus callosum consists of four parts. Fetal development of the corpus callosum is from anterior to posterior. Thus, the rostrum, genu, body, and splenium develop, respectively. The sonographic appearance of the corpus callosum is that of an echogenic band of tissue within the midline of the brain connecting the two cerebral hemispheres. The absence of all or part of the corpus callosum is referred to as **agenesis of the corpus callosum**.

The Cavum Septum Pellucidum

The **cavum septum pellucidum** (CSP) is a midline brain structure located in the anterior portion of the brain

between the frontal horns of the lateral ventricles. It will appear as an anechoic "box-shaped" structure in the axial scan plane (Fig. 24-3). Although the CSP should always be seen between 18 and 37 weeks, the closure of this structure is normal in later gestation and often occurs before birth or shortly thereafter. The CSP does not communicate with the ventricular system, and its absence is associated with multiple cerebral malformations, including agenesis of the corpus callosum.

> 🔊 **SOUND OFF**
> The CSP does not communicate with the ventricular system, and its absence is associated with multiple cerebral malformations, including agenesis of the corpus callosum.

The Thalamus

The **thalamus**, a vital brain structure that has numerous functions, is a significant landmark for sonographers

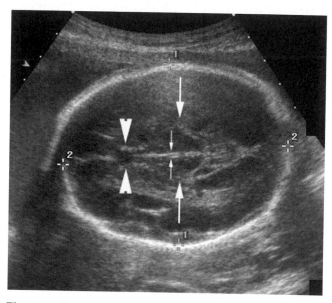

Figure 24-3 Level of the biparietal diameter and occipitofrontal diameter. Axial view of the fetal head, at the level used for measurement of the biparietal diameter, demonstrating the paired thalami (*large arrows*) with the slitlike third ventricle between them (*small arrows*), and the cavum septum pellucidum (*arrowheads*). The falx is the linear bright echo in the midline anterior to the cavum septum pellucidum, separating the cerebral hemispheres. The "+" *calipers* labeled "*1*" are placed on the leading edge of the cranial bone at the near and far sides of the skull (i.e., on the external aspect of the near side and the internal aspect of the far side) to measure the biparietal diameter. The "+" *calipers* labeled "*2*" are placed in the middle of the visible cranial bone anteriorly and posteriorly to measure the occipitofrontal diameter.

to locate within the fetal brain (see Fig. 24-3). The two lobes of the thalamus are located on both sides of the third ventricle. The **massa intermedia** or **interthalamic adhesion** passes through the third ventricle to connect the two lobes of the thalamus. The thalamus should not be confused with the **cerebral peduncles**, which are more inferiorly positioned in the brain.

The Ventricular System

The ventricular system is composed of four ventricles, whose primary function is to provide cushioning for the brain (Fig. 24-4). Each ventricle is lined by a membrane called the **ependyma**. The paired lateral ventricles are located on both sides of the falx cerebri within the cerebral hemispheres. They are frequently referred to as right and left ventricles but may also be called the first and second ventricles. The divisions of lateral ventricles, called the horns of the lateral ventricles, like the lobes of the cerebrum, correlate with the adjacent cranial bones. Thus, each lateral ventricle consists of a frontal, a temporal, and an occipital horn. In addition to the horns, the lateral ventricle also has a segment referred to as the body, which is located between the frontal and occipital horns. The point at which the body, temporal horn, and occipital horn meet is the trigone or atrium of the lateral ventricle. Within the atria of both lateral ventricles lies the echogenic configuration of the **choroid plexus**, the mass of cells responsible for the production of **cerebrospinal fluid** (CSF) in the fetus (Fig. 24-5). Choroid plexus may also be found in the roof of the third and fourth ventricles.

> **◀))) SOUND OFF**
> Choroid plexus, which is mostly located within the atria of the lateral ventricles, is responsible for producing CSF.

Each lateral ventricle communicates with the third ventricle in the midline of the brain at the foramen of Monro, or the paired interventricular foramina. The third ventricle is located between the two lobes of the thalamus. Essentially, part of the thalamus, the interthalamic adhesion or massa intermedia, passes through the third ventricle and can be visualized when enlarged or surrounded by CSF. The third ventricle connects to the fourth ventricle inferiorly by means of a long, tubelike structure called the **aqueduct of Sylvius** or the **cerebral aqueduct**.

The fourth ventricle is located anterior to the cerebellum within the midline of the brain. The fourth ventricle has three apertures or openings through which CSF travels. There are two lateral **apertures** that are also referred to as the foramina of Luschka. These two apertures allow CSF to travel from the fourth ventricle to the **subarachnoid space** around the brain. Another opening of the fourth ventricle, located in the midline, is the median aperture, which is also referred to as the foramen of Magendie. This opening allows CSF to pass from the fourth ventricle to the **cisterna magna** and subarachnoid space.

> **◀))) SOUND OFF**
> The third ventricle connects to the fourth ventricle inferiorly by means of a long, tubelike structure called the aqueduct of Sylvius or the cerebral aqueduct.

The Creation, Flow, and Reabsorption of Cerebrospinal Fluid

The greater part of CSF is produced by the cells of the choroid plexus that are located within the trigone of the lateral ventricles. CSF moves from the lateral ventricles into the third ventricle through the foramina of Monro. From the third ventricle, CSF travels to the

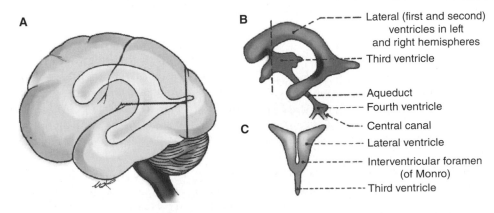

Figure 24-4 Cerebral ventricles. **A.** Sagittal view of the left cerebral hemisphere showing the contour of the lateral ventricles and their relation to the cerebral lobes. **B.** Sagittal outline of the four ventricles. **C.** Coronal section of the lateral and third ventricles at the level of the *dotted line* in (**B**) showing their communicating interventricular foramen.

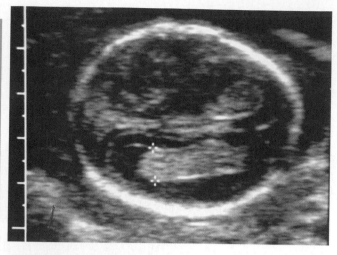

Figure 24-5 Normal choroid plexus. The normal choroid plexus is seen as prominent echogenic structures within each lateral ventricle. In early gestation, the choroid plexus fill the lateral ventricle (between *calipers*).

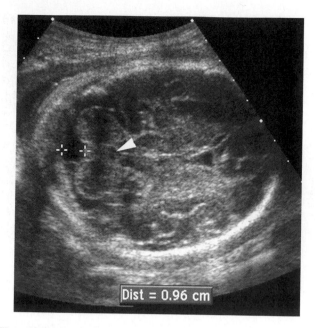

Figure 24-6 Cisterna magna and the fourth ventricle. Axial image demonstrating the cisterna magna (between *calipers*) and the location of the fourth ventricle (*arrowhead*).

fourth ventricle through the cerebral aqueduct. Once in the fourth ventricle, the fluid can exit either through the median aperture or through the lateral apertures. CSF also flows inferiorly and around the spinal cord. **Arachnoid granulations**, also referred to as **arachnoid villi**, are responsible for the reabsorption of CSF into the venous system. This process occurs at the superior sagittal sinus, located along the superior surface of the cerebrum within its midline.

The Cisterna Magna

The cisterna magna, located in the posterior fossa of the cranium, is the largest **cistern** in the head. On sonography, the cisterna magna appears as an anechoic, fluid-filled space, posterior to the cerebellum, between the **cerebellar vermis** and the interior surface of the occipital bone (Fig. 24-6). It is considered common to find some small septations within the cisterna magna.

The Cerebellum

The cerebellum is located in the posterior fossa of the cranium. The cerebellum consists of two hemispheres—right and left—that are coupled at the midline by the cerebellar vermis (Fig. 24-7). The cerebellar tonsils, named for their shape, are located on the undersurface of the cerebellum and become distorted with spina bifida and Arnold–Chiari malformations. The normal cerebellum is a dumbbell-shaped or figure eight–shaped structure noted in the posterior cranium of the fetus. The two hemispheres of the cerebellum should be symmetric, although **hypoplasia** of one cerebellar hemisphere can occur, resulting in the hypoplastic hemisphere appearing smaller than normal.

SOUND OFF
The normal cerebellum is a dumbbell-shaped or figure eight–shaped structure noted in the posterior cranium of the fetus.

FETAL HEAD MEASUREMENTS

Biparietal Diameter

The biparietal diameter (BPD) measurement of the fetal head can be taken after the first trimester has ended, typically starting between 13 and 14 weeks. The BPD is obtained in the axial plane at the level of the CSP, thalamus, and falx cerebri. This is the same level as the third ventricle, which may be seen between the two lobes of the thalamus. The cranial bones must be symmetric on both sides of the head, and the measurement is obtained from the outer table of the proximal parietal bone to the inner table of the distal parietal bone. That means, the measurement is obtained from leading edge to leading edge (Fig. 24-8).

SOUND OFF
The BPD is obtained in the axial plane at the level of the CSP, thalamus, and falx cerebri. This is the same level as the third ventricle, which may be seen between the two lobes of the thalamus.

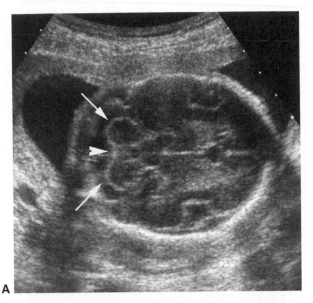
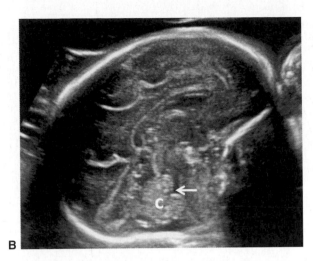

Figure 24-7 Cerebellum. **A.** Axial view of the posterior fossa demonstrating the normal contour of the cerebellum, with rounded cerebellar hemispheres (*arrows*) on either side of the more echogenic cerebellar vermis (*arrowhead*). **B.** Sagittal section of a fetal head in the early third trimester. *Arrow,* fourth ventricle; *c,* cerebellum.

Head Circumference

The head circumference (HC) measurement can be taken at the same time of gestation and at the same level of the cranium as the BPD. Thus, the HC is obtained in the axial plane at the level of the CSP, thalamus, falx cerebri, and a measurement around the entire cranium is obtained (Fig. 24-9). This is the same level as the third ventricle, which may be seen between the two lobes of the thalamus.

The cranial bones must be symmetric on both sides of the head. The HC can also be obtained by measuring the occipitofrontal diameter (OFD) and taking an outer-to-outer diameter measurement at the level of the BPD. Some authors suggest that the HC measurement is typically more accurate than BPD because this measurement is independent of the fetal head shape, consequently providing a more consistent parameter for estimating gestational age.

Occipitofrontal Diameter

The OFD is obtained at the same level of the BPD and HC. For the OFD, one caliper is placed in the anterior midline in the middle of the frontal bone, whereas the other is placed in the middle of the echogenic line of the

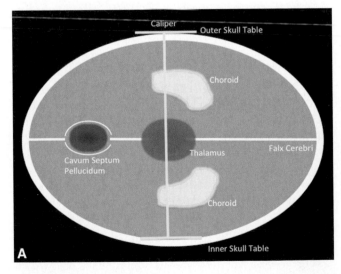
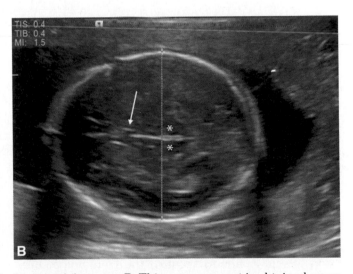

Figure 24-8 Biparietal diameter. **A.** Drawing of the level of the biparietal diameter. **B.** This measurement is obtained on an axial image of the fetal head at the level of the thalami (*asterisk*) and cavum septum pellucidum (*arrow*).

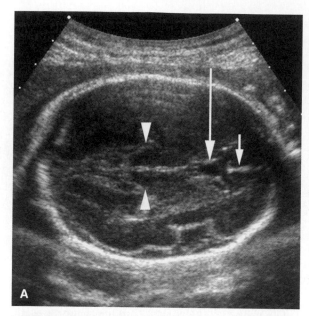

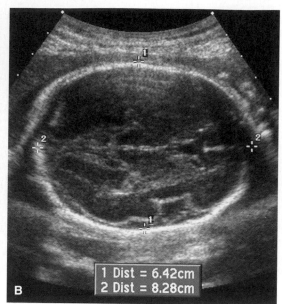

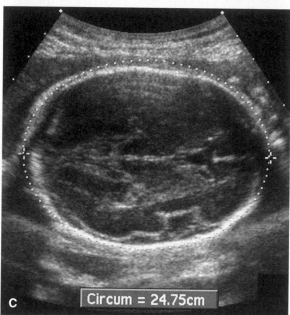

Figure 24-9 Fetal head measurements. **A.** Transverse image of the fetal head at 28 weeks' gestation at the correct level and plane for obtaining measurements. The thalami (*arrowheads*), falx (*short arrow*), and cavum septum pellucidum (*long arrow*) are all visible. **B.** Biparietal diameter (*calipers 1*) is measured from the exterior surface of the skull nearest the transducer to the internal surface of the skull farthest from the transducer. Occipitofrontal diameter (*calipers 2*) is measured from the middle of the anterior skull to the middle of the posterior skull. **C.** Head circumference (*elliptical calipers*) is measured around the outer perimeter of the skull.

occipital bone (see Fig. 24-9). The OFD may also be called the fronto-occipital diameter. The OFD can be used in conjunction with the BPD to obtain the **corrected-BPD**, which represents the BPD of the standard-shaped head of the same cross-sectional area. That means, the corrected-BPD is "shape corrected" and is equivalent to the HC, independent of the shape of the skull. OFD can also be added to the BPD and multiplied by 1.62 to obtain an HC.

> **◀))) SOUND OFF**
> The corrected-BPD is "shape corrected" and is equivalent to the HC, independent of the shape of the skull.

Cephalic Index and Fetal Head Shape

There can be much variability in the shape of the fetal head, and for this reason, the shape of the cranium should be evaluated closely with each examination. The **cephalic index** is a useful tool for indicating the shape of the fetal head. A **brachycephalic** (brachycephaly) head shape is one that is considered round or short and wide, whereas **dolichocephaly**, also referred to as **scaphocephaly**, denotes an elongated, narrow head shape (Fig. 24-10). Other abnormal skull shapes include strawberry, lemon, and cloverleaf. These abnormal shapes are associated with fetal anomalies (Table 24-5). The normal- to medium-sized skull is termed **mesocephalic**. The formula used to calculate the cephalic index considers the BPD and the OFD as

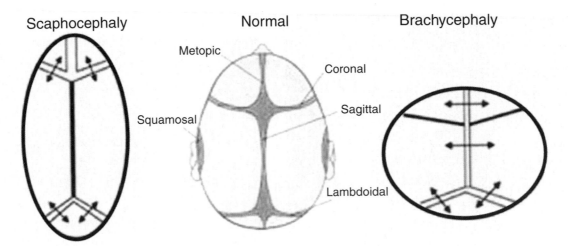

Figure 24-10 Head shapes. Scaphocephaly, which is also referred to as dolichocephaly, is considered to be elongated and narrow. Brachycephaly is described as a round and short head shape.

TABLE 24-5 Fetal head shapes and associated anomalies[a]	
Head Shape	**Associated Anomalies**
Lemon	Chiari II malformation (Fig. 24-11)
Strawberry	**Trisomy 18** (see Fig. 24-11)
Cloverleaf	**Thanatophoric dysplasia**
Microcephaly	**TORCH infections**
	Trisomy 13 and **trisomy 18**
	Meckel–Gruber syndrome
	Fetal alcohol syndrome
Macrocephaly	Hydrocephalus
	Hydranencephaly
	Intracranial tumors
	Familial inheritance
	Beckwith–Wiedemann syndrome
Brachycephaly	Craniosynostosis
	Trisomy 21
	Trisomy 18
Dolichocephaly	Craniosynostosis

[a]Note that this is a condensed list. Other anomalies and syndrome may be present. For review purposes, keep these in mind.

follows: cephalic index = BPD/OFD × 100. Fortunately, the formula is calculated by most of the present-day equipment. A cephalic index of less than 75 denotes a dolichocephalic shape, whereas an index of more than 85 denotes a brachiocephalic shape.

SOUND OFF
A cephalic index of less than 75 denotes a dolichocephalic shape, whereas an index of more than 85 denotes a brachiocephalic shape.

Lateral Ventricle Measurement

The diameter of the lateral ventricle can be easily measured with sonography. The lateral ventricle is measured in the transaxial plane at the level of the atrium (Fig. 24-12). The atrium of the lateral ventricle is the optimal site for measuring the lateral ventricle, because it is the first region where ventricular enlargement occurs. The calipers are placed at the level of the **glomus** of the choroid plexus. The normal lateral ventricle does not typically measure more than 10 mm at the level of the atrium. Enlargement beyond 10 mm is referred to as **ventriculomegaly**.

SOUND OFF
The normal lateral ventricle does not typically measure more than 10 mm at the level of the atrium.

Transcerebellar Measurement

The cerebellum grows at a rate of 1 mm per week between 14 and 21 weeks and thus correlates agreeably with the gestational age of the fetus. That means, the cerebellum of a 16-week fetus will measure approximately 16 mm. The cerebellum is measured in the transverse plane at the same level as the cisterna magna and thalamus (Fig. 24-13). The CSP will also be in the image. This measurement, referred to as the transcerebellar diameter (TCD), will likely lose its accuracy in the presence of chromosomal abnormalities, typically measuring smaller than normal. And though it may be difficult to obtain in later gestation owing to fetal position, it has proven to be useful in several studies as an indicator of growth restriction or large for gestational age when other measurements are lacking.

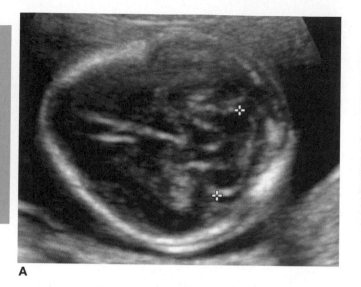

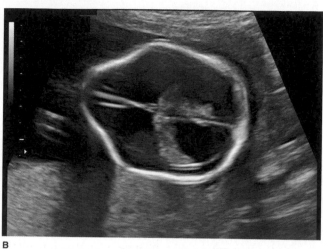

A

B

Figure 24-11 Strawberry skull versus lemon skull. **A.** A strawberry-shaped calvarium in a 19-week fetus with trisomy 18. The cerebellum is measured between the calipers. **B.** Transverse sonogram of the fetal head shows scalloping of the frontal bones, which is consistent with the lemon sign associated with open spina bifida. Note that in **B**, there is dramatic indentation of the frontal bones compared to **A**.

> **SOUND OFF**
> The cerebellum of a 16-week fetus will measure approximately 16 mm in diameter.

Cisterna Magna Measurement

Sonographic measurement of the depth of the cisterna magna can be performed as well (see Fig. 24-13). The depth of the cisterna magna should not measure more than 10 mm or less than 2 mm in the transcerebellar plane. Measurement more than 10 mm is consistent with **mega cisterna magna** and **Dandy–Walker complex**, whereas a measurement of less than 2 mm is worrisome for **Arnold–Chiari II malformation**.

> **SOUND OFF**
> The depth of the cisterna magna should not measure more than 10 mm or less than 2 mm in the transcerebellar plane

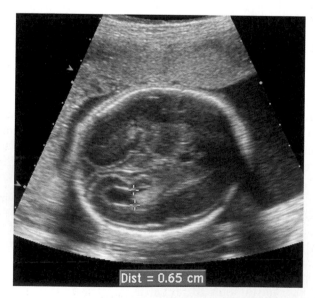

Dist = 0.65 cm

Figure 24-12 Lateral ventricular measurement. Axial view of the head demonstrating measurement of the width of the lateral ventricle at the level of the atrium, with "+" *calipers* placed on the ventricular wall.

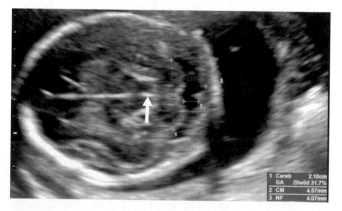

1 Cereb	2.10cm
GA	20w0d 31.7%
2 CM	4.57mm
3 NF	4.07mm

Figure 24-13 Transcerebellar plane—nuchal fold. The landmarks of the transcerebellar plane are the thalamus (*T*), the inferior portion of the third ventricle (*arrow*) near where it joins the aqueduct, and the cisterna magna (*cm*). Measurements, which are routinely made at this level, include the transverse cerebellum (*1*), which in mm approximates the gestational age, the anteroposterior dimension of the cisterna magna (*2*), and the thickness of the nuchal fold (*3*) in the second trimester, which is normal at less than 6 mm.

CEREBRAL MALFORMATIONS

Ventriculomegaly and Hydrocephalus

The abnormal enlargement of the ventricles within the brain is referred to as ventriculomegaly. **Hydrocephalus** refers to dilatation (dilation) of the ventricular system caused by an increased volume of CSF, resulting in increased intraventricular pressure. Hydrocephalus may be reserved for cases of ventriculomegaly that are more severe and are caused by some type of obstruction to the flow of CSF, resulting in a backup of the fluid in the cerebral ventricles. Therefore, obstructive hydrocephalus is the buildup of CSF within the ventricular system secondary to some type of obstruction.

Ventriculomegaly has been cited as the most common cranial abnormality. Suspicion of ventricular dilatation occurs when the atrial diameter measures more than 10 mm. The lateral ventricle that will be readily seen on sonography is most often the ventricle farthest from the transducer. The sonographic finding of the **"dangling choroid" sign** describes the echogenic choroid plexus, hanging limp, and surrounded by CSF, within the dilated lateral ventricle. This finding is exceedingly specific for ventriculomegaly (Fig. 24-14).

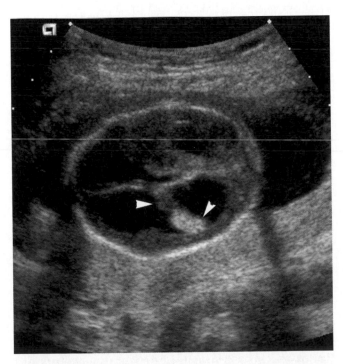

Figure 24-14 Dangling choroid sign. Axial view of the fetal cranium with ventriculomegaly demonstrating choroid plexus (*arrowheads*) dangling within the dilated ventricle.

> ### 🔊 SOUND OFF
> The sonographic finding of the "dangling choroid" sign describes the echogenic choroid plexus, hanging limp, and surrounded by CSF, within the dilated lateral ventricle.

Hydrocephalus can be described further as mild, moderate, or severe. There are two main types of hydrocephalus, communicating and noncommunicating. **Communicating hydrocephalus** is apparent when the obstruction lies outside the ventricular system, whereas **noncommunicating hydrocephalus** is when the obstruction level is located within the ventricular system.

Although hemorrhagic obstruction and the subsequent enlargement of the ventricles can occur in utero, congenital obstruction of the ventricular system, by means of **aqueductal stenosis**, remains the most common cause of hydrocephalus in utero. There are also other etiologies of hydrocephalus, including many chromosomal aberrations and intrauterine infections.

SONOGRAPHIC FINDINGS OF VENTRICULOMEGALY

1. Atrium of the lateral ventricle measures greater than 10 mm
2. Atrial measurement greater than 15 mm is considered moderate to marked ventriculomegaly
3. Dangling choroid sign
4. Dilatation of any part of the ventricular system

Aqueductal Stenosis

Aqueductal stenosis, as stated previously, is the most common cause of hydrocephalus in utero. The cerebral aqueduct (aqueduct of Sylvius), located between the third and fourth ventricles of the brain, may be narrowed, thus preventing the flow of CSF from the third to the fourth ventricle. This obstruction level will cause the third ventricle and both the lateral ventricles to expand, whereas the fourth ventricle remains normal.

SONOGRAPHIC FINDINGS OF AQUEDUCTAL STENOSIS

1. Atrium of the lateral ventricle measures greater than 10 mm
2. Atrial measurement greater than 15 mm is considered moderate to marked ventriculomegaly
3. Dangling choroid sign
4. Dilatation of the lateral ventricles and the third ventricle; the fourth ventricle remains normal

🔊 **SOUND OFF**
Aqueductal stenosis is the most common cause of hydrocephalus in utero.

Hydranencephaly

Hydranencephaly is a fatal condition in which the entire cerebrum is replaced by a large sac containing CSF (Fig. 24-15). With hydranencephaly, the falx cerebri

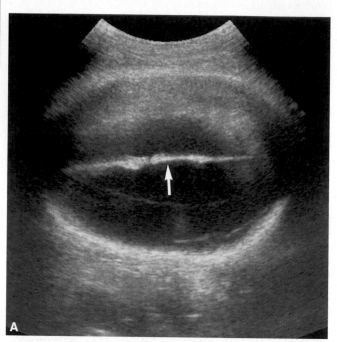

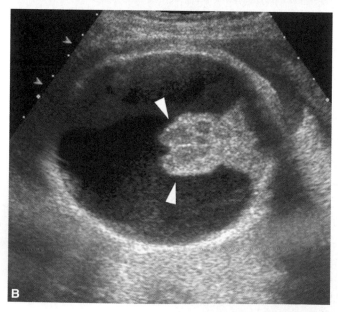

Figure 24-15 Hydranencephaly. **A.** Axial image of a fetus demonstrating a fluid-filled cranium with no visible cerebral cortex. Part of the falx cerebri (*arrow*) is noted within the midline of the brain. All findings are consistent with hydranencephaly. **B.** Hydranencephaly with the thalamus seen (*arrowheads*).

may be partially or completely absent, whereas the **brainstem** and **basal ganglia** are maintained and surrounded by CSF. The thalamus may be seen, but there will be no cerebral cortex identified.

There have been several postulations regarding the cause of hydranencephaly, including bilateral occlusion of the internal carotid arteries with subsequent destruction of the cerebral hemispheres. Another hypothesis is that intrauterine infections such as cytomegalovirus and toxoplasmosis lead to the destruction of the cerebral hemispheres. The brain may appear normal in the first trimester and then reflect hydranencephaly in the second or third trimester. Hydranencephaly can be difficult to differentiate with the sonographic findings of severe ventriculomegaly and **alobar holoprosencephaly**. It is important to note that with both severe ventriculomegaly and **holoprosencephaly**, there will typically be a rim of cerebral tissue maintained, whereas with hydranencephaly, there is no cerebral mantle present. Hydranencephaly is typically a fatal condition, with death occurring in the first year of life.

> **SONOGRAPHIC FINDINGS OF HYDRANENCEPHALY**
>
> 1. Fluid-filled cranium
> 2. Absent or partial absence of the falx cerebri
> 3. Maintained brainstem, basal ganglia, and, perhaps, the thalamus
> 4. No identifiable cerebral cortex

Holoprosencephaly

Holoprosencephaly is a midline brain anomaly that is associated with not only brain aberrations but also atypical facial structures. It may be detected with endovaginal imaging as early as the first trimester. There are three main types of holoprosencephaly: alobar, semilobar, and lobar. With alobar, the cortex can take on three basic shapes, resembling a "pancake," "cup," or "ball" (Fig. 24-16). Although the lobar form can be consistent with life, alobar holoprosencephaly is the most severe form, often resulting in neonatal death. Alobar holoprosencephaly is diagnosed when there is absence of the corpus callosum, CSP, third ventricle, interhemispheric fissure, and falx cerebri. There will also be evidence of a horseshoe-shaped **monoventricle**, and the lobes of the thalamus may be fused and echogenic in appearance (Fig. 24-17; Table 24-6). Conversely, the cerebellum and brainstem remain intact.

🔊 **SOUND OFF**
With holoprosencephaly, there will be evidence of a horseshoe-shaped monoventricle, and the lobes of the thalamus may be fused and echogenic in appearance.

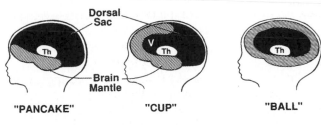

Figure 24-16 Sagittal drawing of pancake, cup, and ball holoprosencephaly morphology. The pancake type is described as having a flattened residual brain mantle at the base of the brain with a correspondingly large dorsal sac. The cup type has more brain mantle, but it does not cover the monoventricle. The dorsal sac communicates widely with the monoventricle. The ball type is described as when the brain mantle completely covers the monoventricle, and a dorsal sac may or may not be present. *Th,* thalami; *V,* ventricle.

TABLE 24-6 Facial anomalies associated with alobar holoprosencephaly

Cyclopia
Hypotelorism
Proboscis
(Median) cleft lip
Anophthalmia
Cebocephaly

Cyclopia, a condition in which the orbits are fused and contain a single eye, and **proboscis**, a false nose situated above the orbits, are two of the most disturbing external findings associated with holoprosencephaly. Other facial anomalies such as **anophthalmia**,

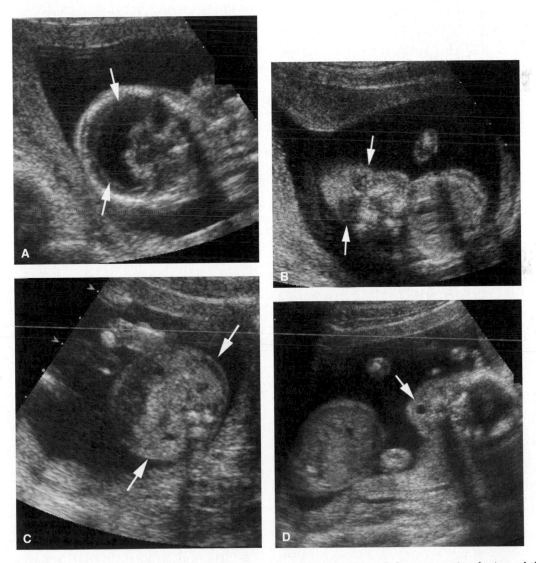

Figure 24-17 Holoprosencephaly and trisomy 13. **A.** Coronal image of fetal head demonstrating fusion of the ventricles into a large monoventricle (*arrows*) and absence of the falx, characteristic of alobar holoprosencephaly. **B.** Coronal image of the face showing the orbits (*arrows*) abnormally close together (hypotelorism). **C.** Transverse image of fetal abdomen demonstrating enlarged, echogenic kidneys (*arrows*). **D.** Coronal image of face showing a midline facial defect (*arrow*).

hypotelorism, **median cleft lip**, and **cebocephaly** may be detected during a fetal sonogram as well. Chapter 25 further discusses facial abnormalities associated with holoprosencephaly. With the less devastating forms of holoprosencephaly, such as lobar, there are varying degrees of fusion of the midline structures. Infants with **lobar holoprosencephaly** may experience severe mental retardation. Trisomy 13, or Patau syndrome, is present in 50% to 70% of fetuses diagnosed with holoprosencephaly.

🔊)) SOUND OFF
Trisomy 13, or Patau syndrome, is present in 50% to 70% of fetuses diagnosed with holoprosencephaly.

SONOGRAPHIC FINDINGS OF ALOBAR HOLOPROSENCEPHALY

1. Horseshoe-shaped monoventricle
2. Fused echogenic thalami
3. Absence of the CSP, interhemispheric fissure, falx cerebri, corpus callosum, and third ventricle
4. Normal cerebellum and brainstem
5. Facial anomalies (e.g., cyclopia, proboscis, cebocephaly, facial clefts, hypotelorism)

Dandy–Walker Malformation and Mega Cisterna Magna

Dandy–Walker malformation (DWM) is actually a classification within a larger group of anomalies referred to as the **Dandy–Walker complex**. Dandy–Walker complex is a spectrum of posterior fossa abnormalities that involve the cystic dilatation of the cisterna magna and fourth ventricle. DWM is thought to be caused by a developmental abnormality in the roof of the fourth ventricle. The sonographic findings of DWM include an enlarged cisterna magna that communicates with a distended fourth ventricle through a defect in the cerebellum (Fig. 24-18). The cerebellar vermis is either completely absent or hypoplastic. As a result, the tentorium, the structure that separates the cerebrum from the cerebellum, is elevated. There are often other midline brain abnormalities present as well. For instance, agenesis of the corpus callosum, ventriculomegaly, holoprosencephaly, and cephaloceles are all associated anomalies of DWM.

Mega cisterna magna, which is the enlargement of the cisterna magna without the involvement of the fourth ventricle, may be confused with DWM. Mega cisterna magna is present when only the cisterna magna is enlarged, measuring more than 10 mm in depth. Consequently, the fourth ventricle is normal with mega cisterna magna and enlarged with DWM. It is important to note that in the early second trimester, the inferior portion of the cerebellar vermis may not be formed, thus making it appear as if the fetus has partial agenesis of the vermis. For this reason, care must be taken to visualize an intact cerebellar vermis. If the cerebellar vermis is absent and the fourth ventricle is enlarged, then DWM must be suspected.

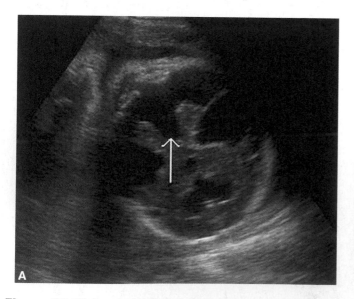
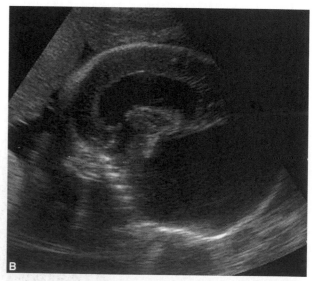

Figure 24-18 Dandy–Walker malformation. **A.** Axial image of Dandy–Walker malformation. The dilated fourth ventricle (*arrow*) is seen between the splayed lobes of the cerebellum, a finding consistent with Dandy–Walker malformation. **B.** Sagittal image of Dandy–Walker malformation. This sagittal image of the fetal cranium demonstrates an enlarged posterior fossa and ventriculomegaly.

SONOGRAPHIC FINDINGS OF DANDY–WALKER MALFORMATION

1. Enlargement of the cisterna magna greater than 10 mm in the anteroposterior dimension
2. Communication of the enlarged cisterna magna with a dilated fourth ventricle
3. Agenesis or hypoplasia of the cerebellar vermis
4. Varying degrees of ventriculomegaly

SONOGRAPHIC FINDINGS OF MEGA CISTERNA MAGNA

1. Enlargement of the cisterna magna greater than 10 mm in the anteroposterior dimension
2. Normal cerebellum and fourth ventricle

SOUND OFF
If the cerebellar vermis is absent and the fourth ventricle is enlarged, then DWM must be suspected.

Agenesis of the Corpus Callosum and Cavum Septum Pellucidum

The corpus callosum is a bridge of tissue located within the midline of the brain that connects the two cerebral hemispheres. It functionally provides a pathway for communication between the hemispheres and is completely formed by 18 weeks. The CSP, located inferior to the corpus callosum, and the corpus callosum develop at the same time. The congenital lack of these structures is termed agenesis, as in agenesis of the corpus callosum, and CSP. There can be partial or complete absence of the corpus callosum. Most often, if the corpus callosum is absent, the CSP will be absent as well. Their nonexistence has been linked to as many as 50 to 200 different syndromes and anomalies such as **Apert syndrome**, holoprosencephaly, DWM, aqueductal stenosis, trisomy 18, **trisomy 8**, and trisomy 13.

There are several distinct sonographic findings consistent with agenesis of the corpus callosum, including the obvious absence of this structure. The "sunburst" manifestation of the sulci is a straightforward and discernible sonographic finding. In the normal brain, the sulci within the cerebrum typically travel parallel to the corpus callosum, but with agenesis of the corpus callosum, they tend to have a more perpendicular or radial arrangement and often appear to have a "spoke-wheel" pattern. This pattern is better imaged in a sagittal plane to the fetal head (Fig. 24-19). **Colpocephaly**, small frontal horns and

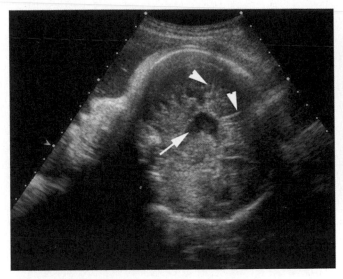

Figure 24-19 Apert syndrome with agenesis of the corpus callosum. Sagittal image of a fetus with Apert syndrome revealing agenesis of the corpus callosum with the typical spoke-wheel or sunburst pattern of the sulci (*arrowheads*) and the elevation and dilation of the third ventricle (*arrow*).

enlarged occipital horns, is often present as well and offers a distinct teardrop shape to the lateral ventricles. In addition, with the absence of the CSP and corpus callosum, the third ventricle tends to migrate more superiorly and appear dilated.

SOUND OFF
With agenesis of the corpus callosum, the sulci tend to have a more perpendicular or radial arrangement and often appear to have a "spoke-wheel" pattern.

SONOGRAPHIC FINDINGS OF AGENESIS OF THE CORPUS CALLOSUM AND CAVUM SEPTUM PELLUCIDUM

1. Partial or complete absence of the corpus callosum and absence of the CSP (after 18 weeks)
2. "Sunburst" sign—radial arrangement of the sulci that produces a "spoke-wheel" pattern
3. Colpocephaly—small frontal horns and enlarged occipital horns (teardrop-shaped lateral ventricles)
4. Elevated and dilated third ventricle

Schizencephaly

Schizencephaly is associated with the development of fluid-filled clefts within the cerebrum. The etiology of schizencephaly is unknown, although there may be an association with intrauterine exposure to some illicit drugs. It may be described as open lip or closed lip, with open lip being more readily identified

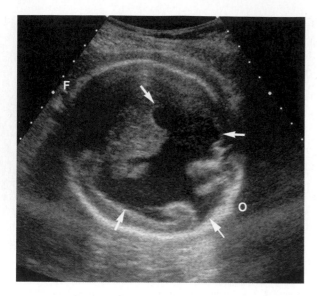

Figure 24-20 Schizencephaly. Axial image of the fetal cranium demonstrating a large irregular asymmetric fluid space (*arrows*) replacing portions of the parietal lobes and occipital lobes on each side, representing large clefts in the brain. F, frontal bone; O, occipital bone

in utero. The sonographic appearance of open lip schizencephaly is that of a cerebrum containing gray matter–lined clefts filled containing anechoic CSF (Fig. 24-20). There are several associated anomalies, such as agenesis of the corpus callosum and CSP, and ventriculomegaly.

SONOGRAPHIC FINDINGS OF SCHIZENCEPHALY

1. Fluid-filled clefts within the cerebrum
2. Agenesis of the CSP and corpus callosum (50% of the time)
3. Ventriculomegaly

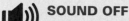 **SOUND OFF**
Schizencephaly is associated with the development of fluid-filled clefts within the cerebrum.

Porencephaly

Porencephaly is a rare condition in which a cyst communicates with the ventricular system. Porencephaly can occur after the fetus has experienced hemorrhage within one or both of the cerebral hemispheres. As the hemorrhage changes states, it will form into a cystic cavity and will eventually communicate with the lateral ventricle of the affected side (Fig. 24-21). This condition may be caused by ischemic events or vascular occlusion within the brain. **Arachnoid cysts** can be confused with porencephaly. It is important to note that arachnoid cysts will not communicate with the ventricular system.

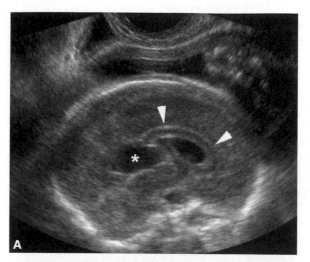

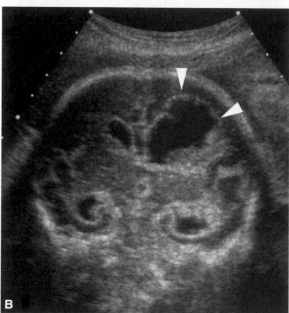

Figure 24-21 Arachnoid cyst versus porencephaly. **A.** An arachnoid cyst (*asterisk*) is seen posterior to the corpus callosum (*arrowheads*) in this sagittal image. **B.** Porencephaly (*arrowheads*) is noted in this coronal image following an intracranial hemorrhage. Note that the porencephalic cyst communicates with the lateral ventricle.

SONOGRAPHIC FINDINGS OF PORENCEPHALY

1. Cystic mass that communicates with the lateral ventricle
2. Most often unilateral

Lissencephaly

Lissencephaly literally means "smooth brain." It is a condition in which there are no gyri within the cerebral cortex. Agyria, and the absence of sulci within the brain, is not typically diagnosed until the third trimester or postnatally and almost always carries a poor prognosis.

1. Lack of sulci and gyri within the cerebrum

Choroid Plexus Cysts

Choroid plexus cysts are cysts located within the choroid plexus of the lateral ventricles. These small cysts are frequently encountered during a routine sonographic examination and typically regress by the end of the third trimester, although there is an association with trisomy 18. A choroid plexus cyst will be located within the choroid plexus of the lateral ventricle, measure more than 2 mm, appear round and anechoic, and have smooth walls (Fig. 24-22).

SONOGRAPHIC APPEARANCE OF A CHOROID PLEXUS CYST

1. Anechoic, round, smooth-walled cyst located within the choroid plexus of the lateral ventricle

SOUND OFF
Choroid plexus cysts often regress, although there is a slight association with trisomy 18.

NEURAL TUBE DEFECTS AND THE BRAIN

Neural tube defects occur when the embryonic neural tube fails to close. Among the list of neural tube defects are cephaloceles, various **spinal dysraphisms**, **anencephaly**, and spina bifida. Anencephaly and spina bifida are the most common neural defects, occurring in 1 per 1,000 pregnancies. Although several causes have been implicated, such as maternal diabetes and the use of valproic acid (seizure medication), chromosomal anomalies, including Edwards syndrome (trisomy 18), Patau syndrome (trisomy 13), and **triploidy**, have all been linked with neural tube defects.

Fortunately, studies have shown that a supplement of 0.4 mg of **folate** (folic acid) in a woman's diet significantly reduces the likelihood of her fetus developing a neural tube defect. Screening for neural tube defects is achieved by a combination of sonography, amniocentesis, and/or maternal serum screening. Maternal serum screening, also referred to as the triple screen, combines the laboratory values of human chorionic gonadotropin, estriol, and maternal serum alpha-fetoprotein (MSAFP), particularly helpful for detecting neural tube defects is the MSAFP component of this test.

Alpha-fetoprotein (AFP) is initially produced by the yolk sac, fetal gastrointestinal tract, and the fetal liver. AFP exits the fetus through an opening in the neural tube if one is present (i.e., an opening in the cranium or spine), thus allowing for a greater amount to pass into the maternal circulation. However, increased levels of AFP may not always indicate that a neural tube defect is present. Elevated levels of AFP are also found with **omphalocele**, **gastroschisis**, multiple gestations, fetal demise, and incorrect gestational dating.

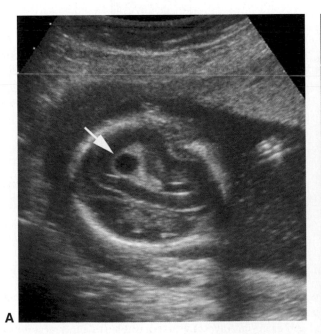
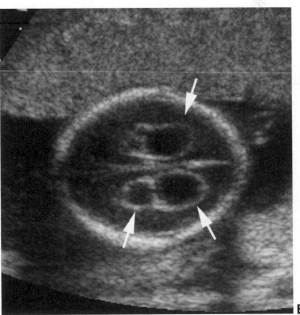

Figure 24-22 Choroid plexus cysts. **A.** Oblique image of fetal head showing single choroid plexus cyst (*arrow*). **B.** Axial image of fetal head showing multiple bilateral choroid plexus cysts (*arrows*).

> ### 🔊 SOUND OFF
> AFP exits the fetus through an opening in the neural tube if one is present (i.e., an opening in the cranium or spine), thus allowing for a greater amount to pass into the maternal circulation.

Acrania (Anencephaly and Exencephaly)

Acrania remains one of the most common neural tube defects. Acrania is defined as the absence of the cranial vault above the bony orbits. It can be further divided into two main subtypes depending on the amount of cerebral tissue present, anencephaly and **exencephaly**. Anencephaly is considered when there are no cerebral hemispheres present, whereas exencephaly denotes a normal amount of cerebral tissue. Nonetheless, the cranium is absent, making this condition fatal. The sonographic appearance of anencephaly has been described as having "froglike" **facies**, or bulging eyes, and the absence of the cranial vault (Fig. 24-23). It is important to note that there may be an active fetal heartbeat and fetal movement as well.

CLINICAL FINDINGS OF ACRANIA/ANENCEPHALY

1. Elevated MSAFP

SONOGRAPHIC FINDINGS OF ACRANIA/ANENCEPHALY

1. Absent cranial vault
2. Some cerebral tissue may be present
3. "Froglike" facies or bulging eyes
4. Possible fetal movement and active fetal heart tones

> ### 🔊 SOUND OFF
> The sonographic appearance of anencephaly has been described as having "froglike" facies, or bulging eyes, and the absence of the cranial vault.

Arnold–Chiari II Malformation and Spina Bifida

Arnold–Chiari II or Chiari II malformation is a group of cranial abnormalities associated with the neural tube defect spina bifida. Spina bifida may result in a mass that protrudes from the spine. This mass can be referred to as a **meningocele** or **myelomeningocele**, depending on its contents. The most common location of spina bifida is within the distal lumbosacral region (Fig. 24-24). Several notable changes occur within the brain and skull with spina bifida. The frontal bones become flattened and will yield a lemon shape to the cranium, which is referred to as the "lemon" sign, often referred to as **scalloping** of the frontal bones (Fig. 24-25). The cerebellum will become displaced inferiorly and posteriorly and appear curved in the presence of

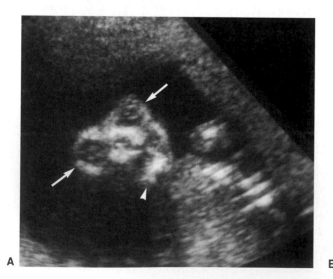

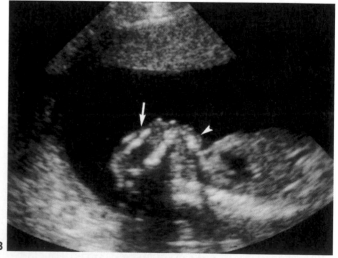

Figure 24-23 Anencephaly. **A.** Coronal image of the fetal face demonstrating the absence of the forehead and cranium with the typical "froglike" facies (*arrows*) of anencephaly. The mandible is normally formed (*arrowhead*). **B.** Sagittal image of the same fetus demonstrating the absence of the forehead and cranium (*arrow*). The mandible (*arrowhead*) and lower face appear normal.

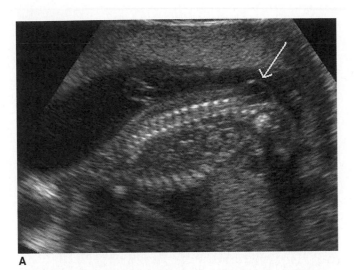

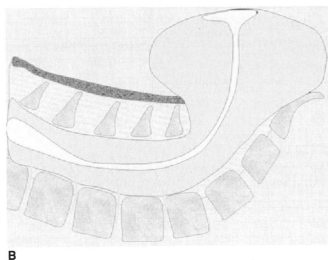

A

B

Figure 24-24 Myelomeningocele. **A.** Sagittal image of the fetal spine demonstrating a myelomeningocele (*arrow*) located in the distal spine. **B.** Sagittal diagram of myelomeningocele.

spina bifida, which is referred to as the "banana" sign (Fig. 24-26). As a result of the cerebellum being displaced inferiorly, the cisterna magna is completely obliterated. Posterior fossa abnormalities and their sonographic findings are provided in Table 24-7. A posterior fossa abnormality such as Chiari II malformation should be suspected if the cisterna magna is not visualized. The lateral ventricles will also be distorted in shape. The frontal horns will be small and slit like, whereas the occipital horns will be enlarged, a condition known as colpocephaly.

SOUND OFF
The cerebellum will become displaced inferiorly and posteriorly and appear curved in the presence of spina bifida, which is referred to as the "banana" sign, whereas the head shape will be shaped like a lemon ("lemon sign"). Remember, when open spina bifida is present, both yellow fruit signs (lemon sign and banana sign) are demonstrated in the skull.

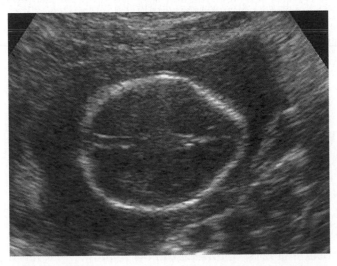

Figure 24-25 Lemon sign. Axial view of the fetal cranium demonstrating the lemon sign found in Arnold-Chairi II malformation and most cases of open spina bifida.

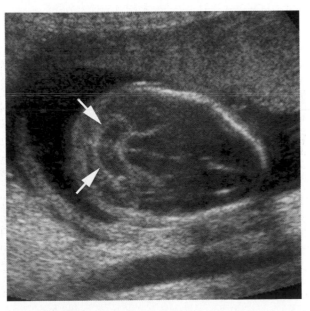

Figure 24-26 Banana sign. Axial image of the posterior fossa revealing a banana-shaped cerebellum (*arrows*) associated with a myelomeningocele. This is consistent with Arnold–Chiari II malformation.

TABLE 24-7 Posterior fossa abnormalities and their sonographic findings

Posterior Fossa Abnormality	Sonographic Findings
Mega cisterna magna	Enlargement of the cisterna magna >10 mm in the anteroposterior dimension Normal cerebellum
Dandy–Walker malformation	Enlargement of the cisterna magna >10 mm in the anteroposterior dimension Absent cerebellar vermis Enlarged fourth ventricle
Arnold–Chiari II malformation	Obliterated cisterna magna Banana-shaped cerebellum Lemon-shaped skull

TABLE 24-8 Different types of cephaloceles and their contents

Type of Cephalocele	Content of the Mass
Meningocele	Meninges only
Encephalocele	Brain tissue only
Encephalomeningocele	Both meninges and brain tissue
Encephalomeningocystocele	Meninges, brain tissue, and lateral ventricle

CLINICAL FINDINGS OF ARNOLD–CHIARI II MALFORMATION

1. Elevated MSAFP

SONOGRAPHIC FINDINGS OF ARNOLD–CHIARI II MALFORMATION

1. Lemon sign—lemon-shaped cranium with flattened or scalloped frontal bones
2. Banana sign—banana-shaped cerebellum
3. Obliterated cisterna magna
4. Colpocephaly
5. Enlarged massa intermedia
6. Hydrocephalus
7. Open spinal defect

Cephaloceles

Cephaloceles are protrusions of intracranial contents through a defect in the skull. Table 24-8 provides a description of the different types of cephaloceles based on their content. Cephaloceles can also be distinguished by their location. The most common location for a cephalocele is in the occipital region (Fig. 24-27). However, cephaloceles may also have frontal and parietal positions. Anterior cephaloceles often lead to hypertelorism. Encephaloceles, which include brain tissue, are common findings in Meckel–Gruber syndrome and have varying sonographic appearances based on their content.

CLINICAL FINDINGS OF CEPHALOCELES

1. Possible elevation of MSAFP

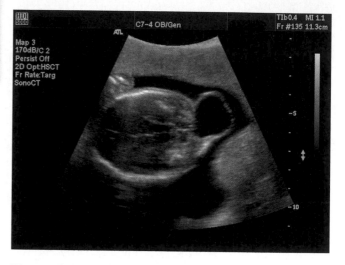

Figure 24-27 Occipital cephalocele. Axial image of the fetal skull revealing a cystic mass protruding from the occipital region, representing a cephalocele.

SONOGRAPHIC FINDINGS OF CEPHALOCELES

1. Open cranial defect (typically posterior in location)
2. Small or obliterated cisterna magna
3. Complex- or simple-appearing mass protruding from the cranium

SOUND OFF
The most common location for a cephalocele is in the occipital region.

THE EFFECTS OF FETAL INFECTIONS ON THE BRAIN

Maternal serum screening for intrauterine infections resulting from **t**oxoplasmosis, **o**ther agents, **r**ubella, **c**ytomegalovirus, and **h**erpes simplex virus (TORCH) can be performed. This is referred to as a TORCH

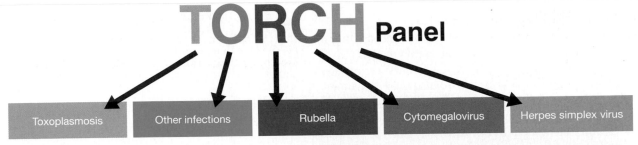

A

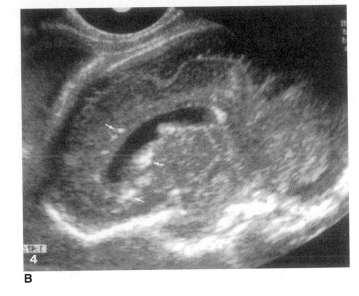

B

Figure 24-28 TORCH and intracranial calcifications. **A.** TORCH acronym defined. **B.** Parasagittal transvaginal sonogram of the fetal brain at 31 weeks' gestation shows abnormal underdeveloped gyri and calcifications (*arrows*) associated with cytomegalovirus.

panel (Fig. 24-28). Although cytomegalovirus has been listed as the most common in utero infection, other infections, such as zika virus, toxoplasmosis, rubella, parvovirus, varicella zoster, and herpes simplex, occur less often but may have devastating effects on the fetus. The sonographic intracranial findings consistent with intrauterine infections are the calcifications around the ventricles (periventricular) and ventriculomegaly. TORCH will be further discussed in Chapter 32.

> **SOUND OFF**
> The sonographic intracranial findings consistent with intrauterine infections are the calcifications around the ventricles and ventriculomegaly.

FETAL INTRACRANIAL TUMORS

The most common intracranial tumor found in utero is the teratoma. Teratomas contain tissues such as hair, sebum, and fat and most often appear as complex masses that distort the normal architecture of the brain. Choroid plexus papillomas are found within the choroid plexus and produce an increase in the production of

CSF, which, in turn, leads to ventriculomegaly. Other sonographic findings associated with brain tumors are macrocephaly and intracranial calcifications. Corpus callosum lipomas may also be present with agenesis of the corpus callosum. A lipoma will appear as a solid echogenic mass.

> **SOUND OFF**
> The most common intracranial tumor found in utero is the teratoma.

FETAL INTRACRANIAL HEMORRHAGE (INTRAVENTRICULAR HEMORRHAGE)

Although **intracranial hemorrhage** is worrisome for premature infants weighing less than 1,500 g and those born before 32 weeks' gestation, it occurs less often in utero. Maternal use of cocaine, trauma, and a history of amniocentesis are all listed as predisposing condition of fetal intracranial hemorrhage; however, the most common risk factor for fetal intrauterine intracranial hemorrhage has been listed as maternal platelet disorders. Most often, the origin of **intracranial hemorrhage**, also referred to as **intraventricular hemorrhage**, is within the **germinal matrix**.

The germinal matrix is a group of thin-walled, pressure-sensitive vessels located in the **subependymal layer** of the ventricles. These vessels are prone to rupture secondary to their thin walls. The hemorrhage can spread into the lateral ventricle, often leading to noncommunicating hydrocephalus, because the clot obstructs the flow of CSF within the narrowed regions of the ventricular system. Hemorrhage can also occur within the **parenchyma** of the brain. Localized areas of hemorrhage within the cerebral hemispheres will eventually lead to the formation of cystic cavities that communicate with the ventricular system, a condition known as porencephaly (see Fig. 24-21).

DOPPLER INTERROGATION OF THE FETAL BRAIN

Doppler of the Middle Cerebral Artery

The normal cerebral circulation typically yields a high-impedance Doppler pattern, with continuous forward flow throughout the cardiac cycle. Doppler assessment of the middle cerebral artery (MCA) has been shown effective at evaluating for potential **hypoxia** in fetuses that are small for dates (Fig. 24-29). When the fetus is starved for oxygen, redistribution of the blood to the vital organs—such as the brain—occurs in order to spare it from damage. This is referred to as the brain-sparing effect. The pulsatility index of the MCA varies with gestational age, but normally decreases as the pregnancy progresses toward term. The resistance pattern of the MCA should be greater than that of the umbilical artery and thus should be compared when fetal shunting is suspected. The MCA/umbilical artery resistive index is normally above 1.0, whereas an index lower than 1.0 is considered abnormal.

SOUND OFF
The resistance pattern of the MCA should be greater than that of the umbilical artery and thus should be compared when fetal shunting is suspected.

Fetal Intracranial Vascular Anomalies

The **vein of Galen aneurysm** is an arteriovenous malformation that occurs within the fetal brain. The sonographic findings of a vein of Galen aneurysm is that of a large, anechoic mass within the midline of the cranium that, when interrogated with color and pulsed Doppler, fills with turbulent venous and arterial flow (Fig. 24-30). The fetus will also have signs **hydrops** and cardiomegaly. Newborns with this condition are prone to suffer from high cardiac output and congestive heart failure in the postnatal period.

CLINICAL FINDINGS OF VEIN OF GALEN ANEURYSM (NEONATAL)

1. Congestive heart failure

SONOGRAPHIC FINDINGS OF VEIN OF GALEN ANEURYSM

1. Anechoic mass within the midline of the brain that contains turbulent arterial and venous flow when interrogated with pulsed and color Doppler
2. Fetal hydrops
3. Cardiomegaly (caused by cardiac overload)

SOUND OFF
The vein of Galen aneurysm is associated with congestive heart failure in the newborn.

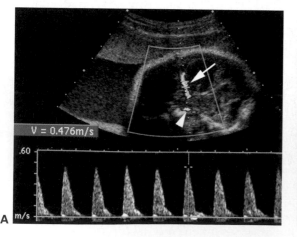
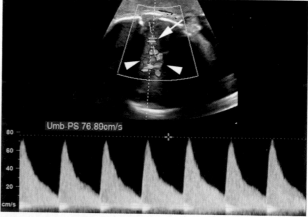

Figure 24-29 Middle cerebral artery Doppler. **A.** Color and spectral Doppler with Doppler gate (*arrow*) placed on the middle cerebral artery and the angle corrected to align with the vessel. The peak systolic velocity is normal for this 28-week fetus at 47.6 cm/s (*caliper*). A small section of the circle of Willis (*arrowhead*) is visible in color Doppler. **B.** Doppler gate on the middle cerebral artery (*arrow*) near its origin from the circle of Willis (*arrowheads*) with angle correction to align with the artery. The peak systolic velocity of 76.89 cm/s (*caliper*) is abnormally elevated in this 31-week fetus with anemia.

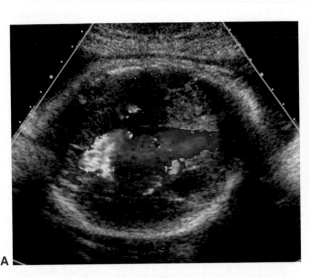

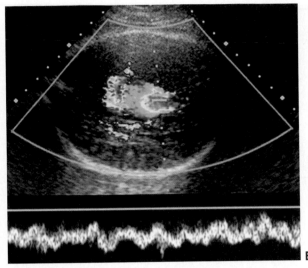

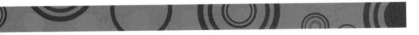

Figure 24-30 Doppler of vein of Galen. **A.** Color Doppler demonstrates high-velocity flow within the dilated vein of Galen. **B.** Color and spectral Doppler confirm the large amount of turbulent flow in this vascular lesion.

REVIEW QUESTIONS

1. The image in Figure 24-31 is indicative of what abnormality?
   a. Ventriculomegaly
   b. Holoprosencephaly
   c. Agenesis of the corpus callosum
   d. Hydranencephaly

3. What is the abnormality noted by the arrow in Figure 24-32?
   a. Subarachnoid hemorrhage
   b. Porencephaly
   c. DWM
   d. Hydranencephaly

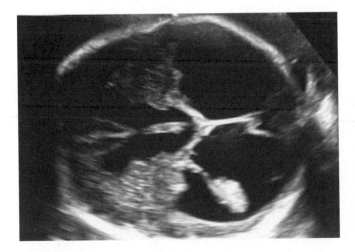

Figure 24-31

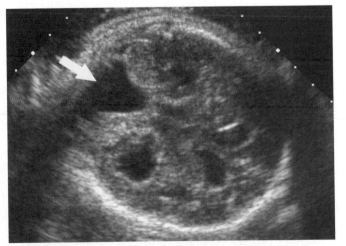

Figure 24-32

2. What is the sonographic sign in Figure 24-31?
   a. Pancake sign
   b. Monoventricle
   c. Dangling choroid
   d. Bilateral choroid plexus cysts

4. Which of the following is the most likely diagnosis for the fetus in Figure 24-33?
   a. Mega cisterna magna
   b. Holoprosencephaly
   c. Apert syndrome
   d. Anencephaly

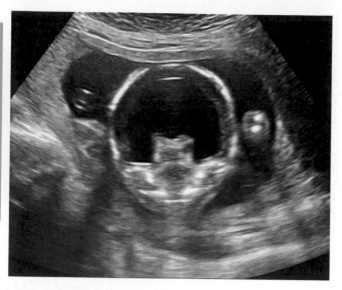

Figure 24-33

5. What sonographic finding is present in Figure 24-33?
   a. Absent cranial vault
   b. Choroid plexus cysts
   c. Colpocephaly
   d. Fused thalami

6. What do the arrows in Figure 24-34 indicate?
   a. Temporal thickening
   b. Ethmoidal enlargement
   c. Scalloped frontal bones
   d. Occipital flattening

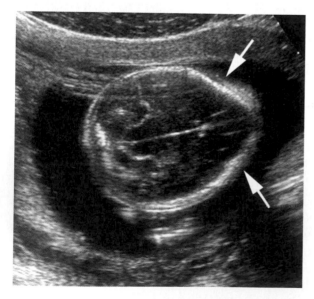

Figure 24-34

7. What is the sonographic sign indicated by the arrows in Figure 24-34?
   a. Lemon sign
   b. Banana sign
   c. Dangling choroid sign
   d. Pancake sign

8. The arrowheads in Figure 24-35 indicate the:
   a. corpus callosum.
   b. CSP.
   c. falx cerebri.
   d. cerebellar vermis.

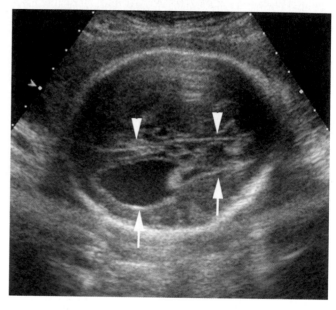

Figure 24-35

9. The arrows in Figure 24-35 are indicating what sonographic finding?
   a. Colpocephaly
   b. Cebocephaly
   c. Schizencephaly
   d. Dangling choroid

10. Which of the following is not part of Apert syndrome?
    a. Craniosynostosis
    b. Aqueductal stenosis
    c. Midline facial hypoplasia
    d. Syndactyly

11. What does the arrowhead in Figure 24-36 indicate?
    a. Cerebral aqueduct
    b. Lateral ventricle
    c. Third ventricle
    d. Fourth ventricle

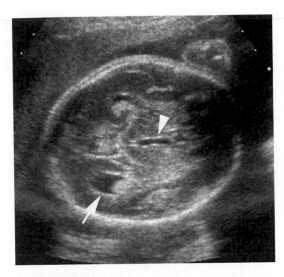

Figure 24-36

12. What part of the lateral ventricle is the arrow indicating in Figure 24-36?
    a. Temporal horn
    b. Body
    c. Anterior horn
    d. Occipital horn

13. Which of the following would be among the list of differential diagnoses for Figure 24-37?
    a. Dandy–Walker variant
    b. Severe ventriculomegaly
    c. Ventriculitis
    d. Mega cisterna magna

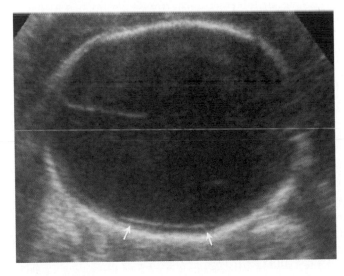

Figure 24-37

14. What abnormality is indicated by the arrow in Figure 24-38?
    a. Holoprosencephaly
    b. Arnold–Chiari II malformation
    c. Acrania
    d. Trisomy 18

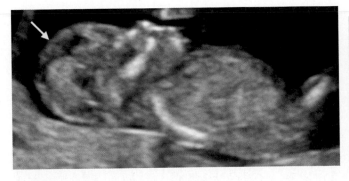

Figure 24-38

15. What does the arrow in Figure 24-39 indicate?
    a. Third ventricle
    b. Fourth ventricle
    c. CSP
    d. Cerebral aqueduct

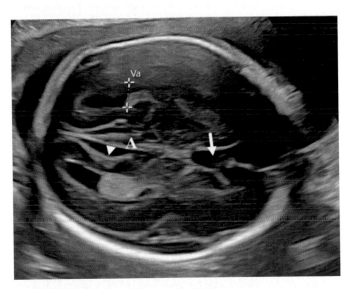

Figure 24-39

16. What part of the lateral ventricle is routinely measured within the fetal cranium?
    a. Atrium
    b. Frontal horn
    c. Temporal horn
    d. Occipital horn

17. What does the drawing in Figure 24-40 represent?
    a. Dolichocephaly
    b. Cloverleaf skull
    c. Brachycephaly
    d. Microcephaly

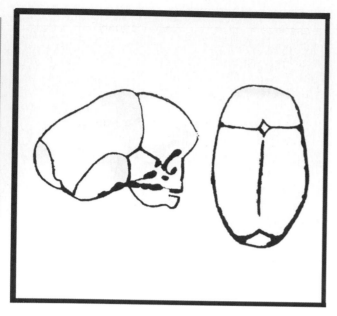

Figure 24-40

18. What measurement is being obtained with caliper #2 in Figure 24-41?
    a. BPD
    b. HC
    c. TCD
    d. OFD

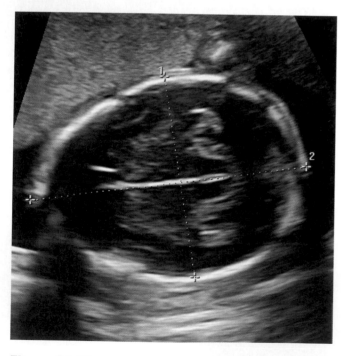

Figure 24-41

19. Which of the following is thought to be caused by bilateral occlusion of the fetal internal carotid arteries?
    a. Hydrocephalus
    b. Holoprosencephaly
    c. DWM
    d. Hydranencephaly

20. Which of the following is typically not seen at the level demonstrated in Figure 24-41?
    a. Thalamus
    b. Fourth ventricle
    c. Area of the third ventricle
    d. CSP

21. With what structure does the posterior fossa cyst associated with DWM communicate?
    a. Fourth ventricle
    b. Third ventricle
    c. Cerebellar vermis
    d. Cerebral aqueduct

22. The choroid plexus cyst could be associated with an increased risk of:
    a. trisomy 13.
    b. trisomy 4.
    c. Arnold–Chiari II malformation.
    d. trisomy 18.

23. All of the following are sonographic findings of Arnold–Chiari II malformation except:
    a. enlarged massa intermedia.
    b. hydrocephalus.
    c. obliteration of the cisterna magna.
    d. strawberry sign.

24. Which of the following is located on both sides of the midline?
    a. Interhemispheric fissures
    b. Third and fourth ventricles
    c. Lateral ventricles
    d. Third ventricle and cerebral aqueduct

25. Which of the following will also typically be absent with agenesis of the corpus callosum?
    a. Cerebellar vermis
    b. CSP
    c. Third ventricle
    d. Fourth ventricle

26. The double fold of dura mater that divides the cerebral hemispheres is the:
    a. cerebellum.
    b. CSP.
    c. corpus callosum.
    d. falx cerebri.

27. The development of fluid-filled cleft within the cerebrum is consistent with:
    a. holoprosencephaly.
    b. lissencephaly.
    c. schizencephaly.
    d. hydranencephaly.

28. The anechoic midline brain structure located between the frontal horns of the lateral ventricles is the:
    a. CSP.
    b. cavum vergae.
    c. corpus callosum.
    d. fourth ventricle.

29. The "sunburst" of the cerebral sulci is a sonographic finding of:
    a. DWM.
    b. agenesis of the corpus callosum.
    c. colpocephaly.
    d. hydranencephaly.

30. Enlargement of the occipital horns and narrowing of the frontal horns is termed:
    a. holoprosencephaly.
    b. DWM.
    c. colpocephaly.
    d. Apert syndrome.

31. The interthalamic adhesion (massa intermedia) passes through the:
    a. third ventricle.
    b. fourth ventricle.
    c. cisterna magna.
    d. CSP.

32. The most severe form of holoprosencephaly is:
    a. lobar.
    b. alobar.
    c. semilobar.
    d. lobular.

33. Which of the following is a genetic disorder that includes craniosynostosis, midline facial hypoplasia, and syndactyly?
    a. Lobar holoprosencephaly
    b. Beckwith–Wiedemann syndrome
    c. Arnold–Chiari II malformation
    d. Apert syndrome

34. The third ventricle is located:
    a. anterior to the thalamus.
    b. anterior to the cerebellar vermis.
    c. between the two lobes of the thalamus.
    d. superior to the corpus callosum.

35. What chromosomal aberration is most often associated with holoprosencephaly?
    a. Anophthalmia
    b. Trisomy 21
    c. Trisomy 13
    d. Trisomy 18

36. Dangling choroid sign is associated with:
    a. ventriculomegaly.
    b. hydranencephaly.
    c. lissencephaly.
    d. Meckel–Gruber syndrome.

37. The third ventricle communicates with the fourth ventricle at the:
    a. foramen of Magendie.
    b. foramen of Luschka.
    c. foramen of Monro.
    d. aqueduct of Sylvius.

38. The fourth ventricle is located:
    a. posterior to the CSP.
    b. between the frontal horns of the lateral ventricles.
    c. anterior to the cerebellar vermis.
    d. medial to the third ventricle.

39. The structure located between the two lobes of the cerebellum is the:
    a. cerebellar vermis.
    b. cerebellar tonsils.
    c. falx cerebri.
    d. corpus callosum.

40. A normal shaped skull is termed:
    a. dolichocephaly.
    b. brachycephaly.
    c. mesocephaly.
    d. scaphocephaly.

41. What is the most accurate head measurement for estimating gestational age in the second trimester?
    a. BPD.
    b. HC.
    c. transcerebellar measurement.
    d. lateral ventricle.

42. The cisterna magna should not exceed ____ in the transcerebellar plane.
    a. 4 mm
    b. 2 mm
    c. 8 mm
    d. 10 mm

43. A strawberry-shaped skull is commonly associated with:
    a. trisomy 21.
    b. trisomy 15.
    c. trisomy 18.
    d. trisomy 13.

44. Which of the following would be the most likely fetal cranial findings with TORCH infections?
    a. Intracranial calcifications
    b. Cerebral atrophy
    c. Porencephaly
    d. Scaphocephaly

45. The band of tissue that allows communication between the right and left cerebral hemispheres is the:
    a. falx cerebri.
    b. corpus callosum.
    c. cerebellar vermis.
    d. CSP.

46. A cloverleaf-shaped skull is related to:
    a. trisomy 18.
    b. Meckel–Gruber syndrome.
    c. trisomy 13.
    d. thanatophoric dysplasia.

47. A lemon-shaped skull is related to:
    a. trisomy 2.
    b. Arnold–Chiari II malformation.
    c. thanatophoric dysplasia.
    d. Beckwith–Wiedemann syndrome.

48. All of the following are sonographic features of alobar holoprosencephaly except:
    a. cyclopia.
    b. monoventricle.
    c. dorsal cyst.
    d. fused thalamus.

49. What cerebral abnormality are atypical facial features most commonly associated with?
    a. DWM
    b. Schizencephaly
    c. Lissencephaly
    d. Holoprosencephaly

50. The absence of the skull is:
    a. hydranencephaly.
    b. schizencephaly.
    c. acrania.
    d. ventriculomegaly.

51. What fetal suture is located within the frontal bone along the midline of the forehead?
    a. Squamosal suture
    b. Sagittal suture
    c. Lambdoidal suture
    d. Metopic suture

52. The most common cause of hydrocephalus in utero is:
    a. cerebral hemorrhage.
    b. holoprosencephaly.
    c. brain tumors.
    d. aqueductal stenosis.

53. The sonographic finding of a fluid-filled cranium with the absence of cerebral tissue is consistent with:
    a. hydrocephalus.
    b. hydranencephaly.
    c. holoprosencephaly.
    d. schizencephaly.

54. The lack of sulci within the fetal cerebrum is a reliable indicator of:
    a. agenesis of the corpus callosum.
    b. lissencephaly.
    c. schizencephaly.
    d. porencephaly.

55. A cisterna magna that measures 15 mm and a normal-appearing cerebellum is most likely:
    a. Arnold–Chiari II malformation.
    b. schizencephaly.
    c. mega cisterna magna.
    d. DWM.

56. What cerebral malformation is as a result of agenesis or hypoplasia of the cerebellar vermis?
    a. Arnold–Chiari II malformation
    b. Schizencephaly
    c. Mega cisterna magna
    d. DWM

57. Which of the following would not be normally located within the midline of the fetal brain?
    a. CSP
    b. Lobes of the thalamus
    c. Third ventricle
    d. Falx cerebri

58. What structures located along the falx cerebri reabsorb CSF into the venous circulation?
    a. Choroid plexus cells
    b. Choroid villi
    c. Arachnoid granulations
    d. Meninges

59. Following an intracranial hemorrhage, a cyst is noted within the cerebrum that communicates with the lateral ventricle. This is referred to as:
    a. schizencephaly.
    b. lissencephaly.
    c. holoprosencephaly.
    d. porencephaly.

60. Which of the following should not be included in the correct level for an HC measurement?
    a. Falx cerebri
    b. Fourth ventricle
    c. Thalamus
    d. CSP

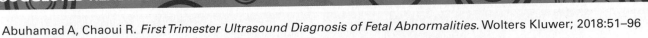

SUGGESTED READINGS

Abuhamad A, Chaoui R. *First Trimester Ultrasound Diagnosis of Fetal Abnormalities*. Wolters Kluwer; 2018:51–96 & 113–144.

Doubilet PM, Benson CB. *Atlas of Ultrasound in Obstetrics and Gynecology: A Multimedia Reference*. 2nd ed. Wolters Kluwer; 2012:49–84.

Gibbs RS, Karlan BY, Haney AF, et al. *Danforth's Obstetrics and Gynecology*. 10th ed. Wolters Kluwer; 2008:113 & 137–164.

Hagen-Ansert SL. *Textbook of Diagnostic Sonography*. 7th ed. Elsevier; 2012:1289–1310.

Haller J. *Textbook of Neonatal Ultrasound*. Parthenon; 1998:1–51.

Henningsen C, Kuntz K, Youngs D. *Clinical Guide to Sonography: Exercises for Critical Thinking*. 2nd ed. Elsevier; 2014:286–303.

Kline-Fath BM, Bulas DI, Lee W. *Fundamental and Advanced Fetal Imaging: Ultrasound and MRI*. 2nd ed. Wolters Kluwer; 2021:9–29 & 405–638.

Norton ME, Scoutt LM, Feldstein VA. *Callen's Ultrasonography in Obstetrics and Gynecology*. 6th ed. Elsevier; 2017:118–131 & 220–242.

Nyberg D, McGaham J, Pretorius D, et al. *Diagnostic Imaging of Fetal Anomalies*. Lippincott Williams & Wilkins; 2003:1–30 & 221–290.

Penny S. Agenesis of the corpus callosum: neonatal sonographic detection. *Radiol Technol*. 2006;78:14–18.

Rumack CM, Wilson SR, Charboneau W, et al. *Diagnostic Ultrasound*. 4th ed. Elsevier; 2011:1197–1244.

Sanders RC, Hall-Terracciano B. *Clinical Sonography: A Practical Guide*. 5th ed. Wolters Kluwer; 2016:295–341.

BONUS REVIEW!

Detailed Midline Brain Anatomy (Fig. 24-42)

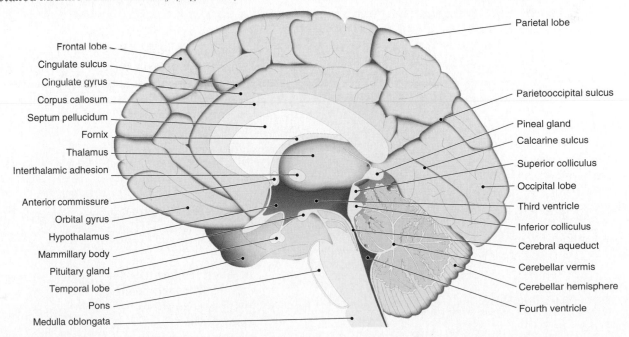

Figure 24-42

(continued)

BONUS REVIEW! (continued)

Three-Dimensional Sonogram of a Fetus with Amniotic Band Syndrome and Anencephaly (Fig. 24-43)

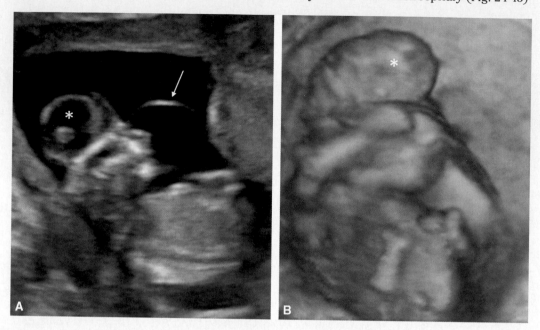

Figure 24-43 Transvaginal two-dimensional (**A**) and three-dimensional sonographic images (**B**) of a fetus at 13 weeks of gestation with severe brain malformation (anencephaly—*asterisk*) resulting from amniotic band syndrome. Note in **A** the presence of a reflective membrane within the amniotic cavity (*arrow*) that is attached to the fetal head. This reflective membrane represents an amniotic band.

The Fetal Face and Neck

Introduction

The astounding resolution and clarity provided by modern sonography equipment has afforded us the opportunity to study in detail the structures of the fetal face and neck. The fetal face may be evaluated using sagittal, axial, and coronal scan planes. Three-dimensional (3D) four-dimensional (4D), and surface rendering sonographic imaging of the face have each made an impact on the sonography profession, providing additional imaging configurations and a better understanding of cleft lip and cleft palate, as well as other features never before noted as clearly in utero. This chapter discusses several significant facial and neck abnormalities that may be discovered during a sonographic examination. In the "Bonus Review" section, a surface rendered image of the face, example of cyclopia, demonstration of fetal breathing, and nasal bone length are provided.

Key Terms

amniotic band syndrome—group of abnormalities associated with the entrapment of fetal parts in the amnion, often resulting in fetal amputations or clefting

anotia—absence of the ear(s)

aneuploidy—a condition of having an abnormal number of chromosomes

anophthalmia—absence of the eye(s)

Beckwith–Wiedemann syndrome—a growth disorder syndrome synonymous with enlargement of several organs, including the skull, tongue, and liver

binocular diameter (distance)—measurement from the lateral margin of one orbit to the lateral margin of the other orbit

branchial cleft cyst—benign congenital neck cysts found most often near the angle of the mandible

canthus—corners of the eyes

cebocephaly—close-set eyes (hypotelorism) and a nose with a single nostril

cleft lip—the abnormal division in the lip

cleft palate—the abnormal development of the soft and/or hard palate of the mouth where there is a division in the palate

cyclopia—fusion of the orbits

cystic hygroma—a mass, typically found in the neck region, that is the result of an abnormal accumulation of lymphatic fluid within the soft tissue

edema—abnormal swelling of a structure as a result of a fluid collection

epignathus—an oral teratoma

ethmocephaly—a condition in which there is no nose and a proboscis separating two close-set orbits; associated with holoprosencephaly

fetal goiter—diffuse enlargement of the fetal thyroid gland

fetal hydrops—an abnormal accumulation of fluid in at least two fetal body cavities

Goldenhar syndrome—rare congenital defect that consists of anophthalmia, abnormal lip and palate, maldevelopment or absence of the ear, and other facial abnormalities

holoprosencephaly—a group of brain abnormalities consisting of varying degrees of fusion of the lateral ventricles, absence of the midline structures, and associated facial anomalies

hypertelorism—increased distance between the orbits; widely spaced orbits

hypotelorism—reduced distance between the orbits

interocular diameter—the length between the orbits; measured from the medial margin of one orbit to the medial margin of the other orbit

macroglossia—an unusual protuberance of the tongue

micrognathia—a small mandible and recessed chin

microphthalmia—a decrease in the size of the eye

microtia—small ear(s)

nuchal—the posterior part or nape of the neck

nuchal fold—a collection of solid tissue on the posterior aspect of the fetal neck

nuchal fold thickness—a measurement taken in the second trimester of the skin on the posterior aspect of the fetal neck

nuchal translucency—the anechoic space along the posterior aspect of the fetal neck

ocular diameter—the measurement from the lateral margin of the orbit to the medial margin of the same orbit

teratoma—a tumor that typically consists of several germ cell layers

thyroglossal duct cyst—benign congenital cysts located within the midline of the neck superior to the thyroid gland and near the hyoid bone

Turner syndrome—a chromosomal aberration where one sex chromosome is absent; may also be referred to as monosomy X

FETAL FACIAL ABNORMALITIES

Holoprosencephaly and Fetal Facial Abnormalities

Whenever any form of **holoprosencephaly** is suspected, a thorough facial evaluation should be performed to assess for the associated facial abnormalities that often accompany this unfortunate brain malformation. Among the list of facial abnormalities that have been linked with holoprosencephaly are **hypotelorism**, **cebocephaly**, **ethmocephaly**, **cyclopia**, and **cleft lip** with or without **cleft palate**. These abnormalities are further discussed in this chapter, and several are demonstrated in Figures 25-1 and 25-2.

((•))) SOUND OFF
Whenever any form of holoprosencephaly is suspected, a thorough facial evaluation should be performed to assess for the associated facial abnormalities that often accompany this unfortunate brain malformation.

Fetal Eyes and Orbital Abnormalities

The globe of the fetal eye appears anechoic, while the lens is readily identifiable sonographically as a hypoechoic, round structure with a thin hyperechoic border in the anterior aspect of the globe. Occasionally, the hyaloid artery can be noted within the globe earlier in gestation. There are three measurements that can be obtained in the transverse plane of the fetal face at the level of the eyes (Fig. 25-3). The corners of the eyes are referred to as the medial **canthus** and the lateral canthus. The **ocular diameter** is a measurement that is obtained from the lateral canthus of the orbit to the medial canthus of the same orbit. This measurement should only be slightly smaller than the **interocular diameter**, which is the length between the orbits. The **binocular diameter** (distance) can also be obtained at

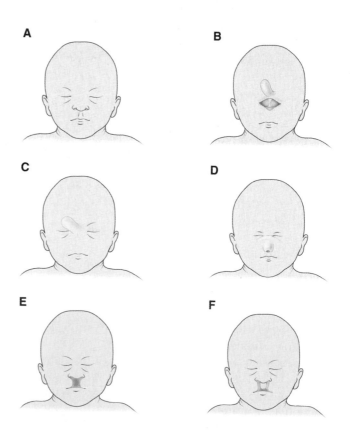

Figure 25-1 Faces of holoprosencephaly. **A.** Normal. **B.** Cyclopia. **C.** Ethmocephaly. **D.** Cebocephaly. **E.** Median cleft lip and palate. **F.** Bilateral cleft lip and palate.

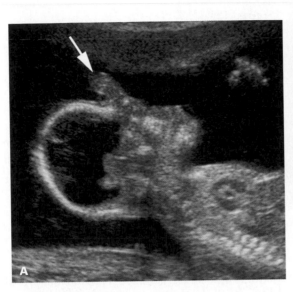

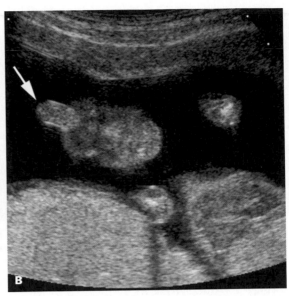

Figure 25-2 Proboscis in a fetus with alobar holoprosencephaly. **A.** Sagittal image of the face demonstrating very abnormal profile with proboscis (*arrow*) extending superiorly from the upper part of the face. Also, note the fluid-filled cranium associated with holoprosencephaly. **B.** Coronal image showing elevated and upward pointing proboscis (*arrow*) instead of a normal nose.

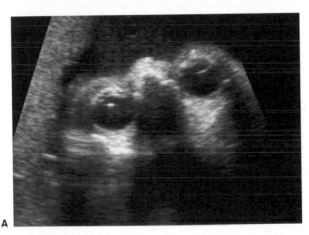

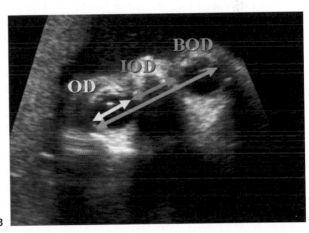

Figure 25-3 Normal orbits. **A.** Transverse view showing normal orbits. **B.** Normal orbital measurements of the ocular diameter (*OD*), interocular diameter (*IOD*), and binocular diameter (*BOD*). (Note the lenses are clearly seen in the anterior aspect of the eyes.)

the same level, and it includes both of the orbits. Thus, the binocular distance is the distance between the lateral canthi of each eye.

Microphthalmia is a decrease in the size of the eye. **Anophthalmia** is the absence of the eye(s). Anophthalmia is diagnosed when the globe and lens of the eye are absent. It results from the failure of the optic vesicle to form and has been linked with multiple abnormalities and chromosomal aberrations, including **Goldenhar syndrome**, trisomy 13, and trisomy 18. An increased distance between the orbits is referred to as **hypertelorism**, a disorder more accurately diagnosed utilizing the interocular diameter. An anterior cephalocele, which displaces the orbits laterally, has been cited as the most common cause of hypertelorism.

Hypertelorism is also associated with craniosynostosis and many chromosomal abnormalities.

A reduction in the distance between the orbits is referred to as hypotelorism (Fig. 25-4). The most common cause of hypotelorism has been cited to be holoprosencephaly, with trisomy 13 being the most frequently associated chromosomal abnormality.

> **SOUND OFF**
> An anterior cephalocele, which displaces the orbits laterally, has been cited as the most common cause of hypertelorism. Holoprosencephaly has been cited as the most common cause of hypotelorism.

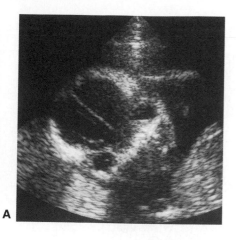

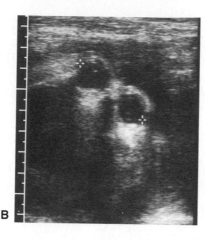

A

B

Figure 25-4 Hypertelorism versus hypotelorism. **A.** Coronal image of the fetal face showing hypertelorism. **B.** Transverse view showing hypotelorism.

Fetal Nasal Bone and Ears

As described in Chapter 23, the fetal nasal bone can be analyzed with sonography. There is a notable link between the absence of the fetal nasal bone and Down syndrome. The nasal bone can also be measured for signs of hypoplasia (see Fig. 23-18). For this reason, some institutions incorporate nasal bone imaging as part of the fetal screening protocol.

The ears can be easily imaged with sonography, and measurements can be taken as well (Fig. 25-5). Anomalies of the ears, including low-set ears, have been noted with trisomies 13, 18, and 21. Small ears, referred to as **microtia**, have a strong link with Down syndrome (trisomy 21). In addition, abnormally shaped ears may be a sign of a more worrisome underlying conditions or syndromes. The fetus may also fail to develop an ear, which is termed **anotia**.

Fetal Mouth, Lip, Mandible, and Maxilla

The fetal lip typically closes between 7 and 8 weeks, whereas the palate closes by 12 weeks. An abnormal closure or incomplete closure of the lip and palate results in cleft lip and cleft palate, respectively. These two abnormalities may exist together or as isolated findings. Cleft lip and cleft palate are among the most common congenital abnormalities and have been associated with many syndromes and congenital anomalies, such as holoprosencephaly, trisomy 13, and **amniotic band syndrome**, although most of the cases are not associated with any other abnormalities. Cleft lip can be unilateral, bilateral, or midline in location (Figs. 25-6 and 25-7). 3D sonography can be used to confirm the diagnosis of facial clefts (Fig. 25-8). Isolated cleft palate is more difficult to diagnose sonographically and may be missed altogether. Nonetheless, coronal and axial imaging of the face have been shown exceedingly effective in discovering these defects.

Macroglossia is defined as an unusual protuberance of the tongue. It is most commonly associated with **Beckwith–Wiedemann syndrome** and Down syndrome (Fig. 25-9). Macroglossia can be difficult to differentiate from **epignathus**, which is a mostly solid-appearing oral **teratoma**. Teratomas most often contain complex tissue, whereas the enlarged tongue of macroglossia is completely solid. Both macroglossia and epignathus can cause obstruction to the normal swallowing and inhalation of amniotic fluid that typically occurs throughout gestation; thus, they may be associated with polyhydramnios.

> 🔊 **SOUND OFF**
> Macroglossia is defined as an unusual protuberance of the tongue. It is most commonly associated with Beckwith–Wiedemann syndrome and Down syndrome.

An additional abnormal presentation of the facial bones takes place in the mandible. **Micrognathia**, a small mandible and recessed chin, is associated with trisomy 13 and trisomy 18 and has been found in several other syndromes and chromosomal aberrations. Micrognathia is best visualized in the sagittal view of the fetal face (Fig. 25-10).

The maxilla, though not often thoroughly analyzed during a sonographic examination, should always be considered for further analysis when fetal abnormalities are present. Of specific relevance is the length of the maxilla and if there are gaps in the bone. The maxilla tends to be short in fetuses with trisomy 21. This is secondary to the fact that the fetus affected with trisomy 21 tends to have flat facial feature with a prominent tongue. A gap in the maxilla in the sagittal plane is also suggestive of facial clefting. The prefrontal space distance can be obtained in these cases. For this measurement, a line is drawn from the anterior aspect of both the mandible and the maxilla and extended toward

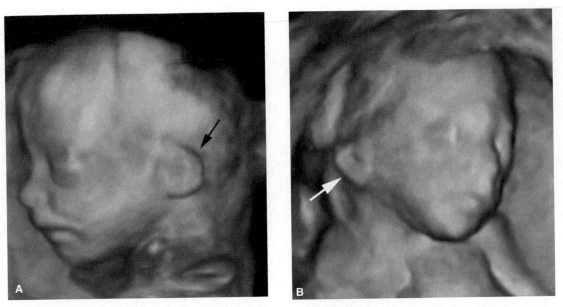

Figure 25-5 Fetal ears. **A.** Three-dimensional (3D) ultrasound of a 20-week fetal face viewed from the left side demonstrating the facial profile and the ear (*arrow*). **B.** Low-set ear with trisomy 21. 3D sonogram of fetal head and face showing abnormal low positioning of the ear (*arrow*).

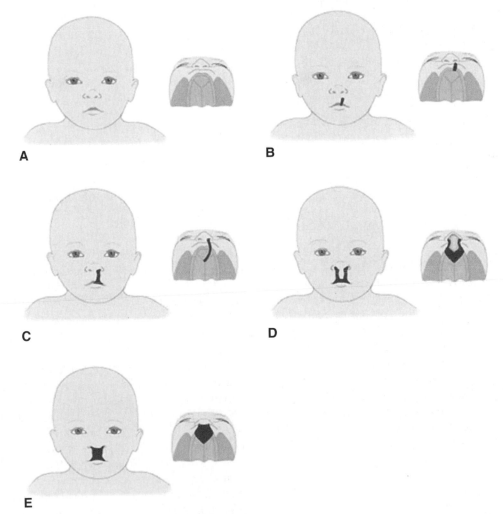

Figure 25-6 Classification of common types of clefts. **A.** Normal. **B.** Unilateral cleft lip (type 1). **C.** Unilateral cleft lip and palate (type 2). **D.** Bilateral cleft lip and palate (type 3). **E.** Median cleft lip and palate (type 4). Not shown are slash-type defects (type 5).

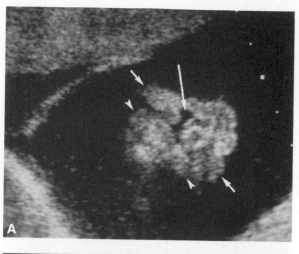

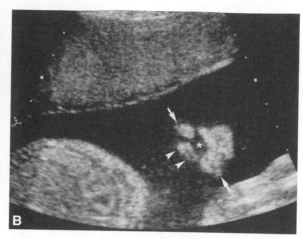

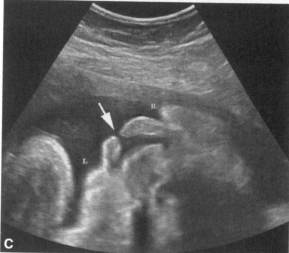

Figure 25-7 Cleft lip. **A.** Coronal image of lower face demonstrating large unilateral defect (*long arrow*) in the upper lip (*short arrows*) extending into the ipsilateral nostril. The lower lip (*arrowheads*) is seen inferior to the cleft. **B.** Coronal image of the same fetus slightly more anterior demonstrating large fluid-filled cleft (*asterisk*) in the upper lip (*arrows*) above the lower lip (*arrowheads*). **C.** Axial image of the upper lip showing defect (*arrow*) on the left. *L*, left; *R*, right.

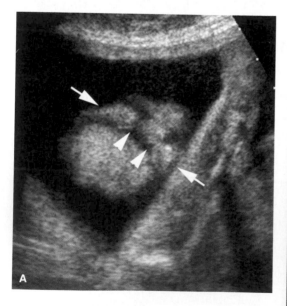

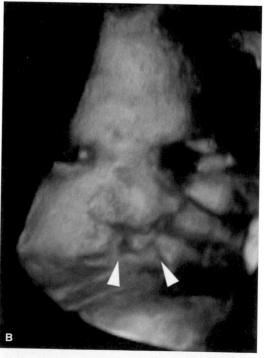

Figure 25-8 Bilateral cleft lip. **A.** Image of bilateral clefts (*arrowheads*) in upper lip (*arrows*). **B.** Three-dimensional image in the same fetus confirming bilateral clefts (*arrowheads*).

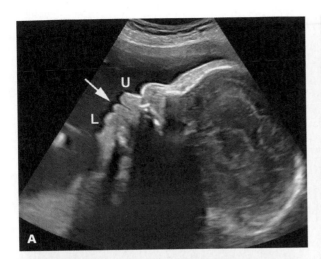

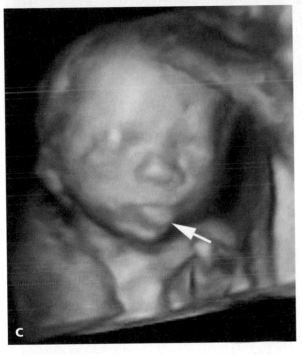

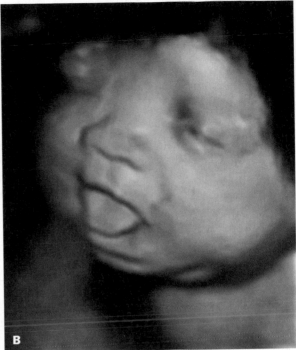

Figure 25-9 Macroglossia. **A.** Sagittal image of face demonstrating large tongue (*arrow*) protruding anteriorly between upper (*U*) and lower (*L*) lips. **B.** Three-dimensional (3D) image of the same fetus showing protruding tongue. **C.** 3D image in a fetus with trisomy 21 and enlarged tongue (*arrow*) seen protruding from the mouth.

the fetal forehead (Fig. 25-11). This analysis is typically performed between 11 and 14 weeks' gestation, and, although it is not a common measurement, it is most often obtained when flattened facial features are present or other facial abnormalities are suspected.

> **◀)) SOUND OFF**
> The maxilla tends to be short in fetuses with trisomy 21.

FETAL NECK ABNORMALITIES

Cystic Hygroma

A **cystic hygroma**, also referred to as a lymphangioma, results in an abnormal accumulation of lymphatic fluid within the soft tissue. The most common location of a cystic hygroma is within the neck, although it may be discovered within the axilla of the fetus or anywhere

lymph nodes can be found. Although they are often related, a cystic hygroma should not be confused with increased **nuchal translucency**, as discussed in Chapter 23, or **nuchal fold** thickening, discussed in the next section of this chapter. The sonographic appearance of a cystic hygroma is that of a cystic neck mass divided in the midline by a thick fibrous band of tissue (Fig. 25-12). The mass may contain smaller cystic areas with internal septations. Cystic hygromas have been found in many syndromes and chromosomal abnormalities, such as **Turner syndrome**, **fetal hydrops**, **aneuploidy**, trisomy 21, trisomy 18, and trisomy 13.

> **SONOGRAPHIC FINDINGS OF A CYSTIC HYGROMA**
>
> 1. Cystic neck mass divided in the midline by a thick fibrous band of tissue
> 2. The mass may contain smaller cystic areas with internal septations

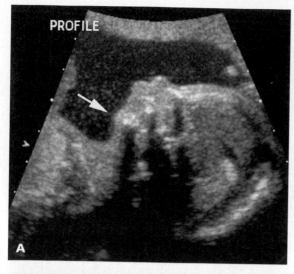

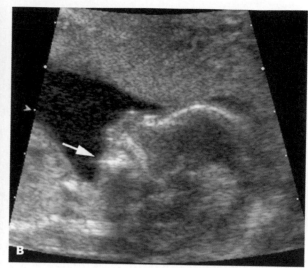

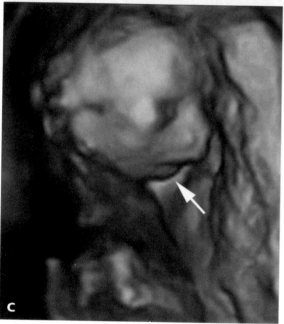

Figure 25-10 Micrognathia. **A.** Sagittal profile of face demonstrating very small mandible and chin (*arrow*). Sagittal image (**B**) and three-dimensional image (**C**) of another fetus with small mandible and chin (*arrow*).

Nuchal Fold Measurement and Nuchal Translucency Measurement

Regardless of the gestational age, the fetal neck should be analyzed for abnormalities. **Nuchal** thickening, **edema**, or redundant skin in the back of the neck is a common finding during the second trimester in fetuses with Down syndrome. The posterior neck can be evaluated and measured starting in the axial plane at the level of the cavum septum pellucidum and angling coronally to include the cerebellum and occipital bone (Fig. 25-13). The calipers are placed from the outer edge of the occipital bone to the outer edge of the skin. A measurement of 6 mm or larger is considered abnormal. **Nuchal fold thickness** measurements are taken later in gestation compared to nuchal translucency measurements. Although protocols may vary, the nuchal fold is typically measured anywhere between 15 and 21 weeks, whereas the nuchal translucency measurement can be taken earlier and is most accurately measured between 11 and 13 weeks 6 days (Fig. 25-14). Nuchal translucency is discussed in Chapter 23. It is important to note that nuchal thickening may completely resolve as the pregnancy progresses.

Prefrontal Space Distance

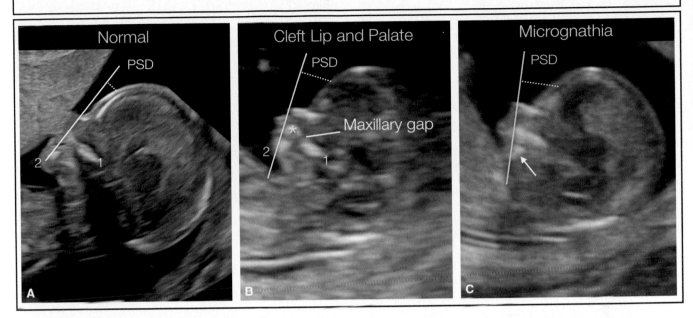

| Normal | Cleft Lip and Palate | Micrognathia |

Figure 25-11 Midsagittal views of the fetal face showing the measurement of the prefrontal space distance in a normal fetus (**A**), in a fetus with cleft lip and palate (**B**), and in a fetus with micrognathia (**C**). The prefrontal space distance (*PSD*) is the distance between the forehead and a line drawn from the anterior aspect of maxilla (*1*) and mandible (*2*). In the normal fetus (**A**), the PSD is quite short. In the presence of a facial cleft (fetus **B**), there is a protrusion of the maxilla (*asterisk*), and the PSD is increased. In the presence of micrognathia (fetus **C**), the mandible is posteriorly shifted (*arrow*), leading to an increased PSD as well. Note in fetus **B** the presence of an interrupted maxilla, called maxillary gap, a midsagittal view sign for the presence of cleft lip and palate.

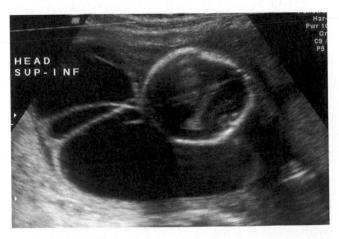

Figure 25-12 Transverse image of the fetal neck revealing a large, septated cystic mass. This is a large cystic hygroma, and the fetus was diagnosed with Turner syndrome.

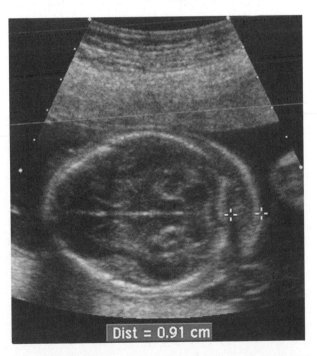

Figure 25-13 Abnormal nuchal fold. Image demonstrating a thickened nuchal fold (between *calipers*) measuring 9.1 mm.

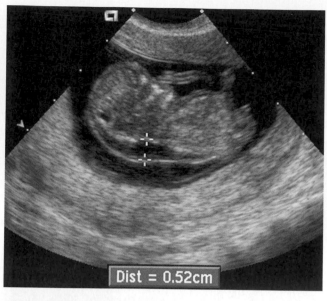

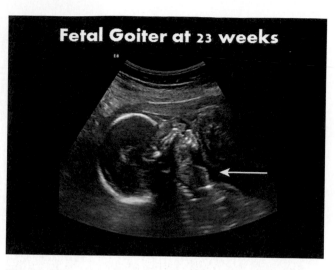

Figure 25-14 Thickened nuchal translucency. This abnormal nuchal translucency measured 5.2 mm.

Figure 25-15 Fetal goiter. *Yellow arrow* shows fetal goiter. Intra-amniotic thyroxine injections slowed progression of goiter growth.

Fetal Goiter and Other Neck Masses

A **fetal goiter** can be the cause of overtreatment of maternal Graves disease, iodine deficiency, or hypothyroidism. Sonographically, a fetal goiter will appear as an anterior fetal neck mass (Fig. 25-15). Other possible solid- or complex-appearing neck masses include the lymphangioma, hemangioma, cervical teratoma, **branchial cleft cyst**, or **thyroglossal duct cyst**. Fetal neck masses can cause compression of the trachea or esophagus and should be noted during a sonographic examination because complication at birth could ensue. Furthermore, fetal swallowing may be inhibited by a neck or oral mass, thus resulting in polyhydramnios.

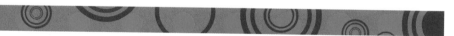

REVIEW QUESTIONS

1. What do the arrows in Figure 25-16 indicate?
   a. Dandy–Walker malformation
   b. Nuchal cord
   c. Cystic hygroma
   d. Turner syndrome

2. What do both the arrows and the arrowheads in Figure 25-16 indicate?
   a. Fetal hydrops
   b. Down syndrome
   c. Edwards syndrome
   d. Turner syndrome

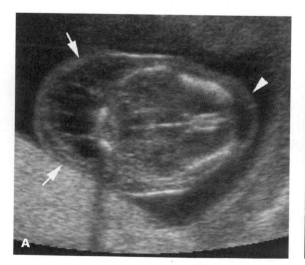

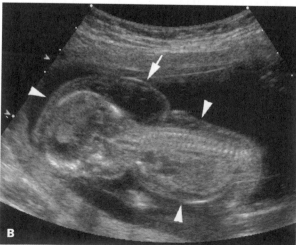

Figure 25-16

3. The profile image in Figure 25-17 demonstrates what abnormality?
   a. Macroglossia
   b. Epignathus
   c. Microtia
   d. Micrognathia

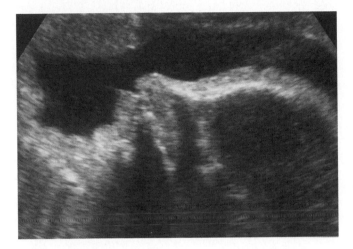

Figure 25-17

4. Figure 25-18 was obtained at the level of the binocular diameter. What finding is evident?
   a. Hypertelorism
   b. Hypotelorism
   c. Anophthalmia
   d. Reduced binocular diameter

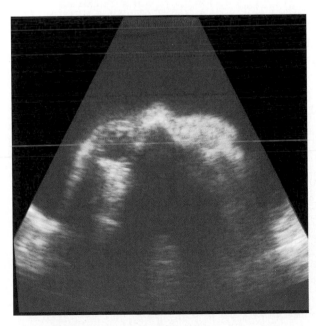

Figure 25-18

5. What does Figure 25-19 depict?
   a. Isolated cleft palate
   b. Median cleft lip
   c. Bilateral cleft lip
   d. Bilateral cleft lip and palate

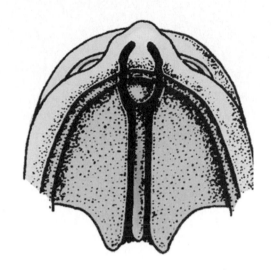

Figure 25-19

6. What is evident in Figure 25-20?
   a. Hypertelorism
   b. Hypotelorism
   c. Anophthalmia
   d. Microphthalmia

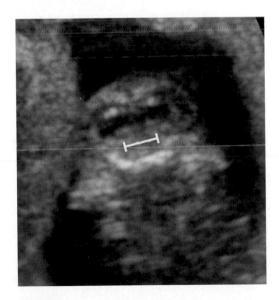

Figure 25-20

7. What is the vessel identified by the arrow in Figure 25-21?
   a. Choroid
   b. Hyaloid
   c. Callosal
   d. Ethmoidal

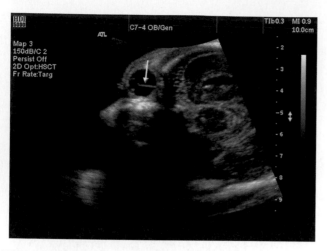

Figure 25-21

8. What facial abnormality does Figure 25-22 depict?
   a. Cebocephaly
   b. Ethmocephaly
   c. Colpocephaly
   d. Cyclopia

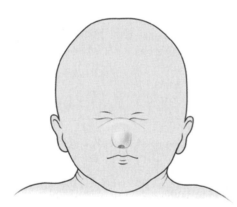

Figure 25-22

9. What facial abnormality does Figure 25-23 depict?
   a. Cebocephaly
   b. Ethmocephaly
   c. Colpocephaly
   d. Cyclopia

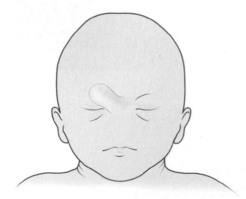

Figure 25-23

10. What facial abnormality does Figure 25-24 depict?
    a. Cebocephaly
    b. Ethmocephaly
    c. Colpocephaly
    d. Cyclopia

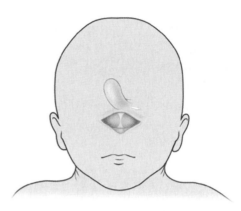

Figure 25-24

11. Which of the following would least likely cause an obstruction to fetal swallowing and thus polyhydramnios?
    a. Fetal goiter
    b. Epignathus
    c. Macroglossia
    d. Anophthalmia

12. Which of the following is being measured in Figure 25-25?
    a. Nuchal fold
    b. Fetal goiter
    c. Nuchal translucency
    d. Epignathus

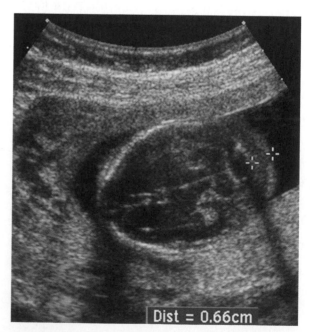

Figure 25-25

13. The term nuchal refers to the:
    a. jaw.
    b. orbit.
    c. neck.
    d. nose.

14. The term for the absence of the ear is:
    a. anophthalmia.
    b. anotia.
    c. cebocephaly.
    d. ethmocephaly.

15. Which of the following may be caused by amniotic band syndrome?
    a. Cleft lip
    b. Microphthalmia
    c. Anophthalmia
    d. Epignathus

16. What scan plane would likely optimize the visualization of a cleft lip?
    a. Oblique
    b. Coronal
    c. Sagittal
    d. Medial

17. Which of the following is not a true statement about the maxilla?
    a. Shortening of the maxilla may result in flattened facial features.
    b. The maxilla is typically long in the fetus with trisomy 21.
    c. A maxillary gap is best noted in the sagittal plane.
    d. The prefrontal space distance can help indicate maxillary abnormalities.

18. Sonographically, you visualize a hypoechoic, round structure with a thin hyperechoic border in the anterior aspect of both fetal eyes. What is the explanation for this finding?
    a. Hyaline arteries
    b. Fetal cataracts
    c. Fetal lenses
    d. Bilateral anophthalmia

19. What does Figure 25-26 depict?
    a. Bilateral cleft lip
    b. Median cleft lip
    c. Median cleft lip and palate
    d. Midline epignathus

20. What does Figure 25-27 depict?
    a. Unilateral cleft lip and palate
    b. Unilateral cleft lip
    c. Unilateral cleft palate
    d. Unilateral epignathus

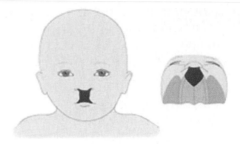

Figure 25-26

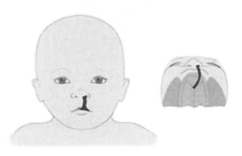

Figure 25-27

21. The isolated enlargement of the fetal thyroid is referred to as:
    a. fetal goiter.
    b. cystic hygroma.
    c. lymphangioma.
    d. cervical teratoma.

22. The absence of the eyes is termed:
    a. agyria.
    b. epignathus.
    c. hypotelorism.
    d. anophthalmia.

23. A reduction in the distance between the orbits is referred to as:
    a. anophthalmia.
    b. micrognathia.
    c. hypertelorism.
    d. hypotelorism.

24. An increased nuchal fold is most likely associated with:
    a. Dandy–Walker syndrome.
    b. trisomy 21.
    c. trisomy 3.
    d. nuchal cord.

25. The most frequently encountered chromosomal abnormality associated with holoprosencephaly is:
    a. triploidy.
    b. trisomy 21.
    c. trisomy 18.
    d. trisomy 13.

26. What is the term for a smaller than normal ear?
    a. Microphthalmia
    b. Micronatia
    c. Microtia
    d. Micrognathia

27. The fetal lip typically closes by:
    a. 18 weeks.
    b. 8 weeks.
    c. 13 weeks.
    d. 6 weeks.

28. The most common cause of hypertelorism is:
    a. Dandy–Walker malformation.
    b. anencephaly.
    c. anterior cephalocele.
    d. holoprosencephaly.

29. Macroglossia is most commonly found with:
    a. anencephaly.
    b. holoprosencephaly.
    c. Beckwith–Wiedemann syndrome.
    d. cystic hygroma.

30. An oral teratoma is referred to as:
    a. macroglossia.
    b. epignathus.
    c. micrognathia.
    d. ethmocephaly.

31. There is a definite link between microtia and what syndrome?
    a. Rays syndrome
    b. VACTERL syndrome
    c. Down syndrome
    d. Fitz-Hugh–Curtis syndrome

32. Which of the following would be most difficult to detect sonographically?
    a. Cleft lip and cleft palate
    b. Isolated cleft lip
    c. Isolated cleft palate
    d. Isolated median cleft

33. An increase distance between the orbits is referred to as:
    a. hypotelorism.
    b. hypertelorism.
    c. anophthalmia.
    d. micrognathia.

34. The optimal scan plane to visualize micrognathia is:
    a. transverse.
    b. axial.
    c. sagittal.
    d. coronal.

35. A cystic hygroma is the result of:
    a. alcohol consumption in the first trimester.
    b. an abnormal development of the roof of the fourth ventricle.
    c. occlusion of the internal carotid arteries.
    d. an abnormal accumulation of lymphatic fluid within the soft tissue.

36. Which of following would most likely involve the development of a cystic hygroma?
    a. Beckwith–Wiedemann syndrome
    b. Hydranencephaly
    c. Turner syndrome
    d. Klinefelter syndrome

37. Which of the following may also be referred to as Turner syndrome?
    a. Down syndrome
    b. Trisomy 15
    c. Trisomy 13
    d. Monosomy X

38. Nuchal thickening is most commonly associated with:
    a. Patau syndrome.
    b. hydranencephaly.
    c. Down syndrome.
    d. cebocephaly.

39. Micrognathia is a condition found in:
    a. Dandy–Walker complex.
    b. hydranencephaly.
    c. Beckwith–Wiedemann syndrome.
    d. trisomy 18.

40. The most common location of a cystic hygroma is within the:
    a. axilla.
    b. neck.
    c. chest.
    d. groin.

41. An absent or hypoplastic nasal bone is most likely associated with:
    a. trisomy 21.
    b. trisomy 15.
    c. trisomy 18.
    d. Turner syndrome.

42. An unusual protuberance of the tongue is termed:
    a. epignathus.
    b. macrognathia.
    c. pharyngoglossia.
    d. macroglossia.

43. Facial anomalies, when discovered, should prompt the sonographer to analyze the brain closely for signs of:
    a. holoprosencephaly.
    b. Dandy–Walker malformation.
    c. schizencephaly.
    d. hydranencephaly.

44. The measurement obtained between the lateral walls of the orbits is referred to as the:
    a. interocular diameter.
    b. binocular diameter.
    c. ocular diameter.
    d. biparietal diameter.

45. Which of the following is a benign congenital neck cysts found most often near the angle of the mandible?
    a. Epignathus
    b. Branchial cleft cyst
    c. Thyroglossal duct cyst
    d. Fetal goiter

46. A large, mostly cystic mass containing a thick, midline septation is noted in the cervical spine region of a fetus. This most likely represents a(n):
    a. sacrococcygeal teratoma.
    b. cystic hygroma.
    c. cephalocele.
    d. anophthalmia.

47. A group of abnormalities associated with the entrapment of fetal parts and fetal amputations is:
    a. cystic hygroma.
    b. Edwards syndrome.
    c. ethmocephaly.
    d. amniotic band syndrome.

48. The growth disorder syndrome synonymous with organ, skull, and tongue enlargement is:
    a. Klinefelter syndrome.
    b. Apert syndrome.
    c. Meckel–Gruber syndrome.
    d. Beckwith–Wiedemann syndrome.

49. Which of the following is also referred to as Patau syndrome?
    a. Trisomy 18
    b. Trisomy 21
    c. Trisomy 12
    d. Trisomy 13

50. Close-set eyes and a nose with a single nostril is termed:
    a. cebocephaly.
    b. cyclopia.
    c. ethmocephaly.
    d. epignathus.

51. Which of the following conditions does not affect the orbits?
    a. Cebocephaly
    b. Cyclopia
    c. Ethmocephaly
    d. Epignathus

52. An abnormal division in the lip is referred to as:
    a. micrognathia.
    b. cleft lip.
    c. anophthalmia.
    d. cebocephaly.

53. At what level is the nuchal fold measurement obtained?
    a. Cavum septum pellucidum
    b. Occipital horns of the lateral ventricle
    c. Brainstem
    d. Foramen magna

54. Fusion of the orbits is termed:
    a. microglossia.
    b. cebocephaly.
    c. cyclopia.
    d. ethmocephaly.

55. Which of the following is also referred to as trisomy 21?
    a. Edwards syndrome
    b. Patau syndrome
    c. Meckel–Gruber syndrome
    d. Down syndrome

56. The thickness of the nuchal fold in the second trimester should not exceed:
    a. 3 mm.
    b. 6 mm.
    c. 10 mm.
    d. 12 mm.

57. A small mandible is termed:
    a. macroglossia.
    b. epignathus.
    c. micrognathia.
    d. ethmocephaly.

58. The condition in which there is no nose and a proboscis separating two close-set orbits is:
    a. ethmocephaly.
    b. epignathus.
    c. micrognathia.
    d. cebocephaly.

The Fetal Face and Neck

59. All of the following are sonographic features of holoprosencephaly except:
    a. cystic hygroma.
    b. proboscis with cyclopia.
    c. fused thalamus.
    d. monoventricle.

60. The nuchal fold measurement is typically obtained:
    a. before 12 weeks 6 days.
    b. between 11 weeks and 13 weeks 6 days.
    c. between 15 weeks and 21 weeks.
    d. after 24 weeks.

SUGGESTED READINGS

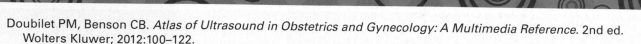

Doubilet PM, Benson CB. *Atlas of Ultrasound in Obstetrics and Gynecology: A Multimedia Reference.* 2nd ed. Wolters Kluwer; 2012:100–122.

Henningsen C, Kuntz K, Youngs D. *Clinical Guide to Sonography: Exercises for Critical Thinking.* 2nd ed. Elsevier; 2014:208 & 291.

Hertzberg BS, Middleton WD. *Ultrasound: The Requisites.* 3rd ed. Elsevier; 2016:383–386.

Kline-Fath BM, Bulas DI, and Lee W. *Fundamental and Advanced Fetal Imaging: Ultrasound and MRI.* 2nd ed. Wolters Kluwer; 2021:549–625.

Norton ME, Scoutt LM, Feldstein VA. *Callen's Ultrasonography in Obstetrics and Gynecology.* 6th ed. Elsevier; 2017:63–72 & 245–262.

Nyberg D, McGaham J, Pretorius D, et al. *Diagnostic Imaging of Fetal Anomalies.* Lippincott Williams & Wilkins; 2003:133–220 (syndromes) & 335–380 (face and neck).

Rumack CM, Wilson SR, Charboneau W, et al. *Diagnostic Ultrasound.* 4th ed. Elsevier; 2011:1166–1196.

Sanders RC, Hall-Terracciano B. *Clinical Sonography: A Practical Guide.* 5th ed. \Wolters Kluwer; 2016:232–260.

Stephenson SR, Dmitrieva J. *Diagnostic Medical Sonography: Obstetrics and Gynecology.* 4th ed. Wolters Kluwer; 2018:467–494 & 805–836.

The Fetal Medicine Foundation. Nasal Bone. https://fetalmedicine.org/fmf-certification-2/nasal-bone Accessed February 2, 2022.

BONUS REVIEW!

Realistic Three-Dimensional and Surface Rendering of the Fetal Face (Fig. 25-28)

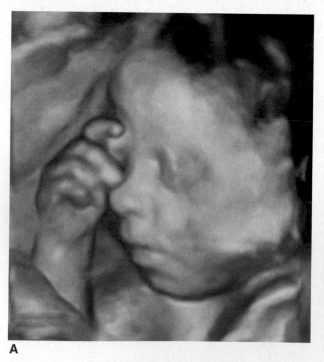

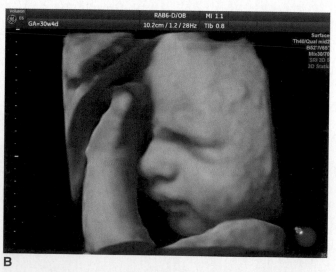

A   **B**

Figure 25-28 Three-dimensional and surface rendering image of the fetal face. **A.** In this surface rendering of the fetal face and arm, the skin—or surface—of the fetus is displayed without displaying the underlying anatomy. **B.** This surface rendering of the fetal face uses a rendering mode intended to provide a more realistic appearance to the fetal face.

Cyclopia with Holoprosencephaly (Fig. 25-29)

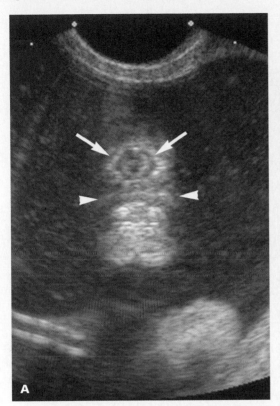
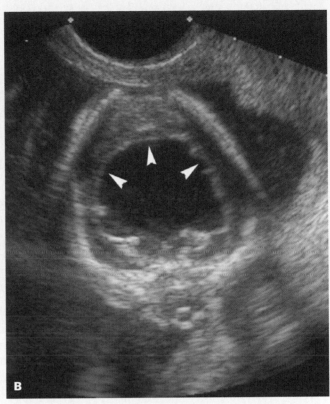

Figure 25-29 Cyclopia with alobar holoprosencephaly. **A.** Coronal image of face demonstrating a single eye (*arrows*) in the middle, above the mouth (*arrowheads*). **B.** Coronal image through cranium demonstrates a monoventricle with fused cerebral tissue (*arrowheads*).

Fetal Breathing Demonstrated with Color Doppler (Fig. 25-30)

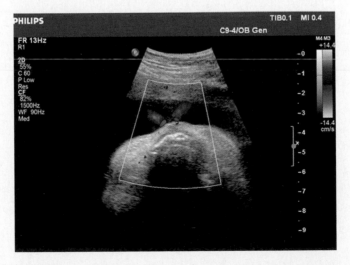

Figure 25-30 Axial view of the fetal face at the level of the nostrils demonstrating fetal breathing through the use of color Doppler.

(*continued*)

BONUS REVIEW! *(continued)*

Fetal Nasal Bone Length (Fig. 25-31)

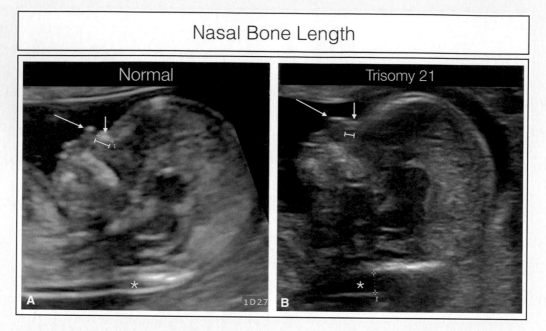

Figure 25-31 Midsagittal views of the fetal face showing the measurement of the nasal bone length in a normal fetus (**A**) and in a fetus with trisomy 21 (**B**). In more than half of the fetuses with trisomy 21, the nasal bone is either completely nonossified or, as in this case, poorly ossified, resulting in a short and thin appearance. Long arrows point to the nose tip and short arrows to the nasal skin. Nuchal translucency measurement is also seen (*asterisk*).

The Fetal Spine and Musculoskeletal System

Introduction

This chapter provides a review of both the fetal skeleton and the fetal spine. The embryologic development and associated abnormalities of the fetal axial and appendicular skeleton are also discussed. The "Bonus Review" section Includes a surface-mode image of the fetal spine in the first trimester, a radiograph of trident hands, and a case of sirenomelia.

Key Terms

achondrogenesis—rare, lethal condition resulting in abnormal development of the bones and cartilage

achondroplasia—a disorder that results in abnormal bone growth and dwarfism

acoustic shadowing—an area where sound has been prohibited to propagate, resulting in a dark shadow projecting posterior to a structure

alpha-fetoprotein—a protein produced by the fetal yolk sac, fetal gastrointestinal tract, and the fetal liver; may also be produced by some malignant tumors

amniotic band syndrome—group of abnormalities associated with the entrapment of fetal parts in the amnion, often resulting in fetal amputations or clefting

anencephaly—neural tube defect that is described as the absence of the cranium and cerebral hemispheres

anhydramnios—no amniotic fluid

appendicular skeleton—includes the bones of the upper extremities, lower extremities, and pelvic girdle

autosomal dominant disorder—a way in which a disorder or trait can be inherited by a fetus; at least one of the parents has to be the carrier of the gene for the disease

axial skeleton—includes the bones of cranium and spine

banana sign—the sonographic sign of the cerebellum being curved in the presence of spina bifida

bilateral renal agenesis—the failure of both kidneys to develop in the fetus

biparietal diameter—a fetal head measurement obtained in the transverse plane at the level of the third ventricle and thalamus; this measurement is obtained from the outer table of the proximal parietal bone to the inner table of the distal parietal bone

caudal regression syndrome—syndrome associated with the absence of the sacrum and coccyx; also referred to as sacral agenesis

cephalocele(s)—protrusions of intracranial contents through a defect in the skull

cerebellum—the portion of the brain located in the inferior posterior part of the skull that is responsible for motor output, sensory perception, and equilibrium

closed spina bifida—see key term spina bifida occulta

cloverleaf skull—the abnormal shape of the cranium caused by premature fusion of the sutures in which there is frontal bossing and a cloverleaf shape to the skull

clubfoot—a malformation of the bones of the foot in which the foot is most often inverted and rotated medially, and the metatarsals and toes lie in the same plane as the tibia and fibula

colpocephaly—the abnormal lateral ventricle shape in which there is a small frontal horn and enlarged occipital horn

629

dwarfism—abnormal short stature

dysplasia—the abnormal development of a structure

encephalocele—protrusion of brain tissue through a defect in the skull

estriol—an estrogenic hormone produced by the placenta

exencephaly—form of acrania in which the entire cerebrum is located outside the skull

femur length—a sonographic measurement of the femoral diaphysis that provides an estimated gestational age

folate—a vitamin that has been shown to significantly reduce the likelihood of a fetus suffering from a neural tube defect; also referred to as folic acid

frontal bossing—the angling of the frontal bones that produces an unusually prominent forehead

gastroschisis—herniation of abdominal contents through a right-sided, periumbilical abdominal wall defect

germ cell tumor—a type of neoplasm derived from germ cells of the gonads; may also be found outside the reproductive tract

hemangioma—a benign tumor composed of blood vessels

hemivertebra—the anomaly of the spine in which there is absence of all or part of a vertebral body and posterior element

heterozygous achondroplasia—most common nonlethal skeletal dysplasia that is characterized by rhizomelia

homozygous achondroplasia—the fatal form of achondroplasia

human chorionic gonadotropin—hormone produced by the trophoblastic cells of the early placenta; may also be used as a tumor marker in nongravid patients and males

hydronephrosis—the dilation of the renal collecting system resulting from the obstruction of the flow of urine from the kidney(s) to the bladder; also referred to as pelvocaliectasis or pelvicaliectasis

kyphoscoliosis—the combination of both scoliosis and kyphosis in the fetus

kyphosis—an abnormal posterior curvature of the spine

lemon sign—the sonographic sign associated with a lemon-shaped cranium; most often found in the fetus with spina bifida

limb–body wall complex—a group of disorders with sonographic findings including a short or absent umbilical cord, ventral wall defects, limb defects, craniofacial defects, and scoliosis

lipoma—a benign fatty tumor

maternal serum alpha-fetoprotein—a screening test that detects the amount of alpha-fetoprotein in the maternal bloodstream

maternal serum screening—blood screening test that evaluates maternal levels of alpha-fetoprotein, estriol, and human chorionic gonadotropin (as well as other labs) during a pregnancy for neural tube defects and chromosomal abnormalities

meninges—the coverings of the brain and spinal cord

meningocele—herniation of the cranial or spinal meninges because of an open cranial or spinal defect; contains cerebrospinal fluid, but no nerve tissue

meningomyelocele—mass that results from open spina bifida that contains the spinal cord and the meninges; also referred to as a myelomeningocele

mermaid syndrome—see key term sirenomelia

myelocele—mass that results from open spina bifida that contains spinal cord only

neural tube—embryologic formation that results from fusion of the two folded ends of the neural plate

oligohydramnios—a lower-than-normal amount of amniotic fluid for the gestational age

omphalocele—an anterior abdominal wall defect where there is herniation of the fetal bowel and other abdominal organs into the base of the umbilical cord

open spina bifida—see key term spina bifida aperta

osteogenesis imperfecta—a group of disorders that result in multiple fractures in utero; caused by decreased mineralization and poor ossification of the bones

polyhydramnios—an excessive amount of amniotic fluid for the gestational age

posterior fossa—posterior portion of the cranium located near the cerebellum and containing the cisterna magna

pregestational diabetes—maternal diabetes that existed before pregnancy; includes both type 1 and 2 diabetes mellitus

radial ray defect—absence or underdevelopment of the radius

rhizomelia—shortening of the proximal segment of a limb

sacral agenesis—the nondevelopment of the sacrum; see key term caudal regression syndrome

sacral dimple—an opening in the skin over the distal spine

scoliosis—an abnormal lateral curvature of the spine

sirenomelia—a fetal abnormality characterized by fusion of the lower extremities, renal agenesis, and oligohydramnios; may also be referred to as mermaid syndrome

spina bifida aperta—most common form of spina bifida; results in open lesions that are typically not covered by skin and a mass that protrudes from the spine; also referred to as open spina bifida

spina bifida occulta—closed spinal lesions that are completely covered by skin and can be difficult to identify sonographically; also referred to as closed spina bifida

spinal dysraphism—a group of neural tube defects that describe some manifestation of incomplete closure of the spine

splay—turned outward

synechiae—adhesions

talipes equinovarus—see key term clubfoot

thanatophoric dysplasia—most common lethal skeletal dysplasia characterized by a cloverleaf skull with frontal bossing and hydrocephalus

trident hand—a wide separation between the middle and ring finger

triple screen—a maternal blood test that typically includes an analysis of human chorionic gonadotropin, alpha-fetoprotein, and estriol

VACTERL association—an acronym for a combination of abnormalities that represent vertebral anomalies, anorectal atresia, cardiac anomalies, tracheoesophageal fistula, renal anomalies, and limb anomalies; may also be referred to as VATER association

EMBRYOLOGY OF THE AXIAL SKELETON

The **axial skeleton** begins to form between the sixth and eighth menstrual weeks. It consists of the bones of the cranium and spine. As bones grow and accumulate minerals, they are said to ossify. It is this ossification that allows sonographers to readily visualize these structures as echogenic reflections that produce **acoustic shadowing**. As the pregnancy progresses, the skull and skeletal bones become more echogenic.

The spine consists of five sections: cervical, thoracic, lumbar, sacrum, and coccyx. The spine is typically imaged in three scan planes: sagittal, transverse, and coronal (Figs. 26-1 to 26-3). Each fetal vertebra consists of three echogenic ossification centers: one **centrum** and two neural processes. The centrum will eventually form the vertebral body, whereas the neural process of each vertebra will become the lamina, pedicle, transverse process, spinous process, and articular process. Between the two laminae and posterior to the centrum lies the vertebral column, the structure that runs the length of the spine and contains the spinal cord. The echogenic laminae are normally angled inward, whereas with **spina bifida**, the defective laminae will be angled outward or be said to **splay**. The spinal cord appears as a hypoechoic linear structure that extends from the base of the cranium to the distal spine.

> 🔊 **SOUND OFF**
> Each fetal vertebra consists of three echogenic ossification centers: one centrum and two neural processes.

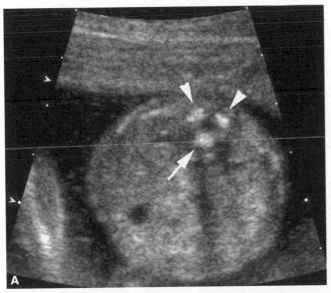
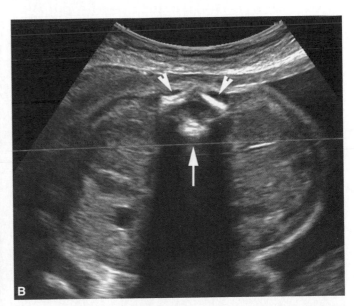

Figure 26-1 Transverse fetal spine. **A.** Transverse fetal spine at 18 weeks demonstrating the three ossification centers: two posterior elements (*arrowheads*) and one anterior element (*arrow*). Skin can be seen clearly covering the spine posteriorly. **B.** Transverse fetal spine at 30 weeks demonstrating more clearly the posterior (*arrowheads*) and anterior (*arrow*) ossification centers.

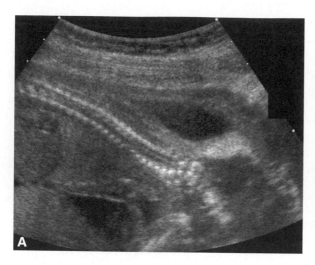

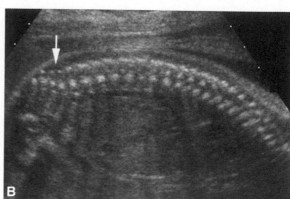

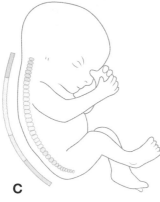

Figure 26-2 Longitudinal fetal spine. **A.** Longitudinal image of the cervical and thoracic spine. **B.** Longitudinal image of the thoracic, lumbar, and sacral spine (*arrow*). **C.** Lateral view of curvature of the fetal vertebral column, showing cervical (*red*), thoracic (*brown*), and lumbar (*yellow*) vertebrae, and the sacrum and coccyx area (*orange*). Note the coccyx is not fully formed by term.

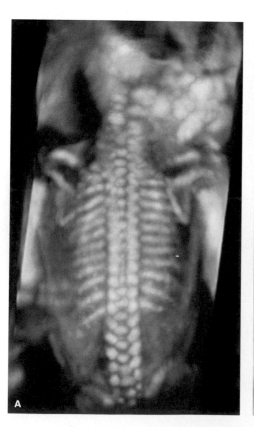

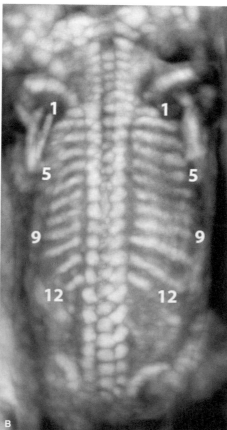

Figure 26-3 Three-dimensional (*3D*) spine and ribs. 3D images at (**A**) 20 weeks and (**B**) 19 weeks of the fetal thorax, with skeletal settings demonstrating one rib on each side of each thoracic vertebral body. The number of ribs can be counted, as in (**B**).

SPINA BIFIDA, ALPHA-FETOPROTEIN, AND FOLIC ACID SUPPLEMENTS

Among the list of **neural tube** defects are **cephaloceles**, **anencephaly**, and spina bifida. Anencephaly and spina bifida are the most common neural defects, occurring in 1 in every 1,000 pregnancies. Recall, **maternal serum screening**, also referred to as the **triple screen**, combines the laboratory values of **human chorionic gonadotropin (hCG)**, **estriol**, and **maternal serum alpha-fetoprotein** (MSAFP). The MSAFP component of this test is particularly helpful for detecting neural tube defects. Reportedly, as many as 80% of spina bifida cases can be detected with **alpha-fetoprotein** (AFP) screening in combination with sonography. AFP is initially produced by the yolk sac, fetal gastrointestinal tract, and the fetal liver. AFP exits the fetus through an opening in the neural tube if one is present, such as with **open spina bifida** and anencephaly, thus allowing a greater amount to pass into the maternal circulation. It is important to note that an elevation in AFP does not necessarily mean that spina bifida is present. Elevated MSAFP is also associated with **omphalocele**, **gastroschisis**, multiple gestations, and fetal death. Moreover, **closed spina bifida** is not associated with elevated MSAFP because of the skin covering. Fortunately, studies have shown that a supplement of just 0.4 mg a day of **folate** (folic acid) in a woman's diet significantly reduces the likelihood of her fetus developing spina bifida and other neural tube defects. In high-risk patients, as much as 4 mg a day may be prescribed.

> **))) SOUND OFF**
> AFP exits the fetus through an opening in the neural tube if one is present, such as with open spina bifida or gastroschisis, thus allowing a greater amount to pass into the maternal circulation.

SPINA BIFIDA

Spina bifida is a neural tube defect that occurs when the embryonic neural tube fails to close. Spina bifida may also be referred to as **spinal dysraphism**, **meningocele**, and **meningomyelocele** (myelomeningocele). There are several ways to classify spina bifida. Essentially, this disorder can be subdivided into two types: **spina bifida occulta** (hidden) and **spina bifida aperta** (open) (Table 26-1). Occult lesions are closed lesions, meaning that they are typically covered by skin and thus can be difficult to identify sonographically in utero. Therefore, with spina bifida occulta, although the vertebrae fail to close, there is no herniation of the spinal contents outside the spinal column. In the

TABLE 26-1 Type of spinal defect and description

Type of Spinal Defect	Description
Spina bifida occulta	Closed defect Skin surface abnormality noted on postnatal physical examination can be a sacral dimple, tuft of hair, hemangioma, or lipoma
Spina bifida aperta	Typically, an open defect May also be referred to as spina bifida cystica Mass is referred to as a meningocele or meningomyelocele (myelomeningocele) depending upon contents

postnatal period, spina bifida occulta is suspected when a **sacral dimple**, **hemangioma**, **lipoma**, or a tuft of hair is identified in the midline of the newborn, directly over the distal spine. Sonography can be highly effective at determining whether the spinal cord is tethered in neonates who present with these clinical findings.

Spina bifida aperta, which is an open lesion, is the most common form of spina bifida and the type more frequently recognized in utero. Open lesions are not covered by skin and will often result in a mass that protrudes beyond the bony defect, making them more readily identifiable with sonography. If the mass only contains spinal cord, it is referred to as a **myelocele**. Meningoceles contain **meninges** only, whereas meningomyeloceles (spina bifida cystic) contain meninges and nerve roots (Figs. 26-4 and 26-5). The most common location of spina bifida is the lumbosacral region, although it can occur anywhere along the spine. It is also important to note that the higher the location of spina bifida, the greater the neurologic impairment.

> **))) SOUND OFF**
> The most common location of spina bifida is the lumbosacral region.

Spina bifida is often initially recognized by its associated cranial findings, a group of abnormalities referred to as Arnold–Chiari II malformation. The pressure of a large mass in the distal spine pulling on the spinal cord causes malformations of the cranium and intracranial contents. The frontal bones

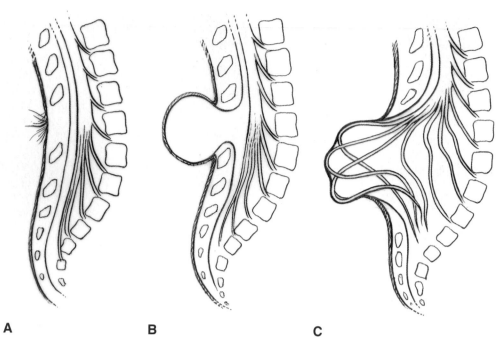

A   **B**   **C**

Figure 26-4 Classifications of spina bifida in sagittal. **A.** Spina bifida occulta is characterized by a defect in one or more vertebrae, but intact skin and no alteration in the spinal cord. **B.** Meningocele is characterized by a protrusion of the meninges and cerebrospinal fluid through the defect in the spine. **C.** Myelomeningocele is characterized by the protrusion of the neural elements as well as the meninges through the spinal defect.

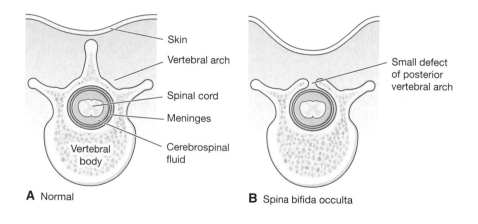

A Normal   **B** Spina bifida occulta

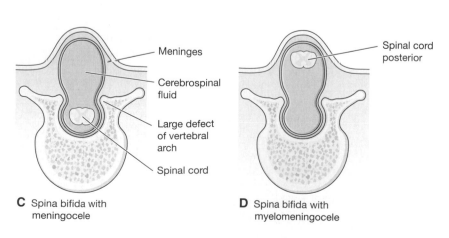

C Spina bifida with meningocele   **D** Spina bifida with myelomeningocele

Figure 26-5 Cross-sectional drawings of the normal and abnormal spine with spina bifida. **A.** Normal vertebra and spinal cord. **B.** In occult spina bifida (spina bifida occulta), the posterior vertebral arch fails to form. It is usually asymptomatic. **C.** In spina bifida with meningocele, the meninges protrude through the defect. **D.** In spina bifida with myelomeningocele, the meninges and spinal cord protrude through the defect.

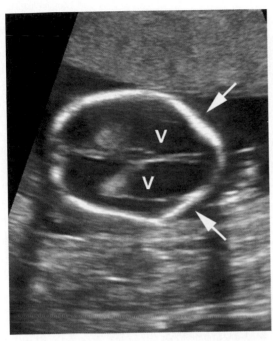

Figure 26-6 Lemon sign. Axial image of the cranium in a fetus with a myelomeningocele demonstrating a concavity in the frontal bones (*arrows*), causing the head to have a lemon shape. This is consistent with Arnold–Chiari II malformation. Ventriculomegaly (*V*) is also noted.

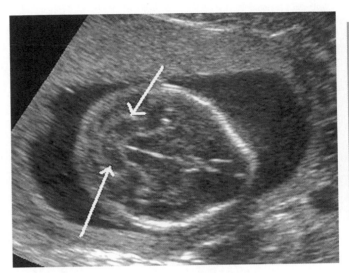

Figure 26-7 Banana sign. Axial view of the cerebellum demonstrating the abnormal banana shape that the cerebellum (between *arrows*) takes in the presence of spina bifida. This is consistent with Arnold–Chiari II malformation.

become flattened (bifrontal concavity) and will yield a lemon-shaped cranium (Fig. 26-6). This "**lemon sign**," often described as scalloping of the frontal bones, presents a distinct finding on sonography.

It is most helpful to analyze the **posterior fossa** of the cranium for abnormalities when a lemon sign is suspected. The **cerebellum** will become displaced inferiorly and posteriorly and appear curved in the presence of spina bifida (Fig. 26-7). This is referred to as the "**banana sign**." As a result of the cerebellum being displaced inferiorly, the cisterna magna is completely obliterated or nonexistent. The lateral ventricles will also be enlarged and distorted in shape. The frontal horns will be small and slit like, whereas the occipital horns will be enlarged, a condition known as **colpocephaly**. The sensitivity of these cranial findings at detecting spina bifida is said to be more than 99%. It is important to note that the fetus with closed spina bifida will lack these intracranial findings. Arnold–Chiari II malformation has also been discussed in Chapter 24.

> ### 🔊 SOUND OFF
> Keep in mind that spina bifida is associated with two yellow fruits—the banana and the lemon.

Once cranial findings are suggestive of spina bifida, a thorough analysis of the spine should be performed. In the presence of spina bifida, the posterior ossification elements or laminae will often appear splayed in the transverse plane (Fig. 26-8). A meningocele will appear as a simple cystic mass protruding from the spine, whereas a myelomeningocele tends to appear more complex (Fig. 26-9). One differential diagnosis of these masses is the sacrococcygeal teratoma (SCT) mentioned later in this chapter. However, it is important to note that the fetus with an SCT will most likely have normal skull and intracranial anatomy, whereas the intracranial anatomy of a fetus with open spina bifida is often altered as described earlier.

With open spina bifida, the exposure of the delicate spinal nerves to the amniotic fluid during fetal life is thought to be one of the causes of neurologic impairment. Open fetal surgery can be performed on the fetus with spina bifida when a mass is identified on the spine, even as early as 16 weeks. The ultimate goal of this procedure is to prevent, or at least minimize, the neurologic deficits associated with spina bifida. During the operation, the uterus, amniotic sac, and fetus are accessed, and the open defect is surgically repaired. After the spinal repair is made, the fetus is placed back into the uterus for continued growth and maturation. In recent years, fetoscopic surgery has presented some promise as a novel approach to fetal spina bifida repair as well. Ultimately, sonography can aid in the detection of spina bifida, the assessment of the level of the defect, and offer postoperative follow-up examinations after fetal surgery.

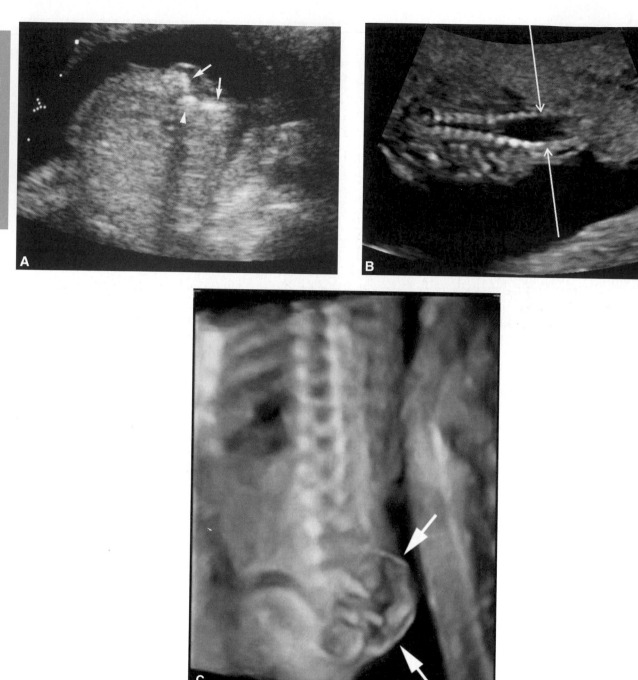

Figure 26-8 Splaying of the posterior ossification centers. **A.** Transverse image of the fetal spine revealing splaying of the two posterior ossification centers (*arrows*). The third ossification (*arrowhead*) represents the vertebral body. **B.** Coronal scan of the fetal lumbosacral spine shows fusiform widening of the spinal canal (between *arrows*). **C.** Three-dimensional images demonstrating a cystic mass (*arrows*) protruding posteriorly from the back of a fetus with a myelomeningocele.

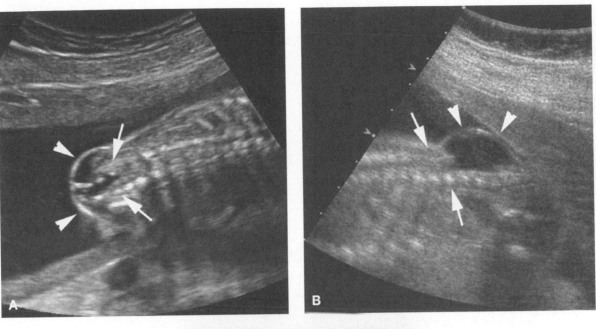

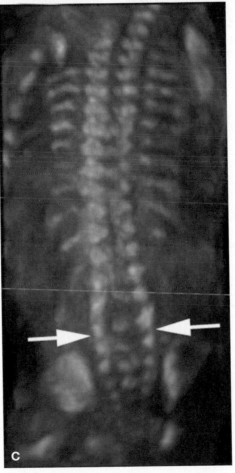

Figure 26-9 Myelomeningocele. **A.** Coronal image of the distal spine (*arrows*) revealing herniation of the spinal cord (*arrowheads*). **B.** A large myelomeningocele (*arrowheads*) is noted protruding from the distal spine (*arrows*) in this image. **C.** Three-dimensional image of the fetal spine demonstrating widening of the distal spine in the area of the defect (between *arrows*).

CLINICAL FINDINGS OF OPEN SPINA BIFIDA APERTA (OPEN)

1. Elevated MSAFP

SONOGRAPHIC FINDINGS OF SPINA BIFIDA APERTA (OPEN)

1. Splaying of the laminae in the area of the defect
2. Cystic mass (meningocele) or complex mass (myelomeningocele) protruding from the spine
3. Lemon sign—lemon-shaped cranium with flattened frontal bones
4. Banana sign—banana-shaped cerebellum
5. Obliterated cisterna magna
6. Colpocephaly
7. Hydrocephalus

CLINICAL FINDINGS OF SPINA BIFIDA OCCULTA

1. In utero—normal laboratory values
2. Postnatal—sacral dimple, hemangioma, lipoma, or excessive hair is identified directly over the distal spine

SCOLIOSIS AND KYPHOSIS

There are several abnormal curvatures that can occur to the spine (Fig. 26-10). **Scoliosis** is a deformity of the spine in which there is an abnormal lateral curvature.

The spine will appear S shaped in the affected region of scoliosis (Fig. 26-11). Scoliosis typically involves the thoracic and upper lumbar spine. **Kyphosis** is an abnormal posterior curvature of the spine. Both of these abnormalities can exist together, a condition known as **kyphoscoliosis**. Although these abnormalities may be the only anomaly noted during a fetal sonogram, distortion of the spine can be seen with **hemivertebrae**, myelomeningoceles, **amniotic band syndrome**, and **limb–body wall complex** (LBWC). Scoliosis and kyphosis are also often associated with additional anomalies in other systems, as seen in **VACTERL association**.

SONOGRAPHIC APPEARANCE OF SCOLIOSIS

1. Lateral curvature of the spine
2. S-shaped spine

SONOGRAPHIC APPEARANCE OF KYPHOSIS

1. Abnormal posterior curvature of the spine

SOUND OFF
Scoliosis is a deformity of the spine in which there is an abnormal lateral curvature, whereas kyphosis is an abnormal posterior curvature of the spine.

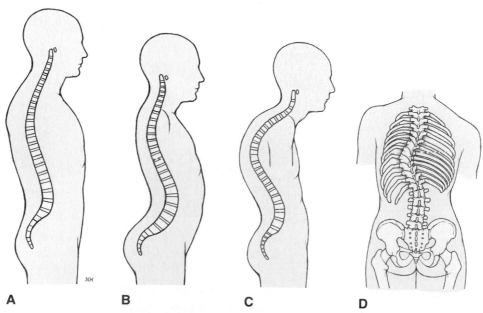

Figure 26-10 Curvatures of the spine. **A.** Normal. **B.** Lordosis. **C.** Kyphosis. **D.** Scoliosis.

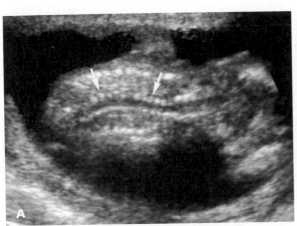
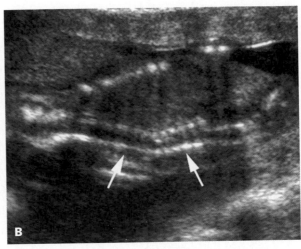

Figure 26-11 Scoliosis. **A.** Coronal image of the spine demonstrating curvature (*arrows*) from scoliosis. This fetus had trisomy 18. **B.** Longitudinal image of spine in another fetus showing mid-thoracic scoliosis (*arrows*).

LIMB–BODY WALL COMPLEX

LBWC, also referred to as body stalk anomaly or short umbilical cord syndrome, is a rare group of fetal defects. There are three postulated causes for this fatal condition: vascular occlusion, amnion rupture, or embryonic dysgenesis. The most common sonographic findings of LBWC are a short or absent umbilical cord, ventral wall defects, limb defects, craniofacial defects (**exencephaly** or **encephalocele**), and scoliosis. The fetus will appear closely connected with the placenta and will have marked scoliosis (Fig. 26-12). Because of the opening in the ventral wall, elevated levels of MSAFP can be detected in the second trimester. **Amniotic band syndrome** has very similar sonographic findings and may actually be seen simultaneously with LBWC.

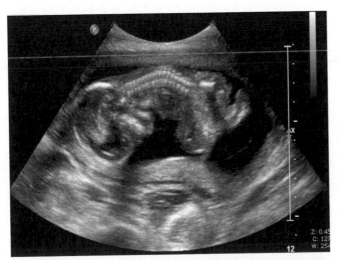

Figure 26-12 Limb–body wall complex (*LBWC*). This fetus had multiple anomalies, including marked scoliosis, neural tube defects, and an anterior abdominal wall defect, and was ultimately diagnosed with LBWC.

CLINICAL FINDINGS OF LIMB–BODY WALL COMPLEX

1. Elevated MSAFP

SONOGRAPHIC FINDINGS OF LIMB–BODY WALL COMPLEX

1. Short or absent umbilical cord
2. Marked scoliosis
3. Various other anomalies including craniofacial and limb defects

◀))) SOUND OFF
A common sonographic finding of LBWC is a short or absent umbilical cord.

FETAL SKELETAL ABNORMALITIES

Overview of Skeletal Dysplasia

Dysplasia denotes the abnormal development of a structure. Skeletal dysplasias exist as a large group of abnormalities of the skeletal system. More than 271 skeletal dysplasias have been identified. The four most common skeletal dysplasias are as **achondroplasia**, **achondrogenesis**, **osteogenesis imperfecta**, and **thanatophoric dysplasia**.

Achondroplasia

Heterozygous achondroplasia is the most common nonlethal skeletal dysplasia. This is a type of **dwarfism** in which the proximal portions of the limbs, the humeri and femurs, are much shorter than the distal portion of the limbs, a condition known as **rhizomelia**. Heterozygous achondroplasia is an **autosomal dominant disorder**, although, many times, it is the result of a spontaneous genetic mutation.

Rhizomelia is typically detected when a notable difference in the gestational age measurements between the **biparietal diameter** and the **femur length** is discovered, typically in the mid to late second trimester. The sonographic findings of achondroplasia include micromelia, macrocrania, **frontal bossing**, flattened nasal bridge, and **trident hand** (Figs. 26-13

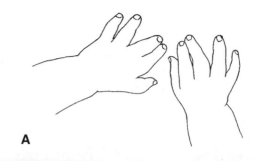

A

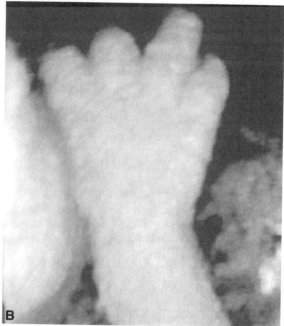

B

Figure 26-14 Trident hand. **A.** Drawing of trident hands. Note the distinct separation between the third and fourth digits. **B.** Three-dimensional image revealing a widening between the third and fourth digits. This is characteristic of a trident hand, often associated with achondroplasia.

and 26-14). Achondroplasia can also be **homozygous**. **Homozygous achondroplasia**, which can occur when both parents are dwarfs, is usually fatal within the first 2 years of life.

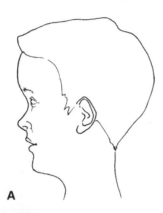

A

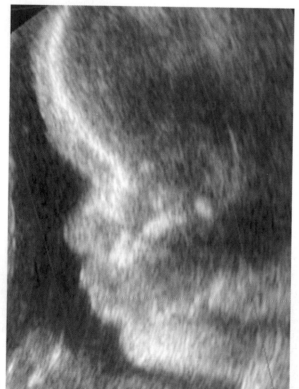

B

Figure 26-13 Achondroplasia and frontal bossing. **A.** Drawing of a child with achondroplasia and frontal bossing. **B.** Facial profile of a 32-week fetus reveals frontal bossing that produces an unusually prominent forehead.

SONOGRAPHIC FINDINGS OF ACHONDROPLASIA

1. Macrocrania
2. Frontal bossing
3. Flattened nasal bridge
4. Micromelia (resulting from rhizomelia)
5. Trident hand

🔊 **SOUND OFF**
Heterozygous achondroplasia is the most common nonlethal skeletal dysplasia.

Achondrogenesis

Achondrogenesis is a rare, lethal condition, resulting in absent mineralization of the skeletal bones. The term achondrogenesis is interpreted "not producing cartilage." There are three types of achondrogenesis—type 1A, type 1B, and type 2. This disorder is apparent when there is deficient ossification of the fetal spine, pelvis, and cranium, ultimately leading to stillbirth or early death. The fetus will suffer from severe limb shortening and may have rib fractures. Sonographic findings include a large skull; severely shortened limbs; demineralization of the fetal skull, spine, pelvis, and limbs; distention of the abdomen; and a narrow chest (Figs. 26-15 and 26-16). **Polyhydramnios** is often present as well.

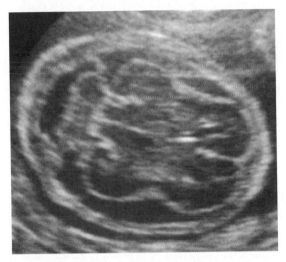

Figure 26-15 Achondrogenesis and the skull. Hypomineralization of the cranium is noted in this image.

SONOGRAPHIC FINDINGS OF ACHONDROGENESIS

1. Severely shortened limbs (micromelia)
2. Absent mineralization of the skull, spine, pelvis, and limbs
3. Large skull
4. Narrow chest and distended abdomen
5. Polyhydramnios

Osteogenesis Imperfecta

Osteogenesis imperfecta, commonly known as brittle bone disease, is a group of disorders that results in multiple fractures that can occur in utero (Fig. 26-17). The fractures are a result of decreased mineralization and poor ossification. There are four different types of osteogenesis imperfecta. Type II, a uniformly fatal form of osteogenesis imperfecta, is the most severe type of the disease. Osteogenesis imperfecta type II results in multiple fractures in utero, skull demineralization (recognized by a lack of posterior shadowing), bell-shaped chest, and decreased fetal movement. One distinctive finding is that when transducer pressure is applied to the skull, the shape of the "soft" skull can be distorted (Fig. 26-18). Types I, III, and IV are typically diagnosed after birth.

SONOGRAPHIC FINDINGS OF OSTEOGENESIS IMPERFECTA

1. Demineralization of the skull (transducer pressure can alter the shape of the skull)
2. Multiple fractures
3. Bell-shaped chest

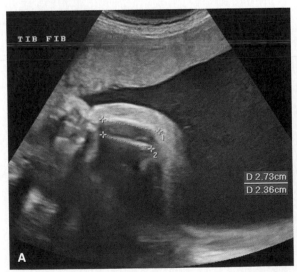

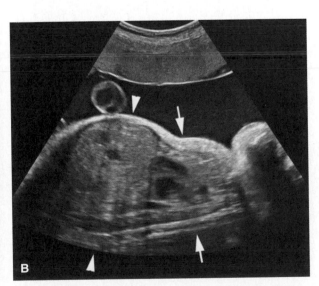

Figure 26-16 Achondrogenesis at 33 weeks' gestation. **A.** Longitudinal image of lower leg showing shortened and poorly ossified tibia and fibula (*calipers*). **B.** Sagittal image of fetus showing very narrow thorax (*arrows*) compared to the abdominal width (*arrowheads*).

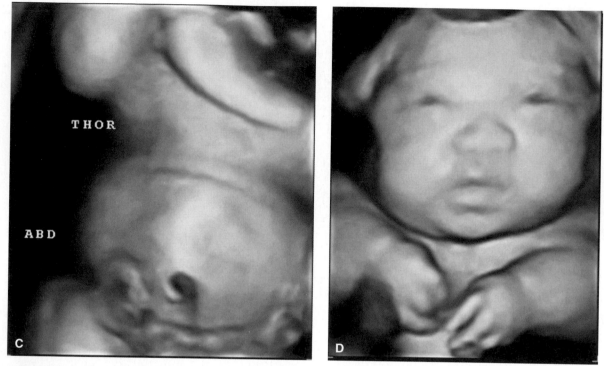

Figure 26-16 (*continued*) **C.** Three-dimensional (*3D*) image of trunk of fetus showing very small thorax (*THOR*) compared to the abdomen (*ABD*). **D.** 3D image of face and upper trunk demonstrating very short upper extremities.

> ### SOUND OFF
> Osteogenesis imperfecta, commonly known as brittle bone disease, is a group of disorders that results in multiple fractures that can occur in utero.

Thanatophoric Dysplasia

Thanatophoric ("death-bearing") dysplasia is the most common lethal skeletal dysplasia. The fetus with thanatophoric dysplasia will have a **cloverleaf skull** with frontal bossing and hydrocephalus (Fig. 26-19). In

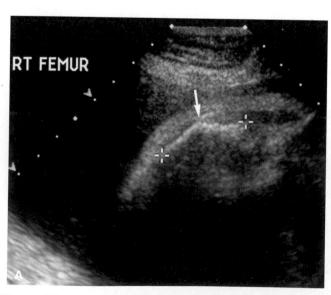

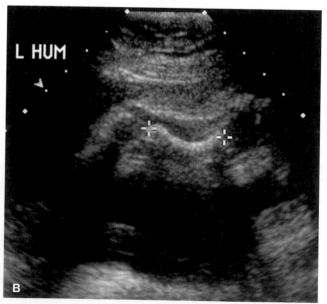

Figure 26-17 Osteogenesis imperfecta type II. **A.** Sonogram of right femur (*calipers*) with a fracture deformity (*arrow*), in a fetus with osteogenesis imperfecta type II. **B.** The left humerus (*calipers*) is bowed.

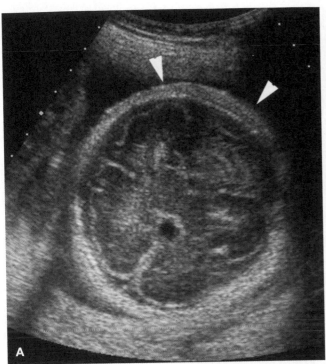
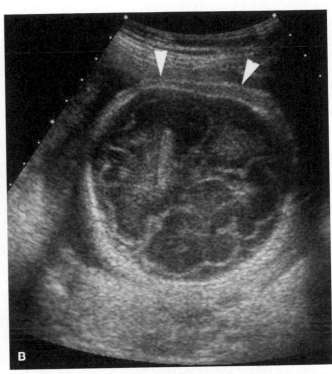

Figure 26-18 Skull with osteogenesis. **A.** Images of the cranium in a 29-week fetus showing poor ossification, making intracranial contents easy to visualize. The skull (*arrowheads*) is very soft, such that when gentle compression was applied for image (**B**), the cranium flattened.

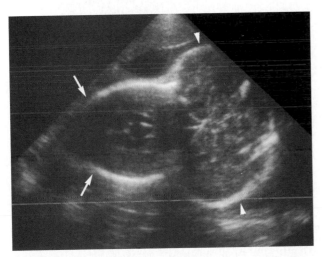

Figure 26-19 Cloverleaf skull. This fetus with thanatophoric dysplasia has a cloverleaf skull with frontal bossing (*arrows*) and lateral protrusion in the region of the temporal bones (*arrowheads*).

addition, the shortened long bones take on a "telephone receiver" shape, because the diaphysis of the long bones will be bowed and have prominent metaphyseal ends (Fig. 26-20). The thoracic and abdominal circumference will be remarkably dissimilar, leading to a bell-shaped chest. Specifically, the thorax will be remarkably narrow, resulting in hypoplasia of the lungs, whereas the abdomen will appear prominent.

This disparity can be best recognized with a sagittal image of the fetus. To document that the chest is much smaller than the abdomen, a thoracic circumference measurement can be obtained. With advancing gestation, redundant soft tissue, especially on the limbs, can also be noted. Fetuses with thanatophoric dysplasia typically die shortly after birth, succumbing most often to respiratory distress as a result of pulmonary hypoplasia.

SONOGRAPHIC FINDINGS OF THANATOPHORIC DYSPLASIA

1. Cloverleaf skull
2. Hydrocephalus
3. Depressed nasal bridge
4. Bell-shaped chest (narrow thorax)
5. Polyhydramnios
6. Redundant soft tissue
7. Telephone receiver–shaped long bones

◀))) SOUND OFF
The fetus with thanatophoric dysplasia will have a cloverleaf skull with frontal bossing and hydrocephalus.

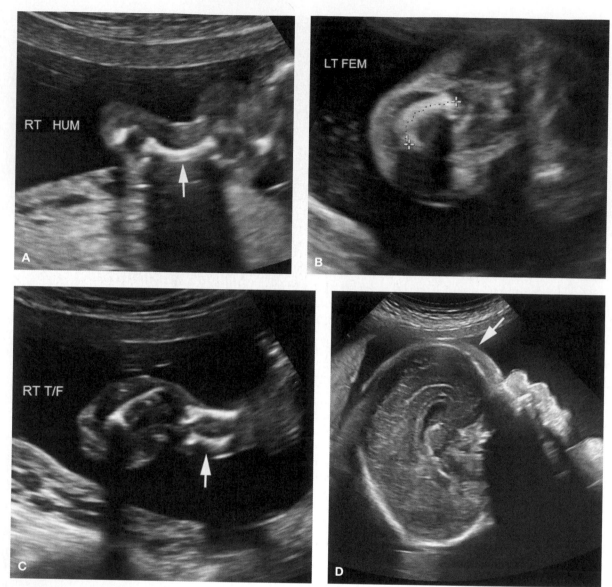

Figure 26-20 Thanatophoric dysplasia. **A.** Humerus (*arrow*). **B.** Femur (*calipers*). **C.** Tibia and fibula (*arrow*) showing the long bones are very short and bowed. **D.** Image of same fetus in the third trimester demonstrating more bulging of the frontal portion of the cranium (*arrow*), called frontal bossing, and characteristic of thanatophoric dysplasia.

CAUDAL REGRESSION SYNDROME

Caudal regression syndrome may also be referred to as **sacral agenesis**. The sonographic findings of caudal regression syndrome are absence of the sacrum (sacral agenesis) and coccyx (coccygeal agenesis) (Fig. 26-21). There may also be defects in the lumbar spine and lower extremities. Uncontrolled maternal **pregestational diabetes** has a strong association with caudal regression syndrome.

CLINICAL FINDINGS OF CAUDAL REGRESSION SYNDROME

1. Uncontrolled maternal pregestational diabetes

SONOGRAPHIC FINDINGS OF CAUDAL REGRESSION SYNDROME

1. Absent sacrum (sacral agenesis) and possibly part of the lumbar vertebra
2. Possible abnormalities in the lower extremities like clubfeet

SIRENOMELIA

Sirenomelia is also referred to as **mermaid syndrome** because of the fusion of the lower extremities that occurs with this disorder. Because **bilateral renal**

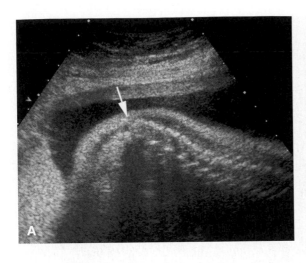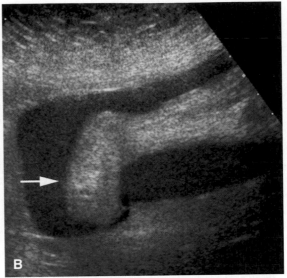

Figure 26-21 Caudal regression syndrome. **A.** Sagittal image of the fetal spine appears to abruptly terminate at the level of the lumbar spine (*arrow*) with absence of the sacrum. **B.** This fetus also had a clubfoot (*arrow*).

agenesis often accompanies this condition, it is almost always lethal. In turn, **oligohydramnios** and many other defects, including cardiac anomalies, genital absence, and a two-vessel cord, may be seen. Again, like caudal regression syndrome, uncontrolled maternal pregestational diabetes seems to play a role in the development of this disorder.

CLINICAL FINDINGS OF SIRENOMELIA

1. Uncontrolled pregestational maternal diabetes

SONOGRAPHIC FINDINGS OF SIRENOMELIA

1. Fusion of the lower extremities
2. Bilateral renal agenesis
3. Oligohydramnios (possibly **anhydramnios**)

🔊 **SOUND OFF**
Sirenomelia is also referred to as mermaid syndrome because of the fusion of the lower extremities that occurs in this disorder.

SACROCOCCYGEAL TERATOMA

An SCT is a **germ cell tumor**. This means that this mass contains elements of the three different germ cell layers: endoderm, mesoderm, and ectoderm.

SCT has been cited as the most common congenital neoplasm and is more frequently found in females. This tumor will typically appear as a complex or solid mass extending posteriorly and inferiorly from the distal fetal spine (Fig. 26-22). An SCT has the potential to grow inside the pelvis and may cause obstruction of the urinary tract and destruction of the sacrum and pelvic bones (Fig. 26-23). Large SCTs have malignant potential. SCTs have been associated with hydrops and may lead to high-output congestive heart failure.

SONOGRAPHIC FINDINGS OF SACROCOCCYGEAL TERATOMA

1. Complex mass extending from the distal fetal spine
2. Mass can be highly vascular
3. **Hydronephrosis** may be present (when mass invades the pelvis)
4. Fetal hydrops may be present
5. Cardiomegaly

EMBRYOLOGY OF THE APPENDICULAR SKELETON

Similar to the axial skeleton, the **appendicular skeleton** begins to form between the sixth and eighth menstrual weeks. The appendicular skeleton includes the bones of the upper extremities, lower extremities, and pelvic girdle. The first sonographic appearances

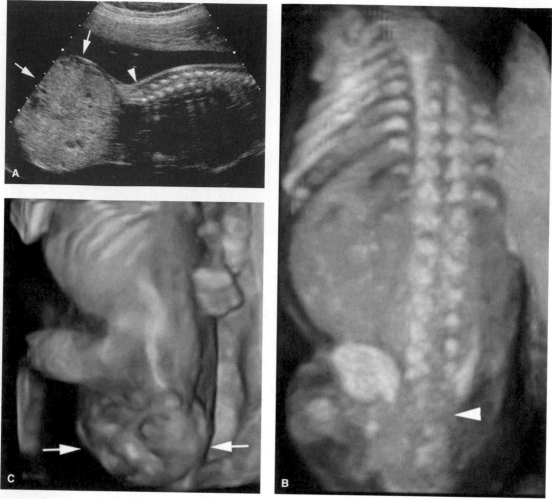

Figure 26-22 Exophytic sacrococcygeal teratoma with erosion of the sacrum. **A.** Sagittal image of lower spine demonstrating large tumor extending inferiorly (*arrows*). The distal spine (*arrowhead*) is not well seen. **B.** Three-dimensional (*3D*) image of the same fetus with skeletal settings showing absence of the sacral vertebrae (*arrowhead*) as a result of tumor invasion. **C.** 3D ultrasound of lower posterior aspect of the fetus showing the outer contour of the mass (*arrows*) extending inferiorly beneath the buttocks.

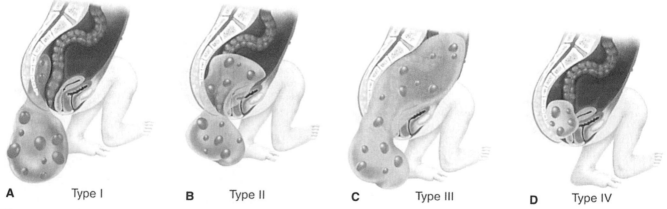

Figure 26-23 The spectrum of sacrococcygeal teratomas. **A.** Type I with predominately cystic teratoma (*arrow*). **B.** Type II teratomas with cystic and solid elements (*arrow*). **C.** Type III solid teratoma. **D.** Type IV teratomas presenting as nonimmune fetal hydrops with a large intra-abdominal mass (*arrow*).

of the fetal limbs are referred to as limb buds. During the second trimester, the fetal limb bones take on more of an adult appearance and appear echogenic and will produce posterior shadowing. The upper extremities include the phalanges (fingers), the metacarpals, carpals, radius, ulna, humerus, clavicle, and scapula. The lower extremities consist of the phalanges (toes), metatarsals, tarsals, tibia, fibula, and femur (see Fig. 14-1).

Measurements of the long bones, especially the femur, are included in an obstetric sonogram. The femur, tibia, fibula, humerus, radius, and ulna can be measured as early as 12 weeks' gestation. Even the clavicles can be measured and correlate nicely in millimeters from 14 weeks to term. The measurement of these long bones should include only the diaphysis of the bones and not the hypoechoic cartilaginous ends. The tibia and fibula end at the same distal location. The tibia is the larger of the two bones, and it is more medial in location. In the forearm, the ulna is longer proximally compared to the radius and is associated with the side of the fifth digit (smallest finger). Thus, in the anatomic position, the radius is located laterally and associated with the thumb.

Shortening of a limb or part of limb can be identified sonographically. The sonographic determination of the shortening of a limb is made when the long bones measure more than four standard deviations below the norm for gestational age. Table 26-2 identifies and defines several terms related to shortening of the limbs and other abnormalities of the appendicular skeleton.

TABLE 26-2 Various limb abnormalities and their description

Type of Limb Abnormality	Description
Acheiria	Absent hand
Acromelia	Shortening of the distal segment of a limb
Amelia	Absent limb
Apodia	Absent foot
Arthrogryposis	Limitation of fetal limb motion as a result of joint contractures; most often affecting the hands and feet
Clinodactyly	Deviation of a finger (e.g., absence of the middle fifth phalanx)
Clubfoot	An inversion of the soles of one foot toward the other; when the metatarsals and toes lie in the same plane as the tibia and fibula; also referred to as talipes equinovarus
Hemimelia	Absent part of an extremity distal to the elbow or knee
Mesomelia	Shortening of the middle segment of a limb
Micromelia	Shortening of an entire limb
Oligodactyly	Having less than the normal number of digits
Phocomelia	Absent long bones with the hands and feet arising from the shoulders and hips
Polydactyly	Having more than the normal number of digits
Rhizomelia	Shortening of the proximal segment of a limb
Rocker-bottom foot	Abnormal curved shape of the sole of the foot
Sandal gap (Fig. 26-24)	Exaggerated distance between the first toe and the second toe
Syndactyly (Fig. 26-25)	Fusion of digits (e.g., webbed toes)
Sirenomelia (mermaid syndrome)	Fusion of the legs
Talipomanus	Clubhand
Trident hand	Increases space between the third finger and the fourth finger

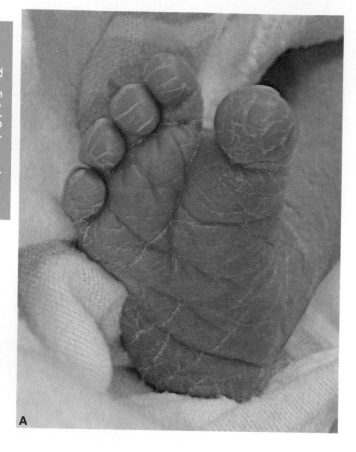

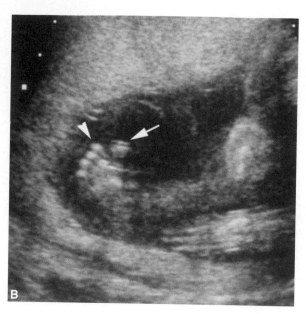

Figure 26-24 Sandal gap foot deformity. **A.** Newborn image of a fetal foot demonstrating sandal gap deformity in a fetus with trisomy 21. **B.** Image of the foot in a fetus with a ventricular septal defect showing abnormally large gap between the great toe (*arrow*) and the second toe (*arrowhead*).

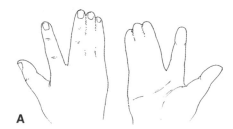

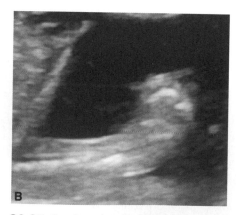

Figure 26-25 Syndactyly. **A.** Webbing of the fingers can be simple or complex. **B.** Sonographic appearance of syndactyly. Right hand shows abnormal clenching of the hand and fingers, with indistinct digits, indicating complete syndactyly, called the "mitten" hand deformity.

RADIAL RAY DEFECT

Radial ray defect is uncommon and described as the absence (aplasia) or underdevelopment (hypoplasia) of the radius. This abnormality can be seen in the presence of trisomy 13, trisomy 18, and several other syndromes. There are often other anomalies present, specifically cardiac abnormalities and possibly a clubhand (talipomanus). There is a link with VACTERL association.

SONOGRAPHIC FINDINGS OF RADIAL RAY DEFECT

1. Absent or hypoplastic radius
2. Various defects in other body systems: cardiac and VACTERL association

CLUBFOOT

Clubfoot, also referred to as talipes or **talipes equinovarus**, is a malformation of the bones of the foot. The foot is most often inverted and rotated

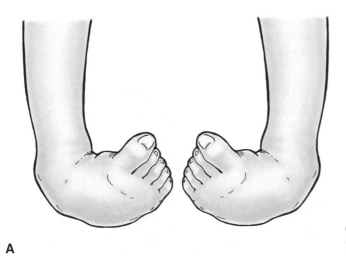

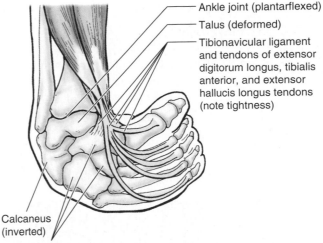

Ankle joint (plantarflexed)

Talus (deformed)

Tibionavicular ligament
and tendons of extensor
digitorum longus, tibialis
anterior, and extensor
hallucis longus tendons
(note tightness)

Calcaneus
(inverted)

Bones of forefoot
(in extreme varus position)

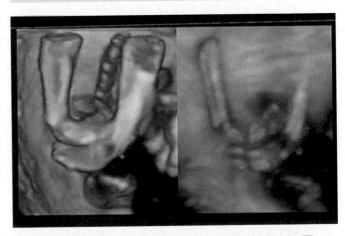

Figure 26-26 Clubfoot. **A.** Drawing of bilateral clubfeet. **B.** Image of the lower leg and knee (*k*) depicting a clubfoot (*arrow*).

medially (Fig. 26-26). The sonographic diagnosis of clubfoot can be made when the metatarsals and toes lie in the same plane as the tibia and fibula. Three-dimensional sonographic imaging can be exceedingly beneficial for proper diagnosis (Fig. 26-27). If an abnormal foot shape is suspected, a foot length measurement can be obtained by measuring from the skin edge of the heel (calcaneus) to the distal end of the longest toe. Foot length has been used for gestational dating as well, and it has been shown to be nearly equivalent to the femur length, resulting in a femur-to-foot ratio of approximately 1.0 after 14 weeks' gestation.

SOUND OFF

Clubfoot results in the metatarsals and toes lying in the same plane as the tibia and fibula.

Figure 26-27 Clubbed feet (21 weeks 5 days). Three-dimensional sonogram demonstrating bilateral clubfeet by surface rendering (*left panel*) and for skeletal structures using maximum intensity projection (*right panel*).

SONOGRAPHIC FINDINGS OF CLUBFOOT

1. Metatarsals and toes lie in the same plane as the tibia and fibula

LIMB REDUCTION AND AMNIOTIC BAND SYNDROME

Limb reduction can be caused by amniotic band syndrome, also referred to as amniotic band sequence. Sticky bands result from the rupture of the amnion. These bands can entrap fetal parts and cause amputation of digits, limbs, and even the skull (Fig. 26-28). Amniotic bands can also lead to peculiar facial clefting. These bands should not be confused with uterine **synechiae**. Amniotic bands may be seen with sonography, though, occasionally, only the results of the bands are seen. Uterine synechiae may be recognized as linear, thin membranes with a broad base crossing the amniotic sac (Fig. 26-29).

SONOGRAPHIC FINDINGS OF AMNIOTIC BAND SYNDROME

1. Amputation of fetal parts or severe edema in the affected area
2. Thin, linear bands may be seen
3. Facial clefting

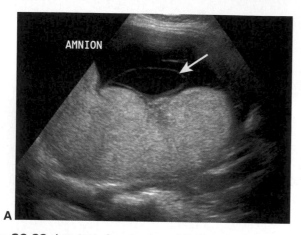
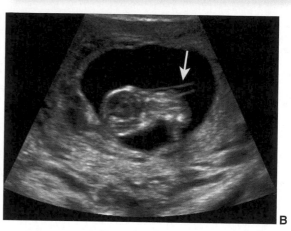

Figure 26-28 Amniotic bands. **A** and **B.** Demonstrating free-floating amniotic bands (*arrows*). The fetus in (**B**) also had scoliosis, limb deformities, and an anterior abdominal wall defect.

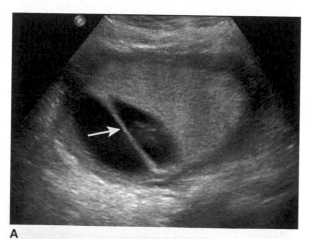
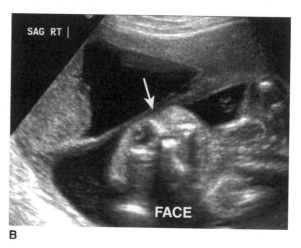
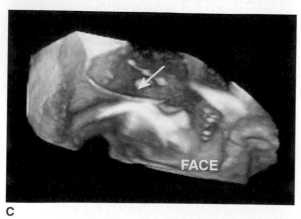

Figure 26-29 Uterine synechia. **A.** Sonographic image lateral to midline demonstrating a thick linear structure continuous with the placenta in a singleton pregnancy, consistent with a uterine synechia (*arrow*). **B.** Oblique sonographic image of a uterine synechia traversing the fetal face (*arrow*). **C.** Three-dimensional surface rendering in the same patient as **B** showing the synechia superior to the fetal face (*arrow*). There was no entrapment of fetal parts, and the pregnancy outcome was normal.

REVIEW QUESTIONS

1. What diagnosis is evident in Figure 26-30?
   a. Spina bifida occulta with Dandy–Walker syndrome
   b. Spina bifida aperta with Arnold–Chiari I malformation
   c. Spina bifida occulta with Arnold–Chiari I malformation
   d. Spina bifida aperta with Arnold–Chiari II malformation

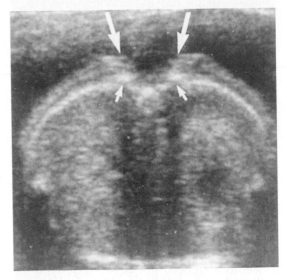

Figure 26-31

4. What abnormality of the lower leg is evident in Figure 26-32?
   a. Amelia
   b. Phocomelia
   c. Clubfoot
   d. Syndactyly

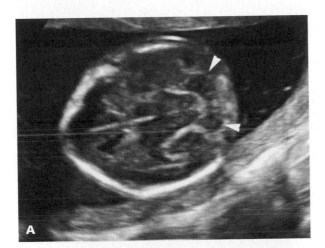

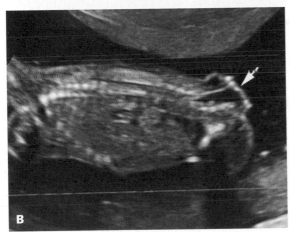

Figure 26-30

2. Which of the following is demonstrated by the large arrows in Figure 26-31?
   a. Spina bifida occulta
   b. Open spinal defect
   c. Kyphosis
   d. Kyphoscoliosis

3. What cranial finding would be least likely associated with Figure 26-31?
   a. Colpocephaly
   b. Hydrocephalus
   c. Enlarged cisterna magna
   d. Flattened frontal bones

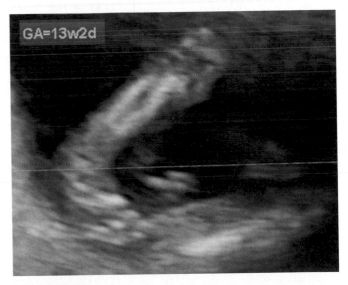

Figure 26-32

5. What abnormality is evident in Figure 26-33?
   a. Lordosis
   b. Kyphosis
   c. Hyphosis
   d. Scoliosis

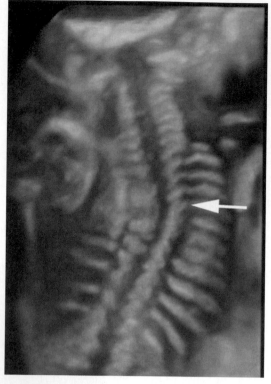

Figure 26-33

6. What finding of the fetal cerebellum would be associated with Figure 26-34?
   a. Lemon shape
   b. Banana shape
   c. Absent
   d. Enlarged

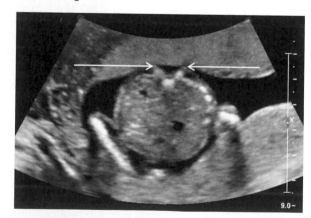

Figure 26-34

7. What does the arrow in Figure 26-35 indicate?
   a. Cervical spine
   b. Thoracic spine
   c. Lumbar spine
   d. Sacral spine

8. What demonstration is Figure 26-35 of the fetal spine?
   a. Transverse
   b. Coronal
   c. Longitudinal
   d. Three-dimensional

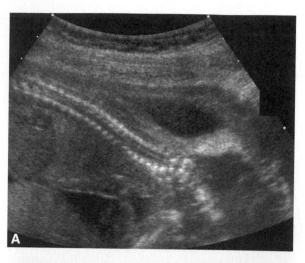

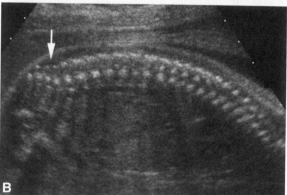

Figure 26-35

9. The neural process of the spine will become all of the following except:
   a. lamina.
   b. pedicle.
   c. vertebral body.
   d. spinous process.

10. What demonstration is Figure 26-36 of the fetal spine?
   a. Transverse
   b. Coronal
   c. Longitudinal
   d. Three-dimensional

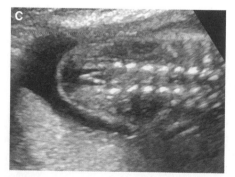

Figure 26-36

11. What is the term defined as the absence of part of an extremity distal to the elbow or knee?
   a. Phocomelia
   b. Amelia
   c. Acromelia
   d. Hemimelia

12. What is the term for absence of a foot?
   a. Amelia
   b. Acheiria
   c. Apodia
   d. Arthrogryposis

13. What is the term for clubhand?
   a. Sirenomelia
   b. Talipomanus
   c. Syndactyly
   d. Rhizomelia

14. Acheiria is absence of the:
   a. hand.
   b. foot.
   c. elbow.
   d. knee.

15. The radius is located on what side of the forearm?
   a. Medial
   b. Lateral

16. What is the larger bone of the lower leg?
   a. Tibia
   b. Fibula

17. Sonographically, you note that the fetal foot has a curved shape of the sole. What is the most likely diagnosis?
   a. Rocker-bottom foot
   b. Sirenomelia
   c. Micromelia
   d. Amelia

18. Which condition is often associated with heterozygous achondroplasia?
   a. Oligodactyly
   b. Mesomelia
   c. Rhizomelia
   d. Phocomelia

19. The brain and spinal cord are covered by the:
   a. meninges.
   b. ependyma.
   c. neural tube.
   d. myelocele.

20. The fetus in Figure 26-37 is suffering from achondroplasia. What is noted in this profile image?
   a. Ventriculomegaly
   b. Frontal bossing
   c. Lemon sign
   d. Cebocephaly

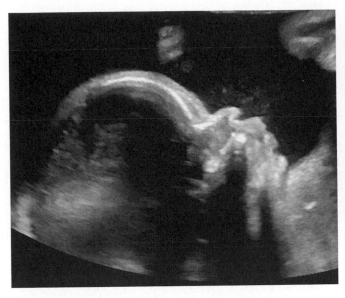

Figure 26-37

21. What is the maternal dietary supplement that has been shown to significantly reduce the likelihood of the fetus suffering from a neural tube defect?
   a. AFP
   b. Estriol
   c. Folate
   d. Pregnancy protein A

22. Talipes equinovarus is associated with:
   a. clubfoot.
   b. syndactyly.
   c. rhizomelia.
   d. rocker-bottom feet.

23. The artifact seen posterior to solid structures such as fetal bone is referred to as:
   a. acoustic shadowing.
   b. posterior enhancement.
   c. reverberation artifact.
   d. edge artifact.

24. What is the anomaly of the spine in which there is absence of all or part of a vertebral body and posterior element?
   a. Kyphosis
   b. Scoliosis
   c. Kyphoscoliosis
   d. Hemivertebra

25. The disorder associated with fetal amputations is:
   a. achondroplasia.
   b. osteogenesis imperfecta.
   c. thanatophoric dysplasia.
   d. amniotic band syndrome.

26. The form of inheritance in which at least one parent has to be a carrier of an abnormal gene for it to be passed to the fetus is:
    a. autosomal recessive.
    b. autosomal dominant.
    c. inherited dominant.
    d. inherited recessive.

27. The condition associated with the absence of the sacrum and coccyx:
    a. limb-body wall complex.
    b. caudal regression syndrome.
    c. thanatophoric dwarfism.
    d. heterozygous achondroplasia.

28. All of the following are characteristics of spina bifida occulta except:
    a. closed defect.
    b. elevated MSAFP.
    c. sacral dimple.
    d. hemangioma.

29. The abnormal lateral ventricle shape in which there is a small frontal horn and enlarged occipital horn is referred to as:
    a. cebocephaly.
    b. banana sign.
    c. colpocephaly.
    d. cephalocele.

30. All of the following are characteristics of spina bifida cystica except:
    a. banana sign.
    b. lemon sign.
    c. enlarged massa intermedia.
    d. normal MSAFP.

31. In VACTERL association, the letter "C" stands for:
    a. cerebellar.
    b. C-spine.
    c. cranial.
    d. cardiac.

32. All of the following are associated with spina bifida except:
    a. splaying of the laminae.
    b. enlarged posterior fossa.
    c. lemon sign.
    d. banana sign.

33. The abnormal lateral curvature of the spine is referred to as:
    a. kyphosis.
    b. scoliosis.
    c. splaying.
    d. achondroplasia.

34. The lemon sign denotes:
    a. an abnormal shape of the fetal skull.
    b. a normal shape of the cerebellum.
    c. an abnormal shape of the cerebellum.
    d. a normal shape of the fetal skull.

35. All of the following are clinical or sonographic findings consistent with LBWC except:
    a. ventral wall defects.
    b. decreased MSAFP.
    c. marked scoliosis.
    d. shortened umbilical cord.

36. A disorder that results in abnormal bone growth and dwarfism is:
    a. osteogenesis imperfecta.
    b. achondroplasia.
    c. radial ray defect.
    d. caudal regression syndrome.

37. Which of the following would increase the likelihood of a fetus developing sirenomelia and caudal regression syndrome?
    a. Previous cesarean section
    b. Preexisting maternal diabetes
    c. Previous ectopic pregnancy
    d. Elevated hCG

38. The group of fetal head and brain abnormalities that often coexists with spina bifida is referred to as:
    a. Dandy–Walker malformation.
    b. Budd–Chiari syndrome.
    c. Arnold–Chiari II malformation.
    d. amniotic band syndrome.

39. In VACTERL association, the letter "L" stands for:
    a. limb.
    b. lung.
    c. liver.
    d. larynx.

40. The most common nonlethal skeletal dysplasia is:
    a. achondrogenesis.
    b. achondroplasia.
    c. thanatophoric dysplasia.
    d. osteogenesis imperfecta.

41. Achondroplasia is associated with all of the following except:
    a. frontal bossing.
    b. flattened nasal bridge.
    c. trident hand.
    d. absent mineralization of the skull.

42. What abnormality results in limitation of the fetal limbs as a result of joint contractures?
    a. Acromegaly
    b. Radial ray defect
    c. Achondrogenesis
    d. Arthrogryposis

43. The thalamic tissue located within the third ventricle of the brain that can become enlarged with Arnold–Chiari II malformation is the:
    a. corpus callosum.
    b. cerebellar vermis.
    c. cavum septum pellucidum.
    d. massa intermedia.

44. Rhizomelia denotes:
   a. long upper extremities.
   b. shortening of an entire limb.
   c. shortening of the proximal segment of a limb.
   d. shortening of the distal segment of a limb.

45. An absent sacrum and coccyx is referred to as:
   a. sirenomelia.
   b. caudal regression syndrome.
   c. achondroplasia.
   d. radial ray defect.

46. Absent long bones with the hands and feet arising from the shoulders and hips describes:
   a. micromelia.
   b. mesomelia.
   c. phocomelia.
   d. arthrogryposis.

47. All of the following are characteristic sonographic findings of achondrogenesis except:
   a. micromelia.
   b. absent mineralization of the pelvis.
   c. multiple dislocated joints.
   d. polyhydramnios.

48. Upon sonographic interrogation of a 28-week pregnancy, you note that when pressure is applied to the fetal skull, the skull can be easily distorted. This is sonographic evidence of:
   a. Arnold–Chiari II malformation.
   b. achondroplasia.
   c. thanatophoric dysplasia.
   d. osteogenesis imperfecta.

49. A bell-shaped chest and multiple fetal fractures are indicative of:
   a. thanatophoric dysplasia.
   b. caudal regression syndrome.
   c. achondrogenesis.
   d. osteogenesis imperfecta.

50. All of the following are signs of Arnold–Chiari II malformation except:
   a. S-shaped spine.
   b. banana sign.
   c. lemon sign.
   d. colpocephaly.

51. All of the following are associated with amniotic band syndrome except:
   a. amputation of fetal parts.
   b. anencephaly.
   c. facial clefting.
   d. synechiae.

52. The exaggerated distance between the first toe and the second toe is:
   a. trident toes.
   b. sandal gap.
   c. phocomelia.
   d. mesomelia.

53. Sirenomelia is commonly referred to as:
   a. radial ray defect.
   b. rhizomelia.
   c. mermaid syndrome.
   d. rocker-bottom feet.

54. Absence of the radius is referred to as:
   a. talipes equinovarus.
   b. clubfoot.
   c. radial ray defect.
   d. phocomelia.

55. Sonographically, you visualize a mass extending from the distal spine of a fetus. This mass could be all of the following except:
   a. SCT.
   b. meningocele.
   c. meningomyelocele.
   d. phocomeningocele.

56. A cloverleaf skull and hydrocephalus is seen with:
   a. achondrogenesis.
   b. osteogenesis imperfecta.
   c. sirenomelia.
   d. thanatophoric dysplasia.

57. What term is defined as fusion of the digits?
   a. Clinodactyly
   b. Polydactyly
   c. Syndactyly
   d. Rhizodactyly

58. A protein produced by the yolk sac and fetal liver that is found in excess in the maternal circulation in the presence of a neural tube defect is:
   a. folate.
   b. hCG.
   c. Estriol.
   d. AFP.

59. What condition is associated with bilateral renal agenesis, oligohydramnios, and fusion of the lower extremities?
   a. SCT
   b. Caudal displacement syndrome
   c. Sirenomelia
   d. Osteogenesis imperfect

60. Which of the following is true for the diagnosis of clubfoot?
   a. The metatarsals and toes lie in the same plane as the tibia and fibula.
   b. The metatarsals are perpendicular to the tibia and fibula.
   c. The carpals and metacarpals lie in the same plane as the tibia and fibula.
   d. The tibia, fibula, and patella are perpendicular to the femur.

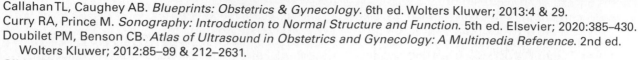

SUGGESTED READINGS

Callahan TL, Caughey AB. *Blueprints: Obstetrics & Gynecology.* 6th ed. Wolters Kluwer; 2013:4 & 29.

Curry RA, Prince M. *Sonography: Introduction to Normal Structure and Function.* 5th ed. Elsevier; 2020:385–430.

Doubilet PM, Benson CB. *Atlas of Ultrasound in Obstetrics and Gynecology: A Multimedia Reference.* 2nd ed. Wolters Kluwer; 2012:85–99 & 212–2631.

Gibbs RS, Karlan BY, Haney AF, et al. *Danforth's Obstetrics and Gynecology.* 10th ed. Wolters Kluwer; 2008:113–114.

Henningsen C, Kuntz K, Youngs D. *Clinical Guide to Sonography: Exercises for Critical Thinking.* 2nd ed. Elsevier; 2014:260 & 295–301.

Kline-Fath BM, Bulas DI, and Lee W. *Fundamental and Advanced Fetal Imaging: Ultrasound and MRI.* 2nd ed. Wolters Kluwer; 2021:639–663 & 879–901.

Norton ME, Scoutt LM, Feldstein VA. *Callen's Ultrasonography in Obstetrics and Gynecology.* 6th ed. Elsevier; 2017:222–225 & 272–345.

Nyberg D, McGaham J, Pretorius D, et al. *Diagnostic Imaging of Fetal Anomalies.* Lippincott Williams & Wilkins; 2003:291–334 & 661–711.

Rumack CM, Wilson SR, Charboneau W, et al. *Diagnostic Ultrasound.* 4th ed. Elsevier; 2011:1245–1272 & 1389–1423.

Sanders RC, Hall-Terracciano B. *Clinical Sonography: A Practical Guide.* 5th ed. Wolters Kluwer; 2016:325–327 & 331–332.

BONUS REVIEW!

Three-Dimensional Surface-Mode Image of the Fetal Spine (Fig. 26-38)

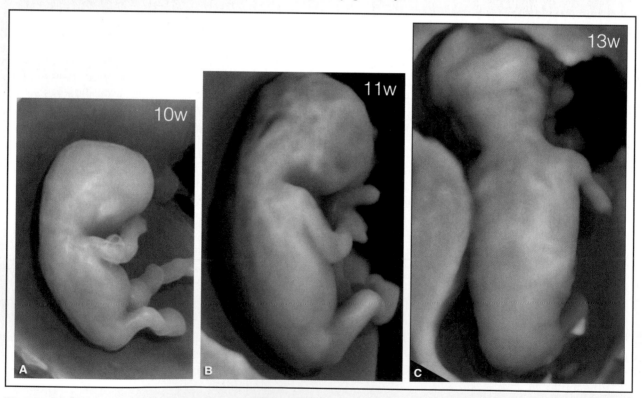

Figure 26-38 Three-dimensional (*3D*) sonogram in surface mode demonstrating the back of three fetuses at 10 (**A**), 11 (**B**), and 13 (**C**) weeks of gestation. Note the absence of a defect in the back, confirming the lack of an open spina bifida. When technically feasible, 3D ultrasound in surface mode allows for an excellent evaluation of the fetal back and spine for open spina bifida.

BONUS REVIEW! (*continued*)

Radiograph of Trident Hands (Fig. 26-39)

Sirenomelia (Fig. 26-40)

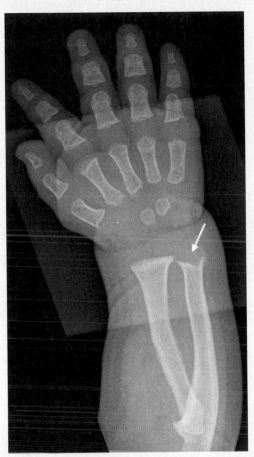

Figure 26-39 Radiograph of a trident hand. Frontal radiograph of the hand demonstrates short, broad, long bones of the forearm and hand. There is a V-shape configuration of the distal ulnar physis (*arrow*) and trident configuration of the hand.

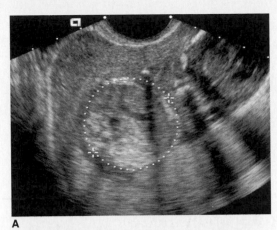

A

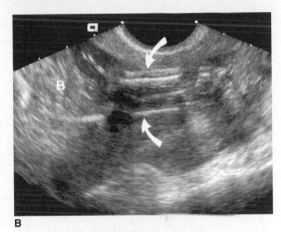

B

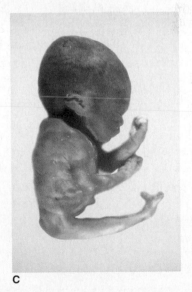

C

Figure 26-40 Sirenomelia. **A.** Transverse view of abdomen showing marked oligohydramnios secondary to renal agenesis. **B.** View of the lower legs showing the tibias and fibulas close to one another (*arrows*). Some cases show absence of one or more bones. **C.** Postnatal image of fetus with sirenomelia.

The Fetal Heart and Chest

Introduction

The primary focus of this chapter is on anomalies detectable on a routine sonographic examination of the fetal heart and chest, although additional anomalies are covered. An overview of embryology of the heart and lungs is also provided. The obstetric sonographer should have a balanced understanding of four-chamber heart anatomy and structural defects that can be detected with this view. With the addition of the outflow tracts, several other anomalies may be distinguished. The "Bonus Review" section includes standard fetal echocardiography color Doppler images, an apical four-chamber view in systole and diastole, and an image of a fetal thoracentesis.

Key Terms

aneuploidy—a condition of having an abnormal number of chromosomes

aortic atresia—abnormality in which there is a small or absent opening between the left ventricle and the aorta

aortic stenosis—abnormal narrowing of the aortic valve

atrioventricular defect—abnormal development of the central portion of the heart; also referred to as endocardial cushion defect

bat-wing sign—the sonographic appearance of a fetal unilateral pleural effusion

biophysical profile—a method of fetal monitoring with sonography to produce a numeric scoring system that predicts fetal well-being

Bochdalek hernia—the herniation of abdominal contents into the chest cavity because of an opening in the left posterolateral portion of the diaphragm

chordae tendineae—tendons within the heart that attach the tricuspid valve in the right ventricle and the mitral valve in the left ventricle to their respective papillary muscle

coarctation of the aorta—the narrowing of the aortic arch

cystic adenomatoid malformation—a mass consisting of abnormal bronchial and lung tissue that develops within the fetal chest

diaphragmatic hernia—the herniation of the abdominal contents into the chest cavity through a defect in the diaphragm

DiGeorge syndrome—a genetic disorder characterized by an absent or hypoplastic thymus, which ultimately leads to impairment of the immune system and susceptibility to infection, as well as cognitive disorders, congenital heart defects, palate defects, and hormonal abnormalities

ductus arteriosus—a fetal shunt that connects the pulmonary artery to the aortic arch

ductus venosus—a fetal shunt that connects the umbilical vein to the inferior vena cava

Ebstein anomaly—the malformation or malpositioning of the tricuspid valve that causes multiple heart defects

ectopic cordis—a condition in which the heart is located either partially or completely outside the fetal chest

endocardial cushion defect—see atrioventricular defect

eventration of the diaphragm—lack of muscle in the dome of the diaphragm

fetal hydrops—an abnormal accumulation of fluid in at least two fetal body cavities

foramen of Bochdalek—an opening located in the left posterolateral portion of the diaphragm

foramen of Morgagni—an opening located right anteromedially within the diaphragm

foramen ovale—an opening within the fetal heart within the atrial septum that allows blood to flow from the right atrium to the left atrium

hypoplastic left heart syndrome—incomplete development of the left ventricle, resulting in a small or absent left ventricle

hypoplastic right heart syndrome—incomplete development of the right ventricle, resulting in a small or absent right ventricle

lecithin-to-sphingomyelin ratio—a test of the amniotic fluid that predicts fetal lung maturity

oligohydramnios—a lower-than-normal amount of amniotic fluid for the gestational age

omphalocele—an anterior abdominal wall defect where there is herniation of the fetal bowel and other abdominal organs into the base of the umbilical cord

papillary muscle—paired muscles in both sides of the heart that hold in place either the mitral or tricuspid valves

pentalogy of Cantrell—a group of anomalies that include an omphalocele, along with ectopic cordis, cleft sternum, anterior diaphragmatic defect, and pericardial defects

pericardial effusion—fluid accumulation around the heart in the pericardial cavity

pleural effusion—the abnormal accumulation of fluid in the pleural space

Potter syndrome—syndrome characterized by bilateral renal agenesis, abnormal facies, pulmonary hypoplasia, and limb abnormalities

pulmonary atresia—the absence of the pulmonary valve, which, in turn, prohibits blood flow from the right ventricle into the pulmonary artery and essentially to the lungs

pulmonary hypoplasia—underdevelopment of the lungs

pulmonary sequestration—a separate mass of nonfunctioning lung tissue with its own blood supply

pulmonary stenosis—the narrowing of the pulmonary valve

rhabdomyoma—a fetal heart tumor found within the myocardium

tetralogy of Fallot—a group of abnormalities consisting of an overriding aortic root, ventricular septal defect, pulmonary stenosis, and right ventricular hypertrophy

thoracentesis—a procedure that uses a needle to drain fluid from the pleural cavity for either diagnostic or therapeutic reasons

transposition of the great vessels—abnormality in which the pulmonary artery arises from the left ventricle and the aorta arises from the right ventricle

tricuspid regurgitation—the leakage of blood back through the tricuspid valve

trisomy 18—chromosomal aberration in which there is a third chromosome 18; also referred to as Edwards syndrome

trisomy 21—chromosomal aberration in which there is a third chromosome 21; also referred to as Down syndrome

tuberous sclerosis—a systemic disorder that leads to the development of tumors within various organs

Turner syndrome—a chromosomal aberration where one sex chromosome is absent; may also be referred to as monosomy X

ventricular septal defect—an opening within the septum that separates the right and left ventricles

THE FETAL HEART

Embryology and Anatomy of the Heart

The embryonic heart begins as two tubes. These two tubes ultimately fuse and fold to form into four chambers, two atria and two ventricles. The heart begins to contract at 36 to 37 days of gestation. It is initially recognized by its motion, which can be seen adjacent to the secondary yolk sac, often before an embryo is distinguishable. A heart rate using M-mode should be sonographically obtainable with endovaginal (EV) imaging when the crown rump length (CRL) measures 4 to 5 mm.

During a **biophysical profile** assessment in the third trimester, an average fetal heart rate is 150 beats per minute (bpm), with a range of 110 to 180 bpm considered normal after the first trimester. An elevation in fetal heart rate is termed tachycardia, whereas a decrease is referred to as bradycardia.

> **◄))) SOUND OFF**
> The embryonic heart begins as two tubes. These two tubes ultimately fuse and fold to form into four chambers, two atria and two ventricles.

Four-Chamber Heart View

The heart, which is fully formed by 10 weeks, is imaged most often in a cross-sectional or axial view of the fetal chest, just above the fetal stomach. This transducer placement will yield the standard four-chamber view of the heart (Figs. 27-1 and 27-2). The apex of the heart will be angled to the left of the midline, with the base closest to the spine. The normal fetal heart will fill approximately one-third of the fetal chest, with its

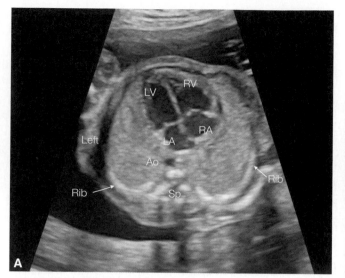

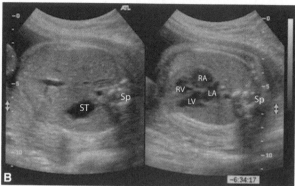

Figure 27-1 Four-chamber heart view. **A.** Axial view of fetal chest at the level of the four-chamber view of heart. Note the appearance of four chambers with right ventricle (*RV*) as most anterior chamber and left atrium (*LA*) as most posterior chamber. Left ventricle (*LV*) and right atrium (*RA*) are also seen. Note the location of descending thoracic aorta (*Ao*) and spine (*Sp*) posteriorly. **B.** The orientation of the heart within the chest in relationship to the fetal stomach (*ST*) is demonstrated in these two images. The apex of the heart is on the same side of the body as the stomach.

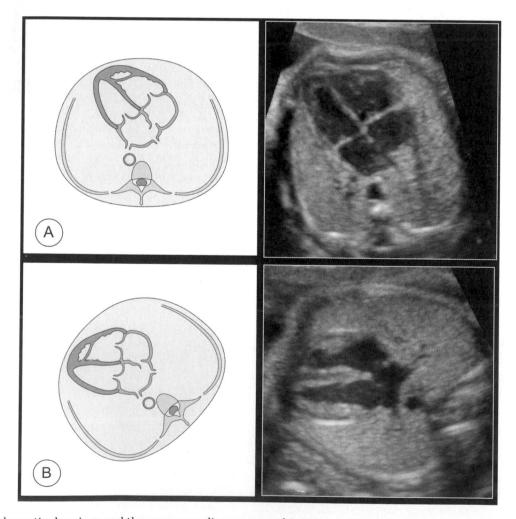

Figure 27-2 Schematic drawings and the corresponding sonographic images of four-chamber views in four fetuses: fetus (**A**) with a posterior spine position, fetus (**B**) with a right lateral spine position, fetus

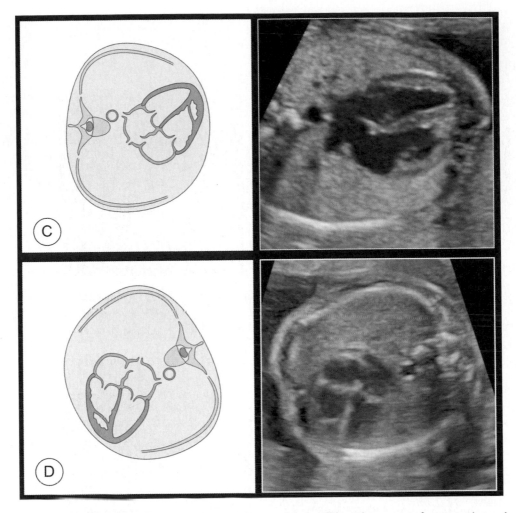

Figure 27-2 *(continued)* (**C**) with a left lateral spine position, and fetus (**D**) with a somewhat anterior spine position.

apex forming a 45-degree angle with the fetal spine. The chamber closest to the fetal spine is the left atrium (Fig. 27-3). If it is suspected that the heart is enlarged, then a cardio/thoracic diameter ratio can be obtained.

> 🔊 **SOUND OFF**
> The normal fetal heart will fill approximately one-third of the fetal chest. If it is suspected that the heart is enlarged, then a cardio/thoracic diameter ratio can be obtained.

The four-chamber view can be used to evaluate the separation of the chambers, structures called septums. The two atria are separated by the atrial septum, and the two ventricles are separated by the ventricular septum. The ventricular septum should be uninterrupted and of equal thickness to the left ventricular wall, whereas the atrial septum is open only at the foramen ovale (Fig. 27-4). Within the right ventricle can be seen the moderator band, a normal structure that appears as an echogenic focus. The left ventricle has much smoother walls compared to the right. Between the right ventricle and the right atrium, one should visualize the tricuspid valve, and between the left ventricle and the left atrium, the mitral valve should be noted. Normally, the tricuspid valve is positioned closer to the cardiac apex than the mitral valve (Fig. 27-5).

Outflow Tracts

Outflow tracts of the fetal heart can be evaluated during the routine screening examination and should be when technically feasible according to the American Institute of Ultrasound in Medicine. The right ventricular outflow tract leads to the pulmonary artery and branches, whereas the left ventricular outflow tract leads to the aorta. One important anatomic finding is that the normal pulmonary artery should be positioned anterior to the aorta and should be visualized crossing over it (Figs. 27-6 through 27-8). That means, the aorta and pulmonary artery normally crisscross each other. There are several other features that should be assessed while imaging the outflow tracts (Table 27-1; Fig. 27-9).

Cardio-Thoracic Diameter

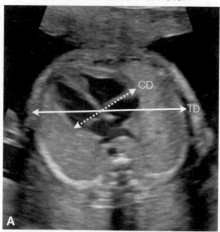

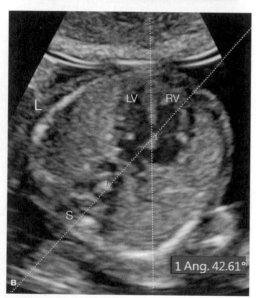

Figure 27-3 Fetal cardiac size. **A.** The diameter of the heart is shown in *double-sided broken arrow* (CD), and the diameter of the thorax is shown in *double-sided solid arrow* (TD). This allows for the calculation of the cardio/thoracic diameter ratio (CD/*TD*). **B.** Normal cardiac axis in a fetus at 13 weeks of gestation.

Three-Vessel and Three-Vessel Tracheal Views

Scanning slowly cephalad from the outflow tracts within the fetus will yield several more vital structures. In Figure 27-9, drawings four through six demonstrate the views that include the three vessels. The three-vessel view (3VV) places the main pulmonary artery, ascending aorta, and superior vena cava in the image (Fig. 27-10). The 3VV is used to detect abnormal vessel number, abnormal vessel caliber, abnormal course or alignment of the vessels, and abnormal flow. The three-vessel trachea view (3VT) is used to evaluate the major vessels in the fetal mediastinum as well. In the 3VT, a "V" is

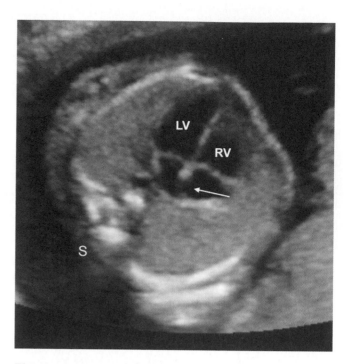

Figure 27-4 Foramen ovale. Normal four-chamber view of the heart in a 21-week fetus. The cardiac apex is directed to the left side of the fetus. The right ventricle (*RV*) is the most anteriorly positioned chamber and is separated from the left ventricle (*LV*) by the interventricular septum. The left atrium is the most posterior chamber, located just anterior to the spine (*S*). The foramen ovale (*arrow*) is seen between the right and left atria.

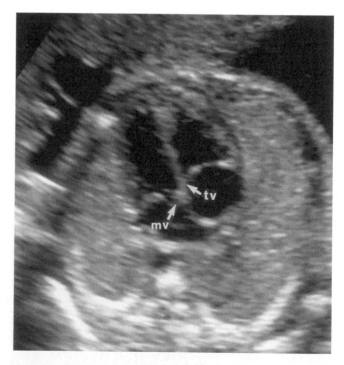

Figure 27-5 Valves seen on the four-chamber view. Normally, the tricuspid valve (*tv*) inserts closer to the apex of the heart compared to the mitral valve (*mv*).

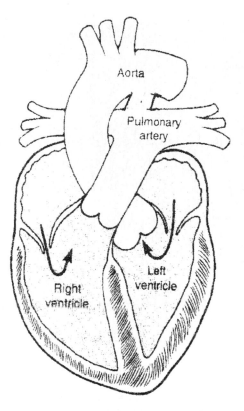

Figure 27-6 Normal crisscrossing of the outflow tracts. Diagram of the heart demonstrating the normal crossing of the pulmonary artery and aorta. The pulmonary artery should be located more anterior than the aorta and be noted crossing over the aorta to originate at the right ventricle.

formed by the merging of the transverse aortic arch and isthmus and the pulmonary trunk and ductus arteriosus (Fig. 27-11). The 3VT is also used to assess the number, size, and alignment of the main pulmonary artery, aorta, and superior vena cava.

FETAL CIRCULATION

It is important for sonographers to have a basic appreciation for fetal circulation (Fig. 27-12). The normal umbilical cord contains two arteries and one vein. The umbilical vein brings oxygen-rich blood from the placenta to the fetus. It travels superiorly and connects to the left portal vein. Half of the blood goes to the liver through the left portal vein, whereas the other half is shunted directly into the inferior vena cava (IVC) via a small branch of the umbilical vein called the **ductus venosus**. The blood that was taken to the liver is used to oxygenate the liver and is then returned back to the IVC by the hepatic veins.

> 🔊 **SOUND OFF**
> Blood is shunted directly into the IVC via a small branch of the umbilical vein called the ductus venosus.

The existing oxygen-rich blood in the IVC travels up to the heart and enters the right atrium. Blood can then travel across the **foramen ovale**, an opening in the lower middle third of the atrial septum and into the left atrium, or it can enter the right ventricle through the tricuspid valve. The blood then leaves the right ventricle through the main pulmonary artery. The main pulmonary artery bifurcates into right and left, thus allowing a small amount of blood to travel to the respective lung. Blood from the right ventricle can also flow through the **ductus arteriosus** and into the descending aorta (Fig. 27-13).

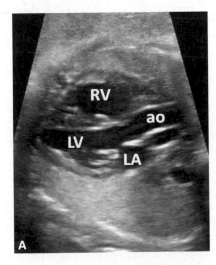
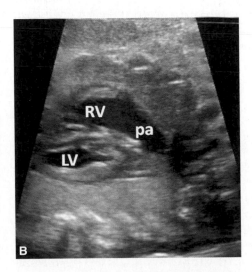

Figure 27-7 Sonogram of outflow tracts. Axial views of the outflow tracts. **A.** Aortic outflow (*ao*) tract exiting from the left ventricle (*LV*). **B.** Pulmonary artery outflow (*pa*) exiting from the right ventricle (*RV*). *LA*, left atrium.

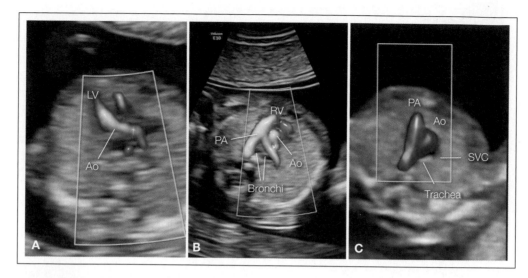

Figure 27-8 Transvaginal sonogram of the outflow tracts in color Doppler in three fetuses between 12 and 13 weeks of gestation showing the five-chamber view (**A**), the short-axis view of the right ventricle (*RV*) (**B**), and the three-vessel trachea view (**C**). *Ao,* aorta; *LV,* left ventricle; *PA,* pulmonary artery; *SVC,* superior vena cava.

T A B L E 27-1 Basic assessment of the fetal outflow tracts
1. The aortic outflow tract originates from the left ventricle.
2. The pulmonary outflow tract originates from the right ventricle.
3. The outflow tracts should be comparable in size.
4. The ascending aorta and the main pulmonary artery are perpendicular to each other because they exit their respective ventricles. They should be seen crossing and not lying in the same plane.

◀))) SOUND OFF
Blood from the right ventricle can flow through the ductus arteriosus and into the descending aorta.

The blood returning from the lungs through the pulmonary veins enters into the left atrium. Blood then travels from the left atrium into the left ventricle via the mitral valve. From the left ventricle, it travels to the ascending aorta and into the aortic arch, where it exits into the brachiocephalic artery, left common carotid artery, and left subclavian artery on its way to the thorax, upper extremities, and head. The blood will return from the head and upper torso via the superior vena cava to the right atrium.

The blood that flows through the ductus arteriosus and into the descending aorta travels inferiorly to either exit the abdomen via the umbilical arteries or travel to the abdomen and lower extremities to replenish those regions. Therefore, the umbilical arteries return the deoxygenated blood from the fetus back to the placenta.

FETAL HEART ABNORMALITIES

Hypoplastic Left Heart Syndrome

Hypoplastic left heart syndrome is a group of anomalies characterized sonographically as a small or absent left ventricle (Fig. 27-14). Hypoplastic left heart syndrome is the leading cause of cardiac death in the neonatal period, with 95% dying within the first month of life if surgery is not performed. This anomaly can be recognized on a four-chamber heart view. To distinguish this anomaly from complete absence of the left side of the heart, a small or normal left atrium must be visualized. When found in girls, **Turner syndrome** should be suspected. There is also a connection with trisomy 18.

SONOGRAPHIC FINDINGS OF HYPOPLASTIC LEFT HEART SYNDROME
1. Absent or small left ventricle
2. No communication between the left atrium and the left ventricle
3. **Aortic atresia** (possibly)
4. **Aortic stenosis** (possibly)
5. **Coarctation of the aorta** (possibly)

Hypoplastic Right Heart Syndrome

Hypoplastic right heart syndrome is sonographically identified as a small or an absent right ventricle (Fig. 27-15). It, like hypoplastic left heart syndrome, is best visualized with the four-chamber heart view. Hypoplastic heart syndrome most often results from **pulmonary stenosis** or **pulmonary atresia**, but it may result from stenosis or atresia of the tricuspid valve.

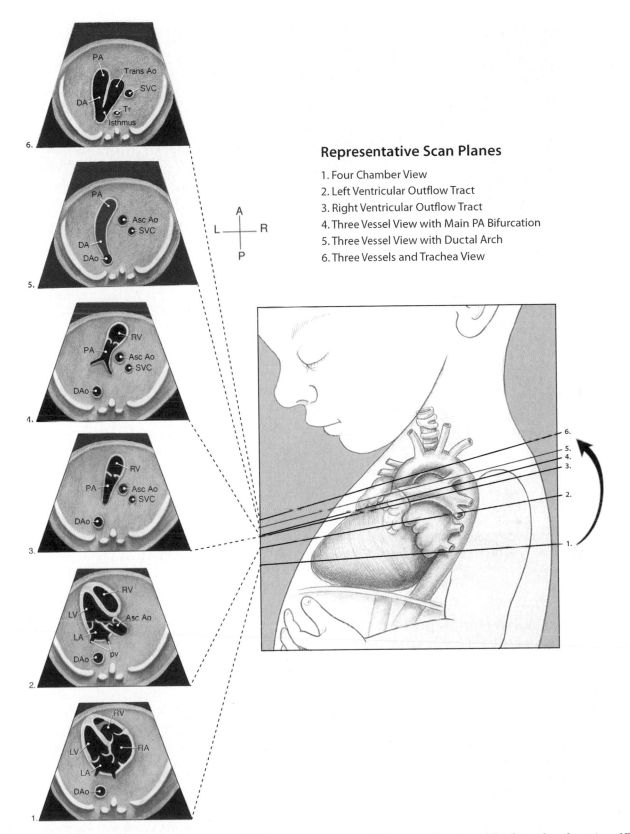

Representative Scan Planes

1. Four Chamber View
2. Left Ventricular Outflow Tract
3. Right Ventricular Outflow Tract
4. Three Vessel View with Main PA Bifurcation
5. Three Vessel View with Ductal Arch
6. Three Vessels and Trachea View

Figure 27-9 Representative scan planes for fetal echocardiography include an evaluation of the four-chamber view (*1*), left and right arterial outflow tracts (*2* and *3*, respectively), two variants of the three-vessel view, one demonstrating the main pulmonary artery bifurcation (*4*) with another more superior plane that demonstrates the ductal arch (*5*), and the three-vessel and trachea view (*6*). Not all views may be seen from a single cephalic transducer sweep without some minor adjustments in the position and orientation of the transducer owing to anatomic variations and the fetal lie. *Asc Ao*, ascending aorta; *DAo*, descending aorta; *LA*, left atrium; *LV*, left ventricle; *PA*, pulmonary artery; *RA*, right atrium; *RV*, right ventricle; *Tr*, trachea.

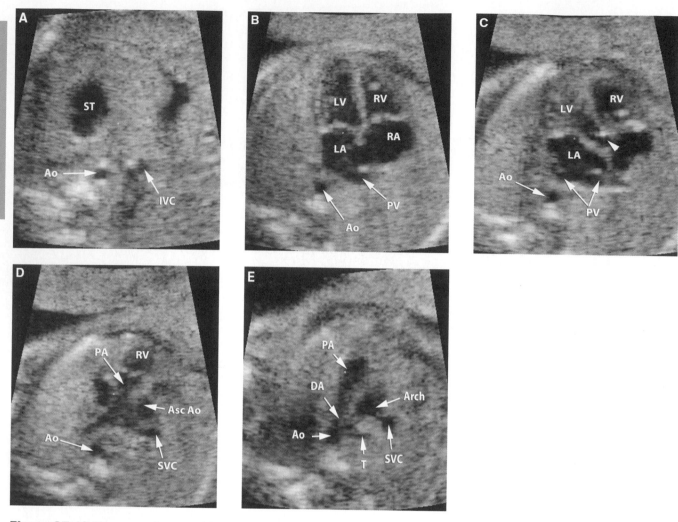

Figure 27-10 Transverse images of the fetus from inferior to superior. **A.** Transverse view of the fetal abdomen; **B.** Four-chamber view; **C.** Five-chamber view; **D.** Three-vessel view; **E.** Three-vessel trachea view. *Ao*, descending aorta; *Asc Ao*, ascending aorta; *DA*, ductus arteriosus; *IVC*, inferior vena cava; *LA*, left atrium; *LV*, left ventricle; *PA*, pulmonary artery; *PV*, pulmonary veins; *RA*, right atrium; *RV*, right ventricle; *Short arrow*: aortic root; *ST*, stomach; *SVC*, superior vena cava; *T*, trachea.

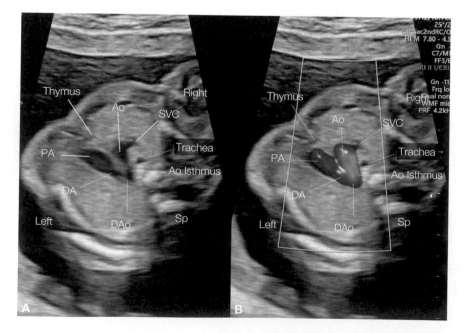

Figure 27-11 Three-vessel trachea view. **A.** Note anterior location of pulmonary artery (*PA*), with ductus arteriosus (*DA*) connecting with descending aorta (*DAo*). The aorta (*Ao*) and *Ao* isthmus are also seen connecting with *DAo*. Superior vena cava (*SVC*) is seen in cross section to the right side of *Ao*. Note that *DA* and *Ao* isthmus are to the left side of trachea, confirming the presence of normal left *Ao* and *DA*. Spine (*Sp*) is seen posteriorly. **B.** Three-vessel trachea view in color Doppler.

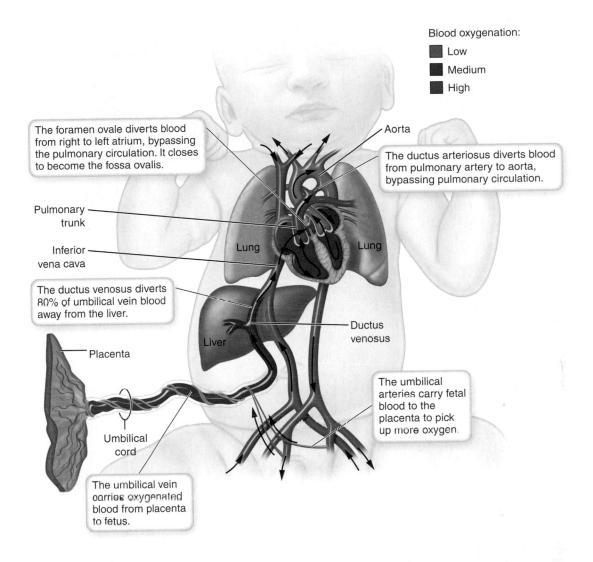

Blood oxygenation:
- Low
- Medium
- High

The foramen ovale diverts blood from right to left atrium, bypassing the pulmonary circulation. It closes to become the fossa ovalis.

Aorta

The ductus arteriosus diverts blood from pulmonary artery to aorta, bypassing pulmonary circulation.

Pulmonary trunk

Inferior vena cava

The ductus venosus diverts 80% of umbilical vein blood away from the liver.

Lung

Lung

Liver

Ductus venosus

Placenta

The umbilical arteries carry fetal blood to the placenta to pick up more oxygen.

Umbilical cord

The umbilical vein carries oxygenated blood from placenta to fetus.

Figure 27-12 Fetal circulation.

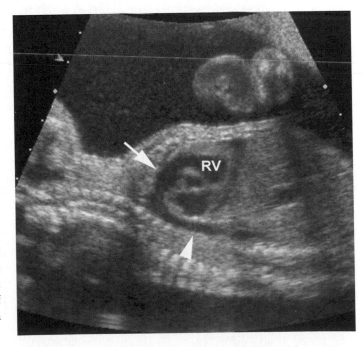

Figure 27-13 Right ventricular outflow tract and ductal arch to the descending aorta. Sagittal image demonstrating the right ventricular (*RV*) outflow tract and ductal arch (*arrow*), representing the connection of the ductus arteriosus to the descending thoracic aorta (*arrowhead*).

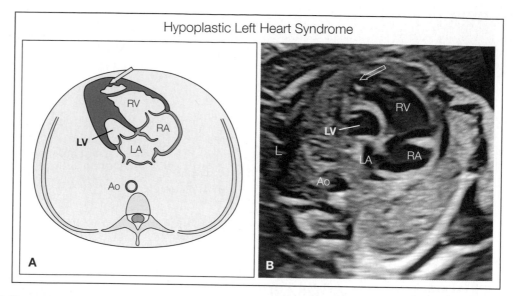

Figure 27-14 Hypoplastic left heart syndrome. Schematic drawing (**A**) and corresponding sonographic image (**B**) of a four-chamber view of a fetal heart with hypoplastic left heart syndrome (*HLHS*) shown in grayscale (**B**). Note the typical features of HLHS with a small globular left ventricle (*LV*) with echogenic walls. The left atrium (*LA*) is often small, as shown in panel **B**. The right ventricle (*RV*) forms the apex of the heart (*arrow*). *Ao*, Aorta; *L*, left; *RA*, right atrium.

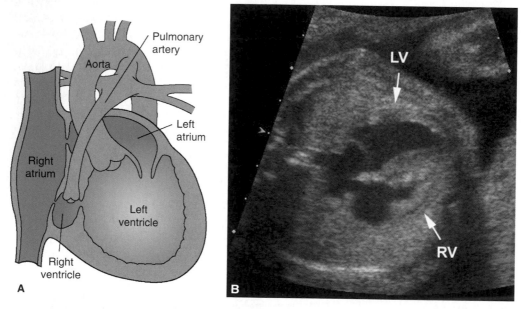

Figure 27-15 Hypoplastic right heart. **A.** Schematic of hypoplastic right heart. **B.** Transverse image of the fetal thorax at the level of the four-chamber view of the heart demonstrating the left ventricle (*LV*) and a small right ventricle (*RV*) with a thickened wall.

SONOGRAPHIC FINDINGS OF HYPOPLASTIC RIGHT HEART SYNDROME

1. Absent or small right ventricle
2. Enlarged left ventricle
3. **Fetal hydrops** (secondary to cardiac failure)
4. Narrowing of the pulmonary valve

Ventricular Septal Defects

A ventricular septal defect (VSD) is an abnormal opening in the septum between the two ventricles of the heart (Fig. 27-16). The VSD is the most common form of cardiac defect. This defect can be isolated, seen in the presence of chromosomal abnormalities, or associated with other cardiac anomalies, including **tetralogy of Fallot**, which is mentioned later in this chapter. Color Doppler can be used to identify the flow within and through the defect.

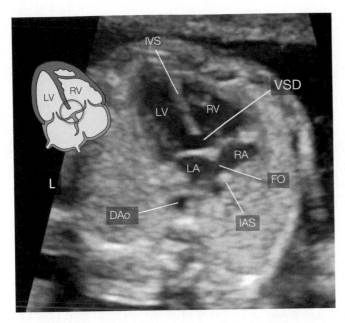

Figure 27-16 Apical four-chamber view in grayscale and the corresponding schematic drawing demonstrating a ventricular septal defect (*VSD*). *DAo*, descending aorta; *FO*, foramen ovale; *IAS*, interatrial septum; *IVS*, interventricular septum; *L*, left; *LA*, left atrium; *LV*, left ventricle; *RA*, right atrium; *RV*, right ventricle.

SONOGRAPHIC FINDINGS OF VENTRICULAR SEPTAL DEFECTS

1. Absence of part of the ventricular septum
2. Color Doppler is helpful at detecting small defects

SOUND OFF
The VSD is the most common form of cardiac defect.

Atrial Septal Defects

An atrial septal defect (ASD) is an abnormal opening in the septum between the two atria of the heart (Fig. 27-17). There are several different types (numbered 1-5) and an ASD can be isolated but may be found in the presence of various syndromes.

SONOGRAPHIC FINDINGS OF ATRIAL SEPTAL DEFECTS

1. Absence of part of the atrial septum
2. Color Doppler is helpful at detecting small defects

Atrioventricular Septal Defects or Atrioventricular Canal

The combination of both ASD and VSD is termed **atrioventricular septal defect** (AVSD) or atrioventricular canal. An AVSD results from the abnormal development of the central portion of the heart. The central portion of the heart is referred to as the "endocardial cushion"; this is the reason why the AVSD may be referred to as an **endocardial cushion defect**. AVSDs are commonly associated with **aneuploidy**, **trisomy 21**, and **trisomy 18**.

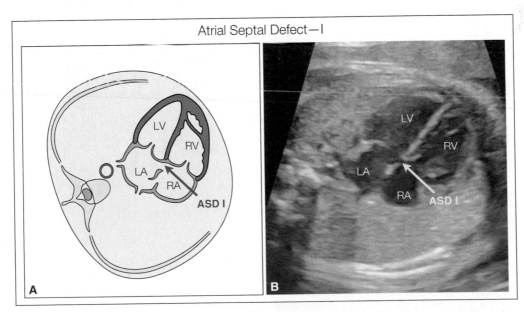

Atrial Septal Defect—I

Figure 27-17 Schematic drawing **(A)** and corresponding sonographic image **(B)** of an apical four-chamber view in a fetus with an atrial septal defect (*arrows*). Note the gap in the atrial part of the heart crux and the linear insertion of the atrioventricular valves. The remaining part of the interatrial septum and foramen ovale region appear normally developed. *LA*, left atrium; *LV*, left ventricle; *RA*, right atrium; *RV*, right ventricle; *ASD 1*, atrial septal defect type 1.

SONOGRAPHIC FINDINGS OF ATRIOVENTRICULAR SEPTAL DEFECTS

1. Absence of the atrial and ventricular septum
2. Color Doppler findings are helpful at showing mixture of flow patterns

Ebstein Anomaly

Malformation or malpositioning of the tricuspid valve results in **Ebstein anomaly** (Fig. 27-18). With this abnormality, the right ventricle is contiguous with the right atrium, a finding referred to as an "atrialized" right ventricle. This anomaly is associated with **tricuspid regurgitation**, ASDs, tetralogy of Fallot, **transposition of the great vessels**, and coarctation of the aorta. The prognosis is poor, with 80% of infants dying in the perinatal period.

SONOGRAPHIC FINDINGS OF EBSTEIN ANOMALY

1. Malpositioned tricuspid valve
2. Right and left atrial shunting
3. Tricuspid regurgitation
4. Enlarged right atrium
5. Deviation of the atrial septum to the left
6. Fetal hydrops (secondary to cardiac failure)

◀))) SOUND OFF
Malformation or malpositioning of the tricuspid valve results in Ebstein anomaly.

Coarctation of the Aorta

Coarctation of the aorta is the narrowing of the aortic arch (Figs. 27-19 and 27-20). The most common location is between the left subclavian artery and the ductus arteriosus. Associated findings consist of right ventricle enlargement, pulmonary artery enlargement, and disproportion in the size of the ventricles in the four-chamber view. This anomaly can be difficult to diagnose in utero during a routine sonographic examination. However, the aforementioned associated findings are most often recognized first, and consequently, further evaluation with fetal echocardiography is typically warranted for official diagnosis. Other common findings include patent ductus arteriosus and VSDs.

SONOGRAPHIC FINDINGS OF COARCTATION OF THE AORTA

1. Narrowing of the aortic arch
2. Right ventricular enlargement
3. Pulmonary artery enlargement

Tetralogy of Fallot

Tetralogy of Fallot is defined as an overriding aortic root, subaortic VSD, pulmonary stenosis, and right ventricular hypertrophy (Figs. 27-21 and 27-22). The right ventricular hypertrophy is not always noted in utero but rather manifests after birth.

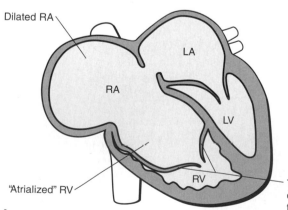

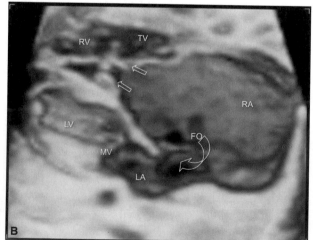

Figure 27-18 Ebstein anomaly. **A.** Schematic drawing of Ebstein anomaly. **B.** Three-dimensional sonography in surface-mode display of the four-chamber view in a fetus with Ebstein anomaly. The large right atrium (*RA*) and the wide foramen ovale (*FO*) are demonstrated (*open curved arrow*). Different levels of attachment of the tricuspid (*TV*) (*open straight arrows*) and mitral valves (*MV*) are noted. *LA*, left atrium; *LV*, left ventricle; *RA*, right atrium; *LV*, left ventricle; *RV*, right ventricle.

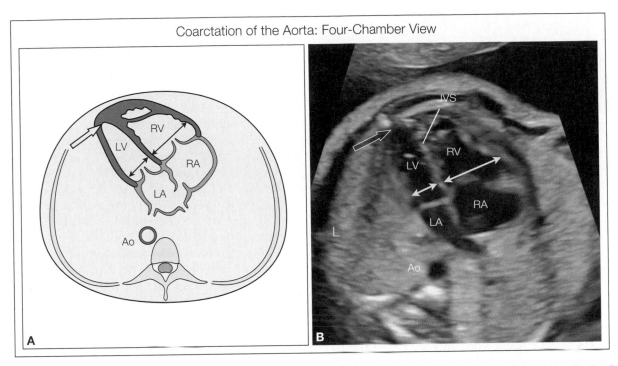

Figure 27-19 Schematic drawing (**A**) and corresponding sonographic image (**B**) of a four-chamber view of a fetal heart with coarctation of the aorta, shown in grayscale (**B**). Primary clue for the presence of coarctation of the aorta is ventricular disproportion (*double arrows*, **A**, **B**), with the left ventricle (*LV*) smaller in width when compared to the right ventricle (*RV*). Another clue, which differentiates coarctation of the aorta from hypoplastic left heart syndrome, is that the *LV* is apex forming in coarctation (*open arrow*). *Ao*, descending aorta; *IVS*, interventricular septum; *L*, left; *LA*, left atrium; *RA*, right atrium.

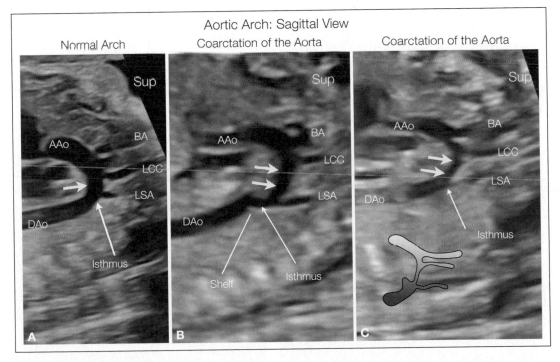

Figure 27-20 Sagittal views of the aortic arch in three fetuses, one with normal aortic arch (**A**) and two fetuses (**B** and **C**) with coarctation of the aorta. Schematic drawing of the arch in fetus **C** is also shown. Fetus B has the coarctation mainly localized to the isthmic region, whereas fetus **C** has tubular hypoplasia of the aortic arch. The schematic drawing (**C**) illustrates the abnormal shape of the arch. *Yellow arrows* indicate the short distal aortic arch in the normal fetus (**A**), compared to a longer distal arch in aortic coarctation in fetuses **B** and **C**. *AAo*, ascending aorta; *BA*, brachiocephalic artery; *DAo*, descending aorta; *LCC*, left common carotid artery; *Sup*, superior; *LSA*, left subclavian artery.

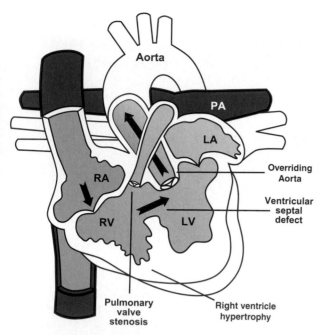

Figure 27-21 Tetralogy of Fallot. The four structural defects of tetralogy of Fallot are a *ventricular septal defect (VSD)*, pulmonary stenosis, an overriding aorta, and right ventricular hypertrophy.

SONOGRAPHIC FINDINGS OF TETRALOGY OF FALLOT

1. Overriding aortic root
2. VSD
3. Pulmonary stenosis
4. Right ventricular hypertrophy

Transposition of the Great Vessels

With transposition of the great vessels, the outflow tracts are reversed. That means, the pulmonary artery abnormally arises from the left ventricle, and the aorta abnormally arises from the right ventricle. Often, the four-chamber view of the heart is normal. However, when the outflow tract images are obtained in a fetus with transposition, instead of the normal crisscross orientation of the outflow tracts, they will be positioned parallel to each other, with the aorta noted anterior and to the right of the pulmonary artery (Figs. 27-23 and 27-24). Occasionally, a VSD or other heart abnormalities may be present. For this reason, if technically feasible, outflow tracts should be attempted during the screening examination. Transposition of the great vessels, which may also be referred to as transposition of the great arteries, has a good prognosis if it is discovered in utero, because corrective surgery can be performed shortly after birth.

SONOGRAPHIC FINDINGS OF TRANSPOSITION OF THE GREAT VESSELS

1. The pulmonary artery abnormally arises from the left ventricle, and the aorta abnormally arises from the right ventricle
2. The outflow tracts will be positioned parallel to each other rather than crisscrossing
3. VSD may be present

🔊)) **SOUND OFF**
Often, the four-chamber view of the heart is normal in the presence of transposition of the great vessels.

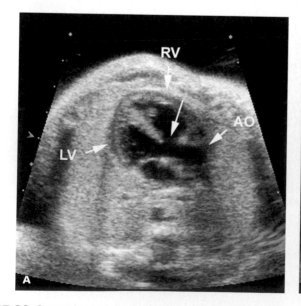
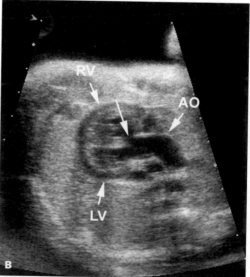

Figure 27-22 Overriding aorta and ventricular septal defect with tetralogy of Fallot. **A** and **B.** Oblique views of the left ventricular outflow tract demonstrating overriding aorta (*AO arrow*) and ventricular septal defect (*long arrow*). *LV arrow*, left ventricle; *RV arrow*, right ventricle.

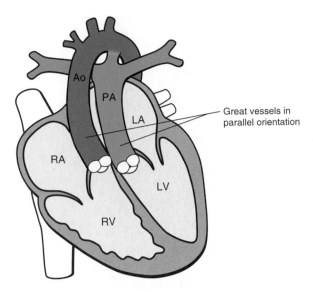

Figure 27-23 Schematic drawing of complete transposition of the great arteries. *Ao*, descending aorta; *LA*, left atrium; *LV*, left ventricle; *PA*, pulmonary artery; *RA*, right atrium; *RV*, right ventricle.

Echogenic Intracardiac Focus

An echogenic intracardiac focus (EIF) is most often seen within the left ventricle of the heart (Fig. 27-25). This is thought to represent the calcification of the **papillary muscle** or **chordae tendineae**. An EIF may be seen in the normal fetus. However, there have been studies that have linked the incidence of an EIF with trisomy 21, particularly if there is more than one EIF detected. The echogenicity of the EIF is comparable to that of the fetal bone.

SONOGRAPHIC FINDINGS OF AN ECHOGENIC INTRACARDIAC FOCUS

1. Echogenic structure most commonly located within the left ventricle

SOUND OFF
An EIF may be seen in the normal fetus. However, there have been studies that have linked the EIF with trisomy 21.

Rhabdomyoma

The most common fetal cardiac tumor is the **rhabdomyoma**. These tumors, located within the myocardium of the heart, are associated with **tuberous sclerosis**, eventual cardiac failure, and subsequent development of fetal hydrops. These tumors are typically echogenic and may be isolated or multiple (Fig. 27-26).

SONOGRAPHIC FINDINGS OF A RHABDOMYOMA

1. Echogenic tumor(s) within the myocardium of the heart

SOUND OFF
The most common fetal cardiac tumor is the rhabdomyoma. It is associated with tuberous sclerosis.

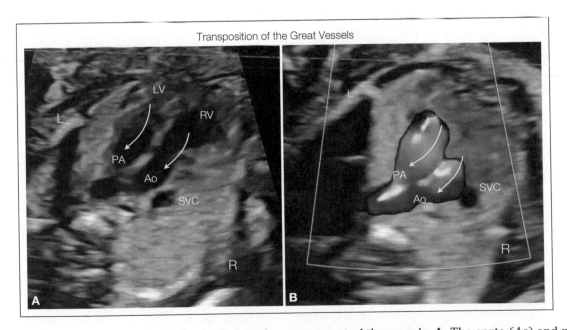

Transposition of the Great Vessels

Figure 27-24 Fetus with a transposition and side-by-side arrangement of the vessels. **A.** The aorta (*Ao*) and pulmonary artery (*PA*) are seen arising from the right (*RV*) and left (*LV*) ventricles, respectively. **B.** Color Doppler helps demonstrate the abnormality. *L*, left; *R*, right; *SVC*, superior vena cava.

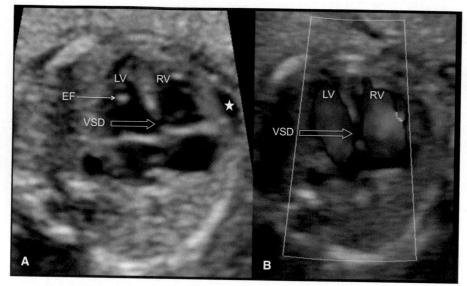

Figure 27-25 Echogenic intracardiac focus. **A.** Echogenic intracardiac focus (*EF*) and pericardial effusion (*star*). Ventricular septal defect (*VSD*) demonstrated on grayscale (**A**, *open arrow*) and color Doppler (**B**, *open arrow*) at the four-chamber view. This fetus was found to have trisomy 21 on karyotypic analysis. *LV*, left ventricle; *RV*, right ventricle.

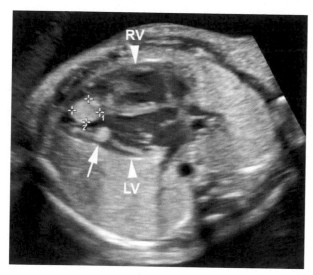

Figure 27-26 Multiple rhabdomyomas. Oblique view of heart demonstrating two homogeneous echogenic masses, one arising from the myocardium in the septum (*calipers*) and the other in the left ventricular wall (*arrow*). *LV arrowhead*, left ventricle; *RV arrowhead*, right ventricle.

Pericardial Effusion

Pericardial effusion is fluid located around the heart. This condition can be isolated or associated with fetal hydrops. The sonographer should evaluate the fetus closely for other signs of fetal hydrops, such as ascites and **pleural effusion** (Fig. 27-27). It is important to note that the normal hypoechoic appearance of the myocardium can mimic the sonographic appearance of small pericardial effusions.

SONOGRAPHIC FINDINGS OF PERICARDIAL EFFUSION
1. Anechoic fluid surrounding the heart

Ectopic Cordis

With **ectopic cordis**, the heart is located either partially or completely outside the chest (Fig. 27-28). **Pentalogy of Cantrell** is a group of anomalies that combine ectopic cordis and an existing **omphalocele**. The prognosis is poor.

SONOGRAPHIC FINDINGS OF ECTOPIC CORDIS
1. Heart located either partially or completely outside the chest

FETAL LUNG DEVELOPMENT AND FUNCTION

The lungs develop in early embryogenesis. However, functional fetal lung tissue does not typically exist until after 25 weeks. Fetal lung maturity can be assessed using the **lecithin-to-sphingomyelin ratio** (L/S ratio). An amniocentesis is performed for this test, and the laboratory findings indicate the levels of lecithin and sphingomyelin within the amniotic fluid. Normally, as the lungs mature, the level of lecithin increases, whereas the level of sphingomyelin decreases.

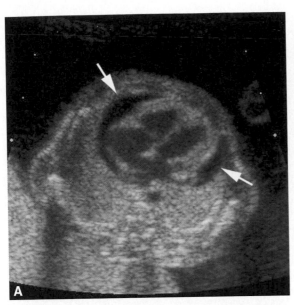
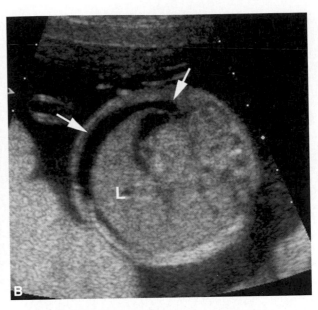

Figure 27-27 Pericardial effusion with hydrops due to anemia. **A.** Transverse image of fetal thorax demonstrating pericardial fluid (*arrows*) around heart. **B.** Transverse image of the abdomen in the same fetus demonstrating moderate amount of ascites (*arrows*) surrounding the liver (*L*).

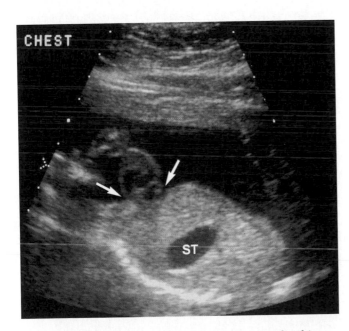

Figure 27-28 Ectopic cordis. Oblique longitudinal image demonstrating a defect in the anterior chest wall (*arrows*) through which the heart has herniated (*ST*, stomach).

FETAL LUNG ABNORMALITIES

Pulmonary Hypoplasia

Pulmonary hypoplasia, or underdevelopment of the lungs, is caused by a decreased number of lung cells, airways, and alveoli. Pulmonary hypoplasia is often associated with major structural and chromosomal abnormalities. The most common lesion that occupies the chest, resulting in pulmonary hypoplasia, is the **diaphragmatic hernia**. Amniotic fluid plays an important role in the development of the fetal lungs; therefore, the fetus, surrounded by little or no amniotic fluid, is at increased risk of pulmonary hypoplasia. Consequently, pulmonary hypoplasia is a common finding with **oligohydramnios**. It is also associated with bilateral renal agenesis and the abnormal facial features in the condition known as **Potter syndrome**.

Pleural Effusion

Fluid surrounding the lungs is referred to as a pleural effusion or hydrothorax. Pleural effusions that occur in utero may spontaneously resolve or may be found in the presence of fetal hydrops, other chest abnormalities, and Turner syndrome. They can be unilateral or bilateral (Fig. 27-29). A pleural effusion will appear sonographically as anechoic fluid within the chest surrounding the fetal lung. The **"bat-wing" sign** has been used to describe the appearance of pleural effusions. Fetal pleural effusions can be treated with an ultrasound-guided **thoracentesis**.

SONOGRAPHIC FINDINGS OF A PLEURAL EFFUSION

1. Anechoic fluid surrounding the fetal lung(s)—"bat-wing" sign
2. Other signs of hydrops may be present

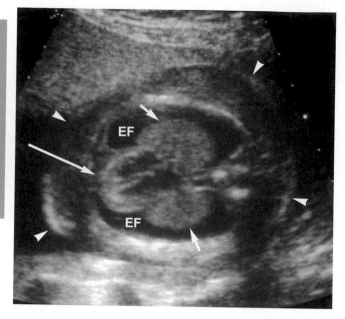

Figure 27-29 Bilateral pleural effusions. Transverse view through the thorax demonstrating moderate-size bilateral pleural effusions (*EF*) surrounding the fetal lungs (*arrows*). This fetus also has subcutaneous edema (*arrowheads*) around the thorax.

Cystic Adenomatoid Malformation

Cystic adenomatoid malformation (CAM), also referred to as congenital cystic adenomatoid malformation (CCAM), is actually a mass consisting of abnormal bronchial and lung tissue. Although there are three types (types 1 to 3), a common sonographic appearance of CAM is that of a mass that has both cystic and solid components. However, it can also appear completely echogenic (type 3) and, therefore, sonographically similar to **pulmonary sequestration** (Fig. 27-30). Most CAMs are unilateral and may resolve spontaneously, although large masses can lead to fetal hydrops and carry a poor prognosis.

SONOGRAPHIC APPEARANCE OF CYSTIC ADENOMATOID MALFORMATIONS

1. Lung mass with varying degrees of cystic and solid components
2. Completely echogenic mass within the lungs
3. Pleural effusion may be present

Pulmonary Sequestration

Pulmonary sequestration, or bronchopulmonary sequestration, is a separate mass of nonfunctioning lung tissue with its own blood supply. The fetal form of this disease is specifically referred to as extrapulmonary sequestration, which denotes its location. The most common sonographic appearance of pulmonary sequestration is an echogenic, triangular-shaped mass, typically located within the left side of the fetal chest. Pulmonary sequestration may resolve spontaneously or lead to the development of fetal hydrops.

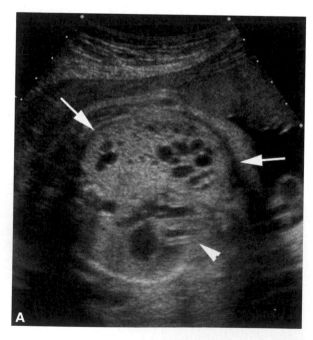
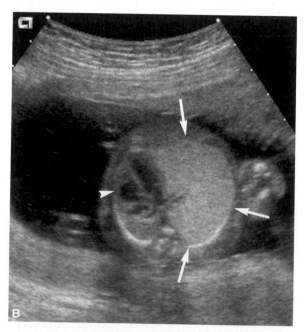

Figure 27-30 Cystic adenomatoid malformation. **A.** Axial image of the chest containing a complex mass with cystic components (*arrows*) that has altered the position of the fetal heart (*arrowhead*). **B.** Echogenic form of cystic adenomatoid malformation of the lung. Transverse view through the fetal chest demonstrating an echogenic mass (*arrows*) in the left hemithorax displacing the heart (*arrowhead*) to the right.

> **SOUND OFF**
> Pulmonary sequestration, or bronchopulmonary sequestration, is a separate mass of nonfunctioning lung tissue with its own blood supply.

Diaphragmatic Hernias

The most common reason for fetal cardiac malposition is the existence of a diaphragmatic hernia. A diaphragmatic hernia results in an abnormal opening in the fetal diaphragm that allows the herniation of abdominal contents into the chest cavity. The most common location of a diaphragmatic hernia is on the left side. This type may also be referred to as a **Bochdalek hernia**. The **foramen of Bochdalek** is located in the left posterolateral portion of the diaphragm. In most cases, the stomach, bowel, and the left lobe of the liver are found within the chest (Fig. 27-31). The **foramen of Morgagni**, which is located right

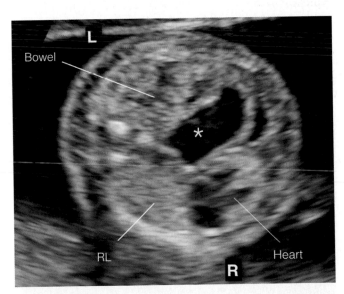

Figure 27-31 Left diaphragmatic hernia. Axial plane of the chest at the level of the four-chamber view at 14 weeks of gestation in a fetus with left-sided congenital diaphragmatic hernia (*CDH*) and chromosomal aneuploidy. Note the severity of the CDH with the heart severely shifted to the right hemithorax and the stomach (*asterisk*) and abdominal content occupying the majority of the right chest. The right lung (*RL*) is compressed. *L*, left; *R*, right.

anteromedially within the diaphragm, may lead to a right-sided diaphragmatic hernia, thus allowing the entire liver to herniate into the chest. Diaphragmatic hernias that are located on the right side may be more difficult to diagnose, given the similar echogenicity of the fetal lungs and fetal liver.

> **SOUND OFF**
> The most common location of a diaphragmatic hernia is on the left side. This type may also be referred to as a Bochdalek hernia.

The sonographic findings of a diaphragmatic hernia include malposition of the heart as a result of the stomach or other abdominal organs being located within the chest. Often, sagittal and coronal imaging at the level of the diaphragm can be helpful to confirm this abnormality. One differential diagnosis of a diaphragmatic hernia is **eventration of the diaphragm**, which is a lack of muscle in the dome of the diaphragm. This will have a similar sonographic appearance to a diaphragmatic hernia and can, therefore, be difficult to distinguish sonographically.

FETAL THYMUS

The thymus gland is located anterior to the mediastinum. It is part of the immune system because it provides a place for the maturation of T cells, which are specialized white blood cells. Although not routinely specifically imaged, the thymus may be seen during a fetal sonogram. Sonographically, it appears as a hypoechoic structure located in the anterior chest at the level of the sternum between the lungs. **DiGeorge syndrome** is a genetic disorder characterized by an absent or a hypoplastic thymus, which ultimately leads to impairment of the immune system and susceptibility to infection, as well as cognitive disorders, congenital heart defects, palate defects, and hormonal abnormalities.

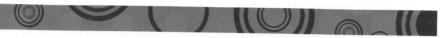

REVIEW QUESTIONS

1. What is the genetic disorder characterized by an absent or a hypoplastic thymus?
   a. DiGeorge syndrome
   b. Ebstein anomaly
   c. Tetralogy of Fallot
   d. Pentalogy of Cantrell

2. The *arrows* in Figure 27-32 indicate the:
   a. pulmonary veins.
   b. pulmonary arteries.
   c. ductus arteriosus and right pulmonary artery.
   d. ductus arteriosus and left pulmonary vein.

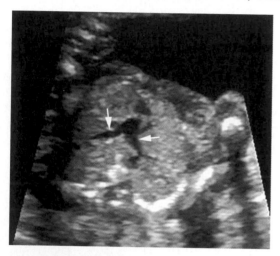

Figure 27-32

3. The *arrowhead* in Figure 27-33 demonstrates a(n):
   a. endocardial cushion defect.
   b. atrioventricular canal.
   c. VSD.
   d. rhabdomyoma.

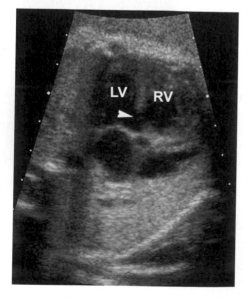

Figure 27-33

4. What abnormality is noted in Figure 27-34?
   a. Pleural effusion
   b. Rhabdomyoma
   c. Pericardial effusion
   d. Ascites

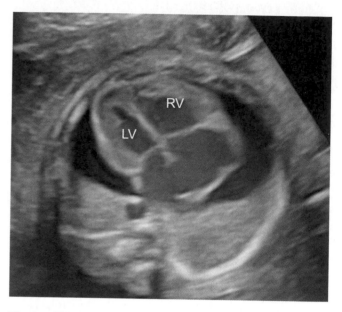

Figure 27-34

5. What abnormality is noted in Figure 27-35?
   a. Pleural effusion
   b. Rhabdomyoma
   c. Pericardial effusion
   d. Ascites

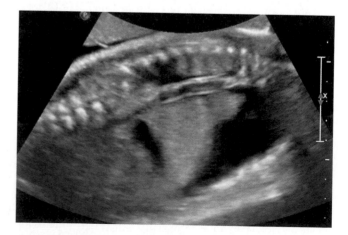

Figure 27-35

6. Which of the following is represented in Figure 27-36?
   a. Calcification of the ventricular wall
   b. Echogenic intracardiac focus
   c. Rhabdomyoma
   d. Echogenic intracardiac atrial appendage

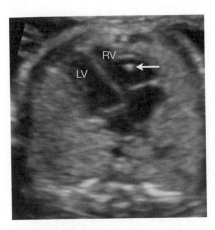

Figure 27-36

7. What does the *arrow* in Figure 27-37 indicate?
   a. EIF
   b. Intracardiac teratoma
   c. Rhabdomyoma
   d. Tuberous sclerosis

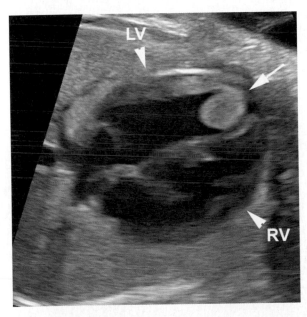

Figure 27-37

8. In Figure 27-38 A, what is the most likely cause of the fetal heart displacement?
   a. Pericardial effusion
   b. Diaphragmatic hernia
   c. CAM
   d. Pleural effusion

9. In Figure 27-38 B, what is the most likely cause of the fetal heart displacement?
   a. Pericardial effusion
   b. Diaphragmatic hernia
   c. CAM
   d. Pleural effusion

10. In Figure 27-38 C, what is the most likely cause of the fetal heart displacement?
    a. Pericardial effusion
    b. Diaphragmatic hernia
    c. CCAM
    d. Pleural effusion

11. What does Figure 27-39 depict?
    a. Tetralogy of Fallot
    b. Coarctation of the aorta
    c. Ebstein anomaly
    d. Pentalogy of Cantrell

12. What is evident in Figure 27-40?
    a. Ebstein anomaly
    b. Tetralogy of Fallot
    c. Hypoplastic left heart
    d. Hypoplastic right heart

13. What does the *arrow* in Figure 27-41 demonstrate?
    a. Ductus venosus
    b. Foramen ovale
    c. Ductus arteriosus
    d. ASD

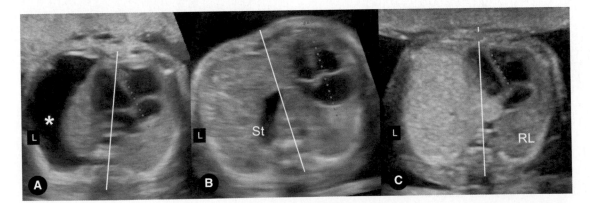

Figure 27-38

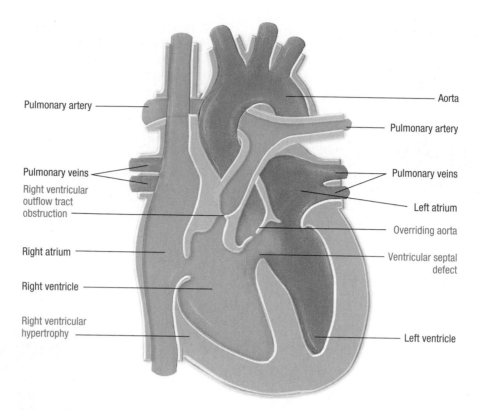

Pulmonary artery

Aorta

Pulmonary artery

Pulmonary veins

Pulmonary veins

Right ventricular outflow tract obstruction

Left atrium

Overriding aorta

Right atrium

Ventricular septal defect

Right ventricle

Right ventricular hypertrophy

Left ventricle

Figure 27-39

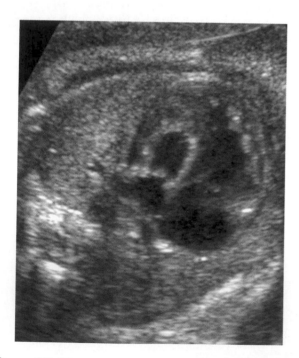

Figure 27-40

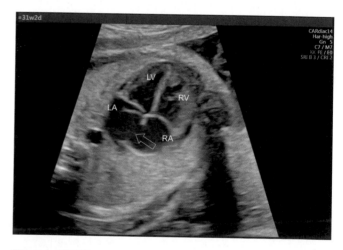

Figure 27-41

14. What is evident in Figure 27-42?
    a. Ebstein anomaly
    b. Tetralogy of Fallot
    c. Hypoplastic left heart
    d. Hypoplastic right heart

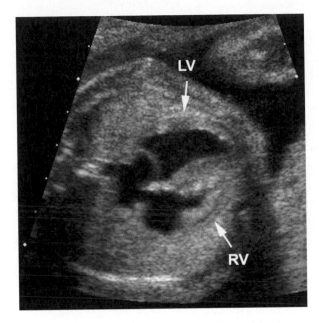

Figure 27-42

15. The thymus gland is part of what system?
    a. Endocrine
    h Fxocrine
    c. Immune
    d. Respiratory

16. Functional fetal lung tissue does not typically exist until after:
    a. 12 weeks.
    b. 20 weeks.
    c. 18 weeks.
    d. 25 weeks.

17. When hypoplastic left heart syndrome is found in girls, what syndrome should be suspected?
    a. Turner syndrome
    b. Patau syndrome
    c. Klinefelter syndrome
    d. Joliet syndrome

18. A heart rate using M-mode should be sonographically obtainable with EV when the CRL measures?
    a. 2 to 3 mm
    b. 1 to 2 mm
    c. 4 to 5 mm
    d. 1.5 to 3.5 mm

19. Blood returning from the head and upper torso enters the heart via the:
    a. abdominal aorta.
    b. IVC.
    c. pulmonary vein.
    d. superior vena cava.

20. Blood returning from the IVC enters the:
    a. left atrium.
    b. left ventricle.
    c. right atrium.
    d. right ventricle.

21. What is the opening located right anteromedially within the diaphragm?
    a. Foramen of Bochdalek
    b. Foramen of Morgagni
    c. Foramen of Monro
    d. Foramen ovale

22. A group of anomalies characterized by a small or an absent left ventricle is:
    a. Turner syndrome.
    b. hypoplastic right heart syndrome.
    c. hypoplastic left heart syndrome.
    d. coarctation of the aorta.

23. What is described as the absence of the pulmonary valve, which, in turn, prohibits blood flow from the right ventricle into the pulmonary artery and essentially to the lungs?
    a. Pulmonary atresia
    b. Pulmonary stenosis
    c. Pulmonary sequestration
    d. Pulmonary effusion

24. A group of anomalies characterized by a small or an absent right ventricle is:
    a. Turner syndrome.
    b. hypoplastic right heart syndrome.
    c. hypoplastic left heart syndrome.
    d. coarctation of the aorta.

25. All of the following are sonographic signs of Ebstein anomaly except:
    a. enlarged right atrium.
    b. fetal hydrops.
    c. narrowing of the aortic arch.
    d. malpositioned tricuspid valve.

26. What is an opening within the septum that separates the right and left ventricles?
    a. Endocardial cushion
    b. Tricuspid regeneration
    c. VSD
    d. ASD

27. The narrowing of the aortic arch is indicative of:
    a. tetralogy of Fallot.
    b. coarctation of the aorta.
    c. Ebstein anomaly.
    d. hypoplastic right heart syndrome.

28. An EIF is most often seen within the:
    a. right atrium.
    b. left atrium.
    c. right ventricle.
    d. left ventricle.

29. What is the term for underdevelopment of the lungs?
    a. Pulmonary atresia
    b. Pulmonary stenosis
    c. Pulmonary agenesis
    d. Pulmonary hypoplasia

30. An EIF would most likely be associated with:
    a. trisomy 21.
    b. trisomy 13.
    c. trisomy 8.
    d. Turner syndrome.

31. The most common fetal cardiac tumor is the:
    a. rhabdomyoma.
    b. chordae tendineae.
    c. cardiomyoma.
    d. CAM.

32. All of the following are sonographic features of pentalogy of Cantrell except:
    a. omphalocele.
    b. gastroschisis.
    c. cleft sternum.
    d. diaphragmatic defect.

33. What is the fetal shunt that connects the pulmonary artery to the aortic arch?
    a. Foramen ovale
    b. Ductus arteriosus
    c. Ductus venosus
    d. Foramen of Bochdalek

34. The accumulation of fluid around the lungs is termed:
    a. ascites.
    b. extracorporeal effusion.
    c. peripleural fluid.
    d. pleural effusion.

35. The normal heart will fill approximately ___ of the fetal chest.
    a. one half
    b. one-fourth
    c. one-fifth
    d. one-third

36. The condition in which the heart is located outside the chest wall is termed:
    a. CAM.
    b. coarctation of the heart.
    c. cardiac sequestration.
    d. ectopic cordis.

37. The most common form of diaphragmatic hernia is the:
    a. foramen of Morgagni.
    b. foramen of Magendie.
    c. foramen of Luschka.
    d. foramen of Bochdalek.

38. The moderator band is located within the:
    a. right atrium.
    b. left atrium.
    c. right ventricle.
    d. left ventricle.

39. The most common cause of cardiac malposition is:
    a. diaphragmatic hernia.
    b. omphalocele.
    c. gastroschisis.
    d. pulmonary hypoplasia.

40. A separate mass of nonfunctioning fetal lung tissue is referred to as:
    a. pulmonary adenomatoid malformation.
    b. pulmonary sequestration.
    c. CAM.
    d. bat-wing sign.

41. The tricuspid valve is located:
    a. between the right atrium and the left atrium.
    b. between the right ventricle and the right atrium.
    c. between the left ventricle and the left atrium.
    d. between the left atrium and the aorta.

42. The most common sonographic appearance of pulmonary sequestration is a(n):
    a. dilated pulmonary artery and hypoechoic chest mass.
    b. pleural effusion and ipsilateral hiatal hernia.
    c. triangular, echogenic mass within the chest.
    d. anechoic mass within the chest.

43. The embryonic heart begins as:
    a. two tubes.
    b. four tubes.
    c. eight folds.
    d. one tube.

44. Tetralogy of Fallot consists of all of the following except:
    a. overriding aortic root.
    b. VSD.
    c. pulmonary stenosis.
    d. left ventricular hypertrophy.

45. Eventration of the diaphragm is best described as:
    a. a lack of muscle in the dome of the diaphragm.
    b. a defect in the anterior lateral wall of the diaphragm.
    c. a defect in the posterolateral wall of the diaphragm.
    d. congenital absence of the diaphragm.

46. The visualization of the fetal stomach within the fetal chest is most indicative of:
    a. pulmonary sequestration.
    b. diaphragmatic hernia.
    c. Turner syndrome.
    d. CAM.

47. The sonographic "bat-wing" sign is indicative of:
    a. pericardial effusion.
    b. pulmonary atresia.
    c. pleural effusion.
    d. endocardial cushion defects.

48. The mitral valve is located:
    a. between the right atrium and the left atrium.
    b. between the right ventricle and the right atrium.
    c. between the left ventricle and the left atrium.
    d. between the left atrium and the aorta.

49. Which statement is true concerning fetal outflow tracts?
    a. The normal pulmonary artery should be positioned posterior to the aorta and should be visualized passing under it.
    b. The normal pulmonary artery should be positioned anterior to the aorta and should be visualized crossing over it.
    c. The right ventricular outflow tract leads to the aorta.
    d. The left ventricular outflow tract leads to the pulmonary artery.

50. Fetal lung maturity can be assessed using the:
    a. L/S ratio.
    b. systolic-to-diastolic ratio.
    c. estriol-to-alpha-fetoprotein ratio.
    d. lung size formula.

51. Which of the following are fetal rhabdomyomas associated with?
    a. Tracheoesophageal fistulas
    b. Tuberous sclerosis
    c. Eventration of the diaphragm
    d. Tuberculosis

52. Which of the following is considered to be the most common cardiac defect?
    a. Hypoplastic right heart syndrome
    b. Transposition of the great vessels
    c. Hypoplastic left heart syndrome
    d. VSD

53. What is the normal opening in the lower middle third of the atrial septum?
    a. Foramen of Magendie
    b. Foramen of Monro
    c. Foramen ovale
    d. Ductus arteriosus

54. What structure shunts blood into the IVC from the umbilical vein?
    a. Ductus venosus
    b. Ductus arteriosus
    c. Foramen ovale
    d. Foramen of Luschka

55. Which of the following is not a true statement about the normal fetal heart?
    a. The ventricular septum should be uninterrupted and of equal thickness to the left ventricular wall.
    b. There is a normal opening within the atrial septum.
    c. Between the right ventricle and the right atrium, one should visualize the tricuspid valve.
    d. The mitral valve is positioned closer to the cardiac apex than the tricuspid valve.

56. The blood returning from the lungs through the pulmonary veins enters into the:
    a. right atrium.
    b. left atrium.
    c. right ventricle.
    d. left ventricle.

57. Which of the following is a true statement about the fetal heart?
    a. The apex of the heart will be angled to the right of the midline.
    b. The apex of the heart is the portion closest to the spine.
    c. The normal fetal heart will fill approximately two-thirds of the fetal chest.
    d. The chamber closest to the fetal spine is the left atrium.

58. The fetal heart is fully formed by:
    a. 2 weeks.
    b. 4 weeks.
    c. 8 weeks.
    d. 10 weeks.

59. A coexisting pericardial effusion and a pleural effusion is consistent with the diagnosis of:
    a. tetralogy of Fallot.
    b. pentalogy of Cantrell.
    c. fetal hydrops.
    d. Potter syndrome.

60. Which of the following best describes transposition of the great vessels?
    a. The aorta arises from the left ventricle, and the pulmonary artery arises from the right ventricle.
    b. The aorta arises from the right ventricle, and the pulmonary artery arises from the left ventricle.
    c. The aortic arch is narrowed and positioned anterior to the pulmonary vein.
    d. The presence of an omphalocele and ectopic cordis is seen.

SUGGESTED READINGS

Curry RA, Prince M. *Sonography: Introduction to Normal Structure and Function*. 5th ed. Elsevier; 2020:385–430.

Doubilet PM, Benson CB. *Atlas of Ultrasound in Obstetrics and Gynecology: A Multimedia Reference*. 2nd ed. Wolters Kluwer; 2012:27–29 & 123–136.

Gibbs RS, Haney AF, Karlan BY, et al. *Danforth's Obstetrics and Gynecology*. 10th ed. Wolters Kluwer; 2008:137–151.

Hagen-Ansert SL. *Textbook of Diagnostic Sonography*. 7th ed. Elsevier; 2012:1311–1322.

Henningsen C, Kuntz K, Youngs D. *Clinical Guide to Sonography: Exercises for Critical Thinking*. 2nd ed. Elsevier; 2014:305–319.

Kline-Fath BM, Bulas DI, and Lee W. *Fundamental and Advanced Fetal Imaging: Ultrasound and MRI*. 2nd ed. Wolters Kluwer; 2021:664–694 & 701–747.

Norton ME, Scoutt LM, Feldstein VA. *Callen's Ultrasonography in Obstetrics and Gynecology*. 6th ed. Elsevier; 2017:346–459.

Nyberg D, McGaham J, Pretorius D, et al. *Diagnostic Imaging of Fetal Anomalies*. Lippincott Williams & Wilkins; 2003:381–506.

Rumack CM, Wilson SR, Charboneau JW, et al. *Diagnostic Ultrasound*. 4th ed. Elsevier, 2011:1273–1326.

Sanders RC, Hall-Terracciano B. *Clinical Sonography: A Practical Guide*. 5th ed. Wolters Kluwer; 2016:358–380.

BONUS REVIEW!

Fetal Echocardiography Examination Images (Fig. 27-43)

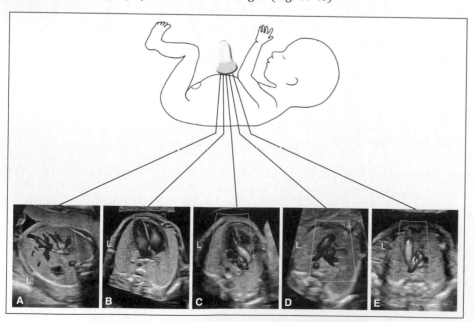

Figure 27-43 Axial planes in color Doppler of the fetal abdomen (**A**) and chest (**B-E**) as part of the performance of the fetal echocardiography examination. These axial planes are obtained at the level of the abdominal circumference (**A**), the four-chamber view (**B**), the five-chamber view (**C**), the three-vessel view (**D**), and the three-vessel trachea view (**E**).

BONUS REVIEW! (*continued*)

Apical Four-Chamber View of the Fetal Heart in Systole and Diastole (Fig. 27-44)

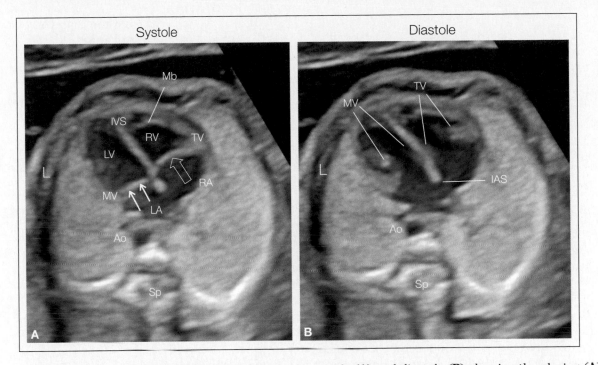

Figure 27-44 Apical four-chamber view of the fetal heart in systole (**A**) and diastole (**B**) showing the closing (**A**) and opening (**B**) of the mitral (*MV*) and tricuspid (*TV*) valves. Note in systole (**A**), the apical displacement of the TV (*open arrow*) as compared to the MV (*two small arrows*). In diastole (**B**), the open valves leaflets are recognized. The intratrial septum (*IAS*) is also best recognized in diastole (**B**) in the region of the crux of the heart. *Ao*, aorta; *IVS*, interventricular septum; *L*, left; *LA*, left atrium; *LV*, left ventricle; *Mb*, moderator band; *RA*, right atrium; *RV*, right ventricle; *Sp*, spine.

Fetal Thoracentesis (Fig. 27-45)

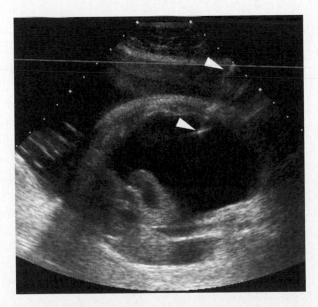

Figure 27-45 Fetal thoracentesis. A needle (*arrowheads*), inserted percutaneously through the maternal anterior abdominal wall, ends in the thorax of a fetus with a large pleural effusion.

The Fetal Gastrointestinal System

Introduction

The gastrointestinal system and abdominal wall defects of the fetus are discussed in this chapter. Most of the fetal abdominal abnormalities can be detected during a routine sonographic examination. While acquiring the abdominal circumference measurements, the sonographer can assess the position of gastrointestinal organs and their size. The sonographic appearance and relationship of the stomach with the fetal heart is an important objective. It is the obligation of the sonographer to utilize critical thinking when abnormalities are discovered in the fetal abdomen, because many of them have multiple associated findings in other systems of the body. The "Bonus Review" section includes an example of Beckwith–Wiedemann syndrome and consecutive axial views of the chest and abdomen in order to prove situs.

Key Terms

abdominal circumference—fetal biometric measurement of the abdomen made in the second and third trimesters; used in conjunction with other measurements to date the pregnancy and size the fetus

anorectal atresia—congenital maldevelopment of the rectum and absence of the anal opening

ascites—excessive fluid in the peritoneal cavity

Beckwith–Wiedemann syndrome—a growth disorder syndrome synonymous with enlargement of several organs, including the skull, tongue, and liver

cholangitis—inflammation of the bile ducts

choledochal cyst—the cystic dilatation of the common bile duct

cystic fibrosis—an inherited disorder in which mucus-secreting organs such as the lungs, pancreas, and other digestive organs produce thick and sticky secretions instead of normal secretions

double bubble sign—classic sonographic sign of duodenal atresia representing the stomach and proximal duodenum

duodenal atresia—congenital maldevelopment or absence of the duodenum

esophageal atresia—congenital absence of part of the esophagus

gastroschisis—herniation of abdominal contents through a right-sided, periumbilical abdominal wall defect

hepatomegaly—enlargement of the liver

Hirschsprung disease—a disease that leads to a functional bowel obstruction because of the lack of nerve cells within the colon wall

intrauterine growth restriction—a fetus that is below the 10th percentile for gestational age (small for gestational age) and whose growth is impeded for some reason

meconium—fetal stool that is composed of fetal skin, hair, amniotic fluid, and bile

omphalocele—an anterior abdominal wall defect where there is herniation of the fetal bowel and other abdominal organs into the base of the umbilical cord

pentalogy of Cantrell—a group of anomalies that include an omphalocele, along with ectopic cordis, cleft sternum, anterior diaphragmatic defect, and pericardial defects

physiologic bowel herniation—the normal developmental stage when the midgut migrates into the base of the umbilical cord

polyhydramnios—an excessive amount of amniotic fluid for the gestational age

portal hypertension—the elevation of blood pressure within the portal venous system

tracheoesophageal fistula—an abnormal connection between the esophagus and the trachea

Turner syndrome—a chromosomal aberration where one sex chromosome is absent; may also be referred to as monosomy X

VACTERL—acronym for associated anomalies; stands for vertebral anomalies, anal atresia, cardiac anomalies, tracheoesophageal fistula or esophageal atresia, renal anomalies, and limb anomalies

NORMAL FETAL GASTROINTESTINAL ANATOMY AND THE ABDOMINAL CIRCUMFERENCE

The fetal gut develops at the end of the fifth menstrual week and can be divided into the foregut, midgut, and hindgut. Abdominal organs, such as the stomach, liver, spleen, gallbladder, pancreas, small intestine, and colon, may all be evaluated during a sonographic examination. The esophagus may be visualized when needed as several parallel echogenic lines within the thorax. Transvaginally, the fetal stomach can be visualized as early as 8 weeks' gestation, but most certainly should be seen by 14 weeks in the left upper quadrant as an anechoic, circular organ. The position of the stomach should be noted in relationship to the fetal heart. Both small bowel and the colon can be examined using sonography. The diameter of small bowel is smaller than the colon and does not typically exceed 5 mm. Differentiating small bowel from the colon is achieved late in gestation, because the colon offers larger loops within the periphery of the abdomen and contains hypoechoic material representing **meconium**.

The **abdominal circumference** is a measurement of the fetal abdomen that is made in the second and third trimesters. The abdominal circumference is made in the axial view of the fetus and should include the fetal stomach, transverse thoracic spine, and intrahepatic portion of the umbilical vein and its junction with the left portal vein (Fig. 28-1). The electronic calipers are placed around the entire outer perimeter of the abdomen. The abdominal diameter measurement is taken at the same level, with two perpendicular caliper sets. The formula for the abdominal diameter is $AC = 1.57 \times (AD_1 + AD_2)$.

SOUND OFF
The abdominal circumference is made in the axial view of the fetus and should include the fetal stomach, transverse thoracic spine, and intrahepatic portion of the umbilical vein.

FETAL GASTROINTESTINAL ABNORMALITIES

Gastrointestinal Abnormalities and Polyhydramnios

Polyhydramnios, or excessive amniotic fluid, can be noted with multiple anomalies. However, sonographers must understand why polyhydramnios results from some gastrointestinal abnormalities. During fetal development, there are several structures that are thought to produce amniotic fluid. Initially, in early embryologic development, the origin of amniotic fluid is thought to result from an osmotic process, because water crosses the amniotic space freely. In later gestation, somewhere around 9 weeks, the fetal kidneys begin to produce urine, a liquid that eventually comprises most of the amniotic fluid.

SOUND OFF
Fetal urine contributes greatly to the amount of amniotic fluid.

Amniotic fluid is a substance that contains valuable proteins that are essential for normal fetal development. The fetus ingests amniotic fluid by swallowing. The fluid passes through the esophagus, into the stomach, and travels through the small bowel and into the colon, where absorption takes place. Polyhydramnios results when there is an obstruction or disturbance to the normal flow and absorption of amniotic fluid. For instance, the fetus that suffers from **esophageal atresia** or **duodenal atresia** cannot transport amniotic fluid into the intestines. The fluid exits back out of the esophagus, and absorption cannot take place. Consequently, there is a buildup of amniotic fluid resulting from the continual production of urine by the fetal kidneys, resulting in polyhydramnios.

SOUND OFF
When polyhydramnios is detected, the sonographers should evaluate the fetal gastrointestinal tract carefully for signs of abnormalities, such as duodenal or esophageal atresia.

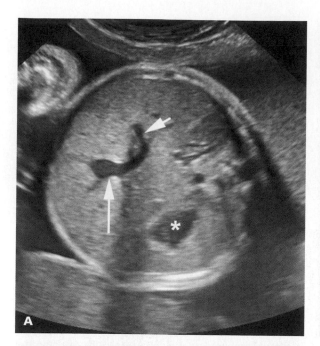

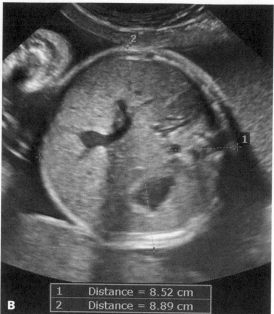

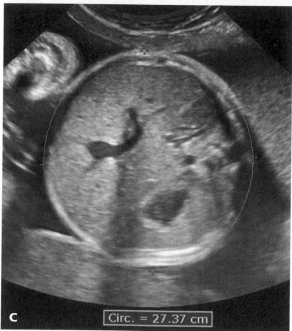

Figure 28-1 Abdominal circumference and abdominal diameter. **A.** Transverse image of the fetal abdomen at 28 weeks' gestation at the correct level and plane for obtaining measurements. The junction of the umbilical vein (*long arrow*) and left portal vein (*short arrow*) is seen, as is the stomach (*asterisk*). **B.** Anteroposterior diameter (*calipers 1*) is measured from the anterior skin surface to the posterior skin surface. Transverse diameter (*calipers 2*) is measured from one lateral skin surface to the opposite skin surface. **C.** Abdominal circumference (*elliptical calipers*) is measured around the outer perimeter of the abdomen.

Esophageal Atresia

The congenital absence of part of the esophagus is termed esophageal atresia. Consequently, the esophagus and the trachea often form an abnormal connection known as a **tracheoesophageal fistula**. This condition is associated with esophageal atresia approximately 90% of the time. The fetal stomach may appear sonographically small or completely absent with esophageal atresia, and there will be evidence of polyhydramnios (Fig. 28-2). Associated anomalies are often present and include duodenal atresia, **VACTERL** association, Down syndrome, **intrauterine growth restriction**, and trisomy 18.

> **SONOGRAPHIC FINDINGS OF ESOPHAGEAL ATRESIA**
>
> 1. Absent or small stomach
> 2. Polyhydramnios
> 3. Intrauterine growth restriction

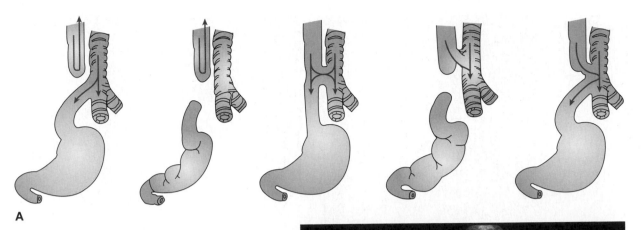

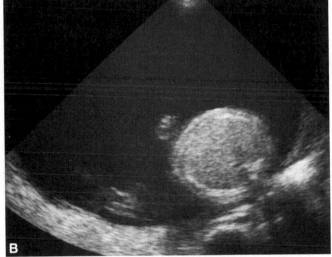

Figure 28-2 Esophageal atresia. **A.** Five variations of esophageal atresia are shown. The most common form is shown on the far left where the esophagus ends in a blind pouch. *Arrows* indicate the flow of food and air. **B.** Transverse view of the fetal abdomen revealing no identifiable stomach and severe polyhydramnios.

Duodenal Atresia

The congenital maldevelopment or absence of the proximal portion of the small bowel, the duodenum, is termed duodenal atresia (Fig. 28-3). Duodenal atresia classically presents sonographically as a dilated, fluid-filled anechoic stomach and an anechoic fluid-filled proximal duodenum, offering the **"double bubble" sign** (Fig. 28-4). Duodenal atresia has a proven association with trisomy 21; thus, additional sonographic markers of trisomy 21 should be aggressively investigated during the examination. Other associated anomalies include esophageal atresia, VACTERL association, intrauterine growth restriction, and cardiac anomalies.

SONOGRAPHIC FINDINGS OF DUODENAL ATRESIA

1. "Double bubble" sign
2. Polyhydramnios
3. Intrauterine growth restriction

◀))) SOUND OFF
Duodenal atresia classically presents as the "double bubble" sign.

Abnormalities of the Fetal Liver, Spleen, Gallbladder, and Biliary Tree

The fetal liver may be evaluated in utero. It is essential to remember that in the fetus, the left lobe of the liver is typically larger than the right lobe. This is secondary to the way in which the fetal circulatory system provides more oxygen to the left lobe in utero. **Hepatomegaly** is the most common abnormality of the fetal liver. Hepatomegaly may occur as a result of intrauterine infections, fetal anemia (Rh incompatibility), or be seen with **Beckwith–Wiedemann syndrome**. Enlargement of the fetal spleen—splenomegaly—can accompany hepatomegaly and may be suggestive of intrauterine infections or Rh incompatibility with hydrops.

Fetal gallstones (cholelithiasis) and sludge within the gallbladder may be noted in utero, most often in

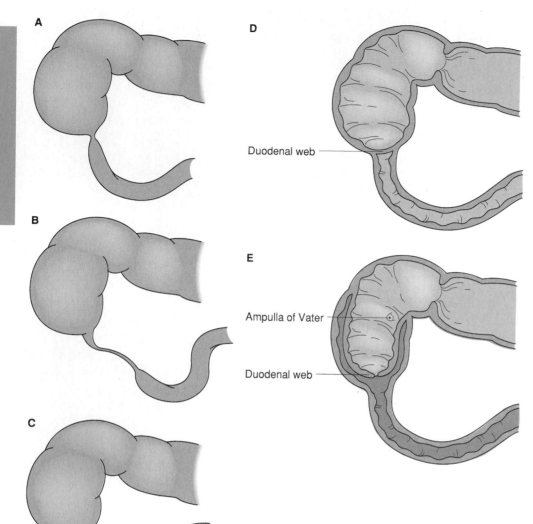

A

B

C

D

Duodenal web

E

Ampulla of Vater

Duodenal web

Figure 28-3 Anatomic forms of duodenal atresia. **A.** Short segment atresia with patent lumen. **B.** Long segment atresia with patent lumen. **C.** Complete atresia with discontinuity. **D.** Distal duodenal web. **E.** Proximal duodenal web.

the third trimester. Gallstones appear sonographically as echogenic foci in the right upper quadrant of the fetus that may or may not produce posterior shadowing (Fig. 28-5). Gallstones that persist postnatally typically resolve spontaneously. An additional rare abnormality of the biliary tree is the **choledochal cyst**. There are four different types of choledochal cysts, with the most common being described as the cystic dilatation of the common bile duct. Choledochal cysts can lead to **cholangitis**, **portal hypertension**, pancreatitis, and liver failure. More information about choledochal cysts can be found in Chapter 4.

> **SOUND OFF**
> Hepatomegaly is the most common abnormality of the fetal liver. It can be associated with intrauterine infection, fetal anemia, or Beckwith–Wiedemann syndrome.

FETAL BOWEL ABNORMALITIES AND THE ABDOMINAL WALL

Echogenic Bowel

The analysis of the echogenicity of the fetal small intestine may be part of the fetal screening examination in some institutions. In general, the echogenicity of the small intestine should not be isoechoic to or greater than that of fetal bone (Fig. 28-6). However, the transducer frequency plays a role in the diagnosis of echogenic bowel. One author suggests that if a higher frequency transducer suggests echogenic bowel, that the sonographer should decrease the frequency to 5 MHz or less and decrease the overall gain. Echogenic bowel has been linked with Down syndrome, **cystic fibrosis**, growth restriction, fetal demise, congenital infections such as cytomegalovirus, and gastrointestinal obstructions.

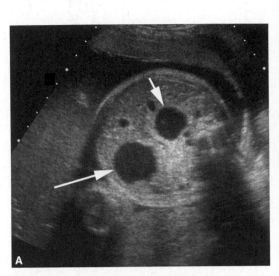

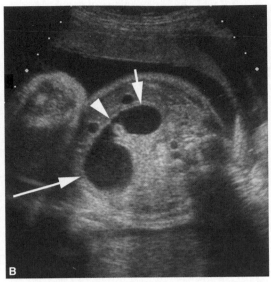

Figure 28-4 Duodenal atresia ("double bubble") in a fetus with trisomy 21. **A.** Transverse view of the fetal upper abdomen demonstrating dilated stomach (*long arrow*) and duodenum (*short arrow*). **B.** Image in a slightly different plane demonstrating the connection (*arrowhead*) between the stomach (*long arrow*) and the duodenum (*short arrow*).

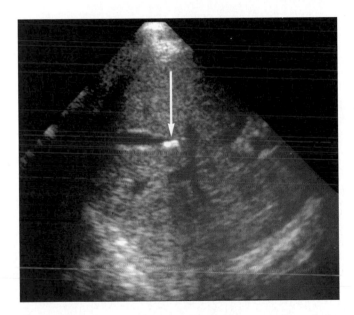

Figure 28-5 Fetal cholelithiasis. Transverse view of the fetal abdomen revealing a gallstone (*arrow*) that produces shadowing.

> **((∘)) SOUND OFF**
> Echogenic bowel has been linked with Down syndrome, cystic fibrosis, growth restriction, fetal demise, congenital infections such as cytomegalovirus, and gastrointestinal obstructions.

Fetal Bowel Obstruction and Anorectal Atresia

Hirschsprung disease, which causes a functional fetal bowel obstruction, is caused by the absence of nerves within the bowel wall. Hirschsprung disease is more common in males, and there is a strong association with trisomy 21. The sonographic finding of dilated loops of bowel within the fetal abdomen is indicative of a fetal bowel obstruction. These dilated loops of bowel should not exceed 7 mm in diameter or measure greater than 15 mm in length. Obstruction of the fetal bowel most often occurs when there is a meconium plug causing the barrier, a condition referred to as meconium plug syndrome. The most common type of colonic atresia that will lead to a bowel obstruction is **anorectal atresia**. This congenital maldevelopment of the rectum and anal opening causes dilation of the bowel. Anorectal atresia may be linked with VACTERL association and chromosomal abnormalities; thus, a thorough analysis of the fetus for other abnormalities is vital. Anorectal atresia will most often lead to the visualization of a dilated fetal rectum.

> **((∘)) SOUND OFF**
> Anorectal atresia will most often lead to the visualization of a dilated fetal rectum.

Abdominal Wall Defects and Alpha-Fetoprotein

Gastroschisis and **omphalocele** are two of the most common ventral abdominal wall defects. As mentioned previously in Chapter 24, alpha-fetoprotein (AFP) exits the fetus through an opening in the neural tube (i.e., an opening in the cranium or spine). AFP may also exit the fetus through an abdominal wall defect, thereby increasing the level of maternal serum alpha-fetoprotein (MSAFP). If an opening is present, a greater amount of

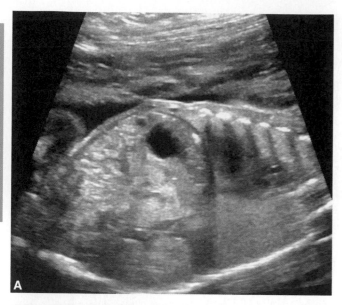
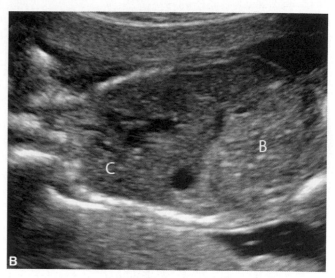

Figure 28-6 Echogenic bowel. **A.** Echogenic bowel at 25 weeks of gestation. Coronal sonogram demonstrates abnormally echogenic bowel in a fetus with cystic fibrosis. **B.** Echogenic bowel is recognized by its abnormal brightness, as noted here in a different fetus at 18 weeks' GA. *B*, bowel; *C*, chest; *GA*, gestational age.

AFP is allowed to pass into the maternal circulation. Although MSAFP screening is not specific for abdominal wall defects, elevated levels of MSAFP are found in the presence of omphalocele and gastroschisis and thus can be used as a reliable screening test for the early detection of these and other abnormalities. Furthermore, it is important to note that MSAFP levels have been shown to be much higher in gastroschisis than in omphalocele.

> **SOUND OFF**
> If the fetus has an abdominal wall defect (opening in the abdomen), then a greater amount of AFP is allowed to pass into the maternal circulation.

Physiologic (Normal) Bowel Herniation

As a part of normal fetal development during the first trimester, the midgut herniates into the base of the umbilical cord; this is termed **physiologic bowel herniation**. The intestines return to the abdomen by the 12th gestational week. Although omphalocele or gastroschisis may be suggested with high-resolution transvaginal imaging in the first trimester, a diagnosis of an abdominal wall defect, such as omphalocele or gastroschisis, may be difficult before 12 weeks and thus follow-up examinations are often required to confirm the diagnosis. This topic is also discussed in Chapter 23 of this book.

Gastroschisis

Gastroschisis is the herniation of abdominal contents through a right-sided, periumbilical abdominal wall

defect (Fig. 28-7). Gastroschisis is thought to be caused by a vascular incident occurring to either the right umbilical vein or the omphalomesenteric artery. Most often, there is herniation of the small intestine, but with larger defects, the stomach and other organs may be found outside the abdomen. The bowel that is exposed to amniotic fluid may become dilated, thick walled, and have decreased peristaltic activity. Gastroschisis, unlike omphalocele, does not have a strong association with chromosomal abnormalities. Although they may suffer from intrauterine growth restriction, the prognosis after surgery for newborns with isolated gastroschisis is much better than for those with omphalocele. Sonographically, normal cord insertion into the abdomen

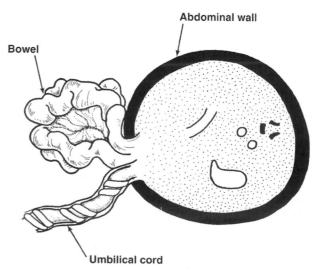

Figure 28-7 Schematic of gastroschisis. Cross-sectional drawing of gastroschisis.

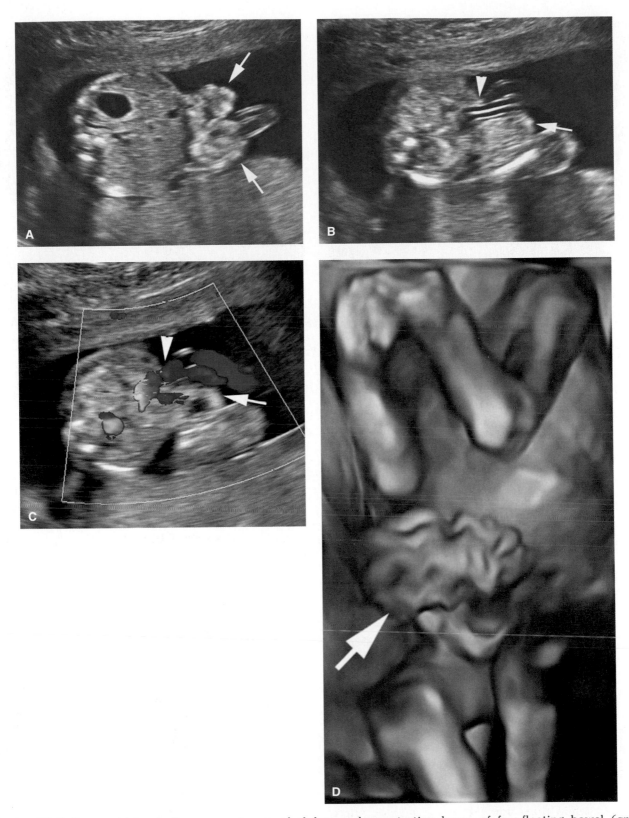

Figure 28-8 Gastroschisis. **A.** Transverse image of abdomen demonstrating loops of free-floating bowel (*arrows*) protruding from anterior abdominal wall. Grayscale (**B**) and color Doppler (**C**) images showing umbilical cord insertion (*arrowhead*) is intact, adjacent to herniated bowel (*arrow*). **D.** Three-dimensional image showing irregular outer contour of gastroschisis (*arrow*) made up of herniated loops of bowel not enclosed by a membrane.

is noted, and most often, the right-sided periumbilical mass will be easily identified (Fig. 28-8). Recognizable loops of bowel are often noted outside of the abdomen floating in the amniotic fluid, and color Doppler should be used to demonstrate the relationship of the mass to the umbilical cord.

CLINICAL FINDINGS OF GASTROSCHISIS

1. Elevated MSAFP

SONOGRAPHIC FINDINGS OF GASTROSCHISIS

1. Normal cord insertion
2. Periumbilical, right-sided mass
3. Recognizable loops of bowel outside the abdomen
4. Intrauterine growth restriction

🔊 **SOUND OFF**
Gastroschisis is the herniation of abdominal contents through a right-sided, periumbilical abdominal wall defect. It generally has a better prognosis than omphalocele.

Omphalocele

The evidence of persistent herniation of the bowel, and potentially other abdominal organs, into the base of the umbilical cord leads to the diagnosis of an omphalocele (Fig. 28-9). An omphalocele is located within the midline of the abdomen. The umbilical cord will insert into this mass. The entire content is contained and covered by peritoneum and amnion. **Ascites** is often noted within an omphalocele, as well as within the abdomen of the fetus. Ascites may be helpful in demarcating the contents of the mass. It is important to note whether the mass contains liver, because a poorer prognosis corresponds with this type of omphalocele.

🔊 **SOUND OFF**
Omphalocele has a more significant risk for heart defects and chromosomal anomalies than gastroschisis.

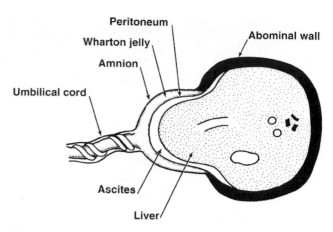

Figure 28-9 Schematic of omphalocele. Cross-sectional drawing of omphalocele containing part of the liver.

The sonographic appearance of an omphalocele is that of a midline abdominal mass that contains bowel, the liver, or other abdominal organs (Fig. 28-10). Omphalocele has a more significant risk for heart defects and chromosomal anomalies than gastroschisis. Trisomy 18, trisomy 13, **Turner syndrome**, and Beckwith–Wiedemann syndrome have all been linked with omphaloceles. **Pentalogy of Cantrell** is another group of anomalies that include an omphalocele, along with ectopic cordis, cleft sternum, anterior diaphragmatic defect, and pericardial defects (Fig. 28-11).

CLINICAL FINDINGS OF OMPHALOCELE

1. Elevated MSAFP

SONOGRAPHIC FINDINGS OF OMPHALOCELE

1. Midline abdominal mass at the base of the umbilical cord that contains bowel, the liver, and/or other abdominal organs
2. Abnormal cord insertion into the midline abdominal mass
3. Multiple associated anomalies

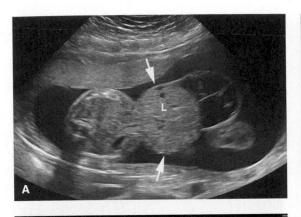

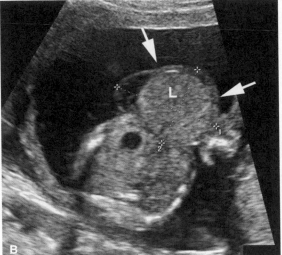

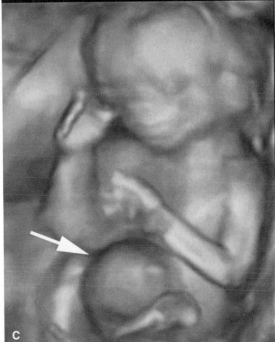

Figure 28-10 Omphalocele containing bowel and liver. A 26-week fetus (**A**) and 21-week fetus (**B**), both with omphaloceles containing bowel and liver (*L*) (*arrows*), shown in transverse view of abdomen. **C.** Three-dimensional image showing smooth outer contour (*arrow*) typical of omphaloceles.

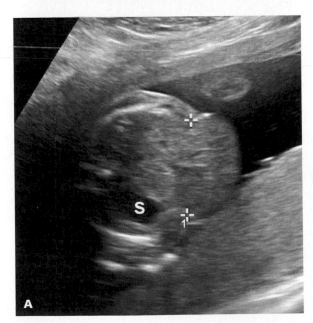

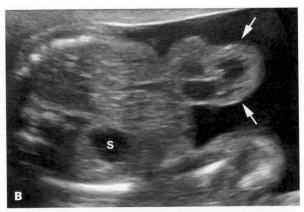

Figure 28-11 Pentalogy of Cantrell. **A.** Transverse image of abdomen in a 22-week fetus with pentalogy of Cantrell showing large defect in anterior abdominal wall (*calipers*) (*S*, stomach). **B.** Transverse image slightly higher than (**A**) showing heart (*arrows*) outside the chest (*S*, stomach).

REVIEW QUESTIONS

1. What do the arrows in Figure 28-12 indicate?
   a. Omphalocele
   b. Gastroschisis
   c. Ectopic cordis
   d. Fetal bowl obstruction

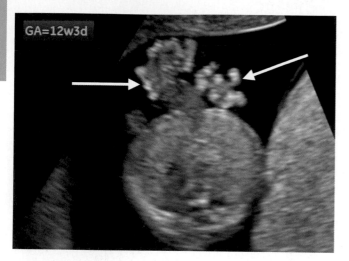

Figure 28-12

2. What does the arrow in Figure 28-13 indicate?
   a. Omphalocele
   b. Gastroschisis
   c. Ectopic cordis
   d. Fetal bowl obstruction

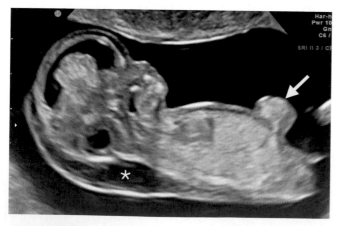

Figure 28-13

3. Figure 28-14 was noted in the presence of polyhydramnios, and there was evidence of other sonographic findings consistent with trisomy 18. What is the most likely diagnosis?
   a. Anorectal atresia
   b. Beckwith–Wiedemann syndrome
   c. Esophageal atresia
   d. Duodenal atresia

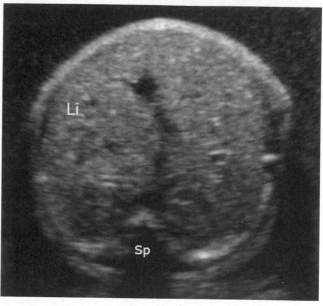

Figure 28-14

4. What do the findings in Figure 28-15 indicate?
   a. Choledochal cyst
   b. Cholangitis
   c. Esophageal atresia
   d. Duodenal atresia

5. What type of amniotic level would most likely be associated with Figure 28-15?
   a. Polyhydramnios
   b. Anhydramnios
   c. Oligohydramnios
   d. Bradyhydramnios

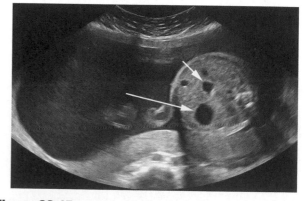

Figure 28-15

6. When do the fetal kidneys begin to produce urine?
   a. 5 weeks
   b. 12 weeks
   c. 20 weeks
   d. 9 weeks

7. Which of the following is not evident in Figure 28-16?
   a. Agenesis of the corpus callosum
   b. Duodenal atresia
   c. Ventriculomegaly
   d. "Double bubble" sign

8. What should the measurement not exceed in Figure 28-16A?
   a. 8 mm
   b. 10 mm
   c. 5 mm
   d. 7 mm

9. Combining the two sonographic findings in Figure 28-16A and B would increase the risk for:
   a. Turner syndrome.
   b. trisomy 18.
   c. trisomy 21.
   d. trisomy 13.

10. What lobe of the liver is typically the largest in the fetus?
    a. Right
    b. Quadrate
    c. Caudate
    d. Left

11. What is the finding consistent with in Figure 28-17?
    a. Choledochal cyst
    b. Cholangitis
    c. Cholelithiasis
    d. Adenomyomatosis of the gallbladder

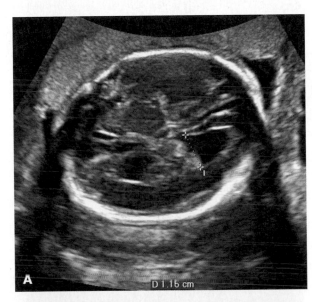

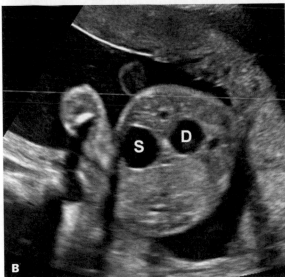

Figure 28-16

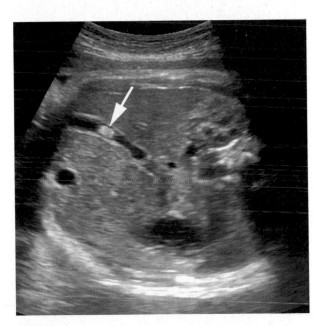

Figure 28-17

12. What does the arrow in Figure 28-18 indicate?
    a. Dilated loop of bowel
    b. Double bubble sign
    c. Hirschsprung disease
    d. Echogenic bowel

13. The arrowhead in Figure 28-19 most likely represents what finding at 10 gestational weeks?
    a. Omphalocele
    b. Physiologic bowel herniation
    c. Gastroschisis
    d. Pentalogy of Cantrell

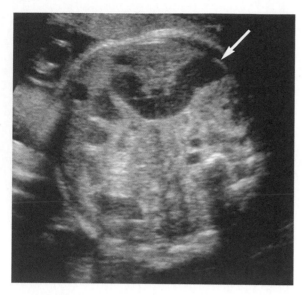

Figure 28-18

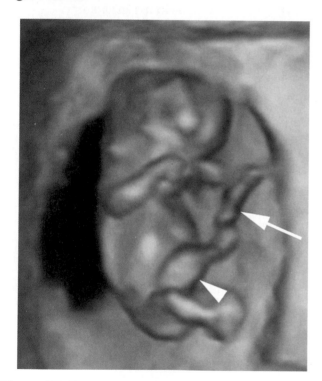

Figure 28-19

14. What does the arrow in Figure 28-19 represent?
    a. Base of the omphalocele
    b. Fetal bowel
    c. Umbilical cord
    d. Lower leg

15. Which of the following could result from a choledochal cyst?
    a. Duodenal atresia
    b. Portal hypertension
    c. Hirschsprung disease
    d. Cystic fibrosis

16. Figure 28-20A is a transverse section through the fetal chest, whereas Figure 28-20B is a transverse section through the umbilical cord site. What is the most likely diagnosis?
    a. Tetralogy of Fallot
    b. Pentalogy of Cantrell
    c. Beckwith–Wiedemann syndrome
    d. Hirschsprung disease

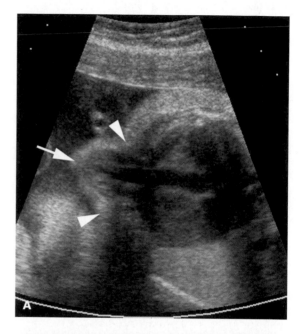

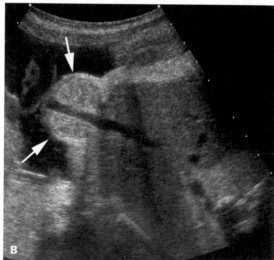

Figure 28-20

17. What is noted in the transverse image of the fetal abdomen in Figure 28-21?
    a. Pleural effusion
    b. Ascites
    c. Splenomegaly
    d. Duodenal atresia

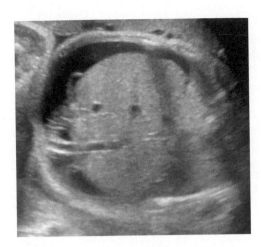

Figure 28-21

18. Fetal bowel loop diameter is abnormal when it exceeds:
    a. 3 mm.
    b. 4 mm.
    c. 7 mm.
    d. 2 mm.

19. Echogenic bowel is associated with all of the following except:
    a. fetal demise.
    b. cytomegalovirus.
    c. growth restriction.
    d. Beckwith–Wiedemann syndrome.

20. The dilated fetal rectum would likely be a sonographic feature of which of the following?
    a. Anorectal atresia
    b. Rectal carcinoma
    c. Cystic fibrosis
    d. Gastroschisis

21. Hepatomegaly would least likely be associated with:
    a. Beckwith–Wiedemann syndrome.
    b. fetal anemia.
    c. intrauterine infections.
    d. gastroschisis.

22. Normally, physiologic bowel herniation resolves by:
    a. 8 weeks.
    b. 10 weeks.
    c. 24 weeks.
    d. 12 weeks.

23. Which of the following is most often associated with duodenal atresia?
    a. Trisomy 21
    b. Trisomy 18
    c. Trisomy 13
    d. Triploidy

24. Hepatomegaly would be seen in conjunction with:
    a. Down syndrome.
    b. Edwards syndrome.
    c. Beckwith–Wiedemann syndrome.
    d. Hirschsprung disease.

25. Pentalogy of Cantrell includes all of the following findings except:
    a. cardiovascular malformations.
    b. diaphragmatic malformations.
    c. omphalocele.
    d. radial ray defect.

26. An excessive amount of amniotic fluid is termed:
    a. polyhydramnios.
    b. oligohydramnios.
    c. esophageal atresia.
    d. amniotic fluid index.

27. The most common abnormality of the fetal liver is:
    a. gallstones.
    b. hepatocellular lymphadenopathy.
    c. cirrhosis.
    d. hepatomegaly.

28. Congenital maldevelopment of the proximal portion of the small intestine is termed:
    a. VACTERL association.
    b. esophageal atresia.
    c. duodenal atresia.
    d. jejunal atresia.

29. A functional bowel disorder within the fetus that is caused by the absence of intestinal nerves is found in:
    a. gastroschisis.
    b. Beckwith–Wiedemann syndrome.
    c. omphalocele.
    d. Hirschsprung disease.

30. Which of the following is associated with echogenic bowel?
    a. Fetal anemia
    b. Cystic fibrosis
    c. Radial ray syndrome
    d. Portal hypertension

31. What chromosomal anomaly is associated with echogenic bowel?
    a. Trisomy 18
    b. Trisomy 13
    c. Trisomy 21
    d. Triploidy

32. The herniation of the bowel into the base of the umbilical cord before 12 weeks is termed:
    a. gastroschisis.
    b. omphalocele.
    c. hernia umbilicus.
    d. physiologic herniation.

33. All of the following are associated with omphalocele except:
    a. trisomy 18.
    b. pentalogy of Cantrell.
    c. intrauterine growth restriction.
    d. Hirschsprung disease.

34. The fetal stomach should be visualized by:
    a. 6 weeks.
    b. 14 weeks.
    c. 20 weeks.
    d. 18 weeks.

35. All of the following are associated with esophageal atresia except:
    a. Down syndrome.
    b. VACTERL association.
    c. Edwards syndrome.
    d. oligohydramnios.

36. An abnormal connection between the esophagus and trachea is termed:
    a. esophageal–duodenal herniation.
    b. double bubble sign.
    c. esophageal atresia.
    d. tracheoesophageal fistula.

37. In what location does gastroschisis occur more often?
    a. Left lateral of the cord insertion
    b. Right lateral of the cord insertion
    c. Just superior to the fetal bladder
    d. Base of the umbilical cord

38. The congenital absence of part of the esophagus is termed:
    a. duodenal atresia.
    b. VACTERL association.
    c. Down syndrome.
    d. esophageal atresia.

39. The "double bubble" sign is indicative of:
    a. esophageal atresia.
    b. duodenal atresia.
    c. hydrocephalus.
    d. anorectal atresia.

40. All of the following are associated with gastroschisis except:
    a. normal cord insertion.
    b. multiple chromosomal abnormalities.
    c. elevated MSAFP.
    d. periumbilical mass.

41. Which of the following laboratory values would be significant in the detection of an abdominal wall defect?
    a. MSAFP
    b. Human chorionic gonadotropin
    c. Maternal serum amylase
    d. Estradiol

42. What is an inherited disorder in which mucus-secreting organs such as the lungs, pancreas, and other digestive organs produce thick and sticky secretions instead of normal secretions?
    a. Hirschsprung disease
    b. Cystic fibrosis
    c. Multiple sclerosis
    d. Turner syndrome

43. What organ(s) produces amniotic fluid after 12 weeks?
    a. Fetal liver and the spleen
    b. Fetal intestines and lungs
    c. Fetal intestines and the liver
    d. Fetal kidneys

44. An omphalocele is associated with all of the following except:
    a. pentalogy of Cantrell.
    b. trisomy 18.
    c. Patau syndrome.
    d. meconium aspiration syndrome.

45. Duodenal atresia and esophageal atresia are associated with:
    a. oligohydramnios.
    b. polyhydramnios.
    c. normal amniotic fluid index.
    d. anhydramnios.

46. The fetal gut develops at the end of the fifth menstrual week and can be divided into all of the following except:
    a. midgut.
    b. foregut.
    c. central gut.
    d. hindgut.

47. Intrauterine growth restriction is defined as:
    a. a small-for-dates fetus.
    b. a fetus that falls below the 10th percentile for gestational age.
    c. a fetus that is immunocompromised and has decreased umbilical cord Doppler ratios for gestational age.
    d. a fetus that fall below the fifth percentile for gestational age.

48. Which of the following best describes a choledochal cyst?
    a. It is the cystic dilatation of the common bile duct.
    b. It is the herniation of the abdominal contents into the umbilical cord.
    c. It is the congenital absence of the cystic duct.
    d. It is the inflammation of the biliary tree caused by extrinsic obstruction.

49. Fetal stool is termed:
    a. plica.
    b. meconium.
    c. laguna.
    d. lanugo.

50. All of the following are associated with omphalocele except:
    a. normal cord insertion.
    b. multiple chromosomal abnormalities.
    c. elevated MSAFP.
    d. periumbilical mass.

51. An omphalocele may contain:
    a. fetal liver.
    b. ascites.
    c. fetal colon.
    d. all of the above.

52. The congenital maldevelopment of the rectum and absence of anal opening is termed:
    a. jejunal atresia.
    b. intussusception.
    c. anorectal atresia.
    d. duodenal atresia.

53. All of the following are associated with duodenal atresia except:
    a. trisomy 21.
    b. esophageal atresia.
    c. VACTERL association.
    d. Turner syndrome.

54. Which of the following would be least likely associated with an elevated MSAFP?
    a. Pentalogy of Cantrell
    b. Anorectal atresia
    c. Gastroschisis
    d. Omphalocele

55. Which of the following is considered to be the most common type of colonic atresia?
    a. Duodenal atresia
    b. Jejunal atresia
    c. Anorectal atresia
    d. Intussusception

56. Fetal meconium typically consists of all of the following except:
    a. skin.
    b. hair.
    c. bile.
    d. blood.

57. Which of the following would be most likely associated with an excessive amount of amniotic fluid?
    a. Duodenal atresia
    b. Hepatomegaly
    c. Bilateral renal agenesis
    d. Physiologic bowel herniation

58. Which of the following would be most likely associated with oligohydramnios?
    a. Duodenal atresia
    b. Hepatomegaly
    c. Bilateral renal agenesis
    d. Physiologic bowel herniation

59. The majority of amniotic fluid is composed of:
    a. fetal blood.
    b. fetal serous fluid.
    c. maternal serous fluid.
    d. fetal urine.

60. All of the following are sonographic findings of esophageal atresia except:
    a. absent stomach.
    b. polyhydramnios.
    c. macrosomia.
    d. intrauterine growth restriction.

SUGGESTED READINGS

Haller J. *Textbook of Neonatal Ultrasound*. Parthenon; 1998:65–92.

Henningsen C, Kuntz K, Youngs D. *Clinical Guide to Sonography: Exercises for Critical Thinking*. 2nd ed. Elsevier; 2014:261–263 & 293–294.

Kline-Fath BM, Bulas DI, Lee W. *Fundamental and Advanced Fetal Imaging: Ultrasound and MRI*. 2nd ed. Wolters Kluwer; 2021:748–799.

Norton ME, Scoutt LM, Feldstein VA. *Callen's Ultrasonography in Obstetrics and Gynecology*. 6th ed. Elsevier; 2017:460–502.

Nyberg D, McGaham J, Pretorius D, et al. *Diagnostic Imaging of Fetal Anomalies*. Lippincott Williams & Wilkins; 2003:507–602.

Rumack CM, Wilson SR, Charboneau JW, et al. *Diagnostic Ultrasound*. 4th ed. Elsevier; 2011:1327–1352.

Stephenson SR, Dmitrieva J. *Diagnostic Medical Sonography: Obstetrics and Gynecology*. 3rd ed. Wolters Kluwer; 2017:575–606.

BONUS REVIEW!

Beckwith–Wiedemann Syndrome (Fig. 28-22)

Beckwith–Wiedemann syndrome

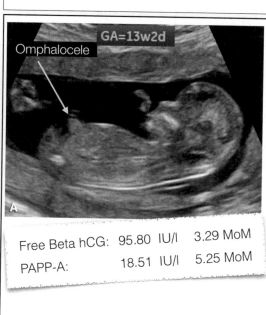
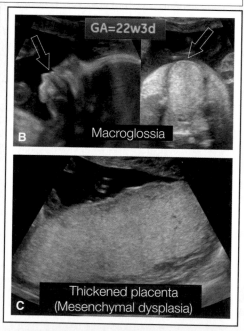

Figure 28-22 Fetus with Beckwith–Wiedemann syndrome. At 13 weeks of gestation, a small omphalocele with bowel content was detected, as shown in a midsagittal plane of the fetus in **A**. In addition, free beta-human chorionic gonadotropin (*hCG*) and pregnancy-associated plasma protein A were elevated. Chorionic villous sampling revealed a normal karyotype. At 22 weeks of gestation, no omphalocele was found, but macroglossia was noted as shown in a midsagittal and coronal planes of the face in **B** (*arrows*). The placenta also appeared thickened at 22 weeks of gestation, suggesting mesenchymal dysplasia (**C**). Sonographic signs were suggestive of Beckwith–Wiedemann syndrome, which was confirmed postnatally with molecular genetics.

Axial View of the Upper Abdomen Shown in a Schematic Drawing and Corresponding Sonographic Image of a Fetus with Normal Situs (Situs Solitus) (Fig. 28-23)

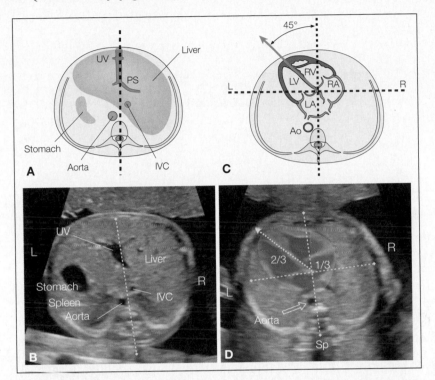

Figure 28-23 Axial view of the upper abdomen shown in a schematic drawing (**A**) and corresponding sonographic image (**B**) of a fetus with normal situs (situs solitus). The vertical line (*A* and *B*) divides the abdomen into right and left sides. The right-sided structures include the gallbladder (not shown), the portal sinus (*PS*), a large part of the liver, and inferior vena cava (*IVC*). The left-sided structures include the descending aorta (*Ao*), the stomach, and the spleen. Axial view of the chest, at the four-chamber view, shown in a schematic drawing (**C**) and corresponding sonographic image (**D**) of a fetus with normal situs. The chest is divided into four equal quadrants by a vertical and horizontal line. Note the position of the heart and the descending *Ao* in the left chest with a normal cardiac axis of 45 degrees. *L*, left; *LA*, left atrium; *LV*, left ventricle; *R*, right; *RA*, right atrium; *RV*, right ventricle; *UV*, umbilical vein.

The Fetal Genitourinary System

Introduction

The most common abnormal findings on a prenatal sonogram are those of the genitourinary system. This chapter provides a review of the normal sonographic findings of the fetal kidneys and bladder. In addition, an overview of the pathology of the fetal genitourinary system is offered. Although the adrenal glands are not part of the genitourinary system, a discussion on the sonographic appearance of the adrenal glands is also provided. The "Bonus Review" section includes images of fetal bladder drainage, OEIS complex, Doppler and three-dimensional (3D) imaging of fetal renal vasculature, and a diagram of urachal development. As a final note, it may behoove the reader to utilize Chapter 7 in this text for partial review as well, especially the topics of renal variants and renal cystic disease within that chapter.

Key Terms

allantois—a membrane that is present during early embryonic development that contributes to urinary bladder formation and development

ambiguous genitalia—a birth defect in which the sex of the fetus cannot be determined

anhydramnios—no amniotic fluid

autosomal dominant—a way in which a disorder or trait can be inherited by a fetus; at least one of the parents has to be the carrier of the gene for the disease

autosomal dominant polycystic kidney disease—an inherited disease that results in the development of renal, liver, and pancreatic cysts late in life; also referred to as adult polycystic kidney disease

autosomal recessive—a way in which a disorder or trait can be inherited by a fetus; both parents must be carriers of the gene for the disease

autosomal recessive polycystic kidney disease—an inherited renal disease that results in bilateral enlargement of the fetal kidneys and microscopic renal cysts; also referred to as infantile polycystic kidney disease

bladder exstrophy—a birth defect in which the bladder is located outside the abdomen

caliectasis—dilation of the calices

clitoromegaly—enlargement of the clitoris

cloaca—the embryonic structure that develops into the normal rectum and urogenital sinus

cloacal exstrophy—birth defect consisting of omphalocele, bladder exstrophy, imperforate anus, and spina bifida; also referred to as OEIS complex

compensatory hypertrophy—enlargement of an organ secondary to an increased workload; often seen when part of an organ has been destroyed or when there is absence or decreased function of paired organs

encephalocele—protrusion of the brain and meninges through a defect in the skull

epispadias—in males, the urethral opening is located on the upper aspect of the penis

horseshoe kidneys—the attachment of the lower poles of the kidneys by a band of renal tissue that crosses the midline of the abdomen

hydrocele—a fluid collection within the scrotum between the two layers of the tunica vaginalis

hydronephrosis—the dilation of the renal collecting system resulting from the obstruction of the flow of urine from the kidney(s) to the bladder; also referred to as pelvocaliectasis or pelvicaliectasis

hydroureter—distension of the ureter with fluid because of obstruction

hypospadias—abnormal ventral curvature of the penis as a result of a shortened urethra that exits on the ventral penile shaft

chordee—the head of the penis curves upward or downward

infantile polycystic kidney disease—an inherited renal disease that results in bilateral enlargement of the fetal kidneys and microscopic renal cysts; also referred to as autosomal recessive polycystic kidney disease

"keyhole" sign—the sonographic appearance of a dilated fetal bladder and urethra in the presence of a bladder outlet obstruction

"lying-down" adrenal sign—the sonographic appearance of the adrenal gland in a parallel position within the abdomen as a result of renal agenesis

macroscopic—large enough to be discerned by the naked eye

Meckel–Gruber syndrome—fetal syndrome associated with microcephaly, occipital encephalocele, polydactyly, and polycystic kidneys

megacystis—an abnormally enlarged urinary bladder

megaureter—an enlarged ureter; can be congenital or acquired

mesoblastic nephroma—the most common solid fetal renal mass

micropenis—an abnormally small penis

microscopic—too small to be seen by the naked eye and thus typically requiring the aid of a microscope

moiety—(renal) refers to a separate collecting system in the upper pole or the lower pole of the kidney in a duplex collecting system

multicystic dysplastic kidney disease—a fetal renal disease thought to be caused by an early renal obstruction; leads to the development of multiple noncommunicating cysts of varying sizes in the renal fossa

neuroblastoma—malignant tumor that can occur within the adrenal gland and anywhere within the sympathetic nervous system

obstructive cystic dysplasia—a fetal disorder caused by an early renal obstruction; leads to small and echogenic kidneys that have cysts located along their margins

OEIS complex—acronym that stands for omphalocele, bladder exstrophy, imperforate anus, and spina bifida; also referred to as cloacal exstrophy

oligohydramnios—a lower-than-normal amount of amniotic fluid for the gestational age

pelvic kidney—a kidney located within the pelvis

pelviectasis—dilation of the renal pelvis; may also be referred to as pyelectasis

pelviureteral junction—see key term ureteropelvic junction

pelvocaliectasis—see key term hydronephrosis

perineum—the region between the external genitalia and the anus

polydactyly—having more than the normal number of fingers or toes

posterior urethral valves—irregular thin membranes of tissue located within the male posterior urethra that does not allow urine to exit the urethra

Potter facies—facial features seen with severe oligohydramnios, including low-set ears, flattened nose, wrinkled skin, and micrognathia

Potter syndrome—physical features of a fetus as a result of oligohydramnios; characterized by bilateral renal agenesis, abnormal facies, pulmonary hypoplasia, and limb abnormalities; also referred to as Potter sequence

prune belly syndrome—syndrome that is a consequence of the abdominal wall musculature being stretched by an extremely enlarged fetal urinary bladder

pulmonary hypoplasia—underdevelopment of the lungs

renal agenesis—failure of the kidney to develop; may be unilateral or bilateral

renal calices—the part of the collecting system that encompasses the apex of the renal pyramids

renal ectopia—refers to an abnormal location of the kidney or kidneys

renal fossa—the region where the kidney is located in the abdomen

renal pelvic diameter—measurement of the fetal renal pelvis; this dimension is obtained from the transverse kidney plane

renal pelvis—the funnel-shaped collecting system in the central portion of the kidney that allows urine to flow from the kidney to the ureter

sirenomelia—a fetal abnormality characterized by fusion of the lower extremities, renal agenesis, and oligohydramnios; may also be referred to as mermaid syndrome

undescended testis—testicles that do not descend into the scrotum; also referred to as cryptorchidism

urachus—canal connecting the fetal bladder with the allantois; normally closes during fetal development and becomes a fibrous cord

ureterocele—an abnormality in which the distal ureter projects into the urinary bladder

ureteropelvic junction—the junction of the ureter and the renal pelvis

ureteropelvic junction obstruction—an obstruction located in the region where the ureter meets the renal pelvis

ureterovesical junction—the junction of the ureter and the urinary bladder

ureterovesical junction obstruction—an obstruction located in the region where the ureter meets the bladder

urethral atresia—the congenital absence of the urethra

VACTERL—acronym for associated anomalies; stands for vertebral anomalies, anal atresia, cardiac anomalies, tracheoesophageal fistula or esophageal atresia, renal anomalies, and limb anomalies

vesicoureteral junction—see key term ureteropelvic junction

vesicoureteral reflux—the retrograde flow of urine from the urinary bladder into the ureter

SONOGRAPHY OF THE FETAL GENITOURINARY SYSTEM

The fetal kidneys develop within the pelvis and ascend into their normal position by 9 weeks. By the 10th week of gestation, fully functional kidneys exist. If the kidneys fail to ascend into the normal position, the result is an ectopic kidney **(renal ectopica)**, most often located within the pelvis (Fig. 29-1). This is referred to as a **pelvic kidney**. The most common renal anomaly is the duplex collecting system, also referred to as a duplicated,

duplex, or double collecting system. In this variant, the kidney is composed of two separate collecting systems, divided into what is termed an upper pole **moiety** and a lower pole moiety. **Horseshoe kidneys** are kidneys that are attached at their lower poles. Initially, the bladder is continuous with the **allantois**, although eventually this channel closes and develops into a fibrous cord referred to as the **urachus**. Thus, the urachus is located between the apex of the bladder and the umbilicus. In newborns, occasionally, the urachus can remain patent or open. The gonads develop in the upper fetal abdomen and descend into the pelvis. The testicles move down into the scrotum during the 7th month of gestation.

> 🔊 **SOUND OFF**
> The urachus is located between the apex of the bladder and the umbilicus.

The kidneys can be sonographically identified as early as 11 weeks with endovaginal imaging and by 12 weeks with transabdominal imaging. Indeed, by the second-trimester fetal anatomy screening examination, the kidneys should be consistently seen adjacent to the fetal spine bilaterally (Fig. 29-2). The renal cortex, medulla, and sinus can be well differentiated within the fetus. The fetal bladder can be seen as early as 12 weeks and should always be seen by 15 weeks and beyond (Fig. 29-3). It is important to note that the fetal urinary bladder normally fills and empties once in every 30 to 45 minutes. Normal fetal ureters are not perceived with sonography. Therefore, visualization of the ureters would indicate some pathologic process. The adrenal

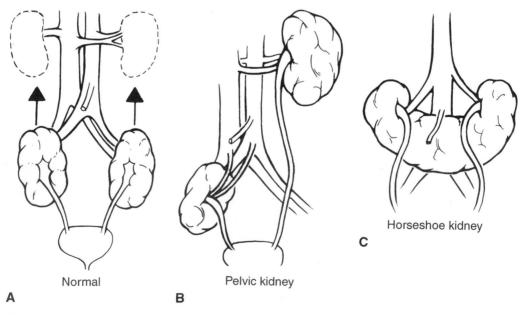

Normal   **A**   Pelvic kidney   **B**   Horseshoe kidney   **C**

Figure 29-1 Normal and abnormal ascension of the kidneys. **A.** The kidneys initially develop in the fetal pelvis and ascend into the upper quadrants. **B.** A kidney that fails to ascend results most often in a pelvic kidney. **C.** If the inferior poles of the kidneys fuse, this is termed a horseshoe kidney.

glands are triangular-shaped hypoechoic structures located superior to the upper pole of the kidneys. They are easily identified within the fetus (Fig. 29-4).

> ### 🔊 SOUND OFF
> The fetal urinary bladder normally fills and empties once in every 30 to 45 minutes.

VACTERL ASSOCIATION

VACTERL stands for **v**ertebral anomalies, **a**nal atresia, **c**ardiac anomalies, **t**racheoesophageal fistula or **e**sophageal atresia, **r**enal anomalies, and **l**imb anomalies (Fig. 29-5). Patients are considered to have this association if three of the organ systems listed have abnormalities. Therefore, if an irregularity is noted

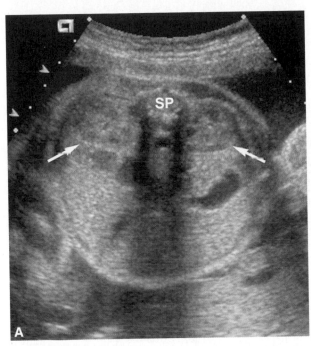

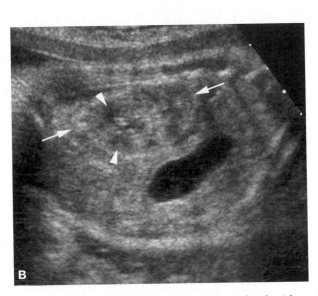

Figure 29-2 Fetal kidneys. **A.** Transverse view of the fetal abdomen revealing the kidneys (*arrows*) on both sides of the spine (*SP*). **B.** Longitudinal image of the fetal kidney (between *arrows*) revealing corticomedullary differentiation, with several identifiable medullary pyramids (*arrowheads*).

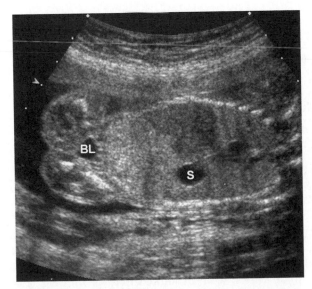

Figure 29-3 Fetal bladder. Longitudinal image of the fetal bladder (*BL*). The fetal stomach (*S*) is also noted in this image.

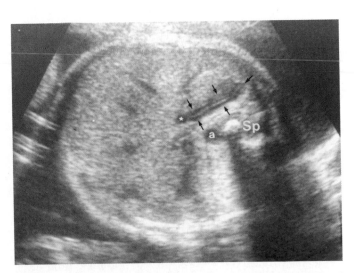

Figure 29-4 Fetal adrenal glands. Transverse view of the fetal abdomen revealing the normal sonographic appearance of the adrenal gland (*arrows*) adjacent to the fetal aorta (*a*) and spine (*Sp*).

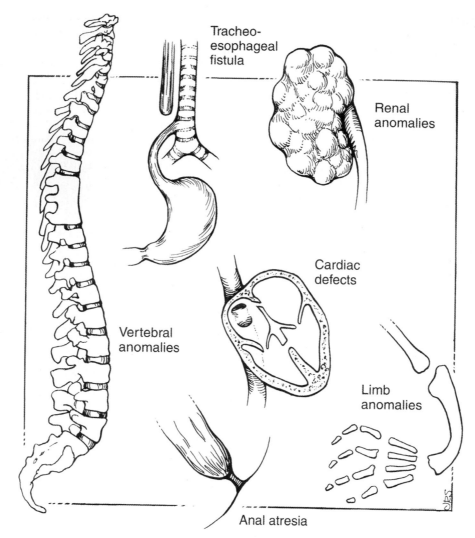

Figure 29-5 The VACTERL association: vertebral anomalies, anal atresia, cardiac defects, tracheoesophageal fistula or esophageal atresia, renal anomalies, and limb anomalies.

within one structure or system, this should prompt the sonographer to further investigate the other systems for associated anomalies. VACTERL association may also be referred to as VATER sequence, VATER, or VACTERL syndrome.

RENAL ABNORMALITIES, OLIGOHYDRAMNIOS, AND PULMONARY HYPOPLASIA

Renal abnormalities are the most frequent cause of **oligohydramnios**. During fetal development, around 9 weeks, the fetal kidneys begin to produce urine. Urine comprises the greater part of amniotic fluid after 14 weeks. Amniotic fluid is a substance that contains valuable proteins that are essential for normal fetal development. It also contributes greatly to normal fetal growth and maturation.

SOUND OFF
Renal abnormalities are the most frequent cause of oligohydramnios. Therefore, if oligohydramnios is discovered, a thorough analysis of the fetal urinary tract is warranted.

The fetus ingests amniotic fluid by swallowing. The fluid passes through the esophagus, into the stomach, and travels through the small bowel and into the colon, where normal absorption takes place. In circumstances in which the fetus has a renal abnormality, specifically those that are linked with bilateral **renal agenesis**, inadequately functioning kidneys, or obstruction of the urinary tract, oligohydramnios will be present, and, in some cases, **anhydramnios** may occur (Fig. 29-6). Therefore, if a normal amount of fluid is noted during a sonogram, one can assume that there is at least one functioning fetal kidney present.

The most worrisome consequence of oligohydramnios is **pulmonary hypoplasia**, or underdevelopment of the lungs. In the upcoming discussion on fetal renal disease, keep in mind that while unilateral conditions carry a better prognosis, bilateral disease often leads to oligohydramnios and is thus related to a poor outcome, in most cases, as a result of pulmonary hypoplasia.

> **SOUND OFF**
> The most worrisome consequence of oligohydramnios is pulmonary hypoplasia, or underdevelopment of the lungs.

Renal Agenesis

Failure of a kidney to form is referred to as renal agenesis. Renal agenesis can be unilateral or bilateral. There are two sonographic findings that are helpful in making the sonographic diagnosis of renal agenesis. First, when the kidney is absent in the abdomen, the adrenal gland can be noted in a parallel, flattened position, a sonographic finding known as the **"lying-down" adrenal sign** (Fig. 29-7). Second, color Doppler can be employed over the renal artery branches of the abdominal aorta. When there is absence of the kidney, there will be no identifiable renal artery branches (Fig. 29-8).

> **SOUND OFF**
> The "lying-down" adrenal sign is associated with renal agenesis.

Bilateral renal agenesis, which results in **Potter syndrome** or Potter sequence, is a fatal condition (Table 29-1; Fig. 29-9). Potter sequence is caused by any condition in which there is a significant lack of amniotic fluid around the fetus as it develops. Though bilateral renal agenesis can cause the typical Potter syndrome features, other conditions, such as an obstructive defect of the urinary tract or amnion rupture, can cause the same issues.

The absence of both the fetal kidneys can be difficult to detect sonographically, secondary to the lack of amniotic fluid surrounding the fetus. Therefore, it is extremely beneficial to utilize color Doppler to investigate the renal area. Nonvisualization of the urinary bladder and kidneys, with associated severe oligohydramnios, is considered to be a trustworthy finding consistent with bilateral renal agenesis. Bilateral renal agenesis may be seen in conjunction with **sirenomelia** and various cardiovascular malformations.

Fortunately, unilateral renal agenesis is much more common than bilateral renal agenesis. Most often, with unilateral renal agenesis, there is an average amount

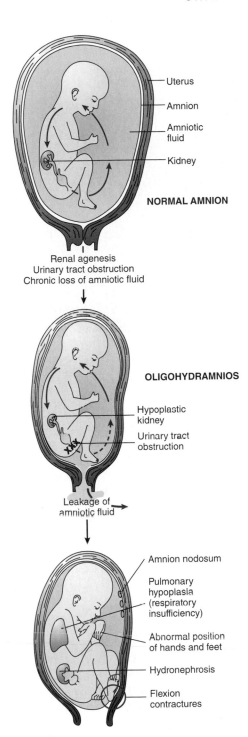

Figure 29-6 Normal amniotic fluid production and cycle. The kidneys produce urine, which comprises the majority of amniotic fluid. The fetus ingests amniotic fluid by swallowing. The fluid passes through the esophagus, into the stomach, and travels through the small bowel and into the colon, where normal absorption takes place. In circumstances in which the fetus has a renal abnormality, specifically those that are linked with bilateral renal agenesis, inadequately functioning kidneys, or obstruction of the urinary tract, oligohydramnios will be present, and in some cases, anhydramnios may occur. Oligohydramnios will also occur when there is leakage of amniotic fluid.

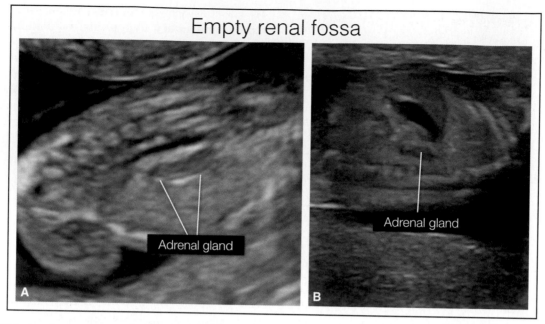

Empty renal fossa

A Adrenal gland

B Adrenal gland

Figure 29-7 Lying-down adrenal sign. Parasagittal plane of the fetal abdomen in two fetuses (**A** and **B**) with empty renal fossa, diagnosed at 12 weeks of gestation in both fetuses. Note the presence of the typical flat adrenal gland (labeled) in **A** and **B**.

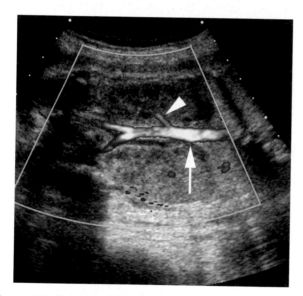

Figure 29-8 Unilateral renal agenesis. Coronal view of the abdomen with color Doppler demonstrates the left renal artery (*arrowhead*) arising from the aorta (*arrow*). No right renal artery is seen.

TABLE **29-1** Features of Potter syndrome or Potter sequence
Bilateral renal agenesis
Abnormal facial features (**Potter facies**)
Pulmonary hypoplasia (small chest)
Limb abnormalities (e.g., clubfeet)
Intrauterine growth restriction
Low-set ears
Oligohydramnios

of amniotic fluid, and the prognosis is good. Before making the conclusion of unilateral renal agenesis, the sonographer should always analyze the fetal pelvis for a pelvic kidney, because this is the most common location of an ectopic kidney. In the presence of unilateral renal agenesis, the contralateral kidney will enlarge, a condition known as **compensatory hypertrophy**.

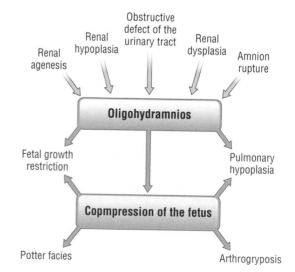

Figure 29-9 Potter sequence. Any abnormality that brings about oligohydramnios, especially severe, can start the sequence referred to as Potter sequence, which ultimately can result in fetal growth restriction, pulmonary hypoplasia, Potter facies, and limb abnormalities.

SONOGRAPHIC FINDINGS OF BILATERAL RENAL AGENESIS

1. Absent kidneys
2. Absent urinary bladder
3. Severe oligohydramnios or anhydramnios
4. Bilateral lying-down adrenal signs
5. Undetectable renal artery branches with color Doppler (bilateral)

SONOGRAPHIC FINDINGS OF UNILATERAL RENAL AGENESIS

1. Absent kidney
2. Compensatory hypertrophy of the contralateral kidney
3. Visible urinary bladder
4. Normal amniotic fluid volume
5. Unilateral lying-down adrenal sign
6. Undetectable renal artery branch with color Doppler (unilateral)

((•))) SOUND OFF
Most often, with unilateral renal agenesis, there is an average amount of amniotic fluid, and the prognosis is good.

Understanding the Nomenclature of Fetal Renal Cystic Disease

There are several distinct categories of fetal renal cystic disease that were formerly described by Potter: **autosomal recessive polycystic kidney disease** (ARPKD), **autosomal dominant polycystic kidney disease** (ADPKD), **multicystic dysplastic kidney** (MCDK) **disease**, and **obstructive cystic dysplasia**. In order for an **autosomal recessive** disease to be passed to the fetus, both parents must be carriers of the disease. Each offspring of parents, who are both carriers of an autosomal recessive disorder, has a 25% chance of being affected and a 50% chance of being a carrier.

In the case of an **autosomal dominant** disease, at least one of the parents has to be the carrier of the disease, and the gene must be dominant. That means, the dominant gene is capable of overriding the normal gene from the parent who is not a carrier. However, this does not indicate that every offspring will be affected. Each offspring of a parent who is a carrier of an autosomal dominant disease has a 50% chance of receiving the gene from their parents. It is important to note that dominant disorders tend to be less severe than recessive disorders (Fig. 29-10).

Autosomal Recessive (Infantile) Polycystic Kidney Disease

ARPKD may also be referred to as autosomal recessive polycystic renal disease or **infantile polycystic kidney disease**. The typical sonographic findings of a fetus affected by ARPKD are bilateral, enlarged, echogenic kidneys, nondetectable urinary bladder, and oligohydramnios (Fig. 29-11). The kidneys may be as large as 3 to 10 times the normal renal size for the gestation. ARPKD would be the most likely cause of enlarged, echogenic kidneys noted in utero.

((•))) SOUND OFF
ARPKD would be the most likely cause of enlarged, echogenic kidneys noted in utero.

One condition associated with ARPKD is **Meckel–Gruber syndrome**, which is a fatal disorder that includes renal cystic disease, occipital **encephalocele**, and **polydactyly** (Fig. 29-12). Fetuses with trisomy 13 and trisomy 18 may also have polycystic kidney disease. Referring to this condition, a renal cystic disease can be puzzling to a sonographer because cysts are not always perceptible with sonography. This is secondary to the size of the cysts because the cysts with ARPKD are often **microscopic** and not **macroscopic**. It is significant to appreciate the differences in the sonographic appearance of ARPKD and MCDK disease. Cysts are typically not identifiable in ARPKD but are evident with MCDK.

SONOGRAPHIC FINDINGS OF AUTOSOMAL RECESSIVE (INFANTILE) POLYCYSTIC KIDNEY DISEASE

1. Bilateral, enlarged echogenic kidneys
2. Absent urinary bladder
3. Oligohydramnios

Autosomal Dominant (Adult) Polycystic Kidney Disease

ADPKD may also be referred to as autosomal dominant polycystic renal disease. The sonographic appearance of fetal kidneys with ADPKD is similar to that of ARPKD in that both kidneys will appear enlarged and echogenic, although the kidneys may appear completely normal. If the kidneys do appear enlarged and echogenic, a distinguishing difference between the two diseases is that in the fetus with ADPKD, the urinary bladder is often present and there is a normal amniotic fluid volume, whereas with ARPKD, the bladder is absent and there is oligohydramnios. However, ADPKD does not typically manifest until approximately the fourth or fifth decade of life, at which time the adult will develop renal cysts and may die from end-stage renal failure. Adult renal cystic disease is also associated with the development of cysts within the liver, pancreas, and spleen.

SONOGRAPHIC FINDINGS OF AUTOSOMAL DOMINANT (ADULT) POLYCYSTIC KIDNEY DISEASE

1. Normal-appearing or bilateral, enlarged echogenic kidneys
2. Visible urinary bladder
3. Normal amniotic fluid volume
4. Cysts often do not manifest until approximately the fifth decade of life

🔊 SOUND OFF
The sonographic appearance of fetal kidneys with ADPKD is similar to that of ARPKD in that both kidneys will appear enlarged and echogenic, although the kidneys may appear completely normal.

Multicystic Dysplastic Renal Disease

Multicystic dysplastic renal disease may also be referred to as multicystic dysplastic kidney (MCDK) disease and multicystic renal dysplasia. MCDK disease is thought to be caused by an early, first-trimester obstruction of the ureter. The sonographic findings of MCDK disease are the identification of unilateral or bilateral multiple, smooth-walled, noncommunicating cysts of varying sizes in the area of the **renal fossa(e)** (Fig. 29-13). There is typically no normal functioning renal tissue present in the kidney affected by MCDK disease. Therefore, MCDK disease is fatal if bilateral, with the consistent associated findings of oligohydramnios and absent bladder. Fortunately, most cases of MCDK disease are unilateral and consequently have a normal amniotic fluid volume. Fetuses with MCDK disease can also have additional related anomalies, such as abnormalities of the gastrointestinal tract and central nervous system, limb anomalies, and further renal abnormalities.

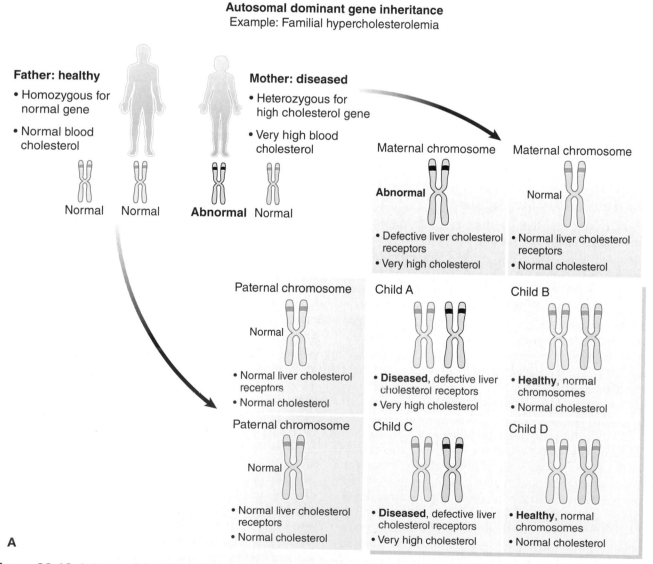

Figure 29-10 Autosomal dominant versus autosomal recessive. **A.** Autosomal dominant inheritance. The dominant gene is present in one affected, unhealthy (diseased) parent. Half of the children will be affected.

The Fetal Genitourinary System

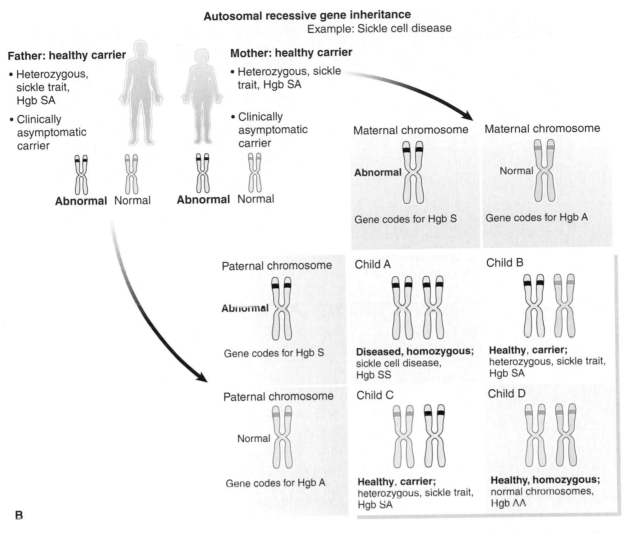

Autosomal recessive gene inheritance
Example: Sickle cell disease

Father: healthy carrier
- Heterozygous, sickle trait, Hgb SA
- Clinically asymptomatic carrier

Abnormal   Normal

Mother: healthy carrier
- Heterozygous, sickle trait, Hgb SA
- Clinically asymptomatic carrier

Abnormal   Normal

Maternal chromosome

Abnormal

Gene codes for Hgb S

Maternal chromosome

Normal

Gene codes for Hgb A

Paternal chromosome

Abnormal

Gene codes for Hgb S

Child A

Diseased, homozygous; sickle cell disease, Hgb SS

Child B

Healthy, carrier; heterozygous, sickle trait, Hgb SA

Paternal chromosome

Normal

Gene codes for Hgb A

Child C

Healthy, carrier; heterozygous, sickle trait, Hgb SA

Child D

Healthy, homozygous; normal chromosomes, Hgb AA

B

Figure 29-10 (continued) **B.** Autosomal recessive inheritance. A recessive gene is present in each healthy, carrier parent. Half of the children will be healthy but carry the gene defect (*Hgb SA*, sickle cell trait); one-fourth will be genetically and clinically normal (*Hgb AA*); and one-fourth will have sickle cell disease (*Hgb SS*).

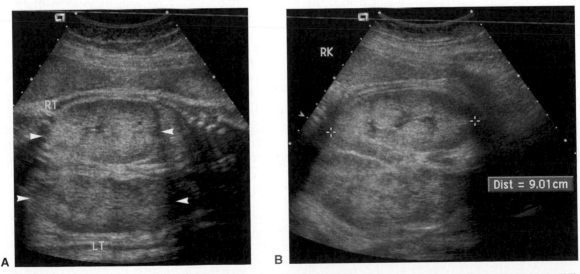

Figure 29-11 Autosomal recessive polycystic kidney disease in the third trimester. **A.** The right (*RT*) and left (*LT*) kidneys (*arrowheads*) are enlarged and have increased echogenicity at 33 weeks. **B.** The right kidney (*RK*) is visualized better and shows signs of increased echogenicity. It is enlarged and measures approximately 9 cm in length (*calipers*). There is also severe oligohydramnios.

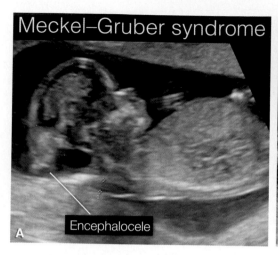

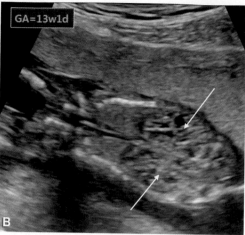

Figure 29-12 Midsagittal plane (**A**) and coronal plane (**B**) of a fetus with Meckel–Gruber syndrome at 13 weeks of gestation. Note in **A** the presence of an occipital encephalocele and in **B** the presence of bilateral polycystic kidneys (*arrows*).

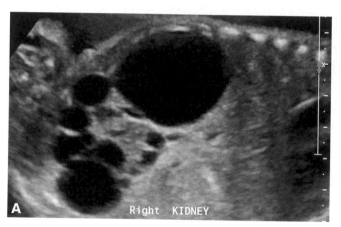

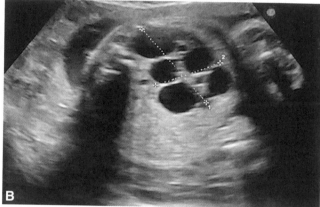

Figure 29-13 Multicystic dysplastic kidney disease. **A.** Multiple cysts of varying sizes are noted within the fetal renal fossa. **B.** Transverse view of a unilateral multicystic dysplastic kidney (between *calipers*).

🔊 SOUND OFF
MCDK disease is fatal if bilateral, but fortunately, most cases of MCDK are unilateral.

SONOGRAPHIC FINDINGS OF BILATERAL MULTICYSTIC DYSPLASTIC RENAL DISEASE

1. Bilateral, smooth-walled, noncommunicating cysts of varying sizes located within the renal fossae
2. Absent urinary bladder
3. Oligohydramnios

SONOGRAPHIC FINDINGS OF UNILATERAL MULTICYSTIC DYSPLASTIC RENAL DISEASE

1. Unilateral, smooth-walled, noncommunicating cysts of varying sizes located within the renal fossae
2. Compensatory hypertrophy of the contralateral kidney
3. Visible urinary bladder
4. Normal amniotic fluid volume

Obstructive Cystic Dysplasia

Obstructive cystic dysplasia, like MCDK disease, is caused by an early renal obstruction. It can be unilateral or bilateral. A **ureterocele**, or a severe bladder outlet obstruction, early in gestation, can lead to bilateral obstructive cystic dysplasia, in which case oligohydramnios will be present. Unilateral obstructive cystic dysplasia is most often caused by a **pelviureteral junction** or **vesicoureteral junction obstruction**. Bilateral cystic dysplasia may be associated with urethral atresia or **posterior urethral valves**. The kidney will appear small and echogenic and have cysts located along its margins. Often, there will be evidence of **hydronephrosis** and a thick-walled urinary bladder.

SONOGRAPHIC FINDINGS OF BILATERAL OBSTRUCTIVE CYSTIC DYSPLASIA

1. Small, echogenic kidneys
2. Peripheral renal cysts
3. Bilateral hydronephrosis
4. Thick-walled urinary bladder
5. Oligohydramnios

Fetal Urinary Tract Obstruction

An obstruction of the fetal urinary tract can lead to distension of the urethra, bladder, ureters, and renal collecting system, depending upon the level of obstruction. Although physiologically fundamental, it is quite imperative for the sonographer to understand the creation and flow of urine through the urinary tract in order to determine the origin of a urinary tract obstruction. Urine is produced by the kidney; exits the kidney by means of the **renal pelvis**; travels down the ureter, into the bladder; and exits the body via the urethra. Any obstruction to this normal succession will result in a backup of urine. For example, if there is an obstruction at the region where the ureter meets the bladder, the **ureterovesical junction (UVJ)**, then those structures that are positioned proximal to the obstruction will be dilated. That means, the entire ureter, the renal pelvis, and the renal calices will be eventually dilated and filled with urine. Conversely, if the obstruction level lies at the point at which the renal pelvis meets the ureter, the **ureteropelvic junction** (UPJ), then the ipsilateral renal pelvis and **renal calices** will be dilated, whereas the ureter and bladder will most likely remain normal, provided that contralateral urine flow is not obstructed in any way (Fig. 29-14).

SOUND OFF
The sonographer must understand the creation and flow of urine through the urinary tract in order to determine the origin of a urinary tract obstruction.

Hydronephrosis is the most common fetal abnormality noted during an obstetric sonogram. Hydronephrosis, or **pelvocaliectasis**, may be described as **pelviectasis** (pyelectasis) or **caliectasis**, depending on which part of the collecting system is dilated. Enlargement of the bladder is called **megacystis**, whereas dilation of the ureter may be referred to as **megaureter** or **hydroureter**.

Fetal pelviectasis, or dilation of the renal pelvis, can be established and measured with sonography by taking a **renal pelvic diameter** (Fig. 29-15). The measurement of the renal pelvis is made in the anteroposterior plane and should not exceed 7 mm before 20 weeks' or 10 mm after 20 weeks' gestation. However, it is important to note that borderline hydronephrosis should be reported because of the possible gradual evolution of this disorder and because of possible chromosomal associations (Table 29-2).

The UPJ, the UVJ, and the urethra are the three most common areas where obstruction occurs. The following sections discuss these causes of fetal hydronephrosis in more detail. It is also important to note that less common causes of hydronephrosis in the fetus include ureterocele, ectopic ureter, **vesicoureteral reflux**, and **urethral atresia**.

Ureteropelvic Junction Obstruction

Ureteropelvic junction obstruction, or UPJ obstruction, is the most common cause of hydronephrosis in the neonate and the most common form of fetal renal obstruction. The UPJ is located at the junction of the renal pelvis and the ureter. The cause of this abnormality

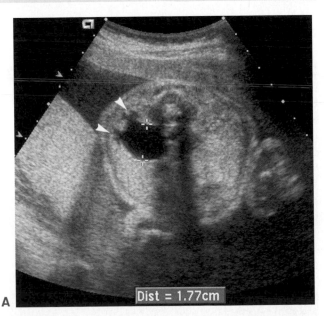

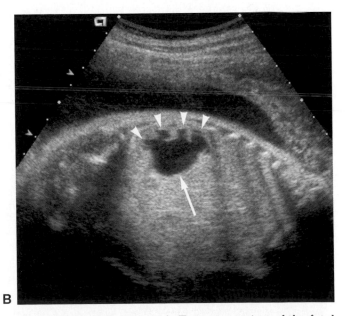

Figure 29-14 Unilateral hydronephrosis caused by a ureteropelvic junction obstruction. **A.** Transverse view of the fetal abdomen demonstrating dilation of the right renal pelvis (*calipers*), measuring 17.7 mm in the anteroposterior diameter, as well as dilation of the calices (*arrowheads*). **B.** Longitudinal view of the abdomen better demonstrating the extent of the dilation, because the calices (*arrowheads*) are clearly visible.

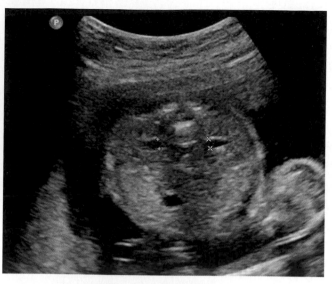

Figure 29-15 Transverse fetal kidneys showing normal anechoic renal pelvis perpendicular to the ultrasound beam. The calipers show proper placement for measurement of the anteroposterior renal pelvic diameter.

TABLE 29-2 Renal pelvis diameter measurements indicative of fetal hydronephrosis

Gestational Weeks	Renal Pelvis Diameter Measurement
20 weeks	≥7 mm (borderline between 4 and 6 mm)
After 20 weeks	≥10 mm (borderline between 5 and 9 mm)

may be due to irregular development of the smooth muscle in the area of the UPJ. Some authors suspect ureteral stenosis or kinks, adhesions, crossing vessels, or abnormal outlet shapes. The disease is usually unilateral and more common in males. The sonographic appearance of a UPJ obstruction is the dilation of the renal pelvis and renal calices (see Fig. 29-14). It is important to note that fetal pyelectasis can be a sonographic marker for Down syndrome.

SONOGRAPHIC FINDINGS OF URETEROPELVIC JUNCTION OBSTRUCTION

1. Hydronephrosis (dilated renal pelvis and calices)
2. Normal ureters (nonvisualization)
3. Normal bladder

◄)) SOUND OFF
It is important to note that fetal pyelectasis can be a sonographic marker for Down syndrome.

Bladder Outlet Obstructions and Posterior Urethral Valves

A bladder outlet obstruction describes the condition in which there is a blockage of the flow of urine out of the urinary bladder. It is especially significant to determine the sex of the fetus once a renal obstruction is identified. For example, posterior urethral valves are a common cause of bladder outlet obstructions in male fetuses. These thin membranes of tissue located within the posterior urethra do not allow urine to exit the urethra. The **"keyhole" sign** is seen when there is dilation of the urinary bladder and the posterior urethra (Fig. 29-16). Posterior urethral valves result in dilation of the bladder, ureters, and renal collecting system. Oligohydramnios and bladder wall thickening will be observed as well.

SONOGRAPHIC FINDINGS OF POSTERIOR URETHRAL VALVES

1. "Keyhole" sign (dilated bladder and urethra)
2. Bilateral hydroureter
3. Bilateral hydronephrosis
4. Oligohydramnios
5. Thickened bladder wall

◄)) SOUND OFF
The "keyhole" sign is seen when there is dilation of the urinary bladder and posterior urethra.

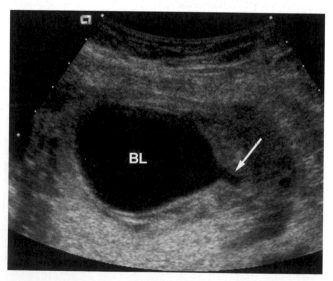

Figure 29-16 The "keyhole" sign. A dilated posterior urethra (*arrow*) and bladder (*BL*) demonstrating the "keyhole" sign in a fetus with posterior urethral valves.

Prune Belly Syndrome

Prune belly syndrome is typically caused by megacystis, a massively dilated urinary bladder. This syndrome is seen mostly in male fetuses and is the result of a urethral abnormality, which, in turn, leads to a bladder outlet obstruction. Prune belly describes the result of the abdominal wall musculature being stretched by the extremely enlarged urinary bladder. The sonographic finding of the "keyhole" sign is also seen with prune belly syndrome. Dilatation of the ureters and the renal collecting systems will occur (Fig. 29-17). The triad of absent abdominal musculature, **undescended testis**, and urinary tract abnormalities is consistent with the diagnosis of prune belly syndrome.

SONOGRAPHIC FINDINGS OF PRUNE BELLY SYNDROME

1. Dilated bladder and, possibly, urethra ("keyhole" sign)
2. Absent abdominal musculature
3. Undescended testis
4. Urinary tract abnormalities (megacystis and hydronephrosis)

🔊))) **SOUND OFF**
The triad of absent abdominal musculature, undescended testis, and urinary tract abnormalities is consistent with the diagnosis of prune belly syndrome.

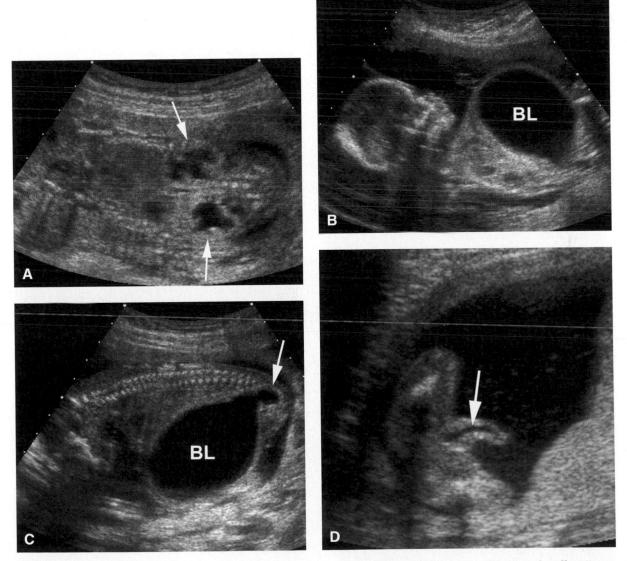

Figure 29-17 Prune belly syndrome. **A.** Bilateral obstruction to the kidneys is noted with dilated collecting systems (*arrows*). **B.** Markedly enlarged urinary bladder (*BL*). **C.** The "keyhole" sign is noted as a dilated bladder (*BL*) and a dilated urethra (*arrow*). **D.** A dilated urethra (*arrow*) is noted as well.

Ureterovesical Junction Obstruction

Ureterovesical junction obstruction, or UVJ obstruction, is the least common cause of hydronephrosis in the fetus. The renal collecting system and ureter will be dilated with a UVJ obstruction. Whereas unilateral UVJ obstructions lead to normal amounts of amniotic fluid, bilateral obstructions lead to oligohydramnios.

> #### SONOGRAPHIC FINDINGS OF URETEROVESICAL JUNCTION OBSTRUCTION
>
> 1. Hydronephrosis
> 2. Dilated ureter
> 3. Normal bladder
> 4. Normal amniotic fluid (if unilateral)

Bladder Exstrophy and Cloacal Exstrophy

Bladder exstrophy is an anomaly wherein the bladder is located outside of the fetal pelvis. After an extended amount of investigation, nonvisualization of the bladder in the presence of a normal amniotic fluid volume and normal kidneys should warrant a search for bladder exstrophy. The sonographic finding of bladder exstrophy is that of a lower abdominal wall mass inferior to the umbilicus (Fig. 29-18).

The **cloaca** is the embryonic structure that develops into the rectum and urogenital sinus. The cloaca can be persistent and result in the combination of the urinary, genitals, and intestinal tract, emptying into a common orifice located on the **perineum**. With **cloacal exstrophy**, also referred to **OEIS complex**, there is an omphalocele, bladder exstrophy, imperforate anus, and spina bifida.

> #### SONOGRAPHIC FINDINGS OF BLADDER EXSTROPHY
>
> 1. Lower abdominal wall mass inferior to the umbilicus
> 2. Absent urinary bladder
> 3. Normal kidneys

> **SOUND OFF**
> OEIS complex stands for omphalocele, bladder exstrophy, imperforate anus, and spina bifida.

Mesoblastic Nephroma

The most common solid fetal renal mass is the **mesoblastic nephroma**, which is essentially a hamartoma of the kidney. This tumor will typically appear as a solid, homogeneous mass within the renal fossa and may completely replace the kidney. However, it may contain cystic components.

> #### SONOGRAPHIC FINDINGS OF THE MESOBLASTIC NEPHROMA
>
> 1. Solid, homogeneous mass within the renal fossa and may completely replace the kidney.

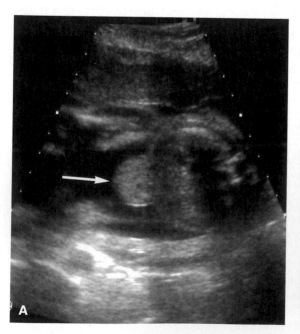
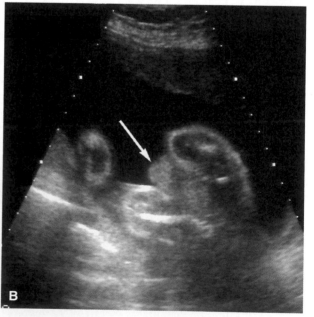

Figure 29-18 Bladder exstrophy. **A** and **B.** A solid, homogeneous mass (*arrow*) is noted in these transverse images just inferior to the umbilicus and extending down to the perineum with no visible bladder seen.

🔊)) **SOUND OFF**
The most common solid fetal renal mass is the mesoblastic nephroma.

SONOGRAPHY OF THE FETAL GENITALIA

The sex of the embryo depends upon the male gamete. The sperm carries either an X or a Y chromosome, whereas the ovary always contributes an X chromosome. An X chromosome from the sperm will yield XX, which is female offspring. The combination of a Y chromosome will yield XY, which is a male offspring. The external genitalia can be visualized and differentiated in the second trimester. Determining the sex of the fetus can offer important diagnostic information. When a urinary tract obstruction is noted, the sonographer should determine the sex of the fetus, because there may be different causes of obstructions specific for each sex. For example, posterior urethral valves are a common cause of urinary obstruction in only the male fetus. Sonography can thus be used to visualize the labia of the female and the penis and scrotum in the male.

ABNORMALITIES OF THE FETAL GENITALIA

Ambiguous genitalia is a birth defect in which the sex of the fetus cannot be determined. Findings of abnormal external genitalia in the male are **micropenis**, **hypospadias**, hypospadias with **chordee**, **epispadias**, and undescended testicles. Fetal **hydroceles** are common findings in utero and may become fairly large (Fig. 29-19). Hypospadias is the abnormal ventral curvature of the penis as a result of a shortened urethra that exits on the ventral penile shaft.

The most common female finding is **clitoromegaly**. Fetal ovarian cysts may be noted in the fetal pelvis, secondary to maternal hormone stimulation (Fig. 29-20). These cysts are most often benign and resolve spontaneously, although if they continue to grow, they can lead to hemorrhage and, possibly, ovarian torsion.

FETAL ADRENAL GLAND ABNORMALITIES

The most common malignant abdominal mass in neonates is the **neuroblastoma**, located primarily within the adrenal gland. Adrenal glands may also spontaneously hemorrhage within the fetus, resembling a mass. Follow-up sonograms are often ordered for an adrenal hemorrhage to determine the level of resolution.

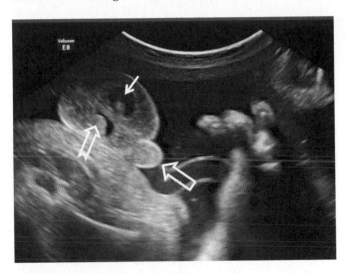

Figure 29-19 A coronal/oblique view of external male genitalia in mid-third trimester. *Notched arrow*, testis; *open arrow*, penis; *solid arrow*, small hydrocele.

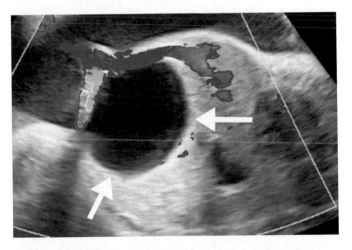

Figure 29-20 Simple ovarian cyst at 32 weeks' gestation. Care must be taken to differentiate an ovarian cyst from the urinary bladder.

REVIEW QUESTIONS

1. The arrowheads in Figure 29-21 indicate the fetal kidney. The ureter and urinary bladder were normal. What is the most likely diagnosis?
   a. UVJ obstruction
   b. UPJ obstruction
   c. Upper pole moiety obstruction
   d. Cystic dysplasia

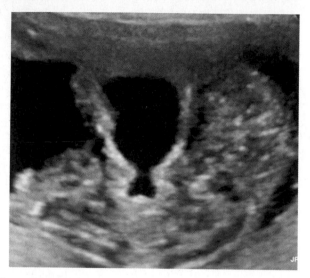

Figure 29-22

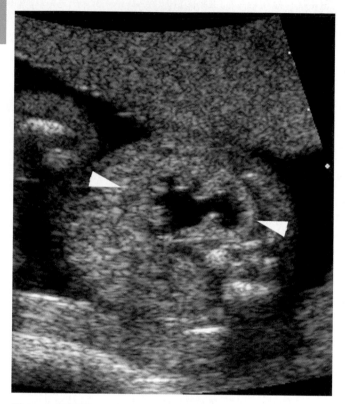

Figure 29-21

2. Figure 29-22 represents what finding of the fetal bladder?
   a. Undescended testicles
   b. Bilateral ureteral obstruction
   c. Keyhole sign
   d. Potter syndrome

3. The findings in Figure 29-23 are consistent with what diagnosis?
   a. ARPKD
   b. Autosomal recessive multicystic kidney disease
   c. Multicystic kidney disease
   d. Autosomal renal cystic dysplasia

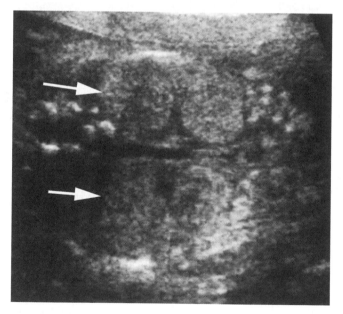

Figure 29-23

4. The fetus in Figure 29-24 had a normal left kidney and a normal amniotic fluid level. What is the most likely diagnosis for this coronal image?
   a. ARPKD
   b. ADPKD
   c. Cystic dysplasia
   d. MCDK

5. What does the asterisk in Figure 29-25 indicate?
   a. Cystitis
   b. Ureterocele
   c. Megacystis
   d. Hydrobladder

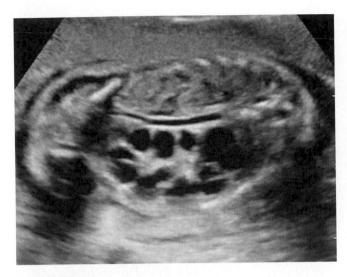

Figure 29-24

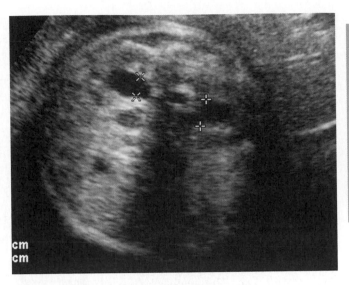

Figure 29-26

6. What does the arrow in Figure 29-25 indicate?
   a. Proximal ureter
   b. Distal ureter
   c. Urethra
   d. Posterior urethral valves

9. What does the arrow indicate within the fetal bladder in Figure 29-27?
   a. Ovarian cyst
   b. Ureterocele
   c. Dilated urethra
   d. Prune belly syndrome

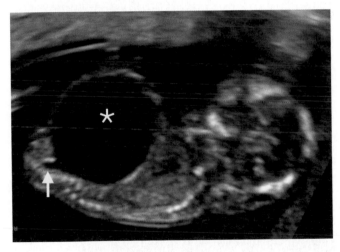

Figure 29-25

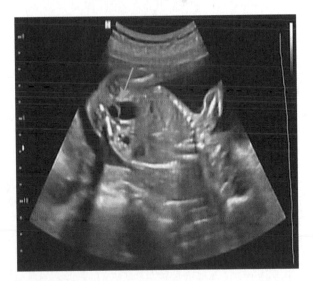

Figure 29-27

7. What abnormality can be noted in Figure 29-26?
   a. Bilateral hydroureter
   b. Bilateral pelviectasis
   c. Unilateral renal agenesis
   d. Bilateral renal cysts

8. Which of the following are being measured in Figure 29-26?
   a. Renal pyramids
   b. Renal arteries
   c. Renal cysts
   d. Renal pelvises

10. What syndrome is indicated by the sonographic findings in Figure 29-28?
    a. Meckel–Gruber syndrome
    b. Prune belly syndrome
    c. OEIS complex
    d. Potter syndrome

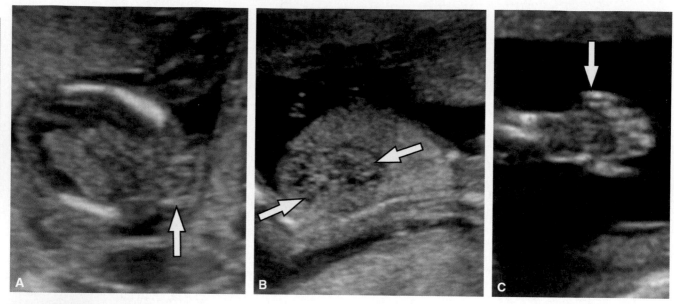

Figure 29-28

11. The fetal urinary bladder fills and empties approximately every:
    a. 10 minutes.
    b. 15 minutes.
    c. 30 minutes.
    d. 60 minutes.

12. What do the arrows indicate in Figure 29-29 at the level of the left kidney?
    a. Renal hypoplasia
    b. Lying-down adrenal sign
    c. Renal dysplasia
    d. ADPKD

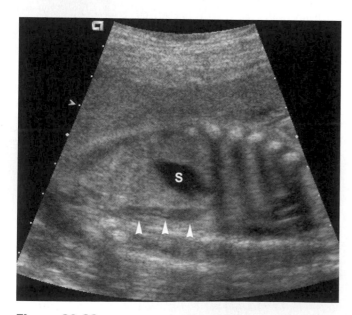

Figure 29-29

13. What is evident in Figure 29-30?
    a. ADPKD
    b. ARPKD
    c. Unilateral renal agenesis
    d. Potter disease

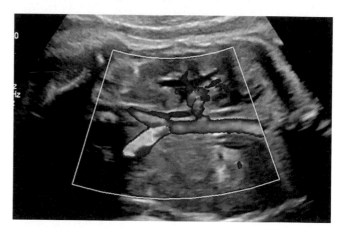

Figure 29-30

14. What is the canal connecting the fetal bladder with the allantois?
    a. Cloaca
    b. Moiety
    c. Urachus
    d. Perineum

15. Which of the following is associated with sirenomelia?
    a. ADPKD
    b. Bilateral renal agenesis
    c. Infantile polycystic disease
    d. MCDK

16. What measurement should the renal pelvis not exceed after 20 weeks' gestation?
    a. 2 mm
    b. 10 mm
    c. 7 mm
    d. 1.2 cm

17. What does the asterisk in Figure 29-31 indicate?
    a. Varicocele
    b. Hypospadias
    c. Hydrocele
    d. Inguinal hernia

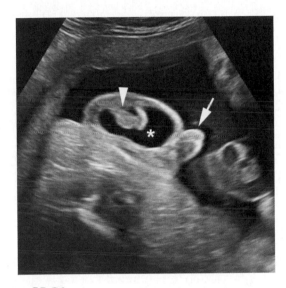

Figure 29-31

18. Which of the following is considered a sonographic marker for Down syndrome?
    a. Megacystis
    b. Urethral atresia
    c. Ureterocele
    d. Pyelectasis

19. Which of the following is not part of Potter syndrome?
    a. Abnormal facial features
    b. Horseshoe kidneys
    c. Pulmonary hypoplasia
    d. Bilateral renal agenesis

20. What is a common cause of a bladder outlet obstruction in the male fetus?
    a. Posterior urethral valves
    b. Hydronephrosis
    c. Urethral atresia
    d. Vesicoureteral reflux

21. During an 18-week sonogram, multiple cysts of varying sizes are noted within the renal fossa of a male fetus. The other kidney appears to be normal. Which of the following would be an associated finding?
    a. Megacystis
    b. Ovarian dysgenesis
    c. Hypospadias
    d. Normal amniotic fluid level

22. The most common malignant adrenal pediatric tumor is the:
    a. nephroblastoma.
    b. pheochromocytoma.
    c. hepatoblastoma.
    d. neuroblastoma.

23. The "keyhole" sign would be seen in all of the following situations except:
    a. urethral atresia.
    b. prune belly syndrome.
    c. autosomal dominant polycystic renal disease.
    d. posterior urethral valves.

24. What is the most common fetal abnormality noted during an obstetric sonogram?
    a. Anencephaly
    b. Spina bifida
    c. Cleft lip
    d. Hydronephrosis

25. The "lying-down" adrenal sign would be seen in all of the following situations except:
    a. unilateral renal agenesis.
    b. bilateral renal agenesis.
    c. Potter syndrome.
    d. pyelectasis.

26. The birth defect in which the sex of the fetus cannot be determined defines:
    a. renal agenesis.
    b. ovarian dysgenesis.
    c. clitoromegaly.
    d. ambiguous genitalia.

27. What measurement should the renal pelvis not exceed before 20 weeks' gestation?
    a. 2 mm
    b. 10 mm
    c. 7 mm
    d. cm

28. Cloacal exstrophy is associated with all of the following except:
    a. omphalocele.
    b. spina bifida.
    c. encephalocele.
    d. imperforate anus.

29. The renal cystic disease that results in the development of cysts late in adulthood is:
    a. multicystic dysplastic renal disease.
    b. autosomal dominant polycystic disease.
    c. autosomal recessive polycystic disease.
    d. obstructive cystic dysplasia.

30. What is the most common cause of hydronephrosis in the neonate and the most common form of fetal renal obstruction?
    a. UVJ obstruction
    b. UPJ obstruction
    c. Vesicoureteral reflux
    d. Urethral atresia

31. Bladder exstrophy describes:
    a. absence of the cloaca.
    b. protrusion of the bladder into the umbilicus.
    c. external position of the bladder.
    d. enlargement of the bladder.

32. Which of the following would result in compensatory hypertrophy?
    a. Unilateral renal agenesis
    b. Bilateral renal agenesis
    c. Pelvic kidney
    d. Horseshoe kidneys

33. Which of the following would cause a bladder outlet obstruction?
    a. Posterior urethral valves
    b. Fetal ovarian cyst
    c. Pelviectasis
    d. Pelvocaliectasis

34. Which of the following is associated with enlarged echogenic kidneys and microscopic renal cysts?
    a. MCDK disease
    b. Obstructive cystic dysplasia
    c. Hydronephrotic syndrome
    d. ARPKD

35. The "lying-down" adrenal sign describes the sonographic findings of:
    a. enlarged bladder and urethra.
    b. renal agenesis.
    c. MCDK disease.
    d. posterior urethral valves.

36. The "I" in OEIS complex stands for:
    a. imperforate anus.
    b. ileal dysfunction.
    c. irregular bladder enlargement.
    d. iniencephaly.

37. Another name for pelvocaliectasis is:
    a. caliectasis.
    b. hydrocele.
    c. hydronephrosis.
    d. pyonephrosis.

38. Which of the following best describes hypospadias?
    a. OEIS complex in the presence of a hydrocele
    b. The chronic obstruction of the renal pelvis and urethra
    c. The underdevelopment of the scrotum in the presence of a hydrocele
    d. An abnormal ventral curvature of the penis

39. The "keyhole" sign describes the sonographic findings of a(n):
    a. enlarged bladder and dilated urethra.
    b. bilateral renal agenesis.
    c. unilateral renal agenesis.
    d. dilation of the renal pelvis and proximal ureter.

40. What is the term for enlargement of the urinary bladder?
    a. Posterior urethral valves
    b. Urethral atresia
    c. Prune belly syndrome
    d. Megacystis

41. Numerous noncommunicating anechoic masses are noted within the left renal fossa of a fetus at 20 weeks' gestation. What is the most likely etiology of these masses?
    a. ARPKD
    b. ADPKD
    c. MCDK
    d. Hydronephrosis

42. Fluid surrounding the fetal testicle is referred to as:
    a. hydroureter.
    b. hydronephrosis.
    c. hydrocele.
    d. hydroscrotum.

43. Fusion of the lower poles of the kidneys describes:
    a. renal agenesis.
    b. horseshoe kidneys.
    c. moiety.
    d. Meckel–Gruber syndrome.

44. The syndrome associated with an occipital encephalocele, cystic renal disease, and polydactyly is:
    a. Meckel–Gruber syndrome.
    b. Potter syndrome.
    c. VACTERL association.
    d. sirenomelia syndrome.

45. Which of the following is not a component of prune belly syndrome?
    a. Megacystis
    b. Undescended testis
    c. Dilated urinary bladder and urethra
    d. Abdominal muscle hypertrophy

46. OEIS complex is also referred to as:
    a. bladder exstrophy.
    b. omphalocele.
    c. Potter syndrome.
    d. cloacal exstrophy.

47. Obstruction at the level of the UPJ would lead to dilation of the:
    a. renal pelvis and bladder.
    b. bladder and ureter.
    c. ureter and renal pelvis.
    d. renal pelvis and calices.

48. The most common location of an ectopic kidney is within the:
    a. lower abdomen.
    b. pelvis.
    c. chest.
    d. contralateral quadrant.

49. Pyelectasis refers to:
    a. enlargement of the urinary bladder, ureter, and renal calices.
    b. dilation of the ureter.
    c. dilation of the renal pelvis.
    d. enlargement of the ureter only.

50. Prune belly syndrome is caused by:
    a. an enlarged bladder.
    b. unilateral renal agenesis.
    c. bilateral renal agenesis.
    d. hypospadias.

51. All of the following would be associated with oligohydramnios except:
    a. bilateral MCDK disease.
    b. unilateral renal agenesis.
    c. bilateral renal agenesis.
    d. ARPKD.

52. What is the most common fetal renal tumor?
    a. Neuroblastoma
    b. Nephroblastoma
    c. Mesoblastic nephroma
    d. Wilms tumor

53. The type of renal cystic disease associated with adult liver and pancreatic cysts is:
    a. MCDK.
    b. ARPKD.
    c. ADPKD.
    d. VATER.

54. Having more than the normal number of digits is:
    a. polydactyly.
    b. clinodactyly.
    c. multidigitopia.
    d. sirenomelia.

55. Cryptorchidism describes:
    a. bilateral pelvic kidneys.
    b. urethral atresia.
    c. undescended testicles.
    d. ovarian dysgenesis.

56. An obstruction at the UVJ would lead to dilation of the:
    a. bladder and urethra.
    b. bladder, urethra, and ureters.
    c. bladder, urethra, ureters, and renal collecting system.
    d. ureter and renal collecting system.

57. Before 9 weeks, the fetal kidneys are located within the:
    a. renal fossae.
    b. pelvis.
    c. chest.
    d. umbilical cord.

58. Which of the following is the most common renal anomaly?
    a. Horseshoe kidneys
    b. Pelvic kidneys
    c. Renal agenesis
    d. Duplex collecting system

59. Failure of the kidneys to form is called:
    a. hydronephrosis.
    b. renal dysplasia.
    c. renal agenesis.
    d. renal ectopia.

60. Which of the following would be the most likely cause of bilateral, enlarged echogenic fetal kidneys and oligohydramnios?
    a. ARPKD
    b. MCDK
    c. Renal cystic dysplasia
    d. ADPKD

SUGGESTED READINGS

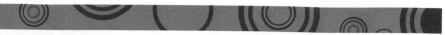

Curry RA, Prince M. *Sonography: Introduction to Normal Structure and Function.* 4th ed. Elsevier; 2020:385–430.

Doubilet PM, Benson CB. *Atlas of Ultrasound in Obstetrics and Gynecology: A Multimedia Reference.* 2nd ed. Wolters Kluwer; 2012:182–211.

Gibbs RS et al. *Danforth's Obstetrics and Gynecology.* 10th ed. Wolters Kluwer; 2008:137–151.

Hagen-Ansert SL. *Textbook of Diagnostic Sonography.* 7th ed. Elsevier; 2012:604–628.

Haller J. *Textbook of Neonatal Ultrasound.* Parthenon; 1998:117–128.

Kline-Fath BM, Bulas DI, and Lee W. *Fundamental and Advanced Fetal Imaging: Ultrasound and MRI.* 2nd ed. Wolters Kluwer; 2021:800–853.

Norton ME, Scoutt LM, Feldstein VA. *Callen's Ultrasonography in Obstetrics and Gynecology.* 6th ed. Elsevier; 2017:503–538.

Nyberg D, McGaham J, Pretorius D, et al. *Diagnostic Imaging of Fetal Anomalies.* Lippincott Williams & Wilkins; 2003:630–660.

Rumack CM, Wilson S, William Charboneau J, et al. *Diagnostic Ultrasound.* 4th ed. Elsevier; 2011:1353–1388.

Siegel MJ. *Pediatric Sonography.* 5th ed. Wolters Kluwer; 2019:346–512.

BONUS REVIEW!

Fetal Bladder Drainage (Fig. 29-32)

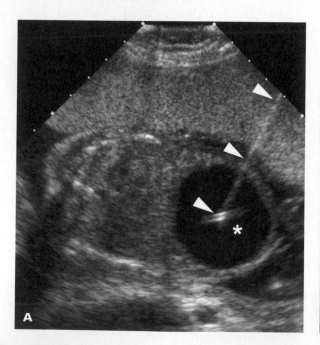
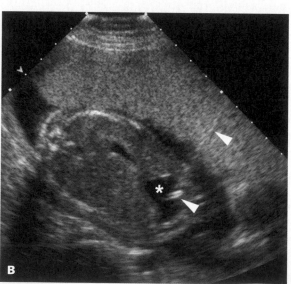

Figure 29-32 Fetal bladder drainage. **A.** A needle (*arrowheads*) has been guided with sonography into a distended fetal bladder (*asterisk*). **B.** After urine has been withdrawn through the needle (*arrowheads*), the bladder (*asterisk*) is considerably smaller.

BONUS REVIEW! (*continued*)

The Urachus (Fig. 29-33)

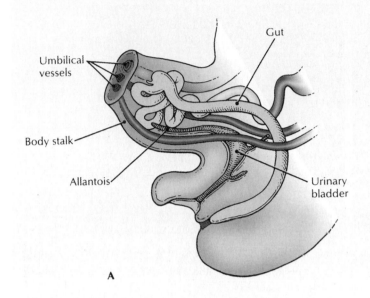

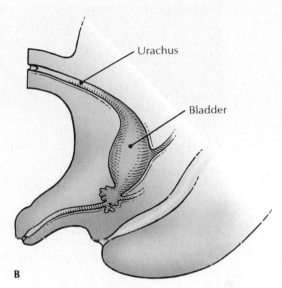

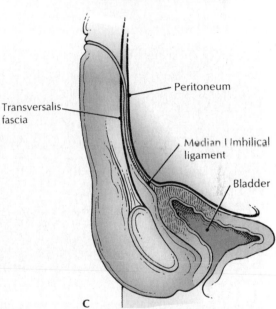

Figure 29-33 The urachus. **A.** At 9 weeks of gestational age showing the allantois extending into the body stalk. **B.** At 3 months' gestation, the urachus connects to the dome of the bladder. **C.** The urachus persisting as the median umbilical ligament in the adult.

(*continued*)

BONUS REVIEW! (*continued*)

OEIS Complex (Fig. 29-34)

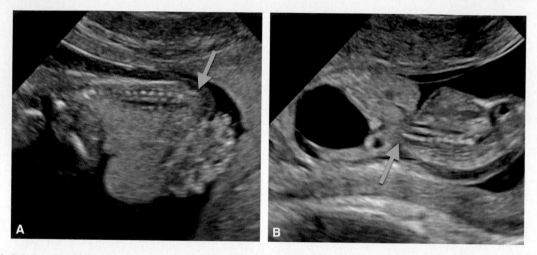

Figure 29-34 Two-dimensional sonogram of two fetuses (11 weeks in **A** and 12 weeks in **B**) with an interrupted spine (*arrow*), abdominal wall defect, and absent bladder and kidneys representing an OEIS complex. OEIS complex include an omphalocele, exstrophy of the bladder, imperforate anus, and spinal defects.

Doppler and Three-Dimensional Image of the Fetal Renal Vasculature (Fig. 29-35)

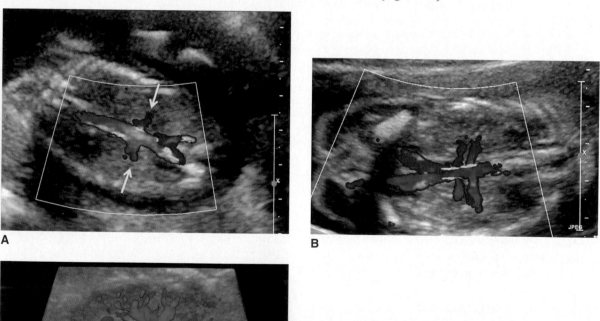

Figure 29-35 Doppler and three-dimensional (*3D*) image of the renal vasculature. **A.** Coronal view of the kidneys, using color Doppler to show the renal arteries (*arrows*) arising from the aorta, just above the iliac arteries. **B.** Coronal image of a fetus with two renal arteries bilaterally. **C.** 3D volume data set of the fetal vasculature (aorta, inferior vena cava [*IVC*], right renal artery [*RRA*], and right renal vein [*RRV*]) demonstrated using a transparency render method to allow all vessels to be displayed simultaneously.

Chromosomal Abnormalities

Introduction

This chapter offers a brief analysis of frequently encountered chromosomal abnormalities and a discussion on the difference between chromosomal abnormalities, anomalies, syndromes, and malformations. An overview of the application of the maternal serum screen, fetal sampling, and fetal karyotyping is also provided. In "Bonus Review" section, sonographic images of facial and cardiac defects in trisomy 21 and more sonographic markers of trisomy 18 are provided.

Key Terms

advanced maternal age—a maternal age of 35 years or older

agenesis of the corpus callosum—the congenital absence of corpus callosum that may be partial or complete

alpha-Fetoprotein—a protein produced by the fetal yolk sac, fetal gastrointestinal tract, and the fetal liver; may also be produced by some malignant tumors

amniocentesis—a surgical procedure in which amniotic fluid is extracted for genetic testing or removed when there is an accumulation of an excessive amount of fluid around the fetus

amnionitis—inflammation of the amniotic sac secondary to infection

aneuploidy—a condition of having an abnormal number of chromosomes

anomaly—a structural feature that differs from the norm

ascites—excessive fluid in the peritoneal cavity

brachycephaly—round skull shape

cell-free DNA—prenatal serum test used to examine fetal cells circulating within the maternal blood; can predict gender and discover evidence of some chromosomal abnormalities

chorionic villi—fingerlike projections of gestational tissue that attach to the decidualized endometrium and allow transfer of nutrients from the mother to the fetus

chorionic villi sampling—prenatal test used that obtains placental tissue for chromosomal analysis

choroid plexus cysts—cysts located within the lateral ventricles of the brain, specifically in the choroid plexus

chromosomal abnormality—an error in either the number or structure of chromosomes

chromosomes—the cellular structures that contain genes

cleft lip—an abnormal division in the lip

cleft palate—the abnormal development of the soft and/or hard palate of the mouth where there is a division in the palate

clinodactyly—the bending of the fifth finger toward the fourth finger

clubfeet—a malformation of the bones of the feet in which the feet are inverted and rotated medially, and the metatarsals lie in the same plane as the tibia and fibula; singular is clubfoot

coarctation of the aorta—the narrowing of the aortic arch

cordocentesis—prenatal test that obtains fetal blood for chromosomal analysis

cyclopia—fusion of the orbits

Dandy–Walker malformation—congenital brain malformation in which there is enlargement of the cisterna magna, agenesis of the cerebellar vermis, and dilation of the fourth ventricle

diaphragmatic hernia—the herniation of the abdominal contents into the chest cavity through a defect in the diaphragm

Down syndrome—see key term trisomy 21

duodenal atresia—congenital maldevelopment or absence of duodenum

Edwards syndrome—see key term trisomy 18

esophageal atresia—congenital absence of part of the esophagus

estriol—an estrogenic hormone produced by the placenta

facies—the features or appearance of the face

fetal karyotyping—an analysis of fetal chromosomes; reveals the morphology and number of chromosomes

gynecomastia—the benign enlargement of the male breast; typically located posterior to the areola

holoprosencephaly—a group of brain abnormalities consisting of varying degrees of fusion of the lateral ventricles, absence of the midline structures, and associated facial anomalies

horseshoe kidneys—the attachment of the lower poles of the kidneys by a band of renal tissue that crosses the midline of the abdomen

human chorionic gonadotropin—hormone produced by the trophoblastic cells of the early placenta; may also be used as a tumor marker in nongravid patients and males

hydrocephalus—the increased volume of cerebrospinal fluid within the ventricular system

hydronephrosis—the dilation of the renal collecting system resulting from the obstruction of the flow of urine from the kidney(s) to the bladder; also referred to as pelvocaliectasis or pelvicaliectasis

hypoplastic—incomplete or arrested development of a structure

hypoplastic left heart—incomplete development of the left ventricle, resulting in a small or absent left ventricle

hypotelorism—reduced distance between the orbits

intrauterine growth restriction—a fetus that is below the 10th percentile for gestational age (small for gestational age) and whose growth is impeded for some reason

macroglossia—enlargement of the tongue

malformation—a structural abnormality that results from an abnormal development

microcephaly—small head

micrognathia—a small mandible and recessed chin

microphthalmia—small eye or eyes

molar pregnancy—also referred to as gestational trophoblastic disease; is associated with an abnormal proliferation of the trophoblastic cells, enlargement of the placenta, and elevated levels of human chorionic gonadotropin

morphology—the form and structure of an organism

monosomy X—see key term Turner syndrome

nonimmune hydrops—fetal hydrops caused by congenital fetal anomalies and infections

nuchal—the posterior part or nape of the neck

nuchal cystic hygroma—a mass found in the neck that is the result of an abnormal accumulation of lymphatic fluid within the soft tissue

nuchal fold—a collection of solid tissue at the back of the fetal neck

nuchal translucency—the anechoic space along the posterior aspect of the fetal neck

omphalocele—an anterior abdominal wall defect where there is herniation of the fetal bowel and other abdominal organs into the base of the umbilical cord

ovarian dysgenesis—imperfect or abnormal development of the ovaries

Patau syndrome—chromosomal aberration in which there is a third chromosome 13; also referred to as trisomy 13

percutaneous umbilical cord sampling—see key term cordocentesis

pericardial effusion—fluid accumulation around the heart in the pericardial cavity

pleural effusion—the abnormal accumulation of fluid in the pleural space

polydactyly—having more than the normal number of fingers or toes

pregnancy-associated plasma protein A—a protein that is produced by the placenta and that can be monitored during pregnancy

pyelectasis—enlargement of the renal pelvis; also referred to as pelviectasis

renal agenesis—failure of the kidney to develop; may be unilateral or bilateral

rocker-bottom feet—abnormal curved shape of the sole of the feet

sandal gap—a large space between the first and second toes

spina bifida—a birth defect in which there is incomplete closure of the spine

spontaneous abortion—the loss of a pregnancy before 20 gestational weeks

subcutaneous edema—a buildup of fluid under the skin

syndactyly—webbed fingers or toes

syndrome—a group of clinically observable findings that exist together and allow for classification

theca lutein cysts—functional ovarian cysts that are found in the presence of elevated levels of human chorionic gonadotropin; also referred to as a theca luteal cysts

triple screen—a maternal blood test that typically includes an analysis of human chorionic gonadotropin, alpha-fetoprotein, and estriol

trisomy—a cell having three copies of an individual chromosome

trisomy 13—chromosomal aberration in which there is a third chromosome 13; also referred to as Patau syndrome; often associated with holoprosencephaly

trisomy 18—chromosomal aberration in which there is a third chromosome 18; also referred to as Edwards syndrome

trisomy 21—chromosomal aberration in which there is a third chromosome 21; also referred to as Down syndrome

trophoblastic cells—the cells that surround the gestation that produce human chorionic gonadotropin

Turner syndrome—a chromosomal aberration where one sex chromosome is absent; may also be referred to as monosomy X

ventriculomegaly—buildup of cerebrospinal fluid that results in an enlargement of one or more of the ventricles within the brain

TABLE 30-1 Often encountered genetic terms and their definitions

Terms Related to Genetics	Definition
Aneuploid	A cell that has an abnormal number of whole chromosomes. The diploid number of 46 chromosomes is altered. There may be too many or too few.
Diploid	A cell having the normal pair of each chromosome. There are 46 chromosomes in this situation. Normal cells are diploid, with the exception of the gametes.
Haploid	A cell having only one member of each pair of chromosomes.
Monosomy	A cell having only one of an individual chromosome.
Mosaic	A situation in which some cells have an abnormal number of chromosomes whereas others do not.
Triploid	A cell having three times the normal haploid number. There are 69 chromosomes.
Trisomy	A cell having three copies of an individual chromosome.

SOUND OFF

Edwards syndrome is an example of a specific type of aneuploid in which there is an additional copy of the chromosome 18. This type of aneuploid is specifically referred to as a trisomy and thus is referred to as trisomy 18.

CHROMOSOMAL ABNORMALITIES, ANOMALIES, SYNDROMES, AND MALFORMATIONS

Chromosomes are the structures, located in each cell in our body, that hold our genes. A **chromosomal abnormality** exists as an error in either the number or structure of chromosomes. The normal cell has 46 chromosomes or two pairs of 23. **Aneuploidy** is a condition in which there are an abnormal number of whole chromosomes. Specifically, an aneuploid has too many or too few chromosomes. **Edwards syndrome** is an example of a specific type of aneuploid in which there is an additional copy of the chromosome 18. This type of aneuploid is specifically referred to as a **trisomy** and thus is referred to as **trisomy 18**. Thus, trisomy 21 or Down syndrome has a third chromosome 21. **Turner syndrome**, also referred to as **monosomy X**, is a different type of chromosomal abnormality in which the fetus has only one sex chromosome. Consequently, this is why it is referred to as a monosomy. Some common genetic terms that you may encounter as you study are listed in Table 30-1.

Structural abnormalities of an individual chromosome may also exist. These can result in deletions, duplications, translocations, and other abnormal configurations. Environmental factors and maternal age have been suspected to increase the likelihood of chromosomal abnormalities.

An **anomaly** is a structural feature that differs from the norm. An example of an anomaly is **agenesis of the corpus callosum** in which there is congenital absence of an important midline brain structure. A **syndrome** is a group of clinically observable findings that exist together and allow for classification. These signs and symptoms are linked to each other in some way. Chromosomal abnormalities often exist when there are multiple defects. For example, **Down syndrome** has clinically identifiable signs such as a flat facial profile and a transverse crease in the palm of the hand. An example of symptoms of Down syndrome would be developmental delays and hearing loss.

A **malformation** is a structural abnormality that results from unusual development. For instance, **Dandy–Walker malformation** is a congenital brain malformation that is thought to be caused by a developmental deviation in the roof of the fourth ventricle.

> ((**SOUND OFF**
> A syndrome is a group of clinically observable findings that exist together and allow for classification.

NONINVASIVE PRENATAL TESTING

As discussed in Chapter 22, the **triple screen** is a maternal blood test that can be helpful in the second trimester for detecting unusual levels of certain proteins or hormones with chromosomal abnormalities. The three laboratory values that typically comprise the triple screen are maternal serum **alpha-fetoprotein** (MSAFP), **estriol**, and **human chorionic gonadotropin** (hCG). AFP is produced in the yolk sac and fetal liver. Estriol and hCG are produced by the placenta. The triple screen has a 60% detection rate for Down syndrome. However, the most common cause of abnormal serum screening tests is incorrect dating of the pregnancy. Atypical first-trimester laboratory findings often lead to follow-up sonographic examinations to date the pregnancy. Two supplementary proteins that can also be monitored are the **pregnancy-associated plasma protein A** (PAPP-A) and the dimeric inhibin A. Both of these proteins are produced by the placenta as well. One of the newer maternal blood test available is **cell-free DNA** testing. This simple blood test can reveal gender and is also highly accurate in detecting chromosomal anomalies, including trisomies 21, 18, and 13 and sex chromosome abnormalities, as early as 9 weeks' gestation. As this chapter progresses, laboratory findings of chromosomal abnormalities are also provided.

> ((**SOUND OFF**
> The three laboratory values that typically comprise the triple screen are MSAFP, estriol, and hCG.

FETAL KARYOTYPING AND GENETIC TESTING

Advanced maternal age is considered to be 35 years or older. Patients with advanced maternal age have

a higher risk of having an abnormal pregnancy or pregnancy failure. **Fetal karyotyping** is an analysis of fetal chromosomes and is frequently recommended for women who are considered to be of advanced maternal age, or when the maternal or paternal history suggests the possibility of fetal abnormalities. Karyotyping is extremely valuable for detecting specific chromosomal abnormalities and the **morphology** of those chromosomes. During pregnancy, a sample of maternal blood, amniotic fluid, or tissue from the placenta can be used for fetal karyotyping. There are three main procedures used to obtain material for fetal karyotyping: (i) **chorionic villi sampling** (CVS), (ii) **amniocentesis**, and (iii) **cordocentesis**.

> ((**SOUND OFF**
> Advanced maternal age is considered to be 35 years or older.

CVS is typically the earliest procedure that can be performed during a pregnancy for fetal karyotyping. With CVS, a small amount of **chorionic villi** is obtained for chromosomal testing. CVS can be performed transabdominally or transvaginally (transcervical) between 10 and 13 gestational weeks. Under sonographic guidance, a needle or plastic catheter is placed into the placental mass for the aspiration of **trophoblastic cells** (Figs. 30-1 and 30-2). Some research links a possible association between CVS performed less than 10 weeks and fetal limb abnormalities.

Amniocentesis is typically used for genetic purposes between 15 and 20 weeks. Some facilities may offer this procedure to patients as early as 10 weeks, although some studies suggest that it should not be done before 15 weeks because of an increase in fetal complications. An amniocentesis is performed transabdominally with sonographic guidance (Fig. 30-3). The physician inserts a 20 to 22G needle through the abdomen and into the amniotic sac to remove amniotic fluid for testing. The most common side effects of this procedure are uterine contractions and cramping. Rarely, patients experience vaginal spotting, amniotic fluid leakage, or **amnionitis**. The fetal loss rate due to miscarriage is between 2% and 3% above the typical loss rate during the sampling weeks. Although some labs produce quicker results, it may take as many as 3 weeks for a complete analysis of the fluid. An amniocentesis may also be performed to assess the fetal lungs for maturity by obtaining fluid and testing the lecithin-to-sphingomyelin ratio (L/S ratio). Also, a therapeutic amniocentesis can be performed to remove excess amniotic fluid or to distend the amniotic cavity with more fluid when scant fluid is noted around the fetus.

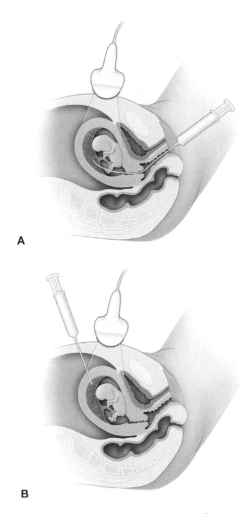

A

B

Figure 30-1 Chorionic villi sampling. Because the villi arise from trophoblast cells, their chromosome structure is the same as the fetus.

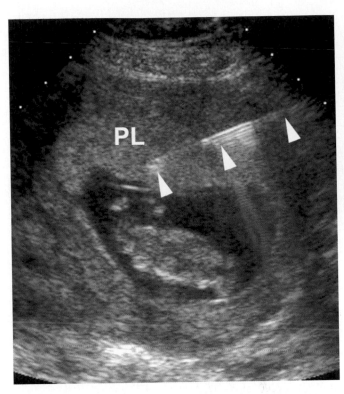

Figure 30-2 Transabdominal chorionic villi sampling. Sonogram of a needle (*arrowheads*) being placed within the placenta (*PL*) during a chorionic villi sampling procedure.

SOUND OFF
Amniocentesis is used for genetic purposes between 15 and 20 weeks.

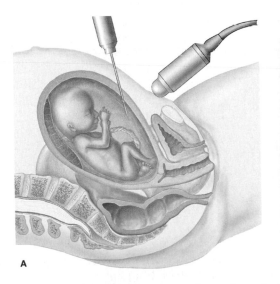

A

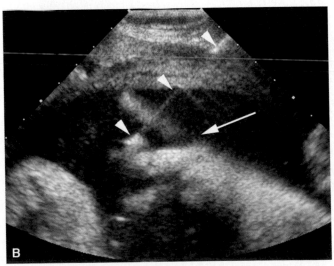

B

Figure 30-3 Amniocentesis. **A.** A genetic amniocentesis is usually performed at around 15 to 20 weeks, obtaining amniotic fluid, which contains fetal cells. Insertion of the amniocentesis needle is under direct sonographic guidance. **B.** Continuous sonographic monitoring of fetal movement during amniocentesis is important. Note that a fetal hand (*arrow*) is in proximity to the needle (*arrowheads*) during amniocentesis.

Cordocentesis, also referred to as **percutaneous umbilical cord sampling** (PUBS) or fetal blood sampling, is performed transabdominally after 17 weeks. A needle is placed through the maternal abdomen and into the umbilical vein. The segment of the cord that is most often accessed is at the cord insertion point into the placenta (Fig. 30-4). A sample of fetal blood is removed. PUBS has been associated with fetal bradycardia and hemorrhage at the sampling site. It also carries a higher fetal loss rate compared to amniocentesis. PUBS allows for rapid detection of chromosomal anomalies, because it requires only 48 to 72 hours for analysis.

> ### 🔊 SOUND OFF
> For PUBS, a needle is placed through the maternal abdomen and into the umbilical vein. The segment of the cord that is most often accessed is at the cord insertion point into the placenta.

COMMON CHROMOSOMAL ABNORMALITIES

Down Syndrome (Trisomy 21)

Down syndrome, or **trisomy 21**, is the most common chromosomal abnormality. It occurs in 1 in 500 to 800 pregnancies. Fetuses with trisomy 21 have an extra chromosome 21. Various sonographic features of Down

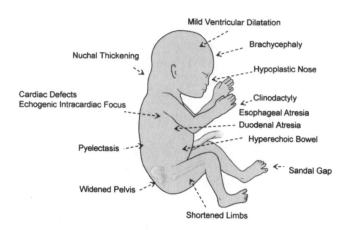

Figure 30-5 Common features of trisomy 21.

syndrome include **duodenal atresia**, thickened **nuchal translucency** in the first trimester or increased **nuchal fold** thickness in the second trimester, **pyelectasis**, and absent or hypoplastic nasal bones (Fig. 30-5). Maternal serum screening outcomes yield evidence of elevated hCG and inhibin A levels, whereas all other laboratory values are reduced.

MATERNAL SERUM SCREENING RESULTS OF DOWN SYNDROME
1. Low MSAFP
2. Low estriol
3. High hCG
4. High inhibin A
5. Low PAPP-A

SONOGRAPHIC FINDINGS OF DOWN SYNDROME
1. Absent nasal bones (**hypoplastic** nose)
2. **Brachycephaly**
3. **Clinodactyly** (Fig. 30-6)
4. Duodenal atresia (Fig. 30-7)
5. Mild **ventriculomegaly** (see Fig. 30-7)
6. Echogenic intracardiac focus
7. Hyperechoic (echogenic) bowel
8. **Macroglossia** (Fig. 30-8)
9. **Nonimmune hydrops**
10. Nuchal thickening 6 mm or larger between 15 and 21 weeks (Fig. 30-9)
11. Thickened nuchal translucency
12. **Pericardial effusion**
13. Pyelectasis
14. **Sandal gap**
15. Shortened limbs (humerus and femur)
16. Ventricular septal defects (VSDs)
17. Widened pelvic angles

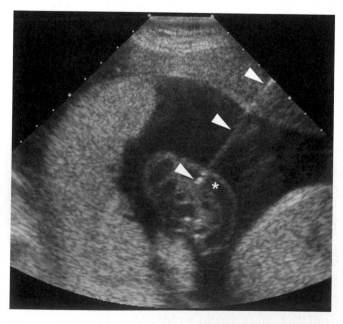

Figure 30-4 Percutaneous umbilical blood sampling. Percutaneous umbilical blood sampling from a free loop of cord. A needle (*arrowheads*) traverses the amniotic cavity and ends in a free loop of the umbilical cord (*asterisk*).

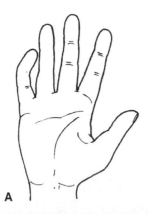

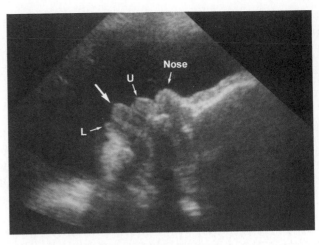

Figure 30-8 Macroglossia. Sagittal image of a fetus with macroglossia revealing the nose, upper lip (*U*), enlarged tongue (*arrow*), and lower lip (*L*).

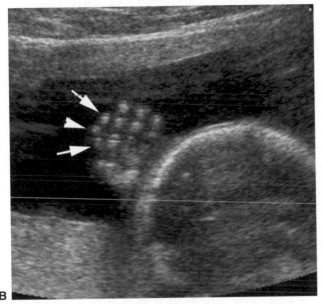

Figure 30-6 Clinodactyly of the fifth digit. **A.** Drawing of clinodactyly. **B.** Sonographic image of the open hand revealing the inward curvature of the fifth digit (*arrows*) caused by a malformed middle phalanx (*arrowhead*).

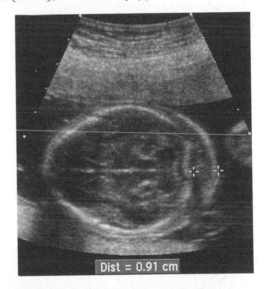

Figure 30-9 Abnormal nuchal fold. Image demonstrating a thickened nuchal fold (between *calipers*) measuring 9.1 mm.

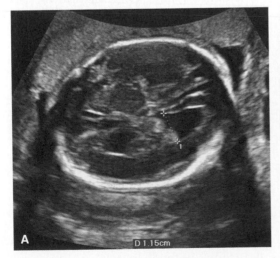

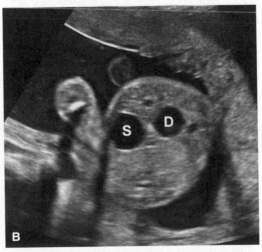

Figure 30-7 Duodenal atresia and ventriculomegaly in a fetus with trisomy 21. **A.** Axial image of fetal head showing dilated lateral ventricle (*calipers*) measuring 1.15 cm. **B.** Axial image of upper abdomen showing two dilated cystic structures, representing the dilated stomach (*S*) and dilated duodenal bulb (*D*), characteristic of duodenal atresia.

🔊 **SOUND OFF**
Down syndrome, or trisomy 21, is the most common chromosomal abnormality.

Edwards Syndrome (Trisomy 18)

Edwards syndrome is the second most common chromosomal abnormality. The majority of fetuses diagnosed with Edwards syndrome, or trisomy 18, die either before birth or shortly after birth. Fetuses with trisomy 18 have an extra chromosome 18. Various sonographic features of Edwards syndrome include a strawberry-shaped skull, **choroid plexus cysts**, **micrognathia**, **rocker-bottom feet**, **omphalocele**, clenched fists, and single umbilical artery (Fig. 30-10). All laboratory values are decreased with Edwards syndrome.

🔊 **SOUND OFF**
The word part *omphalo* means umbilical region.

MATERNAL SERUM SCREENING RESULTS OF EDWARDS SYNDROME

1. Low AFP
2. Low estriol
3. Low hCG
4. Low inhibin A
5. Low PAPP-A

SONOGRAPHIC FINDINGS OF EDWARDS SYNDROME

1. Strawberry-shaped skull (Fig. 30-11)
2. Agenesis of the corpus callosum
3. Choroid plexus cyst (Fig. 30-12)
4. Hypoplastic cerebellum
5. Enlarged cisterna magna
6. **Hydrocephalus**
7. Micrognathia (Fig. 30-13)
8. Small, low-set ears
9. **Esophageal atresia**
10. **Spina bifida**
11. Clenched hands, overlapping index finger, fixed wrists (see Fig. 30-11)
12. Cardiac defects (including VSD and tetralogy of Fallot)
13. Omphalocele
14. Nonimmune hydrops
15. **Diaphragmatic hernia**
16. Renal anomalies
17. Single umbilical artery (Fig. 30-14)
18. Feet abnormalities (rocker-bottom feet, **clubfeet**) (Fig. 30-15)

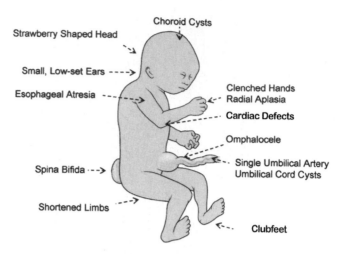

Figure 30-10 Common features of trisomy 18.

🔊 **SOUND OFF**
Edwards syndrome includes a strawberry-shaped skull, choroid plexus cysts, micrognathia, rocker-bottom feet, omphalocele, clenched fists, and single umbilical.

Patau Syndrome (Trisomy 13)

Holoprosencephaly and abnormal **facies** are common findings with **Patau syndrome** or **trisomy 13**. The fetus with Patau syndrome has an extra chromosome 13. Unfortunately, this is almost a uniformly fatal condition, as the newborn typically dies in the neonatal period. Various sonographic features of Patau syndrome include central nervous system aberrations, **cyclopia**, facial clefting, heart defects, and **polydactyly** (Fig. 30-16). Maternal serum screening is not always beneficial in the diagnosis of this condition.

MATERNAL SERUM SCREENING RESULTS OF PATAU SYNDROME

1. Not always beneficial and depends upon the anomaly present (cell-free DNA is helpful)

SONOGRAPHIC FINDINGS OF PATAU SYNDROME

1. **Microcephaly**
2. Polydactyly (Fig. 30-17)
3. Holoprosencephaly (Fig. 30-18)
4. Ventriculomegaly
5. Hydrocephalus
6. Agenesis of the corpus callosum
7. Small, low-set ears
8. Facial anomalies (cyclopia, **cleft lip**, **cleft palate**, **microphthalmia**, **hypotelorism**)
9. Cardiac defects (**hypoplastic left heart** and echogenic intracardiac focus)
10. Omphalocele

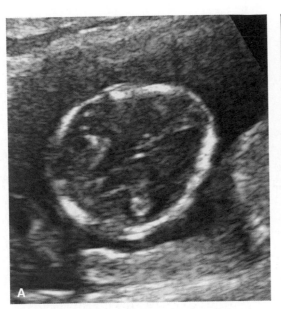

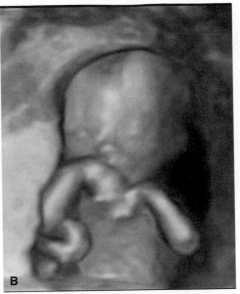

Figure 30-11 Strawberry-shaped skull (**A**) and three-dimensional image of bilateral clinched hands (**B**) in a fetus with trisomy 18.

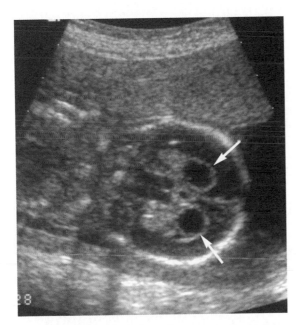

Figure 30-12 Bilateral choroid plexus cysts in a fetus with trisomy 18. Choroid plexus cysts (*arrows*) are identified in both lateral ventricles of this fetus with trisomy 18.

11. Nonimmune hydrops
12. Renal anomalies (**hydronephrosis**, echogenic enlarged kidneys)
13. Single umbilical artery
14. Clubfeet

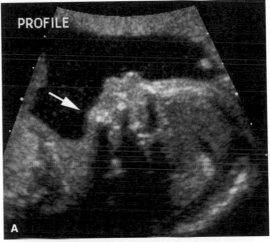

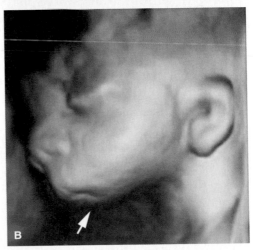

Figure 30-13 Micrognathia. **A.** Sagittal profile of face demonstrating very small mandible and chin (*arrow*). **B.** Three-dimensional image of another fetus with severe hypoplasia of the mandible and chin (*arrow*). Notice the low-set ear as well.

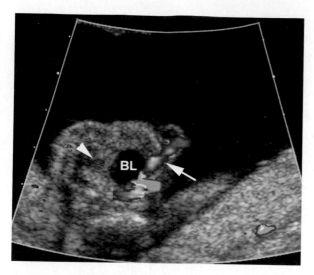

Figure 30-14 Single umbilical artery in pelvis. Color Doppler transverse image of pelvis demonstrating a single umbilical artery (*arrow*) adjacent to one side of the bladder (*BL*). On the contralateral side, no umbilical artery is seen arising from the iliac artery (*arrowhead*).

> **◄)) SOUND OFF**
> Holoprosencephaly and abnormal facies are common findings with Patau syndrome or trisomy 13.

Triploidy

Triploidy is a chromosomal abnormality in which the fetus has 69 chromosomes instead of the normal 46. Specifically, the fetus has three sets of chromosomes instead of the normal two. Because there are multiple major structural anomalies associated with triploidy, most of the fetuses with triploidy die in the first trimester or early second trimester. There are two types of triploidy (type I and type II). Often, a partial **molar pregnancy** is found with a triploid fetus, thus resulting in a markedly elevated hCG level and bilateral ovarian **theca lutein cysts**. Sonographic features of triploidy include small, low-set ears, cardiac defects, **syndactyly**, and **intrauterine growth restriction** (Fig. 30-19).

MATERNAL SERUM SCREENING RESULTS OF TRIPLOIDY

1. Elevated hCG in the presence of a molar pregnancy

FIRST-TRIMESTER SONOGRAPHIC FINDINGS OF TRIPLOIDY

1. Cystic spaces seen within an enlarged placenta (molar pregnancy)
2. Fetal demise
3. Bilateral ovarian theca lutein cysts

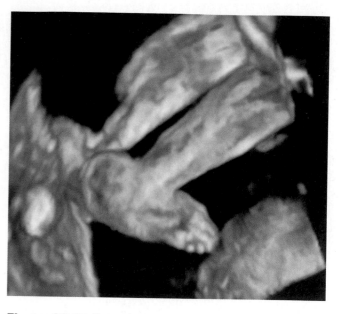

Figure 30-15 Foot abnormalities for Edwards syndrome include rocker-bottom foot, as seen at 23-weeks on this three-dimensional sonogram.

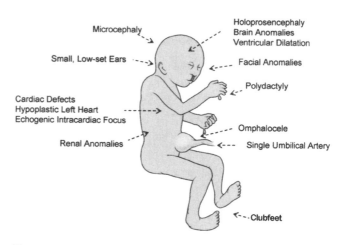

Figure 30-16 Common features of trisomy 13.

SECOND- AND THIRD-TRIMESTER SONOGRAPHIC FINDINGS OF TRIPLOIDY

1. Holoprosencephaly
2. Dandy–Walker malformation
3. Agenesis of the corpus callosum
4. Hydrocephalus
5. Facial abnormalities (microphthalmia and micrognathia)
6. Small, low-set ears
7. Cardiac defects
8. Renal anomalies
9. Intrauterine growth restriction (small abdomen)
10. Omphalocele
11. Syndactyly (third and fourth fingers)
12. Single umbilical artery
13. Clubfeet

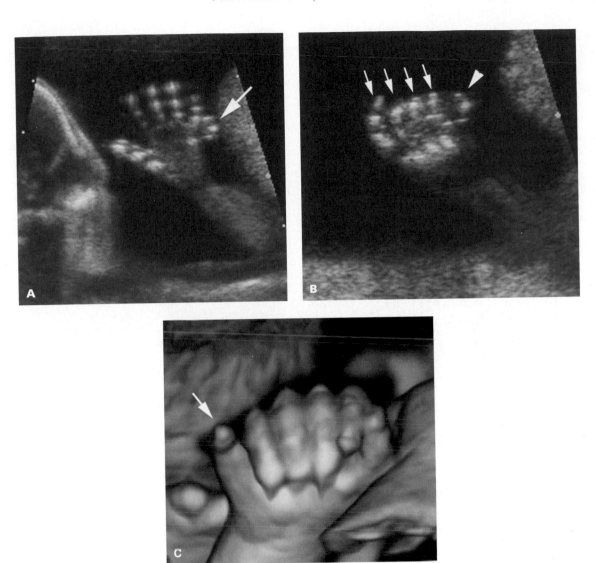

Figure 30-17 Polydactyly. **A.** Image of open hand demonstrating small extra digit (*arrow*) adjacent to the fifth digit. Three bright foci within the extra digit represent small osseous structures. **B.** Close-up of four normal fingers (*arrows*) of hand visible in a fist, with extra digit (*arrowhead*) extending outward next to the small finger. **C.** Three-dimensional sonogram of a different patient with an extra digit (*arrow*) next to the little finger.

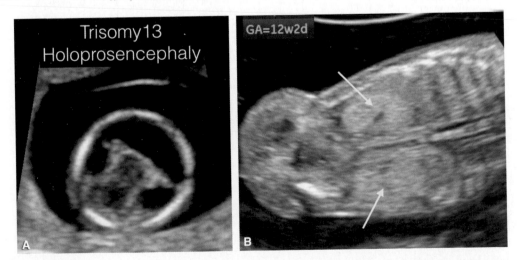

Figure 30-18 Axial view of the head (**A**) and coronal plane of the abdomen (**B**) in a fetus with trisomy 13 at 12 weeks of gestation. Note the presence of holoprosencephaly in **A**. Facial dysmorphism, cardiac anomaly, and other abnormalities were also seen with sonography (not shown). Note in **B**, the presence of hyperechogenic kidneys, a common finding in trisomy 13.

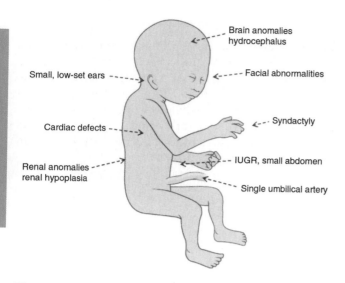

Figure 30-19 Common features of triploidy. IUGR, intrauterine growth restriction.

> 🔊 **SOUND OFF**
> Often, a partial molar pregnancy is found with a triploid fetus, thus resulting in a markedly elevated hCG level and bilateral ovarian theca lutein cysts.

Turner Syndrome

Turner syndrome is a disorder found in females. It may also referred to as 45,X or monosomy X because, most often, the paternal sex chromosome is missing. A fetus with this chromosomal anomaly classically presents with a **nuchal cystic hygroma** and nonimmune hydrops (Fig. 30-20). Nonimmune hydrops is the buildup of fluid within at least two fetal body cavities. Therefore, **ascites**, **pleural effusions**, pericardial effusion, and **subcutaneous edema** are all common findings with Turner syndrome (Fig. 30-21).

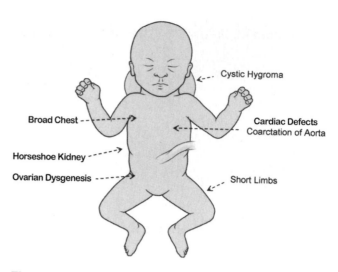

Figure 30-20 Common features of Turner syndrome (45,X).

Turner syndrome is an often-fatal condition that leads to **spontaneous abortion** in the first or second trimester. It does, however, have a reported incidence of 1 in 2,500 to 5,000 live female births. The sonographic diagnosis is initially suspected when there is visualization of a large, septated cystic hygroma located in the neck. Maternal serum screening reveals decreased levels of all laboratory findings when hydrops is present. **Ovarian dysgenesis**, webbed neck, short stature, motor deficits, hearing loss, and renal anomalies are common in those persons who do survive birth and progress into adulthood.

MATERNAL SERUM SCREENING RESULTS OF TURNER SYNDROME

1. Low estriol
2. Low AFP
3. Low hCG (with hydrops)
4. Low inhibin A (with hydrops)
5. Low PAPP-A

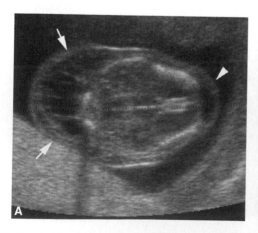
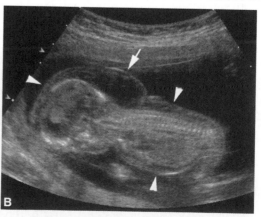

Figure 30-21 Cystic hygroma and subcutaneous edema. **A.** Sonogram of a 15-week fetus with a cystic hygroma (*arrows*) and subcutaneous edema (*arrowhead*). **B.** Sagittal image of fetus with large posterior neck cystic hygroma (*arrow*) and extensive subcutaneous edema (*arrowheads*) posteriorly, anteriorly, and over the top of the head.

SONOGRAPHIC FINDINGS OF TURNER SYNDROME

1. Increased nuchal translucency
2. Cystic hygroma
3. Renal anomalies (**horseshoe kidneys** and **renal agenesis**)
4. Cardiac defects (**coarctation of the aorta**)
5. Nonimmune hydrops

🔊 SOUND OFF
Turner syndrome is a disorder found in females. It may also referred to as 45,X or monosomy X because, most often, the paternal sex chromosome is missing.

Klinefelter Syndrome

Klinefelter syndrome, or 47,XXY, is a male chromosomal anomaly that can result in hypogonadism, small testis, tall stature, long legs and arms, and **gynecomastia**. These individuals also tend to suffer from subnormal intelligence. Although genetic testing may reveal this anomaly, prenatal sonographic imaging may not yield any signs of structural birth defects. Chapter 13 also discusses Klinefelter syndrome.

REVIEW QUESTIONS

1. What is the most likely diagnosis based on the sonographic findings in Figure 30-22?
   a. Trisomy 21
   b. Trisomy 18
   c. Trisomy 13
   d. Turner syndrome

2. What is the syndrome associated with the findings in Figure 30-23?
   a. Patau syndrome
   b. Edwards syndrome
   c. Down syndrome
   d. Turner syndrome

3. What does the arrow in Figure 30-23 indicate?
   a. Cerebellum
   b. Fused thalami
   c. Brainstem
   d. Proboscis

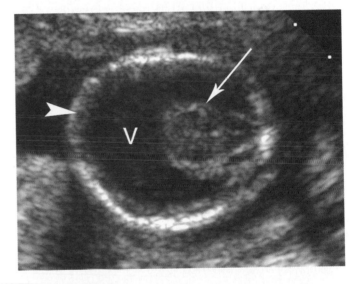

Figure 30-23

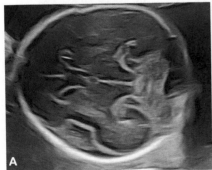

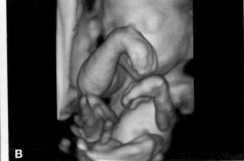

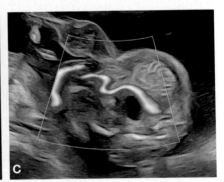

Figure 30-22

4. What cranial abnormality is often associated with Figure 30-23?
   a. Macrocephaly
   b. Anencephaly
   c. Strawberry skull
   d. Microcephaly

5. Which of the following would most likely be associated with Figure 30-24?
   a. Trisomy 13
   b. Monosomy X
   c. Klinefelter syndrome
   d. Meckel–Gruber syndrome

6. A fetus was discovered in Figure 30-25. What chromosomal abnormality would the fetus likely suffer from?
   a. Trisomy 21
   b. Trisomy 18
   c. Triploidy
   d. Turner syndrome

7. The patient in Figure 30-25 had a markedly elevated hCG level. What is the likely diagnosis given the sonographic findings?
   a. Partial molar pregnancy
   b. 45,X
   c. Patau syndrome
   d. Edwards syndrome

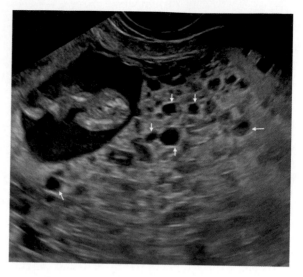

Figure 30-25

8. Figure 30-26 would most likely be associated with which chromosomal abnormality?
   a. Trisomy 21
   b. Turner syndrome
   c. Trisomy 18
   d. Klinefelter syndrome

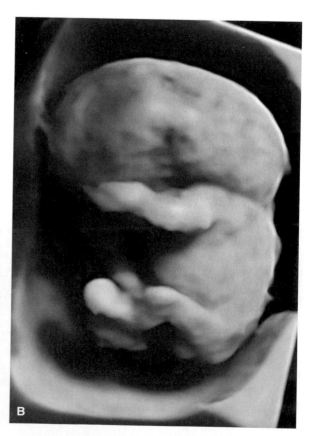

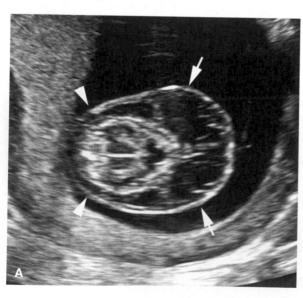

Figure 30-24

9. What abnormality of the fetal foot can be noted in Figure 30-27?
    a. Clubfoot
    b. Sandal gap
    c. Amelia
    d. Rocker-bottom foot

11. What does the arrow in Figure 30-28 indicate?
    a. Nuchal thickening
    b. Cystic hygroma
    c. Turner syndrome
    d. Skin edema

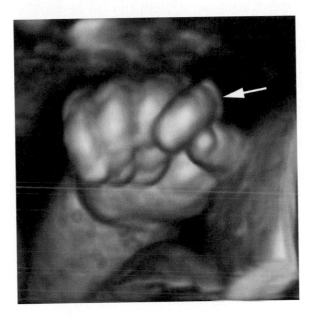

Figure 30-26

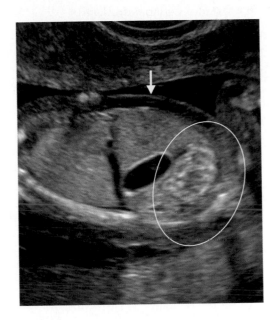

Figure 30-28

10. The abnormality in Figure 30-27 is likely associated with which of the following?
    a. Trisomy 13
    b. Trisomy 21
    c. Trisomy 18
    d. Turner syndrome

12. What does the circled region in Figure 30-28 indicate?
    a. Bowel obstruction
    b. Echogenic bowel
    c. Duodenal atresia
    d. Diaphragmatic hernia

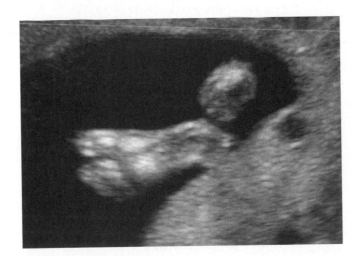

Figure 30-27

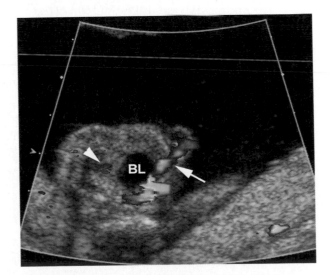

Figure 30-29

13. What does the arrow in Figure 30-29 indicate?
    a. Umbilical vein varices
    b. Nuchal cord
    c. Single umbilical artery
    d. Single umbilical vein

14. Which of the following is the finding in Figure 30-29 most likely associated with?
    a. Trisomy 18
    b. Klinefelter syndrome
    c. Trisomy 8
    d. Turner syndrome

15. The term *omphalo* refers to the:
    a. neck.
    b. cord.
    c. umbilical region.
    d. neck.

16. What is defined as a group of clinically observable findings that exist together and allow for classification?
    a. Syndrome
    b. Chromosomal deviation
    c. Malformation
    d. Congenital association

17. A cell having three copies of an individual chromosome is referred to as a(n):
    a. syndrome.
    b. trisomy.
    c. triploidy.
    d. tetralogy.

18. A situation in which some cells have an abnormal number of chromosomes whereas others do not is defined as:
    a. triploid.
    b. monosomy.
    c. mosaic.
    d. haploid.

19. A cell that has an abnormal number of whole chromosomes is referred to as:
    a. triploid.
    b. mosaic.
    c. haploid.
    d. aneuploid.

20. Which of the following is a maternal serum test that is used to determine the gender, as well as detecting some chromosomal abnormalities?
    a. Cell-free DNA
    b. Cordocentesis
    c. Amniocentesis
    d. CVS

21. Normal diploid cells have:
    a. 46 chromosomes.
    b. 23 chromosomes.
    c. 21 chromosomes.
    d. 69 chromosomes.

22. A 38-year-old pregnant woman presents to the sonography department for an obstetric sonogram with abnormal maternal serum screening. Her AFP and estriol are low, whereas her hCG is elevated. These laboratory findings are most consistent with:
    a. Edwards syndrome.
    b. Patau syndrome.
    c. triploidy.
    d. Down syndrome.

23. The triple screen typically includes:
    a. AFP, estriol, and hCG.
    b. AFP, amniotic fluid index, and hCG.
    c. AFP, estriol, and PAPP-A.
    d. PAPP-A, inhibin A, and hCG.

24. Another name for Patau syndrome is:
    a. trisomy 21.
    b. trisomy 16.
    c. trisomy 18.
    d. trisomy 13.

25. Rounded head shape is referred to as:
    a. dolichocephaly.
    b. brachycephaly.
    c. cebocephaly.
    d. craniosynostosis.

26. Theca lutein cysts would most likely be linked with a molar pregnancy and:
    a. Down syndrome.
    b. intrauterine growth restriction.
    c. triploidy.
    d. monosomy X.

27. With which of the following syndromes is brachycephaly associated most often?
    a. Edwards syndrome
    b. Patau syndrome
    c. Down syndrome
    d. Turner syndrome

28. Advanced maternal age is considered to be:
    a. older than 25 years of age.
    b. older than 30 years of age.
    c. older than 35 years of age.
    d. older than 32 years of age.

29. Which of the following is a sex chromosome anomaly?
    a. Edwards syndrome
    b. Trisomy 13
    c. Down syndrome
    d. 45,X

30. A molar pregnancy, omphalocele, and small, low-set ears are found most often with:
    a. trisomy 21.
    b. trisomy 18.
    c. trisomy 13.
    d. triploidy.

31. With what procedure is placental tissue obtained?
    a. Amniocentesis
    b. Cordocentesis
    c. CVS
    d. Trophoblastic resection technique

32. The bending of the fifth digit toward the fourth digit is called:
    a. syndactyly.
    b. clinodactyly.
    c. polydactyly.
    d. stabodactyly.

33. Webbing of the neck and short stature is found in infertile female patients with a history of:
    a. trisomy 21.
    b. triploidy.
    c. trisomy 13.
    d. Turner syndrome.

34. Pelvocaliectasis refers to:
    a. dilation of the renal pelvis and calices.
    b. enlargement of the fetal pelvis.
    c. ectopic location of the kidney within the pelvis.
    d. dilation of the ureter within the pelvis.

35. The earliest invasive fetal karyotyping technique that can be performed is:
    a. amniocentesis.
    b. cordocentesis.
    c. CVS.
    d. PUBS.

36. A strawberry-shaped skull is associated with:
    a. Edwards syndrome.
    b. Turner syndrome.
    c. Down syndrome.
    d. Patau syndrome.

37. Cleft lip, hypotelorism, and microphthalmia are all sonographic features of:
    a. trisomy 21.
    b. trisomy 18.
    c. trisomy 13.
    d. Turner syndrome.

38. Monosomy X refers to:
    a. Edwards syndrome.
    b. Patau syndrome.
    c. Down syndrome.
    d. Turner syndrome.

39. What are the fingerlike projections of gestational tissue that attach to the decidualized endometrium?
    a. Decidua capsularis
    b. Decidua vera
    c. Chorionic villi
    d. Placental substance

40. A 22-week fetus with clinodactyly, an echogenic intracardiac focus, and hyperechoic bowel is noted during a screening obstetrical sonogram. These findings are most consistent with:
    a. trisomy 21.
    b. trisomy 13.
    c. monosomy X.
    d. trisomy 18.

41. The term for small eyes is:
    a. microphthalmia.
    b. micrognathia.
    c. microcephaly.
    d. microglossia.

42. The maternal serum screening of a mother with a fetus with trisomy 18 will reveal:
    a. decreased hCG, elevated AFP, and normal estriol.
    b. increased hCG, AFP, and estriol.
    c. increased AFP, increased hCG, and decreased estriol.
    d. decreased hCG, AFP, and estriol.

43. Fusion of the orbits and holoprosencephaly is associated with:
    a. Edwards syndrome.
    b. Turner syndrome.
    c. Down syndrome.
    d. Patau syndrome.

44. A structural abnormality that results from an abnormal development describes:
    a. syndrome.
    b. chromosomal deviation.
    c. malformation.
    d. congenital misrepresentation.

45. Absent nasal bones and an increased nuchal fold measurement are most consistent with the sonographic markers for:
    a. trisomy 21.
    b. trisomy 13.
    c. triploidy.
    d. trisomy 18.

46. A large space between the first and second toes is termed:
    a. polydactyly.
    b. clubfoot.
    c. ulnaration.
    d. sandal gap.

47. Bilateral choroid plexus cysts, micrognathia, and rocker-bottom feet are sonographic findings of a 27-week fetus with an omphalocele. These findings are most consistent with:
    a. trisomy 21.
    b. trisomy 13.
    c. trisomy 18.
    d. triploidy.

48. Nonimmune hydrops and ovarian dysgenesis are found in fetuses affected by:
    a. trisomy 21.
    b. trisomy 18.
    c. trisomy 13.
    d. Turner syndrome.

49. What is macroglossia most often associated with?
    a. Trisomy 21
    b. Trisomy 18
    c. Triploidy
    d. Turner syndrome

50. A fetus with a karyotype revealing it has 69 chromosomes and sonographic findings of webbed fingers and intrauterine growth restriction most likely has:
    a. trisomy 21.
    b. trisomy 18.
    c. triploidy.
    d. Turner syndrome.

51. What is another name for the most common chromosomal abnormality?
    a. Edwards syndrome
    b. Triploidy
    c. Down syndrome
    d. Turner syndrome

52. Widened pelvic angles and duodenal atresia are most consistent with the sonographic markers for:
    a. triploidy.
    b. Patau syndrome.
    c. Down syndrome.
    d. Edwards syndrome.

53. Sonographically, you identify a fetus with fusion of the thalami and a monoventricle. Which chromosomal abnormality would be most likely?
    a. Trisomy 8
    b. Trisomy 21
    c. Trisomy 18
    d. Trisomy 13

54. Which protein is not produced by the developing placenta?
    a. AFP
    b. hCG
    c. Estriol
    d. PAPP-A

55. Which of the following laboratory findings would not be consistent with trisomy 21?
    a. High AFP
    b. Low estriol
    c. High hCG
    d. Low PAPP-A

56. Cyclopia would most likely be associated with:
    a. trisomy 8.
    b. trisomy 21.
    c. trisomy 18.
    d. trisomy 13.

57. Webbed fingers or toes are termed:
    a. clinodactyly.
    b. syndactyly.
    c. polydactyly.
    d. Werner syndrome.

58. Which of the following is a sex chromosome anomaly associated with hypogonadism and subnormal intelligence in males?
    a. Down syndrome
    b. Edwards syndrome
    c. Klinefelter syndrome
    d. Turner syndrome

59. Which of the following is not consistent with the diagnosis of nonimmune hydrops?
    a. Hypoplastic mandible
    b. Pleural effusion
    c. Ascites
    d. Subcutaneous edema

60. Echogenic small bowel is most often associated with:
    a. Down syndrome.
    b. Edwards syndrome.
    c. Patau syndrome.
    d. Turner syndrome.

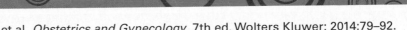

SUGGESTED READINGS

Beckmann CRB, Herbett W, Laube B, et al. *Obstetrics and Gynecology*. 7th ed. Wolters Kluwer; 2014:79–92.

Callahan TL, Caughey AB. *Blueprints: Obstetrics & Gynecology*. 6th ed. Wolters Kluwer, 2013:25–35.

Doubilet PM, Benson CB. *Atlas of Ultrasound in Obstetrics and Gynecology: A Multimedia Reference*. 2nd ed. Wolters Kluwer; 2012:232–252.

Gibbs RS, Karlan BY, Haney AF, Nygaard IE. *Danforth's Obstetrics and Gynecology*. 10th ed. Wolters Kluwer; 2008:88–121.

Henningsen C, Kuntz K, Youngs D. *Clinical Guide to Sonography: Exercises for Critical Thinking*. 2nd ed. Elsevier; 2014:269–285.

Kline-Fath BM, Bulas DI, and Lee W. *Fundamental and Advanced Fetal Imaging: Ultrasound and MRI*. 2nd ed. Wolters Kluwer; 2021:902–947.

Norton ME, Scoutt LM, & Feldstein VA. *Callen's Ultrasonography in Obstetrics and Gynecology*. 6th ed. Elsevier; 2017:24–81.

Nyberg D, McGaham J, Pretorius D, et al. *Diagnostic Imaging of Fetal Anomalies*. Lippincott Williams & Wilkins; 2003:861–944.

Sanders RC, Hall-Terracciano B. *Clinical Sonography: A Practical Guide*. 5th ed. Wolters Kluwer; 2016:232–240, 295–341.

BONUS REVIEW!

Cranial and Facial Markers in Trisomy 21 (Fig. 30-30)

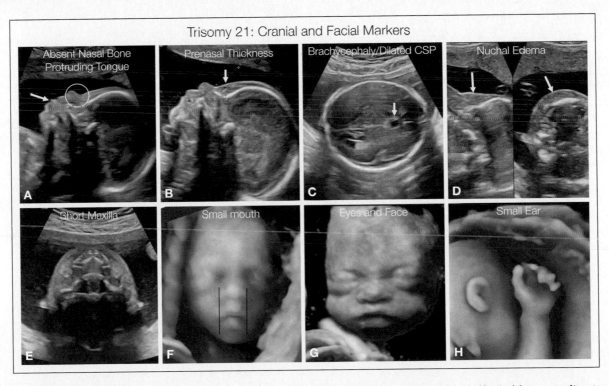

Figure 30-30 Cranial and facial markers in trisomy 21 fetuses including absent nasal bone (**A**-*circle*), protruding tongue with an open mouth (**A**-*arrow*), prenasal thickness (**B**-*arrow*), brachycephaly (**C**), dilated cavum septi pellucidi (*CSP*) (**C**-*arrow*), nuchal edema (**D**-*arrows*), as seen in sagittal (**D**-*left*) or axial (**D**-*right*) view. The midfacial hypoplasia in trisomy 21 is associated with a short maxilla (**E**) and small mouth, as microstoma (**F**). Facial features of trisomy 21 can be recognized on three-dimensional sonography and are shown in panel **G**. A small ear (**H**) can also be found but is not very specific.

(continued)

BONUS REVIEW! (*continued*)

Cardiovascular Abnormalities in Trisomy 21 (Fig. 30-31)

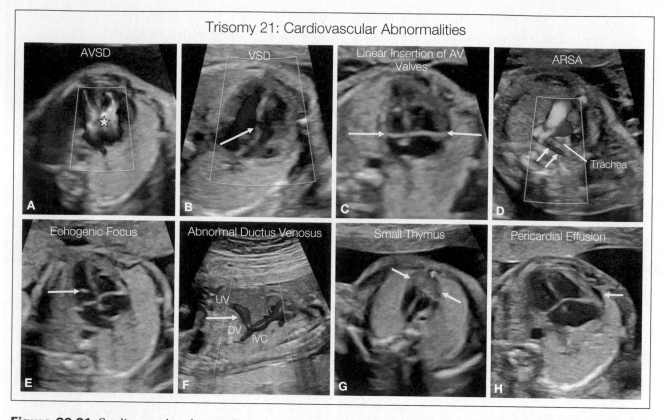

Figure 30-31 Cardiovascular abnormalities in trisomy 21 fetuses typically include an atrioventricular septal defect (*AVSD*) (**A**-*star*), ventricular septal defect (*VSD*) (**B**-*arrow*), linear insertion of the *AV* valves with a cardiac defect (**C**-*arrows*), aberrant right subclavian artery (*ARSA*) (**D**-*arrows*), with the course of the artery behind the trachea, intracardiac echogenic focus (**E**-*arrow*), abnormal course of the umbilical vein (*UV*) with an absent or abnormal connection of the ductus venosus (*DV*) (**F**-*arrow*). The thymus gland (**G**-*arrows*) can be small in fetuses with trisomy 21 with a small thymic-to-thoracic ratio. Pericardial fluid (**H**-*arrow*) can also be found in trisomy 21 fetuses in combination with a cardiac anomaly.

BONUS REVIEW! (*continued*)

Sonographic Markers of Trisomy 18 (Fig. 30-32)

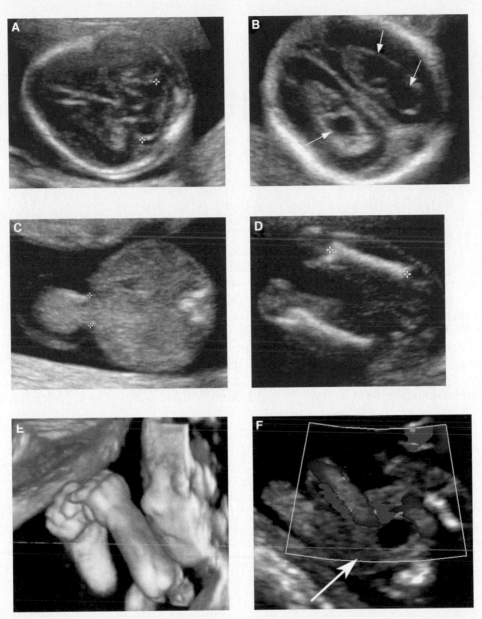

Figure 30-32 Sonographic markers of trisomy 18. **A.** A strawberry-shaped calvarium in a 19-week-gestational age fetus. **B.** Choroid plexus cysts are noted as well-demarcated anechoic spaces within the bulk (*arrows*) of the echogenic choroid. **C.** Small omphaloceles are additional features of this disorder. **D.** Bilateral femurs and remaining long bones are abnormally short. **E.** Clenched hands may be observed by two-dimensional ultrasound and easily seen with three-dimensional sonogram. **F.** A single umbilical artery in isolation is usually of no clinical significance but, with other malformations, contributes to the likelihood of a chromosomal anomaly. *Arrow* indicates the expected location of a nonvisualized umbilical artery.

Multiple Gestations

Introduction

Sonography plays a vital role in the early recognition and follow-up care of multiple gestations. Clinical findings such as large-for-dates or elevated levels of human chorionic gonadotropin may exist as the only clinical indicator at the time of the early sonogram. In the circumstance in which laboratory values and patient history are limited, the sonographer must be capable of evaluating and understanding the distinctiveness of multiple gestations. This chapter provides an overview of the embryology of twinning and other multiple gestations, and several complications that are unique to twins that a sonographer must be aware of. The "Bonus Review" section includes a three-dimensional (3D) image of conjoined twins, cord entanglement, and a Doppler study of acardiac twinning.

Key Terms

acardiac twin—an abnormally developed twin that has an absent upper body and no heart

advanced maternal age—a maternal age of 35 years or older

amnion—the inner sac that contains the embryo and amniotic fluid; echogenic curvilinear structure that may be seen during the first trimester within the gestational sac

amnionicity—relates to the number of amnions in a multiple gestation

amniotic sac—fluid-filled space, created by the amnion, surrounding the developing embryo or fetus

anastomoses—vascular connections

anemia—the condition of having a deficient number of red blood cells

assisted reproductive therapy—techniques used to treat infertility

chorion—the outer membrane of a gestation that surrounds the amnion and developing embryo

chorionicity—relates to the number of chorions and the type of placentation in a multiple gestation

cleavage—the division of a cell

conjoined twins—monoamniotic, monochorionic twins that are attached at the head, thorax, abdomen, or lower body

craniopagus—twins joined at the cranium

delta sign—see key term lambda sign

diamniotic—having two amniotic sacs

dichorionic—having two placentas

dichorionic diamniotic—having two placentas and two amniotic sacs

discordant fetal growth—asymmetric fetal weight between twins

dizygotic—two ova are fertilized by two sperms

endoscopic-guided laser photocoagulation—a treatment that uses lasers to separate abnormal placental vascular connections between twins that are suffering from twin–twin transfusion syndrome

fetus papyraceus—the death of one fetus in a twin pregnancy that is maintained throughout the pregnancy; actually means paperlike fetus

fraternal twins—twins that result from the fertilization of two separate ova and have dissimilar characteristics

heterotopic pregnancy—coexisting ectopic and intra-uterine pregnancies

hydrops (fetal)—an abnormal accumulation of fluid in at least two fetal body cavities

hypoxia—a shortage of oxygen or decreased oxygen in the blood

identical twins—twins that result from the split of a single zygote and share the same genetic structure

lambda sign—a triangular extension of the placenta at the base of the membrane and is indicative of a dichorionic diamniotic pregnancy; also referred to as the delta sign or twin peak sign

monoamniotic—having one amniotic sac

monochorionic—having one chorion

monochorionic diamniotic—having one placenta and two amniotic sacs

monochorionic monoamniotic—having one placenta and one amniotic sac

monozygotic—coming from one fertilized ovum or zygote

morbidity—the relative frequency of occurrence of a disease; condition of suffering from that disease

mortality—the rate of actual deaths

omphalopagus—conjoined twins attached at the abdomen

ovum—an unfertilized egg

parasitic twin—see key term acardiac twin

placentation—formation or structure of a placenta, structural organization, and mode of attachment of fetal to maternal tissues during placental formation

porencephaly—the development of a cystic cavity within the cerebrum; may be the result of an intraparenchymal hemorrhage

preeclampsia—pregnancy-induced maternal high blood pressure and excess protein in the urine after 20 weeks' gestation

pulmonary hypoplasia—underdevelopment of the lungs

pyopagus—conjoined twins joined back-to-back in the sacral region

singleton pregnancy—a single developing fetus

stillborn—dead at birth

stuck twin—when a twin fetus, suffering from twin–twin transfusion syndrome, experiences severe oligo-hydramnios and is closely adhered to the uterine wall

therapeutic amniocentesis—type of amniocentesis used to remove a large amount of amniotic fluid around a fetus suffering from polyhydramnios

thoracopagus—conjoined twins attached at the chest

twin embolization syndrome—when vascular products travel from a demised twin to the surviving twin by means of the common vascular channels within the shared placenta

twin peak sign—see key term lambda sign

twin–twin transfusion syndrome—shunting of venous or arterial blood from one twin to another through placental circulation

twin-reversed arterial perfusion sequence—another name for acardiac twinning

vanishing twin—the death and reabsorption of a twin

zygosity—relates to the number of zygotes (fertilized ova)

zygote—the cell formed by the union of two gametes; the first stage of a fertilized ovum

FACTORS THAT INCREASE THE LIKELIHOOD OF MULTIPLE GESTATIONS

Patients with multiple gestations may present with the clinical indication of large for dates and also an elevated human chorionic gonadotropin blood level compared to a **singleton pregnancy**. When compared with singleton pregnancies, twins have a four times higher risk of fetal **mortality** and a six times higher neonatal **morbidity** rate. There are several factors that influence the frequency of twins and other multiple gestations. A maternal history of multiple gestations, **assisted reproductive therapy** (ART), ovulation induction drugs, **advanced maternal age**, and maternal obesity have all been shown to increase the probability of multiple gestations. It has been reported that as many as 43% of triplets and higher order pregnancies are linked with ART. Thus, patients with a history of ovulation induction drugs or ART should be evaluated systematically, because they are more likely to have not only multiple gestations but also **heterotopic pregnancies**.

> 🔊 **SOUND OFF**
> A maternal history of multiple gestations, ART, ovulation induction drugs, advanced maternal age, and maternal obesity have all been shown to increase the probability of multiple gestations.

TWINS

Zygosity, Chorionicity, and Amnionicity of Twins

The fertilization of a single **ovum** that eventually divides, or the fertilization of several ova, can produce multiple gestations. A fertilized egg is referred to as a

zygote. In multiple gestations, the term **zygosity** refers to the number of eggs that are fertilized. Twins can be either **monozygotic** or **dizygotic**. Monozygotic twins arise from a single zygote, whereas dizygotic twins form from two separate zygotes (Fig. 31-1).

> 🔊 **SOUND OFF**
> Monozygotic twins arise from a single zygote, whereas dizygotic twins form from two separate zygotes.

The **chorion**, the structure that forms the placenta, develops before the **amnion**, the fluid-filled sac containing the embryo. **Chorionicity**, often referred to as **placentation**, relates to how many placentas are present. Twins who have one shared placenta are referred to as **monochorionic**, whereas twins who have two separate placentas are called **dichorionic**.

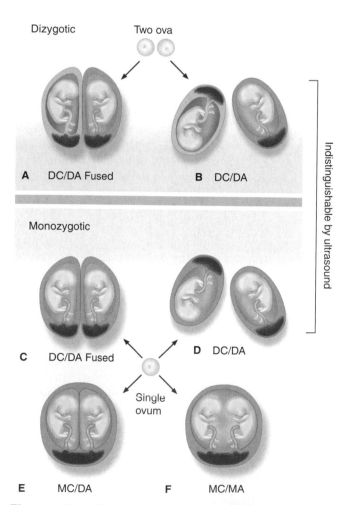

Figure 31-1 Twin development. **A.** Dichorionic diamniotic fused (placentae). **B.** Dichorionic diamniotic. **C.** Dichorionic diamniotic fused (placentae). **D.** Dichorionic diamniotic. **E.** Monochorionic diamniotic. **F.** Monochorionic monoamniotic.

Amnionicity refers to how many amnions or **amniotic sacs** are present. Twins who share the same amniotic sac are referred to as **monoamniotic**, whereas twins who have their own individual amniotic sac are **diamniotic**.

Dizygotic Twinning

Dizygotic twins, the most common form of twinning, arise from two separate fertilized ova. Dizygotic twins are referred to as **fraternal twins** because they have their own genetic structure and can differ from each other in many ways. Dizygotic twinning always results in **dichorionic diamniotic** twins (Table 31-1). That means, if there are two placentas, there must be two amnions. However, in early gestation, the placentas may fuse and appear as one large placenta with sonography.

> 🔊 **SOUND OFF**
> Dizygotic twinning, or fraternal twins, is the most common form of twinning.

Monozygotic Twinning

Monozygotic twins arise from a single zygote that splits. Thus, monozygotic twins are always **identical twins** because they share their design from only one fertilized egg. It depends on the time at which this division, or **cleavage**, takes place as to how many placentas and amnions may be present with monozygotic twins (see Fig. 31-1). There are three categories of monozygotic twins: (i) **monochorionic diamniotic**, (ii) dichorionic diamniotic, and (iii) **monochorionic monoamniotic** (Table 31-2).

TABLE 31-1 Dizygotic twinning

Zygosity	Description	Result	Appearance
Dizygotic	Two separate fertilized ova	Dichorionic diamniotic	Fraternal

TABLE 31-2 Monozygotic twinning

Zygosity	Description	Result	Appearance
Monozygotic	One zygote splits between 4 and 8 d	Monochorionic diamniotic	Identical
Monozygotic	One zygote splits before day 4	Dichorionic diamniotic	Identical
Monozygotic	One zygote splits late	Monochorionic monoamniotic	Identical

Monochorionic diamniotic twins are the most common form of monozygotic twins. Division of the inner cell mass between 4 and 8 days will result in monochorionic diamniotic twinning. In this situation, both twins share a placenta and are positioned within separate amniotic sacs. It is important to note that when two fetuses share the same placenta, complications are more likely to occur. These complications are discussed later in this chapter.

>))) **SOUND OFF**
> Monochorionic diamniotic twins are the most common form of monozygotic twins.

An even earlier division, before day 4, leads to dichorionic diamniotic twins. This means that there are two separate placentas and two separate amnions. However, fusion of the placentas can occur with dichorionic diamniotic twins. The least probable monozygotic twinning to occur is monochorionic monoamniotic twins. A late split, beyond day 8 postconception, will result in monochorionic monoamniotic twins. Because of the shared amniotic sac and this delayed division, monochorionic monoamniotic carries the additional risk of **conjoined twins**.

Sonographic Assessment of Chorionicity and Amnionicity

Sonography can identify the presence of multiple gestations in the first trimester consistently. Determining the number of placentas in a multiple gestation is vital (Fig. 31-2). During the first trimester, dichorionic twins will have a thick membrane separating the two amniotic sacs, whereas monochorionic twins will have a thin membrane or no membrane at all between them (Figs. 31-3 and 31-4).

With monochorionic twins in the first trimester, before 7 weeks, it is helpful to identify the number of yolk sacs. The presence of one yolk sac and two fetuses is indicative of a monoamniotic gestation, whereas the presence of two yolk sacs is indicative of a diamniotic gestation. After this point, the amniotic sacs are readily

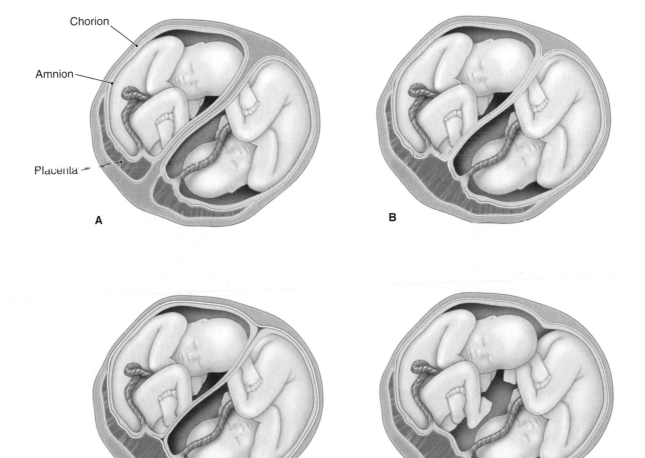

Figure 31-2 Chorionicity in twin pregnancies. **A.** Two placentas, two amnions, two chorions: diamniotic dichorionic. **B.** One placenta (results from fusion of two placentae), two amnions, two chorions: diamniotic dichorionic. **C.** One placenta, two amnions, one chorion: diamniotic monochorionic. **D.** One placenta, one amnion, one chorion: monoamniotic monochorionic.

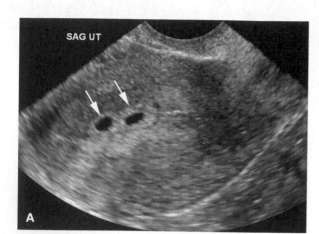

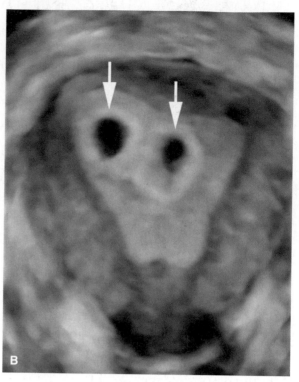

Figure 31-3 Dichorionic twins at 5 weeks diagnosed by counting gestational sacs. **A.** Sagittal view of the uterus demonstrates two intrauterine gestational sacs (*arrows*). **B.** Three-dimensional view of the uterus in another patient reveals two gestational sacs (*arrows*). In both cases, no yolk sac or embryo is identifiable within either sac, and follow-up sonograms revealed twins with heartbeats.

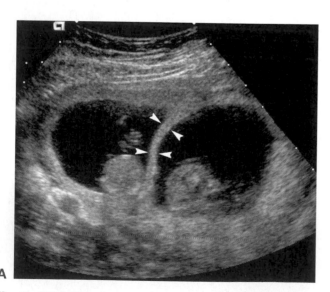

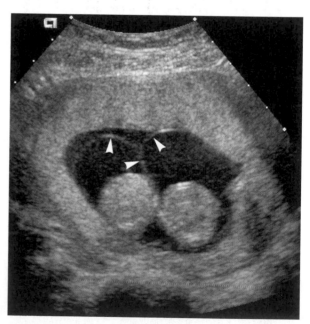

Figure 31-4 Determining chorionicity in the first trimester. **A.** Dichorionicity: sonogram of a twin gestation in which the fetuses are separated by a thick membrane (*arrowheads*), indicating that the twins are dichorionic. **B.** Monochorionicity: sonogram of a twin gestation in which both fetuses lie within a single gestational sac, with no thick band of tissue separating them, indicating that the twins are monochorionic. Each fetus is located within its own separate amnion (*arrowheads*).

visualized and can be counted (Figs. 31-5 and 31-6). If no dividing membrane is seen, the diagnosis of monoamnionicity cannot be ruled out.

> 🔊 **SOUND OFF**
> The presence of one yolk sac and two fetuses is indicative of a monoamniotic gestation, whereas the presence of two yolk sacs is indicative of a diamniotic gestation.

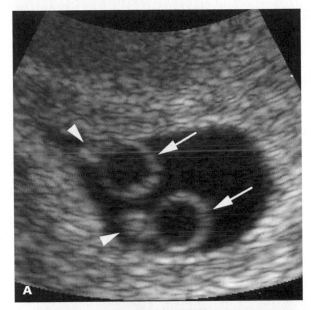

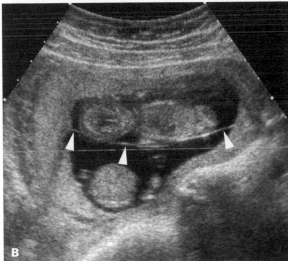

Figure 31-5 Diagnosis of monochorionic diamniotic twins based on two yolk sacs at 6 weeks' gestation. **A.** At 6 weeks' gestation, a single gestational sac contains two yolk sacs (*arrows*) and two embryos (*arrowheads*). The twins can be diagnosed as being monochorionic, but at this gestational age, the amnionicity cannot be determined by direct visualization of the amnions. The presence of two yolk sacs suggests that the twins are diamniotic. **B.** Follow-up sonogram at 12 weeks demonstrates a thin intertwin membrane (*arrowheads*), indicative of a monochorionic diamniotic gestation.

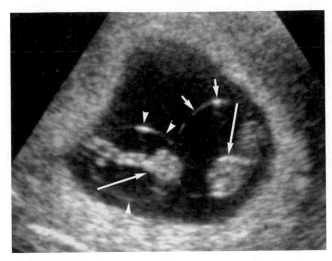

Figure 31-6 Diamniotic twins based on two amniotic sacs at 8 weeks' gestation. There are embryos (*long arrows*), each surrounded by its own amnion (*arrowheads* and *short arrows*).

Chorionicity can be difficult to establish in the second and third trimesters. The membrane separating the twins is not always helpful. If separate placentas are noted, then the pregnancy must be dichorionic diamniotic. In addition, noting a triangular extension of the placenta at the base of the dividing membrane is indicative of a dichorionic diamniotic pregnancy. This is referred to as the **twin peak sign**, **lambda sign**, or **delta sign** (Figs. 31-7 and 31-8). With a monochorionic diamniotic pregnancy, the membrane will be thin and seen separating at the junction point with the placenta, a sonographic sign referred to as the "T sign" (see Figs. 31-7 and 31-9). Determining the sex of the fetuses can be valuable as well. If the twins are different sexes, then one can assume that the twins are dichorionic (Fig. 31-10). Same-sex fetuses that have a single placenta and a thin membrane separating them are almost certainly monochorionic.

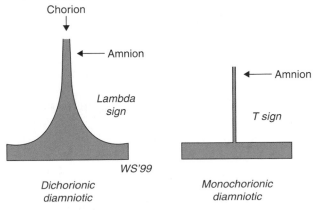

Figure 31-7 Schematic of the lambda, or twin peak, and T signs. The lambda sign is indicative of a dichorionic diamniotic gestation, whereas the T sign is indicative of a monochorionic diamniotic gestation.

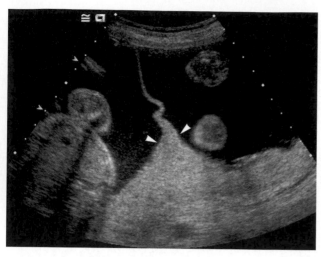

Figure 31-8 Diagnosis of dichorionicity based on the lambda sign. There is a triangular wedge of placental tissue extending into the intertwin membrane (*arrowheads*). This is highly indicative of dichorionicity.

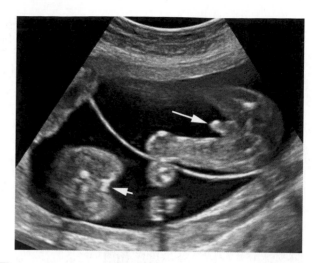

Figure 31-10 Dichorionicity based on different genders. Sonography of the genitalia in the twin gestation revealing a male (*long arrow*) and female (*short arrow*), thus confirming dichorionicity.

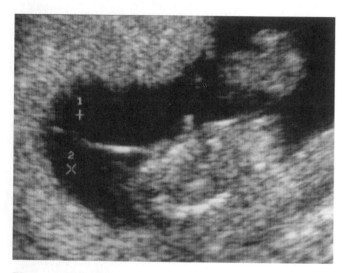

Figure 31-9 Diagnosis of monochorionicity based on the T sign. Transabdominal sonogram of a 12-week monochorionic twin gestation showing the absence of the lambda sign and the presence of the T sign.

🔊)) **SOUND OFF**
With a monochorionic diamniotic pregnancy, the membrane will be thin and seen separating at the junction point with the placenta, a sonographic sign referred to as the "T sign."

TWIN COMPLICATIONS

Twin–Twin Transfusion Syndrome

A complication that carries a high mortality rate for monochorionic twins is **twin–twin transfusion**

syndrome (TTTS). With TTTS, shunting occurs from one twin to the other (Fig. 31-11). The twin that shunts blood to the other is called the "donor" twin and is often smaller than the twin receiving extra blood, the "recipient" twin. The donor twin often suffers from anemia and growth restriction, whereas the recipient experiences **hydrops** and congestive heart failure. The resulting sonogram will reveal **discordant growth**, which is described as a 15% to 25% reduction in the estimated fetal weight of the smaller fetus compared to the larger. Treatment options include **therapeutic amniocentesis** and **endoscopic-guided laser photocoagulation** of the communicating placental vessels. The sonographic findings of TTTS include decreased amniotic fluid

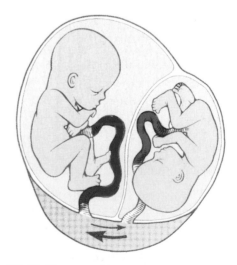

Figure 31-11 Diagram illustrates monochorionic gestation with twin-to-twin transfusion syndrome. The recipient twin is larger and in a polyhydramniotic sac. The donor twin is smaller and in an oligohydramniotic sac.

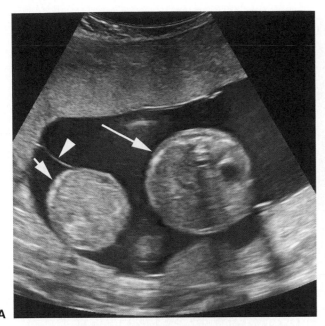

A

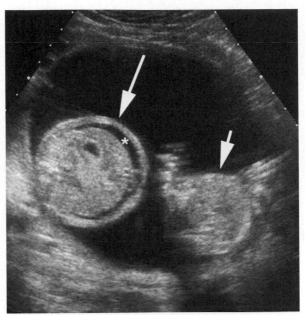

B

Figure 31-12 Twin–twin transfusion syndrome. **A.** The two fetal abdomens differ in size, one smaller (*short arrow*) than the other (*long arrow*), indicating discordant growth. The thin intertwin membrane (*arrowhead*) lies close to the smaller twin, because this twin has oligohydramnios whereas the co-twin has polyhydramnios. **B.** The two fetal abdomens differ in size with these twins also, one smaller (*short arrow*) than the other (*long arrow*), indicating discordant growth. However, there is ascites (*asterisk*) in the abdomen of the larger, recipient twin, indicating possible hydrops.

around the donor twin (Fig. 31-12). **Stuck twin** refers to severe oligohydramnios surrounding a twin that appears to be closely associated with the uterine wall (Fig. 31-13).

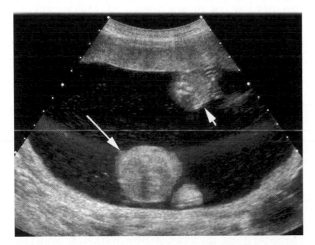

Figure 31-13 Twin–twin transfusion syndrome with a "stuck" twin. The two fetal abdomens differ in size, one smaller (*short arrow*) than the other (*long arrow*), indicating discordant growth. There is a large amount of amniotic fluid. No intertwin membrane is seen, but the unusual location of the smaller twin, adjacent to the anterior wall of the uterus, indicates that it is held there by the membrane. This twin is termed a "stuck twin" because it is pressed against the uterine wall by the membrane and by the severe polyhydramnios in the co-twin's sac.

> **SONOGRAPHIC FINDINGS OF TWIN–TWIN TRANSFUSION SYNDROME**
>
> 1. Monochorionic twinning
> 2. Discordant fetal growth
> 3. Oligohydramnios around donor twin
> 4. Polyhydramnios around recipient twin
> 5. Recipient may be hydropic

> 🔊 **SOUND OFF**
> With TTTS, the twin that shunts blood to the other is called the "donor" twin and is often smaller than the twin receiving extra blood, the "recipient" twin.

Acardiac Twinning

Abnormal **anastomoses** of placental vessels may result in a **parasitic twin** or **acardiac twin**. This is considered to be a severe form of TTTS. Acardiac twinning may also be referred to as **twin-reversed arterial perfusion** (TRAP) sequence or acardiac parabiotic twinning. With acardiac twinning, there is one normal fetus, the "pump twin," and an abnormally developed fetus containing no heart (Fig. 31-14). The normal fetus maintains the growth of the parasitic twin, albeit the growth is considerably irregular, typically resulting in an absence of the head, cervical spine, and upper limbs in the

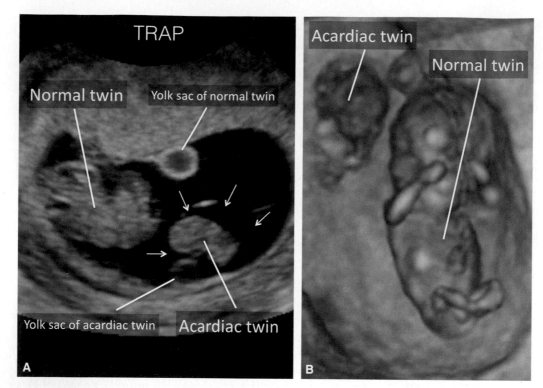

Figure 31-14 TRAP sequence **A.** Grayscale sonogram of an acardiac twin-reversed arterial perfusion (*TRAP*) in a monochorionic twin pregnancy at 9 weeks of gestation. Note the presence of an amorphous mass of tissue with an amniotic membrane covering (*small arrows*) and a yolk sac, representing the acardiac twin. The normal twin is seen with its own yolk sac. **B.** Three-dimensional sonogram in surface mode 2 weeks later showing the amorphous acardiac twin with the TRAP and the adjoining normal fetus.

acardiac twin. Movement of the parasitic twin occurs, so differentiation is achieved through the recognition of other sonographic findings, such as the absence of the heart, severe hydrops, and the absence of the upper body in the acardiac twin (Fig. 31-15). The pump twin has a perinatal mortality of 50% to 55%, secondary to polyhydramnios and prematurity.

SONOGRAPHIC FINDINGS OF ACARDIAC TWIN

1. Normal pump twin
2. Acardiac twin—absent upper body, absent heart, and hydrops

---

🔊 **SOUND OFF**
Acardiac twinning may also be referred to as TRAP syndrome or acardiac parabiotic twinning.

Conjoined Twins

Conjoined twins can result from monochorionic monoamniotic twinning. Conjoined twins can be attached at the head, thorax, abdomen, and the lower part of the body (Figs. 31-16 and 31-17; Table 31-3). The most common forms of conjoined twinning are **thoracopagus** and **omphalopagus**, which is the attachment at the chest

and abdomen, respectively. Conjoined twins may also be joined at the cranium (**craniopagus**) or back-to-back in the sacral region, which is termed **pyopagus**. The prognosis is poor for conjoined twins. They have a 40% chance for being **stillborn**, with many dying within the first 24 hours.

🔊 **SOUND OFF**
Conjoined twins can result from monochorionic monoamniotic twinning.

Vanishing Twin and Twin Embolization Syndrome

It is important to note that follow-up sonograms of twin pregnancies could reveal a decrease in the number of gestational sacs and/or embryos. The death of a twin, and subsequent reabsorption of the embryo during the first trimester, is termed a **vanishing twin** (Fig. 31-18). If the fetus dies in the first trimester and is maintained throughout the pregnancy, it is referred to as **fetus papyraceus**. With dichorionic twins, the surviving twin is rarely affected by the death of the other. However, the death of a monochorionic twin during the first trimester frequently leads to the death of the other twin.

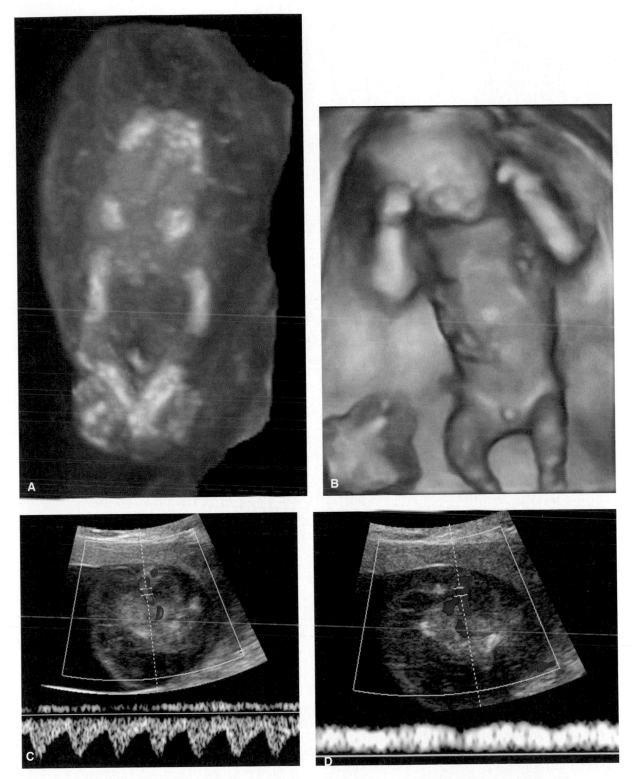

Figure 31-15 Reversed blood flow in umbilical vessels of an acardiac twin. **A.** Three-dimensional (*3D*) sonogram of a massively edematous acardiac twin with absent head and upper extremities. **B.** 3D sonogram of the pump twin, which is normally formed. **C.** Spectral Doppler shows pulsatile blood flow toward the acardiac twin in its umbilical artery, reversal of the normal direction. **D.** Spectral Doppler shows blood flow away from the acardiac twin in its umbilical vein, reversal of the normal direction.

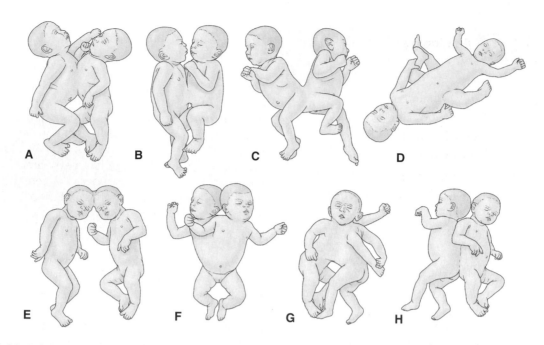

Figure 31-16 Different types of conjoined twins: thoracopagus (**A**), omphalopagus (**B**), pygopagus (**C**), ischiopagus (**D**), craniopagus (**E**), parapagus (**F**), cephalopagus (**G**), rachipagus (**H**).

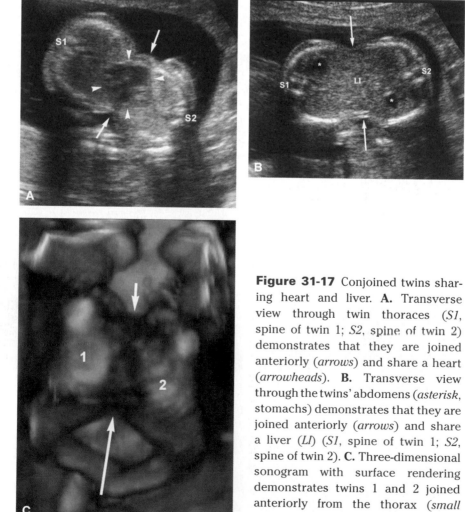

Figure 31-17 Conjoined twins sharing heart and liver. **A.** Transverse view through twin thoraces (*S1*, spine of twin 1; *S2*, spine of twin 2) demonstrates that they are joined anteriorly (*arrows*) and share a heart (*arrowheads*). **B.** Transverse view through the twins' abdomens (*asterisk*, stomachs) demonstrates that they are joined anteriorly (*arrows*) and share a liver (*Ll*) (*S1*, spine of twin 1; *S2*, spine of twin 2). **C.** Three-dimensional sonogram with surface rendering demonstrates twins 1 and 2 joined anteriorly from the thorax (*small arrow*) to the abdomen (*large arrow*).

TABLE 31-3 Terminology associated with conjoined twins	
Conjoined Terminology	**Area of Union**
Craniopagus	Joined at the head
Thoracopagus	Joined at the thorax (chest)
Omphalopagus	Joined at the abdomen
Ischiopagus	Joined at the pelvis
Pyopagus	Joined at the sacral region or back-to-back

The death of a monochorionic twin during the second or third trimester can lead to life-threatening problems in the surviving twin. Potential troubles exist as a consequence of the breakdown of the demised twin. Vascular products, as a result of the breakdown of tissues, travel from the demised twin to the surviving twin by means of the common vascular channels within the shared placenta, a complication known as **twin embolization syndrome**. Particularly, the central nervous system and the kidneys are affected in the surviving twin, with a documented 25% risk of death or neurologic damage for the survivor. Intracranial abnormalities such as hydrocephalus and **porencephaly** are common in the survivor as well (Fig. 31-19).

SOUND OFF
Twin embolization syndrome can result from the death of a monochorionic twin.

BEYOND TWINS

Triplet pregnancies can manifest with different combinations of chorionicity and amnionicity. For example, triplets can be trichorionic triamniotic and dichorionic triamniotic (Fig. 31-20). Most triplet and quadruplet pregnancies result from the use of ovulation induction or in vitro fertilization (Fig. 31-21). Although the sonographic challenge is greatly amplified for the sonographer, the role of sonography remains the same with multiple pregnancies beyond twins. Amnionicity and chorionicity should be determined sonographically so that adequate care can be accessible for the mother and all of her offspring.

Unfortunately, multiple gestations beyond twins have an increased likelihood of discordant growth, miscarriage, and perinatal death. When assisted reproduction is used, resulting in a high number of multifetal pregnancies, multifetal reduction may be used. With sonographic guidance, a needle punctures the fetal heart and potassium chloride is injected.

MATERNAL AND POSTNATAL COMPLICATIONS OF MULTIPLE GESTATIONS

Mothers expecting multiple gestations have an increased risk of developing **preeclampsia** and **anemia**. The risk for preterm delivery is increased 7 to 10 times more compared to a singleton pregnancy, with an associated low birth weight. The median gestational age of delivery for twins is 35 weeks, and for triplets

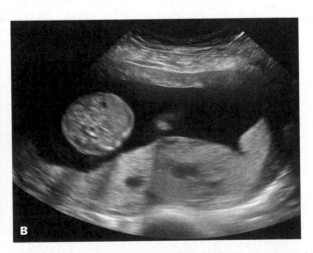

Figure 31-18 Vanishing twin. Death of one twin in the first trimester. **A.** Twin pregnancy at 8 weeks' gestation with one live fetus (*long arrow*) and a smaller demised fetus (*short arrow*). **B.** On a subsequent scan at 16 weeks' gestation, there is no evidence of the demised twin ("vanishing twin").

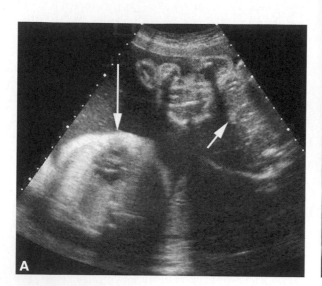
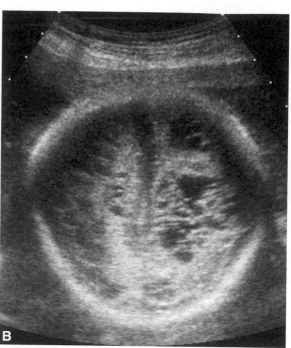

Figure 31-19 Twin embolization syndrome. **A.** A 32-week sonogram revealing a live twin (*long arrow*) and a demised twin (*short arrow*). **B.** One month later, the live twin is suffering from intracranial ischemic damage as a result of twin embolization syndrome.

and beyond, the gestational age of delivery is even earlier. Infants born with low birth weight, and specifically before 32 weeks' gestation, often suffer from **pulmonary hypoplasia** with episodes of **hypoxia**.

Hypoxia at the time of birth can cause tiny, fragile blood vessels within the immature brain to rupture, leading to intracranial hemorrhage and possible irreversible neurologic complications or death.

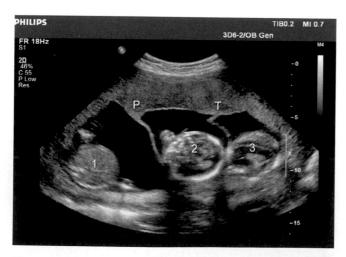

Figure 31-20 A triplet pregnancy demonstrating the placental twin peak sign (*P*) and the T sign (*T*). One abdomen (*1*) and two fetal heads (*2, 3*) confirm the triplet pregnancy.

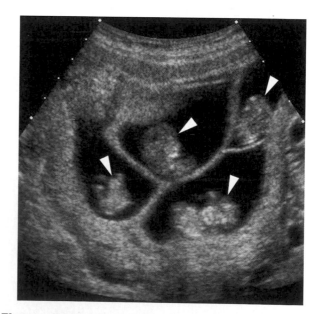

Figure 31-21 Quadruplets. Four fetuses (*arrowheads*) were noted during this 10-week sonogram.

REVIEW QUESTIONS

1. What type of twinning is represented in Figure 31-22?
   a. Monochorionic monoamniotic
   b. Monochorionic diamniotic
   c. Dizygotic
   d. Dichorionic diamniotic

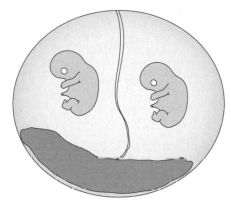

Figure 31-22

2. What sign is present in Figure 31-22?
   a. Win peak sign
   b. Lambda sign
   c. Delta sign
   d. T sign

3. What sign is present in Figure 31-23?
   a. T sign
   b. Lambda sign
   c. Monochorionic sign
   d. Dichorionic sign

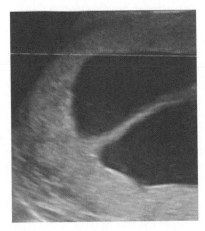

Figure 31-23

4. What is there sonographic evidence of in Figure 31-24?
   a. Fetus papyraceus
   b. Thoracopagus
   c. TRAP sequence
   d. Discordant growth

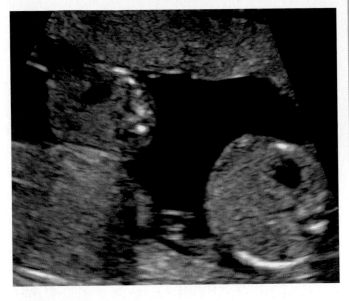

Figure 31-24

5. What would cause the sonographic findings in Figure 31-24?
   a. Dichorionic twinning
   b. Monochorionic twinning
   c. Twin embolization syndrome
   d. Acardiac twinning

6. What does the finding in Figure 31-25 confirm?
   a. Lambda sign
   b. Monoamniotic gestation
   c. Dichorionic gestation
   d. Diamniotic gestation

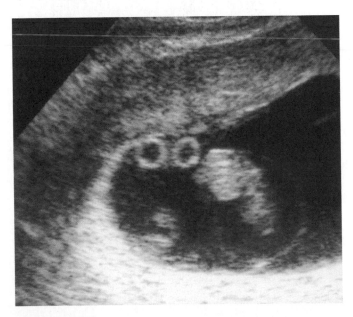

Figure 31-25

7. What type of twinning is evident in Figure 31-26?
   a. Dichorionic monoamniotic
   b. Dichorionic diamniotic
   c. Monochorionic diamniotic
   d. Monochorionic monoamniotic

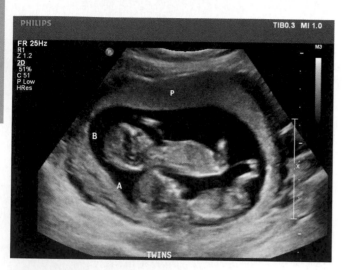

Figure 31-26

8. What does Figure 31-27 depict?
   a. Twin embolization syndrome
   b. Acardiac twinning
   c. TTTS
   d. TRAP

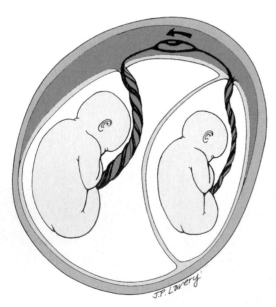

Figure 31-27

9. The arrow in Figure 31-28 indicates an intracranial abnormality noted in a surviving twin. The other twin demised 2 weeks earlier. What is the most likely diagnosis?
   a. Twin embolization syndrome
   b. Acardiac twinning
   c. TTTS
   d. TRAP

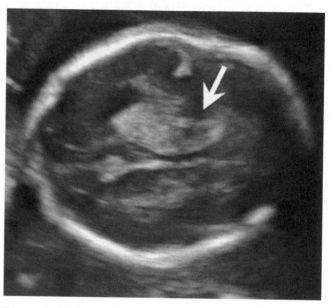

Figure 31-28

10. What is Figure 31-28 the result of?
    a. Diamniotic gestation
    b. Dichorionic gestation
    c. Conjoined twins
    d. Monochorionic gestation

11. What is the intracranial abnormality identified by the arrow in Figure 31-28?
    a. Intracranial teratoma
    b. Twin-reversed arterial aneurysm
    c. Intracranial hemorrhage
    d. Choroid plexus papilloma

12. What does Figure 31-29 depict?
    a. TRAP syndrome
    b. TTTS
    c. Vanishing twin syndrome
    d. Conjoined twins

13. What does the arrow in Figure 31-30 indicate?
    a. Subcutaneous edema
    b. Anasarca
    c. Ascites
    d. Hydrops

Multiple Gestations

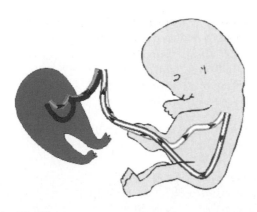

Figure 31-29

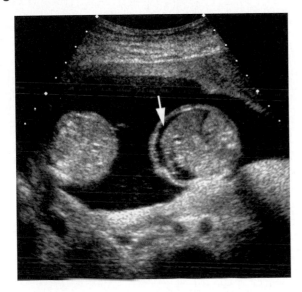

Figure 31-30

14. In Figure 31-31, the monochorionic twin noted was closely associated with the anterior wall of the uterus and did not move. What is the most likely diagnosis?
    a. Discordant growth
    b. Stuck twin
    c. Recipient twin
    d. Twin embolization syndrome

15. What is the term for conjoined twins united at the pelvis?
    a. Omphalopagus
    b. Pelvopagus
    c. Thoracopagus
    d. Ischiopagus

16. Which of the following would result from an intracranial intraparenchymal hemorrhage in a twin?
    a. Porencephaly
    b. Choroid plexus cyst
    c. Arachnoid cyst
    d. Intraventricular hemorrhage

17. What is the median gestational age of delivery for twins?
    a. 25 weeks
    b. 32 weeks
    c. 35 weeks
    d. 38 weeks

18. Preterm twins born with low birth weight are at increased risk to suffer from which of the following?
    a. Preeclampsia
    b. Gestational diabetes
    c. Pulmonary hypoplasia
    d. Neural tube defects

19. If you observe that one fetus is female and one is a male, then you can assume:
    a. dichorionic twinning.
    b. monochorionic twinning.
    c. identical twinning.
    d. increased risk for twin–twin transfusion.

20. What type of twinning is evident in Figure 31-32?
    a. Dichorionic monoamniotic
    b. Dichorionic diamniotic
    c. Monochorionic diamniotic
    d. Monochorionic monoamniotic

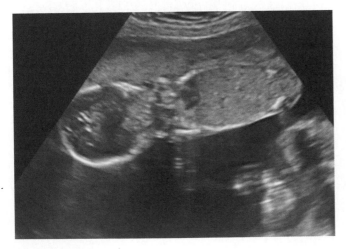

Figure 31-31

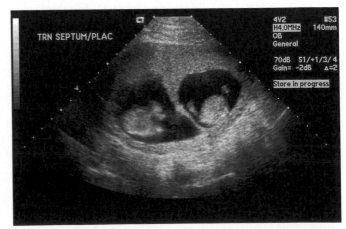

Figure 31-32

21. Which of the following is not a sonographic sign of a dichorionic diamniotic gestation?
    a. Twin peak sign
    b. Lambda sign
    c. Delta sign
    d. T sign

22. Twins that have the threat of being conjoined are:
    a. monochorionic monoamniotic.
    b. monochorionic diamniotic.
    c. dizygotic.
    d. dichorionic diamniotic.

23. Which of the following would a newborn most likely suffer from if they were born before 32 weeks as a result of multiple gestation complications?
    a. Ascites
    b. Pulmonary hypoplasia
    c. Amnionitis
    d. Preeclampsia

24. The inner membrane surrounding the fetus is referred to as the:
    a. placenta.
    b. chorion.
    c. amnion.
    d. yolk sac.

25. Twins that result from the fertilization of two separate ova are called:
    a. diamniotic.
    b. dizygotic.
    c. monozygotic.
    d. monochorionic.

26. What condition is pregnancy-induced maternal high blood pressure and excess protein in the urine after 20 weeks' gestation?
    a. Gestational diabetes
    b. Preeclampsia
    c. Porencephaly
    d. Maternal mirror syndrome

27. The outer membrane of the gestation is referred to as the:
    a. placenta.
    b. chorion.
    c. amnion.
    d. yolk sac.

28. Which of the following would not increase the likelihood of multiple gestations?
    a. Gestational diabetes
    b. Maternal age greater than 40 years
    c. Maternal history of twins
    d. ART

29. Twins whose bodies are connected at some point are said to be:
    a. fraternal.
    b. conjoined.
    c. identical.
    d. stuck.

30. The term that indicates the presence of two separate amniotic sacs is:
    a. dichorionic.
    b. bichorionic.
    c. monoamniotic.
    d. diamniotic.

31. Twins having two placentas and one amniotic sac are referred to as:
    a. monochorionic diamniotic.
    b. monoamniotic dichorionic.
    c. dichorionic monoamniotic.
    d. This does not occur.

32. What is it called when a twin fetus, suffering from TTTS, experiences severe oligohydramnios and becomes closely adhered to the uterine wall?
    a. Acardiac monster
    b. Vanishing twin
    c. Acardiac twin
    d. Stuck twin

33. Which term relates the number of amniotic sacs?
    a. Chorionicity
    b. Placentation
    c. Amnionicity
    d. Embryology

34. Twins having one placenta and one amniotic sac are referred to as:
    a. dichorionic monoamniotic.
    b. dichorionic diamniotic.
    c. monochorionic diamniotic.
    d. monochorionic monoamniotic.

35. Which term relates the number of placentas?
    a. Chorionicity
    b. Zygosity
    c. Amnionicity
    d. Cleavage

36. Identical twins result from:
    a. monozygotic twinning.
    b. dizygotic twinning.
    c. heterotopic pregnancies.
    d. monochorionic pregnancies.

37. The sonographic examination of twins reveals a triangular extension of the placenta at the base of the membrane. This finding is indicative of:
    a. monochorionic monoamniotic twins.
    b. monochorionic diamniotic twins.
    c. dichorionic diamniotic twins.
    d. monochorionic diamniotic twins.

38. Asymmetry in fetal weight between twins is indicative of:
    a. discordant growth.
    b. preeclampsia.
    c. dichorionic diamniotic twinning.
    d. intrauterine infections.

39. Twins having two placentas and two amniotic sacs are referred to as:
    a. monochorionic diamniotic.
    b. biamniotic dichorionic.
    c. dichorionic diamniotic.
    d. dichorionic biamniotic.

40. Typically, the first sonographic manifestation of TTTS is:
    a. oligohydramnios.
    b. polyhydramnios.
    c. dichorionic twinning.
    d. discordant fetal growth.

41. Conjoined twins that are attached at the abdomen are referred to as:
    a. Omphalopagus
    b. Thoracopagus
    c. Ileopagus
    d. Craniopagus

42. Monozygotic twins result from:
    a. a single zygote that splits.
    b. two zygotes that are fertilized by the same sperm.
    c. two morulas.
    d. a single zygote that is fertilized by two sperms.

43. The demise of a twin during the second or third trimester can lead to:
    a. TTTS.
    b. twin embolization syndrome.
    c. twin peak sign.
    d. acardiac twinning.

44. The term that indicates the presence of two separate placentas is:
    a. dichorionic.
    b. bichorionic.
    c. monoamniotic.
    d. diamniotic.

45. What is a treatment that separates abnormal placental vascular connections between twins that are suffering from TTTS?
    a. Cleavage-laser resection treatment
    b. Endoscopic-guided laser photocoagulation
    c. Endemic translocation of placental vessels
    d. Circumvallate resection of shared placental vasculature

46. The shunting of blood from one twin to the other is termed:
    a. TTTS.
    b. twin embolization syndrome.
    c. twin peak sign.
    d. conjoined twins.

47. Factors that increase the likelihood of having multiple gestations include all of the following except:
    a. advanced maternal age.
    b. ovulation induction drugs.
    c. poor nutritional state.
    d. maternal predisposition for twins.

48. TRAP syndrome may also be referred to as:
    a. TTTS.
    b. vanishing twin syndrome.
    c. twin embolization syndrome.
    d. acardiac twinning.

49. Which of the following can occur as a result of dizygotic twinning?
    a. Monochorionic diamniotic twins
    b. Monochorionic monoamniotic twins
    c. Dichorionic diamniotic twins
    d. All of the above

50. The abnormal twin in acardiac twinning is also referred to as the:
    a. pump twin.
    b. parasitic twin.
    c. stuck twin.
    d. vanishing twin.

51. The twin that will appear larger in TTTS is the:
    a. donor.
    b. recipient.
    c. Both will be the same.
    d. Both will be demised.

52. Fraternal twins result from:
    a. monozygotic twinning.
    b. dizygotic twinning.
    c. heterotopic pregnancies.
    d. monochorionic pregnancies.

53. What is the term for conjoined twins attached at the sacral region?
    a. Sacralpagus
    b. Omphalopagus
    c. Pyopagus
    d. Thoracopagus

54. Which of the following can occur as a result of monozygotic twinning?
    a. Monochorionic diamniotic twins
    b. Monochorionic monoamniotic twins
    c. Dichorionic diamniotic twins
    d. All of the above

55. The most common form of monozygotic twins is:
    a. monochorionic diamniotic.
    b. dichorionic monoamniotic.
    c. monochorionic monoamniotic.
    d. none of the above.

56. All of the following complications are associated with multiple gestations except:
    a. preterm delivery.
    b. high birth weight.
    c. maternal anemia.
    d. maternal preeclampsia.

57. Acardiac twinning results from:
    a. poor maternal nutrition.
    b. dizygotic gestations.
    c. abnormal links between the placental vessels.
    d. twin embolization syndrome.

58. Ovulation induction drugs increase the likelihood of not only multiple gestations but also:
    a. maternal diabetes.
    b. ovarian prolapse.
    c. heterotopic pregnancies.
    d. choriocarcinoma.

59. Which form of monozygotic twinning is least common?
    a. Monochorionic diamniotic
    b. Monochorionic monoamniotic
    c. Dichorionic diamniotic
    d. Dichorionic biamniotic

60. The demise of a twin can lead to the development of neurologic complications in the living twin as a result of:
    a. twin embolization syndrome.
    b. TTTS.
    c. TRAP syndrome.
    d. dichorionicity.

SUGGESTED READINGS

Beckmann CRB, Herbett W, Laube B, et al. *Obstetrics and Gynecology*. 7th ed. Wolters Kluwer; 2014:145–149.

Callahan TL, Caughey AB. *Blueprints: Obstetrics & Gynecology*. 6th ed. Wolters Kluwer; 2013:101–104.

Curry RA, Prince M. *Sonography: Introduction to Normal Structure and Function*. 5th ed. Elsevier; 2020:421–430.

Doubilet PM, Benson CB. *Atlas of Ultrasound in Obstetrics and Gynecology: A Multimedia Reference*. 2nd ed. Wolters Kluwer; 2012:298–319.

Gibbs RS, Haney AF, Karlan BY, et al. *Danforth's Obstetrics and Gynecology*. 10th ed. Wolters Kluwer; 2008:220–245.

Kline-Fath BM, Bulas DI, and Lee W. *Fundamental and Advanced Fetal Imaging: Ultrasound and MRI*. 2nd ed. Wolters Kluwer; 2021:352–385.

Norton ME, Scoutt LM, Feldstein VA. *Callen's Ultrasonography in Obstetrics and Gynecology*. 6th ed. Elsevier; 2017:132–156.

Nyberg D, McGaham J, Pretorius D, et al. *Diagnostic Imaging of Fetal Anomalies*. Lippincott Williams & Wilkins; 2003:777–813.

Rumack, CM, Wilson SR, William Charboneau J, et al. *Diagnostic Ultrasound*. 4th ed. Elsevier; 2011:1145–1165.

Conjoined Twins at the Buttocks (Fig. 31-33)

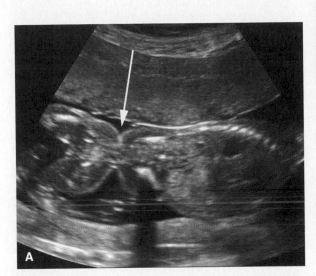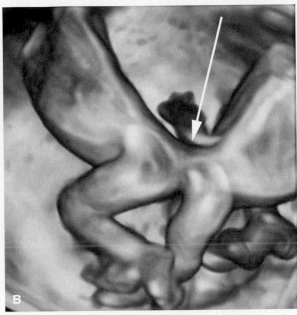

Figure 31-33 Twins conjoined at the buttocks. Two-dimensional (**A**) and three-dimensional (**B**) views of 17-week twins conjoined at the buttocks.

Color Doppler of Cord Entanglement (Fig. 31-34)

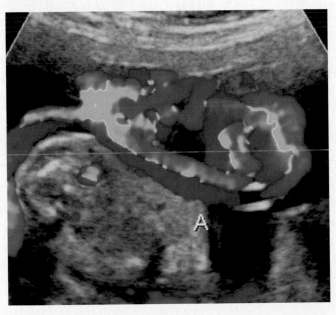

Figure 31-34 Cord entanglement. Color Doppler of monochorionic monoamniotic twin pregnancy with cord entanglement. A, twin A

(continued)

BONUS REVIEW! *(continued)*

Color and Spectral Doppler of Acardiac Twinning (Fig. 31-35)

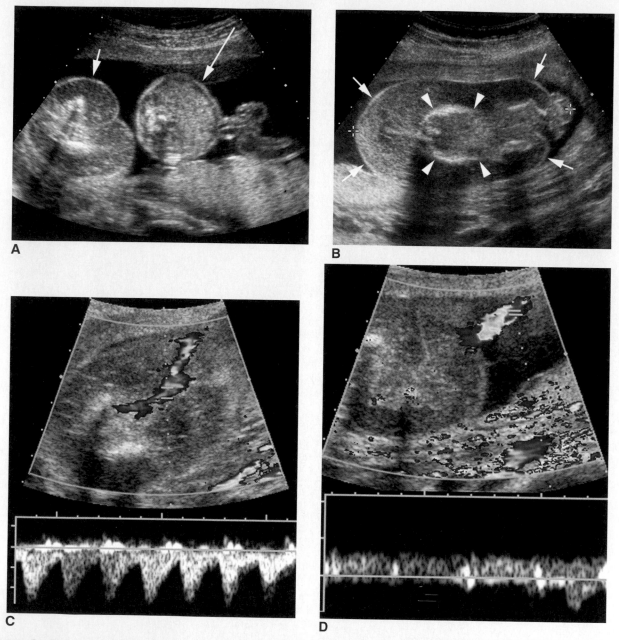

Figure 31-35 Reversed blood flow in umbilical vessels of an acardiac twin. **A.** The edematous body of an acardiac twin (*short arrow*) images next to the normal abdomen of the pump twin (*long arrow*). **B.** Another view of the massively edematous acardiac twin showing marked skin edema (*arrows*) around the body (*arrowheads*). **C.** Spectral Doppler shows pulsatile blood flow toward the acardiac twin in its umbilical artery, reversal of the normal direction. **D.** Spectral Doppler shows blood flow away from the acardiac twin in its umbilical vein, reversal of the normal direction.

Fetal Environment and Maternal Complications

Introduction

This chapter offers a review of the placenta, amniotic fluid, umbilical cord, and cervix. An appraisal of intrauterine growth restriction (IUGR) and maternal complications is also provided. The "Bonus Review" section includes images of calcified retained products of conception, including a three-dimensional (3D) image, as well as images of a cerclage and umbilical venous varix.

Key Terms

abruptio placentae—placental abruption

allantoic cyst—cyst found within the umbilical cord

amniotic fluid index—the amount of amniotic fluid surrounding the fetus; the sum of four quadrant measurements of amniotic fluid

anasarca—diffuse edema

anemia—the condition of having a deficient number of red blood cells

bilateral renal agenesis—the failure of both kidneys to develop in the fetus

bilobed placenta—placenta that consists of two separate discs of equal size

biophysical profile—method of fetal monitoring with sonography to produce a numerical scoring system that predicts fetal well-being

blastocyst—the stage of the conceptus that implants within the decidualized endometrium

cerclage—the placement of sutures within the cervix to keep it closed

cervical incompetence—the painless dilation of the cervix in the second or early third trimester

cesarean section—form of childbirth in which a surgical incision is made through the maternal abdomen to deliver the fetus

chorioangioma—a benign placental tumor

chorion frondosum—the part of the chorion, covered by chorionic villi, that is the fetal contribution of the placenta

chorionic villi—fingerlike projections of gestational tissue that attach to the decidualized endometrium and allow the transfer of nutrients from the mother to the fetus

circumvallate placenta—an abnormally shaped placenta caused by the membranes inserting inward from the edge of the placenta, producing a curled-up placental shape

cotyledons—groups or lobes of chorionic villi

cystic adenomatoid malformation—a mass consisting of abnormal bronchial and lung tissue that develops within the fetal chest

decidua basalis—the endometrial tissue at the implantation site, and the maternal contribution of the placenta

diaphragmatic hernia—the herniation of the abdominal contents into the chest cavity through a defect in the diaphragm

diethylstilbestrol—a drug administered to pregnant women from the 1940s to the 1970s to treat threatened abortions and premature labor that has been linked with uterine malformation in the exposed fetus

duodenal atresia—congenital maldevelopment or absence of the duodenum

erythroblastosis fetalis—condition in which there is an incompatibility between the fetal and maternal red blood cells

estimated fetal weight—the fetal weight based on sonographic measurements

esophageal atresia—congenital absence of part of the esophagus

exsanguination—total blood loss; to bleed out

fetal hydrops—an abnormal accumulation of fluid in at least two fetal body cavities

funneling (cervical)—the result of the premature opening of the internal os and the subsequent bulging of the membranes into the dilated cervix

gastroschisis—herniation of abdominal contents through a right-sided, periumbilical abdominal wall defect

gestational diabetes—diabetes acquired as a result of pregnancy

gestational trophoblastic disease—a disease associated with an abnormal proliferation of the trophoblastic cells during pregnancy; may also be referred to as molar pregnancy

HELLP syndrome—maternal syndrome that stands for hemolysis, elevated liver enzymes, and low platelet count

hemangioma—a benign tumor composed of blood vessels

hydronephrosis—the dilation of the renal collecting system resulting from the obstruction of the flow of urine from the kidney(s) to the bladder; also referred to as pelvocaliectasis or pelvicaliectasis

hypoxia—a shortage of oxygen or decreased oxygen in the blood

idiopathic—from an unknown origin

immune hydrops—fetal hydrops caused by Rh incompatibility

infantile polycystic kidney disease—an inherited renal disease that results in bilateral enlargement of the fetal kidneys and microscopic renal cysts; also referred to as autosomal recessive polycystic kidney disease

intrauterine growth restriction—a fetus that is below the 10th percentile for gestational age (small for gestational age) and whose growth is impeded for some reason

leiomyoma (uterine)—a benign, smooth muscle tumor of the uterus; may also be referred to as a fibroid or uterine myoma

lower uterine segment—the term used for the isthmus of the uterus during pregnancy

macrosomia—an estimated fetal weight of greater than the 90th percentile or the neonate that measures more than 4,500 g

marginal cord insertion—abnormal cord insertion at the edge of the placenta

meconium—fetal stool that is composed of fetal skin, hair, amniotic fluid, and bile

microcephaly—small head

mirror syndrome—a rare disorder in which the mother suffers from edema and fluid buildup similar to her hydropic fetus

multicystic dysplastic kidney disease—a fetal renal disease thought to be caused by an early renal obstruction; leads to the development of multiple noncommunicating cysts of varying sizes in the renal fossa

multiparity—having had several pregnancies

neonatal period—the first 28 days of life

neural tube defects—a group of developmental abnormalities that involve the brain and spine

nongravid—not pregnant

nonimmune hydrops—fetal hydrops caused by congenital fetal anomalies and infections

nuchal cord—condition of having the umbilical cord wrapped completely around the fetal neck

oligohydramnios—a lower-than-normal amount of amniotic fluid for the gestational age

omphalocele—an anterior abdominal wall defect where there is herniation of the fetal bowel and other abdominal organ into the base of the umbilical cord

philtrum—the vertical groove seen between the upper lip and the nasal septum

placenta accreta—the abnormal adherence of the placenta to the myometrium in an area where the decidua is either absent or minimal

placenta increta—invasion of the placenta within the myometrium

placenta percreta—penetration of the placenta through the uterine serosa and possibly into adjacent pelvic organs

placenta previa—when the placenta covers or nearly covers the internal os of the cervix

placentomegaly—enlargement of the placenta

polyhydramnios—an excessive amount of amniotic fluid for the gestational age

posterior urethral valves—irregular thin membranes of tissue located within the male posterior urethra that does not allow urine to exit the urethra

postpartum—time directly after giving birth and extending to about 6 weeks

preeclampsia—pregnancy-induced maternal high blood pressure and excess protein in the urine after 20 weeks' gestation

premature rupture of membranes—the rupture of the amniotic sac before the onset of labor

proteinuria—protein in the urine

retained products of conception—when additional placental tissue remains within the uterus after the bulk of the placenta has been delivered

shoulder dystocia—when the shoulder of the fetus cannot pass through the birth canal during pregnancy

succenturiate lobe—an accessory lobe of the placenta

TORCH—acronym that stands for toxoplasmosis, other infections, rubella, cytomegalovirus, and herpes simplex virus

twin–twin transfusion syndrome—shunting of venous or arterial blood from one twin to another through placental circulation

two-vessel cord—an umbilical cord with one artery and one vein; could possibly be associated with other fetal abnormalities and intrauterine growth restriction

umbilical arteries—two vessels of the umbilical cord that carry deoxygenated blood from the fetus to the placenta

umbilical vein—the vessel of the umbilical cord that carries oxygenated blood from the placenta to the fetus

umbilical vein varix—focal dilatation of the intra-abdominal portion of the umbilical vein

vasa previa—fetal vessels resting over the internal os of the cervix

velamentous cord insertion—the abnormal insertion of the umbilical cord into the membranes beyond the placental edge

venous lakes—pools of maternal blood within the placental substance

vernix—protective fetal skin covering

vitelline duct—the structure that connects the developing embryo to the secondary yolk sac

Wharton jelly—gelatinous material that is located within the umbilical cord around the umbilical vessels

FETAL ENVIRONMENT

The Placenta

The placenta is a vital organ to the fetus during pregnancy (Table 32-1). It normally weighs between 450 and 550 g and has a diameter of 16 to 20 cm. The placenta is derived from both fetal and maternal cells. The **decidua basalis**, the maternal contribution of the placenta, is the endometrium beneath the developing placenta. The **chorion frondosum**, the portion derived from the **blastocyst** and containing the **chorionic villi**, is the fetal contribution to the placenta. The placenta consists of approximately 10 to 30 **cotyledons**, which are groups or lobes of chorionic villi.

TABLE 32-1 Functions of the placenta
Gas transfer
Excretory function
Water balance
pH maintenance
Hormone production
Defensive barrier

◀))) SOUND OFF
The decidua basalis is the maternal contribution of the placenta, and the chorion frondosum is the fetal contribution of the placenta.

The placenta produces human chorionic gonadotropin, which maintains the corpus luteum of the ovary. In later pregnancy, the placenta also produces estrogen and progesterone, taking over that function from the corpus luteum. One major function of the placenta is to act as an excretory organ for the fetus, performing imperative exchanges of waste products and gases with valuable nutrients and oxygen from the mother. The placenta effectively becomes the means of respiration for the fetus.

A definitive placenta may not be identified sonographically until after 10 to 12 weeks. It will appear as an echogenic thickening surrounding part of the gestational sac. As the pregnancy progresses, the placenta becomes more defined (Fig. 32-1). The placenta consists of three parts: (i) the chorionic plate, (ii) the placental substance, and (iii) the basal layer or basal plate. The chorionic plate is the element of the placenta closest to the fetus. The basal layer is the area adjacent to the uterus. The placental substance contains the functional parts of the placenta and is located between the chorionic plate and the basal layer (Fig. 32-2).

There are several normal variants seen within the placental substance that can distort the typical homogeneous appearance of this organ. **Venous lakes**, also referred to as maternal lakes or placental lakes, are pools of maternal blood within the placental substance. They appear as anechoic or hypoechoic areas and may contain swirling blood. These are of little clinical significance.

◀))) SOUND OFF
Venous lakes, also referred to as maternal lakes or placental lakes, are pools of maternal blood within the placental substance.

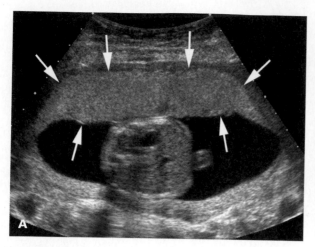
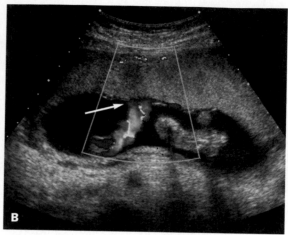

Figure 32-1 Normal placenta at 19-week gestation. **A.** This placenta has a homogeneously echogenic structure (*arrows*) located on the anterior aspect of the gestational sac. **B.** The umbilical cord insertion site into the placenta (*arrow*) is clearly identified using color Doppler.

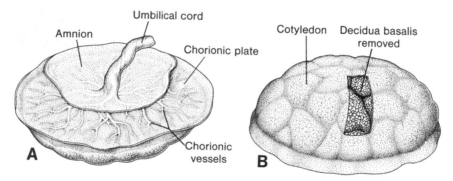

Figure 32-2 A full-term placenta. **A.** Fetal side. The chorionic plate and umbilical cord are covered by amnion. **B.** Maternal side showing the cotyledons. In one area, the decidua has been removed.

The shape of the placenta may vary as well. A **bilobed placenta** consists of two separate discs of equal size. There may also be an accessory lobe or a **succenturiate lobe** of the placenta, which are additional smaller lobes located separate from the main segment of the placenta (Fig. 32-3). Also, a **circumvallate placenta** is an abnormally shaped placenta caused by the membranes inserting inward from the edge of the placenta, producing a curled-up placental contour (Fig. 32-4). A circumvallate placenta may lead to vaginal bleeding and placental abruption, among other complications.

Calcifications may be noted within the placenta, and indentations may be seen within the basal and chorionic plates with advancing gestation. Although it has fallen out of favor in some institutions, grading of the placenta has been performed in the past to predict fetal lung maturity by assessing these indentations and calcifications (Table 32-2; Fig. 32-5). The thickness of the placenta should be evaluated with sonography. It should not exceed 4 cm. Both a thick or large placenta, termed **placentomegaly**, and a thin placenta are associated with maternal and/or fetal abnormalities (Fig. 32-6; Tables 32-3 and 32-4).

SOUND OFF
The thickness of the placenta should be evaluated with sonography. It should not exceed 4 cm.

Placenta Previa

Implantation of the placenta may occur within the **lower uterine segment**. This will often lead to **placenta previa**, which is evident when the placenta covers the internal os of the cervix. Placenta previa is a common cause of painless vaginal bleeding in the second and third trimesters. It is discovered more often in women with a history of **multiparity**, advanced maternal age, previous abortion, and prior **cesarean section** (C-section). The correlation with C-section is theorized to be the result of uterine scar formation from surgery, with the subsequent implantation of the next placenta in that area.

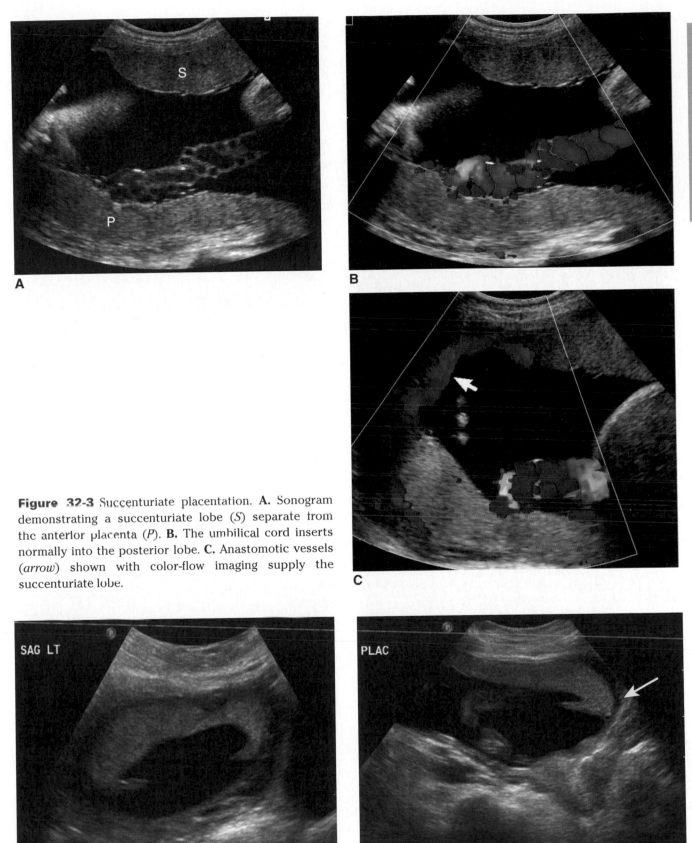

Figure 32-3 Succenturiate placentation. **A.** Sonogram demonstrating a succenturiate lobe (*S*) separate from the anterior placenta (*P*). **B.** The umbilical cord inserts normally into the posterior lobe. **C.** Anastomotic vessels (*arrow*) shown with color-flow imaging supply the succenturiate lobe.

Figure 32-4 Circumvallate placenta. **A.** Sonographic image of a circumvallate placenta demonstrating the characteristic rolled-up placental edge. **B.** Sonographic image of a circumvallate placenta appearing as a linear structure in the amniotic cavity (*arrow*).

TABLE 32-2 Classic placental grading with associated sonographic findings

Placental Grade	Sonographic Findings
Grade 0	Uninterrupted chorionic plate and homogeneous placental substance
Grade I	Subtle indentations on the chorionic plate, with some small calcifications within the placental substance
Grade II	Moderate indentations in the chorionic plate with "comma-like" calcification in the placental substance
Grade III	Prominent indentation in the chorionic plate that extends to the basal layer with diffuse echogenic and anechoic areas noted within the placental substance

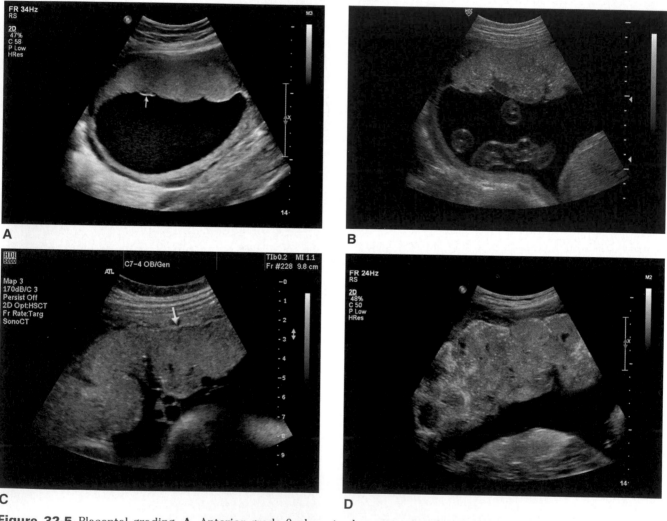

Figure 32-5 Placental grading. **A.** Anterior grade 0 placenta demonstrating the characteristic smooth, homogeneous texture. The perpendicular angle of incidence allows for imaging of the chorionic plate (*arrow*). **B.** This grade I placenta contains scattered calcifications with the beginning of lobulations developing on the fetal side. **C.** In the grade II placenta, lobulations increase with the basal layer (*arrow*) appearing irregular due to small calcifications. **D.** The grade III placenta demonstrates interlobar and septal calcifications.

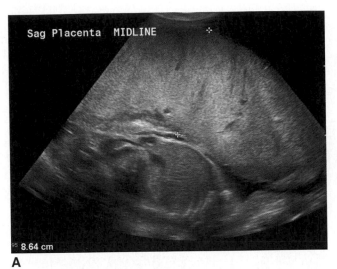

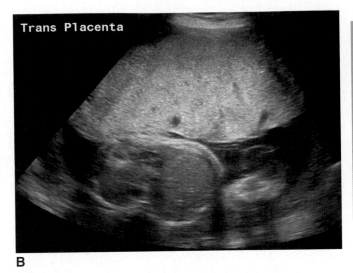

Figure 32-6 Placentomegaly. **A.** Sonographic image of an anterior placenta demonstrating placentomegaly. The electronic calipers denote a maximum thickness exceeding 8 cm. **B.** Sonographic image of an enlarged, thickened anterior placenta associated with nonimmune fetal hydrops.

Placenta previa is not routinely diagnosed until the late second or third trimester. This is secondary to the fact that because of the growth of the uterus, the placenta has the potential to migrate away from the cervix with advancing gestation. The term migration may be misleading, because the placenta does not actually travel but rather the uterine growth shifts the placenta away from the cervix. There are several terms associated with placenta previa that are specific to the location of the placenta in relation to the internal os of the cervix (Table 32-5; Figs. 32-7 and 32-8). Although marginal placenta previa and partial placenta previa are defined separately, they are often difficult to distinguish sonographically.

TABLE 32-3 Possible causes of a thick placenta

Diabetes mellitus

Maternal **anemia**

Infection

Fetal hydrops

Rh isoimmunization

Multiple gestations

TABLE 32-4 Possible causes of a thin placenta

Diabetes mellitus (long standing)

Intrauterine growth restriction

Placental insufficiency

Polyhydramnios

Preeclampsia

Small-for-dates fetus

🔊 **SOUND OFF**
Placenta previa is a common cause of painless vaginal bleeding in the second and third trimesters.

TABLE 32-5 Terms associated with placenta previa

Term Associated with Placenta Previa	Sonographic Description
Complete (total) previa	Placenta covers the internal os completely
Partial previa	Placenta partially covers the internal os
Marginal previa	Placenta lies at the edge of the internal os
Low-lying previa	Placental edge extends into the lower uterine segment but ends >2 cm away from the internal os

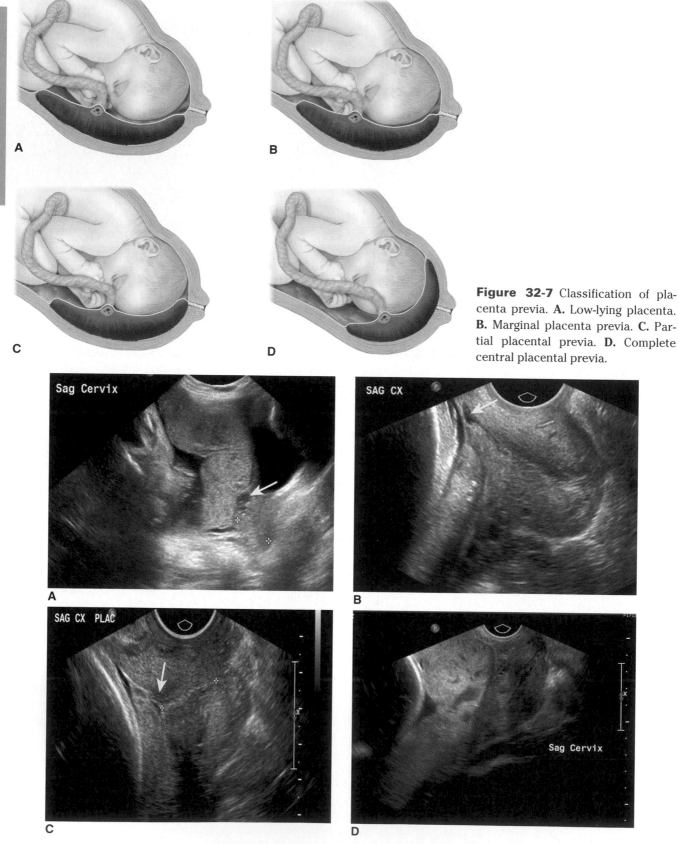

Figure 32-7 Classification of placenta previa. **A.** Low-lying placenta. **B.** Marginal placenta previa. **C.** Partial placental previa. **D.** Complete central placental previa.

Figure 32-8 Placenta previa on sonography. **A.** Sagittal transabdominal image demonstrating the placental tissue covering the internal cervical os. **B.** Endovaginal image demonstrating marginal placenta previa. The *arrow* points to the internal cervical os. **C.** Endovaginal image demonstrating partial placenta. The *arrow* points to the internal cervical os. **D.** Complete central placenta previa with accreta on an endovaginal image.

The placenta should be evaluated for placenta previa after 20 weeks with an empty maternal bladder using a transabdominal approach, because the fully distended bladder may lead to a false-positive diagnosis of placenta previa. Another cause of false-positive placenta previa is painless myometrial contractions that occur in the lower uterine segment. However, these should resolve as the sonographic examination continues.

Transvaginal and translabial or transperineal scanning can be extremely beneficial, especially with advanced gestation when the fetal head or fetal parts obscure the internal os. Translabial scanning is discussed later in this chapter. Because both the patient and the fetus have an increased risk of death with placenta previa, a C-section is the preferred method of delivery.

CLINICAL FINDINGS OF PLACENTA PREVIA

1. Previous C-section or uterine surgery
2. Painless vaginal bleeding
3. Possibly asymptomatic

Vasa Previa

The complication of fetal vessels resting over the internal os of the cervix is referred to as **vasa previa**. These vessels are prone to rupture as the cervix dilates. This, in turn, can lead to **exsanguination** of the fetus. Vasa previa is often associated with **velamentous cord insertion** and, possibly, a succenturiate lobe. The sonographic findings of color Doppler signals over the internal os are sonographically indicative of vasa previa (Fig. 32-9).

SONOGRAPHIC FINDINGS OF VASA PREVIA

1. Identification of vessels over the internal os of the cervix with the use of color Doppler
2. Velamentous cord insertion

Placental Abruption

Placental abruption, also referred to as **abruptio placentae**, is the premature separation of the placenta from the uterine wall before the birth of the fetus, thus causing hemorrhage. It may be further described as complete abruption, partial abruption, marginal abruption, or be defined by its location (Fig. 32-10). A complete abruption, which is the most severe, often results in the development of a retroplacental hematoma, which is located between the placenta and the myometrium (Fig. 32-11). Partial abruption often results in only a few centimeters of separation. Marginal abruption, often referred to as a subchorionic hemorrhage, lies at the edge of the placenta and is the most common placental hemorrhage identified with sonography.

Maternal conditions that are linked to the development of placental abruption include hypertension, preeclampsia, cocaine use, cigarette smoking, poor nutrition, and trauma. Sonography is not always effective

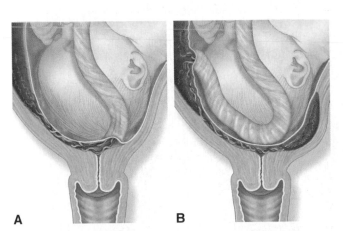

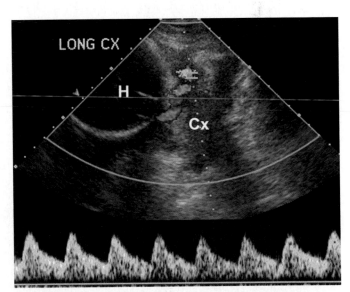

Figure 32-9 Vasa previa is a condition where umbilical vessels run within the membranes near or across the internal cervical os. **A.** Vasa previa in association with velamentous cord insertion into the placenta. **B.** Vasa previa can also occur in cases where there is a succenturiate lobe of the placenta. **C.** Sagittal image of lower uterine segment with color and spectral Doppler showing blood flow in vessels between the fetal head (*H*) and cervix (*Cx*). The spectral Doppler demonstrates an umbilical artery waveform, proving these are umbilical vessels of a vasa previa.

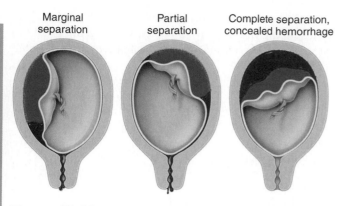

Marginal separation · Partial separation · Complete separation, concealed hemorrhage

Figure 32-10 Types of placental abruption. Note that vaginal bleeding is absent when the hemorrhage is concealed.

CLINICAL FINDINGS OF PLACENTAL ABRUPTION

1. Abdominal pain (often sudden onset)
2. Possible vaginal bleeding
3. Uterine contraction
4. Uterine tenderness

SONOGRAPHIC FINDINGS OF PLACENTAL ABRUPTION

1. Hematoma located either at the edge of the placenta or between the placenta and the myometrium

in identifying placental abruption. A retroplacental hematoma can be identified either between the placenta and myometrium or under the chorionic membrane. Clinically, patients may present with vaginal bleeding, abdominal pain, uterine contractions, and uterine tenderness. Placental abruption is an understandably urgent situation that can lead to fetal death from hypoxia and, possibly, the death of the mother.

> **SOUND OFF**
> Maternal conditions that are linked to the development of placental abruption include hypertension, preeclampsia, cocaine use, cigarette smoking, poor nutrition, and trauma.

Placenta Accreta, Placenta Increta, and Placenta Percreta

Placenta accreta is frequently used as a universal term to describe the condition that is defined as the abnormal adherence of the placenta to the myometrium in an area where the decidua is either absent or minimal (Fig. 32-12). The placenta may attach to a uterine scar following a previous C-section and/or after uterine surgery. This explains the association between anterior placenta previa and placenta accreta. As a result of this abnormal adherence, the placenta does not detach at birth. There are three different terms associated with this abnormality: (i) placenta accreta, (ii) **placenta increta**, and (iii) **placenta percreta** (Table 32-6).

Depending upon the amount of invasion or penetration of the placenta into the myometrium, the patient could suffer from heavy bleeding at delivery and, possibly, uterine rupture. Therefore, an emergency

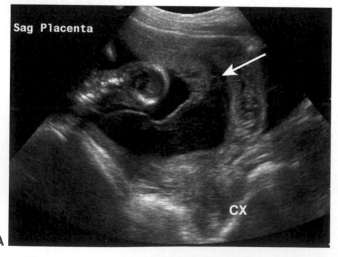

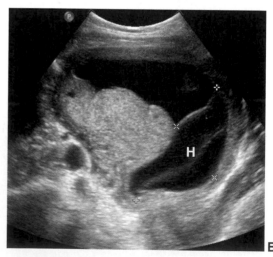

Figure 32-11 Placental abruption with retroplacental hematoma. **A.** Sagittal sonographic image demonstrating partial separation of the placenta from the uterine wall. Note the raised placental edge (*arrow*) with a large accumulation of blood adjacent to the cervix (*CX*). **B.** Sagittal sonographic image of a subchorionic hemorrhage demonstrating the layering of blood products within the clot formation (*H*).

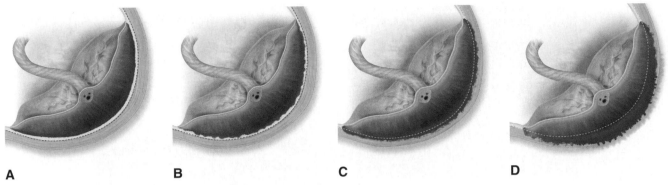

Figure 32-12 Classification of the placenta accreta spectrum. **A.** Normal placentation. **B.** Placenta accreta. **C.** Placenta increta. **D.** Placenta percreta.

hysterectomy may be warranted. The sonographic appearance of placenta accreta is the loss of the normal hypoechoic interface between the placenta and the myometrium (Fig. 32-13). Increta and percreta can be diagnosed based on the amount of invasion and if there is a breach of the serosal layer of the uterus. With placenta percreta, the placenta can even invade the urinary bladder, thus causing urinary complications. Magnetic resonance imaging is a helpful imaging modality to confirm the diagnosis of placenta accreta.

> ◀)) **SOUND OFF**
> Note in Table 32-6 that *accreta* is associated with *adherence*, *increta* is associated with *invasion*, and *percreta* is associated with *penetration* of the placenta.

CLINICAL FINDINGS OF PLACENTA ACCRETA, PLACENTA INCRETA, AND PLACENTA PERCRETA

1. Previous C-section or uterine surgery
2. Painless vaginal bleeding if placenta previa is present
3. Possibly asymptomatic

Chorioangioma

Chorioangioma is the most common placental tumor. Clinically, chorioangiomas are commonly asymptomatic but may produce an elevation in maternal serum alpha-fetoprotein. The most common location of this mass is adjacent to the umbilical cord insertion site at the placenta. They typically do not carry any risks to the fetus or mother, although larger chorioangiomas have been associated with polyhydramnios, intrauterine growth restriction (IUGR), and fetal hydrops. Sonographically, a chorioangioma will appear as a well-circumscribed hypoechoic or hyperechoic mass within the placental substance (Fig. 32-14). Differentials for the chorioangioma include other solid-appearing focal hypoechoic areas within the placenta, that is, the placental infarct and placental fibrin deposits.

SONOGRAPHIC FINDINGS OF PLACENTA ACCRETA, PLACENTA INCRETA, AND PLACENTA PERCRETA

1. Placenta previa (frequent associated finding)
2. Loss of the normal hypoechoic interface between the placenta and the myometrium

TABLE 32-6 Terms associated with placenta accreta

Term Associated with Placenta Accreta	Definition	Sonographic Finding
Placenta *accreta*	Adherence of the placenta to the myometrium	Loss of normal hypoechoic interface between the placenta and the myometrium
Placenta *increta*	Invasion of the placenta within the myometrium	Loss of normal hypoechoic interface between the placenta and the myometrium with invasion into the myometrium
Placenta *percreta*	Penetration of the placenta through the serosa and possibly into adjacent organs	Loss of normal hypoechoic interface between the placenta and the myometrium with penetration beyond the serosa

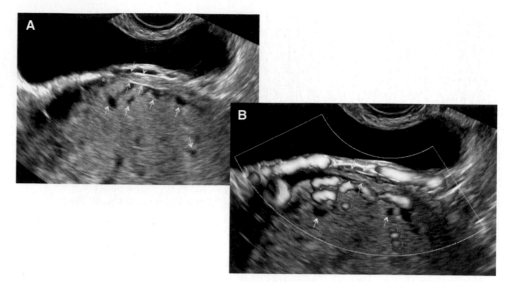

Figure 32-13 Two-dimensional (**A**) and color Doppler (**B**) images of a placenta increta. The placenta bulges into the bladder. The *white arrows* indicate multiple lacunae; thin myometrium is delineated by *yellow arrows*. The myometrium disappears after the thin segment (*asterisk*). Increased vascularity is seen under the bladder using color Doppler.

CLINICAL FINDINGS OF A CHORIOANGIOMA

1. Possible elevation in maternal serum alpha-fetoprotein

SONOGRAPHIC FINDINGS OF A CHORIOANGIOMA

1. Solid hypoechoic or hyperechoic mass within the placenta

Uterine Synechia(e)

Uterine synechiae, also referred to as amniotic sheets, are linear bands of scar tissue within the uterus. These synechiae are the result of intrauterine adhesions, as seen with Asherman syndrome. They can result from uterine surgery. Sonographically, a uterine synechia appears as a linear, echogenic band traversing the uterine cavity (Fig. 32-15). The fetus will be seen to move freely. Although typically isolated, uterine synechiae have been associated with premature rupture of membranes (PROM), premature delivery,

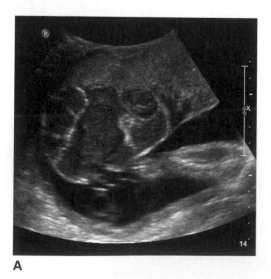

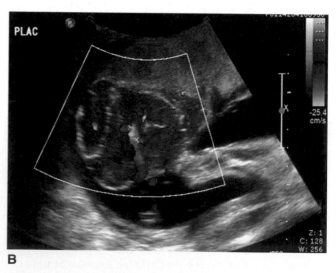

Figure 32-14 Chorioangioma. **A.** Large ovoid mass protruding from fetal surface of the placenta with internal calcifications consistent with a chorioangioma. **B.** As a vascular tumor of the placenta, the chorioangioma demonstrates multiple vascular channels within the mass on color Doppler sonography.

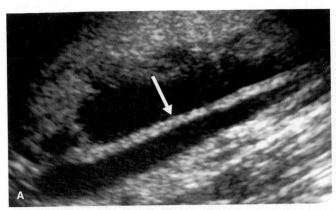
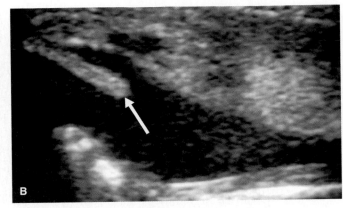

Figure 32-15 Amniotic sheet. **A.** A fibrous band, covered by chorioamniotic membranes (*arrow*), extends across the amniotic cavity. The uterine synechia forms a shelflike structure that partially compartmentalizes the uterine cavity. The fetus has free access to both compartments. **B.** The characteristic free edge (*arrow*) of the amniotic sheet is demonstrated.

and placental abruption. Amniotic bands are typically thinner, or may not be seen, and are associated with fetal anomalies.

SONOGRAPHIC FINDINGS OF UTERINE SYNECHIA(E)

1. Linear, echogenic band of tissue traversing the uterine cavity
2. The band does not involve fetal parts, and the normal fetus appears to move freely

The Umbilical Cord

The umbilical cord, which normally inserts into the middle of the placenta, has two arteries and one vein. These vessels are surrounded by a gelatinous material called **Wharton jelly**, all of which is covered by a single layer of amnion. The cord develops from the fusion of the yolk stalk and the **vitelline duct** (omphalomesenteric duct) early in gestation.

The **umbilical vein**, which carries oxygenated blood from the placenta to the fetus, enters the fetal abdomen and proceeds cephalad to connect to the left portal vein within the liver. The **umbilical arteries** enter the fetal abdomen and carry deoxygenated blood from the fetus to the placenta. The arteries, once they enter the abdomen, proceed caudal around the bladder to connect to the fetal internal iliac arteries. Therefore, color Doppler can establish that there is a three-vessel cord (3VC), by placing the color Doppler box over the fetal bladder and identifying both arteries adjacent to the bladder. A 3VC may also be obtainable in the transverse view of the umbilical cord. A single umbilical artery, or **two-vessel cord** (2VC), has been cited as the

most common abnormality of the umbilical cord. It has been reported in association with abnormalities of all major organ systems and IUGR. Fetuses with a 2VC have an approximate 20% chance of having additional abnormalities, and thus a thorough examination of the fetus for other findings is warranted.

SOUND OFF
Fetuses with a 2VC have an approximate 20% chance of having additional abnormalities, and thus a thorough examination of the fetus for other findings is warranted.

The umbilical cord normally inserts into the central portion of the placenta. Abnormal cord insertion sites are described as either marginal or velamentous. **Marginal cord insertion** is at the edge of the placenta. This is also referred to as a battledore placenta. Velamentous cord insertion denotes the insertion of the umbilical cord into the membranes beyond the placental edge. This type of abnormal insertion is often seen in association with vasa previa (Fig. 32-16).

Occasionally, the umbilical cord may be seen encircling the fetal neck. This is termed **nuchal cord**. A nuchal cord can be confirmed with color Doppler (Fig. 32-17). It does not always indicate fetal distress, even though, on occasion, multiple loops of cord may be noted around the neck. Nonetheless, this abnormality should be documented, particularly if additional signs of fetal distress are evident.

SOUND OFF
Velamentous cord insertion denotes the insertion of the umbilical cord into the membranes beyond the placental edge.

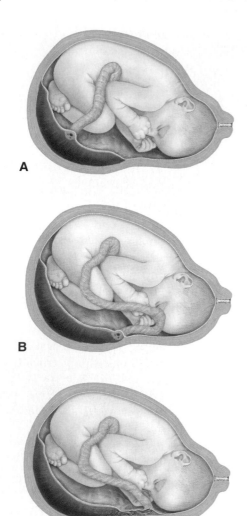

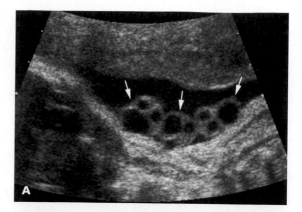

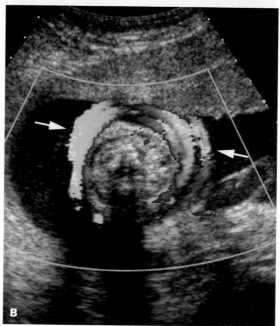

Figure 32-16 Umbilical cord insertions. **A.** Central insertion of cord into placenta. **B.** Battledore insertion. Cord is inserted near the margin or edge of the placenta. **C.** Velamentous insertion. Cord is inserted into chorioamniotic membranes, which extend beyond the placental parenchyma and lie along the uterine wall. Location of this type of insertion near the lower uterine segment can lead to complications such as vasa previa.

Figure 32-17 Triple nuchal cord. **A.** Longitudinal image of fetal neck showing three cross sections of the umbilical cord (*arrows*), each representing a loop of cord around the fetal neck. **B.** Axial color Doppler image showing multiple umbilical vessels (*arrows*) encircling the fetal neck.

Cystic masses of the umbilical cord may be seen with sonography. An **allantoic cyst** is a mass that may be noted in the umbilical cord adjacent to the umbilical vessels. Umbilical cord cysts are most often found near the fetal abdomen and have been seen in connection with omphalocele and aneuploidy, especially if noted in the second or third trimester. Another cystic-appearing mass that may be noted within the abdomen of the fetus, appearing to be adjacent to the umbilical cord, is an **umbilical vein varix**, which is essentially the focal dilatation of the abdominal portion of the umbilical vein. It has been associated with fetal aneuploidy, growth restriction, hydrops, and demise. Color Doppler can be used to prove the vascularity of this abnormality.

The **hemangioma** is the most common tumor of the umbilical cord, although it is exceedingly rare. These masses, unlike allantoic cysts, appear as solid hyperechoic masses and are more often located near the cord insertion site into the placenta.

SONOGRAPHIC FINDINGS OF ALLANTOIC CYSTS

1. Cystic mass within the umbilical cord
2. Most often noted close to the fetal abdomen

SONOGRAPHIC FINDINGS OF HEMANGIOMAS OF THE UMBILICAL CORD

1. Solid hyperechoic mass within the umbilical cord
2. Most often noted close to the cord insertion into the placenta

Umbilical Cord Doppler

Fetal well-being can be evaluated using pulsed Doppler of the umbilical cord by measuring the systolic-to-diastolic ratio (S/D ratio). The S/D ratio assesses the vascular resistance in the placenta by taking a sample of the umbilical artery. It can be performed anywhere along the length of the cord, although a free loop of cord will tend to offer the most accurate measurement. Normally, the S/D ratio will decrease with advancing gestation. Therefore, an elevated S/D ratio is associated with increased placental resistance and an increase in the risk of perinatal mortality and morbidity. Absence or reversal of diastolic flow in the umbilical artery is considered irregular and is associated with an increased incidence of IUGR and oligohydramnios (Fig. 32-18).

> 🔊 **SOUND OFF**
> Normally, the S/D ratio will decrease with advancing gestation. An elevated S/D ratio is associated with increased placental resistance and an increase in the risk of perinatal mortality and morbidity.

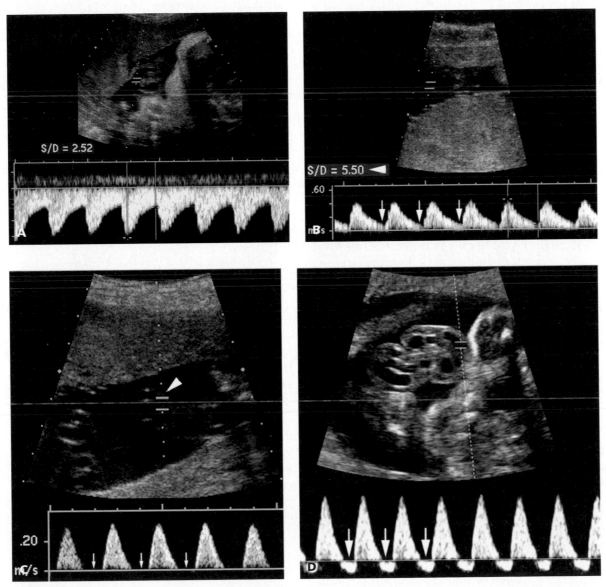

Figure 32-18 Umbilical artery Doppler. **A.** Spectral Doppler of umbilical artery in a 34-week fetus demonstrating a normal waveform with normal end-diastolic flow and normal S/D ratio (*calipers*) of 2.52. **B.** Doppler waveform of an abnormal umbilical artery with elevated S/D ratio to 5.50 (*arrowhead, calipers*), indicating diminished end-diastolic flow (*arrows*). **C.** Doppler interrogation of an abnormal umbilical artery (*arrowhead*) demonstrating absent end-diastolic flow (*arrows*) on the spectral waveform. **D.** Spectral Doppler of an abnormal umbilical artery demonstrating reversed end-diastolic flow (*arrows*), with systolic peaks seen as flow above the baseline and end-diastolic flow below the baseline.

Amniotic Fluid

Amniotic fluid appears sonographically as anechoic fluid surrounding the fetus. Echogenic debris in the amniotic fluid may be **vernix** or **meconium**, with meconium being the least likely to be observed during an otherwise normal examination. Amniotic fluid has a number of important functions, including protecting the fetus from trauma, temperature regulation, musculoskeletal maturity, and normal lung and gastrointestinal development. The fluid that is seen in early gestation is thought to arise from water and various other materials passing freely through the membranes surrounding the embryo. In the second half of the pregnancy, the fetal kidneys and lungs produce the majority of amniotic fluid, with urine being the greatest contributor.

The amount of amniotic fluid, or amniotic fluid volume, can be appraised using several sonographic techniques. The maximum vertical pocket, also referred to as the deepest vertical pocket, may be used. This pocket should contain no fetal parts or umbilical cord and measure at least 2 cm, with a normal range between 2 and 8 cm. The most widely accepted means of evaluating the volume of amniotic fluid is the **amniotic fluid index** (AFI). The AFI is measured using the anteroposterior dimensions obtained from the four quadrants of the amniotic sac and adding them together. Once more, these measurements should not include fetal parts or umbilical cord. Color Doppler can be used to ensure that no cord is included. For the measurement, the transducer must be placed perpendicular to the floor. The "normal" amount of fluid varies with gestation.

◀))) SOUND OFF
The AFI is measured using the anteroposterior dimensions obtained from the four quadrants of the amniotic sac and adding them together. The measurements should not include fetal parts or umbilical cord.

An excessive amount of amniotic fluid is termed polyhydramnios, whereas a deficient amount is termed **oligohydramnios**. When an abnormality is noted in the amount of amniotic fluid, a thorough evaluation of the fetal genitourinary system and gastrointestinal system for abnormalities should be conducted, although other systems may be the reason for the imbalance (Tables 32-7 and 32-8). Because the fetal kidneys produce a significant amount of amniotic fluid, when oligohydramnios is observed, abnormalities of the urinary system should be initially suspected. Amniotic fluid is also constantly being swallowed by the developing fetus and absorbed by the gastrointestinal tract. Therefore, when polyhydramnios is present, abnormalities of the fetal gastrointestinal system should be primarily suspected. Chapters 28 and 29 further stress the significance of understanding these relationships.

TABLE 32-7 Fetal malformation and complications associated with oligohydramnios

Bilateral **multicystic dysplastic kidney disease**

Bilateral renal agenesis

Infantile polycystic kidney disease

Intrauterine growth restriction

Posterior urethral valves

Premature rupture of membranes (PROM)

TABLE 32-8 Fetal malformations and complications associated with polyhydramnios

Cardiac and/or chest abnormalities

Chromosomal abnormalities

Duodenal atresia

Esophageal atresia

Gastroschisis

Neural tube defects

Omphalocele

Rh incompatibility

Twin–twin transfusion syndrome

Fetal Infections and TORCH

TORCH, an acronym that stands for *t*oxoplasmosis, *o*ther infections, *r*ubella, *c*ytomegalovirus, and *h*erpes simplex virus, is a group of infections that can cross the placenta and influence the development of the fetus. Among these, cytomegalovirus is listed as the most common congenital infection. Although additional abnormalities may be present, a common sonographic finding of fetal infections, especially with cytomegalovirus, is the presence of intracranial calcifications. Heart abnormalities, microphthalmia, microcephaly, ventriculomegaly, and hepatosplenomegaly may be noted as well (Fig. 32-19). Recently, the Zika virus has also been linked with microcephaly, decreased brain tissue, and limb abnormalities such as clubfoot.

SONOGRAPHIC FINDINGS OF TORCH

1. Intracranial calcifications
2. **Microcephaly**
3. Microphthalmia
4. Ventriculomegaly
5. Hepatosplenomegaly

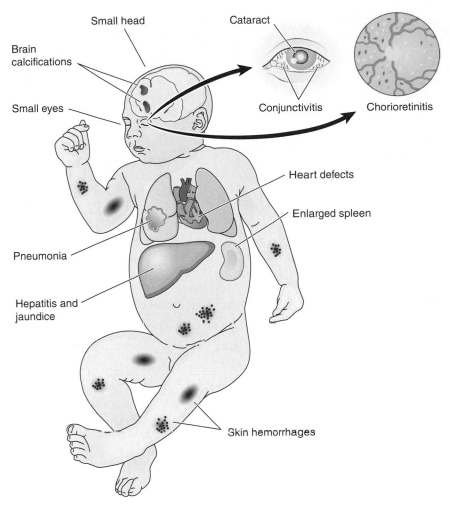

Figure 32-19 TORCH infections. Fetuses infected in the first trimester by toxoplasma, rubella, cytomegalovirus, herpes virus, or other microbes have similar clinical findings as those illustrated in this figure.

SOUND OFF
Cytomegalovirus is listed as the most common congenital infection.

Fetal Alcohol Syndrome

Fetal alcohol syndrome (FAS) includes a wide variety of deleterious effects of alcohol exposure upon the fetus caused by the maternal consumption of alcohol. Children exposed to alcohol in utero have been shown to have an increased risk for growth restriction, mental impairment, physical abnormalities, and immune dysfunction. FAS has been cited as the most common cause of intellectual disability in the United States. Alcohol, which is a teratogen, and its metabolites, have been proven to cross the placenta and inflict irreversible damage on the fetal central nervous system. Sonographic and clinical findings include microcephaly, dysgenesis of the corpus callosum, long round **philtrum**, malformed ears, microphthalmia, heart defects such as ventricular septal defects, and cleft palate (Fig. 32-20).

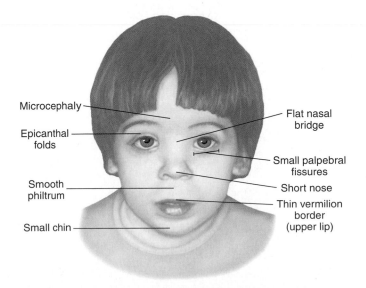

Figure 32-20 Clinical features of fetal alcohol syndrome.

SONOGRAPHIC FINDINGS OF FETAL ALCOHOL SYNDROME

1. Microcephaly
2. Dysgenesis of the corpus callosum
3. Long round philtrum
4. Malformed ears
5. Microphthalmia
6. Cleft palate
7. Heart defects such as ventricular septal defects

🔊 SOUND OFF

Children exposed to alcohol in utero have been shown to have an increased risk of growth restriction, mental impairment, physical abnormalities, and immune dysfunction.

Sonographic Assessment of Intrauterine Growth Restriction

Occasionally, small for dates or large for dates may be suspected clinically during an assessment of the mother's (uterine) fundal height (Fig. 32-21). Sonographic analysis may be requested to investigate for signs of IUGR. IUGR, or fetal growth restriction, is defined as an **estimated fetal weight** (EFW) that is below the 10th percentile at a given gestational age. IUGR typically results from the inadequate transfer of nutrients from the mother to the fetus and thus is the dysfunction of the placenta. The fetus is at risk if the mother suffers from chronic disease, drinks alcohol, smokes cigarettes, has poor nutrition, is younger than 17 or older than 35 years, or has a history of previous pregnancies that were considered growth restricted. IUGR can be either symmetric, in which the entire fetus is small, or asymmetric, wherein the femur length is typically normal while all other measurements are small for gestation. The measurement that should be scrutinized closely in fetuses that are at risk for growth abnormalities is the abdominal circumference (AC), because it carries a sensitivity of greater than 95% for the diagnosis of IUGR. The discrepancy in the AC will yield an abnormal head circumference/AC ratio and a femur length/AC ratio.

The growth-restricted fetus has an increased risk of suffering from physical handicaps and neurodevelopmental delays after birth. Asymmetric and symmetric IUGR appear to have diverse causes (Tables 32-9 and 32-10). The fetus with IUGR can be monitored with sonography by evaluating the flow within the umbilical artery with the S/D ratio mentioned earlier in this chapter. The S/D ratio evaluates the sufficiency of the placenta by means of pulsed Doppler interrogation of the umbilical artery. An abnormally high S/D ratio, resulting from a reversal or absence of diastolic flow within the umbilical artery, is associated with a poor outcome.

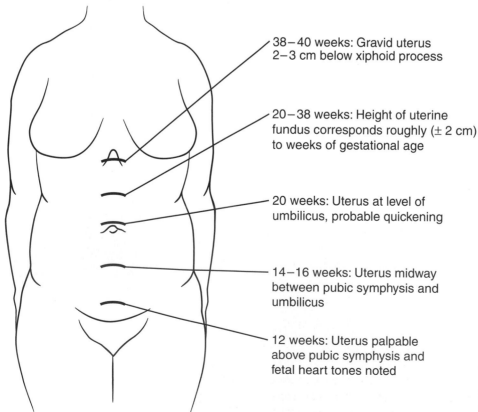

38–40 weeks: Gravid uterus 2–3 cm below xiphoid process

20–38 weeks: Height of uterine fundus corresponds roughly (± 2 cm) to weeks of gestational age

20 weeks: Uterus at level of umbilicus, probable quickening

14–16 weeks: Uterus midway between pubic symphysis and umbilicus

12 weeks: Uterus palpable above pubic symphysis and fetal heart tones noted

Figure 32-21 Uterine size (fundal height).

TABLE 32-9 Suspected causes of symmetric intrauterine growth restriction

Genetic disorders

Fetal infections

Congenital malformations

Syndromes

TABLE 32-10 Suspected causes of asymmetric intrauterine growth restriction

Nutritional deficiency

Oxygen deficiency

🔊 SOUND OFF
IUGR, or fetal growth restriction, is defined as an EFW that is below the 10th percentile at a given gestational age.

When a fetus presents with measurements that lead to suspected small for gestational age, sonography can further assess the pregnancy for signs of IUGR by performing the biophysical profile. A **biophysical profile** combines several fetal monitoring factors to produce a numeric scoring system that predicts fetal well-being. Biophysical profile scoring is discussed further in Chapter 22 of this book.

Doppler assessment of the middle cerebral artery has also been shown effective at evaluating for **hypoxia** in a fetus that is measuring small for dates. Chapter 24 discusses middle cerebral artery Doppler as well. The right and left middle cerebral arteries are branches of the anterior portion of the circle of Willis. Just like umbilical artery Doppler, the pulsatility index of the middle cerebral artery varies with gestational age but normally decreases as the pregnancy progresses toward term. When comparing the two Doppler signals, the middle cerebral artery should generate a higher resistance flow pattern than the umbilical artery.

Maternal uterine artery Doppler may be useful at anticipating the progression of IUGR in high-risk pregnancies. In the first trimester, the uterine artery is analyzed with spectral Doppler before it enters the uterus at the level cervix (Fig. 32-22). Occasional, the portion of the main uterine artery as it crosses over the external iliac artery may be utilized for this sample in the second/third trimester. The normal flow pattern is said to be low resistance. Therefore, an abnormal flow pattern will yield high resistance (high impedance index) within the uterine artery when IUGR is present. Abnormal flow may also be a forewarning of preeclampsia and preterm delivery.

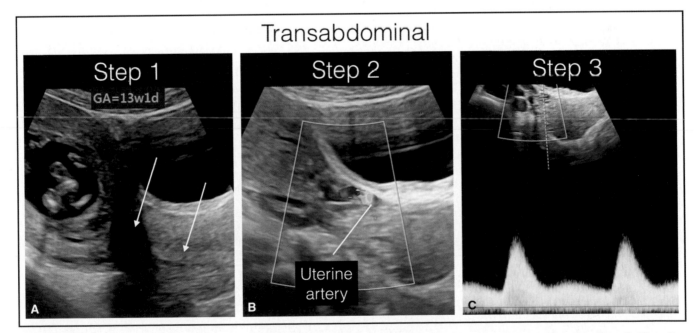

Figure 32-22 Steps for obtaining Doppler waveforms of the uterine artery by the transabdominal route. **Step 1.** Visualize the cervix in a sagittal view on two-dimensional sonography (*arrows*). **Step 2.** Activate color Doppler and tilt the transducer to left or right in a parasagittal plane until visualizing the left or right uterine artery, respectively. The uterine artery is seen crossing over the hypogastric vessels. **Step 3.** Sample the uterine artery with pulsed Doppler.

Large for Dates

The obese fetus is defined as a fetus that has an EFW of greater than the 90th percentile. In the **neonatal period**, **macrosomia** is technically defined as the neonate that measures more than 4,500 g in nondiabetic mothers and 4,000 g in diabetic mothers. Mothers who are prone to have a macrosomic fetus are those who suffer from diabetes, whether pregestational or gestational. A macrosomic fetus is predisposed to **shoulder dystocia** secondary to fetal size and has an increased risk of hypoglycemia and lifelong struggles with obesity. Therefore, they will most often be delivered by means of C-section.

> **SOUND OFF**
> The obese fetus is defined as a fetus that has an EFW of greater than the 90th percentile.

MATERNAL COMPLICATIONS

Translabial Scanning

Occasionally, during the second half of pregnancy, the cervix can be difficult to image with a transabdominal approach. Translabial scanning, also referred to as transperineal scanning, can offer a useful, noninvasive glimpse at the cervix. The sonographer can evaluate the length of the cervix and the proximity of the placenta to the internal os, and for signs of cervical incompetence using a translabial approach.

Translabial scanning should be performed with an empty maternal bladder. The covered transducer, whose size and frequency may vary with institution, is placed against the labia. The cervical length measurement can be obtained with a measurement from the internal os to the external os in the sagittal transducer position, or notch up (Fig. 32-23). The internal os should be observed several times throughout the examination when cervical incompetence is suspected, because the cervix is a dynamic structure whose shape and length can change over time. If the cervix is not seen because of shadowing from the pubic bone, the patient can slightly lift her hips off of the bed for an improved view of the external os. If translabial imaging does not provide optimal images, transvaginal imaging may be performed (Fig. 32-24). It is again important to note that the cervix can undergo dynamic changes and thus cervical length may fluctuate slightly. Therefore, a judicious examination should be conducted and the shortest measurement of the cervix recorded. A cine loop recording may be helpful in this situation as well.

Cervical Incompetence

Cervical incompetence, or an incompetent cervix, is the painless dilation of the cervix in the second or early third trimester. **Funneling** of the cervix is a result of the

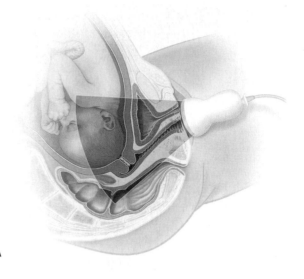

A

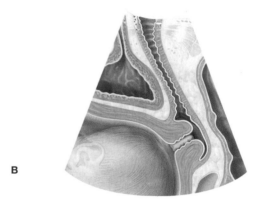

B

Figure 32-23 Translabial scanning. The transducer is covered and placed in a sagittal plane on the surface of labia (**A**). Schematic of the anatomy in the translabial view (**B**).

premature opening of the internal os and the subsequent bulging of the membranes into the dilated cervix. It is an early sign of an incompetent cervix. In cases of PROM, patients may have vaginal bleeding. Patients who are at risk for cervical incompetence include those with uterine malformations, previous pregnancy loss in the second trimester, and intrauterine exposure to **diethylstilbestrol**.

> **SOUND OFF**
> Funneling of the cervix is a result of the premature opening of the internal os and the subsequent bulging of the membranes into the dilated cervix.

A sonographic assessment of the cervix can be performed with transvaginal or translabial imaging as mentioned earlier. There are two measurements of the cervix that can be obtained utilizing these techniques. The most often employed sonographic measurement for the assessment of cervical incompetence is the length

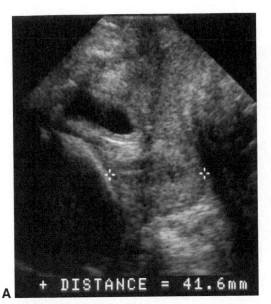

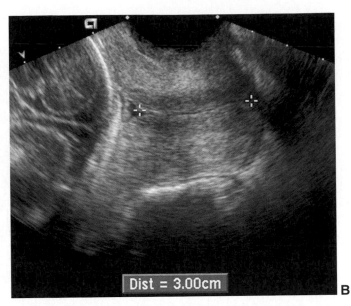

Figure 32-24 Normal cervix. **A.** Translabial demonstrating the cervix (between *calipers*). **B.** Transvaginal cervix (between *calipers*).

measurement taken from the internal os to the external os (Fig. 32-25). The cervical length should measure at least 3 cm. Therefore, the shorter the cervical length, the more likely the patient will suffer from preterm delivery. An additional measurement can be taken of the width of the funnel. The funnel may take on a "U" or "V" shape (Fig. 32-26).

The treatment of an incompetent cervix is a **cerclage**. The two most commonly performed cerclage techniques are the Shirodkar and the McDonald. The suture of the cerclage may be seen during a follow-up

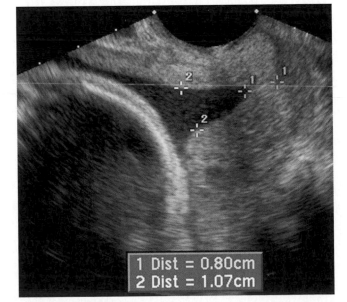

Figure 32-25 Short, funneled cervix. Transvaginal view of the cervix demonstrating that the cervix is 10.7 mm dilated (*#2 calipers*), with a residual cervix of only 8.0 mm (*#1 calipers*).

examination and will appear as echogenic structures within the cervix that may produce some posterior shadowing.

CLINICAL FINDINGS OF CERVICAL INCOMPETENCE
1. Painless dilation of the cervix
2. PROM
3. Vaginal bleeding

SONOGRAPHIC FINDINGS OF CERVICAL INCOMPETENCE
1. Cervical length of less than 3 cm
2. Funneling of the cervix (can produce a "U" or "V" shape)

Fetal Hydrops and Rh Sensitization

Fetal hydrops, also referred to as hydrops fetalis, occurs when there is an accumulation of fluid within at least two fetal body cavities. Fluid can collect within the chest (pleural effusion), the abdomen (ascites), or around the heart (pericardial). Hydrops may also be defined as **anasarca** and fluid in at least one of the previously listed body cavities. Fetal hydrops can be categorized as either immune or nonimmune. **Immune hydrops** is caused by the absence of a detectable circulating fetal antibody against the red blood cells in the mother. This results in incompatibility between the fetal and maternal red blood cells, a condition known as **erythroblastosis fetalis** (Fig. 32-27).

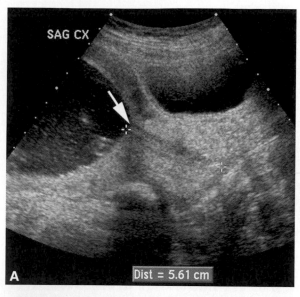

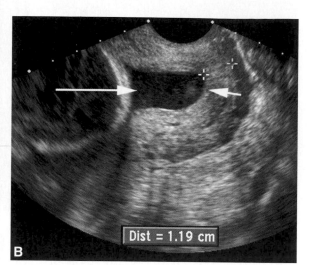

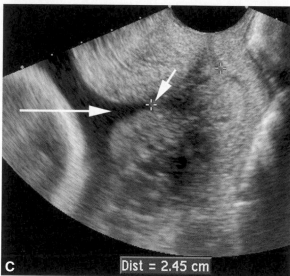

Figure 32-26 Normal cervix and incompetent cervix. **A.** Transabdominal measurement (*calipers*) when the internal os (*arrow*) is closed (i.e., no funneling). **B.** Transvaginal measurement (*calipers*) when the internal os (*long arrow*) is open and there is U-shaped funneling (*short arrow*). **C.** Transvaginal measurement (*calipers*) when the internal os (*long arrow*) is open and there is V-shaped funneling (*short arrow*).

> ((•)) **SOUND OFF**
> Immune hydrops is associated with ery-throblastosis fetalis and Rh isoimmunization.

Maternal Rh sensitization, also referred to as Rh isoimmunization, occurs when the mother has Rh-negative blood and the fetus has Rh-positive blood. Cells from the Rh-positive fetus enter the mother's bloodstream during her first pregnancy. Although antibodies are created in the maternal circulation, this pregnancy will progress normally. With the mother's next pregnancy, the Rh-positive fetus is attacked as a result of the antibodies produced during the first pregnancy. These antibodies cross the placenta and begin to destroy the fetal red blood cells, resulting in fetal anemia, enlargement of the fetal liver and spleen, and the accumulation of fluid within the fetal body cavities.

The prevention of immune hydrops caused by Rh sensitization is the administration of RhoGAM, also referred to as Rh immune globulin, at approximately 28 weeks' gestation. Treatment for fetal hydrops may be conducted via intrauterine transfusion of donor red blood cells to treat the anemic fetus. This is typically performed under sonographic guidance. It is often difficult to determine the cause of fetal hydrops by sonographic findings. Immune and **nonimmune hydrops** may lead to the accumulation of fluid within the abdomen, chest, scrotum, and skin. Table 32-11 provides the causes of nonimmune hydrops.

Maternal **mirror syndrome** is a rare disorder in which the mother suffers from edema and fluid buildup similar to her hydropic fetus. The reason for this syndrome is unknown.

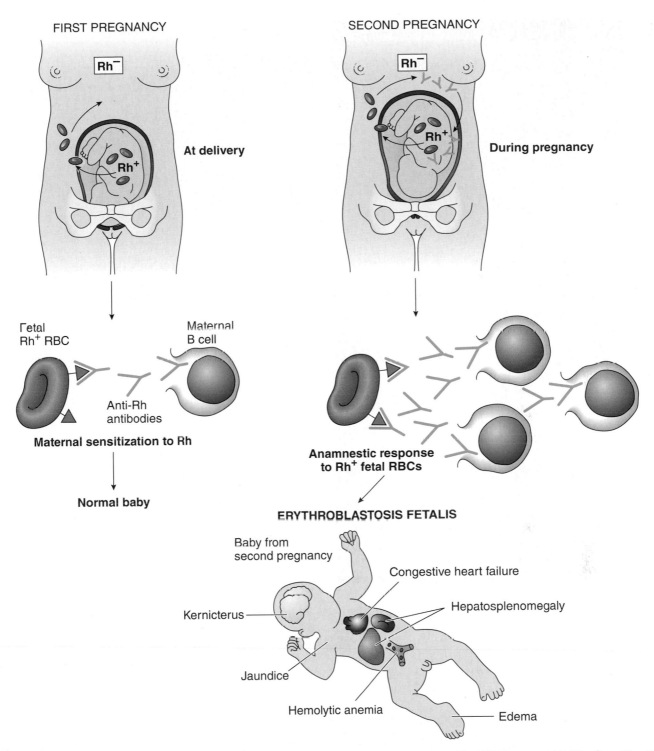

Figure 32-27 Erythroblastosis fetalis. Erythroblastosis fetalis is caused by maternal fetal Rh incompatibility. Sensitization of the Rh− mother with Rh+ RBCs in the first pregnancy leads to the formation of anti-Rh antibodies. These antibodies cross the placenta and damage the Rh+ fetus in subsequent pregnancies. *RBCs*, red blood cells.

TABLE 32-11 Causes of nonimmune hydrops

Chorioangioma

Cystic adenomatoid malformation

Diaphragmatic hernia

Fetal (nonimmune) anemia

Fetal infections

Idiopathic

Structural anomalies of the cardiac and lymphatic systems

Trisomy 13

Trisomy 18

Trisomy 21

Turner syndrome

SONOGRAPHIC FINDINGS OF FETAL HYDROPS

1. Fluid accumulation within at least two fetal body cavities (pleural effusion, ascites, skin edema, pericardial effusion)
2. Fetal hepatosplenomegaly
3. Polyhydramnios
4. Thickened placenta

CLINICAL FINDINGS OF PREECLAMPSIA

1. Maternal hypertension
2. Maternal edema
3. Maternal proteinuria

CLINICAL FINDINGS OF ECLAMPSIA

1. Long-standing, uncontrolled preeclampsia
2. Headaches
3. Seizures

CLINICAL FINDINGS OF HELLP SYNDROME

1. Hemolysis
2. Elevated liver enzymes
3. Low platelet count

SONOGRAPHIC FINDINGS OF PREECLAMPSIA, ECLAMPSIA, AND HELLP SYNDROME

1. Oligohydramnios
2. IUGR
3. Gestational trophoblastic disease
4. Increased risk for placental abruption
5. Elevated S/D ratio
6. Right upper quadrant pain, nausea, and vomiting simulating gallbladder disease with HELLP syndrome

Preeclampsia and Eclampsia

Preeclampsia is defined as the presence of pregnancy-induced hypertension accompanied by **proteinuria**. The mother may also suffer from edema in the hands, face, and legs. Uncontrolled preeclampsia leads to eclampsia, which is potentially fatal. Patients with eclampsia will have headaches and often suffer from convulsions. Those with an increased risk of preeclampsia include advanced maternal age, diabetic patients, and those who have **gestational trophoblastic disease**. **HELLP syndrome**, which stands for hemolysis, elevated liver enzymes, and low platelet count, was said to be a variant of preeclampsia initially, but now it appears to be a separate entity. The sonographic findings for these abnormalities may include oligohydramnios, IUGR, gestational trophoblastic disease, increased risk for placental abruption, or an elevated S/D ratio. Patients with HELLP syndrome may present with right upper quadrant, nausea, and vomiting, which are symptoms similar to gallbladder disease.

Maternal Diabetes

Maternal diabetes can be described as either pregestational diabetes or **gestational diabetes**. With pregestational diabetes, the mother already has a history of diabetes. Gestational diabetes, which is the most common type of diabetes during pregnancy, is pregnancy induced. Women are screened for diabetes at the end of the second trimester, around 26 weeks' gestation. The major risk for the fetus of a mother with gestational diabetes is macrosomia. Sonographically, the placenta may appear enlarged (placentomegaly), measuring greater than 4 cm thick. There may also be polyhydramnios, and the AC typically measures significantly larger than the other measurements. Pregnancy-induced diabetes resolves shortly after birth.

Mothers with pregestational diabetes have a higher risk of miscarriage and toxemia, and the fetus has an increased risk of congenital anomalies, hypoglycemia, respiratory distress, perinatal mortality, and IUGR. The congenital anomalies most often encountered with pregestational diabetes include cardiac defects, neural tube defects, caudal regression syndrome, sirenomelia, and renal anomalies.

🔊 **SOUND OFF**
Mothers with pregestational diabetes have a higher risk of miscarriage and toxemia, and the fetus has an increased risk of congenital anomalies, hypoglycemia, respiratory distress, perinatal mortality, and IUGR.

Bladder Flap Hematoma

A bladder flap hematoma may result from a C-section. This mass can appear anechoic, although it most likely will appear as a complex mass greater than 2 cm. It will be located adjacent to the scar between the lower uterine segment and the posterior bladder wall.

CLINICAL FINDINGS OF BLADDER FLAP HEMATOMA

1. Recent C-section

SONOGRAPHIC FINDINGS OF BLADDER FLAP HEMATOMA

1. Anechoic or complex mass located between the lower uterine segment and the posterior bladder wall

Leiomyoma and Pregnancy

A **leiomyoma**, commonly referred to as a fibroid, is a common benign smooth muscle uterine tumor. They are often asymptomatic during pregnancy, although they may be associated with some pregnancy complications, such as an elevated pregnancy loss rate and increased risk of placental abruption. Occasionally, fibroids can grow during pregnancy secondary to estrogen stimulation and may prevent vaginal delivery if located within the lower uterine segment. Fibroids should be differentiated from normal myometrial contractions. Myometrial contractions typically resolve within 15 to 30 minutes, whereas fibroids will not change in shape.

SONOGRAPHIC FINDINGS OF A LEIOMYOMA

1. Hypoechoic mass within the uterus
2. Posterior shadowing from mass
3. Degenerating fibroids may have calcifications or cystic components
4. Multiple fibroids appear as an enlarged, irregularly shaped, diffusely heterogeneous uterus

Maternal Hydronephrosis

Maternal **hydronephrosis** is common during pregnancy. Dilation of the renal collecting system is most often secondary to the large size of the uterus, with subsequent transient painless obstruction of the ureters. However, maternal hydronephrosis can also be caused by urinary calculi, in which case the patient will suffer from renal colic, flank pain, and hematuria.

Retained Products of Conception

The normal **postpartum** uterus returns to its **nongravid** size 6 to 8 weeks after delivery. Excessive and sustained postpartum vaginal bleeding may be the result of **retained products of conception** (RPOC). Most often, part of the placenta is left behind at the time of delivery. There are several predisposing factors, including adhesions, accessory lobes of the placenta, and placenta accreta.

Sonographically, RPOC may be seen as an echogenic intracavitary mass within the endometrium (Fig. 32-28). Unfortunately, an echogenic blood clot can appear similar and may also be seen after pregnancy. No evidence of an endometrial fluid collection or mass within the endometrium, and an endometrial measurement of less than 10 mm, is less likely to be RPOC. Color Doppler can help prove that retained placental tissue is present, because flow will be noted within the retained placental segment. RPOC is typically treated with dilatation and curettage.

CLINICAL FINDINGS OF RETAINED PRODUCTS OF CONCEPTION

1. Postpartum vaginal bleeding

SONOGRAPHIC FINDINGS OF RETAINED PRODUCTS OF CONCEPTION

1. Echogenic intracavitary mass that may contain some calcifications
2. Color Doppler signals within the retained placental tissue

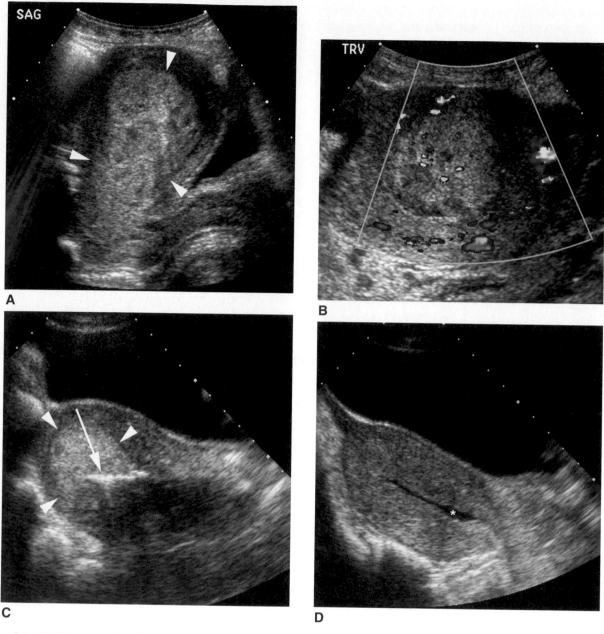

Figure 32-28 Ultrasound-guided evacuation of retained products of conception. **A.** Sagittal transabdominal image of the uterus of a woman who suffered a recent miscarriage demonstrates a soft-tissue mass (*arrowheads*) in the uterine cavity. **B.** Transverse transabdominal view, with blood flow identified within the mass on color Doppler. The mass represents retained products of conception. **C.** A suction device (*arrow*) lies within the retained products of conception (*arrowheads*). **D.** At the end of the procedure, there is a small amount of fluid (*asterisk*) in the uterine cavity, but no abnormal tissue remains.

REVIEW QUESTIONS

1. What does Figure 32-29 demonstrate?
   a. Placental abruption
   b. Complete placenta previa
   c. Partial placenta previa
   d. Incomplete abruption

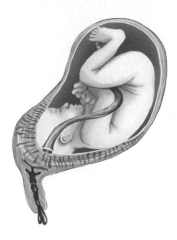

Figure 32-29

2. What is the diagnosis depicted in Figure 32-30?
   a. Complete placenta previa
   b. Low-lying placenta previa
   c. Marginal placenta previa
   d. Normal placental location

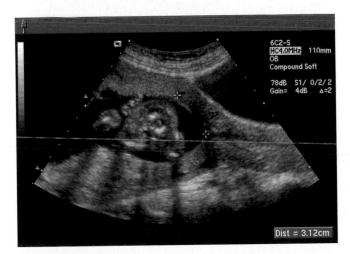

Figure 32-30

3. What does the arrowhead in Figure 32-31 indicate?
   a. Internal os
   b. External os
   c. Vagina
   d. Cervical canal

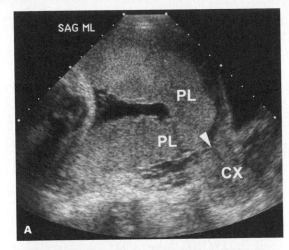

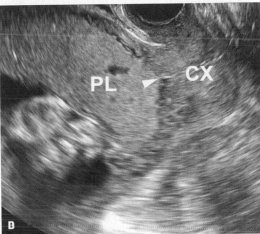

Figure 32-31

4. What does the arrow in Figure 32-32 indicate?
   a. Circumvallate placenta
   b. Synechia
   c. Chorionic villi
   d. Placental abruption

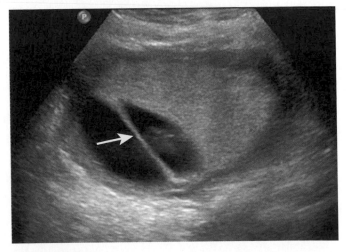

Figure 32-32

5. What sonographic finding is evident in Figure 32-33?
   a. Succenturiate lobe
   b. Bilobed placenta
   c. Circumvallate placenta
   d. Placental abruption

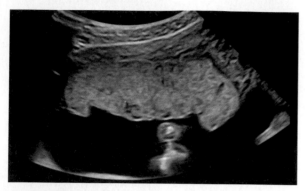

Figure 32-33

6. The hypoechoic regions noted within the placenta in Figure 32-34 most likely represent:
   a. fibrous deposits.
   b. chorioangiomas.
   c. maternal lakes.
   d. hemangiomas.

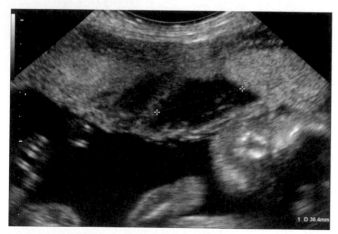

Figure 32-34

7. The mass in Figure 32-35 was noted during a routine sonogram. What is the most likely diagnosis?
   a. Venous lake
   b. Chorioangioma
   c. Choriocarcinoma
   d. Hemangioma

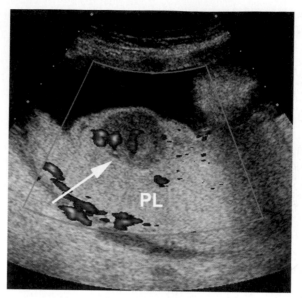

Figure 32-35

8. The patient in Figure 32-36 was suffering from a small amount of vaginal spotting. Which of the following is the likely diagnosis?
   a. Placenta previa
   b. Placenta accreta
   c. Placental abruption
   d. Placenta percreta

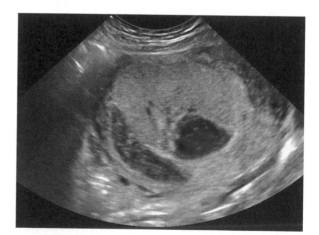

Figure 32-36

9. The patient in Figure 32-37 presented with hematuria and had a history of prior C-section. What is the most likely diagnosis?
   a. Placental abruption
   b. Placenta accreta
   c. Placenta increta
   d. Placenta percreta

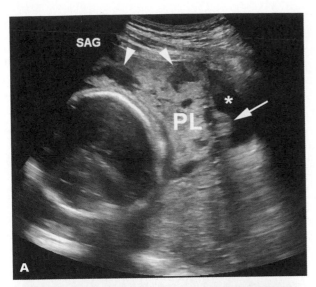

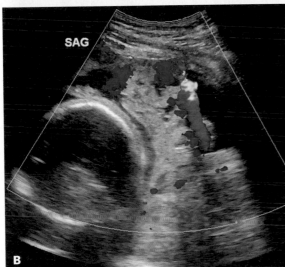

Figure 32-37

10. Figure 32-38 is a transverse image of the cervical spine. What is the most likely diagnosis?
    a. Marginal cord insertion
    b. Umbilical varix
    c. 2VC
    d. Nuchal cord

11. What is evident in Figure 32-39?
    a. 2VC
    b. Umbilical vein varix
    c. Allantoic cyst
    d. Umbilical cord torsion

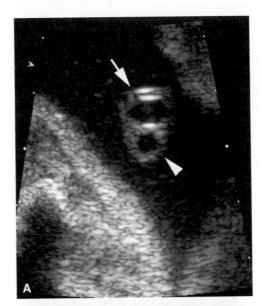

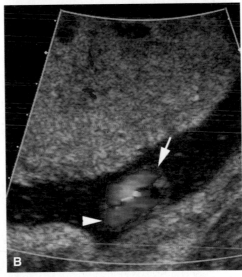

Figure 32-39

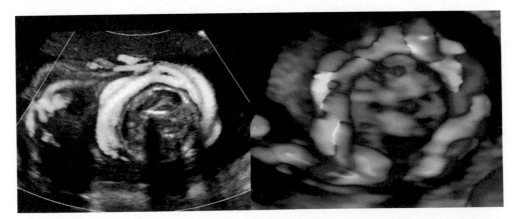

Figure 32-38

12. Which of the following is the most common TORCH infection?
    a. Toxoplasmosis
    b. Zika
    c. Herpes simplex
    d. Cytomegalovirus

13. Protective skin covering that may be sloughed off during pregnancy is referred to as:
    a. vernix.
    b. meconium.
    c. allantoic.
    d. varix.

14. Which of the following is described as the focal dilation of the abdominal portion of the umbilical vein?
    a. Allantoic cyst
    b. Umbilical cord varix
    c. Umbilical cord aneurysm
    d. Umbilical cord berry

15. The umbilical cord forms from the fusion of what two structures?
    a. Placenta and yolk sac
    b. Chorion and amnion
    c. Omphalomesenteric duct and yolk stalk
    d. Decidua basalis and decidua parietalis

16. What is the philtrum?
    a. Nasal tissue between the nostrils
    b. Ear lobe
    c. Vertical groove between the upper lip and the nasal septum
    d. Space between the outer canthus of each eye

17. Which of the following is not associated with FAS?
    a. Cleft palate
    b. Microphthalmia
    c. Malformed ears
    d. Macrocephaly

18. A macrosomic fetus is predisposed to suffer from:
    a. IUGR.
    b. TORCH infections.
    c. shoulder dystocia.
    d. eclampsia.

19. Which of the following is used to surgically treat an incompetent cervix?
    a. Cervical flap
    b. Cerclage
    c. Philtrum
    d. Pessary

20. Which of the following is not included in HELLP syndrome?
    a. Pyuria
    b. Hemolysis
    c. Elevated liver enzymes
    d. Low platelet count

21. Nonimmune hydrops is associated with all of the following except:
    a. RH isoimmunization.
    b. pleural effusion.
    c. Turner syndrome.
    d. fetal infections.

22. The maternal contribution to the placenta is the:
    a. chorionic vera.
    b. decidua vera.
    c. decidua basalis.
    d. chorion frondosum.

23. The placenta releases _____ to maintain the corpus luteum.
    a. human chorionic gonadotropin
    b. follicle-stimulating hormone
    c. luteinizing hormone
    d. gonadotropin-stimulating hormone

24. An anechoic mass is noted within the umbilical cord during a routine sonographic examination. What is the most likely diagnosis?
    a. Hemangioma
    b. Vasa previa
    c. Chorioangioma
    d. Allantoic cyst

25. With Rh isoimmunization, the maternal antibodies cross the placenta and destroy the fetal:
    a. spleen.
    b. red blood cells.
    c. liver.
    d. white blood cells.

26. Mothers with pregestational diabetes, as opposed to gestational diabetes, have an increased risk of a fetus with:
    a. neural tube defects.
    b. proteinuria.
    c. TORCH.
    d. diethylstilbestrol.

27. A succenturiate lobe of the placenta refers to a(n):
    a. bilobed placental lobe.
    b. circumvallate placental lobe.
    c. accessory lobe.
    d. circummarginate placental lobe.

28. Pools of maternal blood noted within the placental substance are referred to as:
    a. accessory lobes.
    b. decidual casts.
    c. chorioangiomas.
    d. maternal lakes.

29. The fetal contribution of the placenta is the:
    a. chorionic vera.
    b. decidua vera.
    c. decidua basalis.
    d. chorion frondosum.

30. Which of the following would be least likely associated with immune hydrops?
    a. Fetal hepatomegaly
    b. Fetal splenomegaly
    c. Anasarca
    d. Leiomyoma

31. The placenta is considered too thick when it measures:
    a. greater than 4 mm.
    b. greater than 4 cm.
    c. greater than 8 mm.
    d. greater than 3.5 cm.

32. All of the following are associated with a thin placenta except:
    a. preeclampsia.
    b. IUGR.
    c. fetal hydrops.
    d. long-standing diabetes.

33. What would be most likely confused for a uterine leiomyoma?
    a. Placental infarct
    b. Chorioangioma
    c. Myometrial contraction
    d. Placenta previa

34. When the placenta completely covers the internal os, it is referred to as:
    a. low-lying previa.
    b. marginal previa.
    c. partial previa.
    d. total previa.

35. One of the most common causes of painless vaginal bleeding in the second and third trimesters is:
    a. spontaneous abortion.
    b. abruptio placentae.
    c. placenta previa.
    d. placenta accreta.

36. All of the following are associated with a thick placenta except:
    a. fetal infections.
    b. Rh isoimmunization.
    c. placental insufficiency.
    d. multiple gestations.

37. Placenta accreta denotes:
    a. the abnormal attachment of the placenta to the myometrium.
    b. the premature separation of the placenta from the uterine wall.
    c. the invasion of the placenta into the myometrium.
    d. the condition of having the fetal vessels rest over the internal os.

38. Doppler sonography reveals vascular structures coursing over the internal os of the cervix. This finding is indicative of:
    a. vasa previa.
    b. placenta previa.
    c. placenta increta.
    d. abruptio placentae.

39. All of the following are clinical features of placental abruption except:
    a. vaginal bleeding.
    b. uterine tenderness.
    c. abdominal pain.
    d. funneling of the cervix.

40. Penetration of the placenta beyond the uterine wall would be referred to as:
    a. placenta accreta.
    b. placenta increta.
    c. placenta previa.
    d. placenta percreta.

41. All of the following are associated with oligohydramnios except:
    a. bilateral renal agenesis.
    b. infantile polycystic kidney disease.
    c. PROM.
    d. duodenal atresia.

42. The most common placental tumor is the:
    a. choriocarcinoma.
    b. maternal lake.
    c. chorioangioma.
    d. allantoic cyst.

43. Pregnancy-induced maternal high blood pressure and excess protein in the urine after 20 weeks' gestation is termed:
    a. preeclampsia.
    b. gestational diabetes.
    c. eclampsia.
    d. gestational trophoblastic disease.

44. The normal umbilical cord has:
    a. one vein and one artery.
    b. two veins and two arteries.
    c. two veins and one artery.
    d. two arteries and one vein.

45. Insertion of the umbilical cord at the edge of the placenta is referred to as:
    a. velamentous cord insertion.
    b. partial cord insertion.
    c. marginal cord insertion.
    d. nuchal cord insertion.

46. Increased S/D ratio is associated with all of the following except:
    a. IUGR.
    b. placental insufficiency.
    c. allantoic cysts.
    d. perinatal mortality.

47. A velamentous cord insertion is associated with which of the following?
    a. Placenta increta
    b. Placental abruption
    c. Vasa previa
    d. Circumvallate placenta

48. The normal umbilical cord insertion point into the placenta is:
    a. central.
    b. superior margin.
    c. inferior margin.
    d. lateral margin.

49. Normally, the S/D ratio:
    a. increases with advancing gestation.
    b. decreases with advancing gestation.
    c. reverses occasionally during a normal pregnancy.
    d. has an absent diastolic component.

50. Fetal TORCH is frequently associated with:
    a. maternal hypertension.
    b. twin–twin transfusion syndrome.
    c. intracranial calcifications.
    d. renal cystic disease.

51. Evidence of polyhydramnios should warrant a careful investigation of the fetal:
    a. genitourinary system.
    b. gastrointestinal system.
    c. extremities.
    d. cerebrovascular system.

52. All of the following are associated with polyhydramnios except:
    a. omphalocele.
    b. gastroschisis.
    c. esophageal atresia.
    d. bilateral multicystic dysplastic kidney disease.

53. IUGR is evident when the EFW is:
    a. above the 90th percentile.
    b. below the 90th percentile.
    c. above the 10th percentile.
    d. below the 10th percentile.

54. The cervix should measure at least _____ in length.
    a. 4 cm
    b. 5 cm
    c. 3 cm
    d. 8 mm

55. The abnormal insertion of the umbilical cord into the membranes beyond the placental edge is termed:
    a. placenta previa.
    b. placental abruption.
    c. marginal insertion.
    d. velamentous insertion.

56. The measurement that should be carefully scrutinized in cases of IUGR is the:
    a. AC.
    b. femur length.
    c. biparietal diameter.
    d. head circumference.

57. Doppler assessment of the middle cerebral artery:
    a. helps to determine whether fetal anorexia is occurring.
    b. is valuable in diagnosing the extent of ventriculomegaly.
    c. can evaluate the fetus for hypoxia.
    d. is important to determine whether TORCH complications are present.

58. Mothers with gestational diabetes run the risk of having fetuses that are considered:
    a. nutritionally deficient.
    b. acromegalic.
    c. microsomic.
    d. macrosomic.

59. Which of the following is described as the situation in which the placental edge extends into the lower uterine segment but ends more than 2 cm away from the internal os?
    a. Low-lying placenta
    b. Marginal previa
    c. Partial previa
    d. Total previa

60. Which of the following would increase the likelihood of developing placenta previa?
    a. Vaginal bleeding
    b. Previous cesarean section
    c. Corpus albicans
    d. Chorioangioma

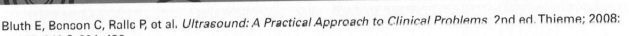

SUGGESTED READINGS

Bluth E, Benson C, Ralls P, et al. *Ultrasound: A Practical Approach to Clinical Problems.* 2nd ed. Thieme; 2008: 307–346 & 394–436.

Curry RA & Prince M. *Sonography: Introduction to Normal Structure and Function.* 5th ed. Elsevier; 2020:385–430.

Doubilet PM, Benson CB. *Atlas of Ultrasound in Obstetrics and Gynecology: A Multimedia Reference.* 2nd ed. Wolters Kluwer; 2012:259–297.

Gibbs RS, Karlan BY, Haney AF, et al. *Danforth's Obstetrics and Gynecology.* 10th ed. Wolters Kluwer; 2008:198–219, 246–275.

Henningsen C, Kuntz K, Youngs D. *Clinical Guide to Sonography: Exercises for Critical Thinking.* 2nd ed. Elsevier; 2014:225–227, 237–241.

Hertzberg BS, Middleton WD. *Ultrasound: The Requisites.* 3rd ed. Elsevier; 2016:469–495.

Hickey J, Goldberg F. *Ultrasound Review of Obstetrics and Gynecology.* Lippincott–Raven; 1996:135–171.

Kline-Fath BM, Bulas DI, Lee W. *Fundamental and Advanced Fetal Imaging: Ultrasound and MRI.* 2nd ed. Wolters Kluwer; 2021:280–351.

Norton ME, Scoutt LM, Feldstein VA. *Callen's Ultrasonography in Obstetrics and Gynecology.* 6th ed. Elsevier; 2017:633–703.

Nyberg D, McGaham J, Pretorius D, et al. *Diagnostic Imaging of Fetal Anomalies.* Lippincott Williams & Wilkins; 2003:85–132.

Rumack CM, Wilson SR, William Charboneau J, et al. *Diagnostic Ultrasound.* 4th ed. Elsevier; 2011:1472–1542.

Sadan O, Golan A, Girtler O, et al. Role of sonography in the diagnosis of retained products of conception. *J Ultrasound Med.* 2005;24:1181–1186.

Sanders RC, Hall-Terracciano B. *Clinical Sonography: A Practical Guide.* 5th ed. Wolters Kluwer; 2016:261–277.

Zika Virus. Microcephaly & other birth defects. https://www.cdc.gov/zika/healtheffects/birth_defects.html. Accessed February 18, 2017.

BONUS REVIEW!

Calcified Retained Products of Conception (Fig. 32-40)

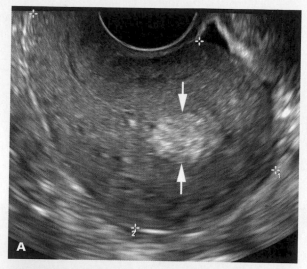

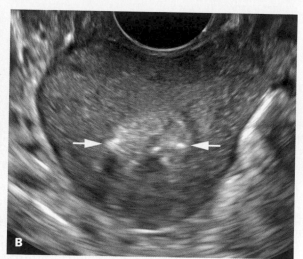

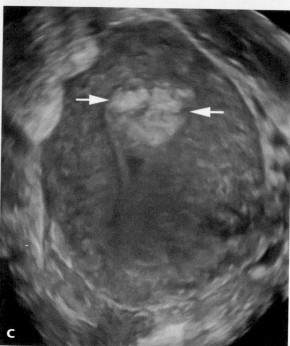

Figure 32-40 Calcified retained products of conception. Longitudinal (**A**) and transverse (**B**) transvaginal views of the uterus in a woman several months postpartum reveals an echogenic mass in the mid-uterus (*arrows*) with areas of calcification. **C.** Three-dimensional coronal rendering showing the echogenic mass (*arrows*) in the upper uterine cavity.

Sonographic Image Following Cerclage Placement (Fig. 32-41)

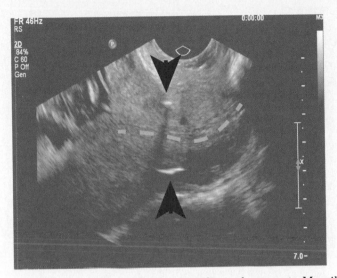

Figure 32-41 Transvaginal sonographic image following cerclage placement. Mersilene, which are sutures, are demonstrated by *red arrows*. Resulting cervical length are marked with *dotted blue line*.

Umbilical Venous Varix (Fig. 32-42)

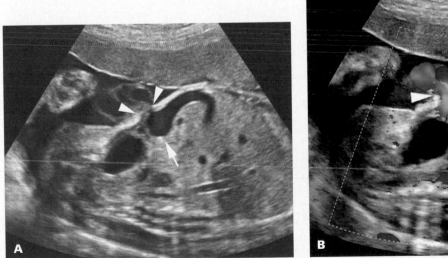
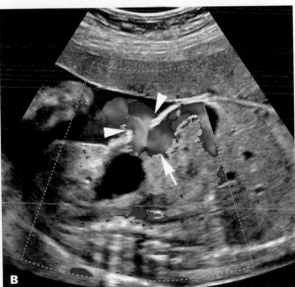

Figure 32-42 Umbilical venous varix. Sagittal grayscale (**A**) and color Doppler (**B**) of 27-week fetal abdomen demonstrating dilatation of the umbilical vein (*arrow*) inside the abdomen near the cord insertion (*arrowheads*).

Answers to Review Questions

Chapter 1	23. C	46. C	8. C
1. B	24. B	47. A	9. A
2. B	25. A	48. B	10. B
3. D	26. C	49. D	11. D
4. A	27. B	50. A	12. A
5. A	28. D	51. C	13. A
6. B	29. B	52. A	14. B
7. C	30. A	53. B	15. D
8. B	31. B	54. D	16. B
9. C	32. A	55. B	17. C
10. C	33. D	56. C	18. A
11. D	34. C	57. C	19. C
12. B	35. B	58. D	20. D
13. A	36. A	59. A	21. D
14. D	37. B	60. B	22. B
15. A	38. A	**Chapter 2**	23. A
16. D	39. C	1. C	24. B
17. C	40. D	2. D	25. C
18. A	41. B	3. A	26. C
19. D	42. D	4. B	27. C
20. B	43. B	5. B	28. D
21. D	44. D	6. C	29. C
22. C	45. A	7. D	30. D

31. A
32. B
33. D
34. B
35. B
36. A
37. D
38. D
39. C
40. D
41. D
42. B
43. A
44. D
45. D
46. C
47. A
48. D
49. A
50. A
51. C
52. C
53. A
54. D
55. B
56. D
57. A
58. B

59. B
60. C

Chapter 3

1. C
2. B
3. C
4. B
5. D
6. C
7. C
8. A
9. A
10. C
11. B
12. D
13. A
14. D
15. C
16. A
17. C
18. A
19. B
20. B
21. A
22. A
23. B
24. B
25. D

26. A
27. C
28. D
29. B
30. C
31. D
32. D
33. C
34. C
35. A
36. C
37. A
38. A
39. C
40. B
41. D
42. A
43. C
44. C
45. A
46. A
47. D
48. D
49. C
50. A
51. C
52. C
53. B

54. A
55. A
56. C
57. D
58. C
59. B
60. A

Chapter 4

1. A
2. C
3. C
4. A
5. B
6. D
7. B
8. C
9. C
10. A
11. D
12. B
13. A
14. A
15. D
16. C
17. C
18. A
19. B
20. A

21. B
22. D
23. C
24. C
25. B
26. A
27. D
28. C
29. D
30. A
31. B
32. D
33. C
34. B
35. C
36. D
37. B
38. D
39. A
40. D
41. C
42. D
43. A
44. C
45. D
46. D
47. A
48. D
49. D

50. A
51. D
52. D
53. C
54. A
55. B
56. A
57. C
58. B
59. A
60. C

Chapter 5

1. A
2. B
3. A
4. B
5. B
6. D
7. C
8. D
9. A
10. C
11. A
12. D
13. B
14. C
15. B
16. A
17. D

18. B
19. C
20. A
21. C
22. C
23. B
24. D
25. D
26. A
27. D
28. C
29. A
30. C
31. A
32. C
33. C
34. D
35. B
36. B
37. A
38. D
39. C
40. A
41. A
42. C
43. D
44. D
45. A
46. B

47. C
48. A
49. B
50. A
51. C
52. A
53. B
54. D
55. A
56. D
57. B
58. C
59. D
60. A

Chapter 6

1. D
2. C
3. B
4. A
5. D
6. A
7. A
8. B
9. B
10. B
11. C
12. A
13. D
14. A

15. A

16. B

17. B

18. A

19. D

20. C

21. C

22. D

23. A

24. A

25. C

26. B

27. D

28. C

29. C

30. A

31. B

32. C

33. B

34. C

35. D

36. A

37. A

38. C

39. B

40. C

41. D

42. C

43. A

44. B

45. D

46. A

47. C

48. B

49. A

50. C

51. A

52. D

53. C

54. C

55. A

56. B

57. B

58. D

59. B

60. C

Chapter 7

1. B

2. A

3. C

4. D

5. D

6. A

7. A

8. D

9. C

10. D

11. B

12. A

13. D

14. B

15. D

16. A

17. C

18. A

19. B

20. C

21. A

22. A

23. B

24. B

25. C

26. D

27. C

28. D

29. C

30. B

31. D

32. B

33. D

34. C

35. B

36. C

37. D

38. A

39. C

40. C

41. D

42. D

43. B

44. A

45. B

46. A

47. A

48. A

49. D

50. B

51. A

52. B

53. C

54. A

55. D

56. B

57. D

58. B

59. B

60. D

Chapter 8

1. A

2. D

3. A

4. B

5. B

6. B

7. C

8. D

9.	B	38.	A	6.	C	35.	C
10.	B	39.	D	7.	A	36.	D
11.	D	40.	C	8.	C	37.	D
12.	A	41.	B	9.	C	38.	C
13.	B	42.	C	10.	A	39.	D
14.	A	43.	D	11.	D	40.	B
15.	C	44.	A	12.	A	41.	D
16.	A	45.	C	13.	D	42.	A
17.	D	46.	C	14.	C	43.	C
18.	B	47.	D	15.	B	44.	C
19.	D	48.	A	16.	A	45.	B
20.	C	49.	C	17.	B	46.	B
21.	C	50.	A	18.	B	47.	D
22.	A	51.	C	19.	D	48.	C
23.	D	52.	A	20.	A	49.	C
24.	C	53.	D	21.	C	50.	B
25.	D	54.	B	22.	C	51.	B
26.	A	55.	A	23.	B	52.	A
27.	D	56.	D	24.	A	53.	A
28.	C	57.	A	25.	B	54.	B
29.	A	58.	B	26.	D	55.	A
30.	D	59.	B	27.	B	56.	D
31.	B	60.	D	28.	A	57.	B
32.	B	**Chapter 9**		29.	D	58.	B
33.	D	1.	A	30.	B	59.	C
34.	C	2.	D	31.	A	60.	A
35.	D	3.	B	32.	D	**Chapter 10**	
36.	B	4.	C	33.	D	1.	B
37.	A	5.	D	34.	A	2.	D

3. C

4. A

5. D

6. B

7. D

8. C

9. B

10. C

11. A

12. B

13. D

14. A

15. A

16. D

17. D

18. D

19. A

20. B

21. D

22. C

23. A

24. A

25. B

26. A

27. B

28. C

29. D

30. D

31. C

32. C

33. D

34. C

35. B

36. C

37. A

38. C

39. A

40. D

41. A

42. D

43. B

44. B

45. C

46. A

47. C

48. C

49. B

50. C

51. B

52. D

53. D

54. A

55. C

56. A

57. A

58. D

59. A

60. B

Chapter 11

1. C

2. B

3. D

4. B

5. B

6. C

7. C

8. D

9. A

10. B

11. B

12. B

13. C

14. D

15. A

16. D

17. C

18. A

19. C

20. A

21. B

22. A

23. C

24. B

25. D

26. C

27. D

28. D

29. A

30. A

31. D

32. C

33. A

34. C

35. B

36. A

37. D

38. A

39. D

40. A

41. C

42. A

43. B

44. C

45. D

46. B

47. A

48. A

49. B

50. A

51. D

52. A

53. C

54. B

55. C

56. A

57. B

58. D

59. D

60. D

Chapter 12

1. B

2. A

3. A

4. C

5. D

6. D

7. B

8. A

9. D

10. B

11. C

12. B

13. A

14. C

15. A

16. D

17. A

18. B

19. D

20. B

21. A

22. C

23. B

24. A

25. A

26. D

27. D

28. C

29. A

30. B

31. B

32. D

33. D

34. B

35. B

36. A

37. D

38. C

39. B

40. C

41. C

42. B

43. B

44. B

45. B

46. A

47. A

48. A

49. D

50. D

51. D

52. D

53. C

54. C

55. B

56. A

57. B

58. A

59. D

60. A

Chapter 13

1. C

2. C

3. A

4. B

5. D

6. C

7. B

8. D

9. A

10. C

11. D

12. C

13. C

14. A

15. B

16. C

17. D

18. B

19. C

20. A

21. A

22. B

23. A

24. B

25. B

26. C

27. C

28. C

29. A

30. D

31. B

32. C

33. D

34. C

35. D

36. C

37. A

38. A

39. A

40. B

41. D

42. B

43. D

44. C

45. D

46. C

47. D

48. D

49. C

50. A

51. A

52. A

53. B

54. C

55. B

56. B

57. A

58. A

59. D

60. D

Chapter 14

1. A

2. B

3. D

4. B

5. A

6. C

7. D

8. C

9. D

10. D

11. B

12. D

13. C

14. C

15. A

16. D

17. A

18. D

19. D

20. B

21. A

22. C

23. A

24. B

25. C

26. A

27. D

28. C

29. C

30. A

31. A

32. B

33. D

34. B

35. A

36. C

37. B

38. D

39. A

40. A

41. C

42. B

43. A

44. D

45. A

46. D

47. A

48. A

49. B

50. C

51. A

52. A

53. A

54. D

55. C

56. D

57. A

58. D

59. B

60. D

Chapter 15

1. D

2. B

3. A

4. C

5. C

6. D

7. A

8. B

9. D

10. A

11. C

12. A

13. B

14. A

15. C

16. D

17. D

18. B

19. C

20. C

21. A

22. C

23. C

24. B

25. A

26. D

27. D

28. B

29. D

30. A

31. D

32. B

33. A

34. D

35. C

36. A

37. C

38. D	5. D	33. C	**Chapter 17**
39. D	6. B	34. D	1. A
40. B	7. C	35. A	2. D
41. D	8. B	36. C	3. C
42. B	9. D	37. B	4. B
43. C	10. A	38. B	5. D
44. D	11. C	39. D	6. C
45. A	12. C	40. A	7. B
46. A	13. B	41. B	8. D
47. B	14. C	42. D	9. A
48. D	15. A	43. D	10. B
49. B	16. D	44. A	11. D
50. A	17. C	45. A	12. C
51. C	18. D	46. D	13. B
52. A	19. A	47. A	14. B
53. D	20. A	48. C	15. C
54. B	21. D	49. B	16. C
55. D	22. B	50. C	17. A
56. D	23. B	51. A	18. D
57. B	24. D	52. A	19. C
58. B	25. A	53. C	20. B
59. A	26. B	54. D	21. A
60. D	27. D	55. A	22. D
Chapter 16	28. C	56. B	23. A
1. D	29. C	57. D	24. B
2. B	30. A	58. A	25. C
3. A	31. D	59. B	26. B
4. B	32. C	60. B	27. C

28. D

29. C

30. D

31. D

32. C

33. D

34. B

35. B

36. D

37. D

38. C

39. B

40. B

41. A

42. C

43. D

44. A

45. C

46. A

47. D

48. B

49. A

50. D

51. C

52. A

53. C

54. D

55. C

56. B

57. C

58. D

59. C

60. B

Chapter 18

1. A

2. C

3. B

4. D

5. D

6. C

7. B

8. D

9. C

10. A

11. D

12. B

13. C

14. B

15. A

16. C

17. C

18. C

19. B

20. B

21. C

22. C

23. C

24. D

25. A

26. A

27. D

28. A

29. B

30. A

31. C

32. C

33. D

34. B

35. C

36. B

37. D

38. B

39. A

40. A

41. D

42. D

43. C

44. C

45. C

46. A

47. D

48. B

49. B

50. B

51. D

52. A

53. B

54. B

55. C

56. B

57. D

58. D

59. B

60. A

Chapter 19

1. C

2. D

3. C

4. C

5. A

6. A

7. D

8. C

9. B

10. C

11. D

12. C

13. A

14. B

15. D

16. D

17. C

18. A
19. C
20. B
21. C
22. B
23. C
24. D
25. D
26. B
27. B
28. B
29. D
30. B
31. A
32. B
33. C
34. C
35. D
36. C
37. C
38. C
39. D
40. C
41. A
42. D
43. B
44. D
45. B

46. C
47. B
48. B
49. A
50. B
51. D
52. A
53. A
54. D
55. D
56. D
57. D
58. C
59. B
60. A

Chapter 20

1. D
2. B
3. A
4. A
5. D
6. B
7. C
8. D
9. A
10. B
11. D
12. C

13. B
14. D
15. D
16. A
17. B
18. C
19. A
20. B
21. A
22. A
23. C
24. B
25. C
26. B
27. C
28. D
29. B
30. D
31. D
32. A
33. A
34. C
35. D
36. D
37. C
38. C
39. D
40. D

41. D
42. D
43. C
44. C
45. A
46. B
47. A
48. B
49. C
50. D
51. C
52. A
53. D
54. C
55. D
56. A
57. D
58. A
59. C
60. D

Chapter 21

1. B
2. C
3. D
4. D
5. B
6. A
7. D

8. A

9. D

10. C

11. A

12. C

13. D

14. D

15. A

16. C

17. B

18. C

19. C

20. D

21. B

22. C

23. D

24. D

25. D

26. B

27. D

28. C

29. B

30. C

31. A

32. A

33. B

34. A

35. D

36. C

37. B

38. A

39. D

40. A

41. D

42. A

43. C

44. C

45. B

46. D

47. A

48. A

49. D

50. D

51. A

52. B

53. D

54. D

55. A

56. A

57. B

58. C

59. D

60. A

Chapter 22

1. C

2. D

3. A

4. B

5. A

6. B

7. C

8. D

9. C

10. A

11. A

12. B

13. D

14. D

15. B

16. D

17. C

18. D

19. A

20. B

21. A

22. B

23. C

24. D

25. A

26. D

27. B

28. A

29. A

30. D

31. C

32. C

33. A

34. B

35. A

36. C

37. B

38. A

39. D

40. D

41. D

42. A

43. B

44. C

45. B

46. C

47. A

48. D

49. B

50. B

51. A

52. B

53. C

54. A

55. C

56. D

57. D

58. C

59. B

60. D

Chapter 23

1. D
2. B
3. C
4. A
5. B
6. C
7. D
8. C
9. C
10. B
11. A
12. A
13. C
14. B
15. D
16. A
17. D
18. C
19. A
20. D
21. A
22. A
23. C
24. D
25. B

26. B
27. D
28. B
29. A
30. D
31. D
32. C
33. B
34. A
35. A
36. B
37. C
38. C
39. A
40. D
41. D
42. C
43. A
44. D
45. D
46. B
47. D
48. A
49. D
50. D
51. D
52. A
53. C

54. D
55. A
56. C
57. B
58. D
59. D
60. D

Chapter 24

1. A
2. C
3. C
4. B
5. D
6. C
7. A
8. C
9. A
10. B
11. C
12. D
13. B
14. C
15. C
16. A
17. A
18. D
19. D
20. B

21. A
22. D
23. D
24. C
25. B
26. D
27. C
28. A
29. B
30. C
31. A
32. B
33. D
34. C
35. C
36. A
37. D
38. C
39. A
40. C
41. B
42. D
43. C
44. A
45. B
46. D
47. B
48. C

49.	D	16.	B	44.	B	11.	D
50.	C	17.	B	45.	B	12.	C
51.	D	18.	C	46.	B	13.	B
52.	D	19.	C	47.	D	14.	A
53.	B	20.	A	48.	D	15.	B
54.	B	21.	A	49.	D	16.	A
55.	C	22.	D	50.	A	17.	A
56.	D	23.	D	51.	D	18.	C
57.	B	24.	B	52.	B	19.	A
58.	C	25.	D	53.	A	20.	B
59.	D	26.	C	54.	C	21.	C
60.	B	27.	B	55.	D	22.	A

Chapter 25

		28.	C	56.	B	23.	A
1.	C	29.	C	57.	C	24.	D
2.	A	30.	B	58.	A	25.	D
3.	D	31.	C	59.	A	26.	B
4.	C	32.	C	60.	C	27.	B
5.	D	33.	B			28.	B

Chapter 26

6.	B	34.	C	1.	D	29.	C
7.	B	35.	D	2.	B	30.	D
8.	A	36.	C	3.	C	31.	D
9.	B	37.	D	4.	C	32.	B
10.	D	38.	C	5.	D	33.	B
11.	D	39.	D	6.	B	34.	A
12.	A	40.	B	7.	B	35.	B
13.	C	41.	A	8.	C	36.	B
14.	B	42.	D	9.	C	37.	B
15.	A	43.	A	10.	C	38.	C

39. A
40. B
41. D
42. D
43. D
44. C
45. B
46. C
47. C
48. D
49. D
50. A
51. D
52. B
53. C
54. C
55. D
56. D
57. C
58. D
59. C
60. A

Chapter 27

1. A
2. B
3. C
4. C

5. A
6. B
7. C
8. D
9. B
10. C
11. A
12. C
13. B
14. D
15. C
16. D
17. A
18. C
19. D
20. C
21. B
22. C
23. A
24. B
25. C
26. C
27. B
28. D
29. D
30. A
31. A

32. B
33. B
34. D
35. D
36. D
37. D
38. C
39. A
40. B
41. B
42. C
43. A
44. D
45. A
46. B
47. C
48. C
49. B
50. A
51. B
52. D
53. C
54. A
55. D
56. B
57. D
58. D

59. C
60. B

Chapter 28

1. B
2. A
3. C
4. D
5. A
6. D
7. A
8. B
9. C
10. D
11. C
12. A
13. B
14. C
15. B
16. B
17. B
18. C
19. D
20. A
21. D
22. D
23. A
24. C

25. D
26. A
27. D
28. C
29. D
30. B
31. C
32. D
33. D
34. B
35. D
36. D
37. B
38. D
39. B
40. B
41. A
42. B
43. D
44. D
45. B
46. C
47. B
48. A
49. B
50. A
51. D

52. C
53. D
54. B
55. C
56. D
57. A
58. C
59. D
60. C

Chapter 29

1. B
2. C
3. A
4. D
5. C
6. C
7. B
8. D
9. B
10. A
11. C
12. B
13. C
14. C
15. B
16. B
17. C

18. D
19. B
20. A
21. D
22. D
23. C
24. D
25. D
26. D
27. C
28. C
29. B
30. B
31. C
32. A
33. A
34. D
35. B
36. A
37. C
38. D
39. A
40. D
41. C
42. C
43. B
44. A

45. D
46. D
47. D
48. B
49. C
50. A
51. B
52. C
53. C
54. A
55. C
56. D
57. B
58. D
59. C
60. A

Chapter 30

1. B
2. A
3. B
4. D
5. B
6. C
7. A
8. C
9. B
10. B

11. D
12. B
13. C
14. A
15. C
16. A
17. B
18. C
19. D
20. A
21. A
22. D
23. A
24. D
25. B
26. C
27. C
28. C
29. D
30. D
31. C
32. B
33. D
34. A
35. C
36. A
37. C
38. D
39. C

40. A
41. A
42. D
43. D
44. C
45. A
46. D
47. C
48. D
49. A
50. C
51. C
52. C
53. D
54. A
55. A
56. D
57. B
58. C
59. A
60. A

Chapter 31

1. B
2. D
3. B
4. D
5. B
6. D
7. C

8. C
9. A
10. D
11. C
12. A
13. C
14. B
15. D
16. A
17. C
18. C
19. A
20. B
21. D
22. A
23. B
24. C
25. B
26. B
27. B
28. A
29. B
30. D
31. D
32. D
33. C
34. D
35. A
36. A

37. C
38. A
39. C
40. D
41. A
42. A
43. B
44. A
45. B
46. A
47. C
48. D
49. C
50. B
51. B
52. B
53. C
54. D
55. A
56. B
57. C
58. C
59. B
60. A

Chapter 32

1. B
2. D
3. A
4. B

5. C	19. B	33. C	47. C
6. C	20. A	34. D	48. A
7. B	21. A	35. C	49. B
8. C	22. C	36. C	50. C
9. D	23. A	37. A	51. B
10. D	24. D	38. A	52. D
11. A	25. B	39. D	53. D
12. D	26. A	40. D	54. C
13. A	27. C	41. D	55. D
14. B	28. D	42. C	56. A
15. C	29. D	43. A	57. C
16. C	30. D	44. D	58. D
17. D	31. B	45. C	59. A
18. C	32. C	46. C	60. B

Glossary

abdominal aorta—major abdominal artery responsible for supplying the abdomen, pelvis, and lower extremities with oxygenated blood

abdominal aortic aneurysm (AAA)—enlargement of the diameter of the abdominal aorta to greater than 3 cm

abdominal circumference—fetal biometric measurement of the abdomen made in the second and third trimesters; used in conjunction with other measurements to date the pregnancy and size the fetus

abnormal uterine bleeding—a change in menstrual bleeding patterns caused by either endocrine abnormalities or lesions within the uterus

abortion—the complete expulsion or partial expulsion of the conceptus

abruptio placentae—placental abruption

acalculous cholecystitis—the inflammation of the gallbladder without associated gallstones

acardiac twin—an abnormally developed twin that has an absent upper body and no heart

accessory spleen—a small, round island of splenic tissue often located near the splenic hilum or near the tail of the pancreas; also referred to as a splenule, a splenunculus, or a supernumerary spleen

acetabulum—the bowl-shaped surface of the pelvis where the head of femur normally rests

Achilles tendon—tendon located along the posterior ankle that connects the calf muscle to the posterior surface of the heel

achondrogenesis—rare, lethal condition resulting in abnormal development of the bones and cartilage

achondroplasia—a disorder that results in abnormal bone growth and dwarfism

acinar cells—the cells of the pancreas that carry out the exocrine function and, therefore, produce amylase, lipase, sodium bicarbonate, and other digestive enzymes

acoustic shadowing—an area where sound has been prohibited to propagate, resulting in a dark shadow projecting posterior to a structure

acquired renal cystic disease—a cystic disease of the kidney that is often the result of chronic hemodialysis

acrania—the absence of the cranial vault above the bony orbits

acute appendicitis—inflammation of the appendix

acute cholecystitis—the sudden onset of gallbladder inflammation

acute pancreatitis—inflammation of the pancreas secondary to the leakage of pancreatic enzymes from the acinar cells into the parenchyma of the organ

acute pyelonephritis—an inflammation of the kidney or kidneys secondary to infection

acute renal failure—a sudden decrease in renal function

acute respiratory distress syndrome—the buildup of fluid within the air sacs or alveoli within the lungs

acute tubular necrosis—damage to the tubule cells within the kidneys that results in renal failure

Addison disease—an endocrine disorder that results from hypofunction of the adrenal cortex

adenocarcinoma—cancer that originates in glandular tissue

adenomyoma—a focal mass of adenomyosis

adenomyomatosis—benign hyperplasia of the gallbladder wall

adenomyosis—the benign invasion of endometrial tissue into the myometrium of the uterus

adhesions—regular bands of tissue

adipose—fat

adnexa—the area located posterior to the broad ligaments and adjacent to the uterus, which contains the ovaries and fallopian tubes

adnexal ring sign—the sonographic sign that describes the appearance of an ectopic pregnancy within the fallopian tube; may be referred to as the tubal ring sign, bagel sign, or blob sign

adrenal adenoma—benign solid mass located within the adrenal glands

adrenal cysts—benign simple cysts located within the adrenal glands

adrenal rest—mass of ectopic adrenal tissue within the testicle; are associated with congenital adrenal hyperplasia or Cushing syndrome

adrenocorticotropic hormone (ACTH)—hormone secreted by the anterior pituitary gland, which controls the release of hormones by the adrenal glands

advanced maternal age—a maternal age of 35 years or older

agenesis—failure of an organ or a structure to grow during embryologic development

agenesis of the corpus callosum—the congenital absence of corpus callosum that may be partial or complete

alcoholic liver disease—liver injury resulting from alcohol abuse

allantoic cyst—cyst found within the umbilical cord

allantois—a membrane that is present during early embryonic development that contributes to urinary bladder formation and development

alobar holoprosencephaly—the most severe form of holoprosencephaly

alpha-fetoprotein—a protein produced by the fetal yolk sac, fetal gastrointestinal tract, and the fetal liver; may also be produced by some malignant tumors

ambiguous genitalia—a birth defect in which the sex of the fetus cannot be determined

amebic hepatic abscess—an abscess that develops from a parasite that grows in the colon and invades the liver via the portal vein

amenorrhea—absence of menstruation

amniocentesis—a surgical procedure in which amniotic fluid is extracted for genetic testing or removed when there is an accumulation of an excessive amount of fluid around the fetus

amnion—the inner sac that contains the embryo and amniotic fluid; echogenic curvilinear structure that may be seen during the first trimester within the gestational sac

amnionicity—relates to the number of amnions in a multiple gestation

amnionitis—inflammation of the amniotic sac secondary to infection

amniotic band syndrome—group of abnormalities associated with the entrapment of fetal parts in the amnion, often resulting in fetal amputations or clefting

amniotic cavity—the cavity that contains simple-appearing amniotic fluid and the developing embryo

amniotic fluid index—the amount of amniotic fluid surrounding the fetus; the sum of four quadrant measurements of amniotic fluid

amniotic sac—fluid-filled space, created by the amnion, surrounding the developing embryo or fetus

ampulla—the longest and most tortuous segment of the fallopian tube

ampulla (fallopian tube)—the longest and most tortuous segment of the fallopian tube; area of the tube in which fertilization takes place and a common location for ectopic pregnancies to implant

ampulla of Vater—the merging point of the pancreatic duct and common bile duct just before the sphincter of Oddi; also referred to as the hepatopancreatic ampulla

amyloidosis—the accumulation of the abnormal protein amyloid in the kidneys and other organs that can lead to organ damage, as well as renal failure

anasarca—diffuse edema

anastomosis—the surgical connection between two structures

androblastoma—see term Sertoli–Leydig cell tumor

androgens—steroid hormones that regulate the development and circulation of secondary male characteristics

anembryonic gestation—an abnormal pregnancy in which there is no evidence of a fetal pole or yolk sac within the gestational sac; also referred to as a blighted ovum

anemia—the condition of having a deficient number of red blood cells

anencephaly—a neural tube defect that is described as the absence of the cranium and cerebral hemispheres

aneuploidy—a condition of having an abnormal number of chromosomes

aneurysm—any dilation of a blood vessel, whether focal or diffuse

angiomyolipoma—a common benign renal tumor that consists of a network of blood vessels, muscle, and fat

angiosarcoma—a rare malignant tumor of the spleen that is derived from blood vessels

angle of insonation—angle at which the sound beams interact with tissue

anhydramnios—no amniotic fluid

annular pancreas—congenital anomaly of the pancreas that results in the maldevelopment of the pancreas in which the most ventral part of the pancreas encases the duodenum and may consequently lead to duodenal obstruction

anomaly—a structural feature that differs from the norm

anophthalmia—absence of the eye(s)

anorectal atresia—congenital maldevelopment of the rectum and absence of the anal opening

anotia—absence of the ear(s)

anovulation—lack of ovulation

anoxia—lack of oxygen supply to the body, organ, or tissue

anteflexion—the uterine body tilts forward and comes in contact with the cervix, forming an acute angle between the body and the cervix

anterior cul-de-sac—peritoneal outpouching located between the bladder and the uterus; also referred to as the vesicouterine pouch

anterior pituitary gland—the anterior segment of the pituitary gland, which is responsible for releasing follicle-stimulating hormone and luteinizing hormone during the menstrual cycle

anteversion—the typical version of the uterus where the uterine body tilts forward, forming a 90-degree angle with the cervix

anticoagulation therapy—drug therapy in which anticoagulant medications are given to a patient to slow down the rate at which that patient's blood clots

aortic atresia—abnormality in which there is a small or absent opening between the left ventricle and the aorta

aortic stenosis—abnormal narrowing of the aortic valve

Apert syndrome—genetic disorder that includes craniosynostosis, midline facial hypoplasia, and syndactyly

aperture(s)—an opening in a structure

appendicolith—a dense, calcified stone within the appendix

appendicular skeleton—includes the bones of the upper extremities, lower extremities, and pelvic girdle

appendix epididymis—the testicular appendage located at the head of the epididymis

appendix testis—the testicular appendage located between the head of the epididymis and the superior pole of the testis

appendix vas—the testicular appendage located between the body and tail of the epididymis

aqueduct of Sylvius—see term cerebral aqueduct

aqueductal stenosis—the abnormal narrowing of the cerebral aqueduct

arachnoid cyst(s)—benign cysts within the brain that do not communicate with the ventricular system

arachnoid granulations—nodular structures located along the falx cerebri that reabsorb cerebrospinal fluid into the venous system

arachnoid membrane—the middle layer of the meninges

arachnoid villi—see term arachnoid granulations

arcuate arteries—peripheral arteries of the uterus that lie at the edge of the myometrium

Arnold–Chiari II malformation—a group of cranial abnormalities associated with spina bifida

arteriovenous fistula—an abnormal passageway between an artery and a vein

arthrogryposis—a congenital disorder associated with severe joint contractures

ascariasis—an infection of the small intestine that is caused by *Ascaris lumbricoides*, a parasitic roundworm

ascites—a collection of abdominal fluid within the peritoneal cavity

Asherman syndrome—a syndrome characterized by endometrial adhesions that typically occur as a result of scar formation after some types of uterine surgery

asplenia—congenital absence of the spleen

assisted reproductive therapy—techniques used to treat infertility

atherosclerosis—a disease characterized by the accumulation of plaque within the walls of arteries

atresia (ovarian follicle)—degeneration of a follicle

atrioventricular defect—abnormal development of the central portion of the heart; also referred to as endocardial cushion defect

atrophy—wasting away of a part of the body

autoimmune disorders—disorders in which the body's immune system attacks and destroys healthy tissues and/or organs

autosomal dominant—a way in which a disorder or trait can be inherited by a fetus; at least one of the parents has to be the carrier of the gene for the disease

autosomal dominant disorder—a way in which a disorder or trait can be inherited by a fetus; at least one of the parents has to be the carrier of the gene for the disease

autosomal dominant polycystic kidney disease—an inherited disease that results in the development of renal, liver, and pancreatic cysts typically late in life; also referred to as adult polycystic kidney disease

autosomal recessive—a way in which a disorder or trait can be inherited by a fetus; both parents must be carriers of the gene for the disease

autosomal recessive polycystic kidney disease—an inherited renal disease that results in bilateral enlargement of the fetal kidneys and microscopic renal cysts; also referred to as infantile polycystic kidney disease

autosplenectomy—the gradual fibrosis and dysfunction of the spleen secondary to a disease

axial skeleton—includes the bones of cranium and spine

azotemia—an excess of urea or other nitrogenous compounds in the blood

bacteremia—presence of bacteria in the blood

bacterial endocarditis—an infection of the surface of the heart that can spread to other organs

bacteriuria—the presence of bacteria in the urine

Baker cyst—a synovial cyst located within the popliteal fossa; may also be referred to as a popliteal cyst

"ball-on-the-wall" sign—when a polyp appears to be a round object, like a ball, that is stuck to the gallbladder wall

banana sign—the sonographic sign of the cerebellum being curved in the presence of spina bifida

barcode sign—abnormal M-mode tracing that indicates the presence of a pneumothorax

bare area—the region of the liver not covered by peritoneum

Barlow test—clinical test for developmental hip dysplasia that is used to evaluate the hip for dislocation

Bartholin duct cyst—a benign cyst that is located in one of the Bartholin glands in the region of the vulva

basal ganglia—a group of nuclei within the brain that function in several ways, including information processing and emotional response

basal layer (endometrium)—the nonfunctional outer layer of the endometrium

bat-wing sign—the sonographic appearance of a fetal unilateral pleural effusion

Beckwith–Wiedemann syndrome—a growth disorder syndrome synonymous with enlargement of several organs, including the skull, tongue, and liver; children with this disorder are prone to several childhood cancers, including within the liver and kidney

"bell-clapper" deformity—the condition in which the patient lacks the normal posterior fixation of the testis and epididymis to the scrotal wall

benign prostatic hyperplasia—the benign enlargement of the prostate gland

bezoars—masses of various ingested materials that may cause an intestinal obstruction

bicornuate uterus—a common uterine anomaly in which the endometrium divides into two horns; also referred to as bicornis unicollis

bilateral renal agenesis—the failure of both kidneys to develop in the fetus

bilateral salpingo-oophorectomy—the surgical removal of both ovaries and fallopian tubes

biliary atresia—a congenital disease described as the narrowing or obliteration of all or a portion of the biliary tree

biliary colic—pain located in the right upper quadrant in the area of the gallbladder

biliary stasis—a condition in which bile is stagnant and allowed to develop into sludge or stones

bilirubin—a yellowish pigment found in bile that is produced by the breakdown of old red blood cells by the liver

biliverdin—a green pigment found in the bile

bilobed placenta—placenta that consists of two separate discs of equal size

biloma—a collection of bile within the abdomen; can be intrahepatic or extrahepatic in location

binocular diameter (distance)—measurement from the lateral margin of one orbit to the lateral margin of the other orbit

biophysical profile—a method of fetal monitoring with sonography to produce a numeric scoring system that predicts fetal well-being

biparietal diameter—a fetal head measurement obtained in the transverse plane at the level of the third ventricle and thalamus; this measurement is obtained from the outer table of the proximal parietal bone to the inner table of the distal parietal bone

bladder diverticulum—an outpouching of the urinary bladder wall

bladder exstrophy—a birth defect in which the bladder is located outside the abdomen

blastocyst—the stage at which the conceptus implants within the decidualized endometrium

blighted ovum—see term anembryonic gestation

blood urea nitrogen—a measure of the amount of nitrogen in the blood in the form of urea

"blue-dot" sign—the appearance of a torsed testicular appendage that can be observed as a blue dot just under the skin surface

blunt trauma—non-penetrating injury to the body

Bochdalek hernia—the herniation of abdominal contents into the chest cavity because of an opening in the left posterolateral portion of the diaphragm

boggy—limp

brachycephalic—round skull shape

bradycardia—a low heart rate

brainstem—the lower part of the brain composed of the pons, midbrain, and medulla oblongata

branchial cleft cysts—benign congenital neck cysts found most often near the angle of the mandible

Brenner tumors—small benign ovarian tumors

broad ligament—pelvic ligament that extends from the lateral aspect of the uterus to the side walls of the pelvis

Buck fascia—deep layer of fascia that covers the corpora cavernosa and corpus spongiosum of the penis

Budd–Chiari syndrome—a syndrome described as the occlusion of the hepatic veins, with possible coexisting occlusion of the inferior vena cava (IVC)

buffalo hump—excessive amount of fat on the back between the shoulders

bulbourethral gland—gland that secretes pre-ejaculate fluid that lubricates the penile urethra before ejaculation; also referred to as the Cowper gland

CA-125—a tumor marker in the blood that can indicate certain types of cancers such as cancer of the ovary, endometrium, breast, gastrointestinal tract, and lungs; stands for cancer antigen 125

caliectasis—dilation of the calices

canthus—corners of the eyes

caput medusae—recognizable dilation of the superficial veins of the abdomen

cardinal ligament—pelvic ligament that extends from the lateral surface of the cervix to the lateral fornix of the vagina and houses the uterine vasculature

Caroli disease—a congenital disorder characterized by segmental dilatation of the intrahepatic ducts

caudal regression syndrome—syndrome associated with the absence of the sacrum and coccyx; also referred to as sacral agenesis

cavernous hemangioma—the most common benign liver tumor

cavum septum pellucidum—a normal midline brain structure identified in the anterior portion of the brain between the frontal horns of the lateral ventricles

cebocephaly—close-set eyes (hypotelorism) and a nose with a single nostril

cell-free DNA—prenatal serum test used to examine fetal cells circulating within the maternal blood; can predict gender and discover evidence of some chromosomal abnormalities

cellulitis—inflammation and infection of the skin and subcutaneous tissues

central dot sign—the presence of echogenic dots in the nondependent part of the dilated duct representing small fibrovascular bundles; seen with Caroli disease

cephalic index—the ratio used for assessing fetal head shape

cephalocele(s)—protrusions of intracranial contents through a defect in the skull

cerclage—the placement of sutures within the cervix to keep it closed

cerebellar vermis—the portion of the cerebellum, located within the midline of the brain, that connects its two hemispheres

cerebellum—the portion of the brain located in the inferior posterior part of the skull that is responsible for motor output, sensory perception, and equilibrium

cerebral aqueduct—the duct that connects the third ventricle of the brain to the fourth ventricle; also referred to as the aqueduct of Sylvius

cerebral peduncles—paired structures located anterior to the cerebral aqueduct

cerebrospinal fluid—the protective and nourishing fluid of the brain and spinal cord produced by the cells of the choroid plexus

cervical incompetence—the painless dilation of the cervix in the second or early third trimester

cervical lymphadenopathy—enlargement of the cervical lymph nodes

cervical polyp—an overgrowth of epithelial cells within the cervix resulting in a broad based or pedunculated mass of tissue

cervicitis—inflammation of the cervix

cervix—the rigid region of the uterus located between the isthmus and the vagina

cervix sign—a sonographic sign associated with pyloric stenosis in the long axis

cesarean section—form of childbirth in which a surgical incision is made through the maternal abdomen to deliver the fetus

champagne sign—the effect of dirty shadowing, reverberation, or ring-down artifact caused by gas or gas bubbles produced by bacteria within the nondependent (typically anterior) gallbladder wall

Charcot triad—fever, right upper quadrant pain, and jaundice associated with cholangitis

chlamydia—a sexually transmitted disease that can lead to an infection of the genital tract in both sexes

chocolate cysts—another name for endometriomas

cholangiocarcinoma—primary bile duct cancer

cholangiography—a radiographic procedure in which contrast is injected into the bile ducts to assess for the presence of disease

cholangitis—inflammation of the bile ducts

cholecystectomy—the surgical removal of the gallbladder

cholecystitis—inflammation of the gallbladder

cholecystokinin—the hormone produced by the duodenum that causes the gallbladder to contract

choledochal cyst—the cystic dilatation of the common bile duct

choledocholithiasis—the presence of a gallstone or gallstones within the biliary tree

cholelithiasis—gallstone(s)

cholesterolosis—a condition that results from the disturbance in cholesterol metabolism and accumulation of cholesterol typically within a focal region of the gallbladder wall; may be diffuse and referred to as a strawberry gallbladder

chordae tendineae—tendons within the heart that attach the tricuspid valve in the right ventricle and the mitral valve in the left ventricle to their respective papillary muscle

chordee—the head of the penis curves upward or downward

chorioangioma—a benign placental tumor

choriocarcinoma—the most malignant form of gestational trophoblastic disease with possible metastasis to the liver, lungs, and vagina

chorionic villi—fingerlike projections of gestational tissue that attach to the decidualized endometrium and allow the transfer of nutrients from the mother to the fetus

chorion frondosum—the part of the chorion, covered by chorionic villi, that is the fetal contribution of the placenta

chorionic cavity—the space between the chorionic sac and the amniotic sac that contains the secondary yolk sac; also referred to as the extraembryonic coelom

chorionic sac—the gestational sac; also see term chorion

chorion—the outer membrane of a gestation that surrounds the amnion and the developing embryo

chorionic villi sampling—prenatal test used that obtains placental tissue for chromosomal analysis

chorionicity—relates to the number of chorions and the type of placentation in a multiple gestation

choroid plexus—specialized cells within the ventricular system responsible for cerebrospinal fluid production

choroid plexus cysts—cysts located within the lateral ventricles of the brain, specifically in the choroid plexus

chromaffin cells—the cells in the adrenal medulla that secrete epinephrine and norepinephrine

chromosomal abnormality—an error in either the number or structure of chromosomes

chromosomes—the cellular structures that contain genes

chronic cholecystitis—cholecystitis that results from the intermittent obstruction of the cystic duct by gallstones

chronic pancreatitis—the recurring destruction of the pancreatic tissue that results in atrophy, fibrosis, scarring, and the development of calcifications within the gland

chronic pyelonephritis—chronic inflammation of the kidney or kidneys

chronic renal failure—the gradual decrease in renal function over time

chyme—partially digested food from the stomach

cilia—hairlike projections within the fallopian tube

cinnamon-bun sign—a sonographic sign associated with the appearance of intussusception

circumvallate placenta—an abnormally shaped placenta caused by the membranes inserting inward from the edge of the placenta, producing a curled-up placental shape

cirrhosis—condition defined as hepatocyte death, fibrosis and necrosis of the liver, and the subsequent development of regenerating nodules

cisterna magna—the largest cistern in the skull; located in the posterior portion of the skull

cistern—a prominent space within the skull that contains cerebrospinal fluid; a cistern is created by the separation of the arachnoid membrane and pia mater

cleavage—the division of a cell

cleft lip—the abnormal division in the lip

cleft palate—the abnormal development of the soft and/or hard palate of the mouth where there is a division in palate

climacteric—another name for menopause

clinical findings—the information gathered by obtaining a clinical history

clinical history—a patient's signs and symptoms, pertinent illnesses, past surgeries, laboratory findings, and the results of other diagnostic testing

clinodactyly—the bending of the fifth finger toward the fourth finger

clitoromegaly—enlargement of the clitoris

cloaca—the embryonic structure that develops into the normal rectum and urogenital sinus

cloacal exstrophy—birth defect consisting of omphalocele, bladder exstrophy, imperforate anus, and spina bifida; also referred to as OEIS complex

Clomid or clomiphene citrate—fertility drug used to treat anovulation

closed spina bifida—see term spina bifida occulta

cloverleaf skull—the abnormal shape of the cranium caused by premature fusion of the sutures in which there is frontal bossing and a cloverleaf shape to the skull

clubfoot—a malformation of the bones of the foot in which the foot is most often inverted and rotated medially, and the metatarsals and toes lie in the same plane as the tibia and fibula

coagulopathies—disorders that result from the body's inability to coagulate or form blood clots; also referred to as bleeding disorders

coarctation of the aorta—the narrowing of the aortic arch

coccygeus—pelvic muscle located posteriorly within the pelvis that helps support the sacrum

cold nodules—the hypofunctioning thyroid nodules seen on a nuclear medicine study that have malignant potential

colloid—the fluid produced by the thyroid that contains thyroid hormones

colpocephaly—the abnormal lateral ventricle shape in which there is a small frontal horn and enlarged occipital horn

columns of Bertin—an extension of the renal cortex located between the renal pyramids

comet-tail artifact—artifact caused by several small, highly reflective interfaces

common iliac arteries—abdominal aortic bifurcation vessels

communicating hydrocephalus—the obstruction of cerebrospinal fluid from a source outside the ventricular system

compensatory hypertrophy—enlargement of an organ secondary to an increased workload; often seen when part of an organ has been destroyed or when there is absence or decreased function of paired organs

compound imaging—ultrasound imaging tool that utilizes electronic beam steering of the transducer array in order to obtain many overlapping scans from varying angles, thus improving image resolution and reducing artifacts; also referred to as compound spatial imaging or SonoCT

compression sonography—operator-applied transducer pressure on a structure during a sonographic examination

computed tomography—an imaging modality that uses X-ray to obtain cross-sectional images of the body in multiple planes; also referred to as CT or computerized axial tomography (CAT scan)

concave—having a rounded inward surface

conception—the combination of a female ovum with a male sperm to produce a zygote; also referred to as fertilization

congenital adrenal hyperplasia—a group of disorders in which there is a deficiency of cortisol production by the adrenal glands, although other hormones produced by the adrenal gland may be deficient as well

congenital cystic adenomatoid malformation—a mass consisting of abnormal bronchial and lung tissue that develops within the fetal chest

congenital hydronephrosis—the dilation of the renal collecting system at birth

congenital malformations—physical defects that are present in a person at birth; may also be referred to as congenital anomalies

conjoined twins—monoamniotic, monochorionic twins that are attached at the head, thorax, abdomen, or lower body

conjugated bilirubin—the water soluble form of bilirubin that is excreted into the intestines in bile and excreted in the stool; also referred to a direct bilirubin

Conn syndrome—a syndrome caused by a functioning tumor within the adrenal cortex that produces excessive amounts of aldosterone

contrast-enhanced (liver) ultrasound—sonographic imaging that includes the injection of a contrast agent intravenously to better enhance the borders of liver lesions and to analyze those lesions for possible signs of malignancy

convex—having a rounded exterior surface

cordocentesis—prenatal test that obtains fetal blood for chromosomal analysis

cornua (uterus)—areas just inferior to the fundus of the uterus where the fallopian tubes are attached bilaterally

coronary heart disease—the buildup of plaque within the arteries that supply the myocardium of the heart

corpora cavernosa—paired erectile tissues of the penis

corpus (uterus)—the uterine body

corpus albicans—the remaining structure of the corpus luteum after its deterioration

corpus callosum—a thick band of white matter that provides communication between the right and left halves of the brain

corpus hemorrhagicum—a temporary structure formed immediately following ovulation as the dominant follicle collapses and fills with blood; after the trauma heals, this becomes the corpus luteum

corpus luteum—the temporary endocrine gland that results from the rupture of the Graafian follicle after ovulation

corpus luteum cyst—physiologic ovarian cyst that develops after ovulation has occurred

corpus luteum of pregnancy—the corpus luteum that is maintained during an early pregnancy for the purpose of producing estrogen and primarily progesterone

corpus spongiosum—component of erectile tissue of the penis that contains the urethra

corrected-BPD—represents the biparietal diameter of a standard-shaped fetal head with the same cross-sectional area

cortical nephrocalcinosis—the accumulation of calcium within the cortex of the kidney

cortical thinning—the thinning of the (renal) cortex

corticomedullary differentiation—the ability to sonographically distinguish between the normal cortex and medullary portions of the kidney

cotyledons—groups or lobes of chorionic villi

Couinaud classification—system used to separate the liver into eight surgical segments; used to describe functional liver anatomy

Courvoisier gallbladder—the clinical detection of an enlarged, palpable gallbladder caused by a biliary obstruction in the area of the pancreatic head; typically caused by a pancreatic head mass

Cowper gland—see term bulbourethral gland

craniopagus—twins joined at the cranium

craniosynostosis—the premature closure of the cranial sutures with subsequent fusion of the cranial bones

creatinine—a chemical waste molecule that is generated from muscle metabolism and excreted in the urine

cremaster muscle—the muscle that raises the testicle

Crohn disease—chronic inflammatory bowel disease that leads to thickening and scarring of the bowel walls, leading to chronic pain and recurrent bowel obstructions

crown rump length—the measurement of the embryo/fetus from the top of the head to the rump

crura of the diaphragm—paired linear muscular sections of the diaphragm that attach to the anterolateral surfaces of the upper lumbar vertebrae

crus of the diaphragm—a tendinous structure that extends from the diaphragm to the vertebral column; there are two crura (plural for crus), a right crus and a left crus

Cruveilhier–Baumgarten syndrome—syndrome characterized by cirrhosis, portal hypertension, and dilation of the umbilical and paraumbilical veins

cryptorchidism—the condition of having an undescended testis or testicles

culling—the splenic process of removing irregular red blood cells from the bloodstream

cumulus oophorus—the structure that contains the developing oocyte

Cushing disease—the presence of a brain tumor in the pituitary gland that increases the release of ACTH, resulting in Cushing syndrome

Cushing syndrome—a syndrome that results from an anterior pituitary gland or adrenal tumor that causes overproduction of cortisol by the adrenal glands

cyclopia—fusion of the orbits

cystic adenomatoid malformation—a mass consisting of abnormal bronchial and lung tissue that develops within the fetal chest

cystic duct—the duct that connects the gallbladder to the common hepatic duct

cystic fibrosis—an inherited disorder in which mucus-secreting organs such as the lungs, pancreas, and other digestive organs produce thick and sticky secretions instead of normal secretions

cystic fibrosis—inherited disorder that can affect the lungs, liver, pancreas, and other organs; this disorder changes how the body creates mucus and sweat

cystic hygroma—a mass, typically found in the neck region, that is the result of an abnormal accumulation of lymphatic fluid within the soft tissue

cystic teratoma—benign ovarian mass that is composed of the three germ cell layers; also referred to as a dermoid cyst

cystitis—inflammation of the urinary bladder

Dandy–Walker complex—a spectrum of posterior fossa abnormalities that involves the cystic dilatation of the cisterna magna and fourth ventricle

Dandy–Walker malformation—congenital brain malformation in which there is enlargement of the cisterna magna, agenesis of the cerebellar vermis, and dilation of the fourth ventricle

dangling choroid sign—a sonographic sign associated with ventriculomegaly when the choroid plexus is noted hanging freely within the dilated lateral ventricle

daughter cyst—a small cyst within a large cyst

decidua basalis—the endometrial tissue at the implantation site, and the maternal contribution of the placenta

decidual reaction—the physiologic effect on the endometrium in the presence of a pregnancy

delta sign—see term lambda sign

dermoid cyst—another name for a cystic teratoma

dermoid mesh—mass of hair within a cystic teratoma

dermoid plug—part of a dermoid tumor that contains various tissues and may produce posterior shadowing during a sonographic examination

detrusor muscle—the muscle that controls the appropriate emptying of the urinary bladder

developmental dysplasia of the hip—a congenital anomaly in which the ball of the hip is prohibited from resting appropriately in the natural socket provided for it on the pelvis

dextroverted uterus—the long axis of the uterus deviating to the right of the midline

diamniotic—having two amniotic sacs

diaphragmatic hernia—the herniation of the abdominal contents into the chest cavity through a defect in the diaphragm

diaphragmatic slip—a pseudomass of the liver seen on sonography resulting from hypertrophied diaphragmatic muscle bundles

dichorionic—having two placentas

dichorionic diamniotic—having two placentas and two amniotic sacs

diethylstilbestrol (DES)—a drug administered to pregnant woman from the 1940s to the 1970s to treat threatened abortions and premature labor that has been linked with uterine malformation in the exposed fetus

DiGeorge syndrome—a genetic disorder characterized by an absent or hypoplastic thymus, which ultimately leads to impairment of the immune system and susceptibility to infection, as well as cognitive disorders, congenital heart defects, palate defects, and hormonal abnormalities

digital rectal examination—the medical procedure that requires the insertion of the finger into the rectum to palpate the prostate gland and lower gastrointestinal tract

dilatation—an enlargement or expansion of a structure

dilation and curettage—a procedure in which the cervix is dilated and the uterine cavity is scraped with a curette

direct groin hernia—acquired inguinal hernia; result from the weakening of the transversalis fascia

dirty shadowing—shadowing seen posterior to gas or air

discordant fetal growth—asymmetric fetal weight between twins

discriminatory zone—the level of human chorionic gonadotropin beyond which an intrauterine pregnancy is consistently visible

diverticulitis—the inflammation of a diverticulum or multiple diverticuli within the digestive tract, most often in the sigmoid colon

diverticulosis—the development of small outpouchings termed diverticuli in the digestive tract, most often in the sigmoid colon

dizygotic—two ova are fertilized by two sperms

dolichocephaly—an elongated, narrow head shape; may also be referred to as scaphocephaly

double bubble sign—classic sonographic sign of duodenal atresia representing the stomach and proximal duodenum

double decidual sign—the normal sonographic appearance of the decidua capsularis and decidua parietalis, separated by the anechoic fluid-filled uterine cavity

double sac sign—see term double decidual sign

double-duct sign—coexisting dilation of the common bile duct and pancreatic duct

double-layer thickness—measurement of the endometrium from basal layer to basal layer excluding both the adjacent hypoechoic myometrium and the intracavitary fluid (if present)

doughnut sign—a sonographic sign associated with pyloric stenosis in the short axis

Down syndrome—see term trisomy 21

duct of Santorini—the accessory duct of the pancreas

duct of Wirsung—the main pancreatic duct

ductus arteriosus—a fetal shunt that connects the pulmonary artery to the aortic arch

ductus (vas) deferens—the tube that connects the epididymis to the seminal vesicles

ductus venosus—a fetal shunt that connects the umbilical vein to the IVC

duodenal atresia—congenital maldevelopment or absence of duodenum

duodenal bulb—the proximal portion of the duodenum closest to the stomach

duodenum—the first segment of the small intestine

duplication of the gallbladder—having two gallbladders that are often, but not always, paired with their own cystic ducts

dura mater—the dense, fibrous outer layer of the meninges

dwarfism—abnormal short stature

dyschezia—difficult or painful defecation

dysentery—infection of the bowel which leads to diarrhea that may contain mucus and/or blood

dysmenorrhea—difficult or painful menstruation

dyspareunia—painful sexual intercourse

dysphagia—difficulty swallowing

dysplasia—the abnormal development of a structure

dyspnea—difficulty breathing

dysuria—painful or difficult urination

Ebstein anomaly—the malformation or malpositioning of the tricuspid valve that causes multiple heart defects

ecchymosis—subcutaneous spot of bleeding

echinococcal cyst—see term hydatid liver cyst

Echinococcus granulosus—a parasite responsible for the development of hydatid liver cysts

echotexture—the sonographic appearance of a structure

eclampsia—a sequela of preeclampsia in which uncontrollable maternal hypertension and proteinuria lead to maternal convulsions and, possibly, fetal and maternal death

ectoderm—the outer germ cell layer of the embryo that develops into the skin, hair, and nails, and other structures

ectopic cordis—a condition in which the heart is located either partially or completely outside the fetal chest

ectopic pregnancy—a pregnancy located outside the endometrial cavity of the uterus

edema—abnormal swelling of a structure as a result of a fluid collection

Edwards syndrome—see term trisomy 18

elastography—a sonographic technique employed to evaluate tissue based on stiffness

embolism—a blockage caused by an abnormal mass (embolus) within the bloodstream that hinders circulation downstream, leading to tissue damage

embryo—term given to the developing fetus before 10 weeks' gestation

embryonic demise—the death of an embryo before 10 weeks' gestation

emphysematous—abnormal distention of an organ with air or gas

emphysematous pyelonephritis—the formation of air within the kidney parenchyma secondary to bacterial infiltration

empyema—the presence or collection of pus

encephalocele—protrusion of the brain and meninges through a defect in the skull

endocardial cushion defect—see term atrioventricular defect

endocrine glands—glands that release their hormones directly into the bloodstream

endoderm—the germ cell layer of the embryo that develops into the gastrointestinal and respiratory tracts

endometrial atrophy—the degeneration of the endometrium with advancing age; most often seen in postmenopausal women

endometrial carcinoma—cancer of the endometrium

endometrial cavity—area that lies between the two layers of the endometrium; may also be referred to as the uterine cavity

endometrial hyperplasia—an increase in the number of endometrial cells

endometrial polyps—small nodules of hyperplastic endometrial tissue

endometrioid tumor—a typically malignant ovarian tumor that is often associated with a history of endometrial cancer, endometriosis, and endometrial hyperplasia

endometrioma—benign, blood-containing tumor that forms from the implantation of ectopic endometrial tissue; tumor associated with endometriosis

endometriosis—functional endometrial tissue located outside the uterus

endometritis—inflammation of the endometrium

endometrium—the inner mucosal layer of the uterus

endoscopic retrograde cholangiopancreatography—endoscopic procedure that utilizes fluoroscopy (radiographic imaging) to evaluate the biliary tree and pancreas

endoscopic-guided laser photocoagulation—a treatment that uses lasers to separate abnormal placental vascular connections between twins that are suffering from twin–twin transfusion syndrome

endoscopy—a means of looking inside of the human body using an endoscope

endovascular aortic stent graft repair—nonsurgical method for treating AAAs

end-stage renal disease—medical condition in which the kidneys fail to function adequately, thus requiring the use of dialysis

ependyma—the lining of the ventricles within the brain

epidermoid cyst—small benign mass within the testicle that contains keratin

epididymal cyst—a cyst located anywhere along the length of the epididymis

epididymis—a coiled structure that is attached to the testicle and the posterior scrotal wall that is responsible for storing sperm

epididymitis—inflammation of all or part of the epididymis

epididymo-orchitis—inflammation of the epididymis and testis

epignathus—an oral teratoma

epispadias—in males, the urethral opening is located on the upper aspect of the penis

Epstein–Barr infection—a herpesvirus that can lead to infectious mononucleosis

Epstein–Barr virus—the virus responsible for mononucleosis and other potential complications

erythroblastosis fetalis—condition in which there is an incompatibility between the fetal and maternal red blood cells

erythropoiesis—the process of making red blood cells

esophageal atresia—congenital absence of part of the esophagus

Essure device—a permanent form of birth control that uses small coils placed into the proximal isthmic segment of the fallopian tubes

estimated date of confinement—the due date of a pregnancy

estimated fetal weight—the fetal weight based on sonographic measurements

estriol—an estrogenic hormone produced by the placenta

estrogen—the hormone released by the ovary that initiates the proliferation and thickening of the endometrium

estrogen replacement therapy—hormone replacement therapy that involves the administration of synthetic estrogen

ethmocephaly—a condition in which there is no nose and a proboscis separating two close-set orbits; associated with holoprosencephaly

eventration of the diaphragm—lack of muscle in the dome of the diaphragm

exencephaly—form of acrania in which the entire cerebrum is located outside the skull

exophthalmos—bulging eyes

exophytic—growing outward

exsanguination—total blood loss; to bleed out

external cephalic version—the manual manipulation by a physician of a fetus that is in breech or transverse position to a cephalic position in order to facilitate vaginal delivery

external iliac arteries—external branches of the common iliac arteries

external os—the inferior portion of the cervix that is in close contact with the vagina

extraembryonic coelom—see term chorionic cavity

extramedullary hematopoiesis—the spleen's hematopoietic function which can return in cases of severe anemia

exudate ascites—a collection of abdominal fluid within the peritoneal cavity that may be associated with cancer

facial telangiectasia—dilated or broken vessels located near the surface of the skin on the face that appears as threadlike red lines; commonly referred to as spider veins

facies—the features or appearance of the face

falciform ligament—ligament that attaches the liver to the anterior abdominal wall

false aneurysm—a contained rupture of a blood vessel that is most likely secondary to the disruption of one or more layers of that vessel's wall

false lumen—the residual channel of a vessel created by the accumulation of a clot within that vessel

false pelvis—superior portion of the pelvis

falx cerebri—a double fold of dura mater located within midline of the brain

fatty liver—a reversible disease characterized by deposits of fat within the hepatocytes; also referred to as hepatic steatosis

fecalith—a stone that consists of feces

femur length—a sonographic measurement of the femoral diaphysis that provides an estimated gestational age

fetal goiter—diffuse enlargement of the fetal thyroid gland

fetal hydrops—an abnormal accumulation of fluid in at least two fetal body cavities

fetal karyotyping—an analysis of fetal chromosomes; reveals the morphology and number of chromosomes

fetor hepaticus—bad breath secondary to end-stage liver disease and the liver's inability to filter toxins; often accompanies cirrhosis, portal hypertension, and hepatic encephalopathy

fetus papyraceus—the death of one fetus in a twin pregnancy that is maintained throughout the pregnancy; actually means paperlike fetus

fibroid—see term leiomyoma

fibroma—an ovarian sex cord–stromal tumor found in middle-aged women

fibromatosis colli—a rare, pediatric fibrous tumor located within the sternocleidomastoid muscle

fimbria—the fingerlike extension of the fallopian tube located on the infundibulum

Fitz-Hugh–Curtis syndrome—a perihepatic infection that results in liver capsule inflammation from pelvic infections such as gonorrhea and chlamydia

flank pain—pain in one side of the body between the upper abdomen and the back

floating gallbladder—a gallbladder that is highly mobile and thus prone to torsion

fluid–fluid level—the distinct layering of fluids within a cyst or cystic structure that is caused by the presence of at least two different fluid compositions

focal fatty infiltration—manifestation of fatty liver disease in which fat deposits are localized

focal fatty sparing—manifestation of fatty liver disease in which an area of the liver is spared from fatty infiltration

focal myometrial contraction—localized, painless contractions of the myometrium in the gravid uterus that should resolve within 20 to 30 minutes

focal nodular hyperplasia—a benign liver mass composed of a combination of hepatocytes and fibrous tissue that typically contains a central scar

folate—a vitamin that has been shown to significantly reduce the likelihood of a fetus suffering from a neural tube defect; also referred to as folic acid

Foley catheter—a catheter placed into the urinary bladder via the urethra that is used to drain urine; it can also be clamped and used to temporarily distend the bladder for pelvic sonography

follicle—small, round groups of cells

follicle-stimulating hormone—hormone of the anterior pituitary gland that causes the development of multiple follicles on the ovaries

follicular aspiration—technique used for in vitro fertilization in which follicles are drained for oocyte retrieval

follicular cyst—ovarian cyst that forms as a result of the failure of the Graafian follicle to ovulate

follicular phase—the first phase of the ovarian cycle

foramen magnum—the opening in the base of the skull through which the spinal cord exits

foramen of Bochdalek—an opening located in the left posterolateral portion of the diaphragm

foramen of Morgagni—an opening located right anteromedially within the diaphragm

foramen ovale—an opening within the fetal heart within the atrial septum that allows blood to flow from the right atrium to the left atrium

fraternal twins—twins that result from the fertilization of two separate ova and have dissimilar characteristics

frontal bossing—the angling of the frontal bones that produces an unusually prominent forehead

functional layer (endometrium)—the functional inner layer of the endometrium that is altered by the hormones of the menstrual cycle

fundus (uterus)—the most superior and widest portion of the uterus

funneling (cervical)—the result of the premature opening of the internal os and the subsequent bulging of the membranes into the dilated cervix

fusiform—shaped like a spindle; wider in the middle and tapering toward the ends

galactocele—a milk-filled breast cyst

gallbladder torsion—the twisting of the vascular supply to the gallbladder

gallstone pancreatitis—form of pancreatitis associated with gallstones and pancreatic duct obstruction

gamete intrafallopian tube transfer—infertility treatment in which oocytes and sperm are placed in the fallopian tube by means of laparoscopy

ganglion cyst—a common cyst found adjacent to a joint or tendon; most often found along the dorsal aspect of the hand, wrist, ankle, or foot

Gartner duct cyst—a benign cyst located within the vagina

gastrin—hormone produced by the stomach lining that is used to regulate the release of digestive acid

gastrinoma—an islet cell tumor found within the cells of the pancreas that may produce an abundance of gastrin

gastroesophageal junction—the junction between the stomach and the esophagus

gastroesophageal reflux—an abnormality in which fluid is allowed to reflux out of the stomach back into the esophagus

gastroschisis—herniation of abdominal contents through a right-sided, periumbilical abdominal wall defect

germ cell tumor—a type of neoplasm derived from germ cells of the gonads; may be found outside the reproductive tract

germinal matrix—a group of thin-walled blood vessels and cells within the subependymal layer of the fetal brain responsible for brain cell migration during fetal development

Gerota fascia—the fibrous envelope of tissue that surrounds the kidney and adrenal gland

gestational age—the way in which a pregnancy can be dated based on the first day of the last menstrual cycle; also referred to as menstrual age

gestational diabetes—diabetes acquired as a result of pregnancy

gestational trophoblastic disease—a disease associated with an abnormal proliferation of the trophoblastic cells during pregnancy; may also be referred to as a molar pregnancy

Glisson capsule—the thin fibrous casing of the liver

glomerular filtration rate—blood test that is used to evaluate the overall function of glomeruli, which are the small blood filters located within the kidney

glomoruli—small blood filters located at the beginning of the nephron

glomerulonephritis—an infection of the kidney glomeruli

glomus (of choroid plexus)—the largest part of the choroid plexus

glucocorticoids—adrenal steroid hormones that include cortisol (hydrocortisone)

goiter—an enlarged, hyperplastic thyroid gland

Goldenhar syndrome—rare congenital defect that consists of anophthalmia, abnormal lip and palate, maldevelopment or absence of the ear, and other facial abnormalities

gonadotropin-releasing hormone—the hormone released by the hypothalamus that stimulates the pituitary gland to release the hormones that regulate the female menstrual cycle

gonorrhea—sexually transmitted disease that leads to infection of the genitals

Graafian follicle—the name for the dominant follicle before ovulation

Graf technique—a technique used to measure the relationship of the femoral head and acetabulum by evaluating the alpha and beta angles created by the relationships of these structures

granulomas—small echogenic calcifications that result from inflammation of the tissue in that area

granulomatous disease—an inherited disease that disrupts the normal immune system and causes it to malfunction, resulting in immunodeficiency; chronic inflammation can lead to the development of granulomas in several organs

Graves disease—the most common cause of hyperthyroidism that produces bulging eyes, heat intolerance, nervousness, weight loss, and hair loss

gravid—pregnant

gravidity—the number of times that a woman has been pregnant

gross hematuria—blood within the urine that is visible to the naked eye

gynecomastia—the benign enlargement of the male breast; typically located posterior to the areola

gyri—folds in the cerebral cortex

harmonics imaging—ultrasound imaging tool that utilizes nonlinear propagation of ultrasound as it travels through the body in order to improve axial and lateral resolution and reduce imaging artifacts; also referred to as tissue harmonic imaging

Hartmann pouch—an outpouching of the gallbladder neck

Hashimoto thyroiditis—the most common cause of hypothyroidism in the United States

HELLP syndrome—maternal syndrome that stands for hemolysis, elevated liver enzymes, and low platelet count

hemangioma—a benign tumor composed of blood vessels

hematemesis—vomiting blood

hematocele—a collection of blood within the scrotum

hematocolpos—blood accumulation within the vagina

hematocrit—a laboratory value that indicates the amount of red blood cells in the blood

hematoma—a localized collection of blood

hematometra—blood accumulation within the uterine cavity

hematometrocolpos—blood accumulation within the uterus and vagina

hematopoiesis—the development of blood cells

hematosalpinx—blood within the fallopian tube

hematospermia—the presence of blood within the semen

hematuria—blood within the urine; can be described as microscopic or gross

hemivertebra—the anomaly of the spine in which there is absence of all or part of a vertebral body and posterior element

hemochromatosis—an inherited disease characterized by disproportionate absorption of dietary iron

hemodialysis—form of dialysis that utilizes a machine that essentially acts as a kidney whereby it extracts the patient's blood, filters it, and returns the filtered blood to the patient

hemolytic anemia—a condition that results in the destruction of red blood cells

hemophiliac—an inherited bleeding disorder that inhibits the control of blood clotting

hemopoiesis—the formation and development of blood cells

hemorrhagic cyst—a cyst that contains blood

hemorrhagic pancreatitis—form of pancreatitis associated with bleeding within or around the pancreas

Henoch–Schönlein purpura—an autoimmune disorder and form of vasculitis associated with purple spots on the skin, gastrointestinal complications, joint pain, and possibly kidney failure; mostly occurs in childhood

hepatic candidiasis—a hepatic mass that results from the spread of fungus in the blood to the liver

hepatic encephalopathy—a condition in which a patient becomes confused or suffers from intermittent loss of consciousness secondary to the overexposure of the brain to toxic chemicals that the liver would normally remove from the body

hepatic jaundice—jaundice resulting from the liver's inability to conjugate bilirubin; may be caused by conditions such as viral hepatitis, toxins, drugs, cirrhosis, and liver cancer

hepatic steatosis—see term fatty liver

hepatitis—inflammation of the liver

hepatization of the gallbladder—situation in which the gallbladder is completely filled with tumefactive sludge, causing the gallbladder to appear isoechoic to the liver tissue

hepatocellular adenoma—a benign liver mass often associated with the use of oral contraceptives

hepatocellular carcinoma—the primary form of liver cancer

hepatofugal—blood flow away from the liver

hepatoma—the malignant tumor associated with hepatocellular carcinoma; primary liver cancer

hepatomegaly—enlargement of the liver

hepatopancreatic ampulla—the level of the biliary tree where the common bile duct and the main pancreatic duct meet; may also be referred to as the ampulla of Vater

hepatopancreatic sphincter—the muscle that controls the emptying of bile and pancreatic juices into the duodenum; may also be referred to as the sphincter of Oddi

hepatopetal—blood flow toward the liver

hepatorenal space—peritoneal space located between the liver and the right kidney; also referred to as Morison pouch

hepatorenal syndrome—the development of renal impairment and possible renal failure because of chronic liver disease

hepatosplenomegaly—concurrent enlargement of the spleen and liver

heterotaxia syndromes—a group of inherited syndromes in which the organs of the chest and abdomen are abnormally arranged; often includes either asplenia or polysplenia and many other anomalies

heterotopic pregnancy—coexisting ectopic and intrauterine pregnancies

heterozygous achondroplasia—most common nonlethal skeletal dysplasia that is characterized by rhizomelia

high-resistance flow—the flow pattern that results from small arteries or arterioles that are contracted, which produces an increase in the resistance to blood flow to the structure that is being supplied

hip joint effusion—buildup of fluid within the hip secondary to inflammation

Hirschsprung disease—a disease that leads to a functional bowel obstruction because of the lack of nerve cells within the colon wall

hirsutism—excessive hair growth in women in areas where hair growth is normally negligible

histoplasmosis—a disease that results from the inhalation of an airborne fungus that can affect the lungs and may spread to other organs

Hodgkin lymphoma—carcinoma of the lymphocytes that has a relatively high recovery rate; cancer of the lymphatic system

holoprosencephaly—a group of brain abnormalities consisting of varying degrees of fusion of the lateral ventricles, absence of the midline structures, and associated facial anomalies

homeostasis—the body's ability or tendency to maintain internal equilibrium by adjusting its physiologic processes

homozygous achondroplasia—the fatal form of achondroplasia

hormone replacement therapy—the medical treatment used to accommodate the reduction of estrogen and progesterone that occurs during menopause

horseshoe kidneys—the attachment of the lower poles of the kidneys by a band of renal tissue that crosses the midline of the abdomen

hot nodules—the hyperfunctioning thyroid nodules seen on a nuclear medicine study that are almost always benign

human chorionic gonadotropin—a hormone produced by the trophoblastic cells of the early placenta; may also be used as a tumor marker in nongravid patients and males

hydatid cyst—a cyst that results from the parasitic infestation of an organ by a tapeworm

hydatid liver cyst—a liver cyst that develops from a tapeworm that lives in dog feces; also referred to as an echinococcal cyst because it originates from the parasite Echinococcus granulosus

hydatidiform mole—the most common form of gestational trophoblastic disease in which there is excessive growth of the placenta and high levels of human chorionic gonadotropin; typically benign

hydranencephaly—a fatal condition in which the entire cerebrum is replaced by a large sac containing cerebrospinal fluid

hydrocele—a fluid collection within the scrotum; most often found between the two layers of the tunica vaginalis

hydrocephalus—the dilatation of the ventricular system caused by an increased volume of cerebrospinal fluid, resulting in increased intraventricular pressure

hydrocolpos—fluid accumulation within the vagina

hydrometrocolpos—fluid accumulation within the uterus and vagina

hydronephrosis—the dilation of the renal collecting system resulting from the obstruction of the flow of urine from the kidney(s) to the bladder; also referred to as pelvocalioctasis or pelvicaliectasis

hydropic gallbladder—an enlarged gallbladder, also referred to as mucocele of the gallbladder

hydrops (fetal)—an abnormal accumulation of fluid in at least two fetal body cavities

hydrosalpinx—the abnormal accumulation of fluid within the fallopian tube

hydroureter—distension of the ureter with fluid because of obstruction

hyperalimentation—the intravenous administration of nutrients and vitamins

hyperamylasemia—elevated amylase

hyperandrogenism—excessive serum androgen levels; produces male characteristics in females

hyperbilirubinemia—elevated levels of serum bilirubin

hypercalcemia—elevated serum calcium

hypercortisolism—high levels of cortisol in the blood

hyperemesis—excessive vomiting

hyperemesis gravidarum—excessive vomiting during pregnancy

hyperemic—an increase in blood flow

hyperkalemia—abnormally high levels of potassium in the blood

hyperlipidemia—abnormally high levels of fats within the blood (i.e., high cholesterol and high triglycerides)

hypernatremia—high levels of sodium in the blood

hypernephroma—carcinoma of the kidney; also referred to as renal cell carcinoma

hyperparathyroidism—the presence of elevated parathyroid hormone

hyperpigmentation—the darkening of the skin

hyperplasia—an increase in the number of cells of a tissue or an organ

hyperplastic cholecystosis—a group of proliferative and degenerative gallbladder disorders, which includes both adenomyomatosis and cholesterolosis

hypersplenism—an overactive spleen; cytopenia caused by splenomegaly

hypertelorism—increased distance between the orbits; widely spaced orbits

hypertension—high blood pressure

hyperthyroidism—a condition that results from the overproduction of thyroid hormones

hypertrophic pyloric stenosis—a defect in the relaxation of the pyloric sphincter that leads to the enlargement of the pyloric muscles and closure of the pyloric sphincter

hypoalbuminemia—abnormal low level of albumin in the blood; albumin is a protein produced in the liver

hypoglycemia—low blood sugar

hypokalemia—low levels of potassium in the blood

hypomenorrhea—decreased or scant menstrual flow; regular timed menses but light flow

hyponatremia—low levels of sodium in the blood

hypoplasia—incomplete growth of a structure or an organ

hypoplastic—incomplete or arrested development of a structure

hypoplastic left heart syndrome—incomplete development of the left ventricle, resulting in a small or absent left ventricle

hypoplastic right heart syndrome—incomplete development of the right ventricle, resulting in a small or absent right ventricle

hypospadias—abnormal ventral curvature of the penis as a result of a shortened urethra that exits on the ventral penile shaft

hypotelorism—reduced distance between the orbits

hypothalamic–pituitary–gonadal axis—the complex interactions that take place between the hypothalamus, pituitary gland, and ovaries as part of the female reproductive cycle

hypothalamus—the area within the brain that is located just beneath the thalamus and controls the release of hormones by the anterior pituitary gland

hypothyroidism—a condition that results from the underproduction of thyroid hormones

hypovolemia—decreased blood volume

hypoxia—a shortage of oxygen or decreased oxygen in the blood

hysterectomy—the surgical removal of the uterus

hysterosalpingography—a radiographic procedure that uses a dye instilled into the endometrial cavity and fallopian tubes to evaluate for internal abnormalities

hysteroscopic uterine septoplasty—the surgical repair of a uterine septum in a septate uterus using a hysteroscopy

hysteroscopy—endoscopy of the uterine cavity

iatrogenic—a condition that is the result of medical treatment; may be due to exposure to a pathogen, toxin, or injury following a treatment or procedure

identical twins—twins that result from the split of a single zygote and share the same genetic structure

idiopathic—from an unknown origin

ileus—bowel obstruction caused by the lack of normal peristalsis

iliopsoas muscles—bilateral muscles located lateral to the uterus and anterior to iliac crest

ilium (pelvis)—the largest and most superiorly located pelvic bone

immune hydrops—fetal hydrops caused by Rh incompatibility

immunocompromised—the state of having an immune system that is impaired for some reason

imperforate hymen—a vaginal anomaly in which the hymen has no opening, therefore resulting in an obstruction of the vagina

implantation bleeding—a bleed that occurs at the time in which the conceptus implants into the decidualized endometrium

in vitro fertilization—fertility treatment that requires that a mature ovum be extracted from the ovary, with fertilization taking place outside the body

incidentaloma—an adrenal mass discovered incidentally during an imaging examination; the term may also be used for incidentally discovered masses in other organs or structures

incontinence—inability to control urination

indirect groin hernia—occurs when the abdominal contents protrude through the deep inguinal ring, lateral to the inferior epigastric vessels and anterior to the spermatic or round ligament

infantile polycystic kidney disease—an inherited renal disease that results in bilateral enlargement of the fetal kidneys and microscopic renal cysts; also referred to as autosomal recessive polycystic kidney disease

inferior vena cava filter—vascular filter placed in the IVC to prevent pulmonary emboli

inferior vena cava web—rare condition characterized by obstruction of the IVC by membranous or fibrous bands; can cause obstruction of the hepatic veins leading to Budd–Chiari syndrome

infertility—inability to conceive a child after 1 year of unprotected intercourse

inflammatory bowel disease—chronic inflammation of the gastrointestinal tract; used as an umbrella term for both Crohn disease and ulcerative colitis

infundibulum—the distal segment of the fallopian tube

inguinal canal—normal passageway in the lower anterior abdominal wall that allows for the passage of the spermatic cord into the scrotum

inguinal hernia—the protrusion of bowel or abdominal contents through the inguinal canal

inhibin A—a peptide hormone secreted by the placenta during pregnancy

innominate bones—pelvic bones that consist of the ilium, ischium, and pubic symphysis

insulinoma—an islet cell tumor found within the beta cells of the pancreas that may produce an abundance of insulin

intercostal sonographic imaging—performing sonographic imaging between the ribs

interhemispheric fissure—groove within the midline of the brain that divides the two cerebral hemispheres

intermenstrual bleeding—bleeding between periods; may be referred to as metrorrhagia

internal iliac arteries—internal branches of the common iliac arteries

internal os—the superior portion of the cervix closest to the isthmus

interocular diameter—the length between the orbits; measured from the medial margin of one orbit to the medial margin of the other orbit

interposition of the gallbladder—rare anomaly of the biliary tree where the main hepatic ducts drain directly into the gallbladder and the gallbladder drains directly into the common bile duct; may lead to childhood jaundice, enlarged gallbladder, and intermittent abdominal pain

interstitial—the segment of the fallopian tube that lies within the uterine horn (cornu)

interstitial edematous pancreatitis—most common form of pancreatitis; associated with inflammation of the pancreas and peripancreatic tissue without necrosis

interthalamic adhesion—the mass of tissue, located in the third ventricle within the midline of the brain, which connects the two lobes of the thalamus; also referred to as the massa intermedia

intimal flap—observation of the intimal layer of a vessel as a result of a dissection

intracavitary (fibroid)—a leiomyoma located within the uterine cavity

intracranial hemorrhage—hemorrhage within the cranium

intradecidual sign—the appearance of a small gestational sac in the uterine cavity surrounded by the thickened, echogenic endometrium

intrahepatic gallbladder—a gallbladder that is completely surrounded by the hepatic parenchyma

intraluminal—located within the lumen or opening of an organ or structure

intramural (fibroid)—location of leiomyoma within the myometrium of the uterus

intraperitoneal—located within the parietal peritoneum

intrauterine contraceptive device—a reversible form of contraception that is manually placed in the uterine cavity to prevent pregnancy; also referred to as an intrauterine device

intrauterine device—a common form of birth control in which a small device is placed within the endometrium to prevent pregnancy; also referred to as an intrauterine contraceptive device

intrauterine growth restriction—a fetus that is below the 10th percentile for gestational age (small for gestational age) and whose growth is impeded for some reason

intraventricular hemorrhage—hemorrhage located within the ventricles of the brain

intussusception—the telescoping of one segment of bowel into another; most often the proximal segment of the bowel inserts into the distal segment

intussusceptum—the proximal segment of the bowel with intussusception

intussuscipiens—the distal segment of the bowel with intussusception

invaginate—to insert

invasive mole—a type of gestational trophoblastic disease in which a molar pregnancy invades into the myometrium and may also invade through the uterine wall and into the peritoneum

ischemic bowel disease—condition that results from decreased blood flow to the intestines resulting in damaged bowel tissue owing to inadequate oxygenation; also referred to as intestinal ischemia

islet cell tumors—tumor found within the islets of Langerhans of the pancreas

islets of Langerhans—small islands of tissue found within the pancreas that produce insulin and glucagon

isthmus (uterus)—area of the uterus between the corpus and the cervix

isthmus (tube)—the segment of the fallopian tube that is located between the interstitial and ampulla; uterus: area of the uterus between the corpus and the cervix

jaundice—broad clinical term referring to the yellowish discoloration of the skin, mucous membranes, and sclerae; found with liver disease and/or biliary obstruction

junctional fold—a fold in the neck of the gallbladder

Kaposi sarcoma—cancer that causes lesions to develop on the skin and other places; often associated with AIDS

Kawasaki disease—a condition associated with vasculitis and can affect the lymph node, skin, and mucous membranes; also referred to as mucocutaneous lymph node syndrome

kernicterus—brain damage from bilirubin exposure in a newborn with jaundice

keyboard sign—sign of small bowel obstruction representing the plicae circulares surrounded by fluid within distended loops of bowel

"keyhole" sign—the sonographic appearance of a dilated fetal bladder and urethra in the presence of a bladder outlet obstruction

Klatskin tumor—a malignant biliary tumor located at the junction of the right and left hepatic ducts

Klinefelter syndrome—a condition in which a male has an extra X chromosome; characteristic features include small testicles, infertility, gynecomastia, long legs, and abnormally low intelligence

Krukenberg tumor—malignant ovarian tumor that metastasizes from most likely the gastrointestinal tract

Kupffer cells—specialized macrophages within the liver that engulf pathogens and damaged cells

kyphoscoliosis—the combination of both scoliosis and kyphosis in the fetus

kyphosis—an abnormal posterior curvature of the spine

lactate dehydrogenase—an enzyme found within the blood that may be used to monitor renal function; may also be used as a tumor marker

lactiferous ducts—the ducts of the breast used to transport milk to the nipple

lactobezoar—a bezoar that consists of powdered milk

lambda sign—a triangular extension of the placenta at the base of the membrane is indicative of a dichorionic diamniotic pregnancy; also referred to as the delta sign or twin peak sign

lecithin-to-sphingomyelin ratio—a test of the amniotic fluid that predicts fetal lung maturity

leiomyoma (uterine)—a benign, smooth muscle tumor of the uterus; may also be referred to as a fibroid or uterine myoma

leiomyosarcoma—the malignant manifestation of a leiomyoma

lemon sign—the sonographic sign associated with a lemon-shaped cranium; most often found in the fetus with spina bifida

lesser sac—a peritoneal cavity located between the stomach and the pancreas where fluid can accumulate

leukocytosis—an elevated white blood cell count

leukopenia—a reduction in the number of leukocytes in the blood

levator ani muscles—hammock-shaped pelvic muscle group located between the coccyx and the pubis consisting of the iliococcygeus, pubourethralis, pubococcygeus, pubovaginalis, and puborectalis

levoverted uterus—the long axis of the uterus deviating to the left of the midline

ligamentum teres—ligament that forms part of the edge of the falciform ligament of the liver, connecting the liver to the umbilicus; a remnant of the left umbilical vein; also referred to as the round ligament of the liver

ligamentum venosum—remnant of the fetal ductus venosus; appears as a hyperechoic linear ligament between the caudate lobe and left lobe of the liver

limb buds—early embryonic structures that will eventually give rise to the extremities

limb–body wall complex—a group of disorders with sonographic findings including a short or absent umbilical cord, ventral wall defects, limb defects, craniofacial defects, and scoliosis

linea alba—the tendonous, fibrous structure that runs along the midline of the abdomen, separating the rectus abdominis muscles

linea terminalis—imaginary line that separates the true pelvis from the false pelvis

lipoma—a benign fatty tumor

lissencephaly—"smooth brain"; condition where there is little to no gyri or sulci within the cerebral cortex

liver fibrosis—the development of scar tissue within the liver as a result of the liver repeatedly trying to repair itself

liver hilum—the area of the liver where the common bile duct exits the liver and portal vein and hepatic artery enter the liver; also referred to as the porta hepatis

lobar holoprosencephaly—the least severe form of the holoprosencephaly

lower uterine segment—the term used for the isthmus of the uterus during pregnancy

low-resistance flow—the flow pattern characterized by persistent forward flow throughout the cardiac cycle

lung consolidation—the replacement of normal air-filled alveoli with fluid, inflammation, blood, or neoplastic cells

luteal phase deficiency—when the endometrium does not develop appropriately in the luteal phase of the endometrial cycle as a result of reduced progesterone production

luteal phase—the second phase of the ovarian cycle

luteinizing hormone—the hormone of the anterior pituitary gland that surges around day 14 of the menstrual cycle, resulting in ovulation

"lying-down" adrenal sign—the sonographic appearance of the adrenal gland in a parallel position within the abdomen as a result of renal agenesis

lymphadenopathy—disease or enlargement of the lymph nodes

lymphangioma—pediatric neck mass that consists of lymphatic fluid secondary to blockage of lymphatic channels; may also be referred to as a cystic hygroma; may occur in other regions of the body where lymphatic tissue exists

lymphedema—buildup of lymph that is most likely caused by the obstruction of lymph drainage

lymphocele—a collection of lymphatic fluid

lysis—destruction or breaking down (i.e., hemolysis, the breaking down of blood components)

macrocephaly—an enlarged head circumference

macroglossia—enlargement of the tongue

macroscopic—large enough to be discerned by the naked eye

macrosomia—an estimated fetal weight of greater than the 90th percentile or the neonate that measures more than 4,500 g

magnetic resonance imaging—a diagnostic modality that utilizes electromagnetic radiation to produce images of the human body in cross-sectional and reconstructed 3D formats

magnetic resonance imaging–guided high-intensity–focused ultrasound—a fibroid treatment that utilizes focused high-frequency, high-energy ultrasound guided by magnetic resonance imaging to heat and destroy fibroid tissue

malaise—feeling of uneasiness

male secondary sex characteristics—sexual characteristics typically attributed to males, such as the growth of body hair on the chest, underarms, abdomen, and face

malformation—a structural abnormality that results from an abnormal development

malignant degeneration—the deterioration of a benign mass into a malignancy

Marfan syndrome—a disorder of the connective tissue characterized by tall stature and aortic and mitral valve insufficiency

marginal cord insertion—abnormal cord insertion at the edge of the placenta

mass effect—the displacement or alteration of normal anatomy that is located adjacent to a tumor

massa intermedia—see term interthalamic adhesion

mastitis—inflammation of the breast

maternal serum alpha-fetoprotein—a screening test that detects the amount of alpha-fetoprotein in the maternal bloodstream

maternal serum screening—blood screening test that evaluates maternal levels of alpha-fetoprotein, estriol, and human chorionic gonadotropin (as well as other labs) during a pregnancy for neural tube defects and chromosomal abnormalities

McBurney point—a point halfway between the anterior superior iliac spine and the umbilicus; the area of pain and rebound tenderness in patients suffering from acute appendicitis

mean sac diameter—the measurement of the gestational sac to obtain a gestational age; achieved by adding the measurements of the length, width, and height of the gestational sac and dividing by 3

mechanical obstruction—a situation in which bowel is physically blocked by something

Meckel diverticulum—a common congenital outpouching of the wall of the small intestine

Meckel–Gruber syndrome—fetal syndrome associated with microcephaly, occipital encephalocele, polydactyly, and polycystic kidneys

meconium—fetal stool that is composed of fetal skin, hair, amniotic fluid, and bile

median cleft lip—a subdivision within the middle of the lip

median raphe—the structure that separates the scrotum into two compartments externally

mediastinum—the central portion of the chest cavity between the pleural sacs of the lungs that contains all of the chest organs but the lungs, including the heart, thymus gland, part of the trachea, esophagus, and many lymph nodes

mediastinum testis—the structure that is formed by the tunica albuginea and contains the rete testis

medullary nephrocalcinosis—the accumulation of calcium within the medulla of the renal parenchyma

medullary sponge kidney—a congenital disorder characterized by the accumulation of calcium within abnormally dilated collecting ducts located within the medulla

mega cisterna magna—an enlargement of the cisterna magna as defined by a depth of more than 10 mm

megacystis—an abnormally enlarged urinary bladder

megaureter—an enlarged ureter; can be congenital or acquired

Meigs syndrome—ascites and pleural effusion in the presence of some benign ovarian tumors

melanoma—a malignant form of cancer found most often on the skin

menarche—the first menstrual cycle

meninges—the coverings of the brain and spinal cord

meningocele—herniation of the cranial or spinal meninges because of an open cranial or spinal defect; contains cerebrospinal fluid, but no nerve tissue

meningomyelocele—mass that results from open spina bifida that contains the spinal cord and the meninges; also referred to as a myelomeningocele

meniscus—thin fibrocartilaginous tissue that is located between the surfaces of two joints

menometrorrhagia—excessive and prolonged menstrual bleeding at irregular intervals

menopause—cessation of menstruation with advanced age

menorrhagia—abnormally heavy and prolonged menstruation

menses—menstrual bleeding

menstrual age—see term gestational age

mermaid syndrome—see term sirenomelia

mesencephalon—the primary brain vesicle also referred to as the midbrain; it eventually becomes the cerebral peduncles, quadrigeminal plate, and cerebral aqueduct

mesentery—a double fold of peritoneum that attaches the intestines to the posterior abdominal wall

mesoblastic nephroma—the most common solid fetal renal mass

mesocephalic—normal head shape

mesoderm—the germ cell layer of the embryo that develops into the circulatory system, muscles, reproductive system, and other structures

metabolic syndrome—condition that includes hypertension, hyperglycemia, excessive body fat around the waist, elevated cholesterol, and nonalcoholic fatty liver disease

metastasis—the spread of cancer from a distant site

methotrexate—a chemotherapy drug used to attack rapidly dividing cells like those seen in an early pregnancy; this drug is often used to manage ectopic pregnancies

metrorrhagia—irregular menstrual bleeding between periods; intermenstrual bleeding

microcephaly—small head

micrognathia—a small mandible and recessed chin

micropenis—an abnormally small penis

microphthalmia—a decrease in the size of the eye

microscopic—too small to be seen by the naked eye and thus requiring the aid of a microscope

microtia—small ear(s)

midgut malrotation—abnormal rotation of the bowel that leads to a proximal small bowel obstruction

mineralocorticoids—adrenal steroid hormones that include aldosterone

Mirena—a small plastic T-shaped intrauterine device

Mirizzi syndrome—a clinical condition when the patient presents with jaundice, pain, and fever secondary to a lodged stone in the cystic duct causing compression of the common duct

mirror syndrome—a rare disorder in which the mother suffers from edema and fluid buildup similar to her hydropic fetus

miscarriage—the spontaneous end of a pregnancy before viability

missed abortion—fetal demise with a retained fetus

mittelschmerz—pelvic pain at the time of ovulation

moiety—division of the duplex collecting system, as in the upper pole moiety and the lower pole moiety

molar pregnancy—also referred to as gestational trophoblastic disease; is associated with an abnormal proliferation of the trophoblastic cells, enlargement of the placenta, and elevated levels of human chorionic gonadotropin

monoamniotic—having one amniotic sac

monochorionic—having one chorion

monochorionic diamniotic—having one placenta and two amniotic sacs

monochorionic monoamniotic—having one placenta and one amniotic sac

mononucleosis—an infectious disease caused by the Epstein–Barr virus

monophasic—vascular flow yielding a single phase

monosomy X—see term Turner syndrome

monoventricle—one large ventricle within the brain associated with holoprosencephaly

monozygotic—coming from one fertilized ovum or zygote

morbidity—the relative frequency of occurrence of a disease

morphology—the form and structure of an organism

Morrison pouch—the space between the liver and the right kidney; also referred to as the posterior right subhepatic space

mortality—the rate of actual deaths

morula—the developmental stage of the conceptus following the zygote

mucoepidermoid carcinoma—the most common malignancy of the salivary glands; typically starts in the parotid gland

Müllerian ducts—paired embryonic ducts that develop into the female urogenital tract

multicystic dysplastic kidney disease—a fetal renal disease thought to be caused by an early renal obstruction; leads to the development of multiple noncommunicating cysts of varying sizes in the renal fossa

multiloculated—having multiple chambers or compartments

multiparity—having had several pregnancies

multiparous—having birthed more than one child

mural nodules—small solid internal projections of tissue originating from the wall of a cyst

Murphy sign—pain directly over the gallbladder with applied probe pressure

mycotic aneurysm—an aneurysm caused by infection

myelocele—mass that results from open spina bifida that contains spinal cord only

myelomeningocele—mass that results from spina bifida that contains the spinal cord and the meninges

myomectomy—the surgical removal of a myoma (fibroid) of the uterus

myometritis—inflammation of the myometrium, the muscular part of the uterus

myometrium—the muscular layer of the uterus

nabothian cysts—benign cysts located within the cervix

natal cleft—area located between the groove of the buttocks

necrosis—death of tissue

necrotizing pancreatitis—severe form of acute pancreatitis in which there is death of the pancreatic tissue

neonatal—the first 4 weeks (28 days) after birth

neonatal period—the first 28 days of life

neoplasm—a mass of tissue that contains abnormal cells; also called a tumor

nephroblastoma—the most common solid malignant pediatric abdominal mass; may also be referred to as Wilms tumor

nephrocalcinosis—an accumulation of calcium within the renal parenchyma

nephrolithiasis—the urinary stones located within the kidney; kidney stones

nephron—the functional unit of the kidney

nephrotic syndrome—a kidney disorder caused by damage to the glomeruli that results in excess amounts of protein in the urine and the swelling of the ankles, face, and feet because of accumulation of excess water

neural plate—the early embryologic structure that develops into the central nervous system

neural tube—embryologic formation that results from fusion of the two folded ends of the neural plate

neural tube defects—a group of developmental abnormalities that involve the brain and spine

neuroblastoma—malignant tumor that can occur within the adrenal gland and anywhere within the sympathetic nervous system

neurogenic bladder—a bladder that is poorly functioning secondary to any type of neurologic disorder

nocturia—frequent urination at night

nonbilious—not containing bile

noncommunicating hydrocephalus—the obstruction of cerebrospinal fluid from a source within of the ventricular system

nongravid—not pregnant

non-Hodgkin lymphoma—carcinoma of the lymphocytes; cancer of the lymphatic system

nonimmune hydrops—fetal hydrops caused by congenital fetal anomalies and infections

nonmechanical obstruction—a situation in which bowel is blocked because of the lack of normal peristalsis of a bowel segment or segments; also referrod to as a paralytic ileus

nonstress test—a noninvasive test performed on the fetus to evaluate fetal movement, heart rate, and reactivity of the heart rate to fetal movement; diagnostic use is to detect signs of fetal distress

nosocomial infections—hospital-acquired infections

nuchal cord—condition of having the umbilical cord wrapped completely around the fetal neck

nuchal cystic hygroma—a mass found in the neck that is the result of an abnormal accumulation of lymphatic fluid within the soft tissue

nuchal—the posterior part or nape of the neck

nuchal fold—a collection of solid tissue on the posterior aspect of the fetal neck

nuchal fold thickness—a measurement taken in the second trimester of the skin on the posterior aspect of the fetal neck

nuchal translucency—the anechoic space along the posterior aspect of the fetal neck

nuclear cystogram—a nuclear medicine examination of the urinary bladder and ureters

nuclear medicine—a diagnostic imaging modality that utilizes the administration of radionuclides into the human body for an analysis of the function of organs or for the treatment of various abnormalities

nulliparity—having birthed no children

nulliparous—never been given birth

nutcracker syndrome—syndrome associated with clinical complications as a result of compression or entrapment of the left renal vein as it passes between the superior mesenteric artery and abdominal aorta

obesity—overweight to the point of causing significant health problems and increased mortality

obstructive cystic dysplasia—a fetal disorder caused by an early renal obstruction; leads to small and echogenic kidneys that have cysts located along their margins

obturator internus muscles—paired pelvic muscles located lateral to the ovaries

occult—hidden

ocular diameter—the measurement from the lateral margin of the orbit to the medial margin of the same orbit

OEIS complex—acronym that stands for omphalocele, bladder exstrophy, imperforate anus, and spina bifida; also referred to as cloacal exstrophy

oligohydramnios—a lower-than-normal amount of amniotic fluid for the gestational age

oligomenorrhea—infrequent or light menstrual periods

oliguria—scant or decreased urine output

olive sign—when the pyloric sphincter muscle is enlarged and palpable on physical examination of the abdomen; often indicative of pyloric stenosis

omentum—a fold of peritoneum

omphalocele—an anterior abdominal wall defect where there is herniation of the fetal bowel and other abdominal organs into the base of the umbilical cord

omphalopagus—conjoined twins attached at the abdomen

oncocytes—large cells of glandular origin

oncocytoma—a benign renal tumor that is often found in men in their 60s

oocyte retrieval—the removal of oocytes from ovarian follicles by aspiration

oogenesis—the creation of an ovum

oophorectomy—surgical removal of the ovary

oophoritis—inflammation of the ovary

open spina bifida—see term spina bifida aperta

orchiopexy—the surgery that moves an undescended testis into the scrotum

orchitis—inflammation of the testis or testicles

Ortolani test—clinical test for developmental hip dysplasia that is used to evaluate the hip for the reduction or relocation of a dislocated hip

osteogenesis imperfecta—a group of disorders that result in multiple fractures in utero; caused by decreased mineralization and poor ossification of the bones

osteomyelitis—bone infection caused by fungus or bacteria

osteopenia—a bone density that is lower than normal

osteoporosis—bone loss that predisposes the individual to fractures

ovarian cystectomy—the surgical removal of an ovarian cyst

ovarian dysgenesis—imperfect or abnormal development of the ovaries

ovarian hyperstimulation syndrome—a syndrome resulting from hyperstimulation of the ovaries by fertility drugs; results in the development of multiple, enlarged follicular ovarian cysts

ovarian ligaments—pelvic ligaments that provide support to the ovary extending from the ovary to the lateral surface of the uterus

ovarian torsion—an abnormality that results from the ovary twisting on its mesenteric connection, consequently cutting off the blood supply to the ovary; may be referred to as adnexal torsion

ovulation—the release of the mature egg from the ovary

ovulation induction—the stimulation of the ovaries by hormonal therapy in order to treat infertility

ovum—an unfertilized egg

pallor—extreme paleness of the skin

palmar erythema—reddening of the palms

pampiniform plexus—the group of veins in the spermatic cord

pancreatic adenocarcinoma—the most common form of pancreatic malignancy, typically found within the head of the pancreas

pancreatic divisum—congenital anomaly of the pancreas that results in a shortened main pancreatic duct that only works to drain the pancreatic head and not the entire pancreas

pancreatic pseudocyst—a cyst surrounded by fibrous tissue that consists of pancreatic enzymes that have leaked from the pancreas

pancreatic steatosis—fatty infiltration of the pancreas; may be classified as alcoholic or nonalcoholic; may also be referred to as a fatty pancreas

pancreaticoduodenectomy—the surgical procedure in which the head of the pancreas, the gallbladder, some of the bile ducts, and the proximal duodenum are removed because of a malignant pancreatic neoplasm; also referred to as the Whipple procedure

pannus—a hanging flap of tissue

papillary carcinoma—the most common form of thyroid cancer

papillary muscle—paired muscles in both sides of heart that hold in place either the mitral or tricuspid valves

papillary projection—a small protrusion of tissue

paracentesis—a procedure that uses a needle to drain fluid from the abdominal cavity for diagnostic and/or therapeutic reasons

ParaGard—intrauterine contraceptive device that utilizes copper in its composition to inhibit sperm transport, or to prevent fertilization or transplantation

parallel tube sign—the enlargement of the common duct to the size of the adjacent portal vein within the porta hepatis

paralytic ileus—see term nonmechanical obstruction

parametritis—inflammation of the connective tissue adjacent to the uterus

parapneumonic effusion—pleural effusion associated with pneumonia

parasitic twin—see term acardiac twin

parenchyma—the functional part of an organ

parietal peritoneum—the portion of the peritoneum that lines the abdominal and pelvic cavities

parity—the total number of pregnancies in which the patient has given birth to a fetus at or beyond 20 weeks' gestational age or an infant weighing more than 500 g

Patau syndrome—a chromosomal aberration in which there is a third chromosome 13; also referred to as trisomy 13

pedunculated—something that grows off a stalk

pedunculated uterine leiomyoma—leiomyoma (fibroid) that extends from the uterus on a stalk

pelvic congestion syndrome—syndrome that results from the compression of the left renal vein at the origin of the superior mesenteric artery; leads to lower abdominal and back pain after standing for long periods of time, dyspareunia, dysmenorrhea, abnormal uterine bleeding, chronic fatigue, and bowel issues

pelvic diaphragm—group of pelvic muscles consisting of the levator ani and coccygeus muscles that provide support to the pelvic organs

pelvic inflammatory disease—an infection of the female genital tract that may involve the ovaries, uterus, and/or the fallopian tubes

pelvic kidney—a kidney located within the pelvis

pelviectasis—dilation of the renal pelvis; may also be referred to as pyelectasis

pelviureteral junction—see term ureteropelvic junction

pelvocaliectasis—see term hydronephrosis

pentalogy of Cantrell—a group of anomalies that include an omphalocele, along with ectopic cordis, cleft sternum, anterior diaphragmatic defect, and pericardial defects

percutaneous umbilical cord sampling—see term cordocentesis

Pergonal—infertility medicine used to stimulate the follicular development of the ovaries

pericardial effusion—fluid accumulation around the heart in the pericardial cavity

pericholecystic fluid—fluid around the gallbladder

perienteric fat—fat around the intestines

perimenopausal—the time before menopause

perimetrium—the outer layer of the uterus; may also be referred to as the serosal layer

perinephric abscess—an abscess that surrounds the kidney

perineum—the region between the external genitalia and the anus

periovulatory phase—another name for the late proliferative phase of the endometrial cycle, which occurs around the time of ovulation

peripheral zone—the largest zone of the prostate and most common location for prostatic cancer

periportal cuffing—an increase in the echogenicity of the portal triads as seen in hepatitis and other conditions

peristalsis—contractions that move in a wavelike pattern to propel a substance

peritoneal dialysis—a form of dialysis that uses a solution that is instilled into the abdomen; uses diffusion and osmosis to filter waste products from the blood

peritonitis—inflammation of the peritoneal lining

Peyronie disease—the buildup of fibrous plaque (scar tissue) and calcifications within the penis that results in a painful curvature

pheochromocytoma—a hyperfunctioning, benign adrenal mass that causes the adrenal gland to release excessive amounts of epinephrine and norepinephrine into the bloodstream, leading to uncontrollable hypertension

philtrum—the vertical groove seen between the upper lip and the nasal septum

phlegmon—the peripancreatic fluid collection that results from the inflammation of the pancreas

Phrygian cap—gallbladder variant when the gallbladder fundus is folded onto itself

physiologic bowel herniation—the normal developmental stage when the midgut migrates into the base of the umbilical cord

phytobezoars—a bezoar that consists of vegetable matter

pia mater—the innermost layer of the meninges

pilonidal cyst—cyst located along the natal cleft that is composed of loose hairs and skin debris

pineal gland—endocrine gland located in the brain that secretes melatonin

piriformis muscles—paired pelvic muscles located posteriorly that extend from the sacrum to the femoral greater trochanter

pitting—the splenic process of cleaning red blood cells of unwanted material

placenta accreta—the abnormal adherence of the placenta to the myometrium in an area where the decidua is either absent or minimal

placenta increta—invasion of the placenta within the myometrium

placenta percreta—penetration of the placenta through the uterine serosa and possibly into adjacent pelvic organs

placenta previa—when the placenta covers or nearly covers the internal os of the cervix

placental abruption—the premature separation of the placenta from the uterine wall before the birth of the fetus

placentation—formation or structure of a placenta, structural organization, and mode of attachment of fetal to maternal tissues during placental formation

placentomegaly—enlargement of the placenta

pleomorphic adenoma—benign and most frequent tumor of the salivary glands; most commonly seen in the parotid gland

pleural effusion—the abnormal accumulation of fluid in the pleural space

plicae circulares—the mucus membrane folds within the inner wall of the small bowel

pneumobilia—air within the biliary tree

pneumothorax—free air within the chest outside the lungs that can lead to lung collapse

polycystic ovary syndrome—a syndrome characterized by anovulatory cycles, infertility, hirsutism, amenorrhea, and obesity; may also be referred to as Stein–Leventhal syndrome

polydactyly—having more than the normal number of fingers or toes

polyhydramnios—an excessive amount of amniotic fluid for the gestational age

polyorchidism—having more than two testicles

polypectomy—the surgical removal of a polyp

polypoid—shaped like a polyp

polysplenia—having many small islands of splenic tissue

porcelain gallbladder—the calcification of all or part of the gallbladder wall

porencephaly—the development of a cystic cavity within the cerebrum; may be the result of an intraparenchymal hemorrhage

porta hepatis—the area of the liver where the portal vein and hepatic artery enter and the hepatic duct exit; also referred to as the liver hilum

portal hypertension—the elevation of blood pressure within the portal venous system

portal triads—an assembly of a small branch of the portal vein, bile duct, and hepatic artery that surround each liver lobule

portal vein thrombosis—the development of clot within the portal vein

posterior cul-de-sac—see term rectouterine pouch

posterior fossa—posterior portion of the cranium located near the cerebellum and containing the cisterna magna

posterior urethral valves—irregular thin membranes of tissue located within the male posterior urethra that do not allow urine to exit the urethra

posthepatic jaundice—elevation in bilirubin caused by an obstruction of bile flow, typically by either a gallstone lodged in the biliary tract or pancreatic mass

postmenopausal—the time after menopause

postmenopausal vaginal bleeding—vaginal bleeding after the onset of menopause

postpartum—the time directly after giving birth and extending to about 6 weeks

postprandial—after a meal

Potter facies—facial features seen with severe oligohydramnios, including low-set ears, flattened nose, wrinkled skin, and micrognathia

Potter syndrome—physical features of a fetus as a result of oligohydramnios; characterized by bilateral renal agenesis, abnormal facies, pulmonary hypoplasia, and limb abnormalities; also referred to as Potter sequence

pouch of Douglas—see term rectouterine pouch

precocious puberty—pubertal development before the age of 8; the early development of pubic hair, breast, or genitals

preeclampsia—pregnancy-induced maternal high blood pressure and excess protein in the urine after 20 weeks' gestation

pregestational diabetes—maternal diabetes that existed before pregnancy; includes both type 1 and 2 diabetes mellitus

pregnancy-associated plasma protein A—a protein that is produced by the placenta and that can be monitored during pregnancy

prehepatic jaundice—when the liver cannot process the amount of hemolysis of the red blood cells, resulting in a buildup of circulating bilirubin in the bloodstream

premature rupture of membranes—the rupture of the amniotic sac before the onset of labor

pretibial myxedema—clinical finding associated with Graves disease in which there is thickening of the skin and edema on the anterior legs

primary amenorrhea—failure to experiencing menarche before age 16

proboscis—fleshy, tongue-like appendage that is typically located within the midline above the orbits in association with cyclopia and holoprosencephaly

progesterone—a hormone that prepares the uterus for pregnancy, maintains pregnancy, and promotes development of the mammary glands; primarily produced by the ovary and placenta

progestin—synthetic progesterone secreted by some intrauterine devices to regulate menstrual flow

progestogen therapy—a hormone replacement therapy that involves administering synthetic progesterone

projectile vomiting—vomiting with so much force that the vomit can travel for quite a distance

prolapse—(uterine prolapse) a condition that results from the weakening of the pelvic diaphragm muscles and allows for the displacement of the uterus, often through the vagina

proliferation—the multiplication of similar forms

proliferative phase—the first phase of the endometrial cycle

prosencephalon—the primary brain vesicle also referred to as the forebrain; it eventually becomes the lateral ventricles, cerebral hemispheres, third ventricle, thalamus, hypothalamus, pineal gland, and pituitary gland

prostate-specific antigen—a protein produced by the prostate gland

prostatitis—inflammation of the prostate gland

proteinuria—protein in the urine

prune belly syndrome—a syndrome that is a consequence of the abdominal wall musculature being stretched by an extremely enlarged urinary bladder

pruritus—severe itchiness of the skin

psammoma bodies—round, punctate calcific deposits

pseudoaneurysm—see term false aneurysm

pseudocirrhosis—nodular appearance of the liver caused by multiple metastatic tumors

pseudogallbladder sign—a sign associated with biliary atresia in children where there is evidence of a cystic structure in the gallbladder fossa without the presence of an actual gallbladder

pseudogestational sac—the appearance of an abnormally shaped false gestational sac within the uterine cavity as a result of an ectopic pregnancy; this often corresponds with the accumulation of blood and secretions within the uterine cavity

pseudomass—false mass

pseudomyxoma peritonei—an intraperitoneal extension of mucin-secreting cells that result from the rupture of a malignant mucinous ovarian tumor or possibly a malignant tumor of the appendix

pseudoprecocious puberty—secondary sexual development induced by sex steroids or from other sources such as ovarian tumors, adrenal tumors, or steroid use

puerperal mastitis—inflammation of the breast that is related to pregnancy

pulmonary atresia—the absence of the pulmonary valve, which, in turn, prohibits blood flow from the right ventricle into the pulmonary artery and essentially to the lungs

pulmonary embolus—blood clot that has traveled to the lungs and is obstructing the pulmonary arterial circulation; most often, the result of a deep venous thrombosis

pulmonary hypoplasia—underdevelopment of the lungs

pulmonary sequestration—a separate mass of nonfunctioning lung tissue with its own blood supply

pulmonary stenosis—the narrowing of the pulmonary valve

punctate—marked with dots

purpura—blood spots under the skin that may appear purple

purulent—an inflammatory reaction that leads to the formation of pus

pyelectasis—enlargement of the renal pelvis; also referred to as pelviectasis

pylorospasm—a temporary spasm and thickening of the pyloric sphincter that can replicate the sonographic appearance of pyloric stenosis

pyocele—a pus collection within the scrotum

pyogenic liver abscess—a liver abscess that can result from the spread of infection from inflammatory conditions such as appendicitis, diverticulitis, cholecystitis, cholangitis, and endocarditis

pyometra—the presence of pus within the uterus

pyonephrosis—the condition of having pus within the collecting system of the kidney

pyopagus—conjoined twins joined back-to-back in the sacral region

pyosalpinx—the presence of pus within the fallopian tube

pyramidal lobe—a normal variant of the thyroid gland in which there is a superior extension of the isthmus

pyuria—pus within the urine

quadrate lobe—the medial segment of the left lobe

quadruple screen—a maternal blood test that includes an analysis of human chorionic gonadotropin, alpha-fetoprotein, estriol, and inhibin A

radial arteries—arteries that supply blood to the deeper layers of the myometrium

radial ray defect—absence or underdevelopment of the radius

radiography—a diagnostic imaging modality that uses ionizing radiation for imaging bones, joints, organs, and some other soft tissue structures

radiolucent—transparent with radiography

rebound tenderness—pain encountered after the removal of pressure; a common clinical finding in patients suffering from acute appendicitis

recanalization—the reopening of canals or pathways

rectouterine pouch—peritoneal outpouching located between the uterus and the rectum; also referred to as the posterior cul-de-sac, pouch of Douglas, and the rectovaginal pouch

rectus abdominis muscles—paired anterior abdominal muscles that extend from the xiphoid process of the sternum to the pubic bone; separated by the linea alba

red currant jelly stool—feces that contains a mixture of mucus and blood; a common clinical finding in patients suffering from intussusception

red pulp—specialized tissue within the spleen that performs its phagocytic function

Reed–Sternberg cells—the cells that indicate the presence of Hodgkin lymphoma

refractive shadowing—acoustic shadowing caused by bending of a sound beam at the edge of a curved reflector; may be referred to as edge artifact or edge shadowing

renal adenoma—a benign renal mass

renal agenesis—failure of the kidney to develop; may be unilateral or bilateral

renal artery stenosis—the narrowing of the renal artery

renal calices—the part of the collecting system that encompasses the apex of the renal pyramids

renal cell carcinoma—the carcinoma of the kidney; also referred to as hypernephroma

renal colic—a sharp pain in the lower back that radiates into the groin and is typically associated with the passage of a urinary stone through the ureter

renal cortex—the outer part of the renal parenchyma that is responsible for filtration

renal ectopia—refers to an abnormal location of the kidney or kidneys

renal fossa—the region where the kidney is located in the abdomen

renal hamartoma—see term angiomyolipoma

renal hemangioma—a benign renal mass that consists of blood vessels

renal hematoma—a collection of blood on or around the kidney that is typically associated with some form of trauma or perhaps an invasive kidney procedure

renal infarction—an area in the kidney that becomes necrotic because of a lack of oxygen; color Doppler most useful at demonstrating a focal or global absence of blood flow

renal lipoma—a fatty tumor on the kidney

renal medulla—the inner part of the renal parenchyma that is responsible for absorption

renal pelvic diameter—measurement of the fetal renal pelvis; this dimension is obtained from the transverse kidney plane

renal pelvis—the funnel-shaped collecting system in the central portion of the kidney that allows urine to flow from the kidney to the ureter

renal pyramids—cone-shaped structures located within the renal medulla that contain part of the nephron

renal sinus—the portion of the kidney containing the minor calices, major calices, renal pelvis, and infundibula

renal vein thrombosis—a blood clot located within the renal vein

renal:aorta ratio—a ratio calculated by dividing the highest renal artery velocity by the highest aortic velocity obtained at the level of the renal arteries

renin—enzyme produced by the kidneys that helps regulate blood pressure

renunculi—the two embryonic parenchymal tissue masses that combine to create the kidney; singular form is renunculus

retained products of conception—when additional placental tissue remains within the uterus after the bulk of the placenta has been delivered

rete testis—a network of tubules that carry sperm from the seminiferous tubules to the epididymis

reticuloendothelial system—phagocytic system of the body that helps remove dead and toxic particles from the blood

retroflexion—the uterine body tilts backward and comes in contact with the cervix, forming an acute angle between the body and the cervix

retroperitoneal—posterior to the peritoneum

retroperitoneal fibrosis—a disease characterized by the buildup of fibrous tissue within the retroperitoneum; this mass may involve the abdominal aorta, IVC, ureters, and sacrum

retroperitoneal hematoma—a bloody tumor located within the retroperitoneum

retroperitoneal lymphadenopathy—the enlargement of the abdominal lymph nodes located within the abdomen

retroversion—the uterine body tilts backward, without a bend where the cervix and body meet

reverberation artifact—an artifact that results from a sound wave interacting with a large acoustic interface that repeatedly bounces back and forth from the interface to the transducer

rhabdomyoma—a fetal heart tumor found within the myocardium

rhizomelia—shortening of the proximal segment of a limb

rhombencephalon—the primary brain vesicle also referred to as the hindbrain; becomes the cerebellum, pons, medulla oblongata, and fourth ventricle

Riedel lobe—a tongue-like extension of the right hepatic lobe

ring-down artifact—artifact seen posterior to air or gas bubbles

rocker-bottom feet—abnormal curved shape of the sole of the feet

Rokitansky–Aschoff sinuses—tiny pockets within the gallbladder wall

Rovsing sign—pain elicited in the right lower quadrant after the left lower quadrant has been palpated; associated with appendicitis

saccular aneurysm—saclike dilation of a blood vessel

sacral agenesis—the nondevelopment of the sacrum; see term caudal regression syndrome

sacral dimple—an opening in the skin over the distal spine

saline infusion sonography—see term saline infusion sonohysterography

saline infusion sonohysterography—a sonographic procedure that uses saline instillation into the endometrial cavity and, possibly, the fallopian tubes to evaluate for internal abnormalities; also referred to as sonohysterography

saliva—fluid produced by the salivary glands that aids in digestion

salpingitis—inflammation of the fallopian tube

sandal gap—a large space between the first and second toes

sandwich sign—the sign associated with abnormal abdominal lymph node enlargement that leads to the compression of the aorta and IVC

sarcoidosis—a systemic disease that results in the development of granulomas throughout the body

scalloping (frontal bones)—indentations on a normally smooth margin of a structure

scaphocephaly—see term dolichocephaly

schistosomiasis—a flatworm that enters humans by penetrating the skin

schizencephaly—a cerebral malformation associated with the development of fluid-filled clefts

scintigraphy (thyroid)—nuclear medicine study in which a radiopharmaceutical is used to examine the thyroid gland

scoliosis—an abnormal lateral curvature of the spine

scrotal pearl—an extratesticular calculus

scrotum—sac of cutaneous tissue that holds the testicles

seashore sign—normal M-mode tracing of lung sliding

sebum—an oily substance secreted by the sebaceous glands

secondary amenorrhea—the cessation of menstruation characteristically diagnosed in the postmenarchal woman who has had 3 to 6 months without a menstrual cycle

secondary yolk sac—the structure responsible for early nutrient transfer to the embryo; the yolk sac seen during a sonographic examination of the early gestation

secretory phase—the second phase of the endometrial cycle

selective reduction—a method of reducing the number of pregnancies in a multiple gestation, whereby certain embryos/fetuses are terminated

semen—a fluid that contains secretions from the testicles, seminal vesicles, and prostate gland

seminal vesicles—small glands located superior to the prostate gland and posterior to the base of the bladder, which secrete an alkaline-based fluid

seminiferous tubules—the location of spermatogenesis within the testicles

seminoma—the most common malignant neoplasm of the testicles

sepsis—a life-threatening condition caused by the body's response to a systemic infection; also referred to as blood poisoning; results in a number of issues including low blood pressure, rapid heart beat, and fever

septate gallbladder—a gallbladder that has one or more septa within its lumen; a gallbladder with several septa; may be referred to as a multiseptate gallbladder

septate uterus—common congenital malformation of the uterus that results in a single septum that separates two endometrial cavities

septation—a partition separating two or more cavities

sequela—an illness resulting from another disease, trauma, or injury

serosal fluid—fluid that is secreted by the serous membranes to reduce friction in the peritoneal and other cavities of the body

serosal layer (uterus)—the outermost layer of the uterus; may also be referred to as the perimetrium

serpiginous—twisted or snake-like pattern

Sertoli–Leydig cell tumor—malignant sex cord–stromal ovarian neoplasm that is associated with virilization

serum lactate dehydrogenase—tumor marker that is elevated in the presence of an ovarian dysgerminoma and other abdominal abnormalities

sex cord–stromal tumors—ovarian tumors that arise from the gonadal ridges

shear wave elastography—elastography technique that utilizes a standard ultrasound transducer with elastography technology to obtain information about the stiffness of tissue as in the case of liver fibrosis or cirrhosis

shotgun sign—the enlargement of the common duct to the size of the adjacent portal vein within the porta hepatis; also referred to as the parallel tube sign

shoulder dystocia—when the shoulder of the fetus cannot pass through the birth canal during pregnancy

sialadenitis—inflammation of the salivary gland or glands

sialadenosis—benign, painless enlargement of a salivary gland or glands

sialolithiasis—salivary duct stones

sickle cell anemia—an inherited disease in which the body produces abnormally shaped red blood cells

sickle cell disease—form of hemolytic anemia typically found in Africans or people of African descent; characterized by dysfunctional sickle-shaped red blood cells

signs—objective proof of a disease such as abnormal laboratory findings and fever

simple cyst—an anechoic, round mass that has smooth walls and demonstrates through transmission (acoustic enhancement)

singleton pregnancy—a single developing fetus

sirenomelia—a fetal abnormality characterized by fusion of the lower extremities, renal agenesis, and oligohydramnios; may also be referred to as mermaid syndrome

situs inversus—condition in which the organs of the abdomen and chest are on the opposite sides of the body (e.g., the liver is within the left upper quadrant instead of the right upper quadrant)

Sjögren syndrome—an autoimmune disease that affects all glands that produce moisture, leading to dysfunction of the salivary glands and severe dryness of the eyes, nose, skin, and mouth

Skene duct cyst—benign cyst that may be noted within the female urethra; may manifest as a Skene gland cyst

small bowel ischemia—a condition resulting in interruption or reduction of the blood supply to the small intestines

sonographic findings—information gathered by performing a sonographic examination

sonohysterogram—a sonographic procedure that uses saline instillation into the endometrial cavity and fallopian tubes to evaluate for internal abnormalities; also referred to as saline infusion sonohysterography

space of Retzius—the space between the urinary bladder and the pubic bone; also referred to as the retropubic space

spermatic cord—the structure that travels through the inguinal canal and contains blood vessels, nerves, lymph nodes, and the cremaster muscle

spermatocele—a common cyst found most often in the head of the epididymis that is composed of nonviable sperm, fat, cellular debris, and lymphocytes

spermatogenesis—the production of sperm

sphincter of Oddi—the muscle that controls the emptying of bile and pancreatic juices into the duodenum; also referred to as the hepatopancreatic sphincter

spider nevi—a cluster of vessels noted on the skin that have a web-like pattern; singular form is nevus

spina bifida—a birth defect in which there is incomplete closure of the spine

spina bifida aperta—most common form of spina bifida; results in open lesions that are typically not covered by skin and a mass that protrudes from the spine; also referred to as open spina bifida

spina bifida occulta—closed spinal lesions that are completely covered by skin and can be difficult to identify sonographically; also referred to as closed spina bifida

spinal dysraphism—a group of neural tube defects that describe some manifestation of incomplete closure of the spine

spiral arteries—tiny, coiled arteries that supply blood to the functional layer of the endometrium

spiral valves of Heister—folds located within the cystic duct that prevent it from collapsing and distending

splanchnic circulation—blood flow to the major gastrointestinal organs including the stomach, liver, spleen, pancreas, and small and large intestines; consists of the celiac artery, superior mesenteric artery, and inferior mesenteric artery

splay—turned outward

splenectomy—surgical removal of the spleen

splenic cleft—a congenital anomaly in which the spleen is divided into two portions by a band of tissue

splenic hamartoma—benign splenic mass that has been associated with Beckwith–Wiedemann syndrome and tuberous sclerosis

splenic infarct—an area within the spleen that has become necrotic owing to a lack of oxygen

splenic lymphangioma—benign tumor composed of lymph spaces

splenic torsion—the twisting of the splenic vasculature causing a disruption in blood supply to the spleen and subsequent ischemia

splenomegaly—enlargement of the spleen

splenosis—the implantation of ectopic splenic tissue possibly secondary to splenic rupture

splenule—an accessory spleen

spontaneous abortion—the loss of a pregnancy before 20 gestational weeks

staghorn calculus—a large urinary stone that completely fills and takes the shape of the renal pelvis

standoff pad—a gel pad that is used to provide some distance between the transducer face and the skin surface, allowing superficial structures to be imaged more clearly

***starry sky* sign**—the sonographic sign associated with the appearance of periportal cuffing in which there is an increased echogenicity of the walls of the portal triads may be associated with hepatitis

steatohepatitis—a type of fatty liver disease that causes inflammation of the liver

Stein–Leventhal syndrome—see term polycystic ovary syndrome

Stensen duct—the main duct of the parotid gland

stillborn—dead at birth

straight arteries—uterine radial artery branch that supplies blood to the basal layer of the endometrium

striae—stretch marks

"string of pearls" sign—sonographic finding that is described as the presence of 10 or more small cysts measuring 2 to 18 mm along the periphery of the ovary

stuck twin—when a twin fetus, suffering from twin–twin transfusion syndrome, experiences severe oligohydramnios and is closely adhered to the uterine wall

subarachnoid space—an area located between the arachnoid membrane and the pia mater

subchorionic hemorrhage—a bleed between the endometrium and the gestational sac at the edge of the placenta

subcutaneous edema—a buildup of fluid under the skin

subependymal (layer)—the area just beneath the ependymal lining the lateral ventricles

subluxation—partial dislocation of the hip

submucosal (fibroid)—a leiomyoma that distorts the shape of the endometrium

subseptate uterus—congenital malformation of the uterus that results in a normal uterine contour with an endometrium that branches into two horns

subserosal (fibroid)—location of a leiomyoma in which the tumor grows outward and distorts the contour of the uterus

subureteric Teflon injection—a treatment method for vesicoureteral reflux disease that uses a bulking agent to elevate the ureteral orifice and distal ureter, allowing for the normal flow of urine from the ureter into the bladder

succenturiate lobe—an accessory lobe of the placenta

sulci—grooves within the brain

superficial epidermal cyst—cysts commonly found in the scalp, face, neck, trunk, or back; they can be congenital, the result of trauma, or the result of an obstructed hair follicle

supernumerary—having above the normal number of a structure; an extra

supine hypotensive syndrome—a reduction in blood return to the maternal heart caused by the gravid uterus compressing the maternal IVC

suppurative cholecystitis—complication of acute cholecystitis characterized by pus accumulation within the gallbladder

suprarenal glands—another name for the adrenal glands

suspensory ligament of the ovary—pelvic ligament that provides support to the ovary and extends from the ovaries to the pelvic side walls

suture (skull)—a flexible, connective tissue that lies between the cranial bones

symptoms—any subjective evidence of a disease such as nausea, weakness, or numbness

syncytiotrophoblastic cells—the trophoblastic cells surrounding the blastocyst that are responsible for producing human chorionic gonadotropin

syndactyly—webbed fingers or toes

syndrome—a group of clinically observable findings that exist together and allow for classification

synechiae—adhesions

tachycardia—abnormally rapid heart rate

talipes equinovarus—see term clubfoot

tamoxifen—a breast cancer drug that inhibits the effects of estrogen in the breast

tardus–parvus—the combination of a slow systolic upstroke and a decreased systolic velocity

tendosynovitis—inflammation of the tendon and synovial tendon sheath

teratogen—something that can cause birth defects or abnormalities within an embryo or fetus; examples include medications, tobacco products, chemicals, alcohol, and certain infections

teratoma—a tumor that typically consists of several germ cell layers

testicular torsion—a condition that results from the arterial blood supply to the testicle being cut off secondary to the twisting of the testicular axis

tetralogy of Fallot—a group of abnormalities consisting of an overriding aortic root, ventricular septal defect, pulmonary stenosis, and right ventricular hypertrophy

thalamus—a brain structure that allows communication between the senses; also performing many other functions

thanatophoric dysplasia—most common lethal skeletal dysplasia characterized by a cloverleaf skull with frontal bossing and hydrocephalus

theca internal cells—cells of the follicle that produce estrogen

theca lutein cysts—functional ovarian cysts that are found in the presence of elevated levels of human chorionic gonadotropin; also referred to as a theca luteal cyst

thecoma—benign ovarian sex cord–stromal tumor that produces estrogen in older women

therapeutic amniocentesis—type of amniocentesis used to remove a large amount of amniotic fluid around a fetus suffering from polyhydramnios

Thompson test—clinical test used to evaluate for a complete tear of the Achilles tendon

thoracentesis—a procedure that uses a needle to drain fluid from the pleural cavity for either diagnostic or therapeutic reasons

thoracopagus—conjoined twins attached at the chest

three-line sign—the periovulatory endometrial sonographic appearance in which the outer echogenic basal layer surrounds the more hypoechoic functional layer, with the functional layer separated by the echogenic endometrial stripe

thromboembolism—the formation of a clot within a blood vessel with the potential to travel to a distant site and cause an occlusion

thrombus—blood clot

thymus gland—gland of the immune and lymphatic system located in the chest

thyroglossal duct—the embryonic duct that is located from the base of the tongue to the midportion of the anterior neck

thyroglossal duct cyst—benign congenital cysts located within the midline of the neck superior to the thyroid gland and near the hyoid bone

thyroid in the belly sign—the sonographic appearance of the hyperechoic edematous connective tissue that surrounds the inflamed appendix

thyroid inferno—the sonographic appearance of hypervascularity demonstrated with color Doppler imaging of the thyroid gland

thyroidectomy—the surgical removal of the thyroid or part of the thyroid

"tip of the iceberg" sign—denotes the sonographic appearance of a cystic teratoma (dermoid) when only the anterior element of the mass is seen, while the greater part of the mass is obscured by shadowing

TORCH—acronym that stands for toxoplasmosis, other infections, rubella, cytomegalovirus, and herpes simplex virus

TORCH infections—an acronym that stands for toxoplasmosis, other infections, rubella, cytomegalovirus, and herpes simplex virus; this group of infections may be acquired by a woman during pregnancy

torsion—twisting

torticollis—twisted neck

total abdominal hysterectomy—the removal of the uterus and cervix

total bilirubin—obtained by adding unconjugated and conjugated bilirubin

total parental hyperalimentation—procedure in which an individual receives vitamin and nutrients through a vein, often the subclavian vein

total parenteral nutrition—the feeding of a person intravenously

trabeculae—muscular bundles

tracheoesophageal fistula—an abnormal connection between the esophagus and the trachea

transient elastography—imaging technique that utilizes a special transducer to assess the liver and other organs for signs of fibrosis and cirrhosis; used to measure the stiffness of tissue

transitional cell carcinoma—a malignant tumor of the urinary tract that is often found within the urinary bladder or within the renal pelvis

transitional zone—the prostatic zone that is the most common site for benign prostatic hyperplasia

transjugular intrahepatic portosystemic shunt (TIPS)— the therapy for portal hypertension that involves the placement of a stent between the portal veins and hepatic veins to reduce portal systemic pressure

translabial sonogram—sonogram that requires the transducer be placed against the labia; often used for imaging of the cervix

transposition of the great vessels—abnormality in which the pulmonary artery arises from the left ventricle and the aorta arises from the right ventricle

transudate ascites—a collection of abdominal fluid within the peritoneal cavity often associated with cirrhosis

transurethral resection of the prostate—surgical procedure performed to treat benign prostatic hyperplasia in which prostatic tissue is removed to relieve urinary complications

transversalis fascia—the fascia that lines the anterolateral abdominal wall and is located between the transversus abdominis muscle and the peritoneum

triangle cord sign—a sign associated with biliary atresia in children that is described as an avascular, echogenic, triangular, or tubular structure anterior to the portal vein, representing the replacement of the extrahepatic duct with fibrous tissue in the porta hepatis

trichobezoars—a bezoar that consists of matted hair

tricuspid regurgitation—the leakage of blood back through the tricuspid valve

trident hand—a wide separation between the middle and ring finger

trigone of the urinary bladder—the area within the urinary bladder where the two ureteral orifices and urethral orifice are located

triphasic—vascular flow yielding three phases

triple screen—a maternal blood test that typically includes an analysis of human chorionic gonadotropin, alpha-fetoprotein, and estriol

triploid—having three sets of each chromosome or 69 total

triploidy—a fetus that has three of every chromosome

trisomy—a cell having three copies of an individual chromosome

trisomy 13—chromosomal aberration in which there is a third chromosome 13; also referred to as Patau syndrome; often associated with holoprosencephaly

trisomy 18—chromosomal aberration in which there is a third chromosome 18; also referred to as Edwards syndrome

trisomy 21—chromosomal aberration in which there is a third chromosome 21; also referred to as Down syndrome

trisomy 8—chromosomal aberration in which there is a third chromosome 8; also referred to as Warkany syndrome 2

trophoblastic cells—the cells that surround the gestation that produce human chorionic gonadotropin

true aneurysm—the enlargement of a vessel that involves all three layers of the wall

true lumen—the true or original channel within a vessel

true pelvis—inferior portion of the pelvis that contains the uterus, ovaries, fallopian tubes, urinary bladder, small bowel, sigmoid colon, and rectum

tubal ligation—a permanent form of female sterilization in which the fallopian tubes are severed

tubal sterilization—see term tubal ligation

tuberous sclerosis—a systemic disorder that leads to the development of tumors (hamartomas) within various organs

tubo-ovarian abscess—a pelvic abscess involving the fallopian tubes and ovaries that is often caused by pelvic inflammatory disease

tubo-ovarian complex—when adhesions develop within the pelvis that leads to the fusion of the ovaries and the dilated tubes as a result of pelvic inflammatory disease

tubular ectasia of the rete testis—the cystic dilation and formation of cysts within the rete testis

tumefactive sludge—thick sludge

tumor markers—biomarkers found in blood, urine, or other body tissues that elevate in response to cancer

tunica adventitia—the outer wall layer of a vessel

tunica albuginea—the dense connective tissue that is closely applied to each testicle; it is also located within the penis

tunica albuginea cysts—cysts located within the tunica albuginea surrounding the testis

tunica dartos—the structure that separates the scrotum into two separate compartments internally

tunica intima—the inner wall layer of a vessel

tunica media—the middle, muscular layer of a vessel

tunica vaginalis—the paired serous coatings of the testis; hydroceles are most often found between the two layers of the tunica vaginalis

Turner syndrome—a chromosomal aberration where one sex chromosome is absent; may also be referred to as monosomy X

twin embolization syndrome—when vascular products travel from a demised twin to the surviving twin by means of the common vascular channels within the shared placenta

twin peak sign—see term lambda sign

twinkle sign—an artifact noted as an increased color Doppler signal posterior to a kidney stone or biliary stone

twin-reversed arterial perfusion sequence—another name for acardiac twinning

twin–twin transfusion syndrome—shunting of venous or arterial blood from one twin to another through placental circulation

two-vessel cord—an umbilical cord with one artery and one vein; could possibly be associated with other fetal abnormalities and intrauterine growth restriction

ulcerative colitis—an inflammatory bowel disease that leads to the development of ulcers within the bowel

umbilical arteries—two vessels of the umbilical cord that carry deoxygenated blood from the fetus to the placenta

umbilical vein—the vessel of the umbilical cord that carries oxygenated blood from the placenta to the fetus

umbilical vein varix—focal dilatation of the intra-abdominal portion of the umbilical vein

uncinate process—a posteromedial extension of the pancreatic head

unconjugated bilirubin—the non–water soluble form of bilirubin that travels to the liver via the bloodstream; eventually converted to conjugated bilirubin by the liver; also referred to as indirect bilirubin

undescended testis—testicles that do not descend into the scrotum; also referred to as cryptorchidism

unicornuate uterus—congenital malformation of the uterus that results in a uterus with one horn

unilocular—having one chamber or compartment

upper genital tract—the uterus, ovaries, and fallopian tubes

urachus—canal connecting the fetal bladder with the allantois; normally closes during fetal development and becomes a fibrous cord

ureteral jets—jets of urine that are the result of urine being forced into the urinary bladder from the ureters; can be demonstrated with color Doppler imaging

ureterocele—an abnormality in which the distal ureter projects into the urinary bladder

ureteropelvic junction—the junction of the ureter and renal pelvis

ureteropelvic junction obstruction—an obstruction located in the region where the ureter meets the renal pelvis

ureterovesicle junction—the junction of the ureter and urinary bladder

ureterovesicular junction obstruction—an obstruction located in the region where the ureter meets the bladder

urethral atresia—the congenital absence of the urethra

urethral caruncle—small benign lesions of the female urethra

urethritis—inflammation of the urethra

urinoma—a localized collection of urine; may appear complex or simple

urolithiasis—a urinary stone

uterine arteries—branches of the internal iliac artery that supplies blood to the uterus, ovaries, and fallopian tubes

uterine artery embolization—procedure used to block the blood supply to a leiomyoma (fibroid)

uterine leiomyoma—a benign, smooth muscle tumor of the uterus; may also be referred to as a fibroid or uterine myoma

uterine myoma—see term leiomyoma

uterus didelphys—congenital malformation of the uterus that results in the complete duplication of the uterus, cervix, and vagina

VACTERL—acronym for associated anomalies; stands for vertebral anomalies, anal atresia, cardiac anomalies, tracheoesophageal fistula or esophageal atresia, renal anomalies, and limb anomalies

VACTERL association—an acronym for a combination of abnormalities that represent vertebral anomalies, anorectal atresia, cardiac anomalies, tracheoesophageal fistula, renal anomalies, and limb anomalies; may also be referred to as VATER association

vaginal atresia—occlusion or imperforation of the vagina; can be congenital or acquired

vaginal cuff—the portion of the vagina remaining after a hysterectomy

vaginal fornices—recesses of the vagina

vaginitis—inflammation of the vagina

Valsalva maneuver—performed by attempting to forcibly exhale while keeping the mouth and nose closed

vanishing twin—the death and reabsorption of a twin

varicocele—a dilated group of veins found within the scrotum

vasa previa—fetal vessels resting over the internal os of the cervix

vasoctomy—a form of male contraception in which the vas deferens is surgically interrupted to prohibit the flow of sperm from the testicles

vein of Galen aneurysm—an arteriovenous malformation that occurs within the fetal brain and is associated with congestive heart failure

velamentous cord insertion—the abnormal insertion of the umbilical cord into the membranes beyond the placental edge

venography—examination of the veins of the legs and pelvis that includes the use of contrast media; can be performed using radiography (fluoroscopy), computed tomography, and magnetic resonance imaging

venous lakes—pools of maternal blood within the placental substance

ventricular septal defect—an opening within the septum that separates the right and left ventricles

ventriculomegaly—buildup of cerebrospinal fluid that results in an enlargement of one or more of the ventricles within the brain

vermiform appendix—a blind-ended tube that is connected to the cecum of the colon

vernix—protective fetal skin covering

verumontanum—an elevated area within the prostatic urethra at which the ejaculatory ducts meet the urethra

vesicoureteral junction—see term ureteropelvic junction

vesicoureteral reflux—the abnormal retrograde flow of urine from the urinary bladder into the ureter and possibly into the kidney(s)

vesicouterine pouch—peritoneal outpouching located between the bladder and the uterus; also referred to as the anterior cul-de-sac

virilization—(female) changes within the female that are typically associated with males; caused by increased androgens and may lead to deepening of the voice and hirsutism

visceral peritoneum—the portion of the peritoneum that is closely applied to each organ

visceromegaly—enlargement of an organ

vitelline duct—the structure that connects the developing embryo to the secondary yolk sac

voiding cystourethrogram—a radiographic examination used to evaluate the lower urinary tract, where a contrast agent is instilled into the urinary bladder by means of urethral catheterization

volvulus—a situation in which a loop of bowel twists upon itself

von Gierke disease—condition in which the body does not have the ability to break down glycogen; also referred to as glycogen storage disease type 1

von Hippel–Lindau disease—a hereditary disease that includes the development of cysts within the pancreas and other organs

von Hippel–Lindau syndrome—an inherited disorder characterized by tumors of the central nervous system and the development of cysts within the kidneys, renal cell carcinoma, and pheochromocytomas

von Willebrand disease—an inherited bleeding disorder that is characterized by low levels of a specific clotting protein in the blood referred to as von Willebrand factor; results in excessive bleeding and specifically vaginal bleeding in women

vulva—collective term for the mons pubis, labia majora and labia minora, vestibule, Bartholin gland, and clitoris

wall–echo–shadow sign—shadowing from the gallbladder fossa produced by a gallbladder that is completely filled with gallstones

wandering spleen—a highly mobile spleen

Wharton duct—the duct that drains the submandibular gland

Wharton jelly—gelatinous material that is located within the umbilical cord around the umbilical vessels

Whipple procedure—see term pancreaticoduodenectomy

Whipple triad—a group of clinical indicators of a functional insulinoma; includes hypoglycemia, low fasting glucose, and relief with intravenous glucose administration

whirlpool sign (gallbladder)—the sonographic sign of gallbladder torsion when color Doppler is applied to the spiraled, twisted cystic artery

whirlpool sign (ovary)—an indicator of the torsed ovarian pedicle adjacent to the ovary, appearing as a round mass with concentric hypoechoic and hyperechoic rings that demonstrates a swirling color Doppler signature

white pulp—specialized lymphatic tissue within the spleen

Wilms tumor—the most common solid malignant pediatric abdominal mass; a malignant renal mass that may also be referred to as nephroblastoma

Wilson disease—a congenital disorder that causes the body to accumulate excess copper

xanthogranulomatous cholecystitis—rare chronic gallbladder infection characterized by intramural accumulation of inflammatory cells; noted sonographically as asymmetrical thickening of the gallbladder wall and intraluminal echogenic debris

xanthogranulomatous pyelonephritis—a rare chronic form of pyelonephritis that is typically the result of a chronic obstructive process

yolk sac tumor—(ovary) malignant germ cell tumor of the ovary

Zinner syndrome—syndrome that consists of unilateral renal agenesis, ipsilateral seminal vesicle cyst, and ejaculatory duct obstruction

Zollinger–Ellison syndrome—the syndrome that includes an excessive secretion of acid by the stomach caused by the presence of a functional gastrinoma within the pancreas

zygosity—relates to the number of zygotes (fertilized ova)

zygote—the cell formed by the union of two gametes; the first stage of a fertilized ovum

zygote intrafallopian transfer—infertility treatment where the zygote is placed into the fallopian tube

Figure Credits

Chapter 1

Figure 1-1. From Kawamura D, Nolan T. *Abdomen and Superficial Structures*. 4th ed. Wolters Kluwer; 2017. (Figure 1-1)

Figure 1-2. From Kawamura D, Nolan T. *Abdomen and Superficial Structures*. 4th ed. Wolters Kluwer; 2017. (Figure 1-3)

Figure 1-3. From Kawamura D, Nolan T. *Abdomen and Superficial Structures*. 4th ed. Wolters Kluwer; 2017. (Figure 1-5)

Figure 1-4A. From Farrell TA. *Radiology 101*. 5th ed. Wolters Kluwer; 2019. (Figure 11-4B)

Figure 1-4B. From Emans SJ. *Emans, Laufer, Goldstein's Pediatric and Adolescent Gynecology*. 7th ed. Wolters Kluwer; 2019. (Figure 37-46A)

Figure 1-4C. From Cardenosa G. *Clinical Breast Imaging: The Essentials*. Wolters Kluwer; 2014. (Figure 7-77B)

Figure 1-5. From Penny SM. *Introduction to Sonography and Patient Care*. Wolters Kluwer; 2015. (Figure 12-1)

Figure 1-6. From Siegel MJ. *Pediatric Sonography*. 4th ed. Wolters Kluwer; 2010. (Figure 2.27)

Figure 1-7. From Siegel MJ. *Pediatric Sonography*. 4th ed. Wolters Kluwer; 2010. (Figure 2.18)

Figure 1-8. From Siegel MJ. *Pediatric Sonography*. 4th ed. Wolters Kluwer; 2010. (Figure 2.22)

Figure 1-9. From Siegel MJ. *Pediatric Sonography*. 4th ed. Wolters Kluwer; 2010. (Figure 2.11)

Figure 1-10. From Siegel MJ. *Pediatric Sonography*. 4th ed. Wolters Kluwer; 2010. (Figure 2.3)

Figure 1-11. From Sanders R. *Clinical Sonography: A Practical Guide*. 4th ed. Lippincott Williams & Wilkins; 2007:630. (Figure 57-3)

Figure 1-12. From Sanders R, Hall-Terracciano B. *Clinical Sonography: A Practical Guide*. 5th ed. Wolters Kluwer; 2015. (Figure 6-26)

Figure 1-13. From Sanders R, Hall-Terracciano B. *Clinical Sonography: A Practical Guide*. 5th ed. Wolters Kluwer; 2015. (Figure 6-9)

Figure 1-14. From Sanders R, Hall-Terracciano B. *Clinical Sonography: A Practical Guide*. 5th ed. Wolters Kluwer; 2015. (Figure 6-13)

Figure 1-15. From Sanders R, Hall-Terracciano B. *Clinical Sonography: A Practical Guide*. 5th ed. Wolters Kluwer; 2015. (Figure 6-19)

Figure 1-16. From Sanders R, Hall-Terracciano B. *Clinical Sonography: A Practical Guide*. 5th ed. Wolters Kluwer; 2015. (Figure 6-22)

Figure 1-17. From Siegel MJ. *Pediatric Sonography*. 4th ed. Wolters Kluwer; 2010. (Figure 2.30)

Figure 1-18. From Siegel MJ. *Pediatric Sonography*. 5th ed. Wolters Kluwer; 2018. (Figure 2-32)

Figure 1-19. From Siegel MJ. *Pediatric Sonography*. 4th ed. Wolters Kluwer Health/Lippincott Williams & Wilkins; 2010. (Figure 2-29)

Figure 1-20. From Shirkhoda A. *Variants and Pitfalls in Body Imaging*. 2nd ed. Wolters Kluwer; 2011. (Figure 22-11B)

Figure 1-21. From Anatomical Chart Company. *The Endocrine System Anatomical Chart*. Wolters Kluwer; 2002.

Figure 1-22. From Rubin P, Hansen JT. *TNM Staging Atlas With Oncoanatomy*. 2nd ed. Wolters Kluwer; 2012. (Figure 50-6A)

Figure 1-23. From Kawamura D, Nolan T. *Abdomen and Superficial Structures*. 4th ed. Wolters Kluwer; 2017. (Figure 3-10)

Figure 1-24. From Bishop M. *Clinical Chemistry*. 8th ed. Wolters Kluwer; 2017. (Figure 32-2)

Figure 1-25. From Shirkhoda A. *Variants and Pitfalls in Body Imaging*. 2nd ed. Wolters Kluwer; 2011. (Figure 24-19B)

Figure 1-26. From Siegel MJ. *Pediatric Sonography*. 5th ed. Wolters Kluwer; 2018. (Figure 2-15A)

Figure 1-27. From Siegel MJ. *Pediatric Sonography*. 5th ed. Wolters Kluwer; 2018. (Figure 2-18)

Figure 1-28. From Shirkhoda A. *Variants and Pitfalls in Body Imaging*. 2nd ed. Wolters Kluwer; 2011. (Figure 8-34C)

Figure 1-29. From Bushberg JT. *The Essential Physics of Medical Imaging*. 4th ed. Wolters Kluwer; 2021. (Figure 14-62)

Figure 1-30. From Siegel MJ. *Pediatric Sonography*. 5th ed. Wolters Kluwer; 2018. (Figure 2-22)

Figure 1-31. From Siegel MJ. *Pediatric Sonography*. 5th ed. Wolters Kluwer; 2018. (Figure 2-19)

Figure 1-32. From Siegel MJ. *Pediatric Sonography*. 5th ed. Wolters Kluwer; 2018. (Figure 2-9)

Figure 1-33. From Sanders RC, Hall-Terracciano B. *Clinical Sonography: A Practical Guide*. 5th ed. Wolters Kluwer; 2015. (Figure 6-24)

Figure 1-34. From Abuhamad A. *A Practical Guide to Fetal Echocardiography*. 2nd ed. Wolters Kluwer; 2010. (Figure 7-3)

Figure 1-35. From Moore KL, Dalley AF, Agur AM, eds. *Clinically Oriented Anatomy*. 8th ed. Wolters Kluwer; 2013. (Figure 4-85)

Chapter 2

Figure 2-1. From Kawamura D, Lunsford B. *Diagnostic Medical Sonography: Abdomen and Superficial Structures*. 3rd ed. Wolters Kluwer; 2012. (Figure 5-4)

Figure 2-2. From Lillemoe KD. *Master Techniques in Surgery: Hepatobiliary and Pancreatic Surgery*. 1st ed. Wolters Kluwer; 2012. (Figure 31-1)

Figure 2-3. From Kawamura D, Lunsford B. *Diagnostic Medical Sonography: Abdomen and Superficial Structures*. 3rd ed. Wolters Kluwer; 2012. (Figure 4-7)

Figure 2-4. From Kupinski AM. *The Vascular System*. 2nd ed. Wolters Kluwer; 2017. (Figure 28-35)

Figure 2-5. From Kupinski AM. *The Vascular System*. 2nd ed. Wolters Kluwer; 2017. (Figure 27-5)

Figure 2-6. From Siegel MJ. *Pediatric Sonography*. 5th ed. Wolters Kluwer; 2018. (Figure 7-13A)

Figure 2-7. From Kawamura D, Nolan T. *Abdomen and Superficial Structures*. 4th ed. Wolters Kluwer; 2017. (Figure 5-15D)

Figure 2-8. From Kawamura D, Nolan T. *Abdomen and Superficial Structures*. 4th ed. Wolters Kluwer; 2017. (Figure 5-21D)

Figure 2-9. From Kawamura D, Nolan T. *Abdomen and Superficial Structures*. 4th ed. Wolters Kluwer; 2017. (Figure 5-21B)

Figure 2-10. From Kawamura D, Nolan T. *Abdomen and Superficial Structures*. 4th ed. Wolters Kluwer; 2017. (Figure 6-6)

Figure 2-13. From Kawamura D, Lunsford B. *Diagnostic Medical Sonography: Abdomen and Superficial Structures*. 3rd ed. Wolters Kluwer; 2012. (Figure 5-7H, I)

Figure 2-14. From Kawamura D, Lunsford B. *Diagnostic Medical Sonography: Abdomen and Superficial Structures*. 3rd ed. Wolters Kluwer; 2012. (Figure 5-7C)

Figure 2-15. From Shirkhoda A. *Variants and Pitfalls in Body Imaging*. 2nd ed. Wolters Kluwer Health/Lippincott Williams & Wilkins; 2010. (Figure 8-38B)

Figure 2-16. From Kawamura D, Nolan T. *Abdomen and Superficial Structures*. 4th ed. Wolters Kluwer; 2017. (Figure 5-28C)

Figure 2-17. From Kawamura D, Lunsford B. *Diagnostic Medical Sonography: Abdomen and Superficial Structures*. 3rd ed. Wolters Kluwer; 2012. (Figure 5.17B)

Figure 2-18. From Kawamura D, Lunsford B. *Diagnostic Medical Sonography: Abdomen and Superficial Structures*. 3rd ed. Wolters Kluwer; 2012. (Figure 5-17D)

Figure 2-19. From Kawamura D, Lunsford B. *Diagnostic Medical Sonography: Abdomen and Superficial Structures*. 3rd ed. Wolters Kluwer; 2012. (Figure 5-17E)

Figure 2-20. From Siegel MJ. *Pediatric Sonography*. 4th ed. Wolters Kluwer; 2010. (Figure 7.45)

Figure 2-21. From Norris TL, Lalchandani R. *Porth's Pathophysiology*. 10th ed. Wolters Kluwer; 2018. (Figure 38-13)

Figure 2-22. From Kawamura D, Lunsford B. *Diagnostic Medical Sonography: Abdomen and Superficial Structures.* 3rd ed. Wolters Kluwer; 2012. (Figure 5-20C)

Figure 2-23. From Klein J, Vinson EN, Brant WE, et al. *Brant and Helms' Fundamentals of Diagnostic Radiology.* 3rd ed. Lippincott Williams & Wilkins; 2006. (Figure 36-6)

Figure 2-24. From Kawamura D, Lunsford B. *Diagnostic Medical Sonography: Abdomen and Superficial Structures.* 3rd ed. Wolters Kluwer; 2012. (Figure 5-20F)

Figure 2-25. From Kawamura D, Nolan T. *Abdomen and Superficial Structures.* 4th ed. Wolters Kluwer; 2017. (Figure 5-36C)

Figure 2-26. From Zierler RE, Dawson DL. *Strandness's Duplex Scanning in Vascular Disorders.* 5th ed. Wolters Kluwer; 2015. (Figure 22-7D)

Figure 2-27. From Kawamura D, Lunsford B. *Diagnostic Medical Sonography: Abdomen and Superficial Structures.* 3rd ed. Wolters Kluwer; 2012. (Figure 5-20O)

Figure 2-28A. Panel A courtesy of Brian Coley, MD.

Figure 2-28B. From Siegel MJ. *Pediatric Sonography.* 4th ed. Wolters Kluwer Health/Lippincott Williams & Wilkins; 2010. (Figure 7-66B)

Figure 2-29. From Siegel MJ. *Pediatric Sonography.* 4th ed. Wolters Kluwer; 2010. (Figure 7.68)

Figure 2-30. From Siegel MJ. *Pediatric Sonography.* 4th ed. Wolters Kluwer; 2010. (Figure 7.64)

Figure 2-31. From Shirkhoda A. *Variants and Pitfalls in Body Imaging.* 2nd ed. Wolters Kluwer; 2011. (Figure 8-20C)

Figure 2-33. From Kupinski AM. *The Vascular System.* 2nd ed. Wolters Kluwer; 2017. (Figure 27-37)

Figure 2-34. From Sanders R, Hall-Terracciano B. *Clinical Sonography: A Practical Guide.* 5th ed. Wolters Kluwer; 2015. (Figure 5-1)

Figure 2-35. From Kawamura D, Lunsford B. *Diagnostic Medical Sonography: Abdomen and Superficial Structures.* 3rd ed. Wolters Kluwer; 2012. (Figure 5-23E,F)

Figure 2-36. From Strayer DS, Saffitz JE, Rubin E. *Rubin's Pathology.* 8th ed. Wolters Kluwer; 2019. (Figure 9-104)

Figure 2-37. From Siegel MJ. *Pediatric Sonography.* 4th ed. Wolters Kluwer; 2010. (Figure 7.49)

Figure 2-38. From Lee E. Pediatric Radiology: Practical Imaging Evaluation of Infants and Children. 1st ed. Wolters Kluwer; 2017. (Figure 14-8A)

Figure 2-39. From Siegel MJ. *Pediatric Sonography.* 4th ed. Wolters Kluwer Health/Lippincott Williams & Wilkins; 2010. (Figure 7-48)

Figure 2-40. From Siegel MJ. *Pediatric Sonography.* 4th ed. Wolters Kluwer; 2010. (Figure 7.48)

Figure 2-41. From Kawamura D, Lunsford B. *Diagnostic Medical Sonography: Abdomen and Superficial Structures.* 3rd ed. Wolters Kluwer; 2012. (Figure 5-30B)

Figure 2-42. From Kawamura D, Lunsford B. *Diagnostic Medical Sonography: Abdomen and Superficial Structures.* 3rd ed. Wolters Kluwer; 2012. (Figure 5-31B)

Figure 2-43. Image courtesy of Robert DeJung, Baltimore, MD.

Figure 2-44. From Sanders R, Hall-Terracciano B. *Clinical Sonography: A Practical Guide.* 5th ed. Wolters Kluwer; 2015. (Figure 32-7)

Figure 2-45. Courtesy of Melanie Willsey, Kettering Health Network, Kettering, OH.

Figure 2-48A. From Kawamura D, Lunsford B. *Diagnostic Medical Sonography: Abdomen and Superficial Structures.* 3rd ed. Wolters Kluwer; 2012. (Figure 5-37A)

Figure 2-48B. From Fischer J. *Fischer's Mastery of Surgery.* 7th ed. Wolters Kluwer; 2018. (Figure 134-4)

Figure 2-49. Used with permission of Elsevier, from Federle MP, Jeffrey RB, Woodward PJ, et al. *Diagnostic Imaging: Abdomen.* 2nd ed. Amirsys; 2009:III 1–115, permission conveyed through Copyright Clearance Center, Inc.

Figure 2-50A. From Kupinski AM. *Diagnostic Medical Sonography: The Vascular System.* 1st ed. Wolters Kluwer Health/Lippincott Williams & Wilkins; 2012. (Figure 22-12)

Figure 2-50B. From Kupinski AM. *Diagnostic Medical Sonography: The Vascular System.* 2nd ed. Wolters Kluwer; 2017. (Figure 27-24)

Figure 2-51A. From Kupinski AM. *The Vascular System.* 2nd ed. Wolters Kluwer; 2017. (Figure 27-25)

Figure 2-51B. From Kupinski AM. *The Vascular System.* 2nd ed. Wolters Kluwer; 2017. (Figure 27-26)

Figure 2-52. From Siegel MJ. *Pediatric Sonography.* 5th ed. Wolters Kluwer; 2018. (Figure 7-91A,B)

Figure 2-53. From Kupinski AM. *The Vascular System.* 2nd ed. Wolters Kluwer; 2017. (Figure 28-39)

Figure 2-54. From Kawamura D, Lunsford B. *Diagnostic Medical Sonography: Abdomen and Superficial Structures.* 3rd ed. Wolters Kluwer; 2012. (Figure 5-36)

Figure 2-55. From Kawamura D, Nolan T. *Abdomen and Superficial Structures.* 4th ed. Wolters Kluwer; 2017. (Figure 5-34B)

Figure 2-56. From Kawamura D, Nolan T. *Abdomen and Superficial Structures.* 4th ed. Wolters Kluwer; 2017. (Figure 5-20G)

Figure 2-57. From Kupinski AM. *The Vascular System.* 2nd ed. Wolters Kluwer; 2017. (Figure 27-15)

Figure 2-58. From Kawamura D, Nolan T. *Abdomen and Superficial Structures.* 4th ed. Wolters Kluwer; 2017. (Figure 5-30A)

Figure 2-59. From Kawamura D, Nolan T. *Abdomen and Superficial Structures.* 4th ed. Wolters Kluwer; 2017. (Figure 5-23E)

Figure 2-60. From Kawamura D, Nolan T. *Abdomen and Superficial Structures.* 4th ed. Wolters Kluwer; 2017. (Figure 5-20P)

Figure 2-61. From Klein J, Vinson EM, Brant WE, et al. *Brant and Helms' Fundamentals of Diagnostic Radiology.* 5th ed. Wolters Kluwer; 2018. (Figure 69-54A)

Figure 2-62. From Torbenson M. *Surgical Pathology of the Liver.* 1st ed. Wolters Kluwer; 2017. (Figure 24-16A,B)

Figure 2-63. From Lee EY. *Computed Body Tomography With MRI Correlation.* 5th ed. Wolters Kluwer; 2019. (Figure 11-72)

Chapter 3

Figure 3-1. From Kawamura D, Lunsford B. *Diagnostic Medical Sonography: Abdomen and Superficial Structures.* 3rd ed. Wolters Kluwer; 2012. (Figure 6-12)

Figure 3-2. From Kawamura D, Nolan T. *Abdomen and Superficial Structures.* 4th ed. Wolters Kluwer; 2017. (Figure 6-3)

Figure 3-4. Modified with permission from Fischer J. *Fischer's Mastery of Surgery.* 7th ed. Wolters Kluwer; 2018. (Figure 110-1)

Figure 3-5. From Gonzales P. *The PA Rotation Exam Review.* Wolters Kluwer; 2019. (Figure 3-6)

Figure 3-6. From Kawamura D, Lunsford B. *Diagnostic Medical Sonography: Abdomen and Superficial Structures.* 3rd ed. Wolters Kluwer; 2012. (Figure 6.23D)

Figure 3-7. From Sanders R, Hall-Terracciano B. *Clinical Sonography: A Practical Guide.* 5th ed. Wolters Kluwer; 2015. (Figure 33-7C)

Figure 3-8. From Siegel MJ. *Pediatric Sonography.* 5th ed. Wolters Kluwer; 2018. (Figure 8-13A)

Figure 3-9. From Sanders R, Hall-Terracciano B. *Clinical Sonography: A Practical Guide.* 5th ed. Wolters Kluwer; 2015. (Figure 33-8A)

Figure 3-10. From Kawamura D, Lunsford B. *Diagnostic Medical Sonography: Abdomen and Superficial Structures.* 3rd ed. Wolters Kluwer; 2012. (Figure 6.20)

Figure 3-11. From Kawamura D, Lunsford B. *Diagnostic Medical Sonography: Abdomen and Superficial Structures.* 3rd ed. Wolters Kluwer; 2012. (Figure 6.18)

Figure 3-12. From Kawamura D, Lunsford B. *Diagnostic Medical Sonography: Abdomen and Superficial Structures.* 3rd ed. Wolters Kluwer; 2012. (Figure 6.35C)

Figure 3-15. From Kawamura D, Lunsford B. *Diagnostic Medical Sonography: Abdomen and Superficial Structures.* 3rd ed. Wolters Kluwer; 2012. (Figure 6.26A,B)

Figure 3-16. From Kawamura D, Lunsford B. *Diagnostic Medical Sonography: Abdomen and Superficial Structures.* 3rd ed. Wolters Kluwer; 2012. (Figure 6.28A,B)

Figure 3-17. From Kawamura D, Lunsford B. *Diagnostic Medical Sonography: Abdomen and Superficial Structures.* 3rd ed. Wolters Kluwer; 2012. (Figure 6.30B)

Figure 3-18. From Kawamura D, Lunsford B. *Diagnostic Medical Sonography: Abdomen and Superficial Structures.* 3rd ed. Wolters Kluwer; 2012. (Figure 6.27C)

Figure 3-20. From Hsu WC, Cummings FP. *Gastrointestinal Imaging: A Core Review.* 1st ed. Wolters Kluwer; 2016. (UnFigure 8-60)

Figure 3-23. From Kawamura D, Nolan T. *Abdomen and Superficial Structures.* 4th ed. Wolters Kluwer; 2017. (Figure 6-29)

Figure 3-24. From Kawamura D, Nolan T. *Abdomen and Superficial Structures.* 4th ed. Wolters Kluwer; 2017. (Figure 6-35A)

Figure 3-25. From Lawrence PF, Bell RM, Dayton MT, et al. *Essentials of General Surgery.* 5th ed. Wolters Kluwer; 2012. (Figure 16-6B)

Figure 3-26A,B. From Fischer J. *Fischer's Mastery of Surgery.* 7th ed. Wolters Kluwer; 2018. (Figure 109-1)

Figure 3-26C. From Irwin RS, Lilly CM, Mayo PH, et al. *Irwin and Rippe's Intensive Care Medicine.* 8th ed. Wolters Kluwer; 2017. (Figure 24-1B)

Figure 3-27. From Britt LD, Peitzman AB, Barie PS, et al. *Acute Care Surgery*. 2nd ed. Wolters Kluwer; 2018. (Figure 7-40)

Chapter 4

Figure 4-1. From Seigel M. *Pediatric Sonography*. 3rd ed. Lippincott Williams & Wilkins; 2002:276. (Figure 7-1A)

Figure 4-2. From Kawamura D, Nolan T. *Abdomen and Superficial Structures*. 4th ed. Wolters Kluwer; 2017. (Figure 6-6)

Figure 4-3. From Cosby K, Kendall J. *Practical Guide to Emergency Ultrasound*. 2nd ed. Wolters Kluwer Health/Lippincott Williams & Wilkins; 2013:227. (Figure 9-41)

Figure 4-4. Figure 3-23. From Kawamura D, Nolan T. *Abdomen and Superficial Structures*. 4th ed. Wolters Kluwer; 2017. (Figure 6-45)

Figure 4-5A. From Blackbourne LH. *Advanced Surgical Recall*. 2nd ed. Baltimore, MD: Lippincott Williams & Wilkins; 2004. (Figure 51-2)

Figure 4-6. Image courtesy of Jillian Platt, Falls Church, VA.

Figure 4-7. From Kawamura D, Nolan T. *Abdomen and Superficial Structures*. 4th ed. Wolters Kluwer; 2017. (Figure 6-52)

Figure 4-8A. From Porrett PM, Drebin JA, Atluri P, et al. *The Surgical Review*. 4th ed. Wolters Kluwer; 2015. (Figure 13-17)

Figure 4-8B. From Brant W. *The Core Curriculum: Ultrasound*. Wolters Kluwer; 2001:63.

Figure 4-11. From Siegel MJ. *Pediatric Sonography*. 4th ed. Wolters Kluwer; 2010. (Figure 8.36B)

Figure 4-12. From Brant W. *The Core Curriculum: Ultrasound*. 1st ed. Lippincott Williams & Wilkins; 2001:59. (Figure 2.63)

Figure 4-13. From Lee E. *Pediatric Radiology: Practical Imaging Evaluation of Infants and Children*. 1st ed. Wolters Kluwer; 2017. (Figure 14-79)

Figure 4-14. From Siegel MJ. *Pediatric Sonography*. 5th ed. Wolters Kluwer; 2018. (Figure 8-45B)

Figure 4-15. From Kawamura D, Nolan T. *Abdomen and Superficial Structures*. 4th ed. Wolters Kluwer; 2017. (Figure 6-18)

Figure 4-16. From Kawamura D, Nolan T. *Abdomen and Superficial Structures*. 4th ed. Wolters Kluwer; 2017. (Figure 6-51)

Figure 4-17A. From Jaffe RA. *Anesthesiologist's Manual of Surgical Procedures*. 5th ed. Wolters Kluwer; 2014. (Figure 13.1-7)

Figure 4-17B. From Hawn M. *Operative Techniques in Foregut Surgery*. 1st ed. Wolters Kluwer; 2015. (Figure 29-6)

Figure 4-17C. From Yamada T, Alpers DH, Laine L, et al. *Textbook of Gastroenterology*. 4th ed. Lippincott Williams & Wilkins; 2003. (Figure 141-2)

Figure 4-18. From Brant WE, Helms CA. *Fundamentals of Diagnostic Radiology*. 4th ed. Wolters Kluwer; 2012. (Figure 26-31)

Chapter 5

Figure 5-1. From Moore KL, Dalley AF II, Agur AMR. *Clinically Oriented Anatomy*. 7th ed. Wolters Kluwer Health/Lippincott Williams & Wilkins; 2013. (Figure 2-22)

Figure 5-2. From Anatomical Chart Company. *Digestive System Anatomical Chart*.

Figure 5-3. Image courtesy of Philips Medical Systems, Bothell, WA.

Figure 5-4. From Sanders R, Winters T. *Clinical Sonography: A Practical Guide*. 4th ed. Lippincott Williams & Wilkins; 2007:57.

Figure 5-5A. From Dimick JB. *Mulholland & Greenfield's Surgery*. 7th ed. Wolters Kluwer; 2021. (Figure 101-54)

Figure 5-5B. From Kawamura D, Lunsford B. *Diagnostic Medical Sonography: Abdomen and Superficial Structures*. 3rd ed. Wolters Kluwer; 2012. (Figure 7-4)

Figure 5-6. From Brant W. *The Core Curriculum: Ultrasound*. Lippincott Williams & Wilkins; 2001:76.

Figure 5-7. From Brant W. *The Core Curriculum: Ultrasound*. Lippincott Williams & Wilkins; 2001:76.

Figure 5-8. From Kawamura D, Lunsford B. *Diagnostic Medical Sonography: Abdomen and Superficial Structures*. 3rd ed. Wolters Kluwer; 2012. (Figure 7.13)

Figure 5-9. Image courtesy of Philips Medical Systems, Bothell, WA.

Figure 5-13. From Siegel MJ. *Pediatric Sonography*. 4th ed. Wolters Kluwer Health/Lippincott Williams & Wilkins; 2010. (Figure 12-38)

Figure 5-14. From Siegel MJ. *Pediatric Sonography*. 5th ed. Wolters Kluwer; 2018. (Figure 12-35)

Figure 5-15. From Lawrence PF. *Essentials of General Surgery and Surgical Specialties*. 6th ed. Wolters Kluwer; 2018. (Figure 21-4)

Figure 5-16. From Kawamura D, Nolan T. *Abdomen and Superficial Structures*. 4th ed. Wolters Kluwer; 2017. (Figure 24-3)

Figure 5-17. From Sanders R, Hall-Terracciano B. *Clinical Sonography: A Practical Guide*. 5th ed. Wolters Kluwer; 2015. (Figure 4-5)

Figure 5-18. From Siegel MJ. *Pediatric Sonography*. 4th ed. Wolters Kluwer Health/Lippincott Williams & Wilkins; 2010. (Figure 12-36)

Figure 5-19. From Kawamura D, Nolan T. *Abdomen and Superficial Structures*. 4th ed. Wolters Kluwer; 2017. (Figure 7-12)

Figure 5-20. From Lee E. *Pediatric Radiology: Practical Imaging Evaluation of Infants and Children*. 1st ed. Wolters Kluwer; 2017. (Figure 15-29A)

Figure 5-21. From Siegel MJ, Coley BD. *Core Curriculum: Pediatric Imaging*. 1st ed. Lippincott Williams & Wilkins; 2005. (Figure 9-30A,B)

Figure 5-22. From Klein J, Vinson EM, Brant WE, et al. *Brant and Helms' Fundamentals of Diagnostic Radiology*. 5th ed. Wolters Kluwer; 2018. (Figure 42-9)

Figure 5-23. From Daffner RH, Hartman M. *Clinical Radiology*. 4th ed. Wolters Kluwer; 2013. (Figure 8-60A)

Chapter 6

Figure 6-1. From Wineski LE. *Snell's Clinical Anatomy by Regions*. 10th ed. Wolters Kluwer; 2018. (Figure 7-61)

Figure 6-2. From Kawamura DM, Nolan TD. *Abdomen and Superficial Structures*. 4th ed. Wolters Kluwer; 2017. (Figure 8-4)

Figure 6-3. From Kawamura D, Lunsford B. *Diagnostic Medical Sonography: Abdomen and Superficial Structures*. 3rd ed. Wolters Kluwer; 2012. (Figure 4-18E)

Figure 6-4. From Sanders R, Hall-Terracciano B. *Clinical Sonography: A Practical Guide*. 5th ed. Wolters Kluwer; 2015. (Figure 36-15)

Figure 6-7. From Siegel MJ. *Pediatric Sonography*. 5th ed. Wolters Kluwer; 2018. (Figure 9-28A,B)

Figure 6-8. From Lee E. *Pediatric Radiology: Practical Imaging Evaluation of Infants and Children*. 1st ed. Wolters Kluwer; 2017. (Figure 15-7A)

Figure 6-10. Image A courtesy of Philips Medical System, Bothell, WA.

Figure 6-11. From Siegel MJ. *Pediatric Sonography*. 4th ed. Wolters Kluwer Health/Lippincott Williams & Wilkins; 2010. (Figure 9-12B)

Figure 6-13. From McConnell TH. *Nature of Disease*. 2nd ed. Wolters Kluwer; 2014. (Figure 7-6)

Figure 6-14. From Lee E. *Pediatric Radiology: Practical Imaging Evaluation of Infants and Children*. 1st ed. Wolters Kluwer; 2017. (Figure 15-20A)

Figure 6-15. From Lee E. *Pediatric Radiology: Practical Imaging Evaluation of Infants and Children*. 1st ed. Wolters Kluwer; 2017. (Figure 15-0A)

Figure 6-16. Image courtesy of Robert DeJong, Baltimore, MD.

Figure 6-17. From Bornemann P. *Ultrasound for Primary Care*. 1st ed. Wolters Kluwer; 2020. (Figure 19-6)

Figure 6-18. From Lee EY, Hunsaker A, Siewert B. *Computed Body Tomography With MRI Correlation*. 5th ed. Wolters Kluwer; 2019. (Figure 17-4B)

Figure 6-19. From Singh A. *Gastrointestinal Imaging: The Essentials*. 1st ed. Wolters Kluwer; 2016. (Figure 11-19)

Chapter 7

Figure 7-1. From Kupinski AM. *The Vascular System*. 2nd ed. Wolters Kluwer; 2017. (Figure 25-2)

Figure 7-2. Image courtesy of Philips Medical Systems, Bothell, WA.

Figure 7-3. From Sanders R, Hall-Terracciano B. *Clinical Sonography: A Practical Guide*. 5th ed. Wolters Kluwer; 2015. (Figure 44-16)

Figure 7-4. From Siegel MJ. *Pediatric Sonography*. 4th ed. Wolters Kluwer; 2010. (Figure 11-10)

Figure 7-6B. Image courtesy of Brian Johnson, North Logan, UT.

Figure 7-7. From Sanders R, Hall-Terracciano B. *Clinical Sonography: A Practical Guide*. 5th ed. Wolters Kluwer; 2015. (Figure 44-3)

Figure 7-8A. From Hannon RA, Porth C. *Porth Pathophysiology*. 2nd ed. Wolters Kluwer; 2017. (Figure 33-2A)

Figure 7-8B. From Brant WE, Helms C. *Fundamentals of Diagnostic Radiology*. 4th ed. Wolters Kluwer; 2012. (Figure 35-58)

Figure 7-9A. From Hannon RA, Porth C. *Porth Pathophysiology*. 2nd ed. Wolters Kluwer; 2017. (Figure 33-2B)

Figure 7-9B. From Klein J, Vinson EM, Brant WE, et al. *Brant and Helms' Fundamentals of Diagnostic Radiology*. 5th ed. Wolters Kluwer; 2018. (Figure 50-59)

Figure 7-10. Images courtesy of Dr. Nakul Jerath, Falls Church, VA.

Figure 7-11. From MacDonald MG, Seshia MK. *Avery's Neonatology*. 7th ed. Wolters Kluwer; 2016. (Figure 40-9B)

Figure 7-12. Images courtesy of Taco Geertsma, MD, Hospital Gelderse Vallei, Ede, The Netherlands.

Figure 7-14. Images courtesy of Dr. Nakul Jerath, Falls Church, VA.

Figure 7-15. Used with permission from Anatomical Chart Company. *Urinary Tract Anatomical Chart.*

Figure 7-16. From Braun C. *Applied Pathophysiology.* 3rd ed. Wolters Kluwer; 2016. (Figure 18-5)

Figure 7-17. From Lee E. Pediatric Radiology: Practical Imaging Evaluation of Infants and Children. 1st ed. Wolters Kluwer; 2017. (Figure 17-13A)

Figure 7-18. From Lee E. Pediatric Radiology: Practical Imaging Evaluation of Infants and Children. 1st ed. Wolters Kluwer; 2017. (Figure 17-72A)

Figure 7-19. From Siegel MJ. *Pediatric Sonography.* 4th ed. Wolters Kluwer; 2010. (Figure 11-72)

Figure 7-20. From Brant W. *The Core Curriculum: Ultrasound.* Wolters Kluwer; 2001:131.

Figure 7-21. From Norris TL. *Porth's Essentials of Pathophysiology.* 5th ed. Wolters Kluwer; 2019. (Figure 33-4)

Figure 7-22. Images courtesy of Philips Medical Systems, Bothell, WA.

Figure 7-23. From Klein J, Vinson EM, Brant WE, et al. *Brant and Helms' Fundamentals of Diagnostic Radiology.* 5th ed. Wolters Kluwer; 2018. (Figure 1-25)

Figure 7-24. From Sanders R, Hall-Terracciano B. *Clinical Sonography: A Practical Guide.* 5th ed. Wolters Kluwer; 2015. (Figure 46-6)

Figure 7-25. From Brant WE, Helms CA. *Fundamentals of Diagnostic Radiology.* 4th ed. Wolters Kluwer; 2012. (Figure 35-62)

Figure 7-26A,B. Images courtesy of Taco Geertsma, MD, Hospital Gelderse Vallei, Ede, The Netherlands.

Figure 7-26C,D. From Kawamura DM, Nolan TD. *Abdomen and Superficial Structures.* 4th ed. Wolters Kluwer; 2017. (Figure 10-27C,D)

Figure 7-27. From Kawamura DM, Nolan TD. *Abdomen and Superficial Structures.* 4th ed. Wolters Kluwer; 2017. (Figure 10-20A)

Figure 7-28. From Kawamura D, Lunsford B. *Diagnostic Medical Sonography: Abdomen and Superficial Structures.* 3rd ed. Wolters Kluwer; 2012. (Figure 10-20IJ)

Figure 7-30. From Zierler RE, Dawson DL. *Strandness's Duplex Scanning in Vascular Disorders.* 5th ed. Wolters Kluwer; 2015. (Figure 24-13B)

Figure 7-31. From Klein J, Vinson EM, Brant WE, et al. *Brant and Helms' Fundamentals of Diagnostic Radiology.* 5th ed. Wolters Kluwer; 2018. (Figure 50-69)

Figure 7-32A. Image courtesy of Dr. Nakul Jerath, Falls Church, VA.

Figure 7-32B. Image courtesy of Rechelle Nguyen, Columbus, OH.

Figure 7-32C-E. From Kawamura DM, Nolan TD. *Abdomen and Superficial Structures.* 4th ed. Wolters Kluwer; 2017. (Figure 20-8C-E)

Figure 7-33B. From Siegel MJ, Coley BD. *Core Curriculum: Pediatric Imaging.* 1st ed. Wolters Kluwer; 2005. (Figure 8-30)

Figure 7-34. From Sadler TW. *Langman's Medical Embryology.* 10th ed. Wolters Kluwer; 2006:239. (Figure 15.15)

Figure 7-35. From Shirkhoda A. *Variants and Pitfalls in Body Imaging.* 2nd ed. Wolters Kluwer; 2011. (Figure 24-18)

Figure 7-36A. Courtesy of Philips Medical Systems, Bothell, WA.

Figure 7-36B,C. From Kawamura D, Lunsford B. *Diagnostic Medical Sonography: Abdomen and Superficial Structures.* 3rd ed. Wolters Kluwer; 2012. (Figure 11-9B,C)

Figure 7-37. From Siegel MJ. *Pediatric Sonography.* 5th ed. Wolters Kluwer; 2018. (Figure 11-28B)

Figure 7-38. From Brant WE, Helms CA. *Fundamentals of Diagnostic Radiology.* 4th ed. Wolters Kluwer; 2012. (Figure 36-47)

Figure 7-39. From Brant W. *The Core Curriculum: Ultrasound.* Wolters Kluwer; 2001:141.

Figure 7-40. From Dunnick R, Sandler C, Newhouse J. *Textbook of Uroradiology.* 5th ed. Wolters Kluwer Health/Wolters Kluwer; 2012. (Figure 7-11)

Figure 7-41. From Brant W. *The Core Curriculum: Ultrasound.* Wolters Kluwer; 2001:119.

Figure 7-42. From Kawamura D, Lunsford B. *Diagnostic Medical Sonography: Abdomen and Superficial Structures.* 3rd ed. Wolters Kluwer; 2012. (Figure 5-23F)

Figure 7-43. From Brant WE, Helms CA. *Brant and Helms Solution.* Wolters Kluwer; 2006. (Figure 36-51)

Figure 7-44. From Dunnick R, Sandler C, Newhouse J. *Textbook of Uroradiology.* 5th ed. Wolters Kluwer Health/Wolters Kluwer; 2012. (Figure 13-3B)

Figure 7-45. Images courtesy of Taco Geertsma, MD, Hospital Gelderse Vallei, Ede, The Netherlands.

Figure 7-46. From Dudek RW, Louis TM. *High-Yield™ Gross Anatomy.* 5th ed. Wolters Kluwer; 2014. (Figure 14-3)

Figure 7-47. From Dunnick R, Sandler C, Newhouse J. *Textbook of Uroradiology.* 5th ed. Wolters Kluwer Health/Wolters Kluwer; 2012. (Figure 7-12)

Figure 7-48. From Lee EY, Hunsaker A, Siewert B. *Computed Body Tomography With MRI Correlation.* 5th ed. Wolters Kluwer; 2019. (Figure 24-87A,B)

Chapter 8

Figure 8-1. Asset provided by Anatomical Chart Co, Philadelphia, PA.

Figure 8-2. Used with permission from Anatomical Chart Company. *Understanding Depression.*

Figure 8-3. From Kawamura DM, Nolan TD. *Abdomen and Superficial Structures.* 4th ed. Wolters Kluwer; 2017. (Figure 13-4)

Figure 8-4. Image courtesy of Dr. Taco Geertsma, Gelderse Vallei, Ede, The Netherlands.

Figure 8-5. From McConnell TH. *Nature of Disease.* 2nd ed. Wolters Kluwer; 2014. (Figure 14-20)

Figure 8-6. From Norris TL. *Porth's Essentials of Pathophysiology.* 5th ed. Wolters Kluwer; 2019. (Figure 41-12)

Figure 8-7. Images courtesy of Dr. Taco Geertsma, Gelderse Vallei, Ede, The Netherlands.

Figure 8-8. From Brant W. *The Core Curriculum: Ultrasound.* Lippincott Williams & Wilkins; 2001:144.

Figure 8-9. Used with permission from SonoSkills.

Figure 8-10. From Sanders R, Hall-Terracciano B. *Clinical Sonography: A Practical Guide.* 5th ed. Wolters Kluwer; 2015. (Figure 39-13)

Figure 8-12. From Brant W. *The Core Curriculum: Ultrasound.* Lippincott Williams & Wilkins; 2001:145.

Figure 8-13. From Brant W. *The Core Curriculum: Ultrasound.* Lippincott Williams & Wilkins; 2001:143.

Figure 8-14. Images courtesy of Dr. Taco Geertsma, Gelderse Vallei, Ede, The Netherlands.

Figure 8-15. From Lee E. Pediatric Radiology: Practical Imaging Evaluation of Infants and Children. 1st ed. Wolters Kluwer; 2017. (Figure 15-59B)

Figure 8-16. From Brant WE, Helms CA. *Fundamentals of Diagnostic Radiology.* 4th ed. Wolters Kluwer; 2012. (Figure 51-61A)

Figure 8-17. Image courtesy of Dr. Taco Geertsma, Gelderse Vallei, Ede, The Netherlands.

Figure 8-18. Image courtesy of Dr. Taco Geertsma, Gelderse Vallei, Ede, The Netherlands.

Figure 8-19. From Siegel MJ, Coley BD. *Core Curriculum: Pediatric Imaging.* 1st ed. Lippincott Williams & Wilkins; 2005. (Figure 9-8)

Chapter 9

Figure 9-1. From Norris TL. *Porth's Essentials of Pathophysiology.* 4th ed. Wolters Kluwer; 2014. (Figure 18-1)

Figure 9-2. From Kupinski AM. *The Vascular System.* 2nd ed. Wolters Kluwer; 2017. (Figure 24-1)

Figure 9-3. From Cosby K, Kendall J. *Practical Guide to Emergency Ultrasound.* 2nd ed. Wolters Kluwer Health/Lippincott Williams & Wilkins; 2013:227. (Figure 10-7B)

Figure 9-4. From Klein J, Vinson EM, Brant WE, et al. *Brant and Helms' Fundamentals of Diagnostic Radiology.* 5th ed. Wolters Kluwer; 2018. (Figure 54-4)

Figure 9-5. Images courtesy of Stephanie Nieport, Kettering College, Kettering, OH.

Figure 9-6. From Darling RC, Ozaki CK. *Master Techniques in Surgery: Vascular Surgery: Arterial Procedures.* 1st ed. Wolters Kluwer; 2015. (Figure 36-1)

Figure 9-7. From Cosby K, Kendall J. *Practical Guide to Emergency Ultrasound.* 1st ed. Lippincott Williams & Wilkins; 2006:227. (Figure 9-12C)

Figure 9-8. From Zierler RE, Dawson DL. *Strandness's Duplex Scanning in Vascular Disorders.* 5th ed. Wolters Kluwer; 2015. (Figure 23-7B)

Figure 9-9. From Cosby K, Kendall J. *Practical Guide to Emergency Ultrasound.* Lippincott Williams & Wilkins; 2006:227.

Figure 9-10. From Brant W. *The Core Curriculum: Ultrasound.* Lippincott Williams & Wilkins; 2001:31.

Figure 9-11. From Sanders R, Hall-Terracciano B. *Clinical Sonography: A Practical Guide.* 5th ed. Wolters Kluwer; 2015. (Figure 38-4)

Figure 9-12. From Zierler RE, Dawson DL. *Strandness's Duplex Scanning in Vascular Disorders.* 5th ed. Wolters Kluwer; 2015. (Figure 24-6A)

Figure 9-14. From Sanders R, Hall-Terracciano B. *Clinical Sonography: A Practical Guide.* 5th ed. Wolters Kluwer; 2015. (Figure 38-8)

Figure 9-15. From Norris TL, Lalchandani R. *Porth's Pathophysiology.* 10th ed. Wolters Kluwer; 2018. (Figure 5-2)

Figure 9-16. From Sanders R, Hall-Terracciano B. *Clinical Sonography: A Practical Guide.* 5th ed. Wolters Kluwer; 2015. (Figure 38-9)

Figure 9-17. From Kupinski AM. *Diagnostic Medical Sonography: The Vascular System.* Wolters Kluwer; 2012. (Figure 18-12)

Figure 9-18. From Zierler RE, Dawson DL. *Strandness's Duplex Scanning in Vascular Disorders.* 5th ed. Wolters Kluwer; 2015. (Figure 16-16A)

Figure 9-19. Images courtesy of Philips Medical System, Bothell, WA.

Figure 9-20. From Siegel MJ. *Pediatric Sonography.* 4th ed. Wolters Kluwer Health/Lippincott Williams & Wilkins; 2010. (Figure 15-64)

Figure 9-21. From Argur AMR, Dalley AF. *Moore's Essential Clinical Anatomy.* 6th ed. Wolters Kluwer; 2019. (Figure 5-66)

Figure 9-23. From Marino PL. *Marino's The ICU Book: Print + Ebook with Updates.* 4th ed. Wolters Kluwer; 2013. (Figure 6-4)

Figure 9-24. From Zierler RE, Dawson DL. *Strandness's Duplex Scanning in Vascular Disorders.* 5th ed. Wolters Kluwer; 2015. (Figure 19-26)

Figure 9-25. From Kupinski AM. *The Vascular System.* 1st ed. Wolters Kluwer; 2012. (Figure 13-8)

Figure 9-26. From Zierler RE, Dawson DL. *Strandness's Duplex Scanning in Vascular Disorders.* 5th od. Wolters Kluwer; 2015. (Figure 32-3)

Figure 9-27. From Zierler RE, Dawson DL. *Strandness's Duplex Scanning in Vascular Disorders.* 5th ed. Wolters Kluwer; 2015. (Figure 22-2B)

Figure 9-28. From Kawamura D, Lunsford B. *Diagnostic Medical Sonography: Abdomen and Superficial Structures.* 3rd ed. Wolters Kluwer; 2012. (Figure 4 13A-F)

Figure 9-29. From Cosby K, Kendall J. *Practical Guide to Emergency Ultrasound.* 2nd ed. Wolters Kluwer Health/Lippincott Williams & Wilkins; 2013:227. (Figure 10-27A,B)

Figure 9-30. From Zierler RE, Dawson DL. *Strandness's Duplex Scanning in Vascular Disorders.* 5th ed. Wolters Kluwer; 2015. (Figure 19-24)

Figure 9-31. From Zierler RE, Dawson DL. *Strandness's Duplex Scanning in Vascular Disorders.* 5th ed. Wolters Kluwer; 2015. (Figure 25-12B)

Figure 9-32. From Higgins CB, de Roos A. *MRI and CT of the Cardiovascular System.* 3rd ed. Wolters Kluwer; 2013. (Figure 34-1)

Figure 9-33. From Leyendecker JR, Brown JJ. *Practical Guide to Abdominal and Pelvic MRI.* 1st ed. Lippincott Williams & Wilkins; 2004. (Figure 2-15)

Figure 9-34. From Britt LD, Peitzman AB, Barie PS, et al. *Acute Care Surgery.* 1st ed. Wolters Kluwer, 2012. (Figure 9-30A)

Chapter 10

Figure 10-2. From Kawamura DM, Nolan TD. *Abdomen and Superficial Structures.* 4th ed. Wolters Kluwer; 2017. (Figure 5-16A)

Figure 10-3. Image courtesy of Philips Healthcare, Bothell, WA.

Figure 10-5. Images courtesy of Philips Medical Systems, Bothell, WA.

Figure 10-6. From Moore KL, Dalley AF II, Agur AMR. *Clinically Oriented Anatomy.* 7th ed. Wolters Kluwer Health; 2013. (Ch 2, Box Image 9)

Figure 10-7A. From Siegel MJ. *Pediatric Sonography.* 4th ed. Wolters Kluwer Health/Lippincott Williams & Wilkins; 2010. (Figure 10-4)

Figure 10-7B. From Penny SM. *Examination Review for Ultrasound.* 1st ed. Wolters Kluwer Health/Lippincott Williams & Wilkins; 2010. (Figure 10-4)

Figure 10-8A. Image modified with permission from Siegel MJ. *Pediatric Sonography.* 4th ed. Wolters Kluwer Health/Lippincott Williams & Wilkins; 2010. (Figure 10-4)

Figure 10-8B. From Penny SM. *Introduction to Sonography and Patient Care.* 1st ed. Wolters Kluwer; 2015. (Figure 8-26C)

Figure 10-9. From Cosby K, Kendall J. *Practical Guide to Emergency Ultrasound.* 2nd ed. Wolters Kluwer Health/Lippincott Williams & Wilkins; 2013:227. (Figure 27-23B)

Figure 10-10A. From Kawamura DM, Nolan TD. *Abdomen and Superficial Structures.* 4th ed. Wolters Kluwer; 2017. (Figure 19-39A)

Figure 10-10B. From Iyer R, Chapman T. *Pediatric Imaging: The Essentials.* 1st ed. Wolters Kluwer; 2015. (Figure 15-13B)

Figure 10-10C. From Kawamura DM, Nolan TD. *Abdomen and Superficial Structures.* 4th ed. Wolters Kluwer; 2017. (Figure 19-39B)

Figure 10-10D. Image courtesy of Rechelle Nguyen, Columbus, OH.

Figure 10-11. From Siegel MJ. *Pediatric Sonography.* 4th ed. Wolters Kluwer Health/Lippincott Williams & Wilkins; 2010. (Figure 10-35)

Figure 10-12. From McConnell TH. *Nature of Disease.* 2nd ed. Wolters Kluwer; 2014. (Figure 11-5)

Figure 10-13. From Bornemann P. *Ultrasound for Primary Care.* 1st ed. Wolters Kluwer; 2020. (Figure 23-6)

Figure 10-14. Images courtesy of Dr. Taco Geertsma, Hospital Gelderse Vallei, Ede, The Netherlands.

Figure 10-15. Image courtesy of Philips Medical Systems, Bothell, WA.

Figure 10-16. Used with permission from Intermountain Healthcare. © 2012 Intermountain Healthcare. All rights reserved.

Figure 10-17. Images courtesy of Dr. Taco Geertsma, Gelderse Vallei, The Netherlands.

Figure 10-19. From Snell RS. *Clinical Anatomy.* 7th ed. Wolters Kluwer; 2003 (Figure 4-40)

Figure 10-20. From Siegel MJ. *Pediatric Sonography.* 5th ed. Wolters Kluwer; 2018. (Figure 10-5A)

Figure 10-21. Farrell TA. *Radiology 101.* 5th ed. Wolters Kluwer; 2019. (Figure 5-47)

Figure 10-22. From Kawamura D, Nolan T. *Abdomen and Superficial Structures.* 4th ed. Wolters Kluwer; 2017. (Figure 5-14A)

Figure 10-23. From Penny SM. *Examination Review for Ultrasound.* 1st ed. Wolters Kluwer Health/Lippincott Williams & Wilkins; 2010. (Figure 10-5)

Figure 10-24. From Lee E. *Pediatric Radiology: Practical Imaging Evaluation of Infants and Children.* 1st ed. Wolters Kluwer; 2017. (Figure 16-64C)

Figure 10-25. From Sherman SC, Ross C, Nordquist E, et al. *Atlas of Clinical Emergency Medicine.* 1st ed. Wolters Kluwer; 2015. (Figure 13-48)

Figure 10-26. From Klein J, Vinson EN, Brant WE, et al. *Brant and Helms' Fundamentals of Diagnostic Radiology.* 5th ed. Wolters Kluwer; 2018. (Figure 69-26)

Figure 10-27. From Shirkhoda A. *Variants and Pitfalls in Body Imaging.* 2nd ed. Wolters Kluwer; 2011. (Figure 17-7B)

Chapter 11

Figure 11-1. From Moore KL, Dalley AF, Agur AM, eds. *Clinically Oriented Anatomy.* 8th ed. Wolters Kluwer, 2013. (Figure 4-33)

Figure 11-2. From Lee E. *Pediatric Radiology: Practical Imaging Evaluation of Infants and Children.* 1st ed. Wolters Kluwer; 2017.

Figure 11-3. Sanders, *Clinical Sonography: A Practical Guide.* 5th ed. Wolters Kluwer; 2015.

Figure 11-4. Bachur RG. *Fleisher & Ludwig's Textbook of Pediatric Emergency Medicine.* 8th ed. Wolters Kluwer; 2020. (Figure 131-12)

Figure 11-5. Herzog E. *Herzog's CCU Book.* Wolters Kluwer; 2017. (Figure 33-4)

Figure 11-6. From Sanders R, Hall-Terracciano B. *Clinical Sonography: A Practical Guide.* 5th ed. Wolters Kluwer; 2015. (Figure 30-17)

Figure 11-7. From Sanders R, Hall-Terracciano B. *Clinical Sonography: A Practical Guide.* 5th ed. Wolters Kluwer; 2015. (Figure 45-2)

Figure 11-8. From Siegel MJ. *Pediatric Sonography.* 4th ed. Wolters Kluwer; 2010. (Figure 12.65)

Figure 11-9. From Kawamura D, Nolan T. *Abdomen and Superficial Structures.* 4th ed. Wolters Kluwer Health; 2017. (Figure 14-10A)

Figure 11-10. Images courtesy of Dr. Taco Geertsma, Gelderse Vallei, Ede, The Netherlands.

Figure 11-11. From Cosby K, Kendall J. *Practical Guide to Emergency Ultrasound.* 2nd ed. Wolters Kluwer Health/Lippincott Williams & Wilkins; 2013. (Figure 5-13)

Figure 11-12. From Kawamura D, Nolan T. *Abdomen and Superficial Structures.* 4th ed. Wolters Kluwer; 2017. (Figure 25-4)

Figure 11-13. From Lee EY. *Computed Body Tomography With MRI Correlation.* 5th ed. Wolters Kluwer; 2019. (Figure 24-90B)

Figure 11-14. From Klein J, Vinson EM, Brant WE, et al. *Brant and Helms' Fundamentals of Diagnostic Radiology.* 5th ed. Wolters Kluwer; 2018. (Figure 10-36)

Chapter 12

Figure 12-1. From Anatomical Chart Company. *Digestive System Anatomical Chart*. Wolters Kluwer; 2000.

Figure 12-2. From Siegel MJ. *Pediatric Sonography*. 4th ed. Wolters Kluwer; 2010. (Figure 4.2)

Figure 12-3. From Siegel MJ. *Pediatric Sonography*. 4th ed. Wolters Kluwer; 2010. (Figure 4.7)

Figure 12-4. From Siegel MJ. *Pediatric Sonography*. 4th ed. Wolters Kluwer; 2010. (Figure 4.8)

Figure 12-5. From Argur AMR, Dalley AF. *Moore's Essential Clinical Anatomy*. 6th ed. Wolters Kluwer; 2019. (Figure SA9.2)

Figure 12-6. From Sanders R, Winters T. *Clinical Sonography: A Practical Guide*. 4th ed. Lippincott Williams & Wilkins; 2007:233.

Figure 12-7. From Kawamura D, Lunsford B. *Diagnostic Medical Sonography: Abdomen and Superficial Structures*. 3rd ed. Wolters Kluwer; 2012. (Figure 15-8)

Figure 12-8. From Porth C. *Essentials of Pathophysiology*. 4th ed. Wolters Kluwer; 2015. (Figure 32-10)

Figure 12-9. Images courtesy of LaNae Holman, Alamosa, Colorado.

Figure 12-10. From Porth C. *Essentials of Pathophysiology*. 4th ed. Wolters Kluwer; 2015. (Figure 32-9)

Figure 12-11. From Siegel MJ. *Pediatric Sonography*. 4th ed. Wolters Kluwer; 2010. (Figure 4.63A,B)

Figure 12-12. From Siegel MJ. *Pediatric Sonography*. 4th ed. Wolters Kluwer; 2010. (Figure 4-54C)

Figure 12-13. From Kawamura D, Lunsford B. *Diagnostic Medical Sonography: Abdomen and Superficial Structures*. 3rd ed. Wolters Kluwer; 2012. (Figure 15-6B)

Figure 12-14. From Braverman LE, Cooper D. *Werner & Ingbar's The Thyroid*. 10th ed. Wolters Kluwer; 2012. (Figure 49-1)

Figure 12-15. From Klingensmith ME. *The Washington Manual of Surgery*. 8th ed. Wolters Kluwer; 2020. (Figure 34-2)

Figure 12-16. From Penny SM. *Introduction to Sonography and Patient Care*. Wolters Kluwer; 2015. (Figure 1-17A,B)

Figure 12-17. From Moore KL, Dalley AF, Agur AM, eds. *Clinically Oriented Anatomy*. 8th ed. Wolters Kluwer; 2013. (Figure 9-31B)

Figure 12-18. From Kawamura DM, Nolan TD. *Abdomen and Superficial Structures*. 4th ed. Wolters Kluwer; 2017. (Figure 15-18B)

Figure 12-19. From Dimick JB, Upchurch GR, Sonnenday CJ, eds. *Clinical Scenarios in Surgery*. Wolters Kluwer; 2012. (Figure 59-4)

Figure 12-20. From Myers J, Hanna E, eds. *Cancer of the Head and Neck*. 5th ed. Wolters Kluwer; 2016. (Figure 18-6)

Figure 12-21A. From Moore KL, Dalley AF, Agur AM, eds. *Clinically Oriented Anatomy*. 8th ed. Wolters Kluwer; 2013. (Figure 8-6A,B)

Figure 12-21B. From Cosby K, Kendall J. *Practical Guide to Emergency Ultrasound*. 2nd ed. Wolters Kluwer Health/Lippincott Williams & Wilkins; 2013:227. (Figure 24-27)

Figure 12-22. From Klein J, Vinson EM, Brant WE, et al. *Brant and Helms' Fundamentals of Diagnostic Radiology*. 5th ed. Wolters Kluwer; 2018. (Figure 70-34)

Figure 12-23. From Bornemann P. *Ultrasound for Primary Care*. Wolters Kluwer; 2021. (Figure 5-7)

Figure 12-24. From Brant W. *The Core Curriculum: Ultrasound*. Lippincott Williams & Wilkins; 2001:357.

Figure 12-25. From Sanelli P. *Neuroimaging: The Essentials*. Wolters Kluwer; 2016. (Figure 23-12A)

Figure 12-26. From Katz MH. *Operative Standards for Cancer Surgery*. Wolters Kluwer; 2019. (Figure 2-1)

Figure 12-27. Lavin M. *Manual of Endocrinology and Metabolism*. 5th ed. Wolters Kluwer; 2019. (Figure 41-2A)

Figure 12-28. From Sanelli P. *Neuroimaging: The Essentials*. Wolters Kluwer; 2016. (Figure 23-17B)

Figure 12-29. From Bornemann P. *Ultrasound for Primary Care*. 1st ed. Wolters Kluwer; 2020. (Figure 18-2)

Figure 12-30. Stocker JT. *Stocker and Dehner's Pediatric Pathology*. 3rd ed. Wolters Kluwer; 2010. (Figure 21-9B)

Chapter 13

Figure 13-1. Rhoades RA. *Medical Physiology*. 4th ed. Wolters Kluwer; 2013. (Figure 36-7)

Figure 13-2. Moore KL, Dalley AF, Agur AM, eds. *Clinically Oriented Anatomy*. 8th ed. Wolters Kluwer; 2013. (Figure 2-21)

Figure 13-3. Kawamura D, Lunsford B. *Diagnostic Medical Sonography: Abdomen and Superficial Structures*. 3rd ed. Wolters Kluwer; 2012. (Figure 17-17)

Figure 13-4A. Anatomical Chart Company. *Infertility Anatomical Chart*. Wolters Kluwer; 2004.

Figure 13-5. Lee E. Pediatric Radiology: Practical Imaging Evaluation of Infants and Children. 1st ed. Wolters Kluwer; 2017. (Figure 18-11)

Figure 13-6. Baskin LS. *Handbook of Pediatric Urology*. 3rd ed. Wolters Kluwer; 2019. (Figure 17-1)

Figure 13-7. Siegel MJ. *Core Curriculum: Pediatric Imaging*. Wolters Kluwer; 2005. (Figure 11-24A,B)

Figure 13-8. Siegel MJ. *Pediatric Sonography*. 4th ed. Wolters Kluwer; 2010. (Figure 14.80)

Figure 13-9. Sanders R, Hall-Terracciano B. *Clinical Sonography: A Practical Guide*. 5th ed. Wolters Kluwer; 2015. (Figure 54-10)

Figure 13-10A. From Anatomical Chart Company. *Atlas of Pathophysiology*. Wolters Kluwer; 2001.

Figure 13-10B. Siegel MJ. *Pediatric Sonography*. 5th ed. Wolters Kluwer; 2018. (Figure 14-72A)

Figure 13-10C. Siegel MJ. *Pediatric Sonography*. 5th ed. Wolters Kluwer; 2018. (Figure 14-172B)

Figure 13-11. Siegel MJ. *Pediatric Sonography*. 4th ed. Wolters Kluwer; 2010. (Figure 14-61A,B)

Figure 13-12. Siegel MJ. *Pediatric Sonography*. 4th ed. Wolters Kluwer; 2010. (Figure 14-64B)

Figure 13-13. Kawamura D, Lunsford B. *Diagnostic Medical Sonography: Abdomen and Superficial Structures*. 3rd ed. Wolters Kluwer; 2012. (Figure 17.34)

Figure 13-14. Lee E. Pediatric Radiology: Practical Imaging Evaluation of Infants and Children. 1st ed. Wolters Kluwer; 2017. (Figure 18-20A)

Figure 13-16. Norris TL. *Porth's Essentials of Pathophysiology*. 4th ed. Wolters Kluwer; 2014. (Figure 6-12)

Figure 13-17. Siegel MJ. *Pediatric Sonography*. 4th ed. Wolters Kluwer; 2010. (Figure 14-19)

Figure 13-18. Waldman S. Comprehensive Atlas of Ultrasound-Guided Pain Management Injection Techniques. 2nd ed. Wolters Kluwer; 2019. (Figure 99-1)

Figure 13-19. Farrell TA. *Radiology 101*. 5th ed. Wolters Kluwer; 2019. (Figure 4-11)

Figure 13-20. Anatomical Chart Company. *Understanding Erectile Dysfunction Anatomical Chart*. Wolters Kluwer; 2003.

Figure 13-21. Sanders R, Hall-Terracciano B. *Clinical Sonography: A Practical Guide*. 5th ed. Wolters Kluwer; 2015. (Figure 56-1)

Figure 13-22A. Anatomical Chart Company. *Male Reproductive System Anatomical Chart*. Wolters Kluwer; 2000.

Figure 13-22B. Sanders R, Hall-Terracciano B. *Clinical Sonography: A Practical Guide*. 5th ed. Wolters Kluwer; 2015. (Figure 56-2B)

Figure 13-23. Shirkhoda A. *Variants and Pitfalls in Body Imaging*. 2nd ed. Wolters Kluwer; 2011. (Figure 32-58A)

Figure 13-24. Anatomical Chart Company. *Prostate Anatomical Chart*. Wolters Kluwer; 2000.

Figure 13-26. Sanders R, Hall-Terracciano B. *Clinical Sonography: A Practical Guide*. 5th ed. Wolters Kluwer; 2015. (Figure 55-2)

Figure 13-27. Sanders R, Hall-Terracciano B. *Clinical Sonography: A Practical Guide*. 5th ed. Wolters Kluwer; 2015. (Figure 55-8)

Figure 13-28. Sanders R, Hall-Terracciano B. *Clinical Sonography: A Practical Guide*. 5th ed. Wolters Kluwer; 2015. (Figure 55-11)

Figure 13-29. Cosby K, Kendall J. *Practical Guide to Emergency Ultrasound*. 2nd ed. Wolters Kluwer; 2013. (Figure 19-16B)

Figure 13-30. Iyer R. *Pediatric Imaging: The Essentials*. Wolters Kluwer; 2015. (Figure 24-5D)

Figure 13-31. Iyer R. *Pediatric Imaging: The Essentials*. Wolters Kluwer; 2015. (Figure 24-10B)

Figure 13-32. Kawamura D, Nolan T. *Abdomen and Superficial Structures*. 4th ed. Wolters Kluwer; 2017. (Figure 17-37)

Figure 13-33. Dunnick NR. *Genitourinary Radiology*. 6th ed. Wolters Kluwer; 2018. (Figure 16-36)

Figure 13-34. Klein J, Vinson EM, Brant WE, et al. *Brant and Helms' Fundamentals of Diagnostic Radiology*. 5th ed. Wolters Kluwer; 2018. (Figure 49-29)

Figure 13-35. Lee E. Pediatric Radiology: Practical Imaging Evaluation of Infants and Children. Wolters Kluwer; 2017. (Figure 18-31)

Figure 13-36A. From Donnelly-Moreno LA. *Timby's Introductory Medical-Surgical Nursing*. 13th ed. Wolters Kluwer; 2022. (Figure 55-7)

Figure 13-36B. Sanders R, Hall-Terracciano B. *Clinical Sonography: A Practical Guide*. 5th ed. Wolters Kluwer; 2015. (Figure 56-5)

Chapter 14

Figure 14-3. Siegel MJ. *Pediatric Sonography*. 5th ed. Wolters Kluwer; 2018. (Figure 15-02A,B)

Figure 14-4. From Beggs I. *Musculoskeletal Ultrasound*. Wolters Kluwer; 2013. (Figure 1-3A,B)

Figure 14-5. Waldman S. Waldman's Atlas of Diagnostic Ultrasound of Painful Foot and Ankle Conditions. Wolters Kluwer; 2017. (Figure 14-33)

Figure 14-6. Cosby KS, Kendall JL. *Practical Guide to Emergency Ultrasound.* 2nd ed. Wolters Kluwer; 2013. (Figure 21-11B)

Figure 14-8. Reprinted with permission from Sanders R, Winters T. *Clinical Sonography: A Practical Guide.* 4th ed. Lippincott Williams & Wilkins; 2007:591.

Figure 14-9. Reprinted with permission from Sanders R, Winters T. *Clinical Sonography: A Practical Guide.* 4th ed. Lippincott Williams & Wilkins; 2007:596.

Figure 14-10. Reprinted with permission from Thordarson D. *Foot & Ankle.* 2nd ed. Wolters Kluwer; 2012. (Figure 2-23)

Figure 14-11. Reprinted with permission from Sanders R, Hall-Terracciano B. *Clinical Sonography: A Practical Guide.* 5th ed. Wolters Kluwer; 2015. (Figure 50-6)

Figure 14-12. Sanders RC, Hall-Terracciano B. *Clinical Sonography: A Practical Guide.* 5th ed. Wolters Kluwer; 2015. (Figure 50-03)

Figure 14-13A. Sanders RC, Hall-Terracciano B. *Clinical Sonography: A Practical Guide.* 5th ed. Wolters Kluwer; 2015. (Figure 50-01)

Figure 14-13B. Sanders RC, Hall-Terracciano B. *Clinical Sonography: A Practical Guide.* 5th ed. Wolters Kluwer; 2015. (Figure 50-02)

Figure 14-15A. Panel A adapted by permission from the Springer: Graf R. Classification of hip joint dysplasia by means of sonography. *Arch Orthop Trauma Surg.* 1984;102(4):248–255. Copyright © 1984 Springer Nature.

Figure 14-15B. Siegel MJ. *Pediatric Sonography.* 4th ed. Wolters Kluwer; 2010. (Figure 15-14B)

Figure 14-16. Sanders RC, Hall-Terracciano B. *Clinical Sonography: A Practical Guide.* 5th ed. Wolters Kluwer; 2015. (Figure 50-15A)

Figure 14-17. Sanders RC, Hall-Terracciano B. *Clinical Sonography: A Practical Guide.* 5th ed. Wolters Kluwer; 2015. (Figure 50-46)

Figure 14-18. Reprinted with permission from Siegel MJ, Coley B. *Core Curriculum: Pediatric Imaging.* Lippincott Williams & Wilkins; 2005. (Figure 12-186A-F)

Figure 14-19. Siegel MJ. *Pediatric Sonography.* 5th ed. Wolters Kluwer; 2018. (Figure 15-46A,B)

Figure 14-20. Dudek RW. *High-Yield™ Gross Anatomy.* 4th ed. Wolters Kluwer; 2011. (Figure 5-2)

Figure 14-21. Reprinted with permission from Kawamura D, Lunsford B. *Diagnostic Medical Sonography: Abdomen and Superficial Structures.* 3rd ed. Wolters Kluwer; 2017. (Figure 16-11)

Figure 14-22. Sanders RC, Hall-Terracciano B. *Clinical Sonography: A Practical Guide.* 5th ed. Wolters Kluwer; 2015. (Figure 53-06)

Figure 14-23. Bornemann P. *Ultrasound for Primary Care.* Wolters Kluwer; 2020. (Figure 16-03)

Figure 14-26. Cardenosa G. *Breast Imaging Companion.* 4th ed. Wolters Kluwer; 2018. (Figure 11-70)

Figure 14-27. Bland KI. *Master Techniques in General Surgery: Breast Surgery.* 2nd ed. Wolters Kluwer; 2019. (Figure 1-11)

Figure 14-28. Siegel MJ. *Pediatric Sonography.* 5th ed. Wolters Kluwer; 2018. (Figure 6-05)

Figure 14-29. Reprinted with permission from Siegel A, Sapru HN. *Essential Neuroscience.* 3rd ed. Wolters Kluwer; 2014. (Figure 15-1A)

Figure 14-30. Bornemann P. *Ultrasound for Primary Care.* Wolters Kluwer; 2020. (Figure 43-02)

Figure 14-31. From Chung KC. *Operative Techniques in Hand and Wrist Surgery.* Wolters Kluwer; 2019. (Figure 71-3)

Figure 14-32. Beggs I. *Musculoskeletal Ultrasound.* Wolters Kluwer; 2013. (Figure 9-50A,B)

Figure 14-33. Beggs I. *Musculoskeletal Ultrasound.* Wolters Kluwer; 2013. (Figure 9-1)

Figure 14-34. From Anatomical Chart Company. *Ligaments of the Joints Anatomical Chart.* Wolters Kluwer; 2004.

Figure 14-35. Beggs I. *Musculoskeletal Ultrasound.* Wolters Kluwer; 2013. (Figure 7-34)

Figure 14-36. From Waldman S. *Waldman's Comprehensive Atlas of Diagnostic Ultrasound of Painful Conditions.* Wolters Kluwer; 2016. (Figure 111-3)

Figure 14-37. From Brant W. *The Core Curriculum: Ultrasound.* Wolters Kluwer; 2001:466.

Figure 14-38A. Bickley LS. *Bates' Guide to Physical Examination and History Taking.* 8th ed. Wolters Kluwer; 2002:435.

Figure 14-38B. From Siegel MJ. *Pediatric Sonography.* 4th ed. Wolters Kluwer; 2010. (Figure 16-26)

Figure 14-39. From Wolfson AB, Cloutier RL, Hendey W, et al. *Harwood-Nuss' Clinical Practice of Emergency Medicine.* 6th ed. Wolters Kluwer; 2014. (Figure 180-1)

Figure 14-40. Bittle MM. *Trauma Radiology Companion.* 2nd ed. Wolters Kluwer; 2012. (Figure 5-53B)

Figure 14-41. Harris JR. *Diseases of the Breast.* 4th ed. Wolters Kluwer; 2010. (Figure 13-11)

Figure 14-42. Kawamura D, Lunsford B. *Diagnostic Medical Sonography: Abdomen and Superficial Structures.* 3rd ed. Wolters Kluwer; 2012. (Figure 23-7)

Figure 14-43. Courtesy of Donna G. Blankenbaker, MD, Department of Radiology, University of Wisconsin.

Figure 14-44. Beggs I. *Musculoskeletal Ultrasound.* Wolters Kluwer; 2013. (Figure 7-43)

Figure 14-45. Greenspan A. *Orthopedic Imaging: A Practical Approach.* 5th ed. Wolters Kluwer; 2011. (Figure 10-71A)

Figure 14-46. Cardenosa G. *Breast Imaging Companion.* 4th ed. Wolters Kluwer; 2018. (Figure 10-49B)

Chapter 15

Figure 15-1. Doubilet PM, Benson CB. *Atlas of Ultrasound in Obstetrics and Gynecology.* 3rd ed. Wolters Kluwer; 2018. (Figure 29.1.5)

Figure 15-2. Bornemann P. *Ultrasound for Primary Care.* Wolters Kluwer; 2020. (Figure 34-02)

Figure 15-3A. From Kawamura DM, Nolan TD. *Abdomen and Superficial Structures.* 4th ed. Wolters Kluwer; 2017. (Figure 1-5B)

Figure 15-3B. Bornemann P. *Ultrasound for Primary Care.* Wolters Kluwer; 2020. (Figure 34-08)

Figure 15-3C. Bornemann P. *Ultrasound for Primary Care.* Wolters Kluwer; 2020. (Figure 34-20)

Figure 15-5. Bornemann P. *Ultrasound for Primary Care.* Wolters Kluwer; 2020. (Figure 34-04)

Figure 15-6. Baggish MS. Hysteroscopy: Visual Perspectives of Uterine Anatomy, Physiology, and Pathology. 3rd ed. Wolters Kluwer; 2008. (Figure 19-17)

Figure 15-7. Stephenson SR. *Diagnostic Medical Sonography: Obstetrics & Gynecology.* 4th ed. Wolters Kluwer; 2015. (Figure 5-58)

Figure 15-8. Cosby KS, Kendall, JL. *Practical Guide to Emergency Ultrasound.* 2nd ed. Wolters Kluwer; 2015. (Figure 2-11B)

Figure 15-9. Siegel MJ. *Pediatric Sonography.* 5th ed. Wolters Kluwer; 2018. (Figure 11-13A)

Figure 15-10. Stephenson SR. *Diagnostic Medical Sonography: Obstetrics & Gynecology.* 4th ed. Wolters Kluwer; 2015. (Figure 10-12)

Figure 15-11. Doubilet PM, Benson CB. *Atlas of Ultrasound in Obstetrics and Gynecology.* 3rd ed. Wolters Kluwer; 2018. (Figure 31.3.3)

Figure 15-12. Doubilet PM, Benson CB. *Atlas of Ultrasound in Obstetrics and Gynecology.* 3rd ed. Wolters Kluwer; 2018. (Figure 20.2.1)

Figure 15-13. Sanders RC, Hall-Terracciano B. *Clinical Sonography: A Practical Guide.* 5th ed. Wolters Kluwer; 2015. (Figure 6-02)

Figure 15-14. From Kawamura DM, Nolan TD. *Abdomen and Superficial Structures.* 4th ed. Wolters Kluwer; 2017. (Figure 3-16)

Figure 15-15. Image courtesy of Philips Medical Systems, Bothell, WA.

Figure 15-16. From Kawamura DM, Nolan TD. *Abdomen and Superficial Structures.* 4th ed. Wolters Kluwer; 2017. (Figure 11-3)

Figure 15-17. Images courtesy of Philips Healthcare, Bothell, WA.

Figure 15-18. Stephenson SR. *Diagnostic Medical Sonography: Obstetrics & Gynecology.* 4th ed. Wolters Kluwer; 2015. (Figure 6-05)

Figure 15-20. Lee EY, Hunsaker A, Siewert B. *Computed Body Tomography With MRI Correlation.* 5th ed. Wolters Kluwer; 2019. (Figure 20-01B)

Chapter 16

Figure 16-1. Detton AJ. *Grant's Dissector.* 17th ed. Wolters Kluwer; 2021. (Online Image 5-30)

Figure 16-2. Moore KL. *Clinically Oriented Anatomy.* 7th ed. Wolters Kluwer; 2014. (Figure 3-1)

Figure 16-3. Tank PW. *Grant's Dissector.* 15th ed. Wolters Kluwer; 2013. (Figure 5-34)

Figure 16-4. Berek JS. *Berek & Novak's Gynecology.* 16th ed. Wolters Kluwer; 2019. (Figure 1-40A)

Figure 16-5A. From Berman M, Cohen H. *Obstetrics and Gynecology.* 2nd ed. Wolters Kluwer; 1997:42.

Figure 16-5B. Bornemann P. *Ultrasound for Primary Care.* Wolters Kluwer; 2020. (Figure 44-05)

Figure 16-7. Stephenson SR. *Diagnostic Medical Sonography: Obstetrics & Gynecology.* 3rd ed. Wolters Kluwer; 2012. (Figure 5-14)

Figure 16-8A. Stephenson SR. *Diagnostic Medical Sonography: Obstetrics & Gynecology.* 4th ed. Wolters Kluwer; 2015. (Figure 5-53)

Figure 16-8B,C. Stephenson SR. *Diagnostic Medical Sonography: Obstetrics & Gynecology.* 4th ed. Wolters Kluwer; 2015. (Figure 5-54A,B)

Figure 16-9. From Doubilet PM, Benson CB. *Atlas of Ultrasound in Obstetrics and Gynecology: A Multimedia Reference.* Wolters Kluwer; 2003:282

Figure 16-10. From Kawamura DM, Nolan TD. *Abdomen and Superficial Structures.* 4th ed. Wolters Kluwer; 2017. (Figure 3-16)

Figure 16-11. Stephenson SR. *Diagnostic Medical Sonography: Obstetrics & Gynecology.* 4th ed. Wolters Kluwer; 2015. (Figure 17-32)

Figure 16-12. From Hickey J, Goldberg F. *Ultrasound Review of Obstetrics and Gynecology.* Wolters Kluwer; 1996:18.

Figure 16-13A. Stephenson SR. *Diagnostic Medical Sonography: Obstetrics & Gynecology.* 4th ed. Wolters Kluwer; 2015. (Figure 5-56A)

Figure 16-13B. Image courtesy of Philips Healthcare, Bothell, WA.

Figure 16-13C. Stephenson SR. *Diagnostic Medical Sonography: Obstetrics & Gynecology.* 4th ed. Wolters Kluwer; 2015. (Figure 6-11C)

Figure 16-13D. Image courtesy of Philips Medical Systems, Bothell, WA.

Figure 16-14. From Hickey J, Goldberg F. *Ultrasound Review of Obstetrics and Gynecology.* Wolters Kluwer; 1996:18.

Figure 16-15. Stephenson SR. *Diagnostic Medical Sonography: Obstetrics & Gynecology.* 4th ed. Wolters Kluwer; 2015. (Figure 5-49)

Figure 16-16. Doubilet PM, Benson CB. *Atlas of Ultrasound in Obstetrics and Gynecology.* 3rd ed. Wolters Kluwer; 2018. (Figure 27.1.1C)

Figure 16-17. Stephenson SR. *Diagnostic Medical Sonography: Obstetrics & Gynecology.* 4th ed. Wolters Kluwer; 2015. (Figure 7-02)

Figure 16-18. Doubilet PM, Benson CB. *Atlas of Ultrasound in Obstetrics and Gynecology.* 2nd ed. Wolters Kluwer; 2011. (Figure 25.2.1)

Figure 16-19. Stephenson SR. *Diagnostic Medical Sonography: Obstetrics & Gynecology.* 4th ed. Wolters Kluwer; 2015. (Figure 17-31)

Figure 16-20. Stephenson SR. *Diagnostic Medical Sonography: Obstetrics & Gynecology.* 4th ed. Wolters Kluwer; 2015. (Figure 5-41)

Figure 16-21. From Barakat R. *Principles and Practice of Gynecologic Oncology.* 6th ed. Wolters Kluwer; 2014. (Figures 11-3C and 11-4A,B)

Figure 16-22. Brant WE, Helms CA. *Fundamentals of Diagnostic Radiology.* 4th ed. Wolters Kluwer; 2012. (Figure 25-5)

Chapter 17

Figure 17-1. Hartwig W. *Fundamental Anatomy.* Wolters Kluwer; 2008. (Figure 5-16)

Figure 17-2. Moore KL, Agur A. *Essential Clinical Anatomy.* 2nd ed. Wolters Kluwer; 2002.

Figure 17-6. Siegel MJ. *Pediatric Sonography.* 5th ed. Wolters Kluwer; 2018. (Figure 13-43A,B)

Figure 17-7. Sanders RC, Hall-Terracciano B. *Clinical Sonography: A Practical Guide.* 5th ed. Wolters Kluwer; 2015. (Figure 14-04A)

Figure 17-8. Agur AM. *Grant's Atlas of Anatomy.* 15th ed. Wolters Kluwer; 2021. (Figure 15-31)

Figure 17-9. Doubilet PM, Benson CB. *Atlas of Ultrasound in Obstetrics and Gynecology: A Multimedia Reference.* Wolters Kluwer; 2003. (Figure 23.1.3A,B)

Figure 17-10. Sanders RC, Hall-Terracciano B. *Clinical Sonography: A Practical Guide.* 5th ed. Wolters Kluwer; 2015. (Figure 14-05)

Figure 17-11A. Bornemann P. *Ultrasound for Primary Care.* Wolters Kluwer; 2020. (Figure 34-10)

Figure 17-11B. Bornemann P. *Ultrasound for Primary Care.* Wolters Kluwer; 2020. (Figure 59-02)

Figure 17-12. Cosby KS, Kendall, JL. *Practical Guide to Emergency Ultrasound.* 2nd ed. Wolters Kluwer; 2015. (Figure 14-08A)

Figure 17-13. Stephenson SR. *Diagnostic Medical Sonography: Obstetrics & Gynecology.* 4th ed. Wolters Kluwer; 2015. (Figure 3-06)

Figure 17-14A. Linn-Watson T. *Radiographic Pathology.* 2nd ed. Wolters Kluwer; 2015. (Figure 7-13)

Figure 17-14B. Doubilet PM, Benson CB. *Atlas of Ultrasound in Obstetrics and Gynecology.* 3rd ed. Wolters Kluwer; 2018. (Figure 29.3.4)

Figure 17-15. Doubilet PM, Benson CB. *Atlas of Ultrasound in Obstetrics and Gynecology: A Multimedia Reference.* Wolters Kluwer; 2003. (Figure 25.3.3)

Figure 17-16. Doubilet PM, Benson CB. *Atlas of Ultrasound in Obstetrics and Gynecology: A Multimedia Reference.* Wolters Kluwer; 2003. (Figure 25.3.2A,B)

Figure 17-17. Speroff L, Fritz M. *Clinical Gynecologic Endocrinology and Infertility.* 7th ed. Wolters Kluwer; 2005. (Figure 14-3)

Figure 17-18. Moore KL. *Clinically Oriented Anatomy.* 7th ed. Wolters Kluwer; 2014 (Figure 3-13)

Figure 17-19. Timor-Tritsch IE, Goldstein SR. *Ultrasound in Gynecology.* 2nd ed. Elsevier; 2007. (Figure 19-7)

Figure 17-20. From Siegel MJ, Coley B. *Core Curriculum: Pediatric Imaging.* Wolters Kluwer; 2005. (Figure 10-30)

Figure 17-21. Image courtesy of Philips Medical Systems, Bothell, WA.

Figure 17-22. Siegel MJ. *Pediatric Sonography.* 5th ed. Wolters Kluwer; 2018. (Figure 13-55A,B)

Figure 17-23. Stephenson SR. *Diagnostic Medical Sonography: Obstetrics & Gynecology.* 4th ed. Wolters Kluwer; 2015. (Figure 11-23)

Figure 17-24. Doubilet PM, Benson CB. *Atlas of Ultrasound in Obstetrics and Gynecology: A Multimedia Reference.* Wolters Kluwer; 2003. (Figure 25.2.1A,B)

Figure 17-25. Doubilet PM, Benson CB. *Atlas of Ultrasound in Obstetrics and Gynecology.* 2nd ed. Wolters Kluwer; 2011. (Figure 26.2.2)

Figure 17-26. Lee EY, Hunsaker A, Siewert B. *Computed Body Tomography With MRI Correlation.* 5th ed. Wolters Kluwer; 2019. (Figure 20-10A)

Figure 17-27A. Hurt KJ. *Pocket Obstetrics and Gynecology.* Wolters Kluwer; 2014. (Figure 6-1)

Figure 17-27B. Guimaraes M. *Embolization Therapy: Principles and Clinical Applications.* Wolters Kluwer; 2016. (Figure 54-1)

Figure 17-28. Doubilet PM, Benson CB. *Atlas of Ultrasound in Obstetrics and Gynecology: A Multimedia Reference.* Wolters Kluwer; 2003. (Figure 25.1.1A-C)

Figure 17-29. Doubilet PM, Benson CB. *Atlas of Ultrasound in Obstetrics and Gynecology.* 2nd ed. Wolters Kluwer; 2011. (Figure 26.1.10)

Figure 17-30. Doubilet PM, Benson CB. *Atlas of Ultrasound in Obstetrics and Gynecology: A Multimedia Reference.* Wolters Kluwer; 2003. (Figure 23.1.2)

Figure 17-31. Doubilet PM, Benson CB. *Atlas of Ultrasound in Obstetrics and Gynecology.* 3rd ed. Wolters Kluwer; 2018. (Figure 29.4.3)

Figure 17-32A. Shirkhoda A. *Variants and Pitfalls in Body Imaging.* 2nd ed. Wolters Kluwer; 2011. (Figure 32-42A)

Figure 17-32B. Stephenson SR. *Diagnostic Medical Sonography: Obstetrics & Gynecology.* 3rd ed. Wolters Kluwer; 2012. (Figure 8-30)

Figure 17-33. Doubilet PM, Benson CB. *Atlas of Ultrasound in Obstetrics and Gynecology.* 3rd ed. Wolters Kluwer; 2018. (Figure 29.4.7)

Figure 17-34. Images courtesy of Philips Healthcare, Bothell, WA.

Figure 17-36. Rubin R. *Rubin's Pathology.* 6th ed. Wolters Kluwer; 2012. (Figure 6-14)

Figure 17-37. Doubilet PM, Benson CB. *Atlas of Ultrasound in Obstetrics and Gynecology.* 2nd ed. Wolters Kluwer; 2011. (Figure 26.1.8)

Figure 17-38. Doubilet PM, Benson CB. *Atlas of Ultrasound in Obstetrics and Gynecology.* 2nd ed. Wolters Kluwer; 2011. (Figure 26.1.7)

Figure 17-39. Doubilet PM, Benson CB. *Atlas of Ultrasound in Obstetrics and Gynecology.* 3rd ed. Wolters Kluwer; 2018. (Figure 29.1.3)

Figure 17-40. Doubilet PM, Benson CB. *Atlas of Ultrasound in Obstetrics and Gynecology.* 2nd ed. Wolters Kluwer; 2011. (Figure 26.2.3)

Figure 17-41. Doubilet PM, Benson CB. *Atlas of Ultrasound in Obstetrics and Gynecology.* 3rd ed. Wolters Kluwer; 2018. (Figure 29.4.6)

Figure 17-42. Dugani S. *Clinical Anatomy Cases.* Wolters Kluwer; 2017. (Figure 4-30)

Figure 17-43. Cosby KS, Kendall, JL. *Practical Guide to Emergency Ultrasound.* 2nd ed. Wolters Kluwer; 2015. (Figure 14-17)

Figure 17-44. Doubilet PM, Benson CB. *Atlas of Ultrasound in Obstetrics and Gynecology.* 3rd ed. Wolters Kluwer; 2018. (Figure 29.1.10)

Figure 17-45A. Berek JS. *Berek & Novak's Gynecology.* 16th ed. Wolters Kluwer; 2020. (Figure 11-8A)

Figure 17-45B. Berek JS. *Berek & Novak's Gynecology.* 16th ed. Wolters Kluwer; 2020. (Figure 11-5B)

Figure 17-46. Images courtesy of Philips Healthcare, Bothell, WA.

Chapter 18

Figure 18-2. Stephenson SR. *Diagnostic Medical Sonography: Obstetrics & Gynecology.* 3rd ed. Wolters Kluwer; 2012. (Figure 5-50A,B)

Figure 18-3. From Wingerd B. *Human Body.* 3rd ed. Wolters Kluwer; 2013. (Figure 17-9)

Figure 18-4. Scott JR. *Danforth's Obstetrics and Gynecology.* 9th ed. Wolters Kluwer; 2004. (Figure 28-10A)

Figure 18-5. Stephenson SR. *Diagnostic Medical Sonography: Obstetrics & Gynecology.* 3rd ed. Wolters Kluwer; 2012. (Figure 5-58)

Figure 18-6. Siegel MJ. *Pediatric Sonography.* 5th ed. Wolters Kluwer; 2018. (Figure 13-07A,B)

Figure 18-7. Stephenson SR. *Diagnostic Medical Sonography: Obstetrics & Gynecology.* 4th ed. Wolters Kluwer; 2015. (Figure 12-08)

Figure 18-8. Doubilet PM, Benson CB. *Atlas of Ultrasound in Obstetrics and Gynecology.* 3rd ed. Wolters Kluwer; 2018. (Figure 31.1.1)

Figure 18-9. Siegel MJ. *Pediatric Sonography.* 4th ed. Wolters Kluwer; 2010. (Figure 13-12)

Figure 18-11. Brant WE, Helms CA. *Fundamentals of Diagnostic Radiology.* 4th ed. Wolters Kluwer; 2012. (Figure 37-5)

Figure 18-12. Brant WE, Helms CA. *Fundamentals of Diagnostic Radiology.* 4th ed. Wolters Kluwer; 2012. (Figure 38-12)

Figure 18-13. Siegel MJ. *Pediatric Sonography.* 4th ed. Wolters Kluwer; 2010. (Figure 13-15)

Figure 18-14. From Anatomical Chart Company. *Atlas of Pathophysiology.* Wolters Kluwer; 2001.

Figure 18-15. Doubilet PM, Benson CB. *Atlas of Ultrasound in Obstetrics and Gynecology.* 2nd ed. Wolters Kluwer; 2011. (Figure 28.3.4)

Figure 18-16. Brant W. *The Core Curriculum: Ultrasound.* Lippincott Williams & Wilkins; 2001:210.

Figure 18-17. Lee EY. Pediatric Radiology: Practical Imaging Evaluation of Infants and Children. Wolters Kluwer; 2017. (Figure 19-31A)

Figure 18-18. Doubilet PM, Benson CB. *Atlas of Ultrasound in Obstetrics and Gynecology: A Multimedia Reference.* Wolters Kluwer; 2003. (Figure 27.4.3A)

Figure 18-19. Doubilet PM, Benson CB. *Atlas of Ultrasound in Obstetrics and Gynecology: A Multimedia Reference.* Wolters Kluwer; 2003. (Figure 27.6.1A,B)

Figure 18-20. Doubilet PM, Benson CB. *Atlas of Ultrasound in Obstetrics and Gynecology.* 2nd ed. Wolters Kluwer; 2011. (Figure 28.4.1)

Figure 18-21. Doubilet PM, Benson CB. *Atlas of Ultrasound in Obstetrics and Gynecology.* 3rd ed. Wolters Kluwer; 2018. (Figure 31.4.2)

Figure 18-22. Doubilet PM, Benson CB. *Atlas of Ultrasound in Obstetrics and Gynecology.* 3rd ed. Wolters Kluwer; 2018. (Figure 31.5.6)

Figure 18-23. Doubilet PM, Benson CB. *Atlas of Ultrasound in Obstetrics and Gynecology: A Multimedia Reference.* Wolters Kluwer; 2003. (Figure 27.5.2B)

Figure 18-24. Doubilet PM, Benson CB. *Atlas of Ultrasound in Obstetrics and Gynecology.* 3rd ed. Wolters Kluwer; 2018. (Figure 31.6.4)

Figure 18-25. Beckmann CR. *Obstetrics and Gynecology.* 5th ed. Wolters Kluwer; 2006. (Figure 3-10)

Figure 18-26. Doubilet PM, Benson CB. *Atlas of Ultrasound in Obstetrics and Gynecology. A Multimedia Reference.* Wolters Kluwer; 2003. (Figure 27.7.1)

Figure 18-27. Benrubi GI. *Handbook of Obstetric and Gynecologic Emergencies.* 4th ed. Wolters Kluwer; 2010. (Figure 28-22)

Figure 18-28A. Geschwind J. *Abrams' Angiography.* 3rd ed. Wolters Kluwer; 2014. (Figure 93-4A)

Figure 18-28B. Stephenson SR. *Diagnostic Medical Sonography: Obstetrics & Gynecology.* 4th ed. Wolters Kluwer; 2015. (Figure 6-19)

Figure 18-29. Stephenson SR. *Diagnostic Medical Sonography: Obstetrics & Gynecology.* 4th ed. Wolters Kluwer; 2015. (Figure 13-18B,C)

Figure 18-30. Daffner RH, Hartman M. *Clinical Radiology.* 4th ed. Wolters Kluwer; 2013. (Figure 10-20A)

Figure 18-31. Farrell TA. *Radiology 101.* 5th ed. Wolters Kluwer; 2020. (Figure 4-22)

Figure 18-32. Doubilet PM, Benson CB. *Atlas of Ultrasound in Obstetrics and Gynecology.* 3rd ed. Wolters Kluwer; 2018. (Figure 17.5.5C)

Figure 18-33. Shirkhoda A. *Variants and Pitfalls in Body Imaging.* 2nd ed. Wolters Kluwer; 2011. (Figure 26-48B)

Figure 18-34. Stephenson SR. *Diagnostic Medical Sonography: Obstetrics & Gynecology.* 3rd ed. Wolters Kluwer; 2012. (Figure 10-19)

Figure 18-35. Iyer RS, Chapman T. *Pediatric Imaging: The Essentials.* Wolters Kluwer; 2016. (Figure 22-08B)

Figure 18-36. Shirkhoda A. *Variants and Pitfalls in Body Imaging.* 2nd ed. Wolters Kluwer; 2011. (Figure 26-58)

Figure 18-37A. Lee EY, Hunsaker A, Siewert B. *Computed Body Tomography With MRI Correlation.* 5th ed. Wolters Kluwer; 2019. (Figure 24-102A)

Figure 18-37B. Britt LD. *Acute Care Surgery.* 2nd ed. Wolters Kluwer; 2019. (Figure 9-3A)

Figure 18-38. Dunnick R. *Textbook of Uroradiology.* 5th ed. Wolters Kluwer; 2013. (Figure 18-18)

Figure 18-39. Farrell TA. *Radiology 101.* 5th ed. Wolters Kluwer; 2020. (Figure 4-29)

Chapter 19

Figure 19-3. Stephenson SR. *Diagnostic Medical Sonography: Obstetrics & Gynecology.* 4th ed. Wolters Kluwer; 2015. (Figure 5-49)

Figure 19-4. From Gibbs RS. *Danforth's Obstetrics and Gynecology.* 10th ed. Wolters Kluwer; 2008. (Figure 30-9A)

Figure 19-5. Doubilet PM, Benson CB. *Atlas of Ultrasound in Obstetrics and Gynecology.* 3rd ed. Wolters Kluwer; 2018. (Figure 28.1.3)

Figure 19-6. Stephenson SR. *Diagnostic Medical Sonography: Obstetrics & Gynecology.* 4th ed. Wolters Kluwer; 2015. (Figure 6-15)

Figure 19-7. Sanders RC, Hall-Terracciano B. *Clinical Sonography: A Practical Guide.* 5th ed. Wolters Kluwer; 2015. (Figure 14-01)

Figure 19-9. Doubilet PM, Benson CB. *Atlas of Ultrasound in Obstetrics and Gynecology.* 2nd ed. Wolters Kluwer; 2011. (Figure 24.2.1B)

Figure 19-10. Doubilet PM, Benson CB. *Atlas of Ultrasound in Obstetrics and Gynecology.* 2nd ed. Wolters Kluwer; 2011. (Figure 24.2.1C)

Figure 19-11. Doubilet PM, Benson CB. *Atlas of Ultrasound in Obstetrics and Gynecology.* 2nd ed. Wolters Kluwer; 2011. (Figure 24.2.1D)

Figure 19-12. Stephenson SR. *Diagnostic Medical Sonography: Obstetrics & Gynecology.* 4th ed. Wolters Kluwer; 2015. (Figure 4-14)

Figure 19-14. Doubilet PM, Benson CB. *Atlas of Ultrasound in Obstetrics and Gynecology: A Multimedia Reference.* Wolters Kluwer; 2003. (Figure 23.2.16)

Figure 19-15. Klein JS, Vinson EM, Brant WE, et al. *Brant and Helms' Fundamentals of Diagnostic Radiology.* 5th ed. Wolters Kluwer; 2018. (Figure 51-01B)

Figure 19-16. Doubilet PM, Benson CB. *Atlas of Ultrasound in Obstetrics and Gynecology.* 2nd ed. Wolters Kluwer; 2011. (Figure 25.1.2)

Figure 19-17. Doubilet PM, Benson CB. *Atlas of Ultrasound in Obstetrics and Gynecology.* 3rd ed. Wolters Kluwer; 2018. (Figure 27-4B)

Figure 19-18. Sanders RC, Hall-Terracciano B. *Clinical Sonography: A Practical Guide.* 5th ed. Wolters Kluwer; 2015. (Figure 63-11)

Figure 19-19. Collins RD. *Differential Diagnosis in Primary Care.* 5th ed. Wolters Kluwer; 2012. (Figure 4-12)

Figure 19-20. Collins RD. *Differential Diagnosis in Primary Care.* 5th ed. Wolters Kluwer; 2012. (Figure 8-33)

Figure 19-21. Collins RD. *Differential Diagnosis in Primary Care.* 5th ed. Wolters Kluwer; 2012. (Figure 8-23)

Chapter 20

Figure 20-1. Doubilet PM, Benson CB. *Atlas of Ultrasound in Obstetrics and Gynecology: A Multimedia Reference.* Wolters Kluwer; 2003. (Figure 23.2.2)

Figure 20-2. Brant WE, Helms CA. *Fundamentals of Diagnostic Radiology.* 4th ed. Wolters Kluwer; 2012. (Figure 37-06)

Figure 20-3A. From Anatomical Chart Company. *Common Gynecological Disorders Anatomical Chart.* Wolters Kluwer; 2007.

Figure 20-3B. Image courtesy of Philips Healthcare, Bothell, WA.

Figure 20-4C. Farrell TA. *Radiology 101.* 5th ed. Wolters Kluwer; 2020. (Figure 4-32)

Figure 20-5. From McConnell TH. *Nature of Disease.* 2nd ed. Wolters Kluwer; 2014. (Figure 17-26)

Figure 20-6A. From Anatomical Chart Company. *Common Gynecological Disorders Anatomical Chart.* Wolters Kluwer; 2007.

Figure 20-6B, C. Doubilet PM, Benson CB. *Atlas of Ultrasound in Obstetrics and Gynecology.* 2nd ed. Wolters Kluwer; 2011. (Figure 27.1.4)

Figure 20-7. Doubilet PM, Benson CB. *Atlas of Ultrasound in Obstetrics and Gynecology.* 2nd ed. Wolters Kluwer; 2011. (Figure 27.1.5)

Figure 20-8. Stephenson SR. *Diagnostic Medical Sonography: Obstetrics & Gynecology.* 3rd ed. Wolters Kluwer; 2012. (Figure 8-05)

Figure 20-9A. Sanders RC, Hall-Terracciano B. *Clinical Sonography: A Practical Guide.* 5th ed. Wolters Kluwer; 2015. (Figure 19-01)

Figure 20-9C. Sanders RC, Hall-Terracciano B. *Clinical Sonography: A Practical Guide.* 5th ed. Wolters Kluwer; 2015. (Figure 19-04)

Figure 20-10B. Kupesic S, Plavsic, BM. 2D and 3D hysterosalpingo-contrast-sonography in the assessment of uterine cavity and tubal patency. *Euro J Obstet Gynecol Reprod Biol.* 2007;133(1):67. With permission from Elsevier.

Figure 20-11A, B. Doubilet PM, Benson CB. *Atlas of Ultrasound in Obstetrics and Gynecology.* 3rd ed. Wolters Kluwer; 2018. (Figure 30.4.2)

Figure 20-11C. From Anatomical Chart Company. *Common Gynecological Disorders Anatomical Chart.* Wolters Kluwer; 2007.

Figure 20-12. Chi D. *Principles and Practice of Gynecologic Oncology.* 7th ed. Wolters Kluwer; 2018. (Figure 10-6B)

Figure 20-13. Doubilet PM, Benson CB. *Atlas of Ultrasound in Obstetrics and Gynecology.* 3rd ed. Wolters Kluwer; 2018. (Figure 30.4.3)

Figure 20-14. Doubilet PM, Benson CB. *Atlas of Ultrasound in Obstetrics and Gynecology.* 3rd ed. Wolters Kluwer; 2018. (Figure 30.2.3)

Figure 20-15. Shirkhoda A. *Variants and Pitfalls in Body Imaging.* 2nd ed. Wolters Kluwer; 2011. (Figure 26-22)

Figure 20-16. Doubilet PM, Benson CB. *Atlas of Ultrasound in Obstetrics and Gynecology.* 3rd ed. Wolters Kluwer; 2018. (Figure 29.1.1)

Figure 20-17. Lee EY, Hunsaker A, Siewert B. *Computed Body Tomography With MRI Correlation.* 5th ed. Wolters Kluwer; 2019. (Figure 20-27A)

Figure 20-18. von Schulthess, GK. *Molecular Anatomic Imaging.* 3rd ed. Wolters Kluwer; 2016. (Figure 52-9)

Figure 20-19. Dunnick R. *Textbook of Uroradiology.* 5th ed. Wolters Kluwer; 2013. (Figure 18-18)

Chapter 21

Figure 21-1. Braun CA. *Pathophysiology.* 2nd ed. Wolters Kluwer; 2011. (Figure 12-13)

Figure 21-2. Callahan T, Caughey A. *Blueprints Obstetrics and Gynecology.* 6th ed. Wolters Kluwer; 2013. (Figure 17-2)

Figure 21-3. Benrubi GI. *Handbook of Obstetric and Gynecologic Emergencies.* 5th ed. Wolters Kluwer; 2019. (Figure 28-22A)

Figure 21-4. Pope TL Jr, Harris JH Jr. *Harris & Harris' The Radiology of Emergency Medicine.* 5th ed. Wolters Kluwer; 2012. (Figure 11-11)

Figure 21-5. Beckmann CR, Herbert W, Laube D, et al. *Obstetrics and Gynecology.* 7th ed. Wolters Kluwer; 2013. (Figure 19-2)

Figure 21-6A. Siegel MJ. *Pediatric Sonography.* 5th ed. Wolters Kluwer; 2018. (Figure 13-34)

Figure 21-6B. Dunnick R. *Textbook of Uroradiology.* 6th ed. Wolters Kluwer; 2018. (Figure 17-23B)

Figure 21-7. Siegel MJ. *Pediatric Sonography.* 4th ed. Wolters Kluwer; 2010. (Figure 13-33)

Figure 21-8. Doubilet PM, Benson CB. *Atlas of Ultrasound in Obstetrics and Gynecology.* 3rd ed. Wolters Kluwer; 2018. (Figure 31.9.3)

Figure 21-10. Berek JS. *Berek & Novak's Gynecology.* 16th ed. Wolters Kluwer; 2020. (Figure 13-1)

Figure 21-11. Doubilet PM, Benson CB. *Atlas of Ultrasound in Obstetrics and Gynecology.* 2nd ed. Wolters Kluwer; 2011. (Figure 28.7.1)

Figure 21-12A. From Anatomical Chart Company. *Infertility Anatomical Chart.* Wolters Kluwer; 2004.

Figure 21-12B. Dunnick R. *Textbook of Uroradiology.* 6th ed. Wolters Kluwer; 2018. (Figure 17-8)

Figure 21-12C. Iyer RS, Chapman T. *Pediatric Imaging: The Essentials.* Wolters Kluwer; 2016. (Figure 22-14B)

Figure 21-13A. Callahan T, Caughey A. *Blueprints Obstetrics and Gynecology.* 7th ed. Wolters Kluwer; 2018. (Figure 26-11)

Figure 21-13B. Doubilet PM, Benson CB. *Atlas of Ultrasound in Obstetrics and Gynecology.* 2nd ed. Wolters Kluwer; 2011. (Figure 31.2.1)

Figure 21-14. Zeind CS. *Applied Therapeutics.* 11th ed. Wolters Kluwer; 2018. (Figure 48-2)

Figure 21-15. Stephenson SR. *Diagnostic Medical Sonography: Obstetrics & Gynecology.* 4th ed. Wolters Kluwer; 2015. (Figure 12-26)

Figure 21-16. Stephenson SR. *Diagnostic Medical Sonography: Obstetrics & Gynecology.* 4th ed. Wolters Kluwer; 2015. (Figure 34-18B)

Figure 21-18. Beckmann CR. *Obstetrics and Gynecology.* 5th ed. Wolters Kluwer; 2006. (Figure 25-5)

Figure 21-19. Bornemann P. *Ultrasound for Primary Care.* Wolters Kluwer; 2020 (Figure 34-33)

Figure 21-20A,B. Cosby KS, Kendall, JL. *Practical Guide to Emergency Ultrasound.* Wolters Kluwer; 2006. (Figure 7-19)

Figure 21-20C. Sanders RC, Hall-Terracciano B. *Clinical Sonography: A Practical Guide.* 5th ed. Wolters Kluwer; 2015. (Figure 20-04)

Figure 21-21. Doubilet PM, Benson CB. *Atlas of Ultrasound in Obstetrics and Gynecology.* 3rd ed. Wolters Kluwer; 2018. (Figure 30.7.2)

Figure 21-22. Doubilet PM, Benson CB. *Atlas of Ultrasound in Obstetrics and Gynecology.* 3rd ed. Wolters Kluwer; 2018. (Figure 30.7.3)

Figure 21-23. Doubilet PM, Benson CB. *Atlas of Ultrasound in Obstetrics and Gynecology: A Multimedia Reference.* Wolters Kluwer; 2003. (Figure 30.2.3)

Figure 21-25. From Siegel MJ, Coley BD. *Core Curriculum: Pediatric Imaging.* Wolters Kluwer; 2005. (Figure 10-21)

Figure 21-26. Doubilet PM, Benson CB. *Atlas of Ultrasound in Obstetrics and Gynecology.* 3rd ed. Wolters Kluwer; 2018. (Figure 29.1.10)

Figure 21-27. Cosby KS, Kendall, JL. *Practical Guide to Emergency Ultrasound.* 2nd ed. Wolters Kluwer; 2015. (Figure 14-26)

Figure 21-28. Doubilet PM, Benson CB. *Atlas of Ultrasound in Obstetrics and Gynecology.* 3rd ed. Wolters Kluwer; 2018. (Figure 30.7.3)

Figure 21-29. Benrubi GI. *Handbook of Obstetric and Gynecologic Emergencies.* 5th ed. Wolters Kluwer; 2019. (Figure 28-22B)

Figure 21-30. Emans L. *Emans, Laufer, Goldstein's Pediatric and Adolescent Gynecology.* 7th ed. Wolters Kluwer; 2020. (Figure 37-29D)

Figure 21-31. Klein JS, Vinson EM, Brant WE, et al. *Brant and Helms' Fundamentals of Diagnostic Radiology.* 5th ed. Wolters Kluwer; 2018. (Figure 51-13)

Chapter 22

Figure 22-1A. Abuhamad A. *A Practical Guide to Fetal Echocardiography.* 3rd ed. Wolters Kluwer; 2015. (Figure 11-04)

Figure 22-1B. Abuhamad A. *A Practical Guide to Fetal Echocardiography.* 3rd ed. Wolters Kluwer; 2015. (Figure 11-05)

Figure 22-2. From Mukherjee D. *Cardiovascular Medicine and Surgery.* Wolters Kluwer; 2021. (Figure 19-2)

Figure 22-3. From Ricci S. *Essentials of Maternity, Newborn, and Women's Health Nursing.* 4th ed. Wolters Kluwer Health; 2016.

Figure 22-4. Bushberg JT. The Essential Physics of Medical Imaging. 4th ed. Wolters Kluwer; 2021. (Figure 14-42A,B)

Figure 22-5. Stephenson SR. *Diagnostic Medical Sonography: Obstetrics & Gynecology.* 4th ed. Wolters Kluwer; 2015. (Figure 25-35)

Figure 22-7. Abuhamad A. *A Practical Guide to Fetal Echocardiography.* 4th ed. Wolters Kluwer; 2022. (Figure 6-02)

Figure 22-8. Casanova R. *Beckmann and Ling's Obstetrics and Gynecology.* 8th ed. Wolters Kluwer; 2019, (Figure 9-6)

Figure 22-10. Stephenson SR. *Diagnostic Medical Sonography: Obstetrics & Gynecology.* 4th ed. Wolters Kluwer; 2015. (Figure 25-34)

Figure 22-11. Kline-Fath B, Bahado-Singh R, Bulas D. *Fundamental and Advanced Fetal Imaging.* Wolters Kluwer; 2015. (Figure 18.c-01a)

Figure 22-12. Neal JM. A Practical Approach to Regional Anesthesiology and Acute Pain Medicine. 5th ed. Wolters Kluwer; 2018. (Figure 3-11A)

Figure 22-13. Kollef M. *The Washington Manual of Critical Care.* 3rd ed. Wolters Kluwer; 2018. (Figure 87-15)

Figure 22-14. Farrell TA. *Radiology 101.* 5th ed. Wolters Kluwer; 2020. (Figure 3-62)

Figure 22-15. Sadler TW. *Langman's Medical Embryology.* 15th ed. Wolters Kluwer; 2023. (Figure 9-9)

Figure 22-16. Doubilet PM, Benson CB. *Atlas of Ultrasound in Obstetrics and Gynecology.* 3rd ed. Wolters Kluwer; 2018. (Figure 31.5.3)

Figure 22-17. Stephenson SR. *Diagnostic Medical Sonography: Obstetrics & Gynecology.* 4th ed. Wolters Kluwer; 2015. (Figure 27-01)

Figure 22-18. Stephenson SR. *Diagnostic Medical Sonography: Obstetrics & Gynecology.* 4th ed. Wolters Kluwer; 2015. (Figure 5-25)

Figure 22-19. Image courtesy of Philips Medical Systems, Bothell, WA.

Figure 22-20. Brant W. *The Core Curriculum: Ultrasound.* Lippincott Williams & Wilkins; 2001:16.

Figure 22-21. Neal JM. A Practical Approach to Regional Anesthesiology and Acute Pain Medicine. 5th ed. Wolters Kluwer; 2018. (Figure 3-10)

Figure 22-22. Modified from Bronshtein M, Gover A, Zimmer EZ. Sonographic definition of the fetal situs. *Obstet Gynecol.* 2002;99(6):1129–1130, with permission.

Figure 22-23. Beckmann CR. *Obstetrics and Gynecology.* 4th ed. Wolters Kluwer; 2003. (Figure 7-6)

Figure 22-24. Kline-Fath B, Bahado-Singh R, Bulas D. *Fundamental and Advanced Fetal Imaging.* Wolters Kluwer; 2015. (Figure 11-19B)

Chapter 23

Figure 23-1. From Anatomical Chart Company. *Atlas of Human Anatomy.* Wolters Kluwer; 2001.

Figure 23-2. From Stephenson SR. *Diagnostic Medical Sonography: Obstetrics & Gynecology,* 4th ed. Wolters Kluwer; 2015. (Figure 8-34)

Figure 23-3. Abuhamad A. *A Practical Guide to Fetal Echocardiography.* 4th ed. Wolters Kluwer; 2022. (Figure 11-35)

Figure 23-4. Doubilet PM, Benson CB. *Atlas of Ultrasound in Obstetrics and Gynecology: A Multimedia Reference.* Wolters Kluwer; 2003. (Figure 1.1.1A)

Figure 23-5. Sadler TW. *Langman's Medical Embryology.* 15th ed. Wolters Kluwer; 2023. (Figure 8-10)

Figure 23-6. Abuhamad AZ, Chaoui, R. *First Trimester Ultrasound Diagnosis of Fetal Abnormalities.* Wolters Kluwer; 2017. (Figure 4-12)

Figure 23-7. Doubilet PM, Benson CB. *Atlas of Ultrasound in Obstetrics and Gynecology: A Multimedia Reference.* Wolters Kluwer; 2003. (Figure 1.1.2)

Figure 23-8A. Abuhamad AZ, Chaoui, R. *First Trimester Ultrasound Diagnosis of Fetal Abnormalities.* Wolters Kluwer; 2017. (Figure 4-06)

Figure 23-8B. Stephenson SR. *Diagnostic Medical Sonography: Obstetrics & Gynecology.* 3rd ed. Wolters Kluwer; 2012. (Figure 13-15)

Figure 23-10. Abuhamad AZ, Chaoui, R. *First Trimester Ultrasound Diagnosis of Fetal Abnormalities.* Wolters Kluwer; 2017. (Figure 4-08)

Figure 23-11. Abuhamad AZ, Chaoui, R. *First Trimester Ultrasound Diagnosis of Fetal Abnormalities.* Wolters Kluwer; 2017. (Figure 2-03)

Figure 23-12. Penny SM. *Introduction to Sonography and Patient Care.* Wolters Kluwer; 2015. (Figure 3-30)

Figure 23-13. Doubilet PM, Benson CB. *Atlas of Ultrasound in Obstetrics and Gynecology: A Multimedia Reference.* Wolters Kluwer; 2003. (Figure 1.2.3A)

Figure 23-14. Doubilet PM, Benson CB. *Atlas of Ultrasound in Obstetrics and Gynecology.* 3rd ed. Wolters Kluwer; 2018. (Figure 1.3.9)

Figure 23-15. Doubilet PM, Benson CB. *Atlas of Ultrasound in Obstetrics and Gynecology.* 2nd ed. Wolters Kluwer; 2011. (Figure 1.3.3)

Figure 23-16. Doubilet PM, Benson CB. *Atlas of Ultrasound in Obstetrics and Gynecology: A Multimedia Reference.* Wolters Kluwer; 2003. (Figure 1.3.4)

Figure 23-17. Doubilet PM, Benson CB. *Atlas of Ultrasound in Obstetrics and Gynecology.* 2nd ed. Wolters Kluwer; 2011. (Figure 7.1.1)

Figure 23-18. Doubilet PM, Benson CB. *Atlas of Ultrasound in Obstetrics and Gynecology.* 2nd ed. Wolters Kluwer; 2011. (Figure 7.1.4)

Figure 23-20. Doubilet PM, Benson CB. *Atlas of Ultrasound in Obstetrics and Gynecology: A Multimedia Reference.* Wolters Kluwer; 2003. (Figure 28.1.1A-C)

Figure 23-21. Courtesy of Maribel U. Lockwood.

Figure 23-22A,B. Doubilet PM, Benson CB. *Atlas of Ultrasound in Obstetrics and Gynecology: A Multimedia Reference.* Wolters Kluwer; 2003. (Figure 26.4.1A,B)

Figure 23-22C. Doubilet PM, Benson CB. *Atlas of Ultrasound in Obstetrics and Gynecology.* 3rd ed. Wolters Kluwer; 2018. (Figure 17.5.5C)

Figure 23-23. Brant WE, Helms CA. *Fundamentals of Diagnostic Radiology.* 4th ed. Wolters Kluwer; 2012. (Figure 37-08)

Figure 23-24. Pope TL. *Harris & Harris' The Radiology of Emergency Medicine.* 5th ed. Wolters Kluwer; 2013. (Figure 16-22)

Figure 23-25. Cosby KS, Kendall, JL. *Practical Guide to Emergency Ultrasound.* 2nd ed. Wolters Kluwer; 2015. (Figure 16-25)

Figure 23-26. Brant WE, Helms CA. *Brant and Helms Solution.* Wolters Kluwer; 2006. (Figure 38-08)

Figure 23-27. Cosby KS, Kendall, JL. *Practical Guide to Emergency Ultrasound.* 2nd ed. Wolters Kluwer; 2015. (Figure 15-16C)

Figure 23-28. Doubilet PM, Benson CB. *Atlas of Ultrasound in Obstetrics and Gynecology.* 3rd ed. Wolters Kluwer; 2018. (Figure 30.5.2)

Figure 23-29. Doubilet PM, Benson CB. *Atlas of Ultrasound in Obstetrics and Gynecology: A Multimedia Reference.* Wolters Kluwer; 2003. (Figure 1.3.3A)

Figure 23-30. Abuhamad AZ, Chaoui, R. *First Trimester Ultrasound Diagnosis of Fetal Abnormalities.* Wolters Kluwer; 2017. (Figure 4-05)

Figure 23-31. Sanders RC, Hall-Terracciano B. *Clinical Sonography: A Practical Guide.* 5th ed. Wolters Kluwer; 2015. (Figure 22-11)

Figure 23-32. Doubilet PM, Benson CB. *Atlas of Ultrasound in Obstetrics and Gynecology.* 3rd ed. Wolters Kluwer; 2018. (Figure 1.2.4)

Figure 23-33. Abuhamad AZ, Chaoui, R. *First Trimester Ultrasound Diagnosis of Fetal Abnormalities.* Wolters Kluwer; 2017. (Figure 8-07C)

Figure 23-34. Sanders RC, Hall-Terracciano B. *Clinical Sonography: A Practical Guide.* 5th ed. Wolters Kluwer; 2015. (Figure 63-11)

Figure 23-35. Dobiesz V. *Manual of Obstetric Emergencies.* Wolters Kluwer; 2021. (Figure 14-4)

Figure 23-36. Kline-Fath B, Bahado-Singh R, Bulas D. *Fundamental and Advanced Fetal Imaging.* Wolters Kluwer; 2015. (Figure 20-01A)

Figure 23-38. Abuhamad AZ, Chaoui, R. *First Trimester Ultrasound Diagnosis of Fetal Abnormalities.* Wolters Kluwer; 2017. (Figure 6-05)

Figure 23-39. Abuhamad A. *A Practical Guide to Fetal Echocardiography.* 4th ed. Wolters Kluwer; 2022 (Figure 25-06)

Figure 23-40. Stephenson SR. *Diagnostic Medical Sonography: Obstetrics & Gynecology.* 4th ed. Wolters Kluwer; 2015. (Figure 15-20)

Chapter 24

Figure 24-1A. Bhatnagar SC. *Neuroscience for the Study of Communicative Disorders.* 5th ed. Wolters Kluwer; 2008. (Figure 2-2)

Figure 24-1B. Kline-Fath B, Bulas D, Lee W. *Fundamental and Advanced Fetal Imaging* Ultrasound and MRI. 2nd ed. Wolters Kluwer; 2021. (Figure 3-03)

Figure 24-2B. Doubilet PM, Benson CB. *Atlas of Ultrasound in Obstetrics and Gynecology.* 3rd ed. Wolters Kluwer; 2018. (Figure 2.1.7)

Figure 24-3. From Doubilet PM, Benson CB. *Atlas of Ultrasound in Obstetrics and Gynecology.* 2nd ed. Wolters Kluwer; 2011. (Figure 2-1.1)

Figure 24-4. Hickey J. *Clinical Practice of Neurological & Neurosurgical Nursing.* 7th ed. Wolters Kluwer; 2013. (Figure 5-12)

Figure 24-5. Brant W. *The Core Curriculum: Ultrasound.* Lippincott Williams & Wilkins; 2001:253.

Figure 24-6. From Doubilet PM, Benson CB. *Atlas of Ultrasound in Obstetrics and Gynecology.* 2nd ed. Wolters Kluwer; 2011. (Figure 2-1.5)

Figure 24-7A. From Doubilet PM, Benson CB. *Atlas of Ultrasound in Obstetrics and Gynecology.* 2nd ed. Wolters Kluwer; 2011. (Figure 2-1.4)

Figure 24-7B. Kline-Fath B, Bulas D, Lee W. *Fundamental and Advanced Fetal Imaging* Ultrasound and MRI. 2nd ed. Wolters Kluwer; 2021. (Figure 3-43)

Figure 24-8. Cosby KS, Kendall, JL. *Practical Guide to Emergency Ultrasound.* 2nd ed. Wolters Kluwer; 2015. (Figure 16-09)

Figure 24-9. Doubilet PM, Benson CB. *Atlas of Ultrasound in Obstetrics and Gynecology.* 3rd ed. Wolters Kluwer; 2018. (Figure 18.1.1)

Figure 24-10. Mongan P. *Practical Approach to Neuroanesthesia.* Wolters Kluwer; 2014. (Figure 18-1)

Figure 24-11A. Kline-Fath B, Bahado-Singh R, Bulas D. *Fundamental and Advanced Fetal Imaging.* Wolters Kluwer; 2015. (Figure 20-07A)

Figure 24-11B. Provenzale JM. *Duke Radiology Case Review.* Wolters Kluwer; 2012. (Figure 9-4C)

Figure 24-12. Doubilet PM, Benson CB. *Atlas of Ultrasound in Obstetrics and Gynecology.* 2nd ed. Wolters Kluwer; 2011. (Figure 2.1.3)

Figure 24-13. Klein JS, Vinson EM, Brant WE, et al. *Brant and Helms' Fundamentals of Diagnostic Radiology.* 5th ed. Wolters Kluwer; 2018. (Figure 52-34)

Figure 24-14. From Doubilet PM, Benson CB. *Atlas of Ultrasound in Obstetrics and Gynecology: A Multimedia Reference.* Wolters Kluwer; 2003:38.

Figure 24-15. From Doubilet PM, Benson CB. *Atlas of Ultrasound in Obstetrics and Gynecology.* 2nd ed. Wolters Kluwer; 2011. (Figure 4-12.2)

Figure 24-16. Modified from McGahn JP, Ellis W, Lindfors KK, et al. Congenital cerebrospinal fluid-containing intracranial abnormalities: sonographic classification. *J Clin Ultrasound.* 1988;16:531–544.

Figure 24-17. From Doubilet PM, Benson CB. *Atlas of Ultrasound in Obstetrics and Gynecology.* 2nd ed. Wolters Kluwer; 2011. (Figure 14-1.1)

Figure 24-19. From Doubilet PM, Benson CB. *Atlas of Ultrasound in Obstetrics and Gynecology.* 2nd ed. Wolters Kluwer; 2011. (Figure 4-17.2C)

Figure 24-20. From Doubilet PM, Benson CB. *Atlas of Ultrasound in Obstetrics and Gynecology.* 2nd ed. Wolters Kluwer; 2011. (Figure 4-10.1)

Figure 24-21. From Doubilet PM, Benson CB. *Atlas of Ultrasound in Obstetrics and Gynecology.* 2nd ed. Wolters Kluwer; 2011. (Figure 4-11.2)

Figure 24-22. From Doubilet PM, Benson CB. *Atlas of Ultrasound in Obstetrics and Gynecology.* 2nd ed. Wolters Kluwer; 2011. (Figure 14-2.4)

Figure 24-23. From Doubilet PM, Benson CB. *Atlas of Ultrasound in Obstetrics and Gynecology: A Multimedia Reference.* Wolters Kluwer; 2003:43.

Figure 24-24B. Zugazaga Cortazar A, Martín Martinez C, Duran Feliubadalo C, et al. Magnetic resonance imaging in the prenatal diagnosis of neural tube defects. *Insights Imaging.* 2013;4:225–237. doi:10.1007/s13244-013-0223-2.

Figure 24-26. From Doubilet PM, Benson CB. *Atlas of Ultrasound in Obstetrics and Gynecology.* 2nd ed. Wolters Kluwer; 2011. (Figure 5-1.4)

Figure 24-27. Image courtesy of Philips Medical Systems, Bothell, WA.

Figure 24-28B. From Malinger G, Lev D, Zahalka N, et al. Fetal cytomegalovirus infection of the brain: the spectrum of sonographic findings. *AJNR Am J Neuroradiol.* 2003;24:28–32. (Figure 4)

Figure 24-29. Doubilet PM, Benson CB. *Atlas of Ultrasound in Obstetrics and Gynecology.* 3rd ed. Wolters Kluwer; 2018. (Figure 18.3.3)

Figure 24-30. Doubilet PM, Benson CB. *Atlas of Ultrasound in Obstetrics and Gynecology.* 3rd ed. Wolters Kluwer; 2018. (Figure 6.8.2)

Figure 24-31. Kline-Fath B, Bahado-Singh R, Bulas D. *Fundamental and Advanced Fetal Imaging.* Wolters Kluwer; 2015. (Figure 12.1-04)

Figure 24-32. Brant WE, Helms CA. *Fundamentals of Diagnostic Radiology.* 4th ed. Wolters Kluwer; 2012. (Figure 37-36)

Figure 24-33. Farrell TA. *Radiology 101*. 5th ed. Wolters Kluwer; 2020. (Figure 4-45)

Figure 24-34. Doubilet PM, Benson CB. *Atlas of Ultrasound in Obstetrics and Gynecology*. 3rd ed. Wolters Kluwer; 2018. (Figure 7.1.6B)

Figure 24-35. Doubilet PM, Benson CB. *Atlas of Ultrasound in Obstetrics and Gynecology*. 2nd ed. Wolters Kluwer; 2011. (Figure 4.6.1)

Figure 24-36. Doubilet PM, Benson CB. *Atlas of Ultrasound in Obstetrics and Gynecology*. 3rd ed. Wolters Kluwer; 2018. (Figure 6.14.4C)

Figure 24-37. Kline-Fath B, Bahado-Singh R, Bulas D. *Fundamental and Advanced Fetal Imaging*. Wolters Kluwer; 2015. (Figure 12.1-09A)

Figure 24-38. Abuhamad AZ, Chaoui, R. *First Trimester Ultrasound Diagnosis of Fetal Abnormalities*. Wolters Kluwer; 2017. (Figure 8-17)

Figure 24-39. Kline-Fath B, Bulas D, Lee W. *Fundamental and Advanced Fetal Imaging Ultrasound and MRI*. 2nd ed. Wolters Kluwer; 2021. (Figure 17.1-02)

Figure 24-40. Kline-Fath B, Bahado-Singh R, Bulas D. *Fundamental and Advanced Fetal Imaging*. Wolters Kluwer; 2015. (Figure 21-20A)

Figure 24-41. Stephenson SR. *Diagnostic Medical Sonography: Obstetrics & Gynecology*. 3rd ed. Wolters Kluwer; 2012. (Figure 16-5)

Figure 24-42. From Olinger AB. *Human Gross Anatomy*. Wolters Kluwer; 2015. (Figure 8-180A)

Figure 24-43. Abuhamad AZ, Chaoui, R. *First Trimester Ultrasound Diagnosis of Fetal Abnormalities*. Wolters Kluwer; 2017. (Figure 15-24)

Chapter 25

Figure 25-1. Kline-Fath B, Bahado-Singh R, Bulas D. *Fundamental and Advanced Fetal Imaging*. Wolters Kluwer; 2015. (Figure 13.2-07)

Figure 25-2. Doubilet PM, Benson CB. *Atlas of Ultrasound in Obstetrics and Gynecology*. 3rd ed. Wolters Kluwer; 2018. (Figure 8.5.2)

Figure 25-3. Nyberg D, McGaham J, Pretorius D, et al. *Diagnostic Imaging of Fetal Anomalies*. Wolters Kluwer; 2003. (Figure 8-07A,B)

Figure 25-4A. Nyberg D, McGaham J, Pretorius D, et al. *Diagnostic Imaging of Fetal Anomalies*. Wolters Kluwer; 2003. (Figure 8-11A)

Figure 25-4B. Nyberg D, McGaham J, Pretorius D, et al. *Diagnostic Imaging of Fetal Anomalies*. Wolters Kluwer; 2003. (Figure 8-10A)

Figure 25-5A. Doubilet PM, Benson CB. *Atlas of Ultrasound in Obstetrics and Gynecology*. 3rd ed. Wolters Kluwer; 2018. (Figure 2.2.5A)

Figure 25-5B. Doubilet PM, Benson CB. *Atlas of Ultrasound in Obstetrics and Gynecology*. 3rd ed. Wolters Kluwer; 2018. (Figure 8.8.4)

Figure 25-6. From Nyberg DA, Sickler GK, Hegge FN, et al. Fetal cleft lip with and without cleft palate: US classification and correlation with outcome. *Radiology*. 1995;195:677–683. (Figure 21-22)

Figure 25-7. From Doubilet PM, Benson CB. *Atlas of Ultrasound in Obstetrics and Gynecology*. 2nd ed. Wolters Kluwer; 2011. (Figure 6-1.1)

Figure 25-8. Doubilet PM, Benson CB. *Atlas of Ultrasound in Obstetrics and Gynecology*. 3rd ed. Wolters Kluwer; 2018. (Figure 8.1.3)

Figure 25-9. Doubilet PM, Benson CB. *Atlas of Ultrasound in Obstetrics and Gynecology*. 2nd ed. Wolters Kluwer; 2011. (Figure 6.2.1)

Figure 25-10. Doubilet PM, Benson CB. *Atlas of Ultrasound in Obstetrics and Gynecology*. 2nd ed. Wolters Kluwer; 2011. (Figure 6.3.1)

Figure 25-11. Abuhamad AZ, Chaoui, R. *First Trimester Ultrasound Diagnosis of Fetal Abnormalities*. Wolters Kluwer; 2017. (Figure 9-17)

Figure 25-13. From Doubilet PM, Benson CB. *Atlas of Ultrasound in Obstetrics and Gynecology*. 2nd ed. Wolters Kluwer; 2011. (Figure 7-2.1)

Figure 25-14. From Doubilet PM, Benson CB. *Atlas of Ultrasound in Obstetrics and Gynecology: A Multimedia Reference*. Wolters Kluwer; 2003:94.

Figure 25-15. MacDonald MG. *Avery's Neonatology*. 7th ed. Wolters Kluwer; 2015. (Figure 10-10)

Figure 25-16. Doubilet PM, Benson CB. *Atlas of Ultrasound in Obstetrics and Gynecology: A Multimedia Reference*. Wolters Kluwer; 2003. (Figure 7.3.5)

Figure 25-17. Kline-Fath B, Bahado-Singh R, Bulas D. *Fundamental and Advanced Fetal Imaging*. Wolters Kluwer; 2015. (Figure 20-28A)

Figure 25-18. Stephenson SR. *Diagnostic Medical Sonography: Obstetrics & Gynecology*. 4th ed. Wolters Kluwer; 2015. (Figure 31-15A)

Figure 25-19. Snell RS. The head and neck. In: *Clinical Anatomy by Regions*. Wolters Kluwer; 2011.

Figure 25-20. Abuhamad AZ, Chaoui, R. *First Trimester Ultrasound Diagnosis of Fetal Abnormalities*. Wolters Kluwer; 2017. (Figure 9-38)

Figure 25-21. Stephenson SR. *Diagnostic Medical Sonography: Obstetrics & Gynecology*. 4th ed. Wolters Kluwer; 2015. (Figure 21-14)

Figure 25-22. Kline-Fath B, Bulas D, Lee W. *Fundamental and Advanced Fetal Imaging Ultrasound and MRI*. 2nd ed. Wolters Kluwer; 2021. (Figure 19-07D)

Figure 25-23. Kline-Fath B, Bahado-Singh R, Bulas D. *Fundamental and Advanced Fetal Imaging*. Wolters Kluwer; 2015. (Figure 13.2-07C)

Figure 25-24. Kline-Fath B, Bahado-Singh R, Bulas D. *Fundamental and Advanced Fetal Imaging*. Wolters Kluwer; 2015. (Figure 13.2-07B)

Figure 25-25. Doubilet PM, Benson CB. *Atlas of Ultrasound in Obstetrics and Gynecology*. 3rd ed. Wolters Kluwer; 2018. (Figure 17.3.2A)

Figure 25-26. From Nyberg DA, Sickler GK, Hegge FN, et al. Fetal cleft lip with and without cleft palate: US classification and correlation with outcome. *Radiology*. 1995;195:677–683. (Figure 21-22E)

Figure 25-27. From Nyberg DA, Sickler GK, Hegge FN, et al. Fetal cleft lip with and without cleft palate: US classification and correlation with outcome. *Radiology*. 1995;195:677–683. (Figure 21-22C)

Figure 25-28A. Doubilet PM, Benson CB. *Atlas of Ultrasound in Obstetrics and Gynecology*. 3rd ed. Wolters Kluwer; 2018. (Figure 2.2.4B)

Figure 25-28B. Sanders RC, Hall-Terracciano B. *Clinical Sonography: A Practical Guide*. 5th ed. Wolters Kluwer; 2015. (Figure 2-19)

Figure 25-29. Doubilet PM, Benson CB. *Atlas of Ultrasound in Obstetrics and Gynecology*. 2nd ed. Wolters Kluwer; 2011. (Figure 6.5.1)

Figure 25-30. Stephenson SR. *Diagnostic Medical Sonography: Obstetrics & Gynecology*. 4th ed. Wolters Kluwer; 2015. (Figure 21-18)

Figure 25-31. Abuhamad AZ, Chaoui, R. *First Trimester Ultrasound Diagnosis of Fetal Abnormalities*. Wolters Kluwer; 2017. (Figure 9-15)

Chapter 26

Figure 26-1. From Doubilet PM, Benson CB. *Atlas of Ultrasound in Obstetrics and Gynecology*. 2nd ed. Wolters Kluwer; 2011. (Figure 2-3.1)

Figure 26-2A,B. From Doubilet PM, Benson CB. *Atlas of Ultrasound in Obstetrics and Gynecology*. 2nd ed. Wolters Kluwer; 2011. (Figure 2-3.2)

Figure 26-3. Doubilet PM, Benson CB. *Atlas of Ultrasound in Obstetrics and Gynecology*. 3rd ed. Wolters Kluwer; 2018. (Figure 2.3.4)

Figure 26-4. Nyberg D, McGaham J, Pretorius D, et al. *Diagnostic Imaging of Fetal Anomalies*. Wolters Kluwer; 2003. (Figure 7-17A-C)

Figure 26-5. Stephenson SR. *Diagnostic Medical Sonography: Obstetrics & Gynecology*. 3rd ed. Wolters Kluwer; 2012. (Figure 19-47A-D)

Figure 26-6. From Doubilet PM, Benson CB. *Atlas of Ultrasound in Obstetrics and Gynecology*. 2nd ed. Wolters Kluwer; 2011. (Figure 5-1.5)

Figure 26-7. Brant W. *The Core Curriculum: Ultrasound*. Lippincott Williams & Wilkins; 2001:253.

Figure 26-8A,B. Daffner RH, Hartman M. *Clinical Radiology*. 4th ed. Wolters Kluwer; 2013. (Figure 10-11B)

Figure 26-8C. Doubilet PM, Benson CB. *Atlas of Ultrasound in Obstetrics and Gynecology*. 3rd ed. Wolters Kluwer; 2018. (Figure 7.1.2C)

Figure 26-9A,B. From Doubilet PM, Benson CB. *Atlas of Ultrasound in Obstetrics and Gynecology*. 2nd ed. Wolters Kluwer; 2011. (Figure 5-1.1)

Figure 26-9C. Doubilet PM, Benson CB. *Atlas of Ultrasound in Obstetrics and Gynecology*. 3rd ed. Wolters Kluwer; 2018. (Figure 7.1.1B)

Figure 26-10. *Stedman's Medical Dictionary*. 28th ed. Courtesy of Neil O. Hardy, Westpoint, CT. Wolters Kluwer; 2005.

Figure 26-11. Doubilet PM, Benson CB. *Atlas of Ultrasound in Obstetrics and Gynecology*. 3rd ed. Wolters Kluwer; 2018. (Figure 7.3.1)

Figure 26-12. Stephenson SR. *Diagnostic Medical Sonography: Obstetrics & Gynecology*. 3rd ed. Wolters Kluwer; 2012. (Figure 18 35A)

Figure 26-13A. Frassica FJ. *5 Minute Orthopaedic Consult*. 2nd ed. Wolters Kluwer; 2006. (Achondroplasia Figure 1)

Figure 26-13B. Nyberg D, McGaham J, Pretorius D, et al. *Diagnostic Imaging of Fetal Anomalies*. Wolters Kluwer; 2003. (Figure 15-24A)

Figure 26-14. From Nyberg D, McGaham J, Pretorius D, et al. *Diagnostic Imaging of Fetal Anomalies*. Wolters Kluwer; 2003:682

Figure 26-15. Stephenson SR. *Diagnostic Medical Sonography: Obstetrics & Gynecology*. 4th ed. Wolters Kluwer; 2015. (Figure 27-12B)

Figure 26-16. Doubilet PM, Benson CB. *Atlas of Ultrasound in Obstetrics and Gynecology*. 3rd ed. Wolters Kluwer; 2018. (Figure 16.1.3)

Figure 26-17. Doubilet PM, Benson CB. *Atlas of Ultrasound in Obstetrics and Gynecology*. 2nd ed. Wolters Kluwer; 2011. (Figure 13.1.2A)

Figure 26-18. Doubilet PM, Benson CB. *Atlas of Ultrasound in Obstetrics and Gynecology*. 3rd ed. Wolters Kluwer; 2018. (Figure 16.1.2G)

Figure 26-19. From Doubilet P, Benson C. *Atlas of Ultrasound in Obstetrics and Gynecology.* Wolters Kluwer; 2003:167.

Figure 26-20. Doubilet PM, Benson CB. *Atlas of Ultrasound in Obstetrics and Gynecology.* 3rd ed. Wolters Kluwer; 2018. (Figure 16.1.1B)

Figure 26-21. From Doubilet PM, Benson CB. *Atlas of Ultrasound in Obstetrics and Gynecology.* 2nd ed. Wolters Kluwer; 2011. (Figure 5-4.2)

Figure 26-22. Doubilet PM, Benson CB. *Atlas of Ultrasound in Obstetrics and Gynecology.* 3rd ed. Wolters Kluwer; 2018. (Figure 7.5.2)

Figure 26-23. Stephenson SR. *Diagnostic Medical Sonography: Obstetrics Gynecology.* 4th ed. Wolters Kluwer; 2015. (Figure 22-14)

Figure 26-24A. Schaaf CP: Angeborene Fehlbildungssyndrome (Congenital malformation syndrome). In: Schaaf CP, Zschocke, eds. *Bassiswissen Humanogenetik (Basic Knowledge of Human Genetics).* Springer; 2018. (Figure 19-2)

Figure 26-24B. Doubilet PM, Benson CB. *Atlas of Ultrasound in Obstetrics and Gynecology.* 3rd ed. Wolters Kluwer; 2018. (Figure 17.6.1)

Figure 26-25A. Frassica FJ. *5-Minute Orthopaedic Consult.* 2nd ed. Wolters Kluwer; 2006. (Syndactyly Figure 1)

Figure 26-25B. Kline-Fath B, Bahado-Singh R, Bulas D. *Fundamental and Advanced Fetal Imaging.* Wolters Kluwer; 2015. (Figure 20-31B)

Figure 26-26. Image courtesy of Philips Medical Systems, Bothell, WA.

Figure 26-27. Doubilet PM, Benson CB. *Atlas of Ultrasound in Obstetrics and Gynecology.* 3rd ed. Wolters Kluwer; 2018. (Figure 16.7.2)

Figure 26-28. Stephenson SR. *Diagnostic Medical Sonography: Obstetrics & Gynecology.* 3rd ed. Wolters Kluwer; 2012. (Figure 18-24B)

Figure 26-29. Stephenson SR. *Diagnostic Medical Sonography: Obstetrics & Gynecology.* 4th ed. Wolters Kluwer; 2015. (Figure 20-23)

Figure 26-30. Courtesy of Dr. Jan Byrne, Department of Obstetrics and Gynecology, University of Utah Health Sciences Center.

Figure 26-31. Eisenberg RL. *An Atlas of Differential Diagnosis.* 4th ed. Wolters Kluwer; 2003. (Figure Sec 9, 1-4)

Figure 26-32. Abuhamad AZ, Chaoui, R. *First Trimester Ultrasound Diagnosis of Fetal Abnormalities.* Wolters Kluwer; 2017. (Figure 14-30B)

Figure 26-33. Doubilet PM, Benson CB. *Atlas of Ultrasound in Obstetrics and Gynecology.* 3rd ed. Wolters Kluwer; 2018. (Figure 7.3.2A)

Figure 26-34. Daffner RH, Hartman M. *Clinical Radiology.* 4th ed. Wolters Kluwer; 2013. (Figure 10-11A)

Figure 26-35. Doubilet PM, Benson CB. *Atlas of Ultrasound in Obstetrics and Gynecology: A Multimedia Reference.* Wolters Kluwer; 2003. (Figure 2.1.9)

Figure 26-36. Kline-Fath B, Bahado-Singh R, Bulas D. *Fundamental and Advanced Fetal Imaging.* Wolters Kluwer; 2015. (Figure 15.2-05C)

Figure 26-37. Kline-Fath B, Bulas D, Lee W. *Fundamental and Advanced Fetal Imaging Ultrasound and MRI.* 2nd ed. Wolters Kluwer; 2021. (Figure 29-13A)

Figure 26-38. Abuhamad AZ, Chaoui, R. *First Trimester Ultrasound Diagnosis of Fetal Abnormalities.* Wolters Kluwer; 2017. (Figure 14-15)

Figure 26-39. From Lee E. *Pediatric Radiology: Practical Imaging Evaluation of Infants and Children.* 1st ed. Wolters Kluwer; 2017. (Figure 21-8A)

Figure 26-40. Stephenson SR. *Diagnostic Medical Sonography: Obstetrics & Gynecology.* 3rd ed. Wolters Kluwer; 2012. (Figure 23-26)

Chapter 27

Figure 27-1A. Abuhamad A. *A Practical Guide to Fetal Echocardiography.* 4th ed. Wolters Kluwer; 2022. (Figure 5-02)

Figure 27-1B. Nyberg D, McGaham J, Pretorius D, et al. *Diagnostic Imaging of Fetal Anomalies.* Wolters Kluwer; 2003. (Figure 10-01)

Figure 27-2. Abuhamad A. *A Practical Guide to Fetal Echocardiography.* 3rd ed. Wolters Kluwer; 2015. (Figure 7-03A)

Figure 27-3A. Abuhamad A. *A Practical Guide to Fetal Echocardiography.* 4th ed. Wolters Kluwer; 2022. (Figure 7-06)

Figure 27-3B. Abuhamad A. *A Practical Guide to Fetal Echocardiography.* 4th ed. Wolters Kluwer; 2022. (Figure 11-06)

Figure 27-4. MacDonald MG. *Avery's Neonatology.* 7th ed. Wolters Kluwer; 2015. (Figure 12-11)

Figure 27-5. Nyberg D, McGaham J, Pretorius D, et al. *Diagnostic Imaging of Fetal Anomalies.* Wolters Kluwer; 2003. (Figure 10-04D)

Figure 27-7. Kline-Fath B, Bahado-Singh R, Bulas D. *Fundamental and Advanced Fetal Imaging.* Wolters Kluwer; 2015. (Figure 1-076A,B)

Figure 27-8. Abuhamad A. *A Practical Guide to Fetal Echocardiography.* 4th ed. Wolters Kluwer; 2022. (Figure 11-21)

Figure 27-9. American Institute of Ultrasound in Medicine. AIUM practice guideline for the performance of fetal echocardiography.

J Ultrasound Med. 2013;32(6):1067–1082. Copyright © 2016 by the American Institute of Ultrasound in Medicine. Reprinted by permission of John Wiley & Sons, Inc.

Figure 27-10. Kline-Fath B, Bulas D, Lee W. *Fundamental and Advanced Fetal Imaging Ultrasound and MRI.* 2nd ed. Wolters Kluwer; 2021. (Figure 7-33)

Figure 27-11. Abuhamad A. *A Practical Guide to Fetal Echocardiography.* 4th ed. Wolters Kluwer; 2022. (Figure 5-05)

Figure 27-12. McConnell T, Hull K. *Human Form, Human Function.* Wolters Kluwer; 2011.

Figure 27-13. From Doubilet PM, Benson CB. *Atlas of Ultrasound in Obstetrics and Gynecology.* 2nd ed. Wolters Kluwer; 2011. (Figure 2-5.6)

Figure 27-14. Abuhamad A. *A Practical Guide to Fetal Echocardiography.* 4th ed. Wolters Kluwer; 2022. (Figure 32-05)

Figure 27-15A. Shaffner DH. *Rogers' Textbook of Pediatric Intensive Care.* 5th ed. Wolters Kluwer; 2016. (Figure 68-18A)

Figure 27-15B. Doubilet PM, Benson CB. *Atlas of Ultrasound in Obstetrics and Gynecology.* 2nd ed. Wolters Kluwer; 2011. (Figure 2.5.6)

Figure 27-16. Abuhamad A. *A Practical Guide to Fetal Echocardiography.* 4th ed. Wolters Kluwer; 2022. (Figure 20-06)

Figure 27-17. Abuhamad A. *A Practical Guide to Fetal Echocardiography.* 4th ed. Wolters Kluwer; 2022. (Figure 19-05)

Figure 27-18A. Abuhamad AZ, Chaoui, R. *First Trimester Ultrasound Diagnosis of Fetal Abnormalities.* Wolters Kluwer; 2017. (Figure 11-26)

Figure 27-18B. Abuhamad A. *A Practical Guide to Fetal Echocardiography.* 3rd ed. Wolters Kluwer; 2015. (Figure 20-10)

Figure 27-19. Abuhamad A. *A Practical Guide to Fetal Echocardiography.* 4th ed. Wolters Kluwer; 2022. (Figure 33-03)

Figure 27-20. Abuhamad A. *A Practical Guide to Fetal Echocardiography.* 4th ed. Wolters Kluwer; 2022. (Figure 33-08)

Figure 27-21. Rosdahl CB, Kowalski MT. *Textbook of Basic Nursing.* 12th ed. Wolters Kluwer; 2021. (Figure 72-10E)

Figure 27-22. Doubilet PM, Benson CB. *Atlas of Ultrasound in Obstetrics and Gynecology.* 2nd ed. Wolters Kluwer; 2011. (Figure 9.7.1)

Figure 27-23. Abuhamad A. *A Practical Guide to Fetal Echocardiography.* 3rd ed. Wolters Kluwer; 2015. (Figure 28-01)

Figure 27-24. Abuhamad A. *A Practical Guide to Fetal Echocardiography.* 4th ed. Wolters Kluwer; 2022. (Figure 37-19)

Figure 27-25. Abuhamad A. *A Practical Guide to Fetal Echocardiography.* 3rd ed. Wolters Kluwer; 2015. (Figure 18-16)

Figure 27-26. Doubilet PM, Benson CB. *Atlas of Ultrasound in Obstetrics and Gynecology.* 3rd ed. Wolters Kluwer; 2018. (Figure 11.11.2)

Figure 27-27. From Doubilet PM, Benson CB. *Atlas of Ultrasound in Obstetrics and Gynecology.* 2nd ed. Wolters Kluwer; 2011. (Figure 9-14.3)

Figure 27-28. From Doubilet PM, Benson CB. *Atlas of Ultrasound in Obstetrics and Gynecology: A Multimedia Reference.* Wolters Kluwer; 2003:121.

Figure 27-29. From Doubilet PM, Benson CB. *Atlas of Ultrasound in Obstetrics and Gynecology: A Multimedia Reference.* Wolters Kluwer; 2003:199.

Figure 27-30. From Doubilet PM, Benson CB. *Atlas of Ultrasound in Obstetrics and Gynecology: A Multimedia Reference.* Wolters Kluwer; 2003:84.

Figure 27-31. Abuhamad AZ, Chaoui, R. *First Trimester Ultrasound Diagnosis of Fetal Abnormalities.* Wolters Kluwer; 2017. (Figure 10-18)

Figure 27-32. Doubilet PM, Benson CB. *Atlas of Ultrasound in Obstetrics and Gynecology.* 3rd ed. Wolters Kluwer; 2018. (Figure 11.8.2B)

Figure 27-33. Doubilet PM, Benson CB. *Atlas of Ultrasound in Obstetrics and Gynecology.* 3rd ed. Wolters Kluwer; 2018. (Figure 11.10.1B)

Figure 27-34. Abuhamad A. *A Practical Guide to Fetal Echocardiography.* 3rd ed. Wolters Kluwer; 2015. (Figure 32-01B)

Figure 27-35. Kline-Fath B, Bulas D, Lee W. *Fundamental and Advanced Fetal Imaging Ultrasound and MRI.* 2nd ed. Wolters Kluwer; 2021. (Figure 31-09)

Figure 27-36. Abuhamad A. *A Practical Guide to Fetal Echocardiography.* 4th ed. Wolters Kluwer; 2022. (Figure 7-19)

Figure 27-37. Doubilet PM, Benson CB. *Atlas of Ultrasound in Obstetrics and Gynecology.* 2nd ed. Wolters Kluwer; 2011. (Figure 9.11.1)

Figure 27-38. Abuhamad A. *A Practical Guide to Fetal Echocardiography.* 3rd ed. Wolters Kluwer; 2015. (Figure 6-08)

Figure 27-39. Kyle. *Essentials of Pediatric Nursing.* 2nd ed. Wolters Kluwer; 2020. (Figure 19-2)

Figure 27-40. Reece EA. *Diabetes and Obesity in Women.* 4th ed. Wolters Kluwer; 2019. (Figure 25-7)

Figure 27-41. Abuhamad A. *A Practical Guide to Fetal Echocardiography.* 3rd ed. Wolters Kluwer; 2015. (Figure 18-10)

Figure 27-42. Doubilet PM, Benson CB. *Atlas of Ultrasound in Obstetrics and Gynecology.* 3rd ed. Wolters Kluwer; 2018. (Figure 11.3.2)

Figure 27-43. Abuhamad A. *A Practical Guide to Fetal Echocardiography.* 4th ed. Wolters Kluwer; 2022. (Figure 13-15)

Figure 27-44. Abuhamad A. *A Practical Guide to Fetal Echocardiography.* 4th ed. Wolters Kluwer; 2022. (Figure 7-10)

Figure 27-45. Doubilet PM, Benson CB. *Atlas of Ultrasound in Obstetrics and Gynecology.* 3rd ed. Wolters Kluwer; 2018. (Figure 26.2.1)

Chapter 28

Figure 28-1. Doubilet PM, Benson CB. *Atlas of Ultrasound in Obstetrics and Gynecology.* 3rd ed. Wolters Kluwer; 2018. (Figure 18.1.2)

Figure 28-2A. LifeART, ©2022, Wolters Kluwer.

Figure 28-2B. From Stephenson SR. *Diagnostic Medical Sonography: Obstetrics & Gynecology.* 3rd ed. Wolters Kluwer; 2012. (Figure 21-23)

Figure 28-3. Mulholland MW, Lillemoe KD, Doherty GM, Maier RV, Upchurch GR, eds. *Greenfield's Surgery.* 4th ed. Wolters Kluwer; 2005. (Figure 110-11)

Figure 28-4. From Doubilet PM, Benson CB. *Atlas of Ultrasound in Obstetrics and Gynecology.* 2nd ed. Wolters Kluwer; 2011. (Figure 10-2.2)

Figure 28-5. From Doubilet PM, Benson CB. *Atlas of Ultrasound in Obstetrics and Gynecology: A Multimedia Reference.* Wolters Kluwer; 2003:133.

Figure 28-6A. Kline-Fath B, Bahado-Singh R, Bulas D. *Fundamental and Advanced Fetal Imaging.* Wolters Kluwer; 2015. (Figure 18.1-02)

Figure 28-6B. Kline-Fath B, Bahado-Singh R, Bulas D. *Fundamental and Advanced Fetal Imaging.* Wolters Kluwer; 2015. (Figure 20-03B)

Figure 28-7. Nyberg D, McGaham J, Pretorius D, et al. *Diagnostic Imaging of Fetal Anomalies.* Wolters Kluwer; 2003. (Figure 12-06B)

Figure 28-8. Doubilet PM, Benson CB. *Atlas of Ultrasound in Obstetrics and Gynecology.* 3rd ed. Wolters Kluwer; 2018. (Figure 13.2.1)

Figure 28-9. Nyberg D, McGaham J, Pretorius D, et al. *Diagnostic Imaging of Fetal Anomalies.* Wolters Kluwer; 2003. (Figure 12-13B)

Figure 28-10. Doubilet PM, Benson CB. *Atlas of Ultrasound in Obstetrics and Gynecology.* 3rd ed. Wolters Kluwer; 2018. (Figure 13.1.2)

Figure 28-11. Doubilet PM, Benson CB. *Atlas of Ultrasound in Obstetrics and Gynecology.* 3rd ed. Wolters Kluwer; 2018. (Figure 11.13.2)

Figure 28-12. Abuhamad AZ, Chaoui, R. *First Trimester Ultrasound Diagnosis of Fetal Abnormalities.* Wolters Kluwer; 2017. (Figure 12-20A)

Figure 28-13. Abuhamad AZ, Chaoui, R. *First Trimester Ultrasound Diagnosis of Fetal Abnormalities.* Wolters Kluwer; 2017. (Figure 12-13)

Figure 28-14. Kline-Fath B, Bahado-Singh R, Bulas D. *Fundamental and Advanced Fetal Imaging.* Wolters Kluwer; 2015. (Figure 20-38D)

Figure 28-15. Doubilet PM, Benson CB. *Atlas of Ultrasound in Obstetrics and Gynecology.* 3rd ed. Wolters Kluwer; 2018. (Figure 12.2.2A)

Figure 28-16. Doubilet PM, Benson CB. *Atlas of Ultrasound in Obstetrics and Gynecology.* 2nd ed. Wolters Kluwer; 2011. (Figure 14.3.1)

Figure 28-17. Doubilet PM, Benson CB. *Atlas of Ultrasound in Obstetrics and Gynecology.* 2nd ed. Wolters Kluwer; 2011. (Figure 10.5.1A)

Figure 28-18. Doubilet PM, Benson CB. *Atlas of Ultrasound in Obstetrics and Gynecology.* 3rd ed. Wolters Kluwer; 2018. (Figure 2.6.8B)

Figure 28-19. Doubilet PM, Benson CB. *Atlas of Ultrasound in Obstetrics and Gynecology.* 2nd ed. Wolters Kluwer; 2011. (Figure 1.3.5C)

Figure 28-20. Doubilet PM, Benson CB. *Atlas of Ultrasound in Obstetrics and Gynecology.* 2nd ed. Wolters Kluwer; 2011. (Figure 9.13.2)

Figure 28-21. Kline-Fath B, Bulas D, Lee W. *Fundamental and Advanced Fetal Imaging Ultrasound and MRI.* 2nd ed. Wolters Kluwer; 2021. (Figure 28.2-19)

Figure 28-22. Abuhamad AZ, Chaoui, R. *First Trimester Ultrasound Diagnosis of Fetal Abnormalities.* Wolters Kluwer; 2017. (Figure 12-18)

Figure 28-23. Abuhamad A. *A Practical Guide to Fetal Echocardiography.* 4th ed. Wolters Kluwer; 2022. (Figure 40-01)

Chapter 29

Figure 29-1. Nyberg D, McGaham J, Pretorius D, et al. *Diagnostic Imaging of Fetal Anomalies.* Wolters Kluwer; 2003. (Figure 14-2)

Figure 29-2. From Doubilet PM, Benson CB. *Atlas of Ultrasound in Obstetrics and Gynecology.* 2nd ed. Wolters Kluwer; 2011. (Figure 2-6.7)

Figure 29-3. From Doubilet PM, Benson CB. *Atlas of Ultrasound in Obstetrics and Gynecology.* 2nd ed. Wolters Kluwer; 2011. (Figure 2-6.9)

Figure 29-4. Nyberg D, McGaham J, Pretorius D, et al. *Diagnostic Imaging of Fetal Anomalies.* Wolters Kluwer; 2003. (Figure 1-37A)

Figure 29-5. Nyberg D, McGaham J, Pretorius D, et al. *Diagnostic Imaging of Fetal Anomalies.* Wolters Kluwer; 2003. (Figure 5-30)

Figure 29-6. Strayer DS. *Rubin's Pathology.* 7th ed. Wolters Kluwer; 2015. (Figure 6-3)

Figure 29-7. Abuhamad AZ, Chaoui, R. *First Trimester Ultrasound Diagnosis of Fetal Abnormalities.* Wolters Kluwer; 2017. (Figure 13-35)

Figure 29-8. Doubilet PM, Benson CB. *Atlas of Ultrasound in Obstetrics and Gynecology.* 3rd ed. Wolters Kluwer; 2018. (Figure 14.1.2C)

Figure 29-10. McConnell TH. *Nature of Disease.* Wolters Kluwer; 2007. (Figure 7-6)

Figure 29-11. From Doubilet PM, Benson CB. *Atlas of Ultrasound in Obstetrics and Gynecology: A Multimedia Reference.* Wolters Kluwer; 2003:156.

Figure 29-12. Abuhamad AZ, Chaoui, R. *First Trimester Ultrasound Diagnosis of Fetal Abnormalities.* Wolters Kluwer; 2017. (Figure 13-31)

Figure 29-13A. MacDonald MG. *Avery's Neonatology.* 7th ed. Wolters Kluwer; 2015. (Figure 40-9A)

Figure 29-13B. Kline-Fath B, Bahado-Singh R, Bulas D. *Fundamental and Advanced Fetal Imaging.* Wolters Kluwer; 2015. (Figure 19.1-20)

Figure 29-14. From Doubilet PM, Benson CB. *Atlas of Ultrasound in Obstetrics and Gynecology: A Multimedia Reference.* Wolters Kluwer; 2003:148.

Figure 29-15. Stephenson SR. *Diagnostic Medical Sonography: Obstetrics & Gynecology.* 4th ed. Wolters Kluwer; 2015. (Figure 26-25)

Figure 29-16. From Doubilet PM, Benson CB. *Atlas of Ultrasound in Obstetrics and Gynecology: A Multimedia Reference.* Wolters Kluwer; 2003:151.

Figure 29-17. From Doubilet PM, Benson CB. *Atlas of Ultrasound in Obstetrics and Gynecology.* 2nd ed. Wolters Kluwer; 2011. (Figure 12-6.1)

Figure 29-18. From Doubilet PM, Benson CB. *Atlas of Ultrasound in Obstetrics and Gynecology.* 2nd ed. Wolters Kluwer; 2011. (Figure 12-3.2)

Figure 29-19. Kline-Fath B, Bulas D, Lee W. *Fundamental and Advanced Fetal Imaging Ultrasound and MRI.* 2nd ed. Wolters Kluwer; 2021. (Figure 3-118)

Figure 29-20. Kline-Fath B, Bahado-Singh R, Bulas D. *Fundamental and Advanced Fetal Imaging.* Wolters Kluwer; 2015. (Figure 18.3-01A)

Figure 29-21. Doubilet PM, Benson CB. *Atlas of Ultrasound in Obstetrics and Gynecology.* 2nd ed. Wolters Kluwer; 2011. (Figure 12.7.4A)

Figure 29-22. Stephenson SR. *Diagnostic Medical Sonography: Obstetrics & Gynecology.* 4th ed. Wolters Kluwer; 2015. (Figure 26-23)

Figure 29-23. Sanders RC, Hall-Terracciano B. *Clinical Sonography: A Practical Guide.* 5th ed. Wolters Kluwer; 2015. (Figure 27-72)

Figure 29-24. Stephenson SR. *Diagnostic Medical Sonography: Obstetrics & Gynecology.* 4th ed. Wolters Kluwer; 2015. (Figure 26-27)

Figure 29-25. Abuhamad AZ, Chaoui, R. *First Trimester Ultrasound Diagnosis of Fetal Abnormalities.* Wolters Kluwer; 2017. (Figure 13-17D)

Figure 29-26. Kline-Fath B, Bahado-Singh R, Bulas D. *Fundamental and Advanced Fetal Imaging.* Wolters Kluwer; 2015. (Figure 20-03D)

Figure 29-27. MacDonald MG. *Avery's Neonatology.* 7th ed. Wolters Kluwer; 2015. (Figure 40-14A)

Figure 29-28. Abuhamad AZ, Chaoui, R. *First Trimester Ultrasound Diagnosis of Fetal Abnormalities.* Wolters Kluwer; 2017. (Figure 8-21)

Figure 29-29. Stephenson SR. *Diagnostic Medical Sonography: Obstetrics & Gynecology.* 3rd ed. Wolters Kluwer; 2012. (Figure 21-32)

Figure 29-30. Stephenson SR. *Diagnostic Medical Sonography: Obstetrics & Gynecology.* 4th ed. Wolters Kluwer; 2015. (Figure 26-09D)

Figure 29-31. Doubilet PM, Benson CB. *Atlas of Ultrasound in Obstetrics and Gynecology.* 3rd ed. Wolters Kluwer; 2018. (Figure 14.15.5A)

Figure 29-32. Doubilet PM, Benson CB. *Atlas of Ultrasound in Obstetrics and Gynecology.* 3rd ed. Wolters Kluwer; 2018. (Figure 26.3.1)

Figure 29-33. Graham SD. *Glenn's Urologic Surgery.* 8th ed. Wolters Kluwer; 2016. (Figure 95.1)

Figure 29-34. Abuhamad AZ, Chaoui, R. *First Trimester Ultrasound Diagnosis of Fetal Abnormalities.* Wolters Kluwer; 2017. (Figure 14-39)

Figure 29-35. Stephenson SR. *Diagnostic Medical Sonography: Obstetrics & Gynecology.* 4th ed. Wolters Kluwer; 2015. (Figure 26-04)

Chapter 30

Figure 30-2. From Doubilet PM, Benson CB. *Atlas of Ultrasound in Obstetrics and Gynecology.* 2nd ed. Wolters Kluwer; 2011. (Figure 22-2.1)

Figure 30-3A. Stephenson SR. *Diagnostic Medical Sonography: Obstetrics & Gynecology.* 4th ed. Wolters Kluwer; 2015. (Figure 34-03)

Figure 30-3B. Doubilet PM, Benson CB. *Atlas of Ultrasound in Obstetrics and Gynecology.* 2nd ed. Wolters Kluwer; 2011. (Figure 22.1.2)

Figure 30-4A. Pillitteri A. *Maternal and Child Health Nursing.* 7th ed. Wolters Kluwer; 2014. (Figure 7-13)

Figure 30-4B. Doubilet PM, Benson CB. *Atlas of Ultrasound in Obstetrics and Gynecology.* 3rd ed. Wolters Kluwer; 2018. (Figure 25.3.3)

Figure 30-5. Stephenson SR. *Diagnostic Medical Sonography: Obstetrics & Gynecology.* 4th ed. Wolters Kluwer; 2015. (Figure 31-30)

Figure 30-6A. Frassica FJ. *5-Minute Orthopaedic Consult.* 2nd ed. Wolters Kluwer; 2006. (Clinodactyly Figure 1)

Figure 30-6B. Scott JR. *Danforth's Obstetrics and Gynecology.* 8th ed. Wolters Kluwer; 1999:192.

Figure 30-7. Doubilet PM, Benson CB. *Atlas of Ultrasound in Obstetrics and Gynecology.* 3rd ed. Wolters Kluwer; 2018. (Figure 17.3.1)

Figure 30-10. Stephenson SR. *Diagnostic Medical Sonography: Obstetrics & Gynecology.* 4th ed. Wolters Kluwer; 2015. (Figure 31-27A)

Figure 30-11. Doubilet PM, Benson CB. *Atlas of Ultrasound in Obstetrics and Gynecology.* 3rd ed. Wolters Kluwer; 2018. (Figure 17.2.3)

Figure 30-13. Doubilet PM, Benson CB. *Atlas of Ultrasound in Obstetrics and Gynecology.* 3rd ed. Wolters Kluwer; 2018. (Figure 8.3.1)

Figure 30-14. Doubilet PM, Benson CB. *Atlas of Ultrasound in Obstetrics and Gynecology.* 3rd ed. Wolters Kluwer; 2018. (Figure 22.1.2)

Figure 30-15. Kline-Fath B, Bahado-Singh R, Bulas D. *Fundamental and Advanced Fetal Imaging.* Wolters Kluwer; 2015. (Figure 20-07G)

Figure 30-16. Stephenson SR. *Diagnostic Medical Sonography: Obstetrics & Gynecology.* 4th ed. Wolters Kluwer; 2015. (Figure 31-25A)

Figure 30-17. Doubilet PM, Benson CB. *Atlas of Ultrasound in Obstetrics and Gynecology.* 3rd ed. Wolters Kluwer; 2018. (Figure 16.5.2)

Figure 30-18. Abuhamad AZ, Chaoui, R. *First Trimester Ultrasound Diagnosis of Fetal Abnormalities.* Wolters Kluwer; 2017. (Figure 13-29)

Figure 30-19. Kline-Fath B, Bahado-Singh R, Bulas D. *Fundamental and Advanced Fetal Imaging.* Wolters Kluwer; 2015. (Figure 20-11)

Figure 30-20. Stephenson SR. *Diagnostic Medical Sonography: Obstetrics & Gynecology.* 4th ed. Wolters Kluwer; 2015. (Figure 31-18)

Figure 30-23. Brant WE, Helms CA. *Brant and Helms Solution.* Wolters Kluwer; 2006. (Figure 38-29)

Figure 30-24. Doubilet PM, Benson CB. *Atlas of Ultrasound in Obstetrics and Gynecology.* 3rd ed. Wolters Kluwer; 2018. (Figure 9.2.5A)

Figure 30-26. Doubilet PM, Benson CB. *Atlas of Ultrasound in Obstetrics and Gynecology.* 3rd ed. Wolters Kluwer; 2018. (Figure 16.6.1C)

Figure 30-27. Kline-Fath B, Bahado-Singh R, Bulas D. *Fundamental and Advanced Fetal Imaging.* Wolters Kluwer; 2015. (Figure 20-04B)

Figure 30-28. Abuhamad AZ, Chaoui, R. *First Trimester Ultrasound Diagnosis of Fetal Abnormalities.* Wolters Kluwer; 2017. (Figure 12-40R)

Figure 30-29. Doubilet PM, Benson CB. *Atlas of Ultrasound in Obstetrics and Gynecology.* 2nd ed. Wolters Kluwer; 2011. (Figure 19.1.2)

Figure 30-30. Abuhamad A. *A Practical Guide to Fetal Echocardiography.* 4th ed. Wolters Kluwer; 2022. (Figure 2-04)

Figure 30-31. Abuhamad A. *A Practical Guide to Fetal Echocardiography.* 4th ed. Wolters Kluwer; 2022. (Figure 2-02)

Figure 30-32. Kline-Fath B, Bulas D, Lee W. *Fundamental and Advanced Fetal Imaging Ultrasound and MRI.* 2nd ed. Wolters Kluwer; 2021. (Figure 30-07A-F)

Chapter 31

Figure 31-1. Stephenson SR. *Diagnostic Medical Sonography: Obstetrics & Gynecology.* 4th ed. Wolters Kluwer; 2015. (Figure 29-01)

Figure 31-2. Snyder R. *Step-Up to Obstetrics and Gynecology.* Wolters Kluwer; 2015. (Figure 19-1). (Based on American College of Obstetricians and Gynecologists. *Having Twins. Patient Education Pamphlet AP092.* Washington, DC: American College of Obstetricians and Gynecologists; 2004.)

Figure 31-3. Doubilet PM, Benson CB. *Atlas of Ultrasound in Obstetrics and Gynecology.* 3rd ed. Wolters Kluwer; 2018. (Figure 23.1.1)

Figure 31-5. Doubilet PM, Benson CB. *Atlas of Ultrasound in Obstetrics and Gynecology.* 3rd ed. Wolters Kluwer; 2018. (Figure 23.2.2)

Figure 31-7. Kline-Fath B, Bahado-Singh R, Bulas D. *Fundamental and Advanced Fetal Imaging.* Wolters Kluwer; 2015. (Figure 11-06)

Figure 31-9. Nyberg D, McGaham J, Pretorius D, et al. *Diagnostic Imaging of Fetal Anomalies.* Wolters Kluwer; 2003. (Figure 18-08)

Figure 31-11. Suresh M. *Shnider and Levinson's Anesthesia for Obstetrics.* 5th ed. Wolters Kluwer; 2013. (Figure 49-1)

Figure 31-12A. Doubilet PM, Benson CB. *Atlas of Ultrasound in Obstetrics and Gynecology.* 3rd ed. Wolters Kluwer; 2018. (Figure 24.1.1)

Figure 31-12B. Doubilet PM, Benson CB. *Atlas of Ultrasound in Obstetrics and Gynecology.* 3rd ed. Wolters Kluwer; 2018. (Figure 24.1.3)

Figure 31-13. Doubilet PM, Benson CB. *Atlas of Ultrasound in Obstetrics and Gynecology.* 3rd ed. Wolters Kluwer; 2018. (Figure 24.1.2)

Figure 31-14. Abuhamad AZ, Chaoui, R. *First Trimester Ultrasound Diagnosis of Fetal Abnormalities.* Wolters Kluwer; 2017. (Figure 7-13)

Figure 31-15. Doubilet PM, Benson CB. *Atlas of Ultrasound in Obstetrics and Gynecology.* 3rd ed. Wolters Kluwer; 2018. (Figure 24.2.3)

Figure 31-16. Kline-Fath B, Bahado-Singh R, Bulas D. *Fundamental and Advanced Fetal Imaging.* Wolters Kluwer; 2015. (Figure 11-39)

Figure 31-17. Doubilet PM, Benson CB. *Atlas of Ultrasound in Obstetrics and Gynecology.* 3rd ed. Wolters Kluwer; 2018. (Figure 24.4.3)

Figure 31-18. Doubilet PM, Benson CB. *Atlas of Ultrasound in Obstetrics and Gynecology.* 3rd ed. Wolters Kluwer; 2018. (Figure 24.5.1)

Figure 31-20. Image courtesy of Philips Healthcare, Bothell, WA. (Figure 29-19)

Figure 31-22. Sanders RC, Hall-Terracciano B. *Clinical Sonography: A Practical Guide.* 5th ed. Wolters Kluwer; 2015. (Figure 26-01)

Figure 31-23. Kline-Fath B, Bahado-Singh R, Bulas D. *Fundamental and Advanced Fetal Imaging.* Wolters Kluwer; 2015. (Figure 11-07)

Figure 31-24. Kline-Fath B, Bahado-Singh R, Bulas D. *Fundamental and Advanced Fetal Imaging.* Wolters Kluwer; 2015. (Figure 11-19A)

Figure 31-25. Kline-Fath B, Bahado-Singh R, Bulas D. *Fundamental and Advanced Fetal Imaging.* Wolters Kluwer; 2015. (Figure 11-05)

Figure 31-26. Stephenson SR. *Diagnostic Medical Sonography: Obstetrics & Gynecology.* 4th ed. Wolters Kluwer; 2015. (Figure 29-03)

Figure 31-27. Stephenson SR. *Diagnostic Medical Sonography: Obstetrics & Gynecology.* 3rd ed. Wolters Kluwer; 2012. (Figure 26-21A)

Figure 31-28. Kline-Fath B, Bahado-Singh R, Bulas D. *Fundamental and Advanced Fetal Imaging.* Wolters Kluwer; 2015. (Figure 11-17A)

Figure 31-29. Kline-Fath B, Bulas D, Lee W. *Fundamental and Advanced Fetal Imaging Ultrasound and MRI.* 2nd ed. Wolters Kluwer; 2021. (Figure 15-31)

Figure 31-30. Doubilet PM, Benson CB. *Atlas of Ultrasound in Obstetrics and Gynecology.* 2nd ed. Wolters Kluwer; 2011. (Figure 21.1.3)

Figure 31-31. Kline-Fath B, Bulas D, Lee W. *Fundamental and Advanced Fetal Imaging Ultrasound and MRI.* 2nd ed. Wolters Kluwer; 2021. (Figure 15-26)

Figure 31-32. Evans AT. *Manual of Obstetric.* 8th ed. Wolters Kluwer; 2015. (Figure 34-1A)

Figure 31-33. Doubilet PM, Benson CB. *Atlas of Ultrasound in Obstetrics and Gynecology.* 3rd ed. Wolters Kluwer; 2018. (Figure 24.4.2)

Figure 31-34. Kline-Fath B, Bahado-Singh R, Bulas D. *Fundamental and Advanced Fetal Imaging.* Wolters Kluwer; 2015. (Figure 11-37A)

Figure 31-35. Stephenson SR. *Diagnostic Medical Sonography: Obstetrics & Gynecology.* 4th ed. Wolters Kluwer; 2015. (Figure 29-04)

Chapter 32

Figure 32-1. Doubilet PM, Benson CB. *Atlas of Ultrasound in Obstetrics and Gynecology.* 2nd ed. Wolters Kluwer; 2011. (Figure 3.3.1)

Figure 32-2. Sadler TW. *Langman's Medical Embryology.* 9th ed. Wolters Kluwer; 2003. (Figure 7-8)

Figure 32-3. Image courtesy of Philips Medical Systems, Bothell, WA.

Figure 32-4. Stephenson SR. *Diagnostic Medical Sonography: Obstetrics & Gynecology.* 4th ed. Wolters Kluwer; 2015. (Figure 20-08)

Figure 32-5. Stephenson SR. *Diagnostic Medical Sonography: Obstetrics & Gynecology.* 4th ed. Wolters Kluwer; 2015. (Figure 19-08)

Figure 32-6. Stephenson SR. *Diagnostic Medical Sonography: Obstetrics & Gynecology.* 4th ed. Wolters Kluwer; 2015. (Figure 20-03)

Figure 32-7. Stephenson SR. *Diagnostic Medical Sonography: Obstetrics & Gynecology.* 3rd ed. Wolters Kluwer; 2012. (Figure 18-09)

Figure 32-8. Stephenson SR. *Diagnostic Medical Sonography: Obstetrics & Gynecology.* 3rd ed. Wolters Kluwer; 2012. (Figure 18-10)

Figure 32-9A,B. Stephenson SR. *Diagnostic Medical Sonography: Obstetrics & Gynecology.* 4th ed. Wolters Kluwer; 2015. (Figure 20-41)

Figure 32-9C. Doubilet PM, Benson CB. *Atlas of Ultrasound in Obstetrics and Gynecology.* 2nd ed. Wolters Kluwer; 2011. (Figure 19.2.3)

Figure 32-11. Stephenson SR. *Diagnostic Medical Sonography: Obstetrics & Gynecology.* 3rd ed. Wolters Kluwer; 2012. (Figure 18-21)

Figure 32-12. Stephenson SR. *Diagnostic Medical Sonography: Obstetrics & Gynecology.* 3rd ed. Wolters Kluwer; 2012. (Figure 18-12)

Figure 32-13. Reece EA. *Clinical Obstetrics.* 4th ed. Wolters Kluwer; 2022. (Figure 19-24)

Figure 32-14. Stephenson SR. *Diagnostic Medical Sonography: Obstetrics & Gynecology.* 4th ed. Wolters Kluwer; 2015. (Figure 20-18)

Figure 32-15. Klein JS, Vinson EM, Brant WE, et al. *Brant and Helms' Fundamentals of Diagnostic Radiology.* 5th ed. Wolters Kluwer; 2018. (Figure 52-30)

Figure 32-16. Stephenson SR. *Diagnostic Medical Sonography: Obstetrics & Gynecology.* 4th ed. Wolters Kluwer; 2015. (Figure 19-02)

Figure 32-17. Doubilet PM, Benson CB. *Atlas of Ultrasound in Obstetrics and Gynecology.* 3rd ed. Wolters Kluwer; 2018. (Figure 22.5.3)

Figure 32-18. Doubilet PM, Benson CB. *Atlas of Ultrasound in Obstetrics and Gynecology.* 3rd ed. Wolters Kluwer; 2018. (Figure 18.3.1)

Figure 32-19. Rubin R. *Rubin's Pathology.* 3rd ed. Wolters Kluwer; 1999. (Figure 6-7)

Figure 32-20. Norris TL. *Porth's Essentials of Pathophysiology.* 5th ed. Wolters Kluwer; 2019. (Figure 5-13)

Figure 32-21. O'Connell CB. *A Comprehensive Review for the Certification and Recertification Examinations for Physician Assistants.* 5th ed. Wolters Kluwer; 2015. (Figure 8-1)

Figure 32-22. Abuhamad AZ, Chaoui, R. *First Trimester Ultrasound Diagnosis of Fetal Abnormalities.* Wolters Kluwer; 2017. (Figure 5-29)

Figure 32-23. Cosby KS, Kendall, JL. *Practical Guide to Emergency Ultrasound.* 2nd ed. Wolters Kluwer; 2015. (Figure 16-06A,B)

Figure 32-24. Stephenson SR. *Diagnostic Medical Sonography: Obstetrics & Gynecology.* 3rd ed. Wolters Kluwer; 2012. (Figure 17-02)

Figure 32-27. Stephenson SR. *Diagnostic Medical Sonography: Obstetrics & Gynecology.* 4th ed. Wolters Kluwer; 2015. (Figure 32-17)

Figure 32-28. Doubilet PM, Benson CB. *Atlas of Ultrasound in Obstetrics and Gynecology.* 2nd ed. Wolters Kluwer; 2011. (Figure 31.3.2)

Figure 32-29. Stephenson SR. *Diagnostic Medical Sonography: Obstetrics & Gynecology.* 3rd ed. Wolters Kluwer; 2012. (Figure 17-20C)

Figure 32-30. Stephenson SR. *Diagnostic Medical Sonography: Obstetrics & Gynecology.* 3rd ed. Wolters Kluwer; 2012. (Figure 17-21)

Figure 32-31. Doubilet PM, Benson CB. *Atlas of Ultrasound in Obstetrics and Gynecology.* 3rd ed. Wolters Kluwer; 2018. (Figure 19.1.1)

Figure 32-32. Stephenson SR. *Diagnostic Medical Sonography: Obstetrics & Gynecology.* 4th ed. Wolters Kluwer; 2015. (Figure 20-23)

Figure 32-33. Kline-Fath B, Bulas D, Lee W. *Fundamental and Advanced Fetal Imaging Ultrasound and MRI.* 2nd ed. Wolters Kluwer; 2021. (Figure 13.1-06A)

Figure 32-34. Kline-Fath B, Bulas D, Lee W. *Fundamental and Advanced Fetal Imaging Ultrasound and MRI.* 2nd ed. Wolters Kluwer; 2021. (Figure 13.1-15)

Figure 32-35. Doubilet PM, Benson CB. *Atlas of Ultrasound in Obstetrics and Gynecology.* 2nd ed. Wolters Kluwer; 2011. (Figure 16.4.1B)

Figure 32-36. Kline-Fath B, Bahado-Singh R, Bulas D. *Fundamental and Advanced Fetal Imaging.* Wolters Kluwer; 2015. (Figure 7-14)

Figure 32-37. Doubilet PM, Benson CB. *Atlas of Ultrasound in Obstetrics and Gynecology.* 3rd ed. Wolters Kluwer; 2018. (Figure 19.3.3)

Figure 32-38. Kline-Fath B, Bulas D, Lee W. *Fundamental and Advanced Fetal Imaging Ultrasound and MRI.* 2nd ed. Wolters Kluwer; 2021. (Figure 13.1-35)

Figure 32-39. Doubilet PM, Benson CB. *Atlas of Ultrasound in Obstetrics and Gynecology.* 2nd ed. Wolters Kluwer; 2011. (Figure 19.1.1)

Figure 32-40. Doubilet PM, Benson CB. *Atlas of Ultrasound in Obstetrics and Gynecology.* 3rd ed. Wolters Kluwer; 2018. (Figure 30.6.3)

Figure 32-41. Belfort M. *Operative Techniques in Obstetric Surgery.* Wolters Kluwer; 2022. (Figure 11.5B)

Figure 32-42. Doubilet PM, Benson CB. *Atlas of Ultrasound in Obstetrics and Gynecology.* 3rd ed. Wolters Kluwer; 2018. (Figure 22.4.2)

Index

Page numbers followed by *f* or *t* indicate material in figures or tables, respectively and those in **bold** indicate definition.

A

AAAs. *See* Abdominal aortic aneurysms
Abdominal aorta, **388**, 396
Abdominal aortic aneurysms (AAAs), **219**, 227–229, 227*f*
   pathology of, 227–229
Abdominal aortic rupture, 229
Abdominal cavity, 23–24
Abdominal circumference, **686**, 687
Abdominal hernias, 259, 259*t*
Abdominal signs, location and description, 30*t*
Abdominal sonography, 1–38. *See also* Body systems; Sonographic abdominal pathology
   clinical history and laboratory findings, gathering, 8–9, 8*t*
   emergency situations, 9
   imaging and Doppler artifacts, 11, 19
   infection control and transducer care, 9–10
      cycle of infection, 10*f*
   instrumentation, 11
   invasive and sterile procedures, 10–11
   patient care, 9
      normal numbers or ranges for, 9*t*
   patient preparation, 6–7
   practice guidelines, 3
   sonographic description of abnormal findings, 5–6, 6*t*. *See also individual entry*
   terminology, 3
Abdominal vasculature, 219–243, 220*f*
   anatomy, 220–225
   aortic dissection, 229
   gonadal arteries, 224–225
   iliac arteries, 225
   inferior mesenteric artery (IMA), 225
   physiology of, 220–225
   pseudoaneurysms, 230
   sonography of, 225–226
   superior mesenteric artery, 223–224
Abdominal wall, 244–266
Abnormal uterine bleeding (AUB), **467**, 475–476
   causes of, 476*t*
Abortion, **549**, 568
   missed, **550**
   spontaneous, **730**
Abruptio placentae, **771**, 779
Acalculous cholecystitis, **82**, 93
Acardiac twin, **750**, 757–758, 758*f*
Accessory spleen, **142**, 145
Acetabulum, **333**, 339
Achilles tendon, **333**, 338–339
   normal, 339*f*
   ruptured, 339*f*
Achondrogenesis, **629**, 641*f*
Achondroplasia, **629**, 639–640
Acinar cells, **121**, 122

Acoustic shadowing, **629**, 631
Acquired renal cystic disease, **159**, 171
Acrania, **579**, 598
ACTH (adrenocorticotropic hormone), 205
Acute appendicitis, **244**, 248–250, **529**, 540
Acute bacterial cholangitis, 108*t*
Acute cholecystitis, **82**, 90
Acute pancreatitis, **103**, 106, 126–128
Acute pyelonephritis, **159**, 174, 175*f*
Acute renal failure (ARF), **159**, 166
Acute respiratory distress syndrome, **503**, 517
Acute tubular necrosis, **159**, 166
Addison disease, **204**, 207
Adenocarcinoma, **244**, 257, **484**, 488
Adenomyoma, **406**, 416
Adenomyomatosis, **82**, 89–90
Adenomyosis, **406**, 416–417, 417*f*, **467**, 476
Adhesions, **484**, 493, 515
Adnexa, **365**, 368, **388**, 391, **434**, 455, **529**, 530
Adnexal ring sign, **549**, 564
ADPKD (autosomal dominant polycystic kidney disease), **26**, 61, **159**, 169, **704**, 711–712
Adrenal adenoma, **204**, 209
Adrenal glands, 204–218
   Addison disease, 207
   adrenal adenoma, 209
   adrenal carcinoma and metastasis, 210–211
   adrenal cysts, **204**, 210, 211*f*
   adrenal hemorrhage, 212, 212*f*
   adrenal rests, **204**, 210
   anatomy, 205–206
   Conn syndrome, 209
   Cushing syndrome, 208
   hormones of, 206*t*
   neuroblastoma, 211–212, 212*f*
   pathology, 207–211
   pediatric adrenal pathology, 211–212
   pheochromocytoma, 209–210, 210*f*
   physiology of, 205–206
   position of, 205*f*, 205*t*
   sonography of, 207
   vascular anatomy of, 206, 206*f*
Adrenal rest, **302**, 315
Adrenocorticotropic hormone (ACTH), **204**, 205
Advanced maternal age, **729**, 732, **750**, 751
Agenesis, **406**, 412
   of the corpus callosum, **579**, **729**, 731
AIDS cholangitis, 108*t*
Alcoholic liver disease, **40**
Aldosterone, 206*t*
Allantoic cyst, **771**, 784
Allantois, **704**, 706
Alobar holoprosencephaly, **579**, 592
Alpha-fetoprotein (AFP), **302**, **365**, 371*t*, **529**, 597, **629**, 633, 691, **729**, 732
Ambiguous genitalia, **365**, 378, **704**, 719
Amebic hepatic abscess, **40**, 63–64

Amenorrhea, **365**, 367*t*, **406**, 415, **484**, 494, **503**, 513
   primary, 468, **468**
   secondary, 468, **468**
American Institute of Ultrasound in Medicine (AIUM), 3, 6*t*
Amniocentesis, **729**, 732
Amnion, **549**, 552, **750**, 752
Amnionicity, **750**, 752
   sonographic assessment, 753–756
   of twins, 751–752
Amnionitis, **729**, 732
Amniotic band syndrome, **611**, 614, **629**, 638, 650
Amniotic cavities, **540**, 556
Amniotic fluid index (AFI), **771**, 786
Amniotic sac, **750**
   diamniotic, 752
   monoamniotic, 752
Amniotic sheets, 782
Ampulla (fallopian tube), **434**, 455, **549**, 551
Ampulla of Vater, **103**, 104
Amyloidosis, **159**, 166
Anasarca, **771**, 791
Anastomoses, **750**
Anastomosis, **40**, 70
Androblastoma, **434**, 452
Androgens, 206*t*, **503**, 513
Anembryonic gestation, **549**, 567
Anemia, **1**, **750**, 761, **771**
Anencephaly, **579**, 597, 598, **629**, 633
Aneuploidy, **529**, 531*t*, **549**, 568, **611**, 617, **658**, **729**, 731
Aneurysm, **219**, 227
Angiomyolipoma, **159**, 173, 181, 181*f*
Angiosarcoma, **142**, 150
Anhydramnios, **629**, **704**, 708
Anisotropy, 11*t*
Annular pancreas, **121**, 125, 125*f*
Anomaly, **729**, 731
Anophthalmia, **579**, 593, **611**, 613
Anorectal atresia, **686**, 691
Anovulation, **484**, 488, **503**, 513
Anovulatory cycle, **467**, 475
Anoxia, **204**, 212
Anteflexion, **406**, 410
Anterior abdominal wall pathology, 257–260
Anterior cul-de-sac, **388**, 391, **434**, 437
Anterior pituitary gland, **467**, 469
   hormones of, 469
Anteversion, **406**, 410
Anticoagulation therapy, **1**
Aortic atresia, **658**
Aortic dissection, 229
Aortic stenosis, **658**
Apert syndrome, **579**, 595
Apertures, 585
Appendicitis, 249*f*
Appendicolith, **244**, 249*f*